In each A group, the number of electrons (#e⁻)
in the outer shell of each element is the same.

In each period, the identifying number (*n*)
for the outer shell of each element is the same.

		3	4	5	6	7	8
							He Helium **2** 4.00
		B Boron **5** 10.81	**C** Carbon **6** 12.01	**N** Nitrogen **7** 14.01	**O** Oxygen **8** 16.00	**F** Fluorine **9** 19.00	**Ne** Neon **10** 20.18
		Al Aluminium **13** 26.98	**Si** Silicon **14** 28.09	**P** Phosphorus **15** 30.97	**S** Sulfur **16** 32.06	**Cl** Chlorine **17** 35.45	**Ar** Argon **18** 39.95
Ni Nickel **28** 58.71	**Cu** Copper **29** 63.55	**Zn** Zinc **30** 65.37	**Ga** Gallium **31** 69.72	**Ge** Germanium **32** 72.59	**As** Arsenic **33** 74.92	**Se** Selenium **34** 78.96	**Br** Bromine **35** 79.90
							Kr Krypton **36** 83.8
Pd Palladium **46** 106.4	**Ag** Silver **47** 107.87	**Cd** Cadmium **48** 112.40	**In** Indium **49** 114.82	**Sn** Tin **50** 118.69	**Sb** Antimony **51** 121.75	**Te** Tellurium **52** 127.60	**I** Iodine **53** 126.90
							Xe Xenon **54** 131.30
Pt Platinum **78** 195.09	**Au** Gold **79** 196.97	**Hg** Mercury **80** 200.59	**Tl** Thalium **81** 204.37	**Pb** Lead **82** 207.2	**Bi** Bismuth **83** 208.98	**Po*** Polonium **84** (210)	**At*** Astatine **85** (210)
							Rn* Radon **86** (222)

Eu Europium **63** 151.96	**Gd** Gadolinium **64** 157.25	**Tb** Terbium **65** 158.93	**Dy** Dysprosium **66** 162.50	**Ho** Holmium **67** 164.93	**Er** Erbium **68** 167.26	**Tm** Thulium **69** 168.93	**Yb** Ytterbium **70** 173.04	**Lu** Lutetium **71** 174.97
Am* Americium **95** (243)	**Cm*** Curium **96** (247)	**Bk*** Berkelium **97** (247)	**Cf*** Californium **98** (251)	**Es*** Einsteinium **99** (254)	**Fm*** Fermium **100** (257)	**Md*** Mendelevium **101** (257)	**No*** Nobelium **102** (255)	**Lr*** Lawrencium **103** (256)

introduction to the chemistry

ureal, Quebec

try

Address orders to:
383 Madison Avenue
New York, NY 10017

Address editorial correspondence to:
West Washington Square
Philadelphia, PA 19105

This book was set in Times Roman by Progressive Typographers.
The editors were John Vondeling, Sally Kusch and Irene Nunes.
The art & design director was Richard L. Moore.
The text design was done by Nancy E. J. Grossman.
The cover design was done by Richard L. Moore.
The new artwork was drawn by Vantage Art.
The production manager was Tom O'Connor.
This book was printed by Von Hoffman.

Cover credit: Wing of a tropical butterfly, © 1974 by Hermann Eisenbeiss.

INTRODUCTION TO THE CHEMISTRY OF LIFE   ISBN 0-03-058516-3

234   032   98765432

CBS COLLEGE PUBLISHING
Saunders College Publishing
Holt, Rinehart and Winston
The Dryden Press

Preface

Introduction to the Chemistry of Life is a completely new textbook for a one-year survey course. It provides a foundation in the molecular concepts needed to understand many of the life processes of the human body, as well as some of the basic techniques of general chemistry, organic chemistry, and biochemistry.

We discuss topics that are accessible to a first-year college student and can be of later use in relating chemical principles to everyday life. Particular care has been taken to include concepts and applications that will prepare *allied health science* students for their future careers. Students who plan to enter fields such as physical education, home economics, agriculture, and the social sciences should also benefit from this approach to chemistry through its impact on human biology.

Expecting the student audience to contain diverse backgrounds and interests, we do not anticipate any particular level of technical preparation. Students with a very limited background in high school chemistry should expect to spend a longer time studying, especially in Chapters 2 to 6, than those coming directly from high school with a strong chemistry background. Our presentation is designed to help each student develop the motivation and enthusiasm that will lead to mastery of chemical skills.

It is quite difficult for a single textbook to meet the needs and interests of every student. An author tends to include what he or she feels the student *should* know and to aim at the highly literate, self-motivated, and extremely capable reader. Unfortunately, such pupils are truly rare. The typical college student needs some help in learning chemistry. The one-year survey course thus poses some very specific challenges, which we attempt to meet with this textbook.

Alternative Chapter Sequences

The most common two-semester sequence using this text might cover Chapters 1 through 12 in the first term and the remainder of the text in the second term. There are several alternative paths through the material. A first-term course that includes only general chemistry might begin with Chapters 1 to 6, then skip to Chapters 10 to 14; the second-term could then include the organic and biochemistry of Chapters 7 to 9 and 15 to 28.

It is possible to use this text in a one-semester or two-quarter course through the judicious elimination of topics that are inessential to a particular student group. The following fifteen chapters might be considered *most essential* to a short course for health science students: 1, 4, 5, 7, 9, 12, 13, 17, 18, 19, 20, 22, 23, 24 and 25. The result would be a course with approximately half of the material in the full text, but with all of the truly important topics for a class studying the chemical background of human physiology. Necessary bridging is minimal and could be carried out in lecture.

A Readable Presentation of Chemistry

Some students are excellent readers; others are not. Any college student should be able to understand a clear, direct presentation. Highly technical discussions, such as we often find in scientific journals, present serious difficulties for some readers. Since our primary objective is to help the student master chemical concepts, we have kept the textual language as coherent and understandable as possible.

As the student progresses from the relatively simple discussions of general and organic chemistry to some of the difficult areas of metabolism, the technical level of the text must inevitably rise. We have tried to avoid "quantum jumps" in reading level and to keep the entire book within the grasp of an average college student.

A Flexible Approach to Chemical Arithmetic

Many students can handle all of the mathematics used in general chemistry, including the calculation of empirical formulas and fractional pH values. Others are prepared to add, subtract, multiply, and divide but are fearful if asked to do much more. In fact, some students settle on biology-related career programs because of an aversion to math!

This text has been organized to allow the instructor to emphasize calculations or to avoid them, depending on the needs and skills of the class. Where calculations are presented, we emphasize the use of *conversion factors* (the dimensional-analysis or unit-factor method) rather than the solution of algebraic equations. Appendix B contains a review of some frequently used mathematical tools, such as the calculation of per cent.

Attention to Mastery of Specific Skills Related to Human Biochemistry

We hope that the student will not only learn some fundamentals of chemistry but will also understand the applications of these principles to a clinical situation. There is a tendency in the allied health field to hope that the student will memorize and retain a tremendous range of information. At the same time, we expect understanding and application of the skills and concepts in diverse situations. Not even our best students can approach this ideal. Choices must be made. There must be an appropriate balance between the learning of concepts and the ability to apply them. Instead of touching superficially on a large number of topics, we have chosen to emphasize mastery of a small but important selection of skills.

In addition, we have tried to emphasize the interrelationships between general and organic chemistry. Some texts begin with the theories, models, and calculations of general inorganic chemistry, followed by a short course in organic nomenclature and reactions. Finally, the student reaches the third "subject," human biochemistry, which may be the only part of the course that will seem relevant and interesting. By that point, the student's enthusiasm and motivation may be weakened, if not entirely evaporated.

We have taken a different approach. The concepts of general chemistry are equally applicable to inorganic and organic compounds, as we have shown by our choice of examples in Chapters 1 to 6. Ionic and covalent compounds work in harmony in the human body. Both types are certainly necessary for life; both types should be well understood.

Thus, instead of providing a "mini-course" in each of the three vast fields of general, organic, and biochemistry, we begin with the simplest aspects of chemistry and gradually proceed to discuss the more complex molecules and reactions of metabolism. Such topics as nutrition, radiation therapy, breathing, and blood pressure are briefly discussed in early chapters. This reminds students that chemical and physical principles underlie many different aspects of life and health.

Of course, there is no way in which our particular selection of topics can possibly meet the needs of every class. Somewhat more material is included in this text than can be learned well during an academic year. If we have included topics that are not needed, then skip those sections. We may have omitted a few subjects that the instructor considers relevant; then by all means provide lectures on such material and bring your own ideas, interests, and enthusiasm directly into the course. A textbook is not a syllabus but a learning resource, to be adapted to the distinct needs of the class.

Study Aids Within Each Chapter

Each chapter section contains *learning goals,* the specific skills or objectives that the student should master. *Self-check questions* are provided right at the end of the chapter section, as an immediate way to verify progress before going on to the next section. Solved *examples* are provided for many techniques that require practice. The student is encouraged to work step by step through these carefully chosen problems. The learning goals, self-checks, and examples work together in each section to steer the student towards mastery of the essentials.

At the end of each chapter, the learning goals are again presented so that the student may use them as a checklist while reviewing for exams. There is a chapter *glossary* of technical terms, with reference to the page on which each term is used in context. A two-column set of *questions and problems* evaluates each learning goal. The left-hand column, with solutions in Appendix A, is for student use. The right-hand column contains equivalent questions, which may be assigned for homework since the answers are provided only in the *instructor's manual.* An unusually large number (1658) of questions are provided so that the instructor may make a judicious selection of those which best suit the needs of the class. Certain starred (*) questions go somewhat beyond the learning goals.

Most self-check and end-of-chapter questions involve situations related to health care and other aspects of modern life. It is important that questions serve not only to measure the student's progress but also to remind the student of the *relevance* of the chemistry that is being learned.

An Attractive Textbook to Motivate Students

We are trying to teach the "TV generation." Some students need some visual impact to focus their attention on what they are learning. A chemistry textbook can be rigorous and effective and also use two-color format, photographs, diagrams, and language in a way that motivates the student. We have attempted to do this.

The Most Important Learning Resource is the Instructor

We have tried to maximize the value of this text for your classes. Some students may learn the material well through self-study. Most, however, enjoy the direct encouragement, insight, and teacher-transmitted enthusiasm that face-to-face instruction can provide. No matter how hard the authors worked to achieve a high level of readability, accuracy, and relevance in the presentation, the true testing ground of our efforts is in your classroom.

The authors welcome communication from instructors who use this text. Which aspects work well? Which chapters could stand some improvement in the next edition? What would you like to see added? deleted?

We have included more than 1000 relevant applications of chemistry to clinical or real-world situations, taken from various sources, such as the *Merck Index*. A few errors of fact or interpretation may have crept in. Please help us correct any such mistakes so that we may better serve your students.

ACKNOWLEDGMENTS

We wish to express our deep appreciation to Professors Lyle Hayes, Melvin Merken, Thomas Record, William Scovell, and Vera Zalkow, who reviewed the entire manuscript, and to Professors Michael Gotto, Edward Peters, and Eleanore Van Norman, who reviewed portions of it, and to Dao Minh Nguyen who checked many of the calculations.

A particular thanks to our publisher, John Vondeling, who patiently saw the manuscript through reviews and revisions to realization; to his assistant, Jeannie Schoch, who was always helpful; to our Copyeditor, Irene Nunes, who refined the entire presentation, to our Project Editor, Sally Kusch, who brought together a very complicated project, and to the others at Saunders College Publishing who were so helpful in bringing this manuscript into print.

PETER P. BERLOW, *Montreal, Quebec, Canada*
DONALD J. BURTON, *Iowa City, Iowa*
JOSEPH I. ROUTH, *Iowa City, Iowa*

To the Student

Chemistry is the study of all substances, the "stuff" or matter that makes up your body, the earth, and all other objects you can feel or taste, smell or see. The chemist wants to know *what* is contained in a particular object and *how* it got there. With this knowledge, the chemist can then classify and name the smallest bits of matter and put them together in the test tubes and flasks of the laboratory to make products that are important in our daily lives.

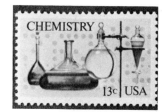

You may be taking this course because you wish to learn more about the chemicals in our environment. Or you may be entering a career that applies chemistry to real-life problems, such as the health professions. As you read through this text, you will see that chemistry affects everyone each day. Knowledge of chemistry is needed to understand food, drugs, metals, plastics, and other materials, living and nonliving. While we introduce you to the scientific principles, we will frequently remind you that these principles are applied every day by real people and are not simply "nice ideas" dreamed up by teachers to make you study.

Whether or not you have previously taken and enjoyed a chemistry course, you *have* the capability to learn this one! Nothing in this text is beyond your grasp. However, you must expect to put in a good deal of hard work. You must plan to organize your study time. This part of *Introduction to the Chemistry of Life* is intended to get you started on the right foot.

STUDYING CHEMISTRY

You already have your own style of learning and your own way of coping with courses and examinations. It is important that you learn how to study chemistry effectively so that this course will be a satisfaction rather than a nightmare.

The most important fact is that **chemistry must be learned actively.** You will not learn much chemistry by simply *listening* to the teacher or only *reading* the textbook. Listening and reading are very important skills. However, they are passive skills; they don't leave very much in your brain!

While you listen to a lecture and while you study a chapter, you should be thinking, challenging, and restating in your own words what is being said. Always have pencil and paper at hand, so you can take notes on what is important. You should also jot down any questions you have so you can get the answers later.

If a new word is presented, write it down, and be sure you know what it means. Try to relate what you are learning now to what you studied last week and a month ago. Try to get an overall picture of what this course is trying to accomplish so that you will understand how each learning goal fits in.

ORGANIZATION OF THIS BOOK

Each of the 28 chapters of this textbook treats a particular theme or topic. Each chapter is divided, to make your studying easier, into several numbered sections, such as Section 23.1, 23.2, 23.3. Each section generally discusses one chemical concept, process, or method.

Your course may not cover every section of every chapter. Don't feel you are being shortchanged. Chemistry is such a vast subject, you can only learn so much of it in one course. If you wish to increase your understanding of chemistry after this course, there are many excellent resources for you to use.

LEARNING GOALS

At the beginning of each section you will find one or more *learning goals*. A learning goal tells you what you should be *able to do* when you finish the section. This can be a tremendous help in studying because you can plan your work to achieve these goals. Naturally, these goals describe almost exactly what kinds of questions you must expect on homework, quizzes, and examinations. If you can "do" the learning goal, you should be able to answer the test question on that same topic.

For example, the first learning goal in this textbook is

LEARNING GOAL 1A: Given the name of any of 25 elements important to the human body, write the symbol; or, given the symbol, write the name.

You thus know, at the beginning of Chapter 1, that you must memorize some names and some symbols. Some of them you probably already know, such as H for hydrogen. Some may be unfamiliar. Your learning task is very clear.

The learning goals in this text are those that the authors felt to be most appropriate for all students. However, your instructor may feel that some other objectives are more important in your particular course. Be alert to any changes, additions, or deletions that your teacher may announce.

SELF-CHECK EXERCISES

At the end of each section, you will find a series of questions called a *self-check*. Think of this as a mini-quiz that acts like a gate in a fence. If you do well on the self-check (compare your answers with those in Appendix A), then pass through the "fence" into the next section. If you have difficulty, go back over the part you have just studied and review the material that you have not yet learned.

Do each self-check with pencil and paper as if you were taking a class-room quiz. Do *not* refer back and forth between the questions and the answers. If a calculation is involved, do all the work before you look at the answer. If you "cheat" here, you injure your own chances of really knowing whether or not you have reached the learning goal. The self-check questions and learning goals are matched very carefully.

MEMORIZATION

Many students (and quite a few teachers) think of "learning chemistry" as involving a lot of memory work. In one sense they are right. Chemistry has a *language* of its own.

If you learn a foreign language, you must repeat certain words to yourself until they are part of your memory. That is how you build a vocabulary so that you can say what you mean in that language. If you cannot find the words to express yourself, you cannot communicate.

However, language is more than a list of memorized words. You must also be able to put those words together to make sentences; the word order must make sense or, again, you will not be able to get your ideas across. You cannot memorize how to form sentences and how to choose the proper words from your list to express each idea. You must *understand* how the language functions. This understanding comes not from memory work but from practice with many different kinds of sentences and situations.

Chemistry works in exactly the same way. You must learn—memorize —a number of terms in each chapter. These terms are given in **boldface** type where they are first discussed and are seen again at the end of the chapter in the glossary. Certain important symbols must also be planted in your memory.

However, that's just the chemical language. To explain what is happening in a chemical process, you must go beyond simple memorization to understand what general principles are being applied.

In the case of a calculation, you should rely on a good deal of practice instead of on memorizing the example. Setting up and solving a problem involving math comes from experience with different kinds of problems.

Some students have very good memories for scientific "facts"; others hate to memorize. Each student must strike a balance between memory work and answering practice questions so that he or she will have both the vocabulary of chemistry and the ability to use it properly.

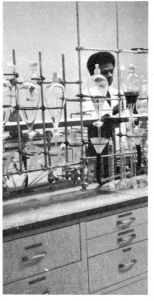

A modern analytical chemistry laboratory, that of the Food and Drug Administration pesticide division. Photograph by Donald D. Dechert.

CHAPTER SUMMARIES

At the end of each chapter, the learning goals are brought together in a checklist so that you can make sure you are ready for a test on that chapter. The glossary contains a simple definition of each new term. Both the learning goals checklist and the glossary contain page references so that you can go back and clarify any doubtful points.

END-OF-CHAPTER QUESTIONS

At the end of each chapter, there are two columns of questions and problems. The questions in the *left*-hand column (color numbers) are answered in the back of this textbook. The right-hand column (black) contains questions generally similar to those in the other column and will probably be used in homework assignments since no answers to these questions are given in this book.

Always write out your own answer completely before you refer to the "book" solution or consult another student.

Most of the end-of-chapter questions are arranged by section and test your performance on the learning goals of that section. Some questions, marked with stars (*), may go a bit beyond the listed goals.

SOME STUDY HINTS

No two students are exactly alike. What works well for your neighbor may not work for you. However, many students have found that the following methods help them complete the course successfully.

1) Outline what your instructor says in class. Do not attempt to copy down every word. Instead, try to take notes on the *main* points. These notes will help you study for exams. In addition, writing something down several times is an excellent way to place it in your memory.
2) Take notes while you study the textbook. Many students write *in* their book; a well-marked book is a sign of a student who knows how to study.
3) Don't try to study chemistry while watching television, talking with friends, or doing a job. Most students learn most effectively if they concentrate in a quiet, comfortable place.
4) Work through every *example* given in the text. Practice makes perfect.
5) When doing calculations (chemical arithmetic), use the simple methods presented in the text or by your instructor. Learn the conversion-factor method (Chapter 2), and use it. Don't panic!
6) Use common sense to check *all* answers.

A typical U.S. college chemistry laboratory of 1869, at the Massachusetts Institute of Technology.

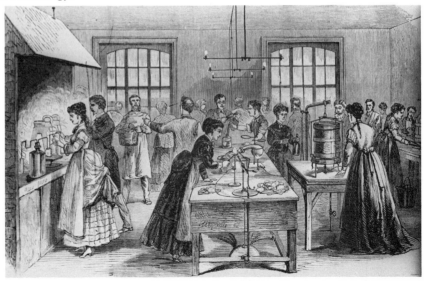

Contents Overview

Contents

The Chemicals of Life

1

The human body is a marvelous chemical factory. Much of this text will be devoted to its operation. You are alive because the chemical reactions in your body are those that sustain life.

What is life? A dictionary is of little help in understanding the subtle difference between living and non-living matter. A biologist can spend a lifetime discovering new aspects of the living cell without really understanding "life" itself. Fortunately, the chemicals and reactions that sustain life inside the body can also be studied in the laboratory. We can study the *nutrients,* the foods that enter the body. We can imitate the body *reactions* that convert these foods to energy and useful tissues. We can then explain what happens in a healthy body, and what may go wrong. Every time a patient undergoes a blood test or urine analysis, we are using this information.

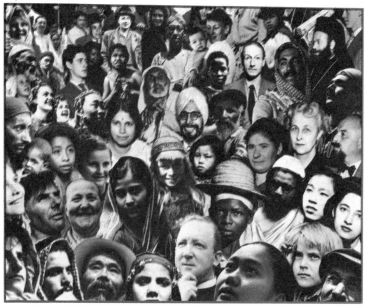

In Chapter 1, we will look at the simplest kinds of substances, the *elements,* and give some examples of how these elements can combine to give chemical *compounds* that are important to human life. We will introduce you to the smallest and simplest "bits" of matter, the *atoms* and *molecules.* Then, through a brief discussion of nutrition, we will give you some idea of what you will learn in the rest of the book.

A *reaction* is a change from one pure substance to another.

If you have already taken a good chemistry course, some of this discussion may be quite familiar. If so, fine. You can complete the chapter very quickly. If this is your first serious exposure to the symbols of the elements and the basic terms used by chemists, plan to spend some time learning this language of chemistry.

1.1 THE ELEMENTS OF THE HUMAN BODY

LEARNING GOAL 1A: *Given the name of any of 25 elements important to the human body, write the symbol; or, given the symbol, write the name.*

1

An **element** is a kind of substance or **matter** that never changes* in the human body or in a chemical laboratory. No matter how we treat such a substance—heat it or cool it, beat it or combine it—it remains the same element. We consider an element to be the simplest kind of pure substance and explain all other substances, no matter how complicated, as being made up of elements, in the same way that all of the millions of words in English, French, Spanish, and many other languages can be formed from the 26 letters of the alphabet.

By the year 1980, scientists had discovered more than 106 different chemical elements. These elements are shown in the **periodic table** inside the front cover of this text. Most of them are found in nature, many in rocks. The others are man-made elements prepared in nuclear laboratories. Look at the periodic table, and notice that there is a number near the top of each box, numbering the elements from #1 to #106. This is called, very logically, the *atomic number* of each element. We will be referring to the periodic table frequently because it contains very useful information about the elements.

You will learn more about *atomic numbers* in Section 2.4.

Some elements were known to the ancients, but most have been discovered within the past 300 years. All of the boxes from #1 to beyond #106 have been filled, although the last few elements to be discovered have not yet been given official names. Scientists are very slowly adding new elements to the end of the list. However, this work is difficult because all of the elements beyond #83 are *radioactive;* they change themselves to other elements in a manner to be discussed in Section 3.5. These changes occur so

FIGURE 1–1 Relative abundance by weight of the most common elements in (a) the earth's outer crust, (b) the whole earth, and (c) the universe. Oxygen is shown in color. It makes up almost two thirds of your body weight.

---

* Nuclear chemistry, discussed in Section 3.5, provides some exceptions to this. Some (radioactive) elements will change by themselves. Others can be prepared in nuclear reactors or cyclotrons, or by cosmic rays. However, in our everyday world, an element should be considered to be an unchanging type of matter.

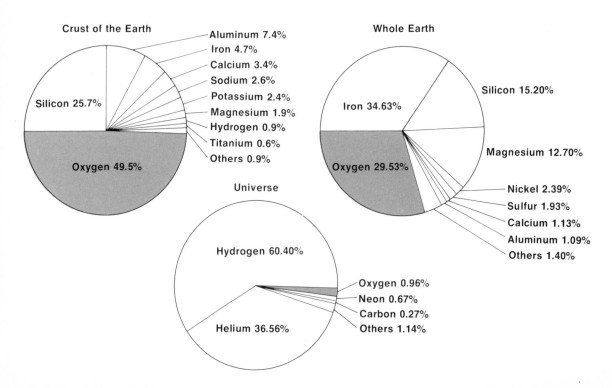

quickly for the elements with very high atomic numbers that the presence of a new element is very difficult to detect.

In the middle of each box of the periodic table is the name of the element. You have heard many of these names, such as aluminum, iron, oxygen, and chlorine. Others like yttrium, osmium, and fermium may be much less familiar. We will not expect you to learn the names of all the elements but will concentrate on those most important to life.

Figure 1–1 shows the relative amounts of the most important elements in the universe, in the whole earth, and in the outer rocks or "crust" of the earth. In every 100 pounds of soil, we find about 49.5 pounds of oxygen and 25.7 pounds of silicon. These two elements make up sand. As we approach the center of the earth, iron and magnesium are found in large amounts. However, in the sun (and stars) hydrogen and helium, the two simplest and lightest elements (#1 and #2), are most important.

Element symbols

Figure 1–2 shows an enlarged box from the periodic table appearing inside the front cover of this book. Along with the atomic number and name of the element (in this case, carbon, the element upon which all life is based), we see a chemical **symbol** and an *atomic weight*.

The symbol of each element is used by scientists in all countries of the world as an international abbreviation for its name, which varies from one language to another. Thus, if you were to pick up a chemical journal from China, Japan, Russia, or Germany, you might not understand the text but you would recognize all of the chemical symbols and all of the formulas and equations that used them.

The symbol is sometimes simply one capital letter, often the first letter of the English name, as for carbon (**C**), hydrogen (**H**), oxygen (**O**), and sulfur (**S**). Most of the elements with one-letter symbols are fairly common and have been known for centuries. Of the 25 elements you must learn to satisfy *Learning Goal 1A*, ten have one-letter symbols.

More often, as you will notice in the periodic table, there is a two-letter symbol, of which the first letter must be a capital and the second must be small (lower-case). Some examples: #2 (**He**, helium); #36 (**Kr**, krypton). Again, many two-letter symbols are easy to match with the English names of the elements.

Some elements, which have been known since ancient times, were given Latin names. Their symbols often come from those early names. Of your important 25, this is true of **K** for potassium (from "kalium"), **Na** for sodium (from "natrium"), **Fe** for iron (from "ferrum"), **Cu** for copper (from "cuprum"), and **Sn** for tin (from "stannum"). You will also notice in the table that the symbols for silver, lead, gold, and mercury (among others) are different from what you might expect from their English names.

Of the more than 106 known elements, only 25 are believed to play a role in life processes. These 25 are listed in Table 1–1.

You may wish to rewrite Table 1–1 in a different way, perhaps in alphabetical order, to help you memorize the names and symbols of the elements. Your instructor may possibly wish you to learn the names and symbols of some additional elements, in which case you should add those to *Learning Goal 1A*. For a while, you may find it useful to refer to the periodic table on the inside front cover each time an element is mentioned. Soon it will no longer be necessary.

Atomic weights **will be further discussed in Section 2.5.**

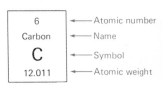

FIGURE 1–2 Each box in the periodic table provides information about a different chemical element.

The Latin name for the metal element lead is *plumbum.* **Since lead was once widely used for pipes, this gave us the English word** *plumbing.* **Pb, the chemical symbol for lead, comes from the Latin name.**

The 25 elements believed to play some role in the chemistry of the human body are shown in colored boxes in the periodic table inside the front cover.

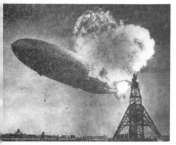

Pure hydrogen will burn in air. Mixtures of hydrogen and air may explode. The airship *Hindenburg,* filled with hydrogen gas, burned over New Jersey in 1937 with the loss of 36 lives. Modern airships use helium gas. (UPI photo.)

TABLE 1–1   NAMES AND SYMBOLS OF ELEMENTS IN THE HUMAN BODY

Hydrogen	H	Silicon	Si	Chromium	Cr	Selenium	Se
Carbon	C	Phosphorus	P	Manganese	Mn	Molybdenum	Mo
Nitrogen	N	Sulfur	S	Iron	Fe	Tin	Sn
Oxygen	O	Chlorine	Cl	Cobalt	Co	Iodine	I
Fluorine	F	Potassium	K	Nickel	Ni		
Sodium	Na	Calcium	Ca	Copper	Cu		
Magnesium	Mg	Vanadium	V	Zinc	Zn		

Elements essential to human life

Four of the elements in Table 1–1 will be seen very frequently in the later chapters of this text. They together make up 96% of your weight.

Hydrogen (#1, **H**) represents 9.3% of your weight. You take in hydrogen in water and every kind of food. However, you never receive *pure* hydrogen, which is actually very rare in nature. Every molecule of biological importance contains a great deal of hydrogen, as we shall see in the next section.

Carbon (#6, **C**) is the element that forms the basis for all living matter. Because carbon atoms can combine with each other to form long chains, there are millions of possible chemical substances containing such chains. Most of this textbook will be concerned with these *organic* substances. Although carbon makes up 19.4% (almost one fifth) of your weight, you contain no *pure* carbon at all. It's all combined with other elements. Pure carbon is found in coal, charcoal, diamond, and the graphite of pencil lead. If you eat any of these, your body will be unable to use the carbon.

Nitrogen (#7, **N**) makes up 5.1% of your weight, mostly in combination with carbon and hydrogen in proteins. You breathe in a large amount of pure nitrogen from the air, but you breathe the same amount out again! Your body cannot use pure nitrogen as a nutrient.

Oxygen (#8, **O**) makes up most of your body weight, 62.8%. You do receive and use pure oxygen from the air. However, this oxygen is soon converted by your body to other substances (in combination with carbon and hydrogen) and especially to water.

These all-important four elements thus make up most of the substances in your body. Remember, however, that there is no pure hydrogen or carbon in your body, and relatively little pure oxygen or nitrogen. These elements combine to form chemical *compounds*.

The remaining 21 elements in Table 1–1 are obtained (in combined form) from foods and are used largely as important structural links in body tissues. For example, **calcium** (#20, **Ca**) is found in bones and teeth; **sulfur** (#16, **S**) is found in proteins (to be discussed in Chapter 19); **phosphorus** (#15, **P**) plays an extremely important role in substances that store and transfer energy (Chapter 21); **sodium** (#11, **Na**) and **chlorine** (#17, **Cl**) are the two elements in table salt and are found throughout the body, as is **potassium** (#19, **K**). These six elements make up 3.3% of your body weight but, again, in combined form, not as pure elements. In fact, five of the six elements just named (all but sulfur) would be extremely poisonous if taken directly into the body.

So you see, the chemistry of the human body involves perhaps 25 elements, of which 4 are extremely important, 6 are present in substantial amounts, and the remainder are present in very small or trace amounts.

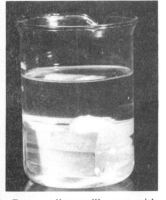

Pure sodium will react with air or water and so must be protected by keeping it under mineral oil.

(These questions allow you to check your mastery of Learning Goal 1A. Answer them after you have studied this section and before you go on to Section 1.2. Do not use the periodic table or Table 1–1, since you should be able to answer from memory. Answers will be found in Appendix A at the end of the textbook.)

1.1)   Write the *symbol* for each element:

sodium	calcium	iron
potassium	phosphorus	chromium

1.2)   Write the *name* of each element whose symbol is given:

H	F
Cu	Cl
Sn	Mg
Si	Co
I	Zn

1.2 SOME COMPOUNDS OF THE HUMAN BODY

LEARNING GOAL 1B: Given a chemical formula, list the elements involved and state how many atoms of each element make up one molecule or formula unit of that substance.

1C: Distinguish between a protein and a carbohydrate or fat by the elements present.

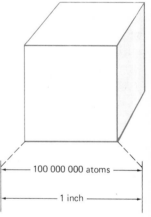

100 000 000 atoms

1 inch

Atoms are very small.

The smallest particle or "bit" of an element is called an **atom**. Atoms cannot be made or destroyed by chemical means. They remain unchanged in a chemical reaction and are extremely small. A 1-inch block of iron metal, which weighs about 4.5 ounces, contains more than a trillion trillion atoms (1.4×10^{24}, to be more exact). Along a 1-inch edge, you will find just about 100 million atoms. Obviously, you can't see each one! Chemists can't either, although we have some interesting photographs that show individual atoms.

The most important thing about atoms is that they rarely exist by themselves. Atoms combine to make *molecules*. A **molecule** is a single particle or "bit" of matter that is made up of two or more atoms. We will not concern ourselves here with exactly *how* atoms bind together to make molecules. The nature of atoms will be discussed in Chapter 2, and the ways atoms bond together and react will be the subject of several chapters. For the moment, it will be simplest to think of the atom as a kind of very small "ball" and to think of a molecule as having several atoms stuck together or joined by hooks or springs.

Molecules of elements

Although the smallest "bit" of a pure element is an atom of that element, the elements found in the pure state in nature usually do not exist as single atoms. Instead, the atoms join together to form molecules. The smallest "bit" of pure hydrogen in nature is not a hydrogen atom but an H_2 molecule.

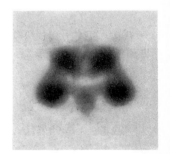

The images of four mercury (Hg) atoms and one sulfur (S) atom are clearly shown in a photograph taken through an electron microscope. Such microscopes can produce pictures that are millions of times as large as the object being viewed.

The chemical formula of a molecule shows the number of atoms of each element that make up that molecule. The prefix "di" means "two."

HCl:

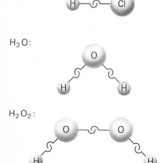

H₂O:

H₂O₂:

CO₂:

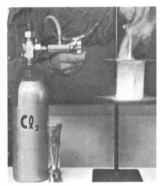

Some early chemists thought of atoms as having hooks that could latch onto other atoms to form molecules.

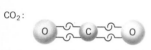

Sodium metal, shown in the beaker, and chlorine gas, in the tank, are both very reactive. They combine to give sodium chloride (table salt), which contains sodium and chlorine in the forms we also find in the human body. From the CHEM Study film, *Chemical Families.*

The subscript (lowered) "2" in the formula H_2 shows that there are *two* atoms of hydrogen in one molecule of hydrogen gas.

The other elements of the human body that are found as pure gases also form two-atom or *diatomic* molecules. We thus have oxygen gas, O_2, which makes up 20% of the air; nitrogen gas, N_2, which makes up most of the rest of the air; and chlorine gas, Cl_2, which is not found free in nature but is prepared in tremendous amounts by the chemical industry for use in making other chemicals and in purifying drinking water.

Gases have very low *density,* as we will see in Chapters 2 and 10. You can pass your hand through a gas without feeling it. Some pure elements form liquids (like water, oil, hot volcano lava) or solids at room temperature. The smallest bit of a liquid may be diatomic, as in the case of bromine (#35, Br_2). For pure elements found as solids, the smallest particle may be diatomic (I_2), or may consist of single atoms (very rare), or may have all atoms linked together in such a way that the whole piece of solid is the smallest unit. We call such a piece of solid a *crystal.* Liquids and solids will be discussed in Chapter 11.

Molecules of compounds

What is the most important molecule in your body? It is doubtless the very small particle that is made up of one oxygen atom and two hydrogen atoms linked or *bonded* together to form water. The formula for water is H_2O. This shows that there are three atoms in one molecule and shows which elements are present and in what amounts. It does *not* necessarily show how each hydrogen atom is connected. In fact, each is bonded to the oxygen atom in the middle. For that information, we must look at a model or picture of the molecule.

Water is a **compound**, a pure substance made up of two or more elements. The **formula** for a compound must show the elements, using the symbols we have already studied. Since the formula for water, H_2O, shows us that there are twice as many atoms of hydrogen as there are of oxygen, we might expect that when water is converted to its pure elements, we will obtain twice as many H_2 molecules as O_2 molecules. Figure 1–3 shows how, in fact, a direct electric current can be used to obtain pure hydrogen gas and pure oxygen gas from H_2O.

Some other common molecules are listed in Table 1–2. Just as the element symbols make up the chemical "alphabet," formulas make up the chemical "words." Each word has a meaning of its own; similarly, each chemical formula refers to a specific compound or element with its own properties.

More complicated formulas

While the substances in Table 1–2 are typical of the simpler chemicals, there are many complex molecules that are important in the human body. For example, one form of vitamin D can be written $C_{28}H_{44}O$. This formula gives you exactly the same kind of information that the formula H_2O gives for water. One such molecule of vitamin D contains 28 carbon atoms, 44 hydrogen atoms, and 1 oxygen atom.

Sometimes the chemist, for a good reason, will write a particular element more than once in a formula. You can still count atoms in the same way,

TABLE 1–2   CHEMICAL FORMULAS OF SOME SIMPLE COMPOUNDS

CO	Carbon monoxide (in air pollution)
CO_2	Carbon dioxide (given off in the lungs)
H_2O	Water (most of the body weight)
H_2O_2	Hydrogen peroxide (used to bleach hair)
NH_3	Ammonia (a cleaning agent)
SO_2	Sulfur dioxide (from smokestack pollution)
H_2S	Hydrogen sulfide (from rotten eggs)
NaCl	Sodium chloride (table salt)
Fe_2O_3	Iron(III) oxide (rust)
$NaHCO_3$	Sodium bicarbonate (baking soda)
CH_4	Methane (natural gas fuel)
C_2H_5OH	Ethyl alcohol (in some beverages)

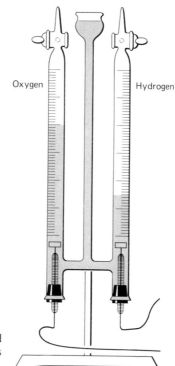

Oxygen   Hydrogen

FIGURE 1–3   Water, H_2O, can be decomposed into hydrogen (H_2) and oxygen (O_2) gases by means of a direct electrical current.

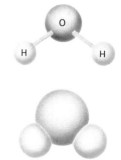

Two views of a molecule of water, H_2O.

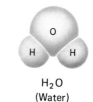

H_2O
(Water)

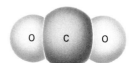

CO_2
(Carbon dioxide)

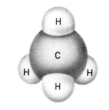

CH_4
(Methane)

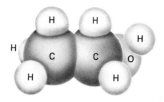

C_2H_5OH
(Ethyl alcohol)

Some examples of common molecules

but be sure to count them all! For example, H_2NNH_2 (hydrazine) has two nitrogen atoms and four hydrogen atoms in one molecule, while C_2H_5OH (ethyl alcohol) has two carbon atoms, one oxygen atom, and *six* hydrogen atoms in each molecule.

Sometimes a molecule may contain several groups of atoms that travel "together." For example, the three atoms "NO_2" are often found in carbon compounds with the nitrogen bonded to a carbon. The highly explosive "TNT" could be written $C_7H_5N_3O_6$. However, the same molecule might be written $C_7H_5(NO_2)_3$. The number "3" here means that everything inside the parentheses is taken three times.

Many substances do not form small molecules at room temperature. For example, sodium chloride (table salt, NaCl) is found in the form of white crystals. The chemical formula in that case shows that for each atom of sodium, one atom of chlorine will be found in the crystal, even though the crystal cannot be broken down into single "NaCl molecules." What then do we call "NaCl," meaning one atom of each element? It is called a **formula unit**, the simplest combination of the element symbols that will show what elements are present and in what proportions. Without knowing something about ionic and covalent bonding (Chapter 4), you will not know whether a given formula represents a molecule or a formula unit. For the purposes of this chapter, it does not matter.

Letters of the alphabet make up words, and words make up sentences. Chemical symbols make up chemical formulas. However, chemical *change* can only be shown if those formulas are put together into chemical *equations*. For the electrolysis of water (shown in Figure 1–3), the reaction is described by the chemical equation

$$2\ H_2O \longrightarrow 2\ H_2 + O_2$$

At this point, you should read this equation as follows: "Two molecules of water react to form two molecules of hydrogen and one molecule of oxygen." In Chapter 5, you will learn how to write many kinds of chemical equations.

Organic compounds of the human body

You have doubtless heard the terms *protein*, *fat*, and *carbohydrate* applied to foods and to diets. These three types of compounds are so important to human chemistry that we devote three chapters (17 to 19) to describing them and four more (20 and 25 to 27) to an explanation of how they are made and used in the body.

These three types of substances are examples of **organic compounds.** There is no point in trying to divide all chemical substances into those that are "purely" organic and those that are inorganic. However, there are many molecules that are clearly of interest to people who call themselves *organic chemists*. These molecules are members of groups of similar carbon-containing compounds. The members of each group tend to have chains of carbon atoms (Chapter 7).

Figure 1–4 shows some organic compounds of the body. You can

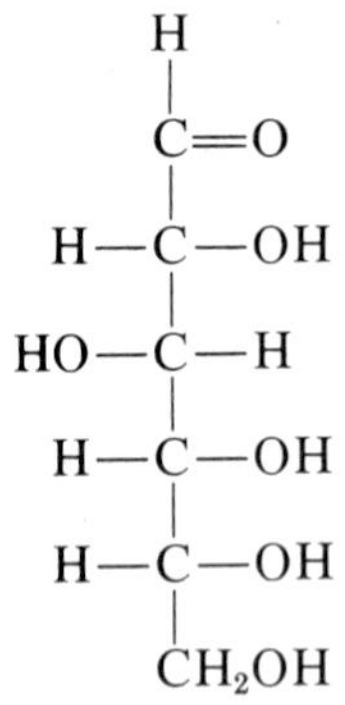

glucose, $C_6H_{12}O_6$,
a carbohydrate (sugar)

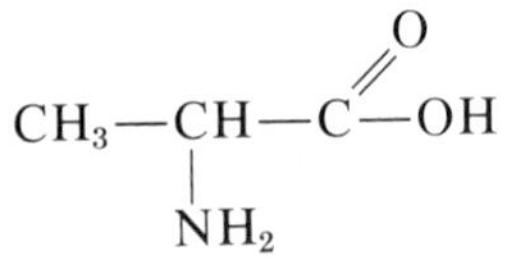

alanine, $C_3H_7NO_2$,
an amino acid

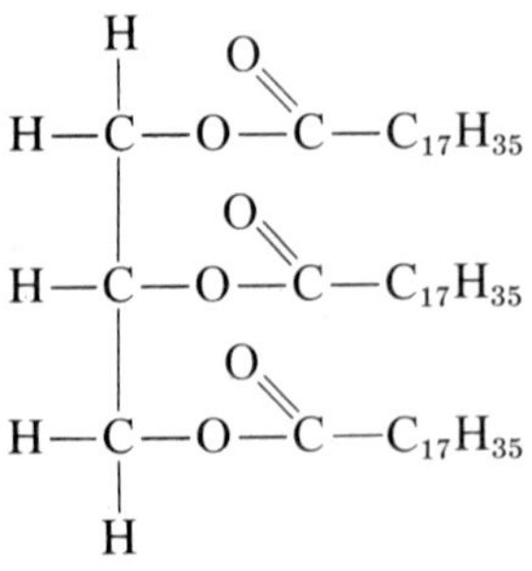

tristearin, $C_{57}H_{110}O_6$, a fat

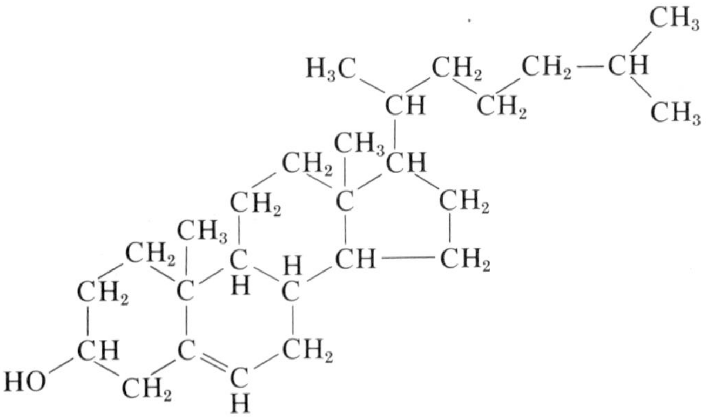

cholesterol, $C_{27}H_{46}O$, a steroid lipid

FIGURE 1–4   Some organic compounds

clearly see the carbon chain or "skeleton," which will be apparent in almost all compounds discussed in the second half of this text. One of the compounds shown in the figure is the famous and controversial substance *cholesterol.*

You see in Figure 1–4 both the molecular formula and a structural formula for each compound. The structural formula shows which atoms are bonded where. You should be able to remember which elements go into carbohydrates and fats (C,H,O) and which go into proteins (C,H,N,O,S).

Approaching chemical formulas

Even from the small taste we have given you of the compounds that will be discussed in this text, you must be wondering how in the world you will be able to memorize so many formulas. The answer is, you *won't* have to. Chemical compounds fall into groups with similar properties, so if you know how to write the formula of one member of the group, you are able to produce many more (Chapters 4 and 7). Right now, you are being asked only to be able to *read* a formula and to count the number of atoms of each element contained in it.

When you do begin to write formulas, remember that chemistry is a very exact science. "Spelling" is very important. If you wish to write carbon monoxide, CO, and instead you write Co, you will have a completely different substance, the element *cobalt.* If you mean to write BI_3 (boron triiodide) and instead write Bi_3, you will have made up a nonexistent molecule containing three atoms of bismuth (#83). Proper use of capital and lower-case letters and proper placement of parentheses, as in $C_7H_5(NO_2)_3$ for TNT, are very important.

SELF-CHECK

1.3)   List the names of the *elements* and count the *number of atoms* of each element in one molecule or formula unit:
a)   ozone, O_3 f)   ammonia, NH_3
b)   marble, $CaCO_3$ g)   rust, Fe_2O_3
c)   hydrogen peroxide, H_2O_2 h)   table sugar, $C_{12}H_{22}O_{11}$
d)   palmitic acid $C_{16}H_{32}O_2$ i)   ammonium nitrate, NH_4NO_3
e)   tyrosine $C_9H_{11}O_3N$ j)   nitroglycerin $C_3H_5O_3(NO_2)_3$
1.4)   Is each of the following formulas possible for a protein segment or for a carbohydrate? Why?
a) $C_5H_{10}O_5$ b) $C_5H_{13}NO_2$

1.3 A BRIEF LOOK AT HUMAN NUTRITION

LEARNING GOAL 1D: Very briefly describe the general function in the human diet of (a) carbohydrates, (b) fats, (c) proteins, (d) mineral elements, (e) vitamins, and (f) water.

The foods we eat contain 42 to 44 important chemical substances, which are consumed as **nutrients.** We must take in each nutrient in the right

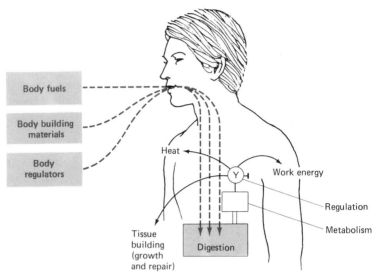

FIGURE 1–5 The varied functions of food nutrients.

amounts if we are to have enough raw materials and energy to grow, reproduce, and lead a full, healthy life. Not too little, or a nutritional deficiency will develop. Not too much, either, for the body functions best when it is in balance.

Foods are generally mixtures of many chemical substances. Each substance can perform one or more of the roles listed in Figure 1–5. There are six general kinds of nutrients:

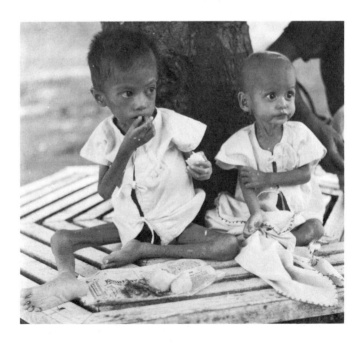

Sad and listless, these children show all the signs of advanced malnutrition. (Courtesy of UNICEF and Mallica Vajrathon. Used with permission.)

1) Carbohydrates or sugars, which are eventually converted to CO_2 and water.
2) Fats, which break down to fatty acids.
3) Proteins, which break down to amino acids.
4) Mineral elements.
5) Vitamins.
6) Water.

Energy nutrients

Carbohydrates, fats, and proteins are often thought of as fuels for the body since they can be used to supply energy. They can all be used by the body as a source of *Calories,* which are a measure of the heat and energy derived from food. If we exercise more, we need more Calories (Chapter 21). Some people seem to need more Calories for the same activities than others of the same size and build.

If a person receives too few Calories from the three energy sources, the body will look to its stored fat and become thin. If intake of Calories continues to be too low, malnutrition will result. If too many Calories of energy are taken in, a person will develop large fat storage deposits and eventually become obese.

Obesity will be discussed in Chapter 26.

That explains why there is no "miracle" way to lose weight. All kinds of Calories count. Furthermore, dieting that eliminates one kind of food and stresses another presents difficulties if continued week after week. The only safe way to lose weight is to simply eat less food in a balanced diet.

Proteins, mineral elements (calcium, magnesium, iron, copper, and others from Table 1–1), and water are necessary for the building and repair of body tissues. Proteins are essentially chains of *amino acids* (described in Chapter 19). The body breaks food proteins down into its amino acids, then uses those amino acids to make new proteins needed by the body. Certain *essential* amino acids must be taken in in food. Some foods are high in some essential amino acids, low in others (Chapter 27). For this reason, nutritionists often recommend certain foods in combination (such as peanut butter with milk) so that there will be no gaps in the nutrient supply.

Mineral elements provide *ions,* which are charged particles, for the proper (electrical) functioning of nerves and muscles, the proper exchange of substances across cell walls, and other body needs. Certain elements, although used in extremely small amounts, play key roles in enzymes (Chapter 23), the substances that permit the body to carry out its chemical processes in a reasonable time. Some vitamins also serve similar roles in connection with enzymes; all are required in small amounts to assure normal body functioning.

The roles of certain trace elements in the human body will be discussed in Sections 3.3 and 3.4.

Water typically makes up 60% of the weight of body cells and is thus essential as a material for new cell growth. However, its role is far more basic. The chemistry of the human body takes place almost entirely in water *solution,* as described in Chapter 12. Without water as a carrier, the chemicals would never get a chance to react. Water serves many other functions, so severe *dehydration* (lack of water) presents many health problems.

All of the required nutrients can be supplied by a normal, balanced diet, such as that described in Table 1–3. A normal person following a good diet has no need of a vitamin or mineral supplement, despite the fact that such supplements are used by millions of people each day.

Food fads and fancies

There are many myths about foods, and as old myths are destroyed ("fish is brain food") new ones are created ("organically grown tomatoes are more nutritious than those grown using chemical fertilizers"). One thing you should remember is that a pure substance has exactly the same properties regardless of where it came from. Vitamin C from a chemical factory is of exactly equal value (as a vitamin) as vitamin C from an orange; no more and no less. Sea salt is of no greater health value than processed salt unless you are an (unusual) individual with an iodine deficiency, in which case you should be using iodized salt, salt with iodine added. Most of the claims about "health food" have been questioned.

One area of controversy is food additives. First of all, the "chemicals in our food" include the foods themselves, as you have seen in this chapter. Additives have generally passed very rigid testing and are probably safer than a variety of "home-brewed" spices and flavorings. However, some food additives subject us to unnecessary and unknown risks, for such questionable benefits as brighter color. There is some evidence that certain people may have reactions (perhaps allergic) to very small amounts of food additives that would not affect others, and that hyperactivity in children is sometimes relieved if food additives are removed from the diet.

The best approach to food claims of all sorts is to view them scientifically. This text will help you to understand the chemical basis of human life and to make intelligent choices regarding the "chemical feast" offered to the consumer.

An outstanding source of detailed information on nutrition and foods is the text *Nutrition and Physical Fitness, 10th edition,* by G.M. Briggs and D.H. Calloway (W.B. Saunders, 1979).

SELF-CHECK

1.5) If a friend recommended that you lose weight with a low-carbohydrate diet (eating as much as you want of proteins and fats), how would you respond?

1.6) Which of the six kinds of nutrients are needed primarily as raw materials for the building of new cells?

TABLE 1-3 DAILY FOOD PLAN BASED ON FOUR FOOD GROUPS

Group and Servings per Day	Role in Diet
1. Grain products—bread, flour, cereals, baked goods (whole-grain preferred). (Four or more servings.)	1. Inexpensive sources of energy and proteins; whole-grain and enriched products carry more iron and B vitamins.
2. Meat and vegetable protein group—meats, poultry, fish, shellfish, eggs; dried beans, peas, nuts. (Two or more servings.)	2. Valuable sources of proteins and amino acids; also furnish minerals (e.g., iron) and B vitamins.
3. Milk group—milk, cheese, yogurt, ice cream. (Four or more glasses or equivalent for teenagers, two for adults.)	3. Valuable sources of protein, calcium, riboflavin, other minerals, and vitamins.
4. Vegetable-fruit group—all fruits, vegetables, potatoes. (Four or more servings, including (a) leafy green and yellow vegetables and (b) citrus fruits, tomatoes, raw cabbage.)	4. Chiefly important as carriers of minerals, vitamins, and fiber; (a) high in iron, vitamin A, folacin; (b) rich in vitamin C.

CHAPTER ONE IN REVIEW ■ The Chemicals of Life

GLOSSARY FOR CHAPTER ONE

atom The smallest particle of an element; can combine with atoms of other elements to form chemical *compounds.* (p. 5)

compound A pure substance made up of two or more *elements;* can be broken down into its elements by chemical changes; represented by a chemical formula. (p. 6)

element A kind of pure substance that cannot be decomposed into simpler pure substances by chemical means; there are over 100 known elements, of which 25 are probably used in the human body. (p. 2)

formula A combination of element *symbols* and subscripts, such as H_2O, to show the *elements* present in a pure substance and the ratio in which the *atoms* of different elements appear. (p. 6)

formula unit The combination of *atoms* represented by a chemical *formula;* may represent a *molecule,* as in H_2O, or an imaginary smallest part of a crystal, as in NaCl. (p. 7)

matter Anything that occupies space; has mass (weight); *elements* and *compounds* are two kinds of matter and are called *pure substances; mixtures* of pure substances are also matter. (p. 2)

molecule A small particle or "bit" of matter that contains more than one *atom;* the smallest particle of a molecular *compound.* (p. 5)

nutrient A pure substance taken into the body to provide energy, building materials, or regulator materials. (p. 9)

organic compound A compound in which carbon is (generally) bonded to other carbon atoms and to hydrogen atoms; often also contains oxygen, nitrogen, and, occasionally, other elements. (p. 8)

periodic table A chart (such as that on the inside front cover of this text) that shows all of the *elements* and their *symbols* in order of *atomic number;* generally also provides the *atomic weight* of each element. (p. 2)

symbol The one-letter or two-letter abbreviation for an *element;* used in writing chemical *formulas* and *equations.* (p. 3)

Note: The terms carbohydrate, fat, protein, vitamin, mineral element, atomic number, and atomic weight will be discussed in later chapters.

All glossary terms should be learned along with the learning goals of each chapter. It is expected that you will be able to use each term correctly.

QUESTIONS AND PROBLEMS FOR CHAPTER ONE ■ The Chemicals of Life

At the end of each chapter, you will find questions and problems to test your understanding. Those marked with a star (*) go somewhat beyond the learning goals listed for the chapter. Your instructor will advise you if such questions are important or optional. Questions 1.1 to 1.6 are in the self-checks.

LEFT-HAND COLUMN OF QUESTIONS:
Answers to these questions will be found in Appendix A at the end of this textbook. Use these questions to check your understanding.

RIGHT-HAND COLUMN OF QUESTIONS:
Answers to these questions are not in the book. The questions may be used for homework.

SECTION 1.1 THE ELEMENTS OF THE HUMAN BODY
(Do the following questions *without* looking at any periodic table or other aid.)

1.7) Write the *symbol* for each element:

oxygen	tin
zinc	magnesium
iron	

1.8) The element *potassium* plays an extremely important role inside every body cell. What is its symbol?

1.9) Write the *name* of each element:

Ni	Si
S	Na
P	Cr

1.10) An element found in the mitochondria of cells, where energy is produced, has the symbol Mn. What is this element?

1.11*) A compound of this element is added to some water supplies to prevent tooth decay in children. Give the name and symbol of this element.

1.12*) Which four elements make up 96% of human body weight?

1.13*) In what *form* does your body contain most of its hydrogen?

1.14*) The earth has a strong magnetic field that allows us to use a compass to determine direction. What element, which we usually associate with magnets, creates this field? See Figure 1–1.

1.29) Write the *symbol* for each element:

hydrogen	vanadium
chlorine	iodine
sodium	

1.30) The element *copper* is needed for normal blood vessels, tendons, and bones. Write its chemical symbol.

1.31) Write the *name* of each element:

Mg	Fe
F	Mo
Ca	Co

1.32) Very low levels of this element are needed to prevent "white muscle disease." It has the symbol Se. What is it?

1.33*) A compound of this element, needed for functioning of the thyroid gland, is sometimes added to table salt. Give the name and symbol of this element.

1.34*) Which one element makes up a greater part of body weight than any other element?

1.35*) In what *form* does your body contain most of its nitrogen?

1.36*) The sun gets its energy from a nuclear *fusion* reaction of a type that mankind hopes to duplicate on earth to obtain cheap power. What elements might be involved? See Figure 1–1.

SECTION 1.2 SOME COMPOUNDS OF THE HUMAN BODY

List the elements that are contained in each of the following compounds, and state how many atoms of each element are in one molecule or formula unit.

1.15) N_2O, laughing gas

1.16) Na_3PO_4, a detergent

1.17) $Ca(OH)_2$, quicklime

1.18) CH_3OH, methyl alcohol

1.19) $(NH_2)_2CO$, urea

1.20) $C_6H_{12}O_6$, glucose sugar

1.21) $C_5H_{10}NO_2$, proline, an amino acid.

1.22) $C_{63}H_{88}CoN_{14}O_{14}P$, a B vitamin

1.23) $(C_{738}H_{1166}FeN_{203}O_{208}S_2)_4$, hemoglobin in red blood cells

1.24) Which of the following elements will you find in a *fat*?

C   O
H   N

1.25*) Which of the following pure elements form diatomic molecules?

a) carbon   c) oxygen
b) hydrogen

1.37) HOCl, found in chlorine bleach.

1.38) $NaHCO_3$, baking soda.

1.39) $Ca_3(PO_4)_2$, found in bone.

1.40) C_6H_5OH, phenol or "carbolic acid."

1.41) $C_7H_5(NO_2)_3$, TNT explosive.

1.42) $C_3H_8O_3$, glycerol.

1.43) $C_6H_{12}N_2O_4S_2$, cystine, an amino acid.

1.44) $C_{27}H_{44}O$, vitamin D.

1.45) $C_{55}H_{72}MgN_4O_5$, plant chlorophyll.

1.46) Which of the following elements will you *not* find in a carbohydrate?

C   O
H   N

1.47*) Which of the following pure elements form diatomic molecules?

a) iron   c) chlorine
b) nitrogen

SECTION 1.3 A BRIEF LOOK AT HUMAN NUTRITION

1.26) Why do we eat carbohydrates?

1.27) Why do we need vitamins?

1.28*) Criticize the following statement: "If the body needs 0.018 grams of iron each day, then it must be fine to take in 18.0 grams daily."

1.48) Why do we eat fats?

1.49) Name two roles of food proteins in the body.

1.50*) Criticize the following statement: "Since the body can get its energy from fats, carbohydrates, and proteins, I might as well cut out the latter two and eat only fats."

2 Matter and Its Measurement

In Chapter 1, you learned about some chemical elements that play a role in human life processes. The *atom* was described as the smallest bit of an element. We estimated (p. 5) that inside a 1-inch cubic block of iron, there are more than 1 000 000 000 000 000 000 000 000 atoms. Along one edge, if you could see all the atoms, you would find about 100 million of them lined up.

This information about atoms that we cannot see with our naked eyes, or even with ordinary microscopes, comes from *measurement*. In this chapter, we will discuss how scientists measure length, volume, mass, and density. You will learn some *uncomplicated, straightforward* ways to do "chemical arithmetic." Finally, we will discuss the sizes and masses of the atoms themselves and of the small particles (electrons, protons, and neutrons) that make up an atom. In this way, you will grow to understand why there are different kinds of atoms with different chemical properties.

2.1 MEASUREMENT OF LENGTH AND VOLUME

LEARNING GOAL 2A: *Convert a length measurement expressed in meters, centimeters, or kilometers to a different metric unit.*

2B: *Convert a volume measurement expressed in cubic centimeters or milliliters to liters; convert liters to milliliters or cubic centimeters.*

2C: *Using a table of conversion factors, convert a length or volume measurement from English units to metric units.*

Length is the most common measurement we make in our daily lives. We estimate distances traveled, heights of people and buildings, lengths of carpet, and widths of pizza. We can then use what we know about the length, width, and height of objects to estimate their volumes, that is, how much they can hold.

Scientists make frequent length measurements. In chemistry, a volume of solution is something that is very often needed in the laboratory, hospital, or even in a police station. In English-speaking countries, the inch, foot, yard, and mile have been in common use as units of length. We measure liquid volumes in pints, quarts, and gallons. Can you relate a volume of one gallon to the size of the container measured in feet? Probably not! How many inches make one mile? The answer is 63 360. Scientists need a better system of units. For example, there are 1 000 000 millimeters in one kilometer.*

SI units and the metric system

In 1793, each country of Europe had its own way of measuring things. The French National Academy of Sciences devised the **metric system** so that everyone would "speak the same language" of weights and measures. In 1960, the International System of Units, or **SI units,** was adopted by most of the countries of the world, and all others (including the United States) have converted to SI or are scheduled to do so.

Scientists, being human, became accustomed to using a variety of units. In theory, we should all learn to use and to write the official SI units. In practice, we are changing our ways slowly. In this textbook, we will use only metric units, and we will teach you to use them, too, since hospitals and laboratories work "in metric."

The meter

The metric (and SI) unit of length is the *metre,* which is generally spelled **meter** in North America. The meter is now defined in terms of a very precise measurement using a beam of light.

The meter is a convenient unit for measuring heights of buildings, lengths of record-breaking home runs, and distances of Olympic track events. However, if you travel from one city to another, you are going a lot of meters. Since a meter is about 39 inches long, from New York to Miami is about 2 million meters.

The metric system has an easy answer for this. Just as there are 100 cents in 1 dollar, we use factors of 100 and 1000 to create new units based on the meter. The convenient unit for road distances is the kilometer, which is a length of 1000 meters. The N.Y.–Miami run is then 2137 kilometers. The legal speed limit on most roads is 92 kilometers/hour.

The word-part or prefix **kilo-** means "a unit 1000 times as great" in the metric system. Other prefixes are used for larger or smaller units. For example, a height might be 5 feet 8 inches, or 68 inches. In meters, this comes to 1.73 meters. People like to think in terms of numbers without fractions or decimals. The metric system has a second prefix, **centi-,** which means "a unit 1/100 as large." The same height can thus be expressed as 173 centimeters. A third very important prefix is **milli-,** meaning "a unit 1/1000 as large" (here, 1730 millimeters).

Table 2–1 shows the metric prefixes, which cover a span from a unit that is 10^{18} meters long (1 exameter = 1 000 000 000 000 000 000 meters) to one smaller than anything known, the attometer.

The prefixes commonly used by chemists are shown in **boldface** type in Table 2–1. You are expected to learn the meanings and symbols of these prefixes. Once you know the symbols, you no longer need to write "1000 meters = 1 kilometer"; you may write "1000 m = 1 km" instead. Notice

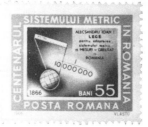

The meter was once defined as 1/10 000 000 of the distance from the equator to the North Pole.

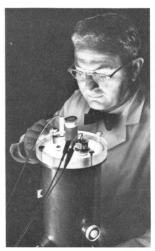

The standard meter is now defined in terms of the wavelength of light emitted by the krypton gas in this apparatus.

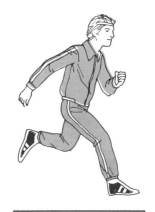

1 m

A meter is about the distance of one long stride.

* Large scientific numbers are now commonly written with spaces rather than commas dividing groups of three digits.

TABLE 2–1   METRIC PREFIXES

Prefix	Symbol	Meaning	Prefix	Symbol	Meaning
exa-	E	10^{18}	atto-	a	10^{-18}
peta-	P	10^{15}	femto-	f	10^{-15}
tera-	T	10^{12}	pico-	p	10^{-12}
giga-	G	$10^9 = 1\ 000\ 000\ 000$	**nano-**	**n**	$10^{-9} = 0.000\ 000\ 001$
mega-	M	$10^6 = 1\ 000\ 000$	**micro-**	**μ**	$10^{-6} = 0.000\ 001$
kilo-	**k**	$10^3 = 1\ 000$	**milli-**	**m**	$10^{-3} = 0.001$
hecto-	h	$10^2 = 100$	**centi-**	**c**	$10^{-2} = 0.01$
deka-	da	$10^1 = 10$	deci-	d	$10^{-1} = 0.1$
(*none*)	—	$10^0 = 1$	(*none*)	—	$10^0\ = 1$

that these symbols do *not* have periods after them (1 km, *not* 1 k.m. or 1 km.) and must be written exactly as shown (1 km, *not* 1 **KM**).

Metric length conversions

We see from Table 2–1 that 1 km = 1000 m. In scientific work, we often have to *convert* a measurement made in one unit, say meters, to a different unit, perhaps kilometers.

You already know the method used, perhaps because you have at some time converted inches to feet. You multiply by the proper **conversion factor.** If your height is 72 inches and you want to find the same measurement in feet, you multiply

$$72 \text{ in.} \times \frac{1 \text{ ft}}{12 \text{ in.}} = 6 \text{ ft}$$

or perhaps you simply divided by 12 in your head. The scientific approach has developed a very good way to insure that you don't multiply when you should divide. We will call this the **conversion-factor method.**†

Each time you set one length measurement equal to the same measurement in a different set of units, you have created a conversion factor. When you divide something by itself, you get exactly one! Since 1 km = 1000 m, what we get when we write

$$\frac{1 \text{ km}}{1000 \text{ m}} \quad \text{or} \quad \frac{1000 \text{ m}}{1 \text{ km}}$$

is a factor that cannot change a measurement.

You choose which conversion factor to use by looking at *units*. In chemical arithmetic, units act somewhat like numbers. They *cancel* out when they appear in both the numerator (top) and denominator (bottom) of a fraction. We can use this fact to convert one length measurement to another.

EXAMPLE 2a: The Mississippi River is 3779 km long. How many meters is this distance?

METHOD: Take the *given quantity* in the problem, which is a length of 3779 km. Choose from the two conversion factors above, 1 km/1000 m or 1000 m/1 km.

---

† This very important skill is used in almost every chemistry class at the college level. It has many names, such as "dimensional analysis," "cancel-unit method," and "unit-factor method."

POSSIBILITY: $3779 \text{ km} \times \dfrac{1 \text{ km}}{1000 \text{ m}} = 3.779 \dfrac{\text{km km}}{\text{m}}$

That's nonsense! The units don't make any sense, and you know very well that the Mississippi River is *not* 3 m long.

POSSIBILITY: $3779 \text{ km} \times \dfrac{1000 \text{ m}}{1 \text{ km}} = 3\,779\,000 \dfrac{\text{km m}}{\text{km}}$

That looks better. Since kilometers are on the top and on the bottom, we can cancel them out to get 3.779 million meters. We often show the canceled units by drawing lines through them.

SOLUTION: $3779 \text{ km} \times \dfrac{1000 \text{ m}}{1 \text{ km}} = 3.779 \times 10^6 \dfrac{\cancel{\text{km}}\,\text{m}}{\cancel{\text{km}}} = \boxed{3.779 \times 10^6 \text{ m}}$

Were you able to see that $3\,779\,000 \text{ m} = 3.779 \times 10^6$ m? If not, the methods of working in scientific notation, with powers of ten, are included in Appendix B at the end of this textbook. You will need this skill if you do much chemical arithmetic.

Let us review the basic principles of the conversion-factor method:

1) Write the *given* measurement with its units.
2) Find a conversion factor that will cancel the units you *don't* want and give you the units you *do* want.
3) Multiply the given measurement by that conversion factor.

EXAMPLE 2b: A piece of typewriter paper is 21.6 cm wide. What is this width in meters? in millimeters?

METHOD: The given measurement is 21.6 cm. From Table 2–1, we find that 100 cm = 1 m and 1000 mm = 1 m. That gives us four possible conversion factors:

$$\frac{1 \text{ m}}{100 \text{ cm}} \quad \frac{100 \text{ cm}}{1 \text{ m}} \quad \frac{1 \text{ m}}{1000 \text{ mm}} \quad \frac{1000 \text{ mm}}{1 \text{ m}}$$

Choose the appropriate one for each conversion.

SOLUTION: i) $21.6 \text{ cm} \times \dfrac{1 \text{ m}}{100 \text{ cm}} = 0.216 \dfrac{\cancel{\text{cm}}\,\text{m}}{\cancel{\text{cm}}} = \boxed{0.216 \text{ m}}$

Using that answer to solve the second problem,

ii) $0.216 \text{ m} \times \dfrac{1000 \text{ mm}}{1 \text{ m}} = 216 \dfrac{\cancel{\text{m}}\,\text{mm}}{\cancel{\text{m}}} = \boxed{216 \text{ mm}}$

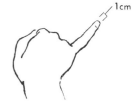

A centimeter is about the width of your little finger.

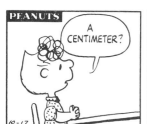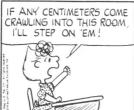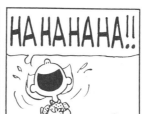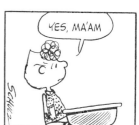

Note that we can use Table 2–1 to make up new conversion factors. If two measurements are equal to a third measurement, they are equal to each other. If 100 cm = 1 m = 1000 mm, then 100 cm = 1000 mm. Part ii can thus be solved:

$$21.6 \text{ cm} \times \frac{1000 \text{ mm}}{100 \text{ cm}} = 216 \frac{\text{cm mm}}{\text{cm}} = \boxed{216 \text{ mm}}$$

The conversion-factor method will work for many different kinds of problems.

EXAMPLE 2c: A bicycle rider finds that he can cover a 25-km distance in one hour. His average speed is 25 km/hr.
i)   How far can he go in two hours?
ii)   What is his average speed in meters per second?

METHOD: Use the principles of the conversion factor method. In problem i, the given measurement is actually 2 hr and the conversion factor we use is 25 km/hr. Thus:

SOLUTION: i) $2 \text{ hr} \times \dfrac{25 \text{ km}}{\text{hr}} = 50 \dfrac{\text{km hr}}{\text{hr}} = \boxed{50 \text{ km}}$

This answer should agree with common sense! For problem ii, we need to change the *time*. We should be able to use one of the two following conversion factors:

$$\frac{1 \text{ hr}}{3600 \text{ sec}} \quad \text{or} \quad \frac{3600 \text{ sec}}{1 \text{ hr}}$$

The given measurement is 25 km/hr. The proper conversion factor will have hours on the *top*. We must *also* go from km to m.

$$\text{ii)} \quad 25 \frac{\text{km}}{\text{hr}} \times \frac{1 \text{ hr}}{3600 \text{ sec}} = 0.00694 \frac{\text{km hr}}{\text{hr sec}} = 0.00694 \frac{\text{km}}{\text{sec}}$$

Then:

$$0.00694 \frac{\text{km}}{\text{sec}} \times \frac{1000 \text{ m}}{\text{km}} = 6.94 \frac{\text{km m}}{\text{sec km}} = \boxed{6.94 \frac{\text{m}}{\text{sec}}}$$

The self-check at the end of this section will give you practice in the use of the conversion-factor method.

Area measurement

On occasion, you may be asked to calculate an area. For a rectangular object, such as a piece of writing paper, the area is width × height. If the units of width and height are cm, the units of area are cm × cm = cm², which is called "square centimeters."

Surface area can become important in life sciences when we must consider gain or loss of heat. For example, if a person falls into very cold water, death can result from hypothermia, a lowering of body temperature. Certain positions of the legs and arms can minimize the amount of body surface area exposed to cold water and thus allow the victim to survive longer.

Volume measurement

Measurement of volume, the total amount of space occupied, is important in describing gases, liquids, and powders. Kitchen recipes often call for "cups," "pints," and "teaspoonsful," all of which are English volume units.

For something in the shape of a cube, where all the sides are of equal length, such as a sugar cube or camera flash cube, the volume is side $\times$ side $\times$ side = $side^3$. For a box or a room, volume is length $\times$ width $\times$ height.

SI uses volume units based on the cubic meter. The metric volume unit of greatest use in the laboratory is the **cubic centimeter,** with symbol cm^3.‡ The volume of a solid object that is a cube 1 cm on each side is 1 cm $\times$ 1 cm $\times$ 1 cm = 1 cm^3. You should be able to use cubic centimeters in calculations.

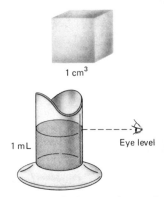

A 1-cm cube has a volume of 1 cm^3, which is exactly the same as a volume of 1 mL.

EXAMPLE 2d: How many cubic centimeters of water will be required to fill a steam sterilizer which is 25.0 cm long by 15.0 cm wide and is to be filled to the 10.0-cm mark?

SOLUTION: 25.0 cm $\times$ 15.0 cm $\times$ 10.0 cm = 3750 cm^3 = $\boxed{3.75 \times 10^3 \ cm^3}$

For many years, chemists have used another unit for gas and liquid volumes, the **liter** (or, internationally, *litre*). The liter is a metric unit, and just as 1000 mm = 1 m, we can divide the liter into 1000 parts such that 1000 **milliliters** = 1 liter. The present official symbol for liter is a capital L and for milliliter mL; up until the late 1970's, the symbols were ℓ and ml. You should be familiar with both sets of symbols.

In clinical chemistry, used in hospitals and medical testing laboratories, the standard volume for blood and urine samples has long been 100 mL, or one **deciliter** (dL), which is 1/10 of a liter. For example, the normal amount of calcium ion in blood serum is considered to be 8.5 to 10.5 mg/dL, which we would read as "milligrams per deciliter." To convert from this common clinical unit to liters, we need only use the conversion factor 10 dL = 1 L. The prefix **deci-** means 1/10.

It is awkward to have two kinds of volume measurements, one based on length (cm^3) and one based on capacity (L, mL, dL). Luckily, the "old" definitions of the milliliter and cubic centimeter differed only slightly, and so the milliliter has been redefined to make it equal to *exactly* one cubic centimeter. Thus,

1 mL = 1 cm^3 = 1 cc = 0.01 dL = 0.001 L (all *exactly*)
1 dL = 100 cm^3 = 100 cc = 100 mL = 0.1 L (all *exactly*)
1 L = 1000 cm^3 = 1000 cc = 1000 mL = 10 dL = 1 dm^3 (all *exactly*)

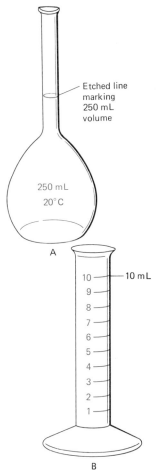

FIGURE 2–1 Two common ways of measuring liquid volume use a volumetric flask (A) or a graduated cylinder (B).

---

‡ Cubic centimeters are still commonly written "cc" or possibly "cu.cm." Although these symbols are unofficial, you should recognize them as having the same meaning as "cm^3" and as "mL" or "ml."

> EXAMPLE 2e: A student prepares a solution in a 250.00-mL volumetric flask, shown in Figure 2–1. i) What is the volume in cm³ (or cc or cu.cm.)? ii) What is the volume in liters? iii) What is the volume in the clinical unit dL?
>
> -
>
> SOLUTION: i) All of these units equal mL. The volume is $\boxed{250.00 \text{ cm}^3}$ = 250.00 cc = 250.00 cu.cm.
>
> ii) Since 1 L = 1000 mL,
>
> $$250.00 \text{ mL} \times \frac{1 \text{ L}}{1000 \text{ mL}} = 0.25000 \frac{\text{L } \cancel{\text{mL}}}{\cancel{\text{mL}}} = \boxed{0.25000 \text{ L}}$$
>
> iii) Since 1 L = 1000 mL = 10 dL,
>
> $$250.00 \text{ mL} \times \frac{10 \text{ dL}}{1000 \text{ mL}} = 2.5000 \frac{\text{dL } \cancel{\text{mL}}}{\cancel{\text{mL}}} = \boxed{2.5000 \text{ dL}}$$

English units of length and volume

Now that you are familiar with the metric units of length and volume, let us look at possible conversions between the traditional (English) units and the metric system.

The English units have quaint origins. The inch, foot, and yard, along with less common units like cubit, hand, and span, were all based on distances between parts of the measurer's body. Distances between towns were estimated in leagues, but no one ever knew exactly how long a league was! It is only in the last few centuries that the British units have had definite and universal meanings.

In the next few years, you will be seeing more and more products and books using the metric units. As a rough guide to *which* metric unit to use in expressing length measurements:

If the thickness of an object has traditionally been given in *mils* (1 mil = 1/1000 of an inch), use *millimeters*.
If the length of an object is expressed in *inches*, use *centimeters*.
If the height of an object is in *feet*, use *meters*.
If a large distance is written in *miles*, you want it in *kilometers*.

Table 2–2 gives the common English units of length and volume and their metric equivalents.

You should be ready to convert any English measurement of length or capacity (volume) to its metric equivalent and vice versa.

> EXAMPLE 2f: One brand of green garbage bags advertises that the plastic is 1.65 mils in thickness. Convert to the appropriate metric unit, using Table 2–2.
>
> -
>
> SOLUTION: $1.65 \, \cancel{\text{mils}} \times \dfrac{0.0254 \text{ mm}}{1 \, \cancel{\text{mil}}} = \boxed{0.0419 \text{ mm}}$ (rather thin!)
>
> EXAMPLE 2g: A runner completed a 1500-m race in 3:34.5 (3 minutes 34.5 seconds). i) What was this distance in miles? ii) What was the runner's average speed in km/hr? in miles/hr?
>
> -

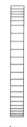

One millimeter is about the thickness of a U.S. dime.

SOLUTION: i) $1500 \, \cancel{m} \times \dfrac{1 \text{ km}}{1000 \, \cancel{m}} = 1.500 \text{ km}$

$1.500 \, \cancel{km} \times \dfrac{1 \text{ mile}}{1.609 \, \cancel{km}} = \boxed{0.932 \text{ mile}}$

ii) $3\!:\!34.5 = (3)(60) + 34.5 = 214.5 \text{ sec}$

Convert to hours: $214.5 \, \cancel{sec} \times \dfrac{1 \text{ hr}}{3600 \, \cancel{sec}} = 0.0596 \text{ hr}$

$\dfrac{1.500 \text{ km}}{0.0596 \text{ hr}} = \boxed{25.2 \text{ km/hr}}$

$\dfrac{0.932 \text{ mile}}{0.0596 \text{ hr}} = \boxed{15.6 \text{ miles/hr}}$

EXAMPLE 2h: One Montreal snowfall measured 39.0 cm. How many inches?

SOLUTION: $39.0 \, \cancel{cm} \times \dfrac{1 \text{ in.}}{2.540 \, \cancel{cm}} = \boxed{15.4 \text{ in.}}$

Note that with these examples we have begun canceling units inside the solution setup.

EXAMPLE 2i: One American soft drink bottle contains 28 fl oz. How many liters are in that bottle?

SOLUTION: $28 \, \cancel{fl oz} \times \dfrac{1 \, \cancel{mL}}{0.0338 \, \cancel{fl oz}} \times \dfrac{1 \text{ liter}}{1000 \, \cancel{mL}} = \boxed{0.83 \text{ L}}$

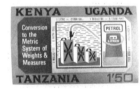

KENYA   UGANDA

Conversion to the Metric System of Weights & Measures

PETROL

TANZANIA   1'50

EXAMPLE 2j: One of the authors recently filled his gas-guzzler with 75.0 liters of fuel at a Montreal service station. How many U.S. gallons went in?

SOLUTION: $75.0 \, \cancel{L} \times \dfrac{1 \text{ U.S. gal}}{3.785 \, \cancel{L}} = \boxed{19.8 \text{ U.S. gal}}$

When members of the British Commonwealth, including Canada, converted to SI volume units, they had to learn to change *gills* and *imperial gallons* to liters. One imperial gallon is 1.20 U.S. gallons, or 4.546 liters.

TABLE 2–2   METRIC UNITS OF LENGTH AND LIQUID VOLUME
WITH ENGLISH EQUIVALENTS

1 km = 1000 m	= 0.6214 mile	= 3281 ft	1 mile	= 1.609 km
1 m	= 3.281 ft	= 39.37 in.	1 ft	= 0.305 m
1 cm = 0.01 m	= 0.3937 in.	= 393.7 mils	1 in.	= 2.540 cm
1 mm = 0.001 m	= 0.03937 in.	= 39.37 mils	1 mil	= 0.0254 mm
$1 \text{ Å} = 1 \times 10^{-8} \text{ cm} = 1 \times 10^{-10} \text{ m} = 3.937 \times 10^{-9}$ in.				

1 L = 1000 mL	= 0.2642 U.S. gal	1 U.S. gal	= 3.785 L
	= 1.0567 U.S. qt	1 U.S. qt	= 0.9463 L
	= 2.1134 U.S. pt	1 U.S. pt	= 0.4732 L
$1 \text{ mL} = 0.001 \text{ L} = 1 \text{ cm}^3$	= 0.0338 fl oz	1 fl oz	= 29.57 mL
	= 16.23 minims	1 minim	= 0.062 mL
$1 \, \mu\text{L} = 10^{-3} \text{ mL} = 10^{-6} \text{ L} = 0.01623$ minims = 1 lambda (λ)			
(approximate: 1 cup $\approx$ 250 mL; 1 tablespoon $\approx$ 15 mL; 1 teaspoon $\approx$ 5 mL)			

Precision of answers

If you are to do any large number of calculations in this course, you will need a simple electronic calculator. An inexpensive one is fine. A memory is a desirable feature.

However, once you start using the calculator, you will begin wondering how many of the digits (numbers) that appear on the display should be used. For example, when we divided 75.0 by 3.785 in Example 2j, the calculator displayed "19.815059." Do we keep all eight digits or round some off?

In all scientific work, the number of digits written down *has* a real meaning. It indicates how much of the answer is known and to what extent the number has been estimated. For example, when we say 1 ft = 0.305 m (Table 2–2), we mean that a foot is larger than 0.304 m and smaller than 0.306 m. **If the quantity has been measured, the last digit written down is considered to be uncertain.**

If you checked your weight on a sidewalk scale and read "133 lb," your weight certainly might be 134 or 132. It would not make sense to write on a medical form that your weight was 133.00 lb.

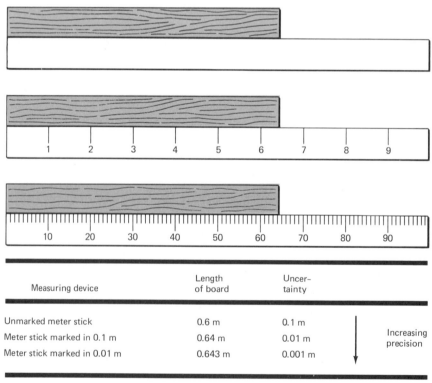

Measuring device	Length of board	Uncertainty	
Unmarked meter stick	0.6 m	0.1 m	
Meter stick marked in 0.1 m	0.64 m	0.01 m	Increasing precision
Meter stick marked in 0.01 m	0.643 m	0.001 m	

If we measure the length of a wooden board with a meter stick, the uncertainty in measurement will depend on the spacing of the markings on the stick. In each case, you are expected to be able to estimate the correct length to within one tenth of one ruler division. With a meter stick marked to the nearest centimeter, you can estimate to the nearest tenth of a centimeter, thus to 1 millimeter. If there are fewer markings on the meter stick, the uncertainty increases. No matter how close to each other one puts the markings on the meter stick, there will always be some uncertainty in the measured length of the board.

On the other hand, when we write 1 km = 1000 m, we are not dealing with a *measured* quantity. We could equally well write "1 km = 1000.0000 m." The 1000 here is defined, not measured. Likewise, 1 dozen = 12.0000 . . . , since we are talking about exactly 12 things being *counted*.

The rules scientists use when writing down the results of scientific measurements and when reporting calculations from those measurements are given in Appendix B. If your instructor requires you to use those detailed procedures, do so. If not, then use the following guidelines:

1) Count the number of **significant digits** in each measurement. A zero that is used simply to "place" the decimal point is not significant. For example, the number 1.65 has *three* significant digits, but 0.0254 also has *three* significant digits, as do 1.38×10^5 and 0.00300 and 17.3!
2) If several measurements enter the calculation, note the one with *fewest* significant digits.
3) Express the answer of a calculation in this course (unless instructed otherwise) to as many significant digits as has the measured number with the *fewest* significant digits given in the problem.

This will often require you to round off your computed answer. A good rule is, if the part of the number to be dropped off is . . . 49999 or less, you drop it. If . . . 50000 or more, then raise the preceding digit by one.§

EXAMPLE 2k: Round off each of the following numbers to the number of significant digits indicated: i) 7.5810287 to three digits. ii) 0.000788132 to two digits.

- -

SOLUTION: i)   7.581 . . . has a "1" in the fourth place. Drop the 1 to leave three digits.

The answer is $\boxed{7.58}$

ii)   0.0007881 . . . has an "8" in the position to be dropped. The previous digit must be increased by one.

The answer is $\boxed{0.00079}$

or, in scientific notation, 7.88132×10^{-4} becomes 7.9×10^{-4}.

EXAMPLE 2l: A young health professional has an annual salary of $20 000.00 and is paid every two weeks. What amount should appear on each of the 26 paychecks?

- -

SOLUTION: When we divide $20 000.00 by 26, we obtain $769.23077! Obviously, a bank cannot honor a paycheck for this amount. The paycheck should read $\boxed{\$769.23}$ so it can be cashed to the nearest cent. In this situation, we use the rules of commerce and common sense rather than scientific principles. However, it illustrates that calculator displays often show meaningless numbers. (The two cents owed to the worker might be added to the last paycheck of the year.)

The conversion-factor method you have learned in this section will be used throughout the course, and perhaps throughout your working life. Remember to apply it properly each time you see a mathematical problem. Some answers in appendix A to the following self-checks and to other

---

§ This simple rule will carry you through the simple calculations of a chemistry course. Some teachers prefer a slightly different manner of rounding off fives.

arithmetic problems in this book have been written out to show each conversion factor involved.

2.1) One of the authors is 173 cm tall. What is his height in a) mm? b) m? c) km? d) in.? e) miles?

2.2) Convert each of these English length measurements to an appropriate metric unit, using Table 2–2.
 a) 3.4 miles   b) 1.5 mil   c) 50 yards

2.3) Convert each of the volumes shown to mL, using Table 2–2.
 a) 5.81 L   b) 45.6 cm³   c) 0.75 U.S. pint

2.4*) An aquarium tank measures 12 in. by 30 in. by 12 in. By converting its volume to cm³, then to mL, then to liters, and finally to U.S. gallons, calculate how many gallons of water will be needed to fill the aquarium.

2.5*) A grocery store is selling A brand apple juice in a 48-fl-oz can for 93¢ and B brand in a 1.50-liter bottle for $1.00. Which brand of apple juice is more economical?

2.6*) The radius of a carbon atom is 0.77×10^{-10} m. Calculate this radius in cm. What is the value in nm (nanometers)? The traditional unit for atomic radii is the angstrom unit (Å), and $1 \text{ Å} = 10^{-8}$ cm. What is the radius of the carbon atom in Å?

2.2 MASS AND WEIGHT

LEARNING GOAL 2D: Explain how an astronaut would distinguish between mass and weight.

2E: Convert a mass measurement from one metric unit (grams, kilograms, milligrams) to another.

2F: Using a table of conversion factors, convert a mass measurement between pounds and grams or kilograms.

Chemists must measure masses even more frequently than they measure volumes. It is by the mass or weight that chemicals and drugs are usually made up and sold. The pain reliever that provides "five grains" and the one that provides "seven grains" compete with each other in providing the greatest mass of active ingredient in each tablet. The lethal dose of a poison is often stated as so many milligrams per kilogram of body weight.

On the surface of the earth, we do not make much distinction between mass and weight. We simply weigh something, record a number, and call that number the mass of the object. So long as the force of gravity is constant, this simple assumption works.

It is possible, however, that you will someday be asked to plan a chemical analysis in the weightless environment of a space platform. The astronauts who have already worked in space and on the moon have experienced the difference between mass and weight. You should know it, too.

The **mass** of an atom is constant and will be discussed later in this chapter. The mass of any object in our daily lives is simply the masses of all its atoms added together. Mass makes something "heavy," hard to push or throw, and hard to stop once it is moving.

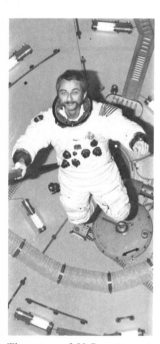
The mass of U.S. astronaut Owen K. Garriot is not zero, but in this picture, his weight is zero because of the lack of gravity inside his space capsule.

Weight, the force with which the earth pulls down on a body, is proportional to mass. If the same object is moved to the moon, where the force of gravity is only one sixth that on earth, the mass will be the same but the weight will be only one sixth as great. The astronauts thus found they could jump higher and farther than on earth.

However, chemical language has developed in such a way that mass and weight are used interchangably. The average *mass* of an atom is commonly described by an atomic *weight*. In the rest of this textbook, we mean "mass" whether we use "mass" or "weight" in our discussion.

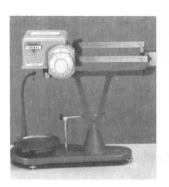

Metric units of mass

The mass units most commonly used by scientists are the **gram** and the **kilogram.** You already know from Table 1–1 that "kilo" means "times 1000." You should thus be able to immediately set up two conversion factors: 1000 g/1 kg and 1 kg/1000 g.

In the medical field, many workers still use "old" symbols for gram, such as "gm." However, in SI "gm" means a gram meter! Use only a single "g" for gram.

Mass conversions

You should be able to carry out conversions of masses in exactly the same fashion as for length and volume, using Table 2-3 as needed.

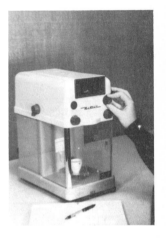

EXAMPLE 2m: What is the weight of a 6-lb-7-oz baby in grams? in kg?

- -

SOLUTION: First change the awkward English measurement to ounces.

$$6 \text{ lb } 7 \text{ oz} = 6 \text{ lb} \times \frac{16 \text{ oz}}{1 \text{ lb}} + 7 \text{ oz} = 96 \text{ oz} + 7 \text{ oz} = 103 \text{ oz}$$

$$\text{Then: } 103 \text{ oz} \times \frac{28.3 \text{ g}}{1 \text{ oz}} = 2.92 \times 10^3 \text{ g}$$

$$2.92 \times 10^3 \text{ g} \times \frac{1 \text{ kg}}{1000 \text{ g}} = \boxed{2.92 \text{ kg}}$$

TABLE 2-3   METRIC UNITS OF MASS AND
ENGLISH EQUIVALENTS

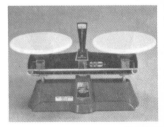

Some common types of laboratory balances, for use in precise mass measurements.

ORDINARY WEIGHTS ("avoirdupois")

1 metric tonne (t) = 1000 kg	= 1.10 (short) U.S. tons	1 ton	= 0.907 t
1 kg = 1000 g	= 2.205 lb	1 lb	= 0.454 kg
1 g	= 0.00221 lb = 0.0353 oz	1 oz	= 28.3 g
1 mg = 0.001 g	= 0.0154 grain	1 grain	= 64.8 mg
1 μg = 0.001 mg = 10^{-6} g	= 1 gamma (γ)		

APOTHECARIES (pharmacy) AND TROY (gold, silver) WEIGHTS

1 kg = 1000 g = 2.68 lb ap = 32.15 oz ap	
1 g	= 0.03215 oz ap = 0.257 dram = 15.4 grains
	= 0.643 pennyweight = 5.00 carats

EXAMPLE 2n: How many pounds of sugar are in a 2.0-kg bag?

SOLUTION: $2.0 \text{ kg} \times \dfrac{1000 \text{ g}}{1 \text{ kg}} \times \dfrac{1 \text{ lb}}{454 \text{ g}} = 4.4 \text{ lb}$

or $\qquad\qquad 2.0 \text{ kg} \times \dfrac{2.205 \text{ lb}}{1 \text{ kg}} = \boxed{4.4 \text{ lb}}$

EXAMPLE 2o: On April 12, 1979, the closing price of gold (Au, #79) on the Hong Kong exchange was \$235.77 (U.S.) per *troy* ounce. What was the cost then of a gram of gold?

SOLUTION: $1.00 \text{ g Au} \times \dfrac{0.03215 \text{ troy oz Au}}{1 \text{ g Au}} \times \dfrac{\$235.77}{1 \text{ troy oz Au}} = \boxed{\$7.58}$

Since gold has gone up considerably in value since then, an interesting exercise would be to make the same calculation at today's prices. Notice that two conversion factors can be included in one setup (as here), or you could first find the mass of gold in troy ounces and then find the cost. Notice also that the substance being measured (gold, Au) has been included in the measurement. This can be very important.

SELF-CHECK

2.7) The heaviest recorded human weighed 1069 pounds in 1958, just before he died at the age of 32. What was his weight in kilograms?

2.8*) Figure 2–2 shows the effect of poor nutrition on body weight. Read from the scales the weights of the well-nourished animal (left) and the vitamin-deficient animal (right).

2.9) The smallest mammal is the fat-tailed shrew, which can, as an adult, weigh as little as 0.090 oz. What is this in grams?

2.10) A typical tablet of the most common pain reliever, acetylsalicylic acid, has 5.0 grains of active ingredient. How many milligrams is this?

2.11) A woman once lifted overhead a weight of 286 lb. That was on the surface of the earth. If she had been on the moon, how much mass could she have lifted? Why? The force of gravity on the moon is one sixth that on earth. (Ignore the fact that the space suit she would be wearing might hinder her.)

2.3 DENSITY AND SPECIFIC GRAVITY

LEARNING GOAL 2G: Given two of the following quantities, calculate the third: (a) mass of a sample; (b) volume of a sample (c) density in g/cm³ or specific gravity.

Density

Length and mass are both quantities we can measure directly, by using a ruler and a balance. If we have an unknown piece of metal, we will not be

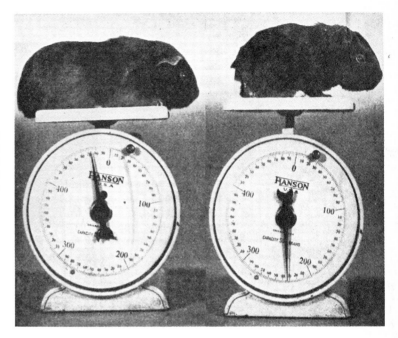

FIGURE 2–2 The guinea pig on the right-hand scale had a diet deficient in Vitamin C. The animal on the left had the same diet plus tomato juice. (Photo from Dr. F.F. Tisdall, Toronto.) Use this picture for Self-Check 2.8.

able to identify it if we simply know its size and mass. With that knowledge, however, we can calculate the **density** of the metal:

$$\text{Density} = \frac{\text{mass}}{\text{volume}}$$

Each pure substance has, at a given temperature, a known density that can be looked up in handbook tables. The density thus can be used to identify what kind of material is present.

Is the following statement true or false? *"Lead is heavier than wood."* Did you say "true"? How about a small piece of lead used on a fishing line compared with the mass of a large tree? Lead may be lighter or heavier than wood, but lead is always *more dense* than wood.

The liter was originally chosen to be extremely close to the volume of 1 kg of water. The density of water at 4°C, slightly above its freezing point, is

Each volume shown—of cork, water, and platinum—contains the *same mass*. Since platinum is more dense than water or cork, it occupies the smallest volume. Will platinum float on water? Will cork? Why?

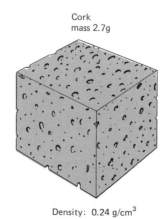

Cork
mass 2.7g

Water
mass 2.7g

Platinum
mass 2.7g

Density: 0.24 g/cm³   1.00 g/cm³   21.5 g/cm³

TABLE 2–4   DENSITIES OF SOME COMMON
SUBSTANCES IN g/cm³ AT 25°C

Hydrogen (H₂) gas	0.000 090	Milk, sea water	1.03
Air	0.001 29	Ebony wood	1.11–1.33
Balsa wood	0.11–0.14	Sugar (sucrose)	1.59
Gasoline	0.66–0.69	Bone	1.7–2.0
Paper	0.70–1.15	Glass	2.4–2.8
Ethyl alcohol	0.79	Aluminum metal	2.7
Potassium metal	0.86	Iron metal	7.9
Ice	0.92	Silver metal	10.5
Olive oil	0.92	Lead metal	11.3
Water (liquid)	1.00	Gold metal	19.3
Urine (normal)	1.01–1.03	Platinum metal	21.5

1.00000 kg/L, more commonly expressed as 1.00000 g/cm³. Remember this value. The density of pure water changes so little in its liquid range (0°C to 100°C) that we generally consider the density to be 1.00 g/cm³ at laboratory temperatures.

The densities of some common substances are shown in Table 2–4. As you would expect from your daily experience, most metals have high density and most types of wood and oil have densities less than 1.00 g/cm³ and thus float on water. Gases are much less dense than liquids and solids. Our units of g/cm³ are not the most convenient to use with gases, so you may see values for gas density in g/L.

EXAMPLE 2p: Dry air has a density of 0.00129 g/cm³. Calculate the same density in g/L (at 25°C).

SOLUTION: $0.00129 \frac{g}{cm^3} \times \frac{1 \ cm^3}{1 \ mL} \times \frac{1000 \ mL}{1 \ L} = \boxed{1.29 \frac{g}{L}}$

The reasons for the low densities of gases will be discussed in Chapter 10. A liquid is usually less dense than the corresponding solid (see Chapter 11), but there are exceptions, such as liquid water and ice.

The calculation of density is straightforward.

EXAMPLE 2q: A cube of magnesium metal 2.00 cm on a side weighs 13.9 grams at 25°C. Calculate the density of Mg. Will it float on water?

SOLUTION: First calculate the volume of the cube. V = 2.00 cm × 2.00 cm × 2.00 cm = 8.00 cm³
Now divide:

$$\frac{13.9 \ g \ Mg}{8.00 \ cm^3} = \boxed{1.74 \ g/cm^3}$$

Mg should not float on water, based on this calculation. Its density is greater than that of water.

The density may be used to calculate mass or volume.

EXAMPLE 2r: Calculate the mass of 76.9 cm³ of Mg metal, at the same temperature as for Example 2q.

SOLUTION: From the previous example, the density of Mg is 1.74 g/cm³. This is a good conversion factor.

$$76.9 \text{ cm}^3 \text{ Mg} \times \frac{1.74 \text{ g Mg}}{1 \text{ cm}^3 \text{ Mg}} = \boxed{134 \text{ g Mg}}$$

EXAMPLE 2s: What volume of ethyl alcohol should we weigh out to get 1.0 kg at 25°C. Use Table 2–4. Answer in liters.

- -

SOLUTION: The conversion factor from Table 2–4 is 0.79 g/cm³. We must use this conversion factor inverted (upside down).

$$1.0 \text{ kg alcohol} \times \frac{1000 \text{ g}}{1 \text{ kg}} \times \frac{1 \text{ cm}^3}{0.79 \text{ g}} \times \frac{1 \text{ mL}}{1 \text{ cm}^3} \times \frac{1 \text{ L}}{1000 \text{ mL}} = \boxed{1.3 \text{ L}}$$

The problem can be done in one series as shown, or you may get an answer after each step.

Specific gravity

At a particular temperature, the **specific gravity** of a substance is calculated as the density of the substance divided by the density of pure water. If we use the almost-universal units of Table 2–4, namely g/cm³, then at 25°C the specific gravity will be density in g/cm³ ÷ 1.00 g/cm³ and will have the same *numeric* value as the density but with no units at all. We can therefore find that, at 25°C, the specific gravity of iron is 7.9; that of olive oil is 0.92, right from a density table such as Table 2–4.

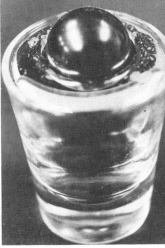

Liquid mercury has a density of 13.6 g/cm³ at 25°C. This picture shows a steel ball floating in mercury. If that appears strange, check the density of iron in Table 2-4. Is it higher or lower than that of mercury?

EXAMPLE 2t: A block of wood measures 2.00 in. × 3.00 in. × 5.00 in. and at 25°C weighs 10.0 oz. Calculate its specific gravity.

- -

SOLUTION: Convert all measurements to the metric system by multiplying each value in inches by 2.54 cm/1 in., and convert the mass in ounces by multiplying by 28.3 g/1 oz, giving the values

$$5.08 \text{ cm} \times 7.62 \text{ cm} \times 12.7 \text{ cm} = 492 \text{ cm}^3 \text{ volume}$$

and 283 grams. The density = 283 g/492 cm³ = 0.575 g/cm³

The specific gravity is thus $\boxed{0.575.}$

Hydrometers

More than 2000 years ago, the Greek inventor Archimedes thought about the force that *pushes up* on an object in water. You have certainly noticed that you can float on water, but not in air. The force holding you up was calculated by Archimedes as equal to the mass of water you displace with your body volume.

For example, suppose a student's body has a mass of 60.0 kg and occupies a volume of 58.0 liters. When it goes underwater, it displaces (pushes out of the way) 58.0 liters of water. In a lake, that water will weigh about 58.0 kg. The body thus has 60.0 kg pulling it down (body weight) and 58.0 kg supporting it. The apparent weight is only 2.0 kg, or less than 5 lb. If the same student swims in the ocean, where the water has a density of 1.03 g/cm³, the upward force will be 59.7 kg and the apparent weight will be almost zero. Floating is easy in that situation.

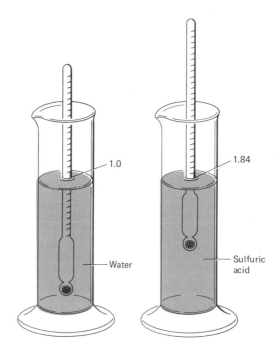

The density of a liquid can be measured with a hydrometer. This particular device shows the density of the sulfuric acid solution in an automobile battery. A similar *urinometer* is used clinically to test the specific gravity of urine samples. The higher the hydrometer tube floats, the less liquid it must displace to equal its own weight and the more dense the solution being measured.

An instrument using this principle to measure the density of a liquid is called a **hydrometer**.

Molarity

In Chapters 12 to 14, where we discuss the properties of water solutions, the amount of substance dissolved in 1 liter of solution is a very important measurement. We will not go into any detail about concentration units here. However, there is a great similarity between density calculations and molarity calculations. If your laboratory program starts early with water solutions, it may be valuable for you to be able to perform calculations of the following type.

The *molarity* of a solution is the number of *moles* (to be defined in Chapter 5) in 1 liter of solution. If you know two of the three amounts (a) moles of dissolved substance, (b) liters of solution, (c) molarity, you can find the third by the same methods we have used for density, replacing "mass" of this chapter with "moles."

EXAMPLE 2u: How many liters of a 3.0 molar solution of hydrochloric acid (HCl) must you take in order to obtain 0.020 moles?

- -

SOLUTION:

$$0.020 \text{ moles HCl} \times \frac{1 \text{ L solution}}{3.0 \text{ moles HCl}} = \boxed{0.0067 \text{ L solution}}$$

Notice the similarity to Example 2s.

You do *not* have to know anything about moles to do this calculation!

2.12) Taken under the proper conditions, the urine of an adult whose kidneys are functioning normally should have a specific gravity between 1.018 and 1.025. A particular urine sample with a volume of 30.00 mL weighed 30.39 g. Is there possible evidence of kidney disease? 2.13) Using the proper density from Table 2–4, calculate the weight in grams of a U.S. quart of milk. See Table 2–2 for the volume conversion factor.

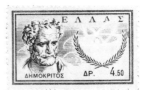

Democritus, born about 460 B.C., was a Greek philosopher who believed in atoms.

2.4 THE ATOM

> *LEARNING GOAL 2H:* *Given a chemical fact or law, such as the Law of Conservation of Mass, discuss its agreement (or lack of it) with Dalton's model of the atom.*
>
> *2I: Distinguish between electrons, protons, and neutrons by describing the charge, relative mass, and position of each in an atom.*
>
> *2J: Define an ion, a cation, and an anion. Given two ions, state whether they attract or repel each other.*
>
> *2K: List and discuss some of the major techniques used in applying the scientific method.*

Hypothesis **is a Greek word meaning "foundation." In science, a hypothesis is a tentative explanation for the observed facts. Eventually, a hypothesis may become a theory.**

If you are a scientist trying to explain the world around you, it is easiest to refer to things you can see, hear, feel, taste, or smell. When he noticed a falling apple, Sir Isaac Newton had eyewitness evidence that some force pulls objects towards the earth. We see more evidence of this fact each time we drop something, fall down, or get rained on. Such direct evidence led to the development of some very important scientific laws several hundred years ago.

Some chemical evidence is similarly "right in front of our eyes." If I fill a balloon with hydrogen gas and heat it with a flame, I will see the flash and hear the sound of an explosion. I might even notice that a new substance, water, has been produced. As a curious person, you have doubtless noticed many chemical events which you could not yet explain, such as the rusting of iron or the rising of a cake in the oven. Until now, you have not yet felt the need to report and explain exactly what happened. A scientist must do so.

The job of science is to make sure the whole world has the facts along with the best possible explanation for the facts. Because atoms are so small, it has taken a long time for people to develop an explanation for the *chemical* facts around us. The story is still being completed, each day. We know enough, however, to draw a pretty good picture of an atom and its parts.

The ancient view of the atom

About 2500 years ago, some Greek philosophers noted that matter can be hot or cold; wet or dry; sweet, sour, or salty; and liquid, solid, or gas. Some of them offered a simple explanation or **hypothesis:** *"All matter consists of four elements: earth, air, fire, and water, mixed together in varying amounts."* Until modern times, we had no better explanation of the chemical world about us.

Some of the early Greeks, notably Democritus, believed that all matter is made up of small pieces which we now call *atoms*. However, the widely respected philospher Aristotle held the opposite view, one that was believed by most educated persons for 2000 years.

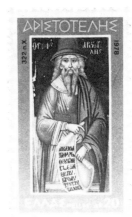

Aristotle (384–322 B.C.) believed not that matter is made up of small bits (atoms), but that it could be subdivided indefinitely. He was so influential that his views were blindly accepted for almost 2000 years.

The earliest "chemists" were more nearly inventors than scientists. They accumulated much useful chemical information in their quest to turn lead into gold or to find eternal youth. These *alchemists,* as well as the very skillful physicians of those days, used a combination of magic and useful chemical knowledge that laid the basis for modern chemical theory.

Boyle's contribution

The Greek "four elements" idea was disproven by the Englishman Robert Boyle (1627–1691), who was the first to explain the difference between a liquid and a solid (which we will discuss in Chapter 11). Boyle's Law, as you will see in Chapter 10, was a major contribution to our understanding of gases.

Boyle was one of the first "natural philosophers" to use the **scientific method.** The use of very carefully planned experiments to obtain information, especially regarding the weights of substances before and after chemical reaction, led to the modern science we are now studying. The results of those experiments had to be reported in a fashion that other scientists could understand and duplicate in their own laboratories. The metric system (Section 2.1) developed largely to avoid misunderstandings about what really happened in an experiment.

Boyle's work was continued in the 1700's by a large group of scientists throughout Europe. The first American chemist may have been Joseph Priestley, an English Unitarian minister who supported the French and American revolutions and who settled in the United States. Priestley was one of the discoverers of oxygen.

Dalton's atomic theory

John Dalton (1766–1844) was one of the most inspired of the early chemists. He put together what was known about gases to generate a theory about how matter is put together. He proposed that elements (such as hydrogen, carbon, oxygen) are made up of atoms, and that

All atoms of a given element have identical properties, such as size, mass, and ability to combine with other elements to form compounds.
Atoms of different elements have different properties.
Chemical changes involve the combination, breaking apart, or rearrangement of groups of atoms, but no atoms are ever created or destroyed in a chemical change.

Dalton drew up a list of symbols for the known elements and then figured out how these might combine into compounds. He felt that the alchemist's dream of turning lead into gold was impossible, since a lead atom cannot become a gold atom in a chemical reaction.

Dalton based his atomic *theory* on known facts about chemical substances. A **theory** is an explanation of *why* nature acts as it does. Scientists always check and recheck a theory, by designing new experiments, to see if the predictions of the theory come true.

Dalton knew that in a given compound a fixed weight (mass) of one element always reacts with a fixed weight of a second element. For example, in carbon dioxide, 3.0 grams of carbon always combine with 8.0 grams of oxygen. This relationship is known as the *Law of Definite Proportions* (or the

An element is made up of atoms, all of which are the same.

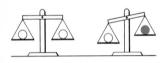

All atoms of one element have the same mass. Atoms of two different elements have different masses. Atoms cannot be destroyed or created.

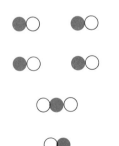

All molecules of a compound are identical. Different combinations of atoms produce different compounds.

Law of Constant Composition). A **law** in science simply states a fact, an observation that has been recorded time after time. Dalton's atomic theory explains this law quite well, as well as a second law of chemical combination, called the *Law of Multiple Proportions*. Both of these laws assume that atoms are neither created or destroyed. This is the *Law of Conservation of Mass*.

Thus, initial experiments were repeated and repeated. The observations led to laws of nature that could be explained in an atomic theory.

We now know that Dalton's atomic theory is a bit too simple to explain all aspects of the atom. Some chemically identical atoms have slightly different weights, as we will discuss under *isotopes* in Section 2.5. Atoms of one element can change to atoms of a different element by *nuclear* change, as described briefly in Section 3.5.

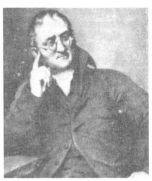

John Dalton (1766–1844) developed the modern concept of the atom and molecules. His first love was the weather; he recorded 200 000 weather observations over 46 years. He was color-blind, possibly a disadvantage in detecting chemical reactions in a laboratory.

The modern view of an atom

Dalton's atom was simply a "ball" that could combine with other similar things to form molecules. Toward the end of the 1800's, there was much evidence that things were more complicated.

First of all, it was possible to change the *charge* on an atom. From the days when Benjamin Franklin (1706–1790) first flew a kite in the middle of a thunderstorm (almost getting himself killed in the process), electricity has fascinated scientists. Eventually, a very small bit of negatively charged matter known as the **electron** was identified as the carrier of electricity. Joseph Thomson (1856–1940) was an English physicist who measured the mass and charge on an electron. He knew that electrons could be easily knocked off neutral atoms and that there must be a positively charged part of the atom left behind.

Experiments in the laboratory of Ernest Rutherford (1871–1937) showed that the positive charges of the atom (equal in number to the number of electrons in the atom) were contained in an extremely small **nucleus** at the center of the atom. This nucleus also accounted for almost all of the mass of the atom. This required an idea different from that of Thomson. In one of the

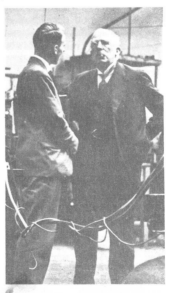

Ernest Rutherford in his laboratory, 1911.

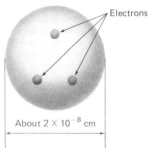

Electrons

About 2 X 10^{-8} cm

Joseph Thomson saw the atom as a ball of uniform positive charge in which electrons were stuck like the raisins in a loaf of raisin bread. Rutherford's discovery of the atomic nucleus made scientists discard the Thomson model.

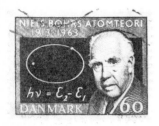

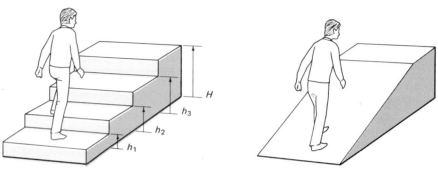

The Bohr–Rutherford model, shown here, was very pleasing to scientists, who like to feel that there is much underlying order in the universe and that both the vast solar system and subatomic particles follow the same laws of nature. Unfortunately, the Bohr model does not correctly predict most atomic properties and is *not* considered a good picture of the atom.

FIGURE 2–3 Quantized electron energy levels are like steps on a staircase. The man at the left can be at heights h_1, h_2, h_3, or H above the ground, but nowhere in between. This corresponds to our modern model of the atom. The man at the right can walk any distance up the ramp; his elevation is *not* quantized.

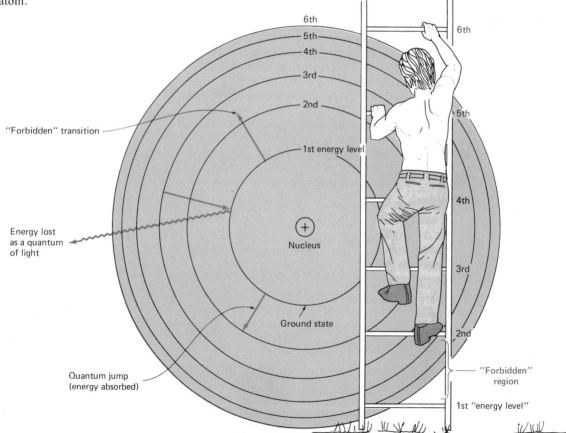

FIGURE 2–4 The energy levels of the hydrogen atom. Electrons may absorb light to gain energy and go to a higher energy level; they then emit light and lose energy to return to the ground state. The electron may *not* have an "in-between" energy.

"flashes of insight" that make science very interesting to study, Rutherford and Niels Bohr (1885–1962) successfully explained some properties of the hydrogen atom by assuming that the atom was, in fact, a kind of miniature sun-and-planets system.

Bohr's theory had to fit some laws of physics. To make the equations work out, Bohr assumed that an electron in the atom cannot simply take "any" position outside the nucleus (as can an artificial earth satellite, for example) but in fact can only occupy one of a fixed series of energy levels (Figure 2–3). We say that such fixed energy levels are **quantized**. The electron cannot take an "in-between" energy.

The hydrogen atom has only one electron. Normally that electron, like any electron, will take the *lowest* energy level available to it, in this case, the first level (Figure 2–4). If light of the proper type hits the atom just right, the electron can gain energy to move into a higher energy level. Eventually, the electron in a higher or *excited* state will lose energy and will return to the first or *ground* state.

To a large extent, this is a very useful model. It provides a basis for understanding why light is given off and absorbed (taken in) by atoms. It is accurate in that it assigns each electron a fixed energy level.

Unfortunately, nature is a bit more complicated than the Bohr model. When the electron is inside the atom, it cannot be treated as a small particle or moon, but instead must be considered in terms of probabilities. According to modern atomic theory:

If we know exactly *where* an electron is, we cannot know which way it is going or how much energy it has.

If we know exactly how much energy an electron has, we cannot find out precisely where it is in the atom.

Any measurement we carry out to look at the electron, such as observing it in a microscope, will necessarily change the electron's position, speed, or direction of travel.

The result is a rather "fuzzy" picture of the electron in an atom, as shown in Figure 2–5.

The atomic nucleus

We will devote the rest of this chapter to discussing the overall size and mass of the atom and leave most of the discussion of the properties of an electron to Chapter 3.

Physicists, working with "atom smashers" of greater and greater energy, have discovered dozens of particles smaller than the atom. Most of those particles exist for only very short periods of time. Chemists are concerned with only three particles that make up the atom: the proton, the neutron, and the electron.

The two most important properties of any particle are its mass and its charge. We already discussed mass in Section 2.2. Most of the mass of matter is made up of the mass of the nuclei, the very small centers of atoms. Since the protons and neutrons of an atom are concentrated in the nucleus, they are responsible for almost all mass in nature.

The property of **charge** may be somewhat less familiar to you. If you have walked across a nylon rug on a dry day, you have built up charge by stripping some atoms of their electrons. This charge may be lost when you

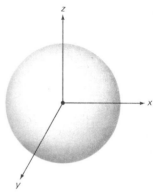

FIGURE 2–5 The cloud model of an electron in an atom. The small atomic nucleus is the black dot in the center. We do not know where the electron is at any one time, but we imagine that it will be found mostly inside this cloud and will tend to "fill" the cloud with constant motion.

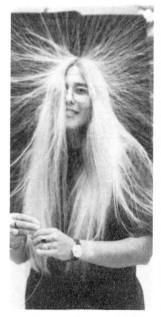

The hair style shown here was created by static charges. The hairs all have the same charge and thus repel each other. This student was so unaware of the charge that she would not believe that her hair was standing on end.

touch a doorknob or another person, and you feel a "shock" as the electrons move, returning to their original atoms. Exactly the same effect, but millions of times stronger, creates the lightning of thunderstorms.

There are two kinds of charge, which we label positive (+) and negative (−). Each electron carries a small negative charge. Our common symbol for an electron (e⁻) shows that charge. The atom as a whole must be electrically neutral, meaning that the number of positive charges must be equal to the number of negative charges. There must therefore be as many positive charges as electrons in an atom. The particle that carries the positive charge is the **proton** (p⁺).

Refer again to the periodic table in the front of this text. The **atomic number** is the number at the top of each box. **The atomic number is the number of protons in an atom of an element.** This number of *protons* is fixed for each element because the nucleus of an atom is not affected by chemical change. Thus carbon, with atomic number 6, has six protons in the nucleus of one atom. That nucleus carries an electrical charge of 6+ units. For the carbon atom to be neutral, there must be six electrons outside the nucleus. Only *electrons* may be gained, lost, or shared by the carbon atom.

The third kind of particle inside an atom is the **neutron**. It has no charge, but it has a mass about equal to that of a proton. It is in the nucleus and contributes to the atomic mass.

Some properties of the three basic particles that make up the atom are shown in Table 2–5. The charge is listed in units of the amount of charge carried by one electron. The mass in grams is, of course, very small. The mass in amu, atomic mass units, will be discussed further in the next section. At this stage, simply note that the mass of each proton and each neutron is approximately 1 amu, while the electron has a much smaller mass, 1/1837 amu.

If we let the number of protons in the nucleus of an atom be Z, which is the atomic number, then **an atom of element #Z consists of a very small nucleus containing Z protons and some number of neutrons. Outside the nucleus are Z electrons.**

The average distance of an electron from the nucleus of an atom is of the order of one to several angstrom units, where 1 Å = 10^{-10} m. The radius of the nucleus is around 10^{-15} m, or only 1/100 000 as great. If the nucleus were the size of a tennis ball, then the outermost electrons in an atom would be found several miles away!

Formation of ions

We have noted that the electrically neutral atom has Z electrons to exactly match the charge of the Z protons of the nucleus. It is possible to strip one or more electrons from an atom. If we do so, there will be more protons than electrons, thus more positive charges than negative charges. The particle will have a net positive charge. We call such a particle a **cation**, or positive **ion**.

The best-known cation is that formed by removing one electron from the sodium atom. The sodium atom ($Z = 11$) has 11 protons in the nucleus and 11 electrons outside. Remove one electron and you have the Na⁺ cation.

TABLE 2–5 PROPERTIES OF PROTONS, NEUTRONS,
AND ELECTRONS

Name	Charge	Mass in grams	Mass in amu	Location in Atom	Common Symbol
Proton	+1	1.673×10^{-24}	1.00728	Inside nucleus	p⁺
Neutron	none	1.675×10^{-24}	1.00867	Inside nucleus	n⁰
Electron	−1	9.107×10^{-28}	0.000549	Outside nucleus	e⁻

The sodium that exists inside the body, and in table salt (NaCl), is in fact entirely in the form of Na$^+$ cations. The neutral Na atom with 11 electrons plays no part in the natural chemistry of our environment. The same is true for most *metals,* both inside and outside the body. Calcium is present not as the neutral atom with 20 electrons, but as the Ca^{2+} cation with 18 electrons and 20 protons. Other positive ions found in the body include K$^+$, Mg^{2+}, and *very* small amounts of some other metal cations, such as Fe^{2+}, Cu^{2+}, and Zn^{2+}.

If we take a neutral atom and *add* an electron, we create a particle with a net negative charge. This is an **anion** or negative ion. The most familiar anion is that formed when a chlorine atom ($Z = 17$) with 17 protons and 17 electrons gains another electron to make 18 e$^-$. The Cl$^-$ ion is found in the body and in table salt. We do not expect to find any neutral Cl atoms, with 17 e$^-$, inside the body.

If two charged particles with the *same* sign approach each other (+ approaches +, or − approaches −), the particles repel (push away) each other. Thus, one Cl$^-$ anion pushes away a second Cl$^-$ anion that gets too close. A Na$^+$ cation and a Ca^{2+} cation that came close together would push away from each other.

When two charged particles of *opposite* sign (+ and −) approach each other, the particles are pulled together. Thus, a Na$^+$ cation and a Cl$^-$ anion are attracted to each other and form an *ionic bond,* as described in Section 4.1.

The existence of cations (positive ions) and anions (negative ions) in the human body is extremely important for the following reasons (among others):

The amount of Na$^+$ in the body is used to control the amount of water retained or lost by the kidneys.
Na$^+$ and K$^+$ ions help move carbohydrates across cell membranes and help keep large protein molecules in solution.
Ca^{2+} ion is involved in the process of muscle contraction.
The information carried by the nervous system is in the form of electrical pulses, carried largely by Na$^+$, K$^+$, and Cl$^-$ ions.

In fact, the correct balance of Na$^+$, K$^+$, Ca^{2+}, and Mg^{2+} ions is critical to the proper functioning of nerves and muscles.

It is not accidental that salt, made up of Na$^+$ and Cl$^-$ ions, is required by the human body. We are electrical systems, and many of our body processes involve the attraction of ions with opposite charges and the repulsion of ions with similar charges.

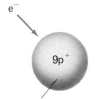

Attracted electron

e$^-$

9p$^+$

Negatively charged cloud of 9 electrons

Fluorine atom

Negatively charged fluoride ion

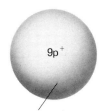

9p$^+$

Negatively charged cloud of 10 electrons

The fluorine atom with nine protons, ten neutrons, and nine electrons can gain an extra electron to form a very stable F$^-$ anion with ten electrons.

SELF-CHECK

2.14)   Graphite and diamond are two forms of the element carbon that look very different. Yet we can burn either of them to make CO_2 gas, and we cannot in any way tell the difference between CO_2 made from diamond and CO_2 made from graphite. Explain in terms of the Dalton atomic theory.
2.15)   Identify the atomic particle(s) having
a)   no charge
b)   very little mass
c)   a special role in determining the atomic number
d)   a location in the nucleus

2.16)   Given the ions Ca^{2+}, K^+, and Cl^-,
a)   which are cations?
b)   which are anions?
c)   which will attract each other?
d)   which will repel each other?
2.17)   Explain where we get a scientific *law*. Can a law be incorrect?
2.18)   What is the role of a scientific *theory?* Can a theory be incorrect?

2.5 THE MASS OF AN ATOM

LEARNING GOAL 2L: Given a nuclear symbol, state the atomic number, the number of protons, the number of neutrons, and the mass number. Given the number of protons and neutrons in the nucleus of an atom, write the nuclear symbol.

2M: Given the per cent natural abundance and the nuclear symbol of each of the naturally occurring isotopes of an element, calculate its atomic weight.

The properties of the electron, proton, and neutron were listed in Table 2–5. Starting with those properties, we can begin to calculate the masses of individual atoms. We could do all of our calculations in grams. However, as you will notice from the information in Table 2–5, we would need to continually write "x 10^{-24}" after each mass.

The atomic mass unit

One solution would be to invent a unit that is 10^{-24} grams. However, that would lead to a large number of uneven masses. The choice of the particular mass that makes one *atomic mass unit* makes a lot of calculations come out even! That makes your studying easier.

The **atomic mass unit** has been chosen so that a particular atom, which we call "carbon-12," has a mass of *exactly* 12.0000000 . . . atomic mass units, or amu.‖ When we do this, then the mass of one proton is almost exactly equal to 1 amu, as is the mass of one neutron (Table 2–5). The mass of any atomic nucleus in amu is just about equal to the total number of protons and neutrons it contains.

The nuclear symbol

If there were only one kind of hydrogen atom, then one symbol, "H," would be enough to tell us everything about it. In fact, there are *three* different kinds or *isotopes* of atoms with atomic number 1.

We can provide the necessary information about an atom by writing a **nuclear symbol,** which consists of the symbol of the element, with two small

‖ The official symbol for an atomic mass unit is "u." While we will write in this text that the atomic weight of carbon is 12.01 amu, officially it would be 12.01 u. Some biochemists call this unit the *dalton.*

numbers before it. A superscript (above) gives the total number (A) of protons *plus* neutrons, which we call the **mass number.** A subscript (below) gives the number of protons, which is the atomic number (Z).

$$\text{EXAMPLE:} \quad {}_1^3H = {}_Z^AH$$

${}_1^1H$ designates an atom with one proton and a total of one particle in its nucleus. There are *no* neutrons. This is normal hydrogen, the type generally found in water.

${}_1^2H$ has one proton and two nuclear particles. It must therefore have one neutron. This is called an atom of *deuterium* or "heavy hydrogen." Less than 1 in every 6000 water molecules contains this kind of atom.

${}_1^3H$ has one proton and three nuclear particles, thus two neutrons. It is not found naturally on earth but can be made in nuclear laboratories and is called *tritium.*

The atomic symbol and the atomic number *must* go together. You cannot have ${}_1He$ or ${}_2H$. Only ${}_1H$ is allowed, since any atom or ion with one proton is hydrogen. Sometimes the atomic number is left out, as in ${}^3H$, for that reason, but, in general, it is a good idea to always write the atomic number.

We noted earlier that the mass of a nucleus in amu is just about equal to the mass number A. Table 2–6 shows that this is true within better than 1%. For example, deuterium actually has a mass of 2.0140 amu. If we assume it to be 2.00 amu, we are making only a small error. As atoms get larger, the error in making this assumption approaches 0.1%, which is negligible for the type of calculations you will be doing in chemistry. So, unless instructed otherwise, assume that the mass number (the total number of protons and neutrons) also gives the weight of an atom in atomic mass units.

Binding Energy

It is interesting to note that, as shown in Table 2–6, the mass of a deuterium atom is not the same as the mass of the three particles that make it up, one proton (1.00728 amu), one neutron (1.00867 amu), and one electron (0.00055 amu). It is *less!* Mass has somehow been lost in converting the three individual particles to a deuterium atom, ${}_1^2H$.

This lost mass has not disappeared. It has been converted to the energy that holds the deuterium nucleus together. Without that energy, the proton and neutron would not stay together in the nucleus but would drift apart. The *binding energy* that glues the deuterium nucleus together can be calculated from the famous Einstein equation $E = mc^2$, where E is the energy produced, m is the mass loss (for ${}_1^2H$, 0.0025 amu), and c is the speed of light in appropriate units.

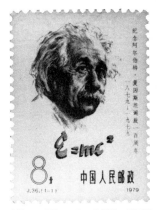

Albert Einstein (1879–1955) made enormous contributions to our understanding of nature. He spent his life trying to unify or "tie together" the various laws of physics and in the process showed that matter and energy are two sides of the same thing.

TABLE 2–6 MASSES OF
HYDROGEN ISOTOPES

Hydrogen ${}_1^1H$	Deuterium ${}_1^2H$	Tritium ${}_1^3H$
Actual mass in amu		
1.00783	2.0140	3.01605
Sum of nuclear particle masses in amu		
$p^+ =$	$p^+ + n^0 =$	$p^+ + 2n^0 =$
1.00783	2.01650	3.02517
Mass defect or binding energy in amu		
—	0.0025	0.00912

This same type of energy conversion is responsible for the awesome effect of an atomic bomb, for the energy produced by the sun, and for the use of nuclear energy to produce electricity (to be discussed in Section 3.5).

Isotopes

You now know that there are three kinds of hydrogen atoms. They all act essentially the same chemically. They all burn in oxygen to form H_2O, and they can all be included in carbohydrates, fats, and proteins. We call the three kinds of hydrogen atoms that differ in weight but not in chemical properties the three **isotopes** of hydrogen.

Every element has many possible isotopes. For example, the element tin ($Z = 50$) has 21 known isotopes, ranging in mass number A from $A = 108$ (58 neutrons) to $A = 128$ (78 neutrons). Another essential element, iodine ($Z = 53$), has 23 known isotopes from $A = 117$ to $A = 139$.

Two atoms represent isotopes of the same element if they have the *same* number of protons (Z) but *different* numbers of neutrons and thus different mass numbers (A).

Atomic weight

You now know that Dalton was somewhat incorrect in one of his assumptions. Atoms of one element are not all alike. Although they act the same chemically, they can have different masses.

If an atom of tin can have any of 21 different masses, from 108 amu to 128 amu, and an atom of iodine can have any of 23 different masses from 117 to 139 amu, how can we determine atomic masses for practical purposes?

Not all known isotopes of an element make up part of the earth's *natural abundance* of that element. Of the 21 tin isotopes, only 9 are found naturally. The other 12 can only be made in "atom smashing" machines or in nuclear reactors. Of the 23 iodine isotopes, only *1* is found in nature. It is only that one isotope, $^{127}_{53}I$, that is used in the human thyroid gland and was once used in an antiseptic called "tincture of iodine." Since there is only one kind of iodine atom, there is only one possible weight for an iodine atom. That weight is shown in the periodic table under the symbol for iodine and is 126.90 amu. This value is the *atomic weight* of iodine.

An **atomic weight** is the average mass in amu of the naturally occurring atoms of an element.

In the case of iodine, the average mass is the *only* mass. In the case of tin, there are nine different masses to be averaged. How do we take an average of nine different things?

Weighted averages

Suppose a group of friends are discussing their families and one decides to find out the average number of brothers and sisters the members of the group have. She asks each person to give a count and gets the following numbers: 0, 2, 2, 5, 1, 3. The average number of siblings is

$$(0 + 2 + 2 + 5 + 1 + 3)/6 \text{ values} = 13/6 = 2.2.$$

Obviously, no one has exactly 2.2 siblings! However, the result, 2.2, is a kind of "middle ground" that can be useful.

Many of your instructors have calculated class averages on tests by adding up all of the marks and dividing by the number of scores. Suppose three students get 50, four get 60, seven have 70, five have 80, and two have 90 on a test. The average is then calculated as follows:

$$\begin{array}{rcl} 3 \text{ students} \times 50 &=& 150 \\ + \ 4 \text{ students} \times 60 &=& 240 \\ + \ 7 \text{ students} \times 70 &=& 490 \\ + \ 5 \text{ students} \times 80 &=& 400 \\ + \ 2 \text{ students} \times 90 &=& \underline{180} \\ \hline 21 \text{ students} && 1460 \end{array}$$

The class average is then total of values/number of values = 1460/21 = 70 on this test. Looking at the marks, that is about what you would expect.

Exactly the same method is used for calculating atomic weights.

EXAMPLE 2v: The element magnesium ($Z = 12$) is found in the human body and in "milk of magnesia" as the Mg^{2+} ion, and as a metal is used in some airplanes. Magnesium has three naturally occurring isotopes, of which $^{24}_{12}Mg$ makes up 78.7%, $^{25}_{12}Mg$ accounts for 10.1%, and $^{26}_{12}Mg$ occurs as 11.2%. What is its atomic weight?

- -

SOLUTION: Make the usual assumption that the mass number A is equal to the atom mass in amu for each isotope, and take a total of 1000 atoms of natural magnesium.

Of the 1000 atoms, 78.7% × 1000 = 787 atoms have mass 24.0 amu;
10.1% × 1000 = 101 atoms have mass 25.0 amu;
and 11.2% × 1000 = 112 atoms have mass 26.0 amu.

Using the same method as for the class average, we see that

$$\text{atomic weight} = \frac{(787 \text{ atoms} \times 24.0 \text{ amu}) + (101 \times 25.0) + (112 \times 26.0)}{1000 \text{ atoms}}$$

$$\text{atomic weight} = \frac{24\ 325}{1000 \text{ atoms}} = \boxed{24.3 \text{ amu}} \text{ (to three significant digits)}$$

That is the *average* mass of a magnesium atom. It agrees with the value that you find in the periodic table at the front of this text (24.31). Remember that *no* magnesium atom actually has a mass of 24.3 amu. This is an average value, useful for calculations with large numbers of magnesium atoms, made up of a mixture of the three isotopes.

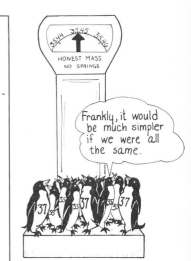

If we take 100 chlorine atoms, some will have mass 35 amu and others will have mass 37 amu. Their total mass will be 3545 amu. The average mass, or atomic weight, is then $\frac{3545}{100}$ = 35.45 amu.

Look over the periodic table. Can you find some other elements that have atomic weights (like that of magnesium) that are uneven? Those must have several natural isotopes. Examples would be lithium ($Z = 3$), boron ($Z = 5$), neon ($Z = 10$), silicon ($Z = 14$), and chlorine ($Z = 17$). Some other atomic weights are almost exact integers. It is *possible* that, like iodine, such elements have only *one* natural isotope. This is true for beryllium ($Z = 4$, at.wt. = 9.01 amu), fluorine ($Z = 9$, at.wt. = 19.00 amu), sodium ($Z = 11$, at.wt. = 22.99 amu), and aluminum ($Z = 13$, at.wt. = 26.98 amu), among others.

The atomic weight, calculated in the manner shown here from the naturally occurring isotopes of an element, is used frequently in many different types of chemical calculations. We will return to the use of atomic weight in Chapter 4.

SELF-CHECK

2.19)   Given each of the following nuclear symbols, write the number of protons, number of neutrons, the name of the element (referring to the periodic table), and the mass number.

a) $^{26}_{11}Na$

d) $^{58}_{26}Fe$

b) $^{28}_{15}P$

e) $^{79}_{35}Br$

c) $^{40}_{20}Ca$

2.20)   Write the nuclear symbol for each of the following atoms. Use the periodic table for the symbols. (*Some hints may be useful.*)
a)   An atom with eight protons and eight neutrons in the nucleus. (*Breathe easily!*)
b)   A neutral atom with 92 electrons and a mass number of 235. (*This one makes quite a blast!*)
c)   An atom with an atomic number of 13 and 17 neutrons. (*It's rather light!*)
d)   An atom with 79 protons and a mass number of 197. (*It glitters!*)

2.21)   Calculate the atomic weight of each of the following elements to the nearest 0.1 amu. Compare your answers with those in the periodic table. Percentage figures are natural abundances.
a)   bromine: 50.54% $^{79}_{35}Br$ and 49.46% $^{81}_{35}Br$
b)   chlorine: 75.53% $^{35}_{17}Cl$ and 24.47% $^{37}_{17}Cl$
c)   phosphorus: 100.00% $^{31}_{15}P$
d)   copper: 69.09% $^{63}_{29}Cu$ and 30.91% $^{65}_{29}Cu$
e)   chromium: 4.31% $^{50}_{24}Cr$, 83.76% $^{52}_{24}Cr$, 9.55% $^{53}_{24}Cr$, and 2.38% $^{54}_{24}Cr$

CHAPTER TWO IN REVIEW ■ Matter and Its Measurement

2F: Using a table of conversion factors, convert a mass measurement between pounds and grams or kilograms.

2G: Given two of the following quantities, calculate the third: (a) mass of a sample; (b) volume of a sample; (c) density in g/cm³ or specific gravity.

2H: Given a chemical fact or law, such as the Law of Conservation of Mass, discuss its agreement (or lack of it) with Dalton's model of the atom.

2I: Distinguish between electrons, protons, and neutrons by describing the charge, relative mass, and position of each in an atom.

2J: Define an ion, a cation, and an anion. Given two ions, state whether they attract or repel each other.

2K: List and discuss some of the major techniques used in applying the scientific method.

2L: Given a nuclear symbol, state the atomic number, the number of protons, the number of neutrons, and the mass number. Given the number of protons and neutrons in the nucleus of an atom, write the nuclear symbol.

2M: Given the per cent natural abundance and the nuclear symbol of each of the naturally occurring isotopes of an element, calculate its atomic weight.

GLOSSARY FOR CHAPTER TWO

anion A negatively charged *ion;* obtained from a neutral atom or group of atoms by adding one or more *electrons;* examples: Cl^-, NO_3^-. (p. 39)

atomic number The number of *protons* in an atom (or ion) of an element; shows the place of that element in the periodic table; equal to the number of *electrons* in a neutral atom; usually symbolized Z. (p. 38)

atomic mass unit (amu) A unit of *mass* used to express the mass of an atom and other very small particles; equal to exactly 1/12 of the mass of a $^{12}_{6}C$ atom: approximately equal to the mass of a *proton* or *neutron.* (p. 40)

atomic weight The average *mass* of an atom of an element, expressed in *amu;* calculated by taking the weighted average of the masses of the naturally occurring *isotopes* of an element; shown on the periodic table. (p. 42)

cation A positively charged *ion;* obtained from a neutral atom or group of atoms by removing one or more *electrons;* examples: Na^+, NH_4^+. (p. 38)

centi- A prefix meaning 1/100 (symbol c) as in centimeter (100 cm = 1 m) or centigram (100 cg = 1 g). (p. 17)

charge, electric A property of matter that is found in two types (positive and negative) of particles; particles with similar charges repel each other; those with unlike charges attract (see *anion, cation, electron, ion, proton*). (p. 37)

conversion factor A ratio of two equivalent measurements; used to multiply a given (known) quantity to find an unknown; examples: 12 in./1 ft, 1 L/1000 mL, 1g H_2O/1 cm³. (p. 18)

conversion-factor method A way of solving numerical problems by multiplying the given measurement by *conversion factors* to obtain the desired answer. (p. 18)

cubic centimeter A unit of volume, equal to the capacity of a container that is 1 cm in each dimension; exactly equal to 1 mL; preferred symbol: cm³. (p. 21)

deci- A prefix meaning 1/10 (symbol d) as in deciliter (10 dL = 1 L). (p. 21)

deciliter One tenth of a liter; a standard clinical volume unit for expressing blood and urine values; 1 dL = 100 mL. (p. 21)

density The *mass* of a substance per unit volume, usually expressed in g/cm³; independent of the amount of substance and can thus be looked up in tables; can be used as a *conversion factor* for determining the mass of a known volume and vice versa. (p. 29)

electron A particle with very low *mass* (0.0005 amu) and the smallest known unit of negative *charge* (symbol e⁻); found outside the *nucleus* of atoms; responsible for all chemical bonding. (p. 35)

gram A metric unit of *mass*, equal to the mass of 1 cm³ of pure water at 4°C; commonly used to express the weight of chemicals. (p. 27)

hydrometer An instrument for measuring the *density* or *specific gravity* of a liquid; one version is called a *urinometer*. (p. 32)

hypothesis An explanation of why an event happened; a scientific hypothesis is one that can be tested many times with different experiments to see if its predictions hold up; if verified, may become a *theory*. (p. 33)

ion A charged particle, such as a *cation* or *anion*. (p. 38)

isotope One of several atoms of the same element that have the same number of protons (same *atomic number*) but different numbers of neutrons (different *mass numbers*), thus have different *nuclear symbols*. (p. 42)

kilo- A prefix meaning 1000 (symbol k) as in kilometer (1 km = 1000 m) or kilogram (1 kg = 1000 g). (p. 17)

kilogram The SI base unit of mass (symbol kg); 1 kg is about equal to 2.2 lb. (p. 27)

law, scientific A natural result that has been repeatedly observed; a "law of nature" that has been checked and rechecked by experiment and still is seen to be true; may be explained by a *hypothesis* or *theory*. (p. 35)

liter The common metric unit of volume or capacity; equal to exactly 1000 cm³ or 0.001 m³; symbol L (formerly ℓ). (p. 21)

mass A property of matter related to the number of atoms of each element contained in a sample; may be measured in amu or grams; on earth, related to the *weight* of an object; the amount of matter. (p. 26)

mass number The total number of protons plus neutrons in a nucleus; shown as a superscript in the nuclear symbol; approximately equal to the mass in amu of the nucleus; (symbol A). (p. 41)

meter The metric base unit of length or distance; symbol m; 1 m is about equal to 39 in. (p. 17)

metric system Units of measurement based on *grams, meters, seconds*, etc., in which all conversions involve powers of ten (see SI). (p. 17)

milli- A prefix meaning 1/1000 (symbol m) as in millimeter (1000 mm = 1 m) or milliliter (1000 mL = 1 L). (p. 17)

milliliter A subunit of volume commonly used in laboratories; 1000 mL = 1 L; equal to 1 cm³. (p. 21)

neutron A small particle with mass of about 1 amu; found in the nucleus; has no charge (symbol n°). (p. 38)

nuclear symbol A symbol showing the *atomic number* (Z), the *mass number* (A), and the element symbol to show exactly which *nucleus* is meant, as in $^{12}_{6}C$; different *isotopes* have nuclear symbols differing only in *mass number.* (p. 40)

nucleus The extremely small and dense collection of protons and neutrons at the center of any atom; holds almost all of the atomic mass and is positively charged. (p. 35)

proton A small particle with a *mass* of 1.0 amu and a positive *charge* equal and opposite to that on the *electron,* found in the *nucleus* (symbol: p^+); the *atomic number* is the number of protons; a hydrogen *cation* would be a single proton. (p. 38)

quantized Allowed to have only one of certain fixed energies and unable to have an "in-between" energy; true of electrons in atoms, which are found only in certain energy levels. (p. 37)

scientific method The way a scientist approaches the investigation and explanation of nature; involves finding the facts through observation, thinking up a *hypothesis,* testing the hypothesis through experiments, and perhaps ultimately devising a *theory* that fits all the natural *laws* and facts. (p. 34)

SI The International System of Units (Système International); the modern version of the *metric system.* (p. 17)

significant digits The numbers used by scientists to express a measurement in such a way that the uncertainty or error in the number is shown; includes all digits that are known for certain plus *one* doubtful figure. (p. 25)

specific gravity The ratio of the *density* of an object to that of water; numerically equal to the density in g/cm^3 (at room temperature) but has no units. (p. 31)

theory A comprehensive explanation of some aspect of nature, often with mathematical equations; can be used to predict the results of many experiments; usually comes from a hypothesis that is very well confirmed. (p. 34)

weight A measure of the force of gravity, which pulls matter down toward the center of the earth; proportional to *mass,* a fact that allows us to use weight measurements to determine the mass of a body. (p. 27)

SUMMARY OF THE MOST IMPORTANT SYMBOLS USED IN CHAPTER TWO

A mass number
amu   atomic mass unit
c   (prefix) centi- = 1/100
cc   cubic centimeter = mL
cg   centigram = 10^{-2} g
cm   centimeter = 10^{-2} m
cm^3 cubic centimeter = mL
d   (prefix) deci- = 1/10
dL   deciliter = 10^{-1} L = 100 mL
dm   decimeter = 10^{-1} m = 10 cm
e^- electron
g   gram
k   (prefix) kilo- = 1000
kg   kilogram = 10^3 g
km   kilometer = 10^3 m

L   or ℓ liter = 10^3 cm^3
m   meter
m   (prefix) milli- = 1/1000
mg   milligram = 10^{-3} g
mL or ml milliliter = 10^{-3} L = 1 cm^3
mm   millimeter = 10^{-3} m
M   (prefix) mega- = 10^6 (1 million)
n° neutron
n   (prefix) nano- = 10^{-9}
p^+ proton
p   (prefix) pico- = 10^{-12}
Z atomic number
μ (prefix) micro- = 10^{-6}
+   positive charge
−   negative charge

QUESTIONS AND PROBLEMS FOR CHAPTER TWO ■ Matter and Its Measuremen

Remember that answers to the questions in the left-hand column are in Appendix A in the back of the text.

SECTION 2.1 MEASUREMENT OF LENGTH AND VOLUME

2.22) Convert each of the following metric lengths to the corresponding distance in *centimeters*.
a) a 100-mm cigarette
b) a 10-km walk
c) a 2.0-m high jump
d) a 145-μm diameter of a fertilized human egg

2.57) Convert each of the following metric lengths to the corresponding distance in *meters*.
a) the 20-Å diameter of a DNA molecule
b) a 500-km journey
c) a 7-μm red blood cell diameter
d) the 3.18-mm length of a 1-month-old human embryo

2.23) A typical U.S. adult human height is 1.72 m; convert this to
a) centimeters
b) kilometers
c) micrometers
d) angstrom units

2.58) The Mbuti pygmies of Zaire have an average adult height of about 135 cm; convert this to
a) meters
b) millimeters
c) nanometers
d) kilometers

The limit to what we can see with a microscope, its *resolving power*, is related to the wavelength of the light we are using. Remembering that $1Å = 10^{-10}$ m, determine the wavelength in *meters* of

2.24) red light of 6500 Å

2.59) blue light of 450 nm

2.25) an electron in an electron microscope at 1.0 nm

2.60) an x-ray at 1.5 Å

The prefixes of the metric system are used for many kinds of measurements. Once you know each prefix, you can understand the measurement. Interpret each of the following statements.

2.26*)
a) Do not touch a 15-*kilo*volt electrical transmission line!
b) Small electrical capacitors are rated in *pico*farads.
c) A current through the body of more than a few *milli*amperes can kill.

2.61*)
a) Home use of electricity is calculated in *kilo*watt-hours.
b) Some lasers emit light in *pico*second pulses.
c) Nuclear weapons are often rated in *mega*tons of TNT equivalent.

2.27) A patient received an injection of 2.5 mL of 2.5% sodium thiopental as an anesthetic. What is that volume in
a) liters?
b) cubic centimeters?
c*) microliters?

2.62) A patient received an injection of 0.50 mL of 0.1% epinephrine solution to help recovery from a bee-sting reaction. Calculate that volume in
a) cubic centimeters
b) liters
c*) microliters

Use Table 2–2 to help you perform the following conversions.

2.28) A 100-yard football field is how many meters long?

2.29) The longest human bone on record was a 29.9-inch femur. How many centimeters long was it?

2.30) One very small instrument for eye surgery has a blade that is 0.078 inches in diameter. How wide in millimeters?

2.31) A recipe calls for 1 cup, or 8.0 fluid ounces, of milk. What is this measurement in
a) U.S. quarts?
b) liters?
c) milliliters?

2.32*) A cubic box exactly 1.0 foot on each side will hold one cubic foot of water. How many liters will fit into the same box?

2.33*) A 750-mL returnable bottle of a soft drink costs 33¢. A quart bottle costs 41¢. Which is the better buy?

SECTION 2.2 MASS AND WEIGHT
2.34) An excellent athlete with a body mass of 70.0 kg can high-jump 2.0 meters. On the moon, that same person would be able to jump farther. Has his mass changed? Explain.

2.63) Angel Falls in Venezuela has a water drop of 3212 feet. How many meters?

2.64) The smallest bone in the human body is the stapes in the middle ear, which may be only 0.10 inch long. What is this length in millimeters?

2.65) The star nearest the sun is 2.52×10^{13} miles away. How far is this in meters?

2.66) A "fifth" of liquor is four fifths of a U.S. quart. What is this amount of alcoholic beverage in
a) fluid ounces?
b) liters?
c) milliliters?

2.67*) How many hogsheads of ale will fit into a cubic box which is 1.0 meter in each direction? (1 hogshead = 63 U.S. gal)

2.68*) A 66-fluid ounce bottle of spring water costs 43¢, but a 2.00-liter bottle costs 48¢. Which is the better buy?

2.69) Spaceships taking off from earth to fly to Mars must carry many times more fuel than the mass of the load. A ship taking off from the moon carrying the same mass needs much less fuel. Why?

2.35 & 2.70) In 100 mL (1 dL) of normal human female blood serum, a laboratory might find the following amounts. Calculate each amount in *grams*.

2.35)
a) 9.5 mg of calcium ion
b) 95 μg of iron ion
c) 65 ng of testosterone
d) 3.55×10^{-4} kg of chloride ion

2.36) 17.5 g = ? kg

2.37) One jeweler's carat is 200 mg. What is the mass in grams of a 0.40-carat diamond?

2.70)
a) 110 μg of copper ion
b) 375 ng of prolactin
c) 33 mg of urea
d) 0.322×10^{-4} kg of sodium ion

2.71) 0.198 g = ? kg

2.72) The commercial metric unit of mass for large objects is the tonne (t), which is 1000 kg. One barrel of oil has the fuel value of 0.20 tonnes of coal. How many grams is this?

2.38 & 2.73)   Use Table 2–3.

2.38) Calculi (stones) in the human gallbladder, bladder, or kidneys can cause great pain. Surgeons once removed a stone weighing 13 pounds 14 ounces. What was that in grams?

2.39*) A lethal dose of the very dangerous street drug *heroin* is 150 mg per kilogram of body weight by injection under the skin (in rabbits). Estimate the lethal dose in grams for a 150-pound person.

2.73) Brain size in humans does *not* relate directly to mental ability. The brain of the Nobel-prize-winning author Anatole France weighed a far-below-normal 35.8 oz. Calculate that mass in grams.

2.74*) The drug strychnine has some medical uses. However, the lethal dose taken orally (by rats) is only 5 mg per kilogram of body weight. Calculate the lethal dose for a 140-pound person taking this drug orally, assuming we function just the way rats do.

SECTION 2.3 DENSITY AND SPECIFIC GRAVITY

Use the densities in Table 2–4 as conversion factors to answer the following questions (at 25°C).

2.40) What is the mass in grams of 1000 cm³ of ice?

2.41) What is the volume in cm³ of one troy ounce (31.1 g) of gold?

2.42) Will all metals sink in water? Can any float? Explain.

2.43) Calculate the volume in mL of 1 lb of olive oil.

2.44) One U.S. gallon of whiskey weighs 7.7 lb. What is its density in g/cm³? What is its specific gravity?

2.75) What is the mass in grams of a 1000-cm³ piece of aluminum?

2.76) What is the volume in cm³ of 1 lb (454 g) of air?

2.77*) Will all kinds of wood float on water? Will any sink? Explain.

2.78) Calculate the volume in cm³ of 1 lb of table sugar.

2.79) One U.S. gallon of the liquid element bromine weighs 26.0 lb. Calculate its density in g/cm³ and its specific gravity.

SECTION 2.4 THE ATOM

2.45) When alcohol burns, the number of carbon atoms produced as carbon dioxide is equal to the number of carbon atoms in the original fuel. Explain in terms of Dalton's theory.

2.46) Describe a neutron in terms of its charge, relative mass, and position in the atom.

2.47) Given the following ions: Na^+ Fe^{3+} OH^-
a) which are cations?
b) which are anions?
c) which will attract each other?

2.80) Under very high pressure, the (very cheap) graphite form of carbon can be converted to useful industrial diamonds. What relationship do you expect between the mass of graphite put in and the mass of diamonds obtained? Explain.

2.81) Describe a proton in terms of its charge, relative mass, and position in the atom.

2.82) Given the following ions: NH_4^+ Br^- S^{2-}
a) which are cations?
b) which are anions?
c) which will repel each other?

2.48) What is meant by a *law* in science? How does one confirm a law?

2.49*) Compare the masses of a calcium atom and a Ca^{2+} ion.

2.50*) Sodium metal would poison the body, but Na^+ ions are essential. Give one reason we must have positive ions in the body.

2.51*) Can you describe the orbit followed by an electron in its travels about the nucleus of an atom? Explain.

2.83) What is meant by a *theory* in science? How does one confirm a theory?

2.84*) Compare the masses of an iodine atom and an I^- ion.

2.85*) Chlorine gas is poisonous but Cl^- ions are essential to humans. Give one reason we must have negative ions in the human body.

2.86*) Which part of the atom do you think is involved in the making of chemical bonds to form compounds? Why?

SECTION 2.5 THE MASS OF AN ATOM

2.52) For each of the following symbols, write the element name, atomic number, mass number, number of protons, and number of neutrons.
a) $^{112}_{50}Sn$ c) $^{52}_{26}Fe$
b) $^{20}_{11}Na$

2.53) An important tool in cancer treatment has a nucleus with 27 protons and 33 neutrons. Write its nuclear symbol, with the aid of a periodic table.

2.54*) Can two different isotopes of iron have the same mass number? Can atoms of two *different elements* have the same mass number?

2.55) Calculate the atomic weight of sulfur if its natural abundances are $^{32}_{16}S$: 95.0%; $^{33}_{16}S$: 0.76%; $^{34}_{16}S$: 4.22%; $^{36}_{16}S$: 0.014%.

2.56*) Knowing that 1 amu = 1.66×10^{-24} grams, calculate the density in g/cm³ of a hydrogen atom if we consider it to be a cube 0.50 Å on each edge.

2.87) For each of the following symbols, write the element name, atomic number, mass number, number of protons, and number of neutrons.
a) $^{18}_{8}O$ c) $^{139}_{53}I$
b) $^{41}_{19}K$

2.88) Very useful radioactive dating can be accomplished by measuring the number of atoms (in a piece of wood or paper) each with six protons and eight neutrons. Write the nuclear symbol of this type of atom.

2.89*) Tellurium ($Z = 52$) has an atomic weight of 127.80 amu, while iodine ($Z = 53$) has an atomic weight of 126.90. Isn't this strange? Explain.

2.90) Calculate the atomic weight of zinc if its natural abundances are $^{64}_{30}Zn$: 48.9%; $^{66}_{30}Zn$: 27.8%; $^{67}_{30}Zn$: 4.1%; $^{68}_{30}Zn$: 18.6%; $^{70}_{30}Zn$: 0.6%.

2.91*) Using the data in Problem 2.56, calculate the density of a proton if we presume it to be a cube 10^{-14} cm on each side.

3 Electrons and the Periodic Table

In Chapter 2, we concentrated on the masses of atoms. You now have some idea of how atomic nuclei are made up and of how their masses compare. The science of chemistry uses atomic weights only as a tool. What really interests chemists is what the *electrons* in atoms do, since it is those electrons that make (and break) chemical bonds and thus form chemical compounds.

In this chapter, we will have a brief look at the modern theory of electrons in atoms and use this theory to explain a few of the properties of elements. In this way, you will understand why the periodic table is placed so prominently inside the front cover of this text. Certain groups of elements behave in a common fashion, and it is these regularities that make the periodic table so important.

The periodic similarities can then be related to another interesting side of chemistry, the properties of radioactive materials.

3.1 ELECTRONS IN ATOMS

LEARNING GOAL 3A: Briefly describe the properties of an electron confined to a particular atomic orbital.

3B: Given a periodic table and given an element among the first 20 elements in the table, write the complete electron configuration for a neutral atom of that element.

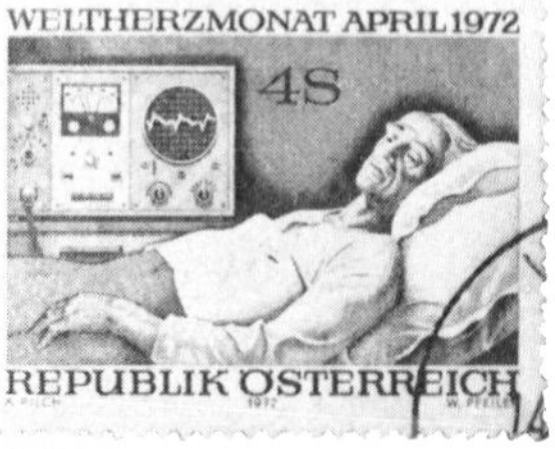

WELTHERZMONAT APRIL 1972

REPUBLIK ÖSTERREICH

An oscilloscope displays the patient's heartbeat in an intensive care unit. Other devices may provide an emergency signal if the patient is in trouble.

Electrons, in many ways, are rather strange objects. When they are free to move in space, they behave like small particles and obey the same laws of motion as do baseballs. Inside a television set, or in the oscilloscope used in hospitals to monitor a patient's heartbeat, there is a beam of electrons hitting a screen. If you imagined millions of little people shooting pebbles at a target, you would not have a bad picture of the electron beam. This is the *particle* picture of an electron.

Inside an atom, however, the electron does not show the type of behavior we expect from a pebble or a particle. Instead, we have to settle for a very abstract, cloudy *wave* picture. As you learned in Section 2.4, we cannot know exactly both where the electron is and what it is doing.

This situation is often frustrating to the student who wants a clear, crisp answer to each question. However, nature does not always provide sharp pictures. We will do our best in this chapter to help you understand some of the mysterious ways of the electron.

The atomic orbital

Some chemists like to compare the electron with a honeybee, flitting from flower to flower collecting pollen but always staying in the general area of the hive. Modern theory tells us that electrons similarly flitter about the atomic nucleus in an unpredictable fashion. The electron never settles down in one place but generally stays near the nucleus.

The extremely complex mathematical description of the electron's behavior boils down to a cloud in which we are likely to find the electron. We call this cloud an **atomic orbital** (Figure 3–1). Each cloud has a particular overall shape in space; the one shown is like a ball or sphere, so we call it a spherical charge cloud.

The more dots shown in a particular region of space, the greater our probability of finding the electron there. The chances of finding the electron shown in Figure 3–1 are fairly good a small distance, say 5×10^{-9} cm, away from the nucleus and fall almost to zero by a distance of 2.5×10^{-8} cm from the nucleus, five times as far.

Associated with each atomic orbital is a very specific energy of the electron. In Section 2.4 we noted that the electron can only have certain very definite amounts of energy. We can thus draw a series of **energy levels** for the electron, as shown in Figure 2–4. Each energy level then corresponds to one or more atomic orbitals.

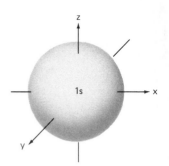

FIGURE 3–1   A typical atomic orbital charge cloud for an electron in an atom. The 1s electron will be found inside this ball or sphere about 90% of the time.

Electrons in the 1s orbital

That's all pretty vague, but we are not being intentionally foggy. Let us take a very specific example, a single electron in a hydrogen atom. We showed the charge cloud of that electron in Figure 3–1. The three axes, x, y, and z, are shown at right angles to each other. This picture looks just like Figure 2–5. We say the electron is in a 1s *atomic orbital* of the hydrogen atom. You might consider "1s" to be the street address of that electron.

The electron can, under the right conditions, leave that orbital (and energy level) and go into a different orbital, the 2s, which will have a different energy. The new orbital will have a charge cloud that is larger than that of the 1s orbital. Eventually, the electron will return to its original home, the 1s orbital.

What do these numbers and letters mean? The "1" in the 1s orbital address means the *lowest* or first *energy level*. We often use the letter "n" to label these levels. For the 1s orbital, $n = 1$. For the 2s orbital, $n = 2$. The higher the value of n, the farther the electron is from the nucleus (on the average), the more "spread out" is the charge cloud, and the higher is the energy.

The "s" in the name of the 1s orbital means that the charge cloud is shaped like a ball or sphere. The 2s orbital has a similar shape.

From our description so far, you realize that an orbital may be empty or may have an electron in it. When the single hydrogen electron is in the 1s orbital, the 2s orbital is empty. In fact, an atomic orbital may have zero, one,

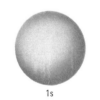

1s

2s

or two electrons in it. (You might think of it as a hotel room with a double bed. At any one time, there may be zero, one, or two guests in the bed.) The helium atom ($Z = 2$, Z being the atomic number we discussed in Section 2.4) has two electrons. Both are normally found in the 1s orbital.

The two helium electrons will thus both be found in the same charge cloud (although, having the same charge, they will repel each other and will presumably be far apart) and have the same description and same energy. Either of them may "jump" to the 2s orbital by gaining energy, although any such *excited* electron rather quickly returns home to the 1s orbital.

Let us now review what we know about these electrons:

1) An electron is found in a particular atomic orbital.
2) The atomic orbital is a region of space in which we are likely to find the electron and is associated with a very definite energy.
3) An atomic orbital may contain zero, one, or two electrons at any one moment.

FILLING ATOMIC ORBITALS— AN ACTIVE EXERCISE

At this point, take a piece of paper and cover the rest of this page, moving the paper down, line by line, to expose the lines you have not yet read. This will help you learn in a painless fashion how electrons fit into atoms.

ORBITAL FILLING EXERCISE

We are going to start with two atomic orbitals, the 1s and the 2s. Each can contain zero, one, or two electrons. We thus have room for up to four electrons. The 1s and 2s orbitals have different energies, shown in the energy level diagram in Figure 3–2a.

The upper line (or it could be a box) shows the room for electrons in the 2s orbital. The lower line represents the 1s orbital. Take out a pencil and copy this diagram <u>four</u> times on a blank sheet of paper.

On your first diagram, you will show one electron. Use an arrow pointing up (↑) to symbolize a single electron. Draw the arrow on the line that represents the <u>lowest</u> energy level. Then uncover the paragraph below.

Your diagram should now look like Figure 3–2b. If it looks like Figure 3–2c, you have placed the electron in a higher energy orbital when a lower energy spot is open to it. This situation is possible, but only for a short time. Put an arrow pointing <u>up</u> in the 1s orbital of all four diagrams.

Now take a <u>second</u> electron, symbolized by an arrow pointing down (↓), and put it in the lowest energy orbital available to it in your second diagram.

Your second diagram should look like Figure 3–2d. The second electron goes into the 1s orbital (not the 2s) in order to have the lowest possible energy.

Put two electrons (↑↓) into the 1s level of your third and fourth diagrams. The two electrons are shown by arrows pointing in different

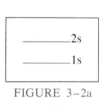

FIGURE 3–2a

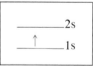

FIGURE 3–2b

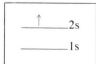

FIGURE 3–2c

directions simply to indicate that they are distinct electrons. They cannot be absolutely identical.*

Now take a third electron, symbolized by (↑), and put it into the remaining space on your third diagram. That drawing should now look like Figure 3–2e.

Did you put the third electron into the 1s orbital with the other two? That won't do! An orbital is filled *when it contains two electrons; no more will fit. The third electron must go into the 2s orbital, even though that level is of higher energy than the 1s, because the 2s is open and the 1s is closed.*

On your fourth diagram, put in a fourth electron (↓). You should now label your four diagrams with the following names: 1) hydrogen, 2) helium, 3) lithium, 4) beryllium.

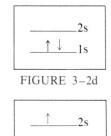

FIGURE 3–2d

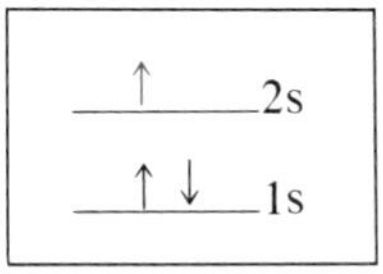

FIGURE 3–2e

Your four energy level diagrams should look like Figure 3–2f.

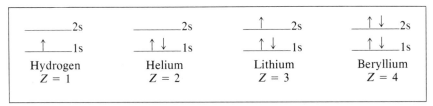

FIGURE 3–2f

What do those four diagrams represent? Hydrogen has only one electron, so it goes in the 1s orbital. Helium has two electrons, both of which go in the 1s orbital and fill it. Lithium with three electrons and beryllium with four electrons use the 2s atomic orbital.

All atoms with more than four electrons have *filled* 1s and 2s atomic orbitals, as shown for beryllium.

Electron configurations

Chemists have a set of abbreviations or "shorthand" for everything that must be written again and again. It would be wasteful to write energy level diagrams each time we wish to show electrons in atomic orbitals. We therefore can equally well represent the orbitals by symbols on a line:

$$1s \quad 2s \quad . \quad . \quad .$$

so that from left to right we have *increasing* energy. The *number of electrons* in an orbital is shown by a superscript written above and to the right of the orbital symbol, such as $1s^2$.

We can therefore write the four energy level diagrams for the first four elements in the following ground-state **electron configurations:**

---

* An arrow pointing up represents an electron with "spin up" and an arrow pointing down shows an electron with "spin down." The property of electron "spin" is not really similar to that of a spinning top or wheel. It is a way of describing a magnetic field created by the motion of the electron. The concept is vague, just like the electron "cloud." You should remember that if two electrons are in the same orbital, one must have "spin up" (↑) and the other must have "spin down" (↓).

Remember from Figure 2–4 that the ground state in the hydrogen atom is the lowest energy level allowed the electron. The ground state for a species with more than one electron has each electron in its lowest possible level. The configuration in Figure 3–2b is a ground state, but Figure 3–2c shows an *excited* state.

hydrogen atom $_1$H: $1s^1$
helium atom $_2$He: $1s^2$
lithium atom $_3$Li: $1s^2\ 2s^1$
beryllium atom $_4$Be: $1s^2\ 2s^2$

A "configuration" is simply an arrangement. It tells what things go in which places. An interior decorator is concerned with the configuration of furniture in a room. We wish to show where electrons are found.

The p atomic orbitals

Starting with five electrons, the description of electrons gets slightly more complex. The next-highest energy level (above 2s) is not 3s yet, but something called 2p.

The "2" in 2p means that we are still talking mathematically about the same broad "level" as for 2s. Yet, 2p does not have the same energy as 2s; its energy is a bit higher. We therefore have to change our terms. We call all orbitals with $n = 2$ the second **principal energy level** and then consider 2s and 2p to be **sublevels** of the $n = 2$ level. Think of the balcony in a theater, which has rows A, B, C, etc., in the same overall level.

The principal energy level $n = 1$ has only one sublevel, the 1s sublevel, which contains only one orbital, the 1s orbital.

The principal energy level $n = 2$ has two different sublevels, the 2s and 2p. The 2s sublevel has only one (2s) orbital, as we have already seen. However, the 2p sublevel has *three* different orbitals, which for convenience we label the $2p_x$, $2p_y$, and $2p_z$ atomic orbitals.

What does "**p**" mean? For our purposes, it means that the shape of the electron charge cloud is not like a ball or sphere but more like a dumbbell, as shown in Figure 3–3. The three dumbbells, $2p_x$, $2p_y$, and $2p_z$, are aimed in three different directions, which you can consider as being along the x, y, and z axes (or as up-down, left-right, and front-back).

The three 2p orbitals all have the *same* energy. That raises the question: Does an electron pair up with a previous one or go into an empty orbital? The rule is: Given the possibility of entering either of two or more orbitals that have exactly the same energy, an electron will go into any orbital that is *empty*.

We are now in a position to draw a more complete energy level diagram, shown in Figure 3–4.

Electron configurations of elements above $Z = 4$

Atomic orbital diagrams and electron configurations for the elements from boron ($Z = 5$) to neon ($Z = 10$) are shown in Figure 3–4. As you can see, it doesn't matter whether we use lines, boxes, or brackets to indicate atomic orbitals.

Notice that with neon both the first principal level ($n = 1$) and the second principal level ($n = 2$) are completely filled. Any new electron could not enter the 1s, 2s, or 2p orbitals since they are filled. It would have to go to a higher energy level, $n = 3$, and into the 3s orbital. Having all of a series of lowest energy sublevels filled lends extra *stability* to an electron configuration, which means it is much more difficult to add or remove an electron from such an arrangement.

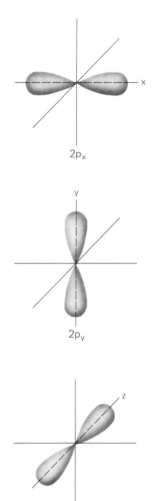

FIGURE 3–3 The three 2p atomic orbitals are turned in directions that are at right angles to each other. Instead of a sphere (as in 1s and 2s orbitals), the electron cloud of a 2p electron has two "lobes" and looks like a balloon squeezed in the middle.

Atom	Orbital diagram					Electron configuration
B	$(\uparrow\downarrow)$	$(\uparrow\downarrow)$	$(\uparrow\ )$	$(\ \ )$	$(\ \ )$	$1s^2 2s^2 2p^1$
C	$(\uparrow\downarrow)$	$(\uparrow\downarrow)$	$(\uparrow\ )$	$(\uparrow\ )$	$(\ \ )$	$1s^2 2s^2 2p^2$
N	$(\uparrow\downarrow)$	$(\uparrow\downarrow)$	$(\uparrow\ )$	$(\uparrow\ )$	$(\uparrow\ )$	$1s^2 2s^2 2p^3$
O	$(\uparrow\downarrow)$	$(\uparrow\downarrow)$	$(\uparrow\downarrow)$	$(\uparrow\ )$	$(\uparrow\ )$	$1s^2 2s^2 2p^4$
F	$(\uparrow\downarrow)$	$(\uparrow\downarrow)$	$(\uparrow\downarrow)$	$(\uparrow\downarrow)$	$(\uparrow\ )$	$1s^2 2s^2 2p^5$
Ne	$(\uparrow\downarrow)$	$(\uparrow\downarrow)$	$(\uparrow\downarrow)$	$(\uparrow\downarrow)$	$(\uparrow\downarrow)$	$1s^2 2s^2 2p^6$
	1s	2s		2p		

FIGURE 3–4 Atomic orbital diagrams for atoms with five to ten electrons. The 2s orbital is of higher energy than the 1s, and 2p is of higher energy than the 2s. Electrons entering the three 2p orbitals, which have equal energy, remain unpaired as long as possible.

All elements with Z greater than ten have, inside their electron configurations, the $1s^2 2s^2 2p^6$ arrangement of neon. We say that each contains a neon **core** of inner electrons, often symbolized by "[Ne]," where [Ne] = $1s^2 2s^2 2p^6$.

Sodium ($Z = 11$) and magnesium ($Z = 12$) use 3s atomic orbitals, and aluminum ($Z = 13$) through argon ($Z = 18$) also use 3p atomic orbitals. You should be able to write orbital diagrams and electron configurations for any of these, given the practice we have had to this point.

EXAMPLE 3a: Write the orbital diagram for sulfur ($Z = 16$), as well as the electron configuration.

SOLUTION: Draw your own energy level diagram, and figure out where the four 3p electrons should go. Your answer should resemble:

$_{16}$S: $(\uparrow\downarrow)$ $(\uparrow\downarrow)$ $(\uparrow\downarrow)(\uparrow\downarrow)(\uparrow\downarrow)$ $(\uparrow\downarrow)$ $(\uparrow\downarrow)(\uparrow)(\uparrow)$ $1s^2 2s^2 2p^6 3s^2 3p^4$
      1s   2s   2p   3s   3p

EXAMPLE 3b: Write the orbital diagram and the electron configuration for the element with atomic number 19. Then write the electron configuration using a *neon core* and an *argon core*.

SOLUTION: Element #19, referring to the periodic table on the inside front cover, is potassium. Its orbital diagram is

$_{19}$K $(\uparrow\downarrow)$ $(\uparrow\downarrow)$ $(\uparrow\downarrow)(\uparrow\downarrow)(\uparrow\downarrow)$ $(\uparrow\downarrow)$ $(\uparrow\downarrow)(\uparrow\downarrow)(\uparrow\downarrow)$ $(\uparrow)$
     1s   2s   2p   3s   3p   4s

The complete electron configuration for $_{19}$K is $1s^2 2s^2 2p^6 3s^2 3p^6 4s^1$. Neon has atomic number 10, so its core configuration is $1s^2 2s^2 2p^6$. Using that neon core, we can write the potassium configuration [Ne] $3s^2 3p^6 4s^1$.

Argon has atomic number 18, thus its configuration is $1s^2 2s^2 2p^6 3s^2 3p^6$. Potassium then can be written [Ar] $4s^1$.

Z	Element	Configuration
1	H	$1s^1$
2	He	$1s^2$
3	Li	$1s^2\ 2s^1$
4	Be	$1s^2\ 2s^2$
5	B	$1s^2\ 2s^2 2p^1$
6	C	$1s^2\ 2s^2 2p^2$
7	N	$1s^2\ 2s^2 2p^3$
8	O	$1s^2\ 2s^2 2p^4$
9	F	$1s^2\ 2s^2 2p^5$
10	Ne	$1s^2\ 2s^2 2p^6$
11	Na	$[Ne]\ 3s^1$
12	Mg	$[Ne]\ 3s^2$
13	Al	$[Ne]\ 3s^2 3p^1$
14	Si	$[Ne]\ 3s^2 3p^2$
15	P	$[Ne]\ 3s^2 3p^3$
16	S	$[Ne]\ 3s^2 3p^4$
17	Cl	$[Ne]\ 3s^2 3p^5$
18	Ar	$[Ne]\ 3s^2 3p^6$
19	K	$[Ar]\ 4s^1$
20	Ca	$[Ar]\ 4s^2$
21	Sc	$[Ar]\ 4s^2\ 3d^1$
22	Ti	$[Ar]\ 4s^2\ 3d^2$
23	V	$[Ar]\ 4s^2\ 3d^3$
24	Cr	$[Ar]\ 4s^1\ 3d^5$
25	Mn	$[Ar]\ 4s^2\ 3d^5$
26	Fe	$[Ar]\ 4s^2\ 3d^6$
27	Co	$[Ar]\ 4s^2\ 3d^7$
28	Ni	$[Ar]\ 4s^2\ 3d^8$
29	Cu	$[Ar]\ 4s^1\ 3d^{10}$
30	Zn	$[Ar]\ 4s^2\ 3d^{10}$
31	Ga	$[Ar]\ 4s^2\ 3d^{10} 4p^1$
32	Ge	$[Ar]\ 4s^2\ 3d^{10} 4p^2$
33	As	$[Ar]\ 4s^2\ 3d^{10} 4p^3$
34	Se	$[Ar]\ 4s^2\ 3d^{10} 4p^4$
35	Br	$[Ar]\ 4s^2\ 3d^{10} 4p^5$
36	Kr	$[Ar]\ 4s^2\ 3d^{10} 4p^6$

FIGURE 3–5   The ground-state electron configurations of neutral gas atoms of elements from $Z = 1$ through $Z = 36$.

TABLE 3–1   KINDS OF ATOMIC ORBITALS

s (1s, 2s, etc.)
Holds up to two electrons in one orbital
p (2p, 3p, etc.)
Holds up to six electrons in three orbitals
d (3d, 4d, 5d, etc.)
Holds up to ten electrons in five orbitals
f (4f, 5f) Holds up to 14 electrons in 7 orbitals

Notice in Example 3b that potassium begins "filling" the 4s atomic orbital. The 4s orbital is a bit lower in energy than the 3d orbital, so elements #19 and #20 have electrons in 4s rather than in 3d. Once the 4s is filled, the next electrons must go into 3d for elements #21 to #30 (scandium through zinc).

The design of the periodic table is directly related to the electron configurations of the elements, as shown in Figure 3–5, which gives the configurations for elements #1 to #36 inside their boxes in the periodic table. You see that elements with similar electron configurations are above and below each other; for example, carbon ($Z = 6$), silicon ($Z = 14$), and germanium ($Z = 32$) all have electron configurations ending in ns^2np^2, where n is the number of the outermost principal energy level that contains electrons.

Notice also that the elements in the first two columns (under H and Be) have incomplete and just-completed s orbitals. The stretch from $Z = 21$ to $Z = 30$ involves d orbitals, and those elements under B, C, N, O, F, and Ne involve p orbitals. These facts will be related in the next section to the chemical properties of these groups of elements.

The elements from $Z = 58$ to $Z = 71$ are those in which electrons are partly filling the seven 4f orbitals, while $Z = 90$ to $Z = 103$ involves the 5f orbitals. The properties of these different kinds of orbitals are summarized in Table 3–1. All of the energy levels for electrons can be placed in an order of "filling" shown in Figure 3–6.

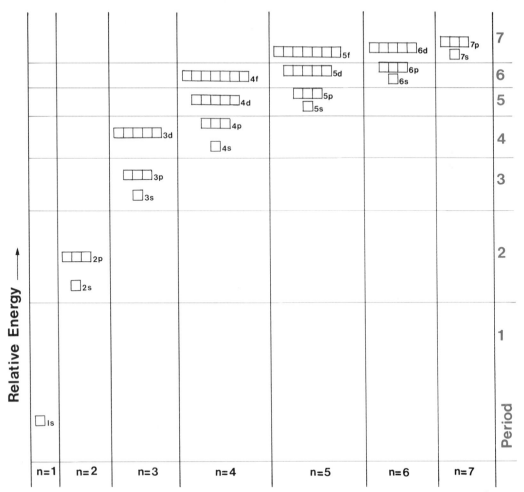

FIGURE 3-6   An energy-level diagram for all of the currently known elements in the periodic table. The periods at the right correspond to the period numbers on the table inside the front cover. Each box (atomic orbital) can hold up to two electrons. There is thus room for two different elements in Period 1, eight in Period 2, eight in Period 3, eighteen in Period 4, etc.

Noble-gas configurations

The electron configurations that include ns^2np^6 are considered very **stable** by chemists. Something is stable if it can be changed only with great difficulty. Elements like helium ($Z = 2$), neon ($Z = 10$), argon ($Z = 18$), and krypton ($Z = 36$) have atoms that resist very strongly any change in the electron configuration. We list those configurations in Table 3–2.

Each noble-gas configuration, with its ns^2np^6 makeup, has *eight* electrons in its outermost principal energy level. This configuration can be reached by other elements if they gain, lose, or share electrons. This search for an octet—eight electrons in the outermost principal level or valence electron level—explains many of the properties of the elements, as you will soon see.

The word "noble" was chosen to describe elements with the ns^2np^6 configuration because they were "aloof" and "would not mix" with the other elements.

TABLE 3–2 THE ELECTRONIC CONFIGURATIONS OF THE NOBLE GASES ALL END IN . . . s^2 . . . p^6

$_2$He	$1s^2$
$_{10}$Ne	$1s^2\,2s^2\,2p^6$
$_{18}$Ar	$1s^2\,2s^2\,2p^6\,3s^2\,3p^6$
$_{36}$Kr	$1s^2\,2s^2\,2p^6\,3s^2\,3p^6\,3d^{10}\,4s^2\,4p^6$
$_{54}$Xe	$1s^2\,2s^2\,2p^6\,3s^2\,3p^6\,3d^{10}\,4s^2\,4p^6\,4d^{10}\,5s^2\,5p^6$
$_{86}$Rn	$1s^2\,2s^2\,2p^6\,3s^2\,3p^6\,3d^{10}\,4s^2\,4p^6\,4d^{10}\,4f^{14}\,5s^2\,5p^6\,5d^{10}\,6s^2\,6p^6$

Some students feel they understand a chemical theory better if they are given a real-life analogy. If you do not like analogies, skim through this one. If they help you understand what we are driving at, read on.

A CAMPING ANALOGY

Suppose 20 little children are attending a summer camp. They are all down by the lake. One by one, they dry themselves off and walk up the path to the cabins to take naps. The cabins are arranged on a hill as shown in Figure 3–7.

In this camp, a child can go to *any* cabin to take a nap. Each cabin contains two beds, one by the window, the other facing the reverse direction.

Since little children are quite tired and lazy after a swim, each child picks the first unoccupied bed that he or she can find that is the *shortest* distance up the hill.

Given the choice, at the same level up the hill, of sharing a cabin or being all alone, these children are instructed to pick a cabin in which there is no other child.

Now, start the children up the hill, and see which beds are used as each child leaves the lake. Your results should be very similar to the electron configurations for elements #1 to #20.

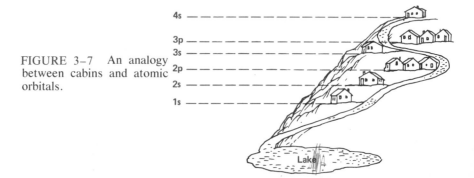

FIGURE 3–7 An analogy between cabins and atomic orbitals.

3.1)   Write a complete electron configuration for each of the following:
a)   carbon ($Z = 6$)
b)   argon ($Z = 18$)
c)   calcium ($Z = 20$)
d)   the element with 13 protons in its nucleus
3.2)   Write an electron configuration using a *neon core* for sulfur ($Z = 16$).
3.3)   Which electron configurations are particularly stable?
3.4)   How does an electron in a 1s orbital differ from one in a 2s orbital?

3.2 FAMILIES OF ELEMENTS

LEARNING GOAL 3C: Given a periodic table, identify each of the main groups or families and describe the valence electron configuration that characterizes each group.
      3D: Given the atomic number or name of an element in one of the representative groups (1 through 8) and given a periodic table, (a) predict the most common monatomic ion that will be formed by that element and (b) write the electron configuration of that ion.
      3E: Write a Lewis electron-dot symbol for a neutral atom or monatomic ion of a representative element.

The following very important chemical properties can be predicted from the electron configurations of most elements:

1)   The kinds of compounds the element will tend to form.
2)   The kind of one-atom or *monatomic ion* that will be formed by an atom of the element through the gain or loss of one or more electrons.
3)   Whether the element will act as a metal or not.
4)   Whether the element will show properties similar to those of other, more common elements, which might lead to an effect on the human body.

Development of the periodic table

About one half of the elements now known were discovered before 1850. Just as biologists classify animals and plants according to their similarities, chemists tried to find some kind of logical order among the chemical elements. As early as 1820, J. W. Dobereiner noticed similarities in the properties of lithium, sodium, and potassium. He also noticed that chlorine, bromine, and iodine are somewhat alike. In 1865, J. A. R. Newlands put the known elements in order of increasing atomic weight. When he did this, elements spaced eight-apart seemed to have characteristics in common.

The Russian scientist D. I. Mendeleyev took Newlands's idea and, in 1869, made a chart that contained eight "families" of elements. There were some gaps in his chart, elements which should exist but were not yet known.

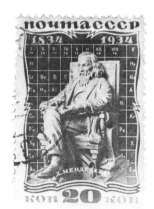

Dmitri Ivanovich Mendeleyev is very important in the history of chemical thought. Behind the statue is an early table showing the periodic groups.

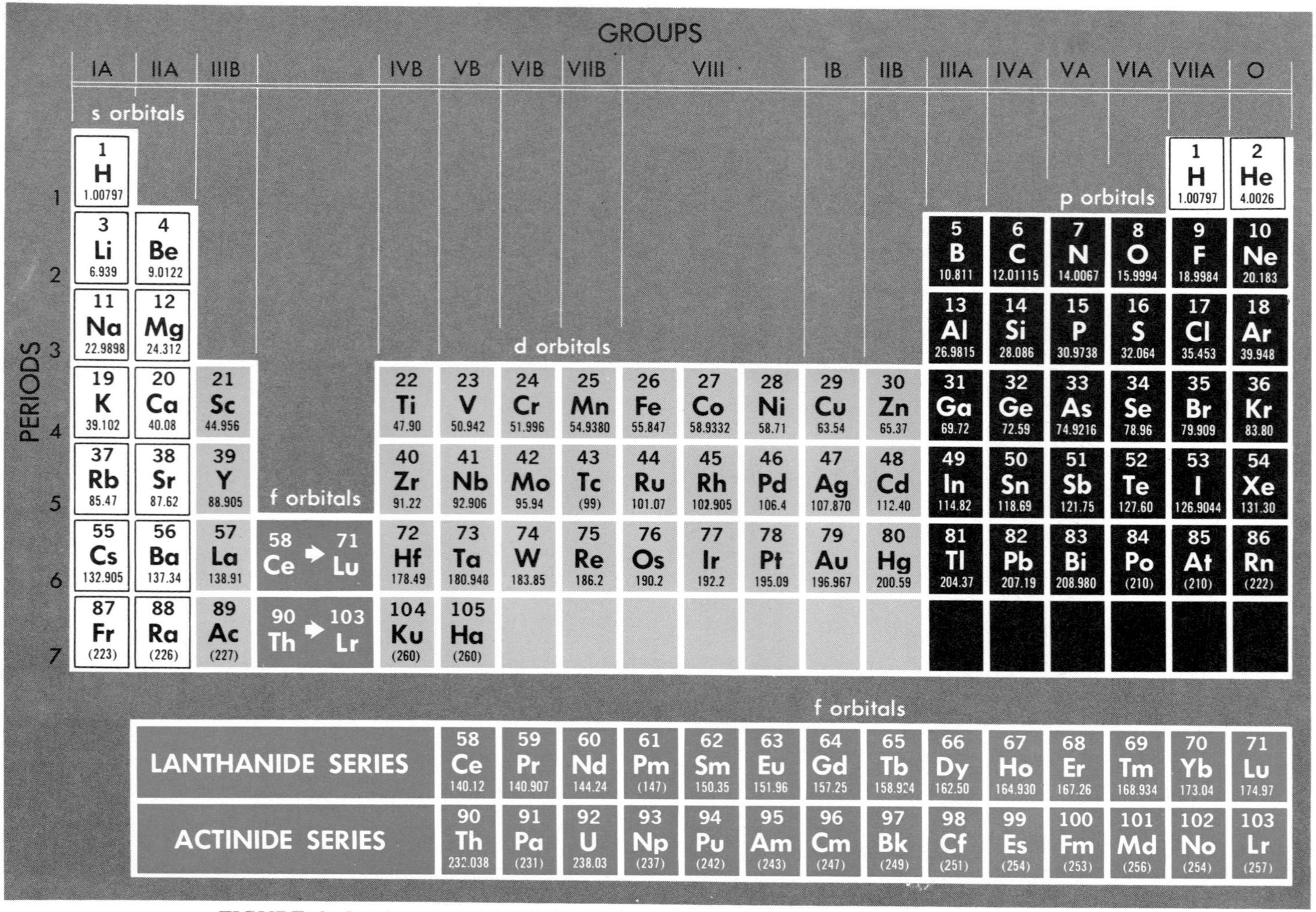

FIGURE 3-8 Arrangement of the periodic table according to energy sublevels. The highest energy sublevels that contain electrons are s sublevels for Groups 1 and 2, p sublevels for Groups 3 through 8, d sublevels for the ordinary transition metals, and f sublevels in the lanthanide and actinide series.

Before the year 1900, three new elements, germanium ($Z = 32$), gallium ($Z = 31$), and scandium ($Z = 21$), were discovered and had exactly the kinds of properties predicted by Mendeleyev from the gaps in his table.

Putting the elements in order of atomic weight, some parts of the table didn't make much sense. Henry Moseley in 1912 found that the number of protons (atomic number) rather than the atomic weight is the key to ordering the elements. The results of those efforts can be seen on the inside front cover and, in terms of electron configuration, in Figure 3–8.

We know from Section 2.5 that the atomic weight of an element depends on which natural isotopes are around. If you look carefully at the numbers in the periodic table, you will see that for elements #27 and #28 (cobalt and nickel), as well as for #52 and #53 (tellurium and iodine), the order of atomic weights does not correspond to the number of protons.

In the modern periodic table (Figure 3–8), the elements are arranged in rows or *periods* and in columns or *groups*. The arrangement corresponds to the electron configurations of the elements. The elements with white backgrounds have ns^1 and ns^2 configurations. Those with black backgrounds are "filling" the p orbitals; those with light-colored backgrounds, the d orbitals; and, at the bottom, those with dark-colored backgrounds are "filling" the f orbitals.

You should notice that from the periodic table you can predict when each energy sublevel (Figure 3–6) will begin to fill.

The **period** of an element in the table is the number to the far left, for example, rubidium ($Z = 37$) begins Period 5. The period number corresponds exactly to the principal energy level number n of the s and p electrons being filled, called the **valence level.** We thus know that Rb is in the process of filling the 5s sublevel.

The **group** of an element is the number at the top of the chart. Figure 3–8 shows these numbered groups of **representative elements** which involve s and p electrons in the filling order, as well as the groups that we call **transition metals** and involve the filling of d orbitals.

The group number (1 through 8) corresponds to the number of outer-level s and p electrons (valence electrons) in an atom of the element. The number is often written in roman numerals (I to VIII) and with "A" groups being representative elements and "B" groups being transition metals.

Lewis electron-dot symbols for the elements

The **valence electrons** of an atom (or ion) are the electrons in the outermost s and p orbitals. The maximum number of valence electrons is eight, made up from a ns^2np^6 configuration of a noble gas like neon ($Z = 10$), argon ($Z = 18$), or krypton ($Z = 36$).

The valence electrons are so important in determining the properties of most elements that chemists have added them to the element symbols in order to show how compounds are formed. An element symbol with dots added to show the valence electrons is called a **Lewis electron-dot symbol.** The Lewis symbols for the elements of the first three periods are shown in Table 3–3.

A noble-gas configuration is indicated if a Lewis symbol has either no electron dots or eight electron dots. The fluorine atom, shown as :$\ddot{\text{F}}$:, needs only one more dot to complete its octet and have the same number of valence electrons as neon. The adding of that one electron turns the fluorine atom into the very stable monatomic (one-atom) ion, the F$^-$ anion.

TABLE 3–3 LEWIS ELECTRON-DOT SYMBOLS

Group	1	2	3	4	5	6	7	8
Period 2	Li·	·Be·	·B·	·C·	·N·	:O·	:F:	:Ne:
3	Na·	·Mg·	·Al·	·Si·	·P·	:S·	:Cl:	:Ar:
4	K·	·Ca·	·Ga·	·Ge·	·As·	:Se·	:Br:	:Kr:

Monatomic ions with noble-gas electron configurations

We earlier (Table 3–2) listed the electron configurations of the noble gases, Group 8, which are particularly stable because both the s and p sublevels of the outermost level are filled. Table 3–4 shows the ions formed from single atoms (**monatomic ions**) of elements neighboring the noble gases. Each type of ion forms a chemical family.

GROUP 1, the **alkali metal family,** forms 1+ cations, since each atom loses one electron from a ns^1 configuration to reach the configuration of the nearest noble gas. You see that lithium ($Z = 3$), sodium ($Z = 11$), potassium ($Z = 19$), and others have this property. Hydrogen is not really in Group 1 because if it loses one electron, it becomes not an ion with a noble-gas-type configuration but a simple proton.

GROUP 2, the **alkaline earth family,** forms 2+ cations. Calcium and magnesium are familiar members of this family.

GROUP 3, generally known as the aluminum family, can in some cases form 3+ cations. However, it takes a lot of energy to remove three electrons. Another member of this family is boron, which does *not* form an ion.

GROUP 4, often called the carbon family, forms few ions.

GROUP 5, the nitrogen family, could not possibly lose five electrons from an atom to form a 5+ cation like the next-lower noble gas. Nitrogen alone can *gain* three electrons (N^{3-}) to have a configuration like that of neon. This group generally does not form monatomic ions.

TABLE 3–4 MONATOMIC IONS WITH NOBLE-GAS CONFIGURATIONS

Period	1	2	3	4	5	6	7	Electron Configuration	Group 8
1							H^-	$1s^2$	$= {}_2He$
2	Li^+	Be^{2+}	—		N^{3-}	O^{2-}	F^-	$1s^2 2s^2 2p^6$	$= {}_{10}Ne$
3	Na^+	Mg^{2+}	Al^{3+}		—	S^{2-}	Cl^-	$1s^2 2s^2 2p^6 3s^2 3p^6$	$= {}_{18}Ar$
4	K^+	Ca^{2+}	Sc^{3+}	—		—	Se^{2-}	Br^-	$[Ar]\,3d^{10}4s^24p^6$ $= {}_{36}Kr$
5	Rb^+	Sr^{2+}	Y^{3+}	—		—	Te^{2-}	I^-	$[Kr]\,4d^{10}5s^25p^6$ $= {}_{54}Xe$
6	Cs^+	Ba^{2+}	La^{3+}						

GROUP 6, the oxygen family, can generally gain two electrons to form anions with a 2− charge. The two most common such ions are oxide (O^{2-}) and sulfide (S^{2-}).

GROUP 7, the **halogens,** exists commonly as the 1− anions. Such an anion is called a *halide,* and the names of the ions all end in *-ide,* as discussed in Section 3.4.

GROUP 8, the **noble gases,** already has atoms with noble-gas configurations and thus does not form ions. As a general rule, such atoms do not associate with others to form molecules or compounds, although some compounds of Xe and Kr have been produced.

The members of Groups 1, 2, and 3 along with the transition metals will be discussed in somewhat more detail in Section 3.3. The nonmetals, Groups 4, 5, 6, and 7, will be reviewed in Section 3.4.

SELF-CHECK

3.5) What valence electron configuration is typical of
a) a halogen?   b) a Group 2 element?   c) a noble gas?

3.6) Give the *name* and *number* of the group to which each of the following elements belongs:
a) potassium   b) chlorine   c) argon

3.7) Write the Lewis electron-dot symbol for
a) a neutral carbon atom   c) a F^- anion
b) a Mg^{2+} cation   d) a neutral calcium atom

3.8) Using a periodic table, predict the charge on the most common monatomic ion formed by
a) magnesium ($Z = 12$)   b) iodine ($Z = 53$)   c) sulfur ($Z = 16$)

3.9) Explain, on the basis of electron configuration, why each of the ions in Question 3.8 is formed.

3.3 SOME IMPORTANT METALS

LEARNING GOAL 3F: List the distinguishing properties of elements that are metals.

3G: Predict from position in the periodic table whether a given element will have a high or low first ionization energy.

3H: Determine the oxidation state of a neutral atom or monatomic ion of an element.

You are already familiar with many properties of metals such as aluminum, iron, and silver. Most metals are solids at room temperature, can be polished to a bright shine, conduct electricity and heat very well, and can be drawn into wires and rolled into sheets or foils. Metals can be mixed with each other to make alloys, such as stainless steel and sterling silver. The everyday materials you think of as **metals** are made up of various neutral atoms of certain elements of Group 3, Group 4, and the transition elements.

Ionization energy

Chemically, a metal has a slightly different definition. It is an element that can easily *lose* one or more electrons to become a cation. The energy re-

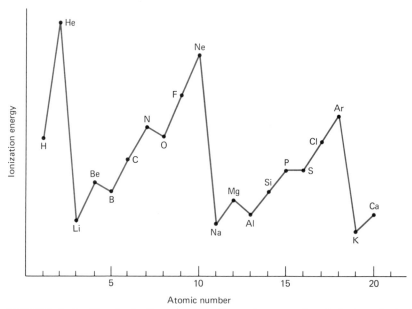

FIGURE 3–9 The ionization energy of an atom can be plotted against atomic number to show the periodic behavior of the elements.

quired to pull one electron off a neutral atom, to make a 1+ ion, is called the **ionization energy** of that atom. All elements with low ionization energies are metals.

The ionization energies of the first 20 elements are graphed in Figure 3–9 so you can see the **periodicity** of the elements. It is clearly easiest to pull an electron off lithium, sodium, and potassium to make the 1+ cations. This fact agrees with what you already know from Section 3.2.

At the other extreme, elements with high ionization energies are very resistant to having an electron removed. The noble gases head the list, but the halogens are also classified as **nonmetals.** A nonmetal tends *not* to lose an electron.

The ionization energies of the elements tend to decrease as you go from the top to the bottom of the periodic table. The $6s^1$ electron in cesium ($Z = 55$) is much farther away from the positive nucleus of the atom than the 2s electron in lithium. Cesium is thus more metallic than lithium.

The ionization energies tend to increase as you scan the periodic table from left to right, since the number of protons in the nucleus increases, holding the outer electrons more tightly. The more metallic elements are at the *left* of the table. These trends are summarized in Figure 3–10.

In Figure 3–10 you see several boxes marked with cross-hatching. These are not clearly metals or nonmetals. They are sometimes called **metalloids.** Boron, silicon, germanium, arsenic, and some other elements may have metallic properties in some situations and nonmetallic properties in others. For example, boron does *not* form a 3+ cation the way aluminum does. However, pure boron will conduct electricity at high temperature, a property of metals.

We are considering here only the *first* ionization energy, that which is needed to remove *one* electron from the neutral atom. The *second* such ionization energy, which is low for a Group 2 element such as Mg or Ca, is the energy needed to remove an electron from the 1+ ion, such as Ca^+, to arrive at the 2+ ion, Ca^{2+}. Aluminum, in Group 3, will have a low *third* ionization energy, since it forms 3+ cations.

Oxidation states

If a neutral atom loses an electron to form a 1+ cation, you know a metal is involved. However, there are many compounds in which electrons have apparently been removed from an atom but without the creation of a positively charged cation. Chemists have therefore assigned **oxidation state** numbers to atoms in order to keep track of electron gain and loss.

Chemical properties are distinct for each different oxidation state of an element. For example, chlorine may be found in oxidation states -1, 0, $+1$, and several others to $+7$. That does not mean that each of these is an ion; a Cl^{7+} ion would be extraordinarily difficult to obtain. However, in going from its -1 to $+7$ oxidation state, electrons have somehow been lost to other atoms. The chloride ion, Cl^-, is familiar in table salt and other compounds. The properties of the -1 oxidation state of chlorine are very different from those of the 0 oxidation state, which is the poisonous gas Cl_2.

As we proceed with more detailed chemical explanations, we will often discuss oxidation states. Let us start very simply by using two definitions:

The oxidation state of a pure element is *zero*.

Thus, the oxidation state of oxygen in O_2, hydrogen in H_2, sodium in the pure sodium metal, or chlorine in Cl_2 gas is zero.

The oxidation state in a monatomic ion is equal to the charge on the ion.

The oxidation state of sodium in Na^+ is $+1$. The oxidation state of oxygen in the O^{2-} anion is -2.

Oxidation states will be further discussed and used in Chapter 8, which deals with oxidation-reduction reactions. At this stage, we will add only one

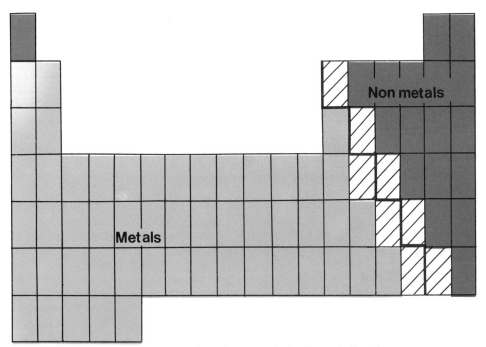

FIGURE 3–10 The metals and nonmetals in the periodic table.

more small thing for you to learn. We can show the oxidation state of an element by writing a Roman numeral after its name. Iron in the +3 oxidation state (as in rust) may be shown as "iron(III)."

The alkali metals—Group 1

Each alkali metal, such as sodium ($Z = 11$) or potassium ($Z = 19$), reacts violently when put in water. After all the sparks have died down, the solution that remains is a strong *alkali* or base (like lye), hence the name of the group. The pure metals thus do not exist in nature and are rarely used.

All animals and plants contain large amounts of sodium and potassium cations dissolved in water. Both ions are often accompanied by the chloride ion, since there must be an equal number of positive and negative charges in any small region.

The potassium ion is generally found *inside* the cell, while sodium ion is mostly in the fluids surrounding the cell. Since both ions tend to migrate (move) into regions where they are scarce, living cells have developed amazing means, called *active transport* (Chapter 18) to kick Na^+ ions back out of the cell and bring K^+ ions into the cell. A large number of body processes depend not only on the presence of Na^+ and K^+ ions, but on the proper balance being maintained between them.

Lithium ($Z = 3$) is occasionally used to treat mental illness in the form of one of its compounds. Taking in too much Li^+ over a long period of time can cause kidney damage.

Rubidium ($Z = 37$) and cesium ($Z = 55$) are quite rare. Francium ($Z = 87$) is a member of Group 1 that is found naturally only in trace amounts. It is naturally radioactive, as are all elements above $Z = 83$. (We will discuss radioactivity in Section 3.5.)

The alkaline earth metals—Group 2

Calcium ($Z = 20$) ions, Ca^{2+}, make up about 2% of our body weight, almost entirely in the bones and teeth. A proper level of calcium in the body fluids is needed for nerve response, muscle contraction (including heart pumping), and even the maintenance of correct body temperature. Ca^{2+} ions must also be present for the clotting of blood.

Magnesium ($Z = 12$) ions, Mg^{2+}, are also essential to the body, especially for nerve impulses and muscle contraction. There are many enzymes, substances that speed up chemical reactions of the body, that include Mg^{2+} as part of their structure. The plant molecule *chlorophyll* includes magnesium(II).

The hydroxides of these two metals, $Ca(OH)_2$ and $Mg(OH)_2$, are widely used. The former is lime, used largely in building materials. Magnesium hydroxide, $Mg(OH)_2$, is sold (as *milk of magnesia*) as a solid suspended in water. A small dose works as an antacid, a larger amount is used as a laxative.

Barium ($Z = 56$) is a heavy metal whose ions are poisonous. However, barium sulfate, $BaSO_4$, does not dissolve in water and is very useful in taking x-rays of the digestive system. Beryllium ($Z = 4$) is rare and very poisonous, either as a pure element or in the form of Be^{2+} salts. Strontium is rare. Radium is a famous radioactive element discovered by Pierre and Marie Curie.

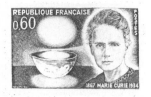

Marie Sklodowska Curie (1867–1934) and her husband were awarded the Nobel Prize in physics in 1903 for studies of nuclear radiation. Her discovery of the elements radium ($Z = 88$) and polonium ($Z = 84$) earned her the Nobel Prize in chemistry in 1911.

The aluminum group—Group 3

The most important element in Group 3 is aluminum ($Z = 13$), which we encounter every day as a structural metal. It is the third most abundant element (as the Al^{3+} ion) in the earth's crust. None of the Group 3 elements seems to play a role in the human body. Aluminum hydroxide, $Al(OH)_3$, is found in many antacids.

Gallium ($Z = 31$) shares with mercury the distinction of being found as a liquid metal at room temperature.

Table 3–4 shows how the most common metals of Groups 1, 2, and 3 ionize to form monatomic cations.

Transition metals in the human body

Below and between magnesium and aluminum in the periodic table are elements in Periods 4, 5, 6, and 7, in which d orbitals are being filled. These are the transition metals. Although the differences among transition metals are due to differing numbers of d electrons, their basic chemical properties come from their *valence* electrons.

The most common oxidation state for transition metals is the $+2$ state, but many of these elements also have $+1$ states. These states are often seen in monatomic ions, such as the two cations of copper ($Z = 29$), the Cu^+ and Cu^{2+} ions. Both states are due to loss of s (not d) electrons.

Since there are 30 transition metals whose properties are well known, we can only give a brief account here. Most of them tend to form colored compounds and solutions. Nine of them are listed in Table 1–1 as required by the human body. We shall concentrate our discussion on these.

Iron ($Z = 26$) is perhaps the most essential transition metal, both in everyday life, where so many physical objects are made of steel, and in the body, where an iron-containing molecule called *hemoglobin* carries oxygen from the lungs to the rest of the body. The actual need for iron is very low, only about 1 to 1.5 mg per day for a normal person. About ten times as much must be taken in in our food, however, because not all of the iron that passes through the body is absorbed. Small amounts of iron are found in every tissue cell in molecules that use oxygen. About 3% of the iron in the body is in muscle cells in a molecule called *myoglobin*. There are two common forms of iron in its compounds, iron(II) or "ferrous" (Fe^{2+}) and iron(III) or "ferric" (Fe^{3+}). Both are involved in the energy-producing processes described in Chapter 22.

Copper ($Z = 29$) is required for a variety of roles in the body, several of which are connected to the use of iron. Although the total amount of copper in the body is less than 3% of the amount in a penny coin, deficiency of copper will result in weak blood vessels and bones as well as nerve damage.

Manganese (Mn, $Z = 25$) should not be confused with the similar-sounding element magnesium (Mg, $Z = 12$). Manganese is a common metal and is used in making steel. Although a deficiency of Mn is almost impossible to have, and thus we are not absolutely sure what symptoms would result, we do know that Mn has many essential functions in every cell.

Zinc ($Z = 30$) as a metal is widely used as a coating or "galvanizing" on iron as protection from rust. It is also widely used in brass and in batteries. Inside the body, zinc is essential (as Zn^{2+}) for normal growth of genital organs, wound healing, and general growth of all tissues. It is also associated

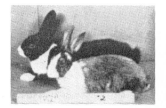

The rabbit in the back received sufficient copper in its diet. The rabbit in the front displays smaller size and depigmentation after six weeks on a copper-deficient diet. (From Hunt, C. E., and Carlton, W. W.: *J. Nutr.*, 87:385, 1965.)

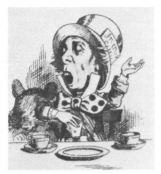

An example of mercury poisoning (?)—the "Mad Hatter" of *Alice in Wonderland*. A hundred years ago, mercury was used in making felt hats. The workers suffered from shaking, loss of hair and teeth, and sometimes premature death.

with the hormone *insulin*, which is used to treat diabetes. Oysters are an unusually rich source of zinc.

Cobalt ($Z = 27$) is an essential part of one molecule, vitamin B_{12}. Like iron (Fe^{2+}) in hemoglobin, Co^{2+} serves to hold the large vitamin molecule together and to make it function properly.

Molybdenum ($Z = 42$) is part of several important enzymes. We are not sure if a deficiency is possible or what symptoms would result.

Chromium ($Z = 24$) is best known for automobile bumpers. Its requirement in the human body was only determined in 1959. We now know that Cr^{3+} serves a variety of roles.

Nickel ($Z = 28$) and vanadium ($Z = 23$) are included in our list of essential elements on the basis of their requirement by some animals other than humans. No deficiency of either is likely to be seen, and in the absence of very clear evidence of how these two elements work in the human body, some authors leave them off the list of essential elements. They are both needed by chickens.†

As research continues, it is possible that additional elements may be shown to play a role in living animal cells.

Some other transition metals

One element that concerns many health workers is mercury ($Z = 80$). It is quite unusual in its pure liquid state and is widely used in barometers and thermometers, as well as in dental fillings. Mercury compounds released into water supplies can cause serious poisoning, with the most famous case being that of Minamata disease.

Silver ($Z = 47$), gold ($Z = 79$), platinum ($Z = 78$), and palladium ($Z = 46$) are transition metals commonly used for jewelry and high-value coins. They tend to be very expensive but are also resistant to chemical change.

Tungsten ($Z = 74$) is the wire used inside light bulbs. It will not melt, even at temperatures above 3000°C, but will glow and give off light when carrying electric current.

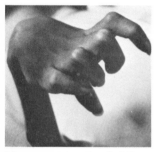

Mercury poisoning in Minamata disease. In the early 1950's, a plastics firm released large amounts of waste mercury compounds into a Japanese bay. The mercury level built up in the fish. People eating the fish were stricken with muscle weakness, poor vision, mental retardation, and sometimes paralysis and death. (Photo by W. Eugene Smith.)

The elements with atomic numbers 58–71 and 90–103 are special types of transition metals since they are "filling" 4f and 5f orbitals. Elements #104 and beyond are again filling d orbitals. However, the naming of such elements has become controversial. For example, we have labelled element #104 as rutherfordium, with symbol Rf. That's the unofficial U.S. version, based on the name of a famous Western scientist (Section 2.4). Others have called element 104 "kurchatovium" after an important Soviet scientist, since the U.S.S.R. claims to have discovered it first, in 1964. To remove national pride from this, official names have recently been assigned to elements 104 to 106 which are based entirely on the Greek form of the *atomic number*. Element 104 is unnilquadium (Unq), 105 is unnilpentium (Unp) and 106 is unnilhexium (Unh), although these names have not yet been universally accepted. None of these elements plays an important role in the chemistry of life.

SELF-CHECK

3.10)   What can you say about the ionization energies of elements that are classified as metals?

3.11)   What do you know about the oxidation states of elements that are classified as metals?

---

† See Briggs, G.M., and Calloway, D., *Bogert's Nutrition and Physical Fitness*, 10th edition, Philadelphia, W.B. Saunders Company, 1979, Chapter 12.

3.12) Which would you expect to be *more* metallic,
a) Sb ($Z = 51$) or Pb ($Z = 82$)?
b) S ($Z = 16$) or F ($Z = 9$)?
c) Cs ($Z = 55$) or Ba ($Z = 56$)?
3.13) Write the oxidation state of the element in each of the following species:
a) Mg   b) Ca^{2+} c) H_2 d) Fe^{3+} e) Cl^-

3.4 SOME IMPORTANT NONMETALS

LEARNING GOAL 3I: List the distinguishing properties of elements that are nonmetals.

    3J: Explain, using an example from this chapter, how an element can be considered both essential to life and poisonous to life.

The elements toward the upper right of the periodic table are the nonmetals. While metals will have only positive and zero oxidation states (and only positive ions), nonmetals will often be found in negative oxidation states forming negative ions.

The carbon family—Group 4

Most of this textbook will be devoted to the chemistry of carbon compounds. No compound has much to do with pure carbon, found in coal, graphite, and diamonds. A much more important substance is carbon dioxide, CO_2, which is produced by animals and taken in by plants. The plants then use the CO_2, with water and with the help of sunlight and nutrients from the soil, to make the gigantic number of organic compounds we find in the plant world.

When not enough oxygen is available for the complete burning of carbon (as discussed in Chapter 5), carbon monoxide, CO, is produced. This is a poisonous gas. Other compounds that contain carbon and oxygen include the carbonates, such as washing soda (Na_2CO_3), baking soda ($NaHCO_3$), and limestone ($CaCO_3$).

Silicon ($Z = 14$) is of great importance in the electronics industry. As a metalloid (neither metal nor nonmetal), it has the properties of a *semiconductor*, which make possible various types of transistors and solar cells. Silicon has been shown to be an essential element in the chick and rat, and thus presumably essential in humans. Our greatest use of the element is in glass, which is largely sand containing SiO_2. Silicon is generally found in the $+4$ oxidation state.

Germanium ($Z = 32$) is used in semiconductors of various types. It is otherwise quite rare. Tin ($Z = 50$) is common in construction and other metal uses. It seems to be required by rats and thus probably by humans. Lead ($Z = 82$) is a very dense metal that finds uses in lead weights and shielding against radiation. Lead was once widely used for water pipes and in paints. We now know that Pb^{2+} is extremely poisonous. Intake of more than 0.001 gram per day is considered dangerous; children living in low-income areas sometimes eat paint flaking from walls and become poisoned.

One advantage of no-lead gasolines to the general population is the lower level of Pb^{2+}.

The nitrogen family—Group 5

Nitrogen is one of the most important elements for life. The simple molecule NH_3, ammonia, is important not only for washing windows but also in our internal chemistry. Often found as part of organic molecules is the NH_2 group, typical of an *amine* and found in amino acids and proteins, to be seen in Chapter 13.

Although there is plenty of nitrogen in the air, it is mostly present there as *pure* nitrogen, N_2. Neither animals nor plants (with a few bacteria as exceptions) can use nitrogen in its zero oxidation state. To be absorbed into a living cell, N_2 must be converted to ammonia or to a nitrate such as saltpeter, KNO_3. Some of these inorganic nitrogen compounds will be seen in Chapter 4.

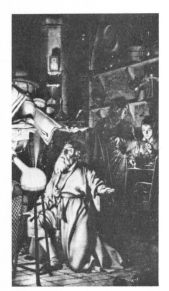

FIGURE 3–11 The medieval alchemist Hennig Brand searched for the "philosopher's stone" of eternal life. He discovered phosphorus in a sample of urine. (Bettman Archives.)

Phosphorus ($Z = 15$) is a very important element of life. It was first identified in urine by an alchemist in 1669 (Figure 3–11). In its free form, P_4, it glows in the dark and is extremely poisonous. In its combined form, mostly as phosphates (like Na_3PO_4), it has a $+5$ oxidation state and acts in many key roles in the body. Among other functions, phosphates are involved in the energy transfer processes described in Chapter 22.

Arsenic ($Z = 33$) is mainly known as a murder weapon; most forms of arsenic are indeed poisonous, although a bit slow. However, arsenic may possibly be the next element to be identified as required by the body. Rats, pigs, and poultry seem to benefit from a diet that contains arsenic in very small amounts. Arsenic like antimony ($Z = 51$) below it is a metalloid, with -3, $+3$, and $+5$ oxidation states. Bismuth ($Z = 83$) is a metal with occasional uses.

The oxygen family—Group 6

We are all aware of the importance of oxygen, the third most common element in the universe. In its role as the central atom in water, oxygen provides most of your body weight. We have already in this chapter run across many oxygen-containing compounds and ions, such as nitrates (NO_3^-), carbonates (CO_3^{2-}), and phosphates (PO_4^{3-}). In Chapter 4, we shall discuss how these oxygen-containing negative ions combine with positive ions like Na^+, Ca^{2+}, and Al^{3+}.

Oxygen is required for all types of *combustion,* or burning. It combines with many metals to form an *oxide* layer in which oxygen is in its -2 oxidation state (in the form of an O^{2-} anion), as in rust (Fe_2O_3). It is, in fact, from this very process that we obtain our word *oxidation.* The more general meaning of oxidation, losing electrons, will be discussed in Chapter 8. You should be aware that we breathe oxygen molecules (O_2) from the air and transport these molecules in the blood to cells of the body.

A second type of pure oxygen, with *three* atoms linked together is *ozone* (O_3). This can be made from O_2 by an electric spark or by the ultraviolet rays in sunlight. Although some people seem to think ozone is beneficial, it is actually poisonous and irritating to the lungs. It can cause difficulty for some passengers on high-flying aircraft, since the upper layers of the atmosphere contain much ozone. This ozone screens out some of the high-energy ultraviolet rays from the sun, which otherwise would cause considerable amounts of skin cancer. Our recent heavy use of aerosol spray cans has been criticized because certain propellant chemicals inside the can eventually find their way to the upper atmosphere, where they react with the ozone and reduce our protection against ultraviolet rays.

It is possible to produce compounds called peroxides, which have oxygen in the -1 state. The most common is a solution of hydrogen peroxide, H_2O_2, used for bleaching and as a disinfectant.

Sulfur ($Z = 16$) is part of the human body, found in protein molecules. Sulfur, in fact, forms much of the "bridge" structure that holds protein molecules together. We often think of sulfur as "brimstone," a foul-smelling stuff associated with the devil. That is because sulfur burns to form the irritating oxides SO_2 and SO_3. Since coal and oil naturally contain some sulfur, the SO_2 pollution coming out of smokestacks presents a serious health problem in many areas. When the SO_3 molecule is dissolved in water, we get sulfuric acid, H_2SO_4, which has thousands of uses, but kills wildlife when it falls in "acid rain."

One of the most poisonous gases known is H_2S, hydrogen sulfide. It carries the odor of "rotten eggs." Luckily, we can smell H_2S long before it can kill us.

In Table 1–2 you saw the formula of ethyl alcohol, C_2H_5OH, found in alcoholic beverages. Ethyl alcohol contains oxygen. Sulfur and oxygen are both in Group 6. We may then expect sulfur to have some chemical properties similar to those of oxygen, and thus perhaps to form a compound C_2H_5SH. Indeed it does. This is ethyl mercaptan, with an odor similar to that of skunks! You can detect one part of this compound in 50 billion parts of air.

The remaining elements of Group 6 are much less common. However, it was recently learned that selenium ($Z = 34$) is just as important a nutrient for humans as the transition metals zinc, iron, and copper. Selenium seems to work in coordination with vitamin E. A deficiency in one may be partly made up by an excess of the other. If neither is available, poor growth and liver damage result, as well as a kind of muscular dystrophy.

On the other hand, too much selenium is harmful because, as a Group 6 element very similar to sulfur, selenium can replace sulfur in body compounds. In fact, selenium is *more* toxic (in terms of amount needed to cause damage) than mercury or lead. Animals grazing in areas where the soil contains large amounts of selenium develop the "blind staggers" and die.

The body's need for a very specific amount of selenium illustrates a general fact about many different kinds of nutrients. Too much is as injurious as too little, but in a different way.

Tellurium ($Z = 52$) is very rare. Its claim to fame is the fact that its analog (compound similar in composition) to water, H_2Te, is the worst-smelling inorganic compound known.

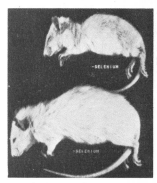

A selenium-deficient diet fed to a rat produces smaller size (top) than a diet adequate in this Group 6 element. (From Hunt, H. D., Cary, E. E., and Visek, W. J.: *J. Nutr.* 101:761, 1976.)

The halogens—Group 7

The most "nonmetallic" of the common elements are the halogens, which all form 1− anions called *halides*.

Fluorine ($Z = 9$) accepts an electron extremely readily. We say that its *electron affinity* is the highest in the periodic table. It reacts readily with al-

Electron affinity is the energy given off when an electron is added to a particle, for example when the fluorine (F) atom gains an electron to form the F− anion. Electron affinities are generally difficult to measure.

most all elements to form the fluoride ion, F^-. Hydrogen fluoride, HF, can be dissolved in water to form a solution that will etch glass.

The fluoridation of water supplies is a very controversial subject because, as with selenium, too much fluoride can be as injurious as too little. If the F^- level in water supplies is about 1 part per million by weight (or about 1 gram/ton), tooth decay in children is cut in half compared with water supplies deficient in fluoride. If the levels reach 2 parts per million, discoloration or mottling of teeth occurs. At slightly higher levels (4 to 8 parts per million), there is some evidence that fluoride can actually strengthen bones and prevent loss of calcium from them. At high levels, representing a daily intake of more than 0.25 grams of NaF, muscle and nerve damage can result. The lethal (death-dealing) dose is considered to be 4 grams of NaF. There is no scientific evidence that F^- is linked with cancer.

Fluorine also plays a part in medical implants. Compounds of carbon with fluorine are safe to use in the body. One of these compounds, C_2F_4, can combine with itself or *polymerize* (Chapter 16) to form *Teflon,* a plastic material that is used to make heart valves.

Chlorine ($Z = 17$) is the most familiar halogen, but in the form of Cl^- salts called chlorides. The chloride ion is the major anion of the human body.

Stomach acid is needed for proper digestion. It is a solution (Chapter 12) of hydrochloric acid, HCl. A more concentrated (stronger) HCl solution is sold as muriatic acid to clean tiles and brickwork.

As a pure element, chlorine is used to kill bacteria in drinking water. Two million tons of Cl_2 are produced each year. One factory doing this uses more electricity than a city of one million people. Chlorine can have oxidation states from -1 (Cl^-) through zero (Cl_2) to $+7$. The positive states are not common except for the $+1$ state, seen in the hypochlorite ion, ClO^-. This is the active ingredient in chlorine bleaches.

Bromine ($Z = 35$) is named from a Greek word meaning "stench" or awful odor. Pure Br_2 is a liquid at room temperature and is dangerous to touch or inhale. Bromide ion, Br^-, can be obtained from sea water. It was once commonly used (as NaBr or KBr) in sleeping pills. However, overuse of such drugs can upset the chloride ion balance in the body and cause mental disturbances.

Iodine ($Z = 53$), like chlorine but unlike bromine, is essential to life. It is part of the molecule *thyroxine,* a thyroid gland hormone that controls growth. Seafood contains adequate amounts of I^- to supply the body's needs. People living far from the sea may develop *goiter* as a result of iodine deficiency. To prevent this, a small amount of I^- is added to most brands of table salt. Pure I_2 is poisonous, both to people and to bacteria. One way to make drinking water safe is to add the right amount of solid iodine, enough to kill the bacteria but too little to affect your health. Pure iodine dissolved in alcohol was once widely used as an antiseptic for cuts. However, it was found to damage the skin tissues around the cuts and should not be used.

Astatine ($Z = 85$) is radioactive and very rare. It may possibly amount to less than one ounce in the entire earth!

The four major halogens can form many different compounds with carbon, many of which are used as refrigerants. Some of the halogenated hydrocarbons will be discussed in Chapter 4.

The noble gases—Group 8

Our voyage across the periodic table ends with the group of elements with the very stable ns^2np^6 electron configuration in the neutral atom. For many years, it was assumed that these elements were only good for filling balloons (helium, $Z = 2$) and filling light bulbs and tubes for signs (neon, $Z = 10$, and argon, $Z = 18$). Compounds of these elements were considered impossible to make.

However, chemical theory is occasionally wrong. Neil Bartlett produced in 1962 several compounds that combine xenon ($Z = 54$) with fluorine ($Z = 9$). We now know the properties of a number of xenon compounds, such as XeF_2, XeF_4, XeF_6, XeO_3, and H_4XeO_6. A few compounds of krypton ($Z = 36$) and radon ($Z = 86$) have also been prepared, but all are relatively unstable. Note that these few compounds have been made using the more *metallic* of the noble gases, those closest to the bottom of the table.

Radon is a gas that is produced by the disintegration (breaking up) of uranium nuclei (Section 3.5) in rocks. It is thus present to a slight extent in building materials and contributes to the natural "background" radiation to which humans have been exposed for millions of years.

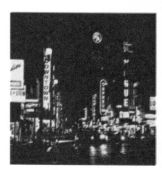

Noble gases, such as neon ($Z = 10$) can be used for commercial lighting.

SELF-CHECK

3.14) What can you say about the ionization energies of elements that are classified as nonmetals? Are they high or low?

3.15) Are nonmetals more likely to be found in negative or positive oxidation states?

3.16) Which three elements would you expect to have the neutral atoms with the greatest tendency to *gain* electrons? Explain.

3.17) Could we live in a world without iodine? Could we live in a world in which our drinking water contains large amounts of iodine? Explain.

3.18) Match each group of the periodic table (left) with its name (right).

Group 1	transition metals
Group 2	halogens
Group 7	alkaline earth metals
Group 8	noble gases
	alkali metals

3.19) Write the electron configuration and Lewis electron-dot symbol that is typical of
a) a neutral atom of a member of the nitrogen family
b) a monatomic ion formed by a halogen

3.5 RADIOACTIVITY

LEARNING GOAL 3K: Identify or describe the three main types of natural radiation, the alpha, beta, and gamma rays.

> *3L: Describe how emissions from radioactive substances can affect gases and living cells.*
>
> *3M: Explain how radioisotopes may be used in medical diagnosis and cancer treatment.*
>
> *3N: Predict from family resemblances in the periodic table how a particular radioisotope will affect the human body.*
>
> *3O: Use Table 3.6 to estimate the probable health effect of a given radiation dose.*
>
> *3P: Describe or illustrate what is meant by the half-life of a radioactive isotope.*

In addition to the chemical properties we have discussed in this chapter, each atom has nuclear properties that are related to the relative numbers of protons and neutrons in its nucleus.

Review what was said in Section 2.5 about the isotopes of the elements, recalling that the atomic weight of an element is a weighted average of the masses of the atoms of the *naturally occurring* isotopes of an element. For example, cobalt ($Z = 27$) has only one natural isotope. Its nuclear mass is 58.93 amu, and it contains 27 protons and 32 neutrons.

However, an important medical tool for the treatment of cancer is the cobalt-60 ($^{60}_{27}$Co) isotope. Since an atom of cobalt-60 has the same number of protons and electrons as natural $^{59}_{27}$Co, it has exactly the same chemical properties. However, the one extra neutron makes the nucleus of the $^{60}_{27}$Co atom unstable and capable of changing to a $^{60}_{28}$Ni nucleus. In the process it gives off a very high-energy electron called a *beta* (β) particle as well as electromagnetic radiation, like light rays or x-rays, which we call *gamma* (γ) rays. These radiations can kill normal cells. However, they are particularly likely to kill living cells that are dividing rapidly, such as cancer cells.

Hundreds of different radioactive isotopes, or **radioisotopes,** are available for use not only in medicine but also in agriculture, food sterilization, industrial quality control, and scientific research. Many homes are now protected by ionization-type smoke detectors, each of which contains a tiny chip of $^{241}_{95}$Am, an element not found in nature.

However, you are well aware that there is another side to the story. Nuclear radiation can kill living organisms, cause sterility and cancer, and create genetic defects. The proliferation of nuclear weapons and the capability of building them raise fears of total destruction of the human race. Our planned reliance on nuclear power to provide electricity for the 1990's while fossil fuels (oil, coal, natural gas) run short angers many citizens who see the dangers far outweighing the benefits. Safety questions, related to the operation of nuclear reactor power stations and to the adequate transportation and disposal of fuel and highly radioactive waste products, have not been completely answered.

In this short section, we can only scratch the surface of this fundamental topic.

Types of radioactivity

Radioactivity is the spontaneous emission of radiation resulting from the decay (falling apart) of an atomic nucleus. "Spontaneous" means it happens all by itself, regardless of the world around it. If a nucleus is going to decay in the next second, then nothing we can do to the substance will stop it. No one can make it decay any faster or slower, no matter where we put it or what temperature we subject it to. On the other hand, in a large sample of radioactive material, some atoms will decay right now and others will wait a long time to decay. We cannot predict, for a particular atom, when it will emit radiation.

There are three kinds of natural radioactive rays or emissions:

1) **Alpha rays** (α-rays), which are helium nuclei, $^4_2He^{2+}$, shot out at high speed from nuclei of decaying atoms.
2) **Beta rays** (β-rays), which are high-energy electrons traveling at almost the speed of light.
3) **Gamma rays** (γ-rays), which are like ordinary visible light beams but of much higher "punch" or energy effect.

As shown in Figure 3–12, alpha particles are so massive that they are stopped by a few sheets of tissue paper or the dead cells on the surface of human skin. Beta particles, being electrons, are faster and lighter. They can penetrate up to 4 mm into skin. Gamma radiation (like the similar but lower-energy x-rays used in medical diagnosis) will pass right through the body.

Effect of radiation

When an alpha, beta, or gamma ray hits an atom or molecule, some of its energy may be transferred. A common result is that the ray ionizes the target by knocking an electron out of its orbital and creating a cation. The energies of these particles are far greater than the ionization energy of even a fluorine atom.

Because of this effect, radioactive rays are often called *ionizing radiation,* in contrast to visible light, which is incapable of ionizing most atoms or molecules. If the radiation from nuclear decay strikes a molecule in a vulnerable spot, a bond may be broken. If that bond happens to lie inside a gene of the chromosomal material in a cell, the cell may die or become changed (mutated) and possibly become cancerous. If a sperm or ovum (egg cell) is struck and later forms the nucleus of a new living organism, that animal may have a built-in genetic defect, as described in Chapter 28.

Alpha-particle emitters are less dangerous outside the body (where the skin will stop the rays) than if they are inhaled or eaten and can attack in-

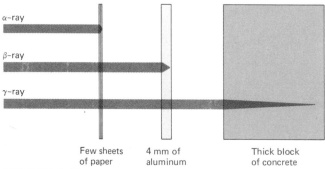

FIGURE 3–12 Penetration power of radioactive emissions.

ternal organs directly. If an alpha emitter is absorbed into the bloodstream, it will behave chemically in the same manner as a nonradioactive substance and do its damage in a particular part of the body.

For example, watch dials in the early years of this century were painted with a material that contained radium, so they would glow in the dark. The workers who applied the paint used their tongues and lips to put the fine points on their brushes needed to apply the very small spots of paint. A high proportion of those workers suffered bone cancer, leukemia, and other damage to the bone marrow. Why the bones? Radium is a Group 2 metal, like calcium. The Ra^{2+} ions are therefore carried to the bones as if they were Ca^{2+} ions and deposited there to do their damage by alpha-particle radiation.

When ionizing radiation strikes air, it ionizes some of the gas molecules, producing, for example, N_2^+ and O_2^+ ions. If the air is between two charged plates, an electric current may pass across the plates. In a common measuring device called a Geiger-Muller counter, there is a click each time a current passes across the gap. The counter thus "counts" how many times the gas has been ionized. The same principle in reverse operates the home smoke detector. If the ionization of air is disrupted by a smoke particle, the alarm goes off.

Radioisotopes in medicine

Table 3–5 lists some of the isotopes that are useful for diagnosis of illnesses (especially cancer) and for treatment of cancer. The diagnosis

TABLE 3–5   SOME MEDICALLY IMPORTANT RADIOISOTOPES

Element Isotope	Nuclear Symbol	Emissions	Half-life	Some Uses for Diagnosis and Treatment
Tritium	^3_1H	β	12 years	Measure water in body
Carbon-14	$^{14}_6C$	β	5730 years	Studies of metabolism
Sodium-24	$^{24}_{11}Na$	β, γ	15 hours	Blood studies; locate clots
Phosphorus-32	$^{32}_{15}P$	β	14 days	Treat bone and skin cancers; detect brain tumors; eye studies
Sulfur-35	$^{35}_{16}S$	β	88 days	Study protein metabolism
Calcium-47	$^{47}_{20}Ca$	β, γ	4.5 days	Study calcium in body
Chromium-51	$^{51}_{24}Cr$	γ	28 days	Study red blood cells
Iron-59	$^{59}_{26}Fe$	β, γ	45 days	Red blood cells, iron use
Cobalt-57	$^{57}_{27}Co$	γ	270 days	Vitamin B_{12} use in body
Cobalt-60	$^{60}_{27}Co$	β, γ	5.3 years	Treat cancer
Gallium-67	$^{67}_{31}Ga$	γ	78 hours	Detect hidden cancers
Arsenic-74	$^{74}_{33}As$	Varies	18 days	Locate brain tumors
Selenium-75	$^{75}_{34}Se$	β, γ	120 days	Pancreas scan
Strontium-90	$^{90}_{38}Sr$	β	28 years	Study bone formation
Technetium-99m	$^{99}_{43}Tc$	γ	6 hours	Scans of brain and many other organs
Iodine-131	$^{131}_{53}I$	β, γ	8.1 days	Thyroid diagnosis and cancer treatment; many other studies
Gold-198	$^{198}_{79}Au$	β, γ	2.7 days	Treat lung cancer and leukemia
Mercury-203	$^{203}_{80}Hg$	β, γ	47 days	Scan brain and kidney
Radium-226	$^{226}_{88}Ra$	α, γ	1600 years	Treat cancer

(Note: With some exceptions, these elements are used in the form of compounds [such as H_2O, NaCl, $CaCl_2$, NaI] that are readily taken in by the human body.)

method is to use the radioactive elements as *tracers*. Each kind of element will collect in a certain point of the body, and the amount of radiation given off can provide very useful information to the medical team. In 1970, about 8 million diagnoses were made in the United States on the basis of such data, using about 30 different isotopes. Recent developments have included computer analysis of radiation measurements in brain-scan and body-scan procedures.

Radioactive isotopes used as *tracers* are injected into the bloodstream and the progress of the molecules followed by detectors.

CAT scanning

For many years, x-rays have been used in medical diagnosis because they can show damage to bones and some internal organs. One disadvantage of x-ray photographs is the fact that they compress onto a two-dimensional picture what is actually present in the body in three dimensions. Much detail is thus lost.

The 1979 Nobel Prize in physiology or medicine was awarded to Allan M. Cormack, a medical physicist, and Godfrey N. Hounsfield, an electronics engineer, for the development of an x-ray scanning technique that uses a computer to provide three-dimensional information about the body. In a typical scanning system, called CAT for *computerized axial tomography*, a source of x-rays (along with a detector) is rotated completely around the body of the patient. The computer then provides "cross section" pictures of internal organs, pictures that are extremely useful in diagnosis.

For more information and good illustrations of the CAT method, see Gordon, R., Herman, G.T., and Johnson, S.A., "Image Reconstruction from Projections," *Scientific American* 233(4):cover, 56 (October 1975).

PET scanning

One disadvantage of CAT scans is their failure to show how the body responds to specific compounds. They can only show the relative densities of various tissues. By the time a disease shows up on a CAT scan, it may be well advanced.

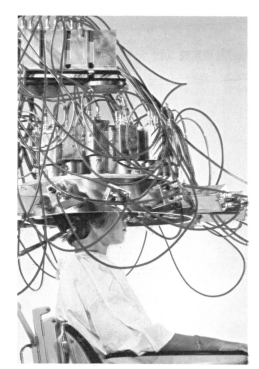

Radioisotopes injected into the body emit radiation that permits this instrument to locate brain tumors.

A newer technique combines computerized image reconstruction, as in CAT, with the techniques of radioactive tracer diagnosis. Certain novel radioisotopes are used which emit not alpha, beta, or gamma rays, but *positrons*, particles like electrons but with 1+ charges. Positrons are then converted by the body to gamma rays, which can be detected as in CAT.

As of 1980, PET (*positron-emission tomography*) was in use at 40 major medical centers throughout the world. It can detect exactly when, and to what extent, injected biochemical substances enter organs of the body. It has shown particular promise in detecting biochemical problems with the brain. There is, in fact, some early evidence that patients with such mental diseases as schizophrenia may show PET scans that are different from those of persons without such brain malfunctions.

See also Ter-Pogossian, M.M., Raichle, M.E., and Sobel, B.E., "Positron-Emission Tomography," *Scientific American* 243(4):170 (October 1980).

PET scans are also of great use in detecting the specific type of damage to the heart muscle in coronary artery disease. The PET scan can follow the progress of a biochemical process (metabolism), which gives it a wide range of uses.

Measurement of radiation

There are several different kinds of measuring units available to assess the amount of radiation emitted by a source or received by a patient. The simplest unit is the **curie** (symbol *Ci*), which is equal to 3.7×10^{10} nuclear disintegrations per second. That tells you very little about the health effect of radiation since it is the amount of radiation received in the tissues that counts. This will vary according to the distance of the body from the source and the type of radiation being emitted.

For our purposes, the most useful unit is the **rem,** which stands for *r*oentgen *e*quivalent *m*an. The rem tells you the biological effect of radiation, no matter what the source (including medical x-rays). If a group of test animals is given a 500-rem dose of radiation, it is estimated that about 50% of the group will die within 30 days.‡

---

‡ Living organisms do not all react in the same way to a given dose of radiation or poison. A "lethal" dose is often expressed as $LD_{50}/30$, a dose that will leave about 50% of the victims dead after 30 days.

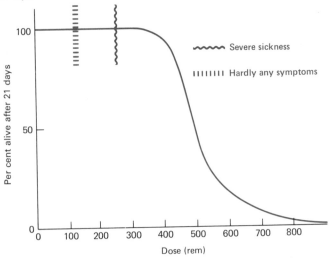

Effect of a radiation dose on health. This curve shows the approximate relationship between the amount of radiation received by an animal (in rem) through x-rays, gamma rays, or beta rays and the per cent of the exposed animals who survive at least three weeks. (From *American Scientist* 57:206, 1969. Copyright 1969 by Sigma Xi National Science Honorary.)

TABLE 3–6   EFFECT OF EXPOSURE TO A SINGLE
                     DOSE OF RADIATION

Dose (rems)	Probable Effect
0 to 25	No observable effect
25 to 50	Small decrease in white blood cell count
50 to 100	Lesions, marked decrease in white blood cells
100 to 200	Nausea, vomiting, loss of hair
200 to 500	Hemorrhaging, ulcers, possible death
500+	Fatal

Table 3–6 shows the probable effect on a normal person of exposure to a single dose of radiation. As a comparison, the background radiation provided by nature through cosmic rays, natural uranium and radon, and other isotopes ranges from 0.08 to 0.20 rem/year. A single chest x-ray is 0.20 rem; a series of x-rays in fluoroscopy of the gastrointestinal tract is about 22 rem. The present operation of nuclear power plants adds about 0.001 rem/year, and the home smoke detector level is so low that one would receive less than 0.0001 rem if you stood 1 m away from it continuously for a year.

However, no level of radiation is absolutely "safe." Even one ionization can cause a cell to become cancerous, just as one bit of soot from a fireplace might possibly be related to the appearance of lung cancer 25 years later. Airplanes, automobiles, and kitchen stoves have their level of danger also. The scientist's job is to minimize the dangers to the population from each of these benefits of modern technology while recognizing that it is impossible to be in a totally safe environment.

Half-lives of radioactive isotopes

Some samples of radioactive materials will decay almost completely within a few seconds. Others may take billions of years. One convenient way to measure the rate at which decay occurs is the **half-life,** the time required for one half of the atoms in a sample to disintegrate.

Each radioisotope has its own distinctive half-life, which is constant, no matter what the time, place, or other conditions, and is symbolized by $t_{1/2}$. Most of the uranium in rocks is $^{238}_{92}U$, with a half-life of 4.5 billion years. When it decays, it becomes $^{234}_{90}Th$, which turns within days to $^{234}_{91}Pa$, which in turn decays within minutes to $^{234}_{92}U$. Two more steps along is the $^{226}_{88}Ra$ isotope discovered by the Curies, followed by $^{222}_{86}Rn$, found to some extent in building materials. After a number of further decays, the end product is $^{206}_{82}Pb$, which is stable and not radioactive. Thus, much of the lead ($Z = 82$) now present on the earth was probably once uranium. The heat released in this decay series is believed by many scientists to have heated the earth's crust and perhaps made human life possible.

The half-life can be used as a measure of decay rate because the number of atoms decaying within a certain period of time is proportionate to the number present at the start. The result is shown as a graph in Figure 3–13.

Most of the carbon atoms in living matter are of the isotope $^{12}_{6}C$. However, carbon-14 ($^{14}_{6}C$) is produced when cosmic rays from outer space collide with air molecules. The carbon-14 becomes part of the carbon dioxide in the air and is absorbed by plants. In a living organism, there is one atom of $^{14}_{6}C$ (which is radioactive) for every trillion (10^{12}) atoms of $^{12}_{6}C$. Once the

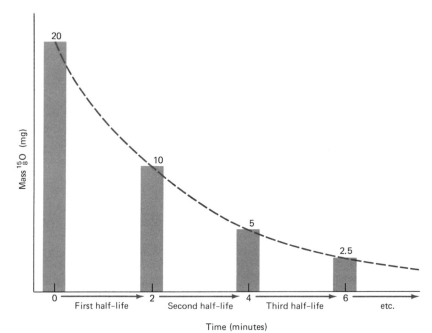

FIGURE 3–13 The decay of a given amount of a radioactive substance, such as 20 mg of the $^{15}_{8}O$ isotope. For each half-life, the amount present is reduced by one half.

organism dies, no more carbon-14 is taken in. The remaining amounts decay by beta emission with a half-life of 5730 years.

For a living plant, the carbon-14 contained in 1 gram of pure carbon will emit an average of 14 rays/minute. After 5720 years, the rate would be only 7 disintegrations/minute. After 11 000 years, about 3.5 decays/minute, and after 17 000 years about 1.8 decays/minute. By counting the decay rate from the carbon-14 contained in an object made from a plant or wood (such as the Dead Sea Scrolls), we can determine the age of the object. This procedure is called *radiochemical dating*.

Other naturally radioactive isotopes are contained in rocks and can be used by geologists to estimate the ages of the different rock layers.

Fission

Radioactive decay happens by itself. However, certain very heavy nuclei will break apart if struck by a high-energy particle, such as a neutron. If the nucleus that breaks apart can itself release more neutrons, we have the possibility of a *chain reaction* of the type used in the atomic bomb. If the chain reaction is very strictly controlled by spacing the fissionable material and by putting neutron "catchers" in the way, we can generate heat to produce steam in an electrical power plant.

When the large nucleus **fissions** and breaks into several smaller nuclei, it liberates energy. The total mass at the end is less than that at the beginning. Mass has been converted into energy, as predicted by Einstein (Section 2.5).

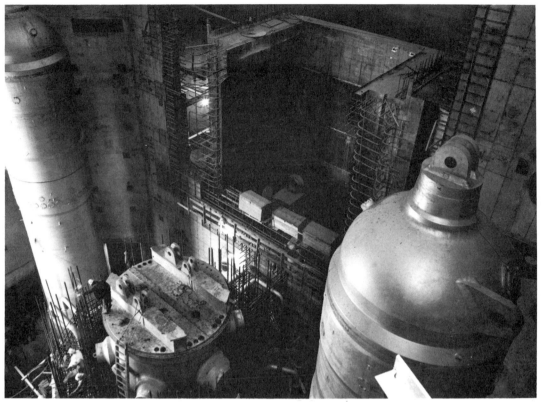

A nuclear reactor being installed between the two steam generators it will operate. The steam then produces electricity for consumers. (Courtesy of Duke Power Company.)

Fusion

In the sun, at a temperature of several million degrees, small nuclei can collide and form larger nuclei, again with a loss of energy. This **fusion** energy provides us with the heat and light that makes life possible on earth.

Several scientific teams are hoping to be able to duplicate this kind of reaction on earth. If they succeed, then within about 50 years it may be possible to replace much of our present reliance on fossil fuels and nuclear reactors with a process that uses deuterium, which is in unlimited supply in sea water. The process would be relatively free from pollution or radiation hazards. However, the high temperature required has been sustained for the required length of time in only one situation so far, inside a hydrogen bomb. We will know in a few decades if the technical problems can be overcome so our descendants may be assured of adequate energy supplies.

SELF-CHECK

3.20)   Of the three types of natural radiation, alpha, beta, and gamma rays,
a) which does *not* involve a particle with mass?
b) which shoots out atomic nuclei at high speeds?
c) which is very similar to x-rays?

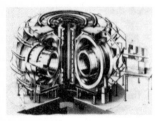

This "fusion machine" is designed to build up a very high gas temperature, using strong magnetic fields. No ordinary container can be used to hold gas heated to the temperatures required for fusion, of the order of 1 million degrees.

d)   which is like the cathode ray hitting the screen of a TV set?
e)   which can pass right through the human body?

3.21)   When a gamma ray passes through a human body cell, what happens that can cause cancer?

3.22)   Patients are sometimes asked to inhale air mixed with radioactive xenon-133 gas, to examine lung function. How can this provide useful information about the lungs?

3.23)   Radioactive gold-198, a beta emitter, is sometimes administered to treat widespread abdominal cancer. It has a half-life of 2.7 days.
a)   How can it kill cancer cells?
b*)   Would the gold be removed after treatment is complete?

3.24)   Astatine ($Z = 85$) is a radioactive element that is extremely poisonous in very small amounts. Looking at the periodic table, predict where the body would absorb astatine and state why it would be particularly dangerous.

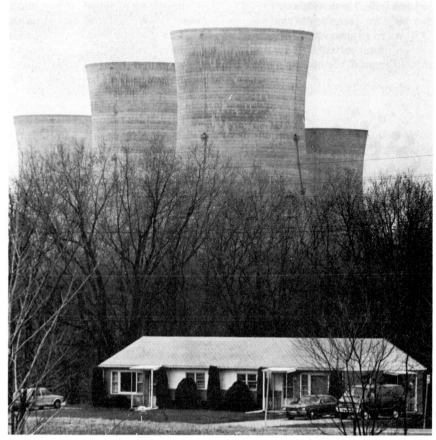

Living with nuclear energy. The cooling towers of the nuclear generating plant at Three Mile Island, near Middletown, Pennsylvania, loom over a home. A crisis at this plant was narrowly averted in March and April of 1979. (Photo by Laurie Usher.)

3.25)   A neighbor is complaining about his hair falling out and blames it on x-rays coming from his TV set. You find out that the maximum dosage he could be receiving from the set is 1.0 millirem/year. Could this be the cause of his hair problem? Consult Table 3–6.

3.26)   Copper acetate, $Cu(C_2H_3O_2)_2$, containing radioactive copper-64 is used to study Wilson's disease. The Cu-64 isotope has a half-life of 12.8 hours. If 1 millicurie is used at midnight,
a)   how many millicuries would be left at 12:48 the next afternoon?
b)   how many millicuries would be left 64 hours after administration?

3.27*)   At one stage in the crisis at the Three Mile Island nuclear power plant near Harrisburg, Pennsylvania, there was some fear that radioactive iodine might be emitted from the plant. Emergency supplies of potassium iodide (dissolved in water) were quickly prepared but were never used by the population. Why would taking KI orally provide some protection against injury from radioactive iodine in the air?

CHAPTER THREE IN REVIEW ■ Electrons and the Periodic Table

3.5 RADIOACTIVITY   Page 75

3K: Identify or describe the three main types of natural radiation, the alpha, beta, and gamma rays.

3L: Describe how emissions from radioactive substances can affect gases and living cells.

3M: Explain how radioisotopes may be used in medical diagnosis and cancer treatment.

3N: Predict from family resemblances in the periodic table how a particular radioisotope will affect the human body.

3O: Use Table 3–6 to estimate the probable health effect of a given radiation dose.

3P: Describe or illustrate what is meant by the half-life of a radioactive isotope.

GLOSSARY FOR CHAPTER THREE

alkali metal   An element in *Group 1* of the periodic table, such as sodium or potassium; has a ns^1 outer *electron configuration*, which permits a neutral atom to easily lose one electron to become a 1+ cation like Na^+. (p. 64)

alkaline earth metal   An element in *Group 2* of the periodic table, such as calcium or magnesium; has a ns^2 outer *electron configuration*, which permits a neutral atom to easily lose two electrons to become a 2+ cation like Ca^{2+}. (p. 64)

alpha (α) ray   A type of *radioactive* emission that consists of high-speed helium nuclei ($_2^4He^{2+}$); this type of radiation has low penetrating power. (p. 77)

atomic orbital   A mathematically described region of space outside the nucleus of an atom in which an electron with a particular energy may be found; may contain zero, one, or two electrons; may be of the type called "s," "p," "d," or "f" for the known elements; may be described by an electron cloud drawing. (p. 53)

beta (β) ray   A type of *radioactive* emission that consists of high-speed electrons (e^-); this type of radiation has medium penetrating power. (p. 77)

core, noble gas   An *electron configuration* ending in ns^2np^6, which is typical of the noble-gas family and which may be considered to make up a highly stable group of valence electrons; may thus be used (symbolized like "[Ar]") to shorten the work of writing a complete electron configuration. (p. 57)

curie (Ci)   A *radioactivity* unit, equal to an amount of material that will emit 3.7×10^{10} particles/second. (p. 80)

electron configuration   The arrangement of electrons in the atomic orbitals of an atom or ion, written showing each sublevel and its population of electrons; example: $1s^22s^22p^2$ for the neutral carbon atom with six electrons. (p. 55)

energy level   An energy that an electron in an atom is allowed to have; corresponds to one or more orbitals; energy levels are quantized (Chapter 2). (p. 53)

fission, nuclear   The breaking up of an atomic nucleus into smaller nuclei, accompanied by the liberation of very large amounts of energy; happens spontaneously (all by itself) or can be caused by absorption of a particle; found in atomic bombs and nuclear reactors. (p. 82)

fusion, nuclear   The combining of two very small atomic nuclei into one larger nucleus, accompanied by the liberation of very large amounts of energy; requires very high temperatures; found in the sun and stars and in hydrogen bombs; a possible energy source for humans if it can be controlled. (p. 83)

gamma (γ) ray A type of *radioactive* emission that consists of electromagnetic radiation like that in x-rays or visible light, but of extremely high penetrating power. (p. 77)

group The elements in a vertical (up-and-down) column of the periodic table, which have similar chemical properties because of similar valence level electron configurations; a chemical family such as the *alkali metals* or *halogens*. (p. 63)

half-life The time required for one half of a sample of *radioactive* material to decay; constant for each isotope; may vary from a small fraction of a second to more than 10^{17} years. (p. 81)

halogen An element in *Group 7* of the periodic table, such as fluorine or chlorine; forms $1-$ ions easily because of an ns^2np^5 electron configuration. (p. 65)

ionization energy The amount of energy required to pull off one electron from a neutral atom; a periodic property of the elements, low for *metals* and high for *nonmetals*. (p. 66)

Lewis electron-dot symbol The symbol of an element surrounded by a number of dots equal to the number of *valence electrons* in an atom or monatomic ion; will be used in later chapters to show bonding. (p. 63)

metal An element with a low *ionization energy;* tends to form monatomic cations; as the pure element, shows "metallic" properties such as luster and conductivity. (p. 65)

metalloid An element on the borderline between metals and nonmetals; may show some metallic properties. (p. 66)

monatomic ion A cation or anion formed from a single atom through loss or gain of electrons; for the *representative elements*, generally an ion with a noble-gas configuration. (p. 64)

noble gas An element in *Group 8* of the periodic table; rarely or never forms chemical compounds owing to a particularly stable electron configuration in the neutral atom. (p. 65)

nonmetal One of the elements in the upper right of the periodic table that does not show metallic properties; includes carbon, nitrogen, oxygen, sulfur, and the halogens; only nonmetals are likely to form monatomic anions. (p. 66)

oxidation state A number assigned to each element in a chemical formula by a set of rules; two different oxidation states of an element have distinctly different chemical properties, for example, Na (0 oxidation state) is a metal, Na^+ ($+1$ oxidation state) is found in various salts; also called oxidation number; may be shown in a compound or monatomic ion name by a Roman numeral in parentheses, for example, "iron(III)" means iron in its $+3$ oxidation state. (p. 67)

p atomic orbital An orbital in a p sublevel of the second or higher principal energy level; one of three orbitals with the same energy oriented at right angles to each other; directed somewhat along a line in space. (p. 56)

period A horizontal (left-to-right) row of the periodic table; along a period the representative elements are all "filling" the same valence level; for example, the third period consists of elements sodium ($Z = 11$) to argon ($Z = 18$). (p. 63)

periodicity The tendency of the chemical and physical properties of the elements to recur in cycles; for example, each eighth element among the first 20 has similar properties; the basis of the periodic table. (p. 66)

principal energy level One of the main groups of energy levels within an atom; ranked using a "quantum number" n; for $n = 2$ and above, divided into several (s, p, d . . .) sublevels with different energies; shown by the numbers in the electron configuration (e.g., the

"2" in 2s or 2p means $n = 2$); has the greatest effect on the electron energy; corresponds somewhat to the periods of the periodic table. (p. 56)

radioactivity The ability of an atom to transform itself (or be artificially changed) into an atom of a different isotope through changes in the number of protons and/or neutrons in the nucleus; most often involves emission of gamma rays as well as alpha or beta rays. (p. 76)

radioisotope An isotope that is radioactive; often used in medicine for diagnosis and/or cancer treatment. (p. 76)

rem A unit measuring the biological effect of a radiation dosage of any kind on the human body, taking into account the type of radiation involved. (p. 80)

representative element An element in one of the main groups (1 to 8) of the periodic table in which the *valence electrons* determine the chemical properties almost exclusively; any element other than a *transition metal*. (p. 63)

s atomic orbital The only orbital in the s sublevel of any principal energy level; has an electron cloud

shaped somewhat like a ball or sphere. (p. 53)

stable Difficult to change; a stable electron configuration is one that tends to resist addition or removal of electrons. (p. 59)

sublevel An energy level within a *principal energy level*, described by the letters s, p, d, f . . . , in which all of the electrons (of an isolated atom or monatomic ion) have the same energy; can hold two electrons (s), or six electrons (p), or ten electrons (d), etc. (p. 56)

transition metal One of the elements other than the *representative elements;* d or f atomic orbitals are involved in situating it in the periodic table; elements #21 to 30, 39 to 48, 57 to 80, and 89 to 112. (p. 63)

valence electron An electron in the outermost s or p sublevel of an atom or monatomic ion; the most easily lost or gained electron; tends to determine the bonding properties of an element; an electron in a *valence level*. (p. 63)

valence level The s and p *sublevels* of an atom or monatomic ion that are outermost and incompletely or completely filled; contains the *valence electrons;* fills with eight electrons (p. 63)

QUESTIONS AND PROBLEMS FOR CHAPTER THREE ■

Electrons and the Periodic Table

SECTION 3.1 ELECTRONS IN ATOMS

3.28) What is wrong with saying "The electron travels about the atomic nucleus just as a planet moves around the sun"?

3.29) How many electrons can be added to an atomic orbital that already contains one electron?

3.30*) Draw an atomic orbital filling diagram (with arrows ↑↓) for the neutral aluminum atom ($Z = 13$).

3.61) How do we describe the position of an electron in a 1s atomic orbital?

3.62) How many electrons can be added to a 4s orbital that is empty?

3.63*) Draw an atomic orbital filling diagram (with arrows ↑↓) for the neutral potassium atom ($Z = 19$).

For the following electron configurations, we will consider only situations in which the electrons all occupy the *lowest* available energy levels (the *ground state*).

3.31) Write complete electron configurations for the following neutral atoms:
a) lithium ($Z = 3$)
b) silicon ($Z = 14$)
c) fluorine ($Z = 9$)

3.32) Using an *argon* core, write electron configurations for
a) potassium ($Z = 19$)
b) calcium ($Z = 20$)
c*) arsenic ($Z = 33$)

3.33*) What is *wrong* with each of the following electron configurations?
a) $_2$He: $1s^2 2s^1$
b) $_{19}$K: $1s^2 2s^2 2p^6 3s^2 3p^7$
c) $_{10}$Ne: $1s^2 2s^2 2s^2 2p^4$

3.64) Write complete electron configurations for the following neutral atoms:
a) beryllium ($Z = 4$)
b) sulfur ($Z = 16$)
c) neon ($Z = 10$)

3.65) Using a *neon* core, write electron configurations for
a) chlorine ($Z = 17$)
b) sodium ($Z = 11$)
c) argon ($Z = 18$)

3.66*) What is *wrong* with each of the following electron configurations?
a) $_3$Li: $1s^3$
b) $_7$C: $1s^2 2s^2 2p^3$
c) $_{13}$Al: $1s^2 2s^2 2p^6 2d^3$

SECTION 3.2 FAMILIES OF ELEMENTS

3.34) Which group of the periodic table
a) has outer electron configuration $ns^2 np^1$?
b) forms 2+ ions easily?
c) forms 1− ions easily?

3.67) Which group of the periodic table
a) has outer electron configuration $ns^2 np^3$?
b) forms 2− ions easily?
c) forms 1+ ions easily?

Use the imaginary periodic table shown in Figure 3–14 to answer Questions 3.35 and 3.68. Answer with the letters (A, G, X, Z, etc.) on that table.

3.35) Give the letters for those elements that are
a) halogens
b) alkali metals
c) in Period 4 of the table
d) *not* representative elements

3.68) Give the letters for those elements that are
a) alkaline earth metals
b) noble gases
c) in Period 3 of the table
d) likely to form 1+ ions

You may use the periodic table inside the front cover to answer the remaining questions of this chapter.

3.36) Predict the charge on the monatomic ion formed by
a) magnesium
b) sulfur
c) iodine

3.37) Name each of the following ions:
a) Na^+
b) O^{2-}
c) Te^{2-}

3.69) Predict the charge on the monatomic ion formed by
a) lithium
b) radium
c) nitrogen

3.70) Name each of the following ions:
a) K^+
b) Se^{2-}
c) Ca^{2+}

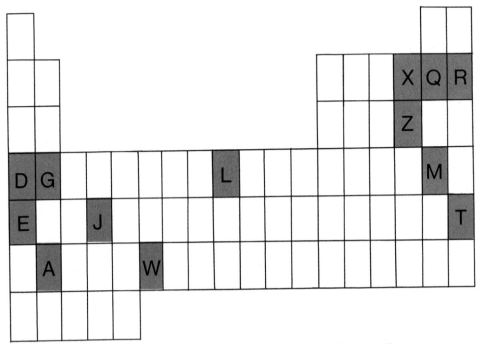

FIGURE 3–14   Periodic chart for Questions 3.35 and 3.68.

3.38) Write the Lewis electron-dot symbol for
a)   a carbon atom
b)   a potassium atom
c)   a Br^- ion
d)   a Ca^{2+} ion

3.39*) Why is carbon *not* likely to form 4+ cations?

SECTION 3.3 SOME IMPORTANT METALS

3.40) If you know an element is a *metal,* what can you predict about
a)   the *sign* of the charges on its monatomic ions?
b)   the relative position of that element in the periodic table?
c)   the relative ionization energy of that element?
d)   the *sign* of the most common oxidation state of that element

3.41*) Which Group 1 cation is found mostly *inside* body cells?

3.71) Write the Lewis electron-dot symbol for
a)   an aluminum atom
b)   a fluorine atom
c)   a Na^+ ion
d)   a O^{2-} ion

3.72*) Why is aluminum *not* likely to form 5 − anions?

3.73) If you know an element is a *nonmetal,* what can you predict about
a)   the *sign* of the charges on its monatomic ions?
b)   the relative position of that element in the periodic table?
c)   the relative ionization energy of that element?
d)   the sign of the most common oxidation state of that element?

3.74*) Which Group 1 cation is found mostly in the fluids *outside* the cells?

3.42*) Which Group 2 cation is found in plant chlorophyll?

3.43) Which of the following elements is a transition metal?
a) Ca
b) Co
c) Cl
d) C
e) Mg

3.44*) Which transition metal is found in muscles and red blood cells?

3.45) Write the oxidation state of each of the following elements in the form shown.
a) Al^{3+}
b) O_2
c) I^-

3.75*) Which Group 2 cation is found in large amounts in bone and teeth?

3.76) Which of the following elements is a transition metal?
a) Al
b) N
c) Na
d) Ni
e) Ne

3.77*) Which transition metal is found in vitamin B_{12}?

3.78) Write the oxidation state of each of the following elements in the form shown.
a) Fe^{2+}
b) S^{2-}
c) Cl_2

SECTION 3.4 SOME IMPORTANT NONMETALS

3.46*) Which Group 4 element is found in almost every compound of the human body?

3.47*) Can nitrogen from the air be used by the human body for compound formation?

3.48) Which of the following elements is essential to the human body but can be poisonous if taken directly?
a) oxygen
b) chlorine
c) nitrogen

3.49*) What is probably the main role of fluorine in the body?

3.79*) Which Group 4 element often causes poisoning in children?

3.80*) Is phosphorus found in its elemental form in the human body? If not, in what form is it found?

3.81) Which of the following elements is essential to the human body but can be poisonous if taken directly?
a) hydrogen
b) iodine
c) sulfur

3.82*) What is the main role of iodine in the body?

SECTION 3.5 RADIOACTIVITY

3.50) For an alpha particle,
a) is the mass comparatively high or low?
b) what is the charge?
c) is the particle more dangerous inside or outside the body? why?

3.51) How can radiation kill a living cell?

3.83) For a beta particle,
a) is the mass comparatively high or low?
b) what is the charge?
c) compare its penetrating power to that of an alpha particle.

3.84) What effect does radiation have on air?

Use Table 3–5 as necessary to answer the remaining questions of this chapter.

3.52) Phosphate ion, PO_4^{3-}, entering the body tends to be absorbed by the bones. Radioactive P-32 is used to treat chronic leukemia, since the cancer is related to bone tissue. What particles are emitted by the phosphate ions containing P-32?

3.85) Radium-226 was once commonly used to treat cancers, although it has now been largely replaced by Co-60 and other sources. What particles are emitted by Ra-226?

3.53*) Radioactive iodine-131 may be used both to detect *and* to treat cancers of the thyroid gland. Explain how one isotope can serve *both* functions. It is administered in the form of sodium iodide, NaI.

3.54) Radioactive sodium-24 in the form of sodium chloride, NaCl, may be used to see how sodium is used by the body. Explain.

3.55) Doctors may use radioactive chromium-51, which sticks to red blood cells, to find the exact position of the placenta in a pregnant woman. How might this work? What emissions would be detected?

3.56) In radioactive fallout from atomic bomb tests or in possible leakage from nuclear power plants, the three most dangerous radioisotopes that may be detected are strontium-90 (Z = 38), cesium-137 (Z = 55), and iodine-131 (Z = 53). In *which part of the body* is each of these isotopes likely to do its damage and possibly cause cancer? Use periodic properties if useful.

3.57) What is the probable health effect of the x-rays used in a "GI series" to look at the esophagus, stomach, and intestines. The total exposure is about 22 rem. You may use Table 3–6.

3.58) A hospital has a cobalt-60 source for cancer therapy that is rated at 16.0 curies on a particular day. Approximately how much will be left of the original cobalt after 5.3 years? after 10.6 years? Use Table 3–5.

3.59*) Which is a better measurement unit for estimating how many alpha particles are being emitted by a radium implant to treat cancer, *curies* or *rem?* Explain.

3.86*) Phosphorus-32 may be used both to detect skin cancer (since it is absorbed more by cancerous cells than by normal cells) and to treat skin cancer. Explain.

3.87) Radioactive iron-59 may be used in the form of its sulfate, $FeSO_4$, to see how iron is used in the body. Explain.

3.88) One of the functions of the liver is to remove foreign matter from the blood stream. If a dye containing I-131 is injected into the body, it travels to the liver and can be used to assess possible liver damage. Explain.

3.89) Since long before mankind discovered atomic energy, animal life has been subjected to radiation from natural radioactive isotopes such as potassium-40 (Z = 19), radon-222 (a noble gas, Z = 86), and radium-226 (Z = 88). In *which part of the body* is each of these radioisotopes likely to do its damage and possibly cause cancer? Use periodic properties if useful.

3.90) If an industrial worker were found to have been exposed to about 150 rem in the course of a year, what kinds of health effects might be seen? Would this exposure be likely to kill the worker? Could cancer result? You may use Table 3–6.

3.91) A 10-millicurie sample of technetium-99m is injected into a patient's vein as sodium pertechnate, $NaTcO_4$, at 10:00 AM, so a brain scan can be performed to look for a possible brain tumor. How much activity will be left at 4:00 PM? at 10:00 PM? at 10:00 AM the following day?

3.92*) Which is a better measurement unit for the radiation to which a hospital nucleography technician has been exposed, *curies* or *rem?* Explain.

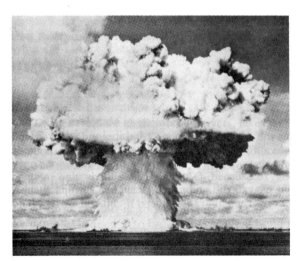 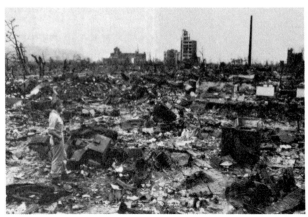

The perils of uncontrolled nuclear energy: (*left*) a hydrogen bomb explosion; (*right*) Hiroshima, Japan, on August 6, 1945. (Courtesy of Compix, United Press International.)

3.60*) Suppose you were to be exposed externally to one of two radiation sources as described below, for a period of one hour. *Which* would be *less likely* to cause serious health damage? Assume all factors are identical except for those mentioned. Explain your answer.

a) a beta source or an alpha source? (equal *curies* at equal distance)

b) an uncovered source or one with a layer of lead between it and you?

c) cobalt-57 or cobalt-60 (equal number of *atoms* of each; assume the only difference is in half-life).

3.93*) Some books say that strontium-90 is particularly dangerous because it has a relatively long half-life (28.1 years) and thus may be stored in a person's bones throughout a whole life.

a) Suppose an equal number of atoms of phosphorus-32 and strontium-90 go into the same bone tissue. Which will cause the most damage after 1 year? After 30 years?

b) Suppose an equal number of *curies* of radium-226 and strontium-90 go into the same bone tissue. Again compare the effect after 1 year and after 30 years.

What do you conclude about statements such as the one at the start of this problem?

4 Chemical Formulas

Chapter 3 was concerned with the chemical elements and some of their properties. In this chapter, we will discuss how compounds are formed from chemical elements. The compounds are represented by chemical *formulas*. If the symbols of the chemical elements are the "letters" of the alphabet, then the chemical formulas are the "words" chemists use to express what is happening in nature.

There are two major ways in which atoms of chemical elements can combine to form molecules or formula units of compounds. Atoms may first form ions, the charged particles we discussed in Chapter 3, and then form compounds through the attraction of a positively charged metal ion, such as Na^+, to a negatively charged nonmetal ion such as Cl^-. We call such attractions *ionic bonds,* and they will be discussed in Sections 4.1 and 4.2.

A more common way for atoms to combine is by the sharing of electrons between atoms. Such *covalent bonds* will be discussed in Sections 4.3 and 4.4. They are typical of almost all organic molecules, as well as many inorganic substances.

The molecules of life—those we will be discussing in the chapters on metabolism—involve *both* ionic and covalent bonding. The long carbon chains in proteins, for example, are held together by covalent bonds, but the three-dimensional structure of proteins involves ionic bonding, as will be discussed in Chapter 19. It is thus important in understanding the chemistry of life to become familiar with both types of bonds: ionic and covalent.

The formula of a chemical compound provides useful information about the mass of a molecule or formula unit (discussed in Section 4.5).

4.1 FORMATION OF IONIC SALTS

LEARNING GOAL 4A: *Explain why an ionic bond forms between a cation and an anion.*

4B: *Given the formulas of a cation and an anion, predict the formula of the ionic compound that can be formed by combining the two ions.*

Chapter 3 gave us a series of monatomic cations (of metallic elements) and anions (of nonmetals), all of which have very stable noble-gas electron configurations. We know from Section 2.4 that cations, carrying positive charge, and anions, with a net negative charge, attract each other. The strong attraction between a cation and an anion is called an **ionic bond.**

Nature works in such a way that electrical neutrality is preserved, that is, the number of positive charges in any region of space becomes equal to the number of negative charges. When cations and anions come together, they form compounds that are electrically neutral. Therefore, the number of positive charges must be equal to the number of negative charges. The compound formed when cations and anions come together is generally called an **ionic salt.**

You should be able to combine the proper number of cations and anions to make the formula of the salt electrically neutral.

EXAMPLE 4a: Write the formula of the ionic salt formed by combining the Na^+ cation and the Cl^- anion to make ordinary table salt.

- -

SOLUTION: Since each ion has a single charge, the compound has equal numbers of Na^+ and Cl^- ions in each region of space. The formula for this ionic salt is $\boxed{NaCl}$.

Note that when we write the *formula* of the compound, we do not indicate the charges. If we were to draw a picture of the NaCl formula unit, we would perhaps write, using Lewis electron-dot symbols for the two ions:

$$Na^{\oplus} \overset{\ominus}{:}\overset{..}{Cl}:$$

EXAMPLE 4b: Write the formulas of the ionic salts formed by combining the Ca^{2+} cation with i) the S^{2-} anion and ii) the Cl^- anion.

- -

SOLUTION: i) Each ion has a double charge. Neutrality is preserved if there are equal numbers of Ca^{2+} and S^{2-} ions in each region. The formula of the ionic salt is $\boxed{CaS}$.

ii) The charges on the ions are 2+ for Ca^{2+} and 1− for Cl^-. Neutrality thus requires twice as many chloride ions in each region of space as Ca^{2+} cations. Or, we can calculate the requirement to make the charge on the formula go to zero: $(2\ Cl^- \times -1) + (1\ Ca^{2+} \times +2) = 0$. The formula is thus $\boxed{CaCl_2}$.

Remember that Ca^{2+} and S^{2-} have equal charges, so they go together one-to-one as CaS. The one Ca^{2+} and two Cl^- go to make the ionic salt $CaCl_2$, not $Ca^{2+}2Cl^-$ or $Ca^{2+}Cl_2^{2-}$ or Ca2Cl.

EXAMPLE 4c: Write the formula of the ionic salt formed by combining the monatomic aluminum $(Z = 13)$ ion with the sulfate anion, SO_4^{2-}.

- -

SOLUTION: First we must find the cation. Aluminum is in Group 3 and loses three electrons to reach the neon electron configuration. The cation is Al^{3+}. The anion is polyatomic (many atoms) in this case, but the principles are exactly the same; it is a 2− anion. We must combine a 3+ cation and a 2− anion in such a way that the compound will be electrically neutral. There are various ways to "juggle" the charges, but the simplest is to multiply $3 \times 2 = 6$ and try to get six charges of each kind. That will require *two* Al^{3+} cations and *three* SO_4^{2-} anions. The formula of this ionic salt is thus $\boxed{Al_2(SO_4)_3}$.

This seems to be a complicated formula, but the procedure for reaching it is exactly the same as for Examples 4a and 4b. Remember to put the parentheses around the *entire* sulfate group.

Properties of ionic salts

You will find that ionic compounds have certain things in common. With rare exceptions, they are solids at room temperature, forming very orderly crystals (Chapter 11). When dropped into water, most (but not all) of these crystals dissolve, in the way that table salt (NaCl) dissolves in soup (Chapter 12 on solutions). The water solution formed when an ionic salt dissolves is a good conductor of electricity (a fact that finds many applications in the health sciences, including the technique for taking electrocardiograms), and so a dissolved salt will actually be found in the form of its ions, surrounded by water molecules, as discussed in Section 14.4.

SELF-CHECK

4.1) Explain why a Mg^{2+} cation and a O^{2-} anion will attract each other to form an ionic bond.

4.2) Write the chemical formula for the ionic salt produced by combining each of the following cation-anion pairs:

(A common use of each compound is mentioned.)
a) K^+ and I^- (used to treat asthma)
b) Sn^{2+} and F^- (the stannous fluoride used in some toothpastes)
c) Ca^{2+} and SO_4^{2-} (plaster casts for bone fractures)
d) NH_4^+ and CO_3^{2-} (an expectorant to treat coughs; the ammonium ion, NH_4^+, is the only important *positive* polyatomic ion)
e) Fe^{3+} and PO_4^{3-} (an iron supplement found in enriched bread)
f) Zr^{4+} and O^{2-} (an ointment used to treat poison ivy)
g) Zn^{2+} and P^{3-} (a rat poison)

4.2 NAMES AND FORMULAS OF IONIC COMPOUNDS

LEARNING GOAL 4C: Given the name of any cation in Table 4–1 or anion in Table 4–2, write its formula; given the formula, write the name of the ion.
4D: Given the names of a cation and an anion, write the name and formula of an ionic salt that can be produced by those ions.

(NOTE: Your instructor may supply you with lists of cations and anions to supplement or replace those in Tables 4-1 and 4-2.)

You now know how to combine cations and anions in such a way that the charges balance so that the formula unit for the ionic salt that results has a net charge of zero. Section 4.2 will give you a vocabulary for writing the formulas of those inorganic compounds that are formed through ionic bonding between cations and anions.

You have seen from Question 4.2 of the self-check of Section 4.1 that ionic salts may be used in medicine, food additives, garden supplies, and other preparations. For example, one type of whole wheat cracker contains sodium chloride, ammonium bicarbonate, sodium bicarbonate, and calcium acid phosphate. By the time you complete this section, you should be able to write the chemical formula for each of those compounds.

Cations

You learned about many monatomic cations in Chapter 3. There is no need to repeat all of those shown in Table 3–4 (p. 64). Remember that such an atom may form a monatomic cation by gaining or losing enough electrons to attain the electron configuration of a noble gas. Table 4–1 lists only those cations that you will frequently run across, along with some transition metal cations that cannot be predicted simply by knowledge of the representative groups of the periodic table.

The name of a cation is generally the name of the element followed by the word "ion." If there are two or more different cations formed by the same element (as for iron, which forms both Fe^{2+} and Fe^{3+} cations), the "official" systematic name is given and the common name follows in parentheses. The ammonium ion, NH_4^+, behaves much like a Group 1 element cation, such as Na^+ or K^+.

Anions

Table 3–4 contains a number of monatomic negative ions (anions) with 3-, 2-, and 1- charges. We have used several many-atom (polyatomic) anions in earlier examples. In ions such as sulfate, SO_4^{2-}, nitrate, NO_3^-, phosphate, PO_4^{3-}, or carbonate, CO_3^{2-}, the negative charge is spread out over a group of atoms.

Table 4–2 includes some of the most important anions. There are many more. Each organic acid described in Chapters 9 and 13 forms *carboxylate* anions, and there are thousands of organic acids. We have included only three of them in Table 4–2: the acetate ion (from the acetic acid found in vinegar), the benzoate ion (often used as a food preservative), and the stearate ion (often found in soap).

As with cations, there are systematic names for the anions as well as common names shown in color. You should notice that hydrogen can join with one anion, such as SO_4^{2-}, to make a different anion (in this case, HSO_4^-). The added hydrogen acts somewhat as though it were a H^+ ion (a proton), although in reality the H^+ is always bonded to some larger molecule, such as water. Compounds containing an H^+ that can be transferred to water are called *acids* (Chapter 13). The anions containing hydrogen are thus often called "acid anions."

On bottle labels and in textbooks, the extremely important anion HCO_3^- (found in the bloodstream) may be called "bicarbonate ion," "hydrogen carbonate ion," or "acid carbonate ion." The HPO_4^{2-} and $H_2PO_4^-$ ions play important roles inside living cells.

Most anions without oxygen have names ending in *-ide*. The many anions that contain oxygen usually have names ending in *-ate* or *-ite*.

TABLE 4–1 SOME IMPORTANT CATIONS

Symbol	Name
Na^+	Sodium ion
K^+	Potassium ion
Cu^+	Copper(I) ion (cuprous)
Ag^+	Silver ion
NH_4^+	Ammonium ion
Mg^{2+}	Magnesium ion
Ca^{2+}	Calcium ion
Ba^{2+}	Barium ion
Mn^{2+}	Manganese(II) ion
Fe^{2+}	Iron(II) ion (ferrous)
Cu^{2+}	Copper(II) ion (cupric)
Zn^{2+}	Zinc ion
Al^{3+}	Aluminum ion
Fe^{3+}	Iron(III) ion (ferric)

TABLE 4–2 SOME IMPORTANT ANIONS

Symbol	Name
F^-	Fluoride
Cl^-	Chloride
Br^-	Bromide
I^-	Iodide
NO_3^-	Nitrate
OH^-	Hydroxide
CN^-	Cyanide
ClO^-	Hypochlorite
MnO_4^-	Permanganate
CH_3COO^- or $C_2H_3O_2^-$	Acetate
$C_6H_5COO^-$	Benzoate
$C_{17}H_{35}COO^-$	Stearate
HCO_3^-	Hydrogen carbonate (bicarbonate)
HSO_4^-	Hydrogen sulfate (bisulfate)
$H_2PO_4^-$	Dihydrogen phosphate (biphosphate)
O^{2-}	Oxide
S^{2-}	Sulfide
$C_2O_4^{2-}$	Oxalate
SO_4^{2-}	Sulfate
CO_3^{2-}	Carbonate
$Cr_2O_7^{2-}$	Dichromate
HPO_4^{2-}	Monohydrogen phosphate
PO_4^{3-}	Phosphate

SELF-CHECK

4.3) Name each of the following ions according to the official or systematic names provided in Tables 4–1 and 4–2.

a) K^+

b) OH^-

c) NH_4^+

d) CO_3^{2-}

e) Fe^{3+}

f) $H_2PO_4^-$

g) Zn^{2+}

h) $C_2O_4^{2-}$

i) Mn^{2+}

j) S^{2-}

4.4) Write the formula of each of the following ions.
a) silver ion
b) copper(II)
c) bromide
d) phosphate
e) manganese(II)
f) magnesium ion
g) aluminum ion
h) cyanide
i) hydrogen sulfate ion
j) acetate

4.5*) Write the formula of each of the following useful ions (common names are given).
a) bicarbonate
b) ferric
c) cuprous

4.6) Using the methods shown in Section 4.1, write the name and formula of the compound formed by combining the ions named.
a) iron(II) and sulfate (treats iron-deficiency anemia)
b) aluminum and hydroxide (a common antacid tablet)
c) potassium and oxalate (permits the storage of whole blood)
d) magnesium and benzoate (has been used to treat rheumatism)
e) zinc and chloride (a common antiseptic)
f) zinc and phosphate (used in dental cements)
g) mercury (II) and chloride (surgical hand wash)
h) sodium and hydrogen carbonate (baking soda)
i) ammonium and nitrate (to acidify the urine; Chapter 24)

4.3 INTRODUCTION TO COVALENT BONDS

LEARNING GOAL 4E: Explain how a covalent bond may be formed between two neutral atoms.

4F: Given several elements, write the Lewis electron-dot symbol for a neutral atom of each element and predict the formula of a simple covalent compound that can be formed by combining those elements.

In the examples of Section 4.1, we considered an ionic bond to be formed by combining a positively charged cation with a negatively charged anion.

There is another way of looking at an ionic bond, such as that formed by the attraction between Na^+ and Cl^- in table salt. We know from Figure 3–9 (p. 66) that the sodium atom has a very low ionization energy—it easily loses one electron. The chlorine atom, with a $3s^2\ 3p^5$ electron configuration, readily accepts an electron to achieve the electron configuration of a noble gas; chlorine will receive the electron lost by sodium in order to become a Cl^- ion. We can thus look upon the formation of NaCl as involving an exchange of electrons from Na atoms to Cl atoms.

Electron sharing

We cannot use this same explanation for the poisonous gas that is chlorine in its natural state which consists of Cl_2 molecules. A chlorine molecule cannot consist of a Cl^+ cation attracting a Cl^- anion. The ionization energy of Cl atoms is too high to permit the formation of Cl^+ ions in any large amounts. Each chlorine atom is, in fact, in search of one electron to change

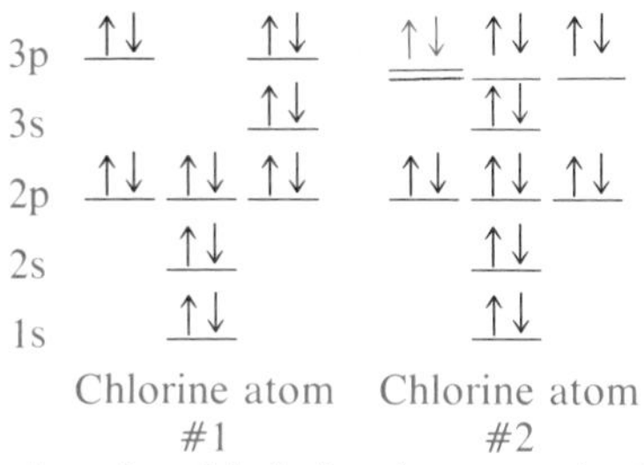

3p ↑↓   ↑↓   ↑↓ ↑↓ ↑↓   ↑↓ ↑↓ ↑↓

3s   ↑↓   ↑↓

2p ↑↓ ↑↓ ↑↓   ↑↓ ↑↓ ↑↓

2s   ↑↓   ↑↓

1s   ↑↓   ↑↓

Chlorine atom   Chlorine atom
      #1   #2

FIGURE 4–1   Atomic orbitals for the atoms in the Cl_2 molecule.

its valence level electron configuration from $3s^2\ 3p^5$ to the much more stable $3s^2\ 3p^6$.

If the chlorine atoms are quite close together, then it is possible to imagine a situation in which two electrons can team up to fill the needs of *both* chlorine atoms. Remember from Table 3–3 (p. 64) that the Lewis electron-dot symbol for the chlorine atom is

$$\overset{\cdot\cdot}{\underset{\cdot\cdot}{:Cl}}\cdot$$

If we now write the two chlorine atom symbols together, we obtain

$$\overset{\cdot\cdot}{\underset{\cdot\cdot}{:Cl}}\cdot + \cdot\overset{\cdot\cdot}{\underset{\cdot\cdot}{Cl}}: \longrightarrow \overset{\cdot\cdot}{\underset{\cdot\cdot}{:Cl}}:\overset{\cdot\cdot}{\underset{\cdot\cdot}{Cl}}:$$

Each dot represents an electron in the valence level. The electron pair right *between* the chlorine atoms, shown in color, makes a **covalent bond.** Each chlorine atom has an octet, eight electrons around it (count them!), because two of the electrons are *shared* by the atoms.

We can draw orbital diagrams for the two chlorine atoms as shown in Figure 4–1. As the two atoms move close together, it is possible for two electrons to fill the 3p sublevel of chlorine atom #1 and at the same time fill the 3p sublevel of chlorine atom #2. A total of 14 valence electrons can thus make both atoms more stable.

Covalent bonding is electron sharing in such a way that each atom gains a more stable electron configuration.

This approach, called the *valence bond* theory, allows us to predict with very good accuracy whether two atoms will form bonds with each other. Once the Cl—Cl bond is formed, the electrons in the covalent bond are held relatively tightly, so the molecule Cl_2 has the electron cloud shown in Figure 4–2.

The pair of dots shown in color indicates two electrons that are shared by the atoms on either side to form a covalent bond. The other electrons shown around the chlorine atoms may be considered to remain in their original atomic orbitals as in Table 3–4.

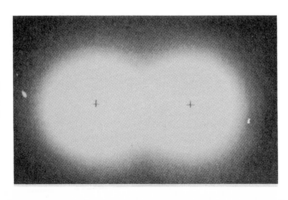

FIGURE 4–2   The electron cloud of the Cl_2 molecule. Note that both sides have equal electron charge.

Let us consider some more examples. Each of two neutral hydrogen atoms has a $1s^1$ electron configuration. Each would be more stable with a $1s^2$ configuration. We can therefore form a covalent bond between two hydrogen atoms by having them share both electrons:

$$H \cdot + \cdot H \longrightarrow H : H$$

The electron cloud of the H_2 molecule has the same general shape as that shown in Figure 4–2, although it is much smaller.

If we combine hydrogen gas and chlorine gas, we find that a covalent bond can be formed between hydrogen and chlorine. We can again write the covalent bond:

$$H : \overset{\cdot\cdot}{\underset{\cdot\cdot}{C}l} :$$

In this case, hydrogen fills its 1s orbital at the same time as chlorine fills its 3p energy level. The electron cloud for this molecule, hydrogen chloride, is shown in Figure 4–3. This cloud is shifted towards the chlorine atom, as will be discussed in Section 6.4. The result is a *polar* covalent bond.

Covalence numbers

The covalence number is the number of unpaired valence electrons in the neutral atom. It is therefore also the number of extra electrons needed to achieve a noble-gas electron configuration. This same number then tends to indicate how many covalent bonds will be formed by an atom through providing one electron to each bond.

Hydrogen with a $1s^1$ electron configuration can gain one electron through covalent bonding to achieve the helium ($1s^2$) stable situation. The halogens, with s^2p^5 electron configurations, need one more electron for each atom to reach the noble-gas s^2p^6 configuration.

A convenient method for writing the formulas of covalently bonded molecules, which works most of the time, is to recall *how many* electrons are needed to complete the valence level of an atom of each element. For example, hydrogen needs one electron to convert $1s^1$ to the stable $1s^2$. We say that hydrogen has a **covalence number** of one. The H atom tends to form only *one* bond.

Chlorine needs only one electron to convert $3s^23p^5$ to the stable $3s^23p^6$. Chlorine also has a covalence number of *one* and generally forms only one bond per atom. An element with a covalence number of one will fill its valence level when it shares two electrons, as we have seen in the examples of Cl_2, H_2, and HCl. It resists forming additional bonds.

We know from this discussion that elements with a covalence number of *one* will form diatomic (two-atom) molecules. Since hydrogen and the halogens each need one electron per atom to arrive at a noble-gas electron configuration, we would expect these 15 stable molecules to form: H_2, F_2, Cl_2, Br_2, I_2, HF, HCl, HBr, HI, ClF, BrF, IF, BrCl, ICl, and BrI.

An element in Group 6 of the periodic table, such as oxygen or sulfur, has an electron configuration of the form ns^2np^4. Each such atom needs *two*

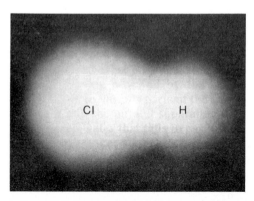

FIGURE 4–3 The electron cloud of the HCl molecule. The chlorine side has a larger electron cloud, as will be discussed in Section 6.4.

electrons to complete its valence level and arrive at ns^2np^6. These elements thus have covalence numbers of *two*. Oxygen generally forms *two* bonds when it joins with other elements to make covalent molecules.

For example, in water, we can write

$$H \cdot + \cdot \overset{\cdot\cdot}{\underset{\cdot\cdot}{O}} \cdot + \cdot H \longrightarrow H : \overset{\cdot\cdot}{\underset{\cdot\cdot}{O}} : H$$

There are two hydrogen atoms for each oxygen atom. It should be no surprise to learn that the following molecules can also be found: H_2S, F_2O, Cl_2O, and Br_2O.

Lewis electron-dot diagrams

A **Lewis diagram** shows the bonding between the atoms in a molecule. It is made from the Lewis symbols for the elements (as in Table 3–3) with the electron dots arranged to show which electrons are shared to form covalent bonds. The diagrams we have drawn for Cl_2, H_2, HCl, and H_2O are all Lewis electron-dot diagrams.

While Lewis diagrams generally do *not* show the real directions of the bonds in space, they are very useful for deciding which atoms go where, especially if we consider the covalence numbers of the elements.

We know, in fact, that water, with the formula H_2O, *cannot* have the arrangement

$$H : H : \overset{\cdot\cdot}{O} :$$

because of covalence numbers. Hydrogen only forms one bond, and oxygen generally forms two bonds. The above diagram gives the central hydrogen four electrons, but there is only room for two in its 1s orbital. It also gives oxygen only six electrons, but it needs eight to complete its valence level.

Nitrogen and carbon

A Group 5 element, such as nitrogen or phosphorus, needs three electrons to complete its valence level. The covalence number for N and for P is thus *three*.

This leads us to the formula for the very important compound, for both the human body and the chemical industry, *ammonia*, NH_3:

$$H : \overset{\cdot\cdot}{\underset{\cdot\cdot}{N}} : H$$
$$\overset{\cdot\cdot}{H}$$

Other stable compounds that agree with what we have said about covalence numbers include NF_3, NCl_3, NI_3, PH_3, PF_3, PCl_3, PBr_3, and PI_3.

It is very hard for an atom to gain three electrons to form a 3- ion. The nitride ion, N^{3-}, and the phosphide ion, P^{3-}, are quite rare. Instead, these elements tend to form covalent compounds, sharing electrons to reach the stable noble-gas configuration.

Carbon, in Group 4, cannot form a 4+ ion. Instead, it almost always shares four electrons to reach a noble-gas configuration. The Group 4 elements thus can have a covalence number of *four*, and when they form covalent molecules (as the nonmetals carbon and silicon do), they form *four* bonds.

TABLE 4–3 COVALENCE
NUMBERS OF COMMON
ELEMENTS

Hydrogen	H	1
Chlorine	Cl	1
Oxygen	O	2
Sulfur	S	2
Nitrogen	N	3
Phosphorus	P	3
Carbon	C	4

When carbon forms a molecule with hydrogen, the simplest result is thus CH_4. This is methane, which we will discuss in more detail in the next section.

Now you are in a position to predict some chemical formulas by assuming that each element will form the number of bonds given by its covalence number. These covalence numbers are listed in Table 4–3. You should be able to memorize them very easily by relating the covalence numbers to the groups of the periodic table.

(For various reasons, compounds are formed that do not correspond to these covalence numbers. The most important, from a biochemical point of view, are those in which phosphorus forms *five* bonds, rather than three.)

EXAMPLE 4d: Predict the formula of a compound formed between phosphorus and bromine.

- -

SOLUTION: Bromine forms one bond, and phosphorus normally three. We expect the formula to be PBr_3. Check this by writing the Lewis electron-dot diagram.

$$:\overset{..}{\underset{..}{Br}}:\overset{..}{P}:\overset{..}{\underset{..}{Br}}:$$
$$:\overset{..}{\underset{..}{Br}}:$$

EXAMPLE 4e: Predict the formula of a compound formed between carbon and chlorine.

- -

SOLUTION: Chlorine forms one bond, and carbon four. We expect the formula to be CCl_4. This is, in fact, the formula of carbon tetrachloride, once a common dry cleaning solvent and fire extinguisher fluid but now banned because it causes liver damage and may cause cancer.

$$:\overset{..}{\underset{..}{Cl}}:$$
$$:\overset{..}{\underset{..}{Cl}}:\overset{}{C}:\overset{..}{\underset{..}{Cl}}:$$
$$:\overset{..}{\underset{..}{Cl}}:$$

EXAMPLE 4f: Alcoholic beverages contain ethyl alcohol, a compound whose formula is C_2H_6O. By using the rules for covalence numbers, write a suitable Lewis electron-dot diagram for ethyl alcohol.

- -

SOLUTION: Although this seems quite complicated, we can eliminate several possibilities. Carbon forms four bonds, oxygen two, and hydrogen one. It is impossible, for example, for the proper Lewis diagram to be

$$\begin{array}{cc} H & H \\ C:C:H:\overset{..}{\underset{..}{O}}:H \\ H & H \end{array}$$

because that would involve one carbon having only three bonds and one hydrogen having two bonds.

If you work out the possibilities, you will be left with two Lewis diagrams that obey the rules we have set out. One turns out to be the correct diagram for ethyl alcohol:

$$H \quad H$$
$$H : \overset{..}{\underset{..}{C}} : \overset{..}{\underset{..}{C}} : \overset{..}{\underset{..}{O}} : H$$
$$H \quad H$$

The other possible diagram, which at this stage you should consider to be a correct answer to the question, given the limited information provided, is

$$H \quad \quad H$$
$$H : \overset{..}{\underset{..}{C}} : \overset{..}{\underset{..}{O}} : \overset{..}{\underset{..}{C}} : H$$
$$H \quad \quad H$$

This is the correct diagram for a different compound, dimethyl ether, used in refrigeration and chemically similar to the type of ether used in anesthesia and in biology laboratories. This situation, in which two different compounds can result from the same formula, is common in organic chemistry and will be treated in Chapter 7 when we discuss *isomers*.

In the next section, we will discuss some common covalently bonded compounds in greater detail. The theory of covalent bonding will be treated in Chapter 6, which also considers the shapes of molecules.

SELF-CHECK

4.7) Explain how two neutral iodine atoms can combine through formation of a covalent bond to form an I_2 molecule.

4.8) Predict the molecular formula and write a simple Lewis electron-dot diagram for a covalent compound that contains the elements shown. Assume that the covalence numbers used in this chapter do apply.
a) fluorine only
b) hydrogen and bromine
c) hydrogen and sulfur
d) oxygen and chlorine
e) nitrogen and iodine
f) *one* carbon atom, with hydrogen
g) *two* carbon atoms, with hydrogen
h) *one* carbon atom, one oxygen atom, and hydrogen

4.4 SOME SIMPLE COVALENT MOLECULES

LEARNING GOAL 4G: Given the formula of an inorganic binary molecule, write its name according to the system described in this section; given the name of such a compound, write its molecular formula.

   4H: Given the common name (or formula) of any compound in Table 4–4, write its molecular formula (or name).

As a general rule, the compounds formed by *metals* with *nonmetals* are ionic and follow the rules we discussed in Section 4.1. Compounds between two metals do not really exist in the manner that we have been describing. Metals do combine to form *alloys* (Table 11–9), but in varying combinations, so there is no fixed formula for steel, brass, or sterling silver.

Compounds between two nonmetals involve covalently bonded molecules. For our purposes, we will consider hydrogen and carbon to be nonmetals, along with nitrogen, phosphorus, oxygen, sulfur, and the halogens. Compounds of these elements are thus covalent compounds.

Covalent binary compounds

A **binary** compound contains *two* elements; the prefix "bi-" means "two." Binary compounds between a metal and a nonmetal such as NaF, $FeCl_2$, or Al_2O_3 are named, according to the methods of Section 4.2, sodium fluoride, iron(II) chloride, and aluminum oxide, respectively.

One method for naming binary covalent compounds is based on the same type of system that gives us "iron(II)" or "copper(I)" in Table 4–1. In this method, the oxidation state (p. 67) of the more metallic element is shown in parentheses after its name.

Remembering that oxygen is almost always found combined in its −2 oxidation state, we can apply this rule to such compounds as CO_2, *carbon (IV) oxide;* CO, *carbon(II) oxide;* and N_2O, *nitrogen(I) oxide.* This method will be easier to apply after you learn more about oxidation and reduction in Chapter 8. The systematic names are only rarely used for the compounds that most interest us.

A second naming method comes from some "common names" that have been passed down through the years, such as "water" for H_2O, "ammonia" for NH_3, and "laughing gas" or "nitrous oxide" for N_2O. In the most obvious cases, we keep these traditional names.

The most commonly used method for distinguishing between binary covalent compounds comes from counting the atoms of each element. The most metallic element is named first, and in front of its name, we put a prefix that shows how many atoms of it are present in one molecule, according to the following Greek roots:

One atom: *mono-* (from the Greek *monos*) or no prefix at all
Two atoms: *di-* (from the Greek *dis,* meaning twice)
Three atoms: *tri-* (from the Greek *tris,* meaning three times)
Four atoms: *tetra-* (from the Greek *tetras,* having four parts)
Five atoms: *penta-* (from the Greek *pentas,* having five parts)
Six atoms: *hexa-* (from the Greek *hexas,* having six parts)

The prefixes that mean seven (hepta-), eight (octa-), nine (nona-), and ten (deca-) are also fairly common and will be learned in Chapter 7.

Memorize this list. The same prefixes are used to name many different kinds of compounds, including the hydrocarbons to be considered in Chapter 7. We have already run across the *mono*hydrogen phosphate ion HPO_4^{2-} and the *di*hydrogen phosphate ion $H_2PO_4^-$ in Table 4–2. Now apply these prefixes to the number of atoms present.

EXAMPLE 4g: Count the number of atoms of the *first* element present in each of the following formulas, and apply the correct prefix to the element name.

a) N_2O b) C_3S_2 c) P_4S_7 d) Si_2F_6

- -

SOLUTION:
a) two nitrogens: *dinitrogen*
b) three carbons: *tricarbon*
c) four phosphorus: *tetraphosphorus*
d) two silicons: *disilicon*

If only one atom of the first element in the formula is present in each molecule, the prefix *mono-* is usually left out.

Now count the atoms of the second element in the molecular formula, and apply the proper prefix to the -ide ending of that element (oxide, sulfide, chloride, nitride, etc.).

EXAMPLE 4h: Write the name of each of the following covalent binary compounds, using Greek prefixes to indicate number of atoms.

a) CO_2 d) P_2O_5 g) N_2O
b) C_3S_2 e) SO_3 h) CCl_4
c) CO f) Si_2F_6 i*) P_4S_7

- -

SOLUTION:
a) one carbon, two oxygens: *carbon dioxide* (the gas we exhale)
b) three carbons, two sulfurs: *tricarbon disulfide*
c) one carbon, one oxygen: *carbon monoxide* (poisonous)
d) two phosphorus, five oxygen: *diphosphorus pentoxide* (often simply called "phosphorus pentoxide")
e) one sulfur, three oxygens: *sulfur trioxide* (in smokestack pollution)
f) two silicon, six fluorine: *disilicon hexafluoride*
g) two nitrogen, one oxygen: *dinitrogen monoxide* ("laughing gas")
h) one carbon, four chlorine: *carbon tetrachloride*
i*)   four phosphorus, seven sulfur: *tetraphosphorus heptasulfide.*
Note that if the name of the element begins with a vowel (a, e, i, o, u), we may cut one letter from the prefix. We get carbon *mon*oxide, not "*mono*oxide"; diphosphorus *pent*oxide, not "*penta*oxide."

It is easy to see from Example 4h that the covalence numbers we have been using to predict some formulas of covalent compounds do not necessarily predict *all* such formulas.

Hydrocarbons

In Table 1–2 (p. 7), we listed some simple compounds, most of which we have discussed in this chapter. Methane and ethyl alcohol from that table will be considered in this section. Figure 1–4 (p. 8) showed, in contrast, some of the more complicated types of compounds found in the human body. All of the compounds in Figure 1–4 have in common a central chain of carbon atoms, which is arranged in different ways. This illustrates the most important fact about organic compounds—carbon atoms can bond together (by covalent bonding) to form long chains.

For example, the glucose molecule shown in Figure 1–4 has a chain of six carbon atoms bonded together. Various atoms and groups of atoms are then connected to this central chain.

We will discuss the formation and naming of organic compounds in detail in Chapter 7. Here, we will discuss several compounds of great importance.

Hydrocarbons are compounds of hydrogen and carbon; they are *binary* compounds. Knowing that hydrogen always forms one bond (it has a covalence number of one) and carbon forms four bonds, we can write some Lewis electron-dot diagrams for the simplest organic compounds.

We will be using structural formulas for these compounds. The structural formula for the hydrocarbon with six carbons in a continuous chain is

$$
\begin{array}{ccccccc}
 & H & H & H & H & H & H \\
 & | & | & | & | & | & | \\
H- & C- & C- & C- & C- & C- & C-H \\
 & | & | & | & | & | & | \\
 & H & H & H & H & H & H
\end{array}
$$

This compound is hexane, with a molecular formula C_6H_{14}. Notice that each carbon indeed has four bonds around it; we have replaced the two dots that represent a bond in an electron-dot diagram with a straight line. Each hydrogen atom similarly has one bond. A **structural formula** is thus an electron-dot diagram that uses a straight line for each covalent bond. Valence electron pairs that belong entirely to individual atoms may or may not be shown; there are none in hexane.

The glucose molecule has the structural formula shown in Figure 1–4 and may be considered a *derivative* of hexane, since both molecules have six-carbon continuous chains.

Methane

While hexane, C_6H_{14}, is quite typical of hydrocarbons, it is rarely encountered in our homes. The most common hydrocarbon is also the simplest. It is methane, the molecule formed by one atom of carbon with four atoms of hydrogen, CH_4. It is the most important fuel in natural gas, used to heat homes and for stoves and ovens.

Methane can be represented by diagrams as follows:

$$
\begin{array}{cc}
\begin{array}{c}
H \\
\cdot\cdot \\
H:C:H \\
\cdot\cdot \\
H
\end{array}
&
\begin{array}{c}
H \\
| \\
H-C-H \\
| \\
H
\end{array} \quad \text{Methane}
\end{array}
$$

Lewis electron-dot   Structural
diagram   formula

You see that a covalent bond may be shown by either two dots or a line. However, these diagrams are only good for showing which atoms are bonded together. They are not intended to show the actual shape of the molecule, which *is* shown in Figure 4–4. This ball-and-stick model does not pretend to show exactly where the electron clouds are located around the nuclei, but it does show the relative positions of the atoms. Instead of the "square" implied by the structural formula, methane actually has a shape that we call a *tetrahedron,* which will be described further in Section 6.3.

To summarize the three ways we can now describe a covalent molecule:

A molecular formula tells us how many atoms of each element are in one molecule, as in the formula for methane, CH_4.

A structural formula shows which atoms are connected by covalent bonds.

A three-dimensional picture or model, as in Figure 4–4, shows how the atoms are distributed in space.

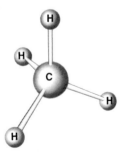

FIGURE 4–4 The three-dimensional structure of methane, CH_4.

Some other simple hydrocarbons

Suppose we remove one hydrogen from a methane molecule. That leaves the molecule-part or fragment

$$
\begin{array}{c}
\text{H} \\
\text{H}\!:\!\ddot{\text{C}}\cdot \\
\text{H}
\end{array}
\qquad \text{Methyl group}
$$

which is called a *methyl* group.

If we combine two methyl groups by a carbon-carbon bond, we obtain the two-carbon hydrocarbon C_2H_6, which is **ethane.**

Ethane has the structural formula

$$
\begin{array}{c}
\text{H}\quad\text{H} \\
|\qquad| \\
\text{H}-\text{C}-\text{C}-\text{H} \\
|\qquad| \\
\text{H}\quad\text{H}
\end{array}
\qquad \text{Ethane}
$$

and makes up between five and ten per cent of natural gas.

If we remove a hydrogen atom from ethane, we obtain a fragment called an *ethyl* group:

$$
\begin{array}{c}
\text{H}\quad\text{H} \\
|\qquad| \\
\text{H}-\text{C}-\text{C}\cdot \\
|\qquad| \\
\text{H}\quad\text{H}
\end{array}
\qquad \text{Ethyl group}
$$

If we combine an ethyl group with a methyl group, we end up with a hydrocarbon with three carbons in its chain, called propane, C_3H_8.

$$
\begin{array}{c}
\text{H}\quad\text{H}\quad\text{H} \\
|\qquad|\qquad| \\
\text{H}-\text{C}-\text{C}-\text{C}-\text{H} \\
|\qquad|\qquad| \\
\text{H}\quad\text{H}\quad\text{H}
\end{array}
\qquad \text{Propane}
$$

Figure 4–5 shows photographs of models of the methane (CH_4), ethane (C_2H_6), and propane (C_3H_8) molecules. The space-filling models give a better idea of the electron clouds around the molecule but make it much more difficult to see exactly which way each bond is arranged.

If we continue the process of adding carbon atoms to the chain, we obtain C_4H_{10}, butane:

$$
\begin{array}{c}
\text{H}\quad\text{H}\quad\text{H}\quad\text{H} \\
|\qquad|\qquad|\qquad| \\
\text{H}-\text{C}-\text{C}-\text{C}-\text{C}-\text{H} \\
|\qquad|\qquad|\qquad| \\
\text{H}\quad\text{H}\quad\text{H}\quad\text{H}
\end{array}
\qquad \text{Butane}
$$

Propane and **butane** are commonly used fuels for camp stoves, cigarette lighters, and the torches used by electricians and plumbers.

Adding one more carbon will make pentane, C_5H_{12}. Note the use of the Greek prefix *penta,* which means "five." Earlier in this section, the same prefix was used in naming inorganic binary compounds. In organic chemistry, it is used when there are five carbon atoms in a chain. You may be able

The naming of these continuous-chain hydrocarbons is quite systematic, as will be discussed in Section 7.1.

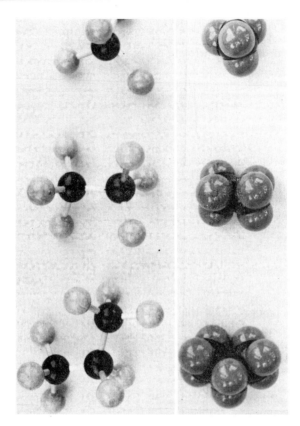

FIGURE 4–5 Ball-and-stick and "space-filling" molecular models for methane (top), ethane (middle), and propane (bottom). Organic chemistry laboratories often have such models available for student use. (Photographs by Janice Peters.)

to remember this prefix if you can relate it to the shape of the *Penta*gon building in Washington, D.C., which has five sides.

If we add a sixth carbon, we arrive at the compound hexane, C_6H_{14}, which we have already seen.

Derivatives of methane

There are over 3 million organic compounds. Many of them can be obtained by replacing one or more hydrogen atoms on a carbon chain by other *functional groups*. Let us use methane as an example.

If we replace a hydrogen on CH_4 with a chlorine atom, we obtain

$$H-\overset{\displaystyle H}{\underset{\displaystyle H}{C}}-Cl \qquad \text{Methyl chloride}$$

If, instead, we replace the hydrogen by an —OH, as in self-check 4.8h, we obtain

$$H-\overset{\displaystyle H}{\underset{\displaystyle H}{C}}-OH \qquad \text{Methyl alcohol}$$

If the —OH group replaces hydrogen not on methane but on ethane, we get

$$H-\underset{\underset{H}{|}}{\overset{\overset{H}{|}}{C}}-\underset{\underset{H}{|}}{\overset{\overset{H}{|}}{C}}-OH \qquad \text{Ethyl alcohol}$$

Methyl alcohol (wood alcohol) is widely used in industry. Ethyl alcohol is used in beverages and in commercial applications. Both will be discussed further in Section 9.2 on alcohols.

If two hydrogens on methane are removed and replaced by one double bond to oxygen, we obtain H_2CO, formaldehyde:

$$H-\underset{}{\overset{\overset{H}{|}}{C}}=O \qquad \text{Formaldehyde}$$

Formaldehyde is found in biology laboratories (in a water solution called *formalin*), where it is used to preserve specimens. It will be described further in Section 9.3, along with other aldehydes and ketones. Note that the covalence-number rules apply to formaldehyde because of the double bond. Such bonds will be further discussed in Section 6.2.

These compounds will be discussed systematically in Chapters 7 and 9. At this stage, you should note that

1) There is often a logical relationship between the common *name* of a compound, such as *meth*yl chloride, CH_3Cl, and the name of the hydrocarbon with the same number of carbon atoms, *meth*ane. The word stems are

   if one carbon atom: *meth-*
   if two carbon atoms: *eth-*
   if three carbon atoms: *prop-*
   if four carbon atoms: *but-*
   if five or more carbon atoms: same stem as for inorganic nomenclature (*pent-, hex-, hept-, oct-* for five, six, seven, and eight carbons)

2) Many organic compounds of interest can be related to simple hydrocarbons. For this reason, basic organic chemistry is relatively easy to understand, even though there are so many compounds.

3) The carbon chain in an organic molecule is arranged not in a straight line (the way we show it in a structural formula), but in a zigzag fashion as shown for propane in Figure 4–5.

Some of the organic compounds discussed in this section will be used to illustrate the calculation of molecular weights (Section 4.5), the balancing of chemical equations (Section 5.2), and the prediction of shapes of molecules (Section 6.3). For the upcoming chapters, you should learn the names and formulas of the simple organic compounds listed in Table 4–4.

Alkyl Halides

Since we began this chapter with several kinds of chlorides that involved ionic bonding, we should also note the numerous organic compounds that involve chlorine and the other halogens. Although such compounds are generally not found in the human body, they have major applications in fields like plastics (particularly in the manufacture of Teflon and PVC, polyvinyl chloride), refrigeration, and anesthetics for surgery.

We have already discussed the simplest such compound, methyl chloride (CH_3Cl). Unlike the compounds of chlorine with metals, such as $NaCl$, $CaCl_2$, or $AlCl_3$, which involve ionic bonding, organic chlorine compounds form covalent molecules. Each halogen has a covalence number of one.

TABLE 4–4 NAMES AND FORMULAS OF SOME SIMPLE ORGANIC COMPOUNDS

Methane	CH_4
Ethane	C_2H_6
Propane	C_3H_8
Butane	C_4H_{10}
Methyl alcohol	CH_3OH
Ethyl alcohol	C_2H_5OH
Formaldehyde	$HCHO$

A halogen atom (F, Cl, Br, or I) can replace one hydrogen on a hydrocarbon. Some useful products of this type include

CH_3Cl methyl chloride (a refrigerant)
CH_3Br methyl bromide
C_2H_5Cl ethyl chloride (a local anesthetic)
C_2H_5Br ethyl bromide (once an inhalation anesthetic for surgery)
C_2H_5I ethyl iodide (used in determination of heart output)
C_4H_9Cl butyl chloride (used to kill worms in dogs and cats)

Each of these compounds is derived from one of the simple hydrocarbons we have discussed (methane, ethane, or butane) by replacement of one hydrogen by a halogen atom. Replacement can continue until two, three, or more hydrogens are removed and similar or different halogen atoms are added. Some resulting compounds are

CH_2Cl_2 methylene chloride (an organic solvent)
$CHCl_3$ chloroform (formerly an inhalation anesthetic, but damages the liver and may cause cancer)
CCl_4 carbon tetrachloride (formerly a dry-cleaning solvent; same dangers as $CHCl_3$)
$CFCl_3$, CF_2Cl_2, freons (used in refrigeration and as spray-can propellants)
$CHBr_3$ bromoform (a medical sedative)
CHI_3 iodoform (an antiseptic)
$C_2HBrClF_3$ halothane (a modern inhalation anesthetic for surgery)

Some halogenated hydrocarbons have been used by ''glue sniffers'' to obtain temporary ''highs.'' This is extremely dangerous because some of these compounds can cause death from heart stoppage as well as damage to kidneys and liver. Many of these substances can be absorbed through the skin. While they can be beneficial to humans by allowing us to transport and store food in refrigerators and freezers, the excessive use of spray-can propellants has opened a new danger, that of removing the ozone barrier in the upper atmosphere that protects us from some of the dangerous rays of the sun.

The production of plastics, such as Teflon and PVC, from such compounds will be discussed in Chapter 16.

SELF-CHECK

4.9) Write the name, using Greek prefixes, of each of the following.
a) NO_2 (very poisonous gas widely used in industry)
b) P_2S_5 (used in the production of safety matches)
c) $SiCl_4$ (has been used to produce smoke screens in warfare)
d) ICl (has been used as a medical antiseptic)
e) P_2O_3
f*) IF_7
4.10) Write the molecular formula of
a) diiodine pentoxide (used in respirators to prevent CO poisoning by converting this poisonous gas to CO_2)
b) carbon disulfide (common organic solvent)
c) chlorine trifluoride (used in processing nuclear reactor fuel)
d) sulfur hexafluoride (used in electrical circuit breakers)
e) trisilicon tetranitride
4.11) Write the common name of
a) CH_4
b) C_3H_8
c) C_2H_5OH

4.12)   Write the molecular formula of
a)   methyl alcohol
b)   butane
c)   formaldehyde

4.5 FORMULA WEIGHTS

LEARNING GOAL 4I: Given a periodic table and the chemical formula of any substance, calculate the formula weight in atomic mass units.

4J: Given a periodic table and a chemical formula, calculate the percent by weight of each element contained in the compound.

4K: Given adequate information about a molecular substance, distinguish between its simplest formula and its correct molecular formula.

Now that we have learned how to write a large number of chemical formulas, we can use these formulas to determine the average weight of one molecule (for a covalent substance) or of one formula unit (for an ionic substance).

The average weight of one atom of an element was discussed in Section 2.5 (p. 42). We can read it from the periodic table. For example, the average mass (or weight) of one carbon atom is 12.01 amu. For our purpose in calculating the weights of molecules and formula units, you may round off any atomic weight to the nearest 0.1 amu. Some very commonly used atomic weight values are listed in Table 4–5.

Molecular weights

You are continuously breathing oxygen gas from the air. However, you are not drawing individual oxygen atoms into your lungs. The oxygen in the atmosphere is almost all in the form of O_2 molecules.

The Law of Conservation of Mass tells us that when two oxygen atoms, weighing 16.0 amu each, combine to make an oxygen molecule, no mass may be lost. The oxygen molecule thus weighs 2×16.0 amu $= 32.0$ amu. This mass, the sum of the weights of the atoms in the molecule, is called the **molecular weight** of oxygen gas.

TABLE 4–5   SOME ATOMIC WEIGHTS FOR USE IN CALCULATING FORMULA WEIGHTS

Element	Atomic Weight, amu
H	1.0
C	12.0
N	14.0
O	16.0
F	19.0
Na	23.0
Mg	24.3
Al	27.0
P	31.0
S	32.1
Cl	35.5
K	39.1
Ca	40.1
Br	79.9
Ag	108
I	127

EXAMPLE 4i: Calculate the molecular weight of
a)   methane   b)   tricarbon disulfide   c)   formaldehyde

- -

SOLUTION: You must add together the atomic weights of the atoms in each molecule. Methane is CH_4. Tricarbon disulfide is C_3S_2. Formaldehyde is HCHO. The atomic weights from the periodic table inside the front cover or from Table 4–5 are
H: 1.0 amu   C: 12.0 amu   O: 16.0 amu   S: 32.1 amu

a)   for CH_4,   mass   of   1 C + 4 H = (1) (12.0 amu) + (4) (1.0 amu) =
16.0 amu

b) for C_3S_2, mass of 3 C + 2 S = (3) (12.0 amu) + (2) (32.1 amu) = 100.2 amu (we will normally round this off to three figures: $\boxed{100 \text{ amu}}$)

c) for HCHO, mass of 1 C + 2 H + 1 O = (12.0) + (2) (1.0) + (16.0) = $\boxed{30.0 \text{ amu}}$

Formula weights

The **formula weight** of any substance is the sum of the atomic weights of all of the atoms that make up one *formula unit* of that substance.

For a covalent substance, the formula unit corresponds to the formula for one molecule, the molecular formula. The formula weight *is* therefore the molecular weight.

For an ionic substance, the *formula unit* is simply the simplest way we can express the relative proportions of the elements present. For sodium chloride, the formula unit NaCl simply tells us that one atom of chlorine is present for each atom of sodium. (Remember, there is *no* NaCl molecule this small.)

For either an ionic or molecular substance, therefore, we can calculate a formula weight by adding together atomic weights.

Some books use the term for-mula weight only for ionic compounds and molecular weight for all covalent com-pounds. We will use the term formula weight for both kinds of substances in this text.

EXAMPLE 4j: Calculate the following formula weights.
a) carbon dioxide   b) potassium iodide   c) propane

– –

SOLUTION: The method is the same as we used in Example 4i for calcu-lation of molecular weights. In fact, two of these three formula weights *are* molecular weights. Recall from earlier sections of Chapter 4 that our three compounds have the formulas a) CO_2 b) KI c)C_3H_8

a) for CO_2, mass of 1 C + 2 O = (12.0) + (2) (16.0) = $\boxed{44.0 \text{ amu}}$

b) for KI, mass of 1 K + 1 I = (39.1) + (127) = $\boxed{166 \text{ amu}}$ (again, we generally round off to three digits)

c) for C_3H_8, mass of 3 C + 8 H = (3) (12.0) + (8) (1.0) = $\boxed{44.0 \text{ amu}}$

Exactly the same method is used for more complicated formulas. However, you must remember to include every atom in each formula.

EXAMPLE 4k: Calculate the following formula weights.
a) aluminum sulfate   b) cholesterol, $C_{27}H_{46}O$

– –

SOLUTION: First determine the formula of aluminum sulfate, which is $Al_2(SO_4)_3$. If you have difficulty with this, see Section 4.2. Then follow the same procedure as before, remembering that the subscript "3" at the end of the aluminum sulfate formula means 3 sulfurs and 12 oxygens.

a) for $Al_2(SO_4)_3$, mass of 2 Al + 3 S + 12 O = (2) (27.0) + (3) (32.1) + (12) (16.0) = $\boxed{342 \text{ amu}}$

b) for $C_{27}H_{46}O$, mass of 27 C + 46 H + O = (27) (12.0) + (46) (1.0) + (16.0) = $\boxed{386 \text{ amu}}$

Percentage composition

You may have noticed on breakfast cereal boxes some information about the *composition* of the cereal. For example, one very popular and relatively nutritious dry cereal has a label that indicates that in each 100 grams of cereal, there are 20.1 grams of protein, 0.60 grams of fat, and 72.8 grams of carbohydrates, as well as smaller amounts of some vitamins and minerals. Since "per cent" means "parts in 100 parts," this same information could have been written: "20.1% protein, 0.60% fat, 72.8% carbohydrate." Such information allows a nutritionist to compare the food value of that cereal with the food value of other breakfast foods.

Similarly, the chemist is often interested in the element composition or "makeup" of a given compound. We express the **percentage composition** of a substance in terms of the number in grams of each element in 100 grams of the substance. This can also be written

If you have difficulty working with per cents, see Appendix B of this text.

$$\text{Percent by weight of an element in a given compound} = \frac{\text{weight of element}}{\text{total weight of compound}} \times 100\%$$

EXAMPLE 41: Calculate the per cent by weight of each element in
a) carbon dioxide   b) aluminum sulfate

- -

SOLUTION: The formula weights of these substances were calculated in Examples 4j and 4k. We may use the information from those examples.
a) for CO_2, mass of carbon in one molecule = (1) (12.0 amu) = 12.0 amu
        mass of oxygen in one molecule = (2) (16.0 amu) = 32.0 amu
        total mass of one molecule   = 44.0 amu

Then for carbon we have $\dfrac{12.0 \text{ amu C}}{44.0 \text{ amu total}} \times 100\% = \boxed{27.3\% \text{ carbon}}$

and for oxygen we have $\dfrac{32.0 \text{ amu O}}{44.0 \text{ amu total}} \times 100\% = \boxed{72.7\% \text{ oxygen}}$

$$\text{total} = 27.3\% + 72.7\% = 100.0\%$$

Because of rounding off, the total per cent may be slightly more or less than exactly 100%.
b) For $Al_2(SO_4)_3$, in one formula unit of this ionic substance, we have mass of aluminum = (2) (27.0) = 54.0 amu Al
        mass of sulfur = (3) (32.1) = 96.3 amu S
        mass of oxygen = (12) (16.0) = 192   amu O
                           342 amu total mass
Then to calculate the composition of this compound:
for aluminum we have $\dfrac{54.0 \text{ amu Al}}{342 \text{ amu total}} \times 100\% = \boxed{15.8\% \text{ Al}}$

for sulfur we have $\dfrac{96.3 \text{ amu S}}{342 \text{ amu total}} \times 100\% = \boxed{28.2\% \text{ S}}$

for oxygen we have $\dfrac{192 \text{ amu O}}{342 \text{ amu total}} \times 100\% = \boxed{56.1\% \text{ O}}$

$$\text{total} = 15.8\% + 28.2\% + 56.1\% = 100.1\% \approx 100\%$$

Use of composition data

Information regarding per cent by weight of each element can be used to tell us how much of each element goes into a given mass of compound, or how much could be removed.

EXAMPLE 4m: How many grams of carbon are contained in 10.0 grams of butane?

- -

SOLUTION: First of all, butane is C_4H_{10}. Determine the composition in per cent by weight.

$$\text{for carbon: 4 atoms C} \times 12.0 \text{ amu} = 48.0 \text{ amu C}$$
$$\text{for hydrogen: 10 atoms H} \times 1.0 \text{ amu} = \underline{10.0 \text{ amu H}}$$
$$\text{total mass of one molecule: } 58.0 \text{ amu}$$

We then have for carbon $\dfrac{48.0 \text{ amu C}}{58.0 \text{ amu total}} = 82.8\%$ C

The composition of any compound is constant, no matter how much we take. If we start with 58.0 amu of compound (one molecule), then 82.8% of 58.0 amu = 48.0 amu will be carbon. If we start with 1000 amu of butane, then 82.8% of 1000 amu = 828 amu will be carbon.

Similarly, we can use *any* units of mass. In 1000 tons of butane, 82.8% × 1000 tons = 828 tons will be carbon. In this particular problem, we have 10.0 grams of butane, so

$$10.0 \text{ g} \times 82.8\% = 10.0 \text{ g butane} \times \frac{82.8 \text{ g C}}{100 \text{ g butane}} = \boxed{8.28 \text{ g C}}$$

Simplest formulas

We can take an unknown substance and find, through what the chemists call *quantitative analysis,* the per cent by weight of each element present. For example, for the hydrocarbon acetylene, which is used as a fuel for welding torches, we find that each molecule contains 92.3% carbon and 7.7% hydrogen. The weight of carbon in the molecule is 92.3/7.7 = 12.0 times the weight of hydrogen. Since one atom of carbon itself weighs 12 times as much as an atom of hydrogen, there must be an equal number of atoms of carbon and of hydrogen in each molecule of acetylene.

If we analyze benzene, a common organic solvent that will be discussed in detail in Chapter 15, we find that it also contains 92.3% carbon and 7.7% hydrogen. There are equal numbers of atoms of carbon and of hydrogen in benzene also.

Knowing this, we would be tempted to say that the chemical formula of acetylene, and of benzene, was "CH." That formula certainly agrees with the information we have been given regarding the compositions of these two compounds. We call such a formula the **simplest formula** or *empirical formula* for acetylene and for benzene.

The word empirical *means "from an experiment."*

For various reasons, we know that the formula "CH" simply cannot describe either the acetylene molecule or the benzene molecule. If we try to write a Lewis electron-dot diagram for "CH," we soon find that it contains an odd number (five) of valence electrons and cannot possibly satisfy the rules we have been using. In addition, the chemical and physical properties of acetylene and benzene are completely different; they cannot be the same molecule.

Our problem is solved if we find a way to determine the formula weight of acetylene (26.0 amu) and the formula weight of benzene (78.0 amu). Since one carbon atom has a mass of 12.0 amu and one hydrogen atom has a mass of 1.0 amu, acetylene must contain *two* carbons and *two* hydrogens in each molecule. The molecular formula for acetylene is C_2H_2. Acetylene will be discussed further in Section 7.2.

Similarly, the benzene molecule must contain *six* carbons and *six* hydrogens to obtain a total mass of 78.0 amu. Benzene is described in Section 15.1.

We can summarize this situation as follows:

1) Data from chemical analysis, giving the percent-by-weight composition of each element in a compound, gives the ratio of the atoms of the elements and thus the simplest formula for the compound.
2) The actual molecular formula may be the same as the simplest formula or may consist of a number of atoms that is two times, three times, four times, etc., the number of atoms in the simplest formula.
3) To find the real molecular formula, we must know the formula weight.

Looking at a real molecular formula, you should be able to figure out what its simplest formula would be.

EXAMPLE 4n: Determine the simplest formula (from chemical analysis) for

a) ethane
b) methane

c) hydrogen peroxide, H_2O_2
d) glucose, $C_6H_{12}O_6$

- -

SOLUTION: Find the simplest ratio of atoms.
a) For C_2H_6, the simplest ratio is one C to three H's; thus CH_3.
b) For CH_4, the simplest ratio is one C to four H's; thus CH_4 (in this case, the simplest formula is also the molecular formula).
c) For H_2O_2, the simplest ratio is one H to one O; thus HO.
d) For $C_6H_{12}O_6$, the simplest ratio is one C to two H's to one O; thus CH_2O. This is also the simplest formula (and the molecular formula) for formaldehyde!

For an ionic compound, the formula unit is already a simplest formula, since there is no "real" molecular formula at all.

Calculating the simplest formula from analytical data

The procedure for obtaining the simplest formula is not very difficult, provided you draw a mental picture. The steps are

1) Pick a convenient total amount of compound, such as 100 amu.
2) Applying the percent-by-weight figures, find the mass of each element.
3) Using the atomic weight of each element, find the number of atoms of each element present in the total mass.
4) Find the simplest ratio of atoms.

EXAMPLE 4o: The hydrocarbon ethene is known to be composed of 85.6% carbon and 14.4% hydrogen. Find its simplest formula.

- -

SOLUTION: Take 100 amu of total compound for convenience in doing the calculation. Remember that the amount taken doesn't really matter, since the per cents by weight apply to any amount.

$$\text{Mass of carbon} = 100 \text{ amu ethene} \times \frac{85.6 \text{ amu C}}{100 \text{ amu ethene}} = 85.6 \text{ amu C}$$

$$\text{Mass of hydrogen} = 100 \text{ amu ethene} \times \frac{14.4 \text{ amu H}}{100 \text{ amu ethene}} = 14.4 \text{ amu H}$$

$$\text{Atoms of carbon present: } 85.6 \text{ amu C} \times \frac{1 \text{ atom C}}{12.0 \text{ amu C}} = 7.13 \text{ atoms C}$$

$$\text{Atoms of hydrogen present: } 14.4 \text{ amu H} \times \frac{1 \text{ atom H}}{1.0 \text{ amu H}} = 14.4 \text{ atoms H}$$

Within experimental error, we have two atoms of hydrogen for each atom of carbon, so the simplest formula is $\boxed{CH_2}$.

Once we know the simplest formula, information about the molecular weight will permit us to find the true molecular formula.

EXAMPLE 4p: The compound ethene is better known as ethylene and is one of the most important organic substances used in industry. Polyethylene, a common plastic (Chapter 16) is made from this compound. If the molecular weight of ethene is 28.0 amu, find its molecular formula.

- -

SOLUTION: From Example 4o, we know that there is one atom of carbon for two atoms of hydrogen. These three atoms together weigh 14.0 amu. Since the weight of one ethene molecule is 28.0 amu, we must have two atoms of carbon and four atoms of hydrogen: $\boxed{C_2H_4}$.

SELF-CHECK

4.13) Using Table 4–5 or the periodic table inside the front cover, calculate the formula weight, in atomic mass units, for
a) butane   d) iron(II) phosphate
b) sodium chloride   e) dinitrogen monoxide
c) ethyl alcohol
4.14) Which of the formula weights in Question 4.13 are also molecular weights?
4.15) Using information from Question 4.13, calculate the percent-by-weight composition of each element in
a) ethyl alcohol   b) iron(II) phosphate
4.16*) If all of the oxygen in 10.0 grams of ethyl alcohol were removed as pure elemental oxygen, how many grams of oxygen would be obtained?

4.17) Which of the following real molecular formulas are also simplest formulas? For any that are *not* simplest formulas, write the simplest formula.
a) C_6H_{14} (hexane)
b) $C_{51}H_{98}O_6$ (a typical fat)
c) CH_3COOH (acetic acid, in vinegar)
d) N_2O_4 (dinitrogen tetroxide, widely used in industry)
e) $C_{18}H_{22}O_2$ (estrone, a female sex hormone)
f) $C_{19}H_{28}O_2$ (testosterone, a male sex hormone)
4.18*) Find the simplest formula for each compound.
a) 23.8 C, 5.9% H, and 70.3% Cl
b) naphthalene, 93.7% C and 6.3% H
c) morphine, 71.6% C, 6.72% H, 4.91% N
4.19*) A certain drug contains aspirin as its major ingredient. Aspirin (acetylsalicylic acid) is $C_9H_8O_4$. Chemical analysis shows that each *tablet* contains 25.0% carbon, and all of the carbon comes from the aspirin. What is the percentage of *aspirin* in each tablet?

CHAPTER FOUR IN REVIEW ▪ Chemical Formulas

4.1 FORMATION OF IONIC SALTS   Page 94
4A: Explain why an ionic bond forms between a cation and an anion.
4B: Given the formulas of a cation and an anion, predict the formula of the ionic compound that can be formed by combining the two ions.

4.2 NAMES AND FORMULAS OF IONIC COMPOUNDS   Page 96
4C: Given the name of any cation in Table 4–1 or anion in Table 4–2, write its formula; given the formula, write the name of the ion.
4D: Given the names of a cation and an anion, write the name and formula of an ionic salt that can be produced by those ions.

4.3 INTRODUCTION TO COVALENT BONDS   Page 98
4E: Explain how a covalent bond may be formed between two neutral atoms.
4F: Given several elements, write the Lewis electron-dot symbol for a neutral atom of each element and predict the formula of a simple covalent compound that can be formed by combining those elements.

4.4 SOME SIMPLE COVALENT MOLECULES   Page 103
4G: Given the formula of an inorganic binary molecule, write its name according to the system described in this section; given the name of such a compound, write its molecular formula.
4H: Given the common name (or formula) of any compound in Table 4–4, write its molecular formula (or name).

4.5 FORMULA WEIGHTS   Page 111
4I: Given a periodic table and the chemical formula of any substance, calculate the formula weight in atomic mass units.

4J: Given a periodic table and a chemical formula, calculate the per cent by weight of each element contained in the compound.
4K: Given adequate information about a molecular substance, distinguish between its simplest formula and its correct molecular formula.

GLOSSARY FOR CHAPTER FOUR

binary Containing two elements. (p. 104)

butane The hydrocarbon C_4H_{10}, often used as a fuel. (p. 107)

composition, percentage A way of showing the relative mass of each element in a compound; the number of grams of each element in 100 grams of compound; may be used to calculate the simplest formula. (p. 113)

covalence number A measure of the number of covalent bonds usually formed by an element through equal sharing of electrons, e.g., four for carbon, one for hydrogen. (p. 100)

covalent bond A chemical link holding two atoms together in a molecule or ion, produced by sharing electrons in the region between the two atoms. (p. 99)

ethane The hydrocarbon C_2H_6, often used as a fuel. (p. 107)

formula weight The sum of the atomic weights of the atoms in any chemical formula; the molecular weight or mass of a formula unit in atomic mass units. (p. 112)

hydrocarbon A compound containing only carbon and hydrogen. (p. 105)

ionic bond A chemical link between a cation and an anion, formed by the attraction of opposite charges; found in ionic salts. (p. 95)

ionic salt A compound consisting of cations and anions held together by ionic bonds; at room temperature, usually a crystalline solid such as NaCl. (p. 95)

Lewis electron-dot diagram A drawing of the atoms in a molecule or ion that shows the distribution of electrons (as dots) on individual atoms or in covalent bonds; incorporates the Lewis symbol for each element; does not necessarily show the shape of the molecule; see structural formula. (p. 101)

methane The simplest hydrocarbon, CH_4. (p. 106)

molecular weight The formula weight of a molecular substance: the sum of the atomic weights of the atoms in a molecule. (p. 111)

propane The hydrocarbon C_3H_8, used as a fuel. (p. 107)

simplest formula A formula that shows the ratio of the number of atoms of each element in a compound but does not necessarily give the number of atoms in each molecule. (p. 114)

structural formula Like a Lewis electron-dot diagram, but uses lines to indicate covalent bonds; the most common way of showing the bonding in an organic molecule. (p. 106)

QUESTIONS AND PROBLEMS FOR CHAPTER FOUR ■ Chemical Formulas

SECTION 4.1 FORMATION OF IONIC SALTS *and*
SECTION 4.2 NAMES AND FORMULAS OF IONIC COMPOUNDS

In the following questions, if an ion is listed in Table 4–1 or 4–2, you will be expected to know its name and formula.

4.20) Why does an ionic bond form in the compound ammonium cyanide? Write the formula for this salt.

4.21) Predict the *formula* of the ionic compound formed by combining
a) sodium and benzoate ions (used as a food preservative)
b) manganese(II) and sulfate ions (poultry feed additive)
c) calcium and hydroxide ions (to treat oxalic acid poisoning)
d) ammonium and hydrogen sulfate ions (in hair-waving preparations)
e) potassium and dichromate ions (an external antiseptic)
f) copper(II) and phosphate ions (used in fertilizers)

4.22) Write the *name* of the ionic compound with each of the following formulas.
a) Cu_2O (a fungicide)
b) Na_3PO_4 (dishwashing detergent)
c) $Ba(MnO_4)_2$ (used in dry-cell batteries)
d) $Al(NO_3)_3$ (an antiperspirant)
e) $Fe(OH)_3$ (used in purifying water)

4.23) Write the formulas of the ionic compounds with the following names.
a) silver bromide (used in photography)
b) magnesium monohydrogen phosphate (a laxative)
c) iron(II) carbonate (used to treat anemia)
d) zinc sulfide (used on TV screens)
e) sodium stearate (a soap)
f) ammonium acetate (preserves meat)

4.24*) Titanium dioxide, TiO_2, is a white coloring matter often used in eye makeup. From the formula of the salt, write the formula of the cation and give its name.

4.45 Why does an ionic bond form in the compound calcium oxalate? Write the formula for this salt.

4.46) Predict the *formula* of the ionic compound formed by combining
a) silver and nitrate ions (drops used in eyes of babies)
b) sodium and hypochlorite ions (antiseptic, chlorine bleach)
c) magnesium and sulfate ions (Epsom salts, a cathartic drug)
d) ammonium and monohydrogen phosphate ions (fireproofing paper and wood)
e) iron(II) and phosphate ions (used in ceramics)
f) zinc and stearate ions (used in ointments)

4.47) Write the name of the ionic compound with each of the following formulas.
a) AgI (used in rain-making)
b) Na_2S (sometimes found in mascara coloring agents; may cause blindness if it gets into the eyes)
c) CuC_2O_4 (used in some dental anticaries agents)

4.48) Write the formulas of the ionic compounds with the following names.
a) copper(I) cyanide (an insecticide)
b) potassium hydrogen carbonate (an antacid)
c) barium carbonate (used in rat poisons)
d) manganese(II) acetate (used to dry paints)
e) aluminum chloride (an antiperspirant)
f) iron(III) oxide (rust)
g) sodium dihydrogen phosphate (used in baking powder)

4.49*) A chromium oxide with formula Cr_2O_3 is used as a green dye in U.S. paper money. From the formula of the salt, write the formula of the cation and give its name.

4.25*) Potassium cyanate, KNCO, has been used very successfully to treat sickle cell anemia. From the formula of the salt, write the formula of the cyanate anion.

4.50*) Sodium nitrite, $NaNO_2$, is commonly used in packaged meat products (like sliced ham) to prevent spoiling. However, nitrites are suspected of possibly reacting with foods to give cancer-causing substances called nitrosamines, such as H_2NNO. From the formula of the sodium nitrite salt, determine the formula of the nitrite anion.

For a salt consisting of a *single* kind of cation bonded to a single kind of anion, it is easy to write a name and formula. However, in nature, we often run across more complicated ionic compounds. The next few questions illustrate this.

4.26*) Bones and teeth are made up largely of a solid, hydroxyapatite, which can be written $Ca_{10}(PO_4)_6(OH)_2$. Show that this formula obeys the rules we have been using for a neutral ionic salt by adding the charges on the cations and on the anions.

4.51*) The substance in Question 4.26 is softer than another solid, fluorapatite, $Ca_{10}(PO_4)_6F_2$. Add up the charges on the cations and on the anions of this formula to show that it is a valid ionic salt. Then explain briefly why adding fluoride ion, F^-, to teeth results in strengthening them!

4.27*) A compound containing two different cations is $KAg(CN)_2$, which has in the past been used in an antiseptic wash. What ions are contained in this compound? What is its name? Would you expect it to be a safe substance to use?

4.52*) Calcium ferrous citrate, $FeCa_2(C_6H_5O_7)_2$, is used to treat iron-deficiency anemia. It contains two different cations. From the name and formula of this compound, write the formula and charge of the citrate anion.

SECTION 4.3 INTRODUCTION TO COVALENT BONDS

4.28) Explain how a covalent bond differs from an ionic bond.

4.53) Explain how two atoms may be held together by a covalent bond, as in Cl_2.

4.29) What kinds of elements do *not* have covalence numbers? Explain why they do not.

4.54) What is a covalence number? How do you use it in predicting the formula of a covalently bonded compound?

4.30) Draw a Lewis electron-dot diagram for each of the following covalent compounds.
a) Br_2 d) CF_4
b) HI
c) NCl_3

4.55) Draw a Lewis electron-dot diagram for each of the following covalent compounds.
a) I_2 c) PF_3
b) HCl   d) $SiCl_4$

4.31) Draw a Lewis electron-dot diagram for a reasonable covalently bonded compound formed from each of the following sets of atoms.
a) one P and several Br atoms
b) one Si and several H atoms
c) three C and several F atoms

4.56) Draw a Lewis electron-dot diagram for a reasonable covalently bonded compound formed from each of the following sets of atoms.
a) one S and several Cl atoms
b) one N and several I atoms
c) two C, two O, and several H atoms.

SECTION 4.4 SOME SIMPLE COVALENT MOLECULES

4.32) Write a correct name for each of the following binary covalent compounds.
a) NO (used to bleach rayon)
b) CF_4
c) ClO_2 (used to purify water)
d) ClF_3 (a rocket fuel)
e) IF_5
f) As_2O_5 (as is arsenic, $Z = 33$)

4.33) Write the molecular formula for each of the following compounds.
a) sulfur dioxide (pollutes air)
b) disilicon hexabromide
c) trimanganese carbide
d) diphosphorus tetriodide
e) bromine monofluoride
f) molybdenum pentachloride

4.34*) Which of the following compounds are *hydrocarbons?*
a) CH_4 d) $C_{10}H_8$
b) CaC_2 e) $C_6H_{12}O_6$
c) C_2H_5OH

4.35) Write the common names of the following compounds.
a) C_2H_6 c) NH_3
b) C_3H_8 d) CH_3OH

4.36) Write the formulas of the following compounds.
a) ethyl alcohol c) formaldehyde
b) butane   d) methane

4.37*) What is the major use of the *Freon* compounds, such as CF_2Cl_2?

SECTION 4.5 FORMULA WEIGHTS (Use a periodic table.)

4.38) Calculate the formula weight of each of the following compounds, which we have seen before.
a) ethane
b) $Al_2(CO_3)_3$
c) methyl alcohol
d) NH_4NO_3
e) C_4H_9Cl
f) $C_{28}H_{44}O$ (vitamin D)
g) $C_3H_7NO_2$ (alanine)

4.39) Using the information gained from doing Problem 4.38, calculate the per cent by weight of *carbon* in
a) methyl alcohol
b) C_4H_9Cl
c) vitamin D
d) alanine
e) aluminum carbonate

4.57) Write a correct name for each of the following binary covalent compounds.
a) N_2S_5
b) CBr_4
c) NO_3
d) BrCl
e) TeF_6 (Te is tellurium, $Z = 52$)
f) B_4C (B is boron, $Z = 5$)

4.58) Write the molecular formula for each of the following compounds.
a) carbon monoxide (poisonous)
b) tetrasulfur tetranitride
c) selenium disulfide
d) iodine tribromide
e) oxygen difluoride
f) diuranium trisulfide (uranium is U, $Z = 92$)

4.59*) Which of the following compounds are *hydrocarbons?*
a) HCHO   d) $C_{12}H_{26}$
b) CO_2 e) C_4H_8
c) CH_3OH

4.60) Write the common names of the following compounds.
a) C_4H_{10} c) HCHO
b) C_2H_5OH d) CH_4

4.61) Write the formulas of the following compounds.
a) ammonia   c) methyl alcohol
b) propane   d) ethane

4.62*) Is it completely safe to inhale spray-can propellants?

4.63) Calculate the formula weight of each of the following compounds, which we have seen before.
a) butane
b) $Ca_3(PO_4)_2$
c) ammonia
d) NH_4CN
e) $NaHCO_3$
f) $C_2HBrClF_3$ (halothane)
g) $C_{51}H_{98}O_6$ (a lipid)

4.64) Using the information gained from doing Problem 4.63, calculate the per cent by weight of *carbon* in
a) butane
b) ammonium cyanide
c) sodium hydrogen carbonate
d) halothane
e) the lipid of the previous problem

4.40) Would the simplest formula of each compound in Problem 4.38 be the *same* as that given? Determine the simplest formula for any cases that are not.

4.41*) How many grams of oxygen are contained in 10.0 grams of aluminum carbonate? Use information from Problem 4.38.

4.42*) Calculate the simplest formula of amphetamine sulfate from the following composition data: 46.3% carbon, 6.0% nitrogen, 6.5% hydrogen, 13.8% sulfur, and 27.5% oxygen.

4.43*) When marihuana passes through the body, one product contains 76.4% carbon, 9.2% hydrogen, and 14.5% oxygen. What is the simplest formula of this product?

4.44*) The compound in Problem 4.43 actually has a formula weight of 330 amu. What is its true molecular formula?

4.65) Would the simplest formula of each compound in Problem 4.63 be the *same* as that given? Determine the simplest formula for any cases that are not.

4.66*) How many grams of oxygen are contained in 25.0 grams of calcium phosphate? Use information from Problem 4.63.

4.67*) Calculate the simplest formula of an organic compound from the following composition data: 47.3% carbon, 10.6% hydrogen, and 42.0% sulfur.

4.68*) An organic compound called TCDD has 44.3% carbon, 2.47% hydrogen, 9.82% oxygen, and 43.5% chlorine. What is its simplest formula?

4.69*) The compound in Problem 4.68 actually has a formula weight of 326 amu. What is its true molecular formula?

Chemical Reactions and Equations

5

In previous chapters we concentrated on the mass and makeup of the formula unit of a pure substance. Now that you know how to write chemical formulas, we can discuss some chemical changes and begin writing chemical equations.

Let us first review in a systematic fashion the way a chemical formula is written. It is important now to put each number and letter in just the right place because other numbers called *coefficients* will be added when we write chemical equations.

If we write the formula for calcium phosphate, which is found in bone and in some kidney and bladder stones, we should have

$$\underset{a}{Ca}\ \underset{b}{_3}\ \underset{c}{(}\ \underset{}{P}\ \underset{}{O}\ \underset{d}{_4}\ \underset{c}{)}\ \underset{e}{_2}$$

Notice that

a) The chemical symbol for the more metallic element comes first in the formula. No number goes in front of it because that's the spot for equation coefficients.

b) A subscript shows how many calcium atoms (three) are in one formula unit of calcium phosphate. This number is never changed.

c) Parentheses are used to show that the *whole* phosphate anion, PO_4^{3-}, appears two times in the chemical formula.

d) The chemical symbols for the calcium cation and the phosphate anion appear without their charges. Charges are generally not shown in formulas.

e) A subscript shows how many whole phosphate groups (two) are in one formula unit. This number cannot be changed in the process of balancing a chemical equation.

There are several *wrong* ways to write formulas. Avoid them!

Not $3Ca^{2+}2PO^{3-}_4$ The number of calcium or phosphate ions must be written as a *subscript* (below the line) *after* the symbol and charges are not to be shown.*

---

* Do not confuse the formula of the compound with the formulas of the individual ions. We shall see later that in water solution we can write an equation for the dissociation of calcium phosphate in which ionic charges will appear:

$$Ca_3(PO_4)_2 \longrightarrow 3\ Ca^{2+} + 2\ PO_4^{3-}$$

Not $(Ca_3PO_4)_2$ That would double the number of calcium atoms to six, as well as provide two phosphates. The charges would then not balance. Everything inside the parentheses is multiplied by the subscript following.

Not $CA_3(Po_4)_2$ The symbol for calcium is Ca, not CA. Oxygen is O, not o.

Not $Ca_3P_2O_8$ While this contains the correct numbers of atoms, there is no indication that phosphate ions, PO_4^{3-}, are involved.

Now we are ready to start writing chemical equations.

5.1 BALANCING A CHEMICAL EQUATION

> *LEARNING GOAL 5A: Given a chemical equation, explain its meaning in terms of formula units of reactants and products.*
>
> *5B: Given the formulas of the reactants and products of a simple chemical equation, balance the equation.*

A **chemical equation** is a symbolic way of showing that one chemical substance has changed into another. Chemists often distinguish between physical change and chemical change.

Chemical and physical change

A **physical change** affects the shape, size, smoothness, or some other features of a substance without changing its composition, that is, its chemical formula. For example, cutting, polishing, freezing, melting, boiling, and expanding are physical changes. A small change in temperature affects some physical properties of a substance, such as density, but generally leaves chemical formulas unchanged. Dissolving sugar in water may be considered a physical change since the same sugar formula unit, $C_{12}H_{22}O_{11}$, exists both in the white powder and in the solution.

A **chemical change** results in a change in chemical formula. Paper burns; iron rusts; milk sours; a cake batter rises because a gas has been produced inside it. Each of these is a chemical change. We can often tell that a chemical change has occurred because we can see, smell, or feel a new substance. A change in color or the formation of a solid or gas from a clear solution provides evidence that a chemical change has probably occurred.

Coefficients

If you have used a hydrogen peroxide solution to bleach hair or disinfect a cut, you may have noticed some foaming. A gas is formed from hydrogen peroxide. The chemical equation to represent this is

$$2\ H_2O_2 \longrightarrow 2\ H_2O + O_2$$

We read this equation in English as "two hydrogen peroxide molecules decompose to give two water molecules and one oxygen molecule."

The "2" in front of the formulas for hydrogen peroxide and water is an **equation coefficient.** It tells you the ratio of water (two molecules) to oxygen (one molecule) in the products of this chemical change. If a coefficient is "1" (as for the oxygen), it is not shown.

The substances on the left-hand side of the equation, which *react,* are called the **reactants.** The substances on the right-hand side, those that are *produced,* are called **products.** The arrow pointing to the right shows that the reactant (H_2O_2) is disappearing and that the products (H_2O, O_2) are being made in this chemical reaction.

To show this clearly:

$$2\ H_2O_2 \longrightarrow 2\ H_2O + O_2$$

reactants   change to   products

Coefficients

We could write the same process with different coefficients:

$$30\ H_2O_2 \longrightarrow 30\ H_2O + 15\ O_2$$

but we would not be saying anything new. There is no reason to write coefficients of 30 and 15 because coefficients only show ratios, not the actual number of molecules involved. To give a ratio of 30/15 is simply a complicated way of writing 2/1. We therefore always use the *lowest* possible coefficients that properly give the formula unit ratios of the substances involved.*

Do not make the common mistake of thinking that the coefficient in an equation is telling you how much of that substance you have in a particular reaction. Writing "2 H_2O_2" does not give you any hydrogen peroxide at all! Equation coefficients are only good for determining reaction *ratios.*

Conservation of mass

Recall from Chapter 1 that an element is a kind of substance that never changes in an ordinary chemical reaction. An atom is the smallest particle of an element. The atomic nucleus thus does not change in any way during a chemical process. The number of atoms of each element going into the reaction as reactants must be the same as the number of atoms of each element coming out as products. In the hydrogen peroxide equation, there are four hydrogen atoms and four oxygen atoms on each side.

This must be true for every balanced chemical equation. **For each element involved, the number of atoms of that element on the two sides of the equation must be equal.**

Since the nucleus of an atom contains almost all of the atom's mass and since nuclei are not changed during a chemical process, it follows that the total mass of reactants must equal the total mass of products. This is another way of stating the *Law of Conservation of Mass* discussed in Section 2.4.

What does happen in a chemical change? *Electrons* are gained, lost, and shuffled around. Chemical bonding involves electrons. Bonds are broken and made; atoms that were once neighbors (having been bonded together) are now complete strangers. Chemical change thus involves the breaking apart and combination of groups of atoms, with no atoms being created or destroyed.

Writing and balancing equations

We are now ready to convert a *word description* of a chemical change to an equation. There are two important steps.

---

* Sometimes there are two ways to write an equation, depending on whether you insist that every coefficient be a whole number or will accept fractions. In this text, we will use only whole-number coefficients.

1) Write the correct chemical formula for each reactant to the left of the arrow and the chemical formula for each product to the right of the arrow. **Do not change any of these formulas.** Each symbol and subscript mean something and cannot be juggled. **Do not add any new formulas or remove any formulas.**

2) Using *coefficients* only, balance the number of atoms of each element. If you simply leave the formulas alone, you will find the balancing of chemical equations to be a relatively simple task. Here are some examples.

EXAMPLE 5a: Calcium metal reacts with carbon to give calcium carbide, CaC_2. Write a balanced equation that shows this.

– –

ANSWER: You first write an *unbalanced* equation that contains all of the reactants and products, with their correct formulas.

$$\text{Unbalanced:} \quad Ca + C \longrightarrow CaC_2$$

Now you count atoms on the left and right sides:
calcium: one on left = one on right
carbon: one on left $\neq$ two on right
We must adjust the coefficients so the number of carbon atoms comes out equal. Since the number of calcium atoms is already balanced, don't change the coefficient of any substance containing calcium. That leaves only one coefficient, that of carbon.

$$\text{Balanced:} \quad \boxed{Ca + 2\ C \longrightarrow CaC_2}$$

As a final check, count again to make sure there are equal numbers of atoms of each element and recheck that the reactants and products are indeed those given in the problem.

EXAMPLE 5b: Potassium solid reacts violently with water to give hydrogen gas and a solution of potassium hydroxide. Write the equation.

– –

ANSWER: Reactants are K and H_2O. The products are hydrogen gas, not H atoms but H_2, and potassium hydroxide, which you know from Section 4.2 to be KOH. (The reaction is shown in Figure 5–1.)

$$\text{Unbalanced:} \quad K + H_2O \longrightarrow H_2 + KOH$$

Now count atoms on the right and left sides. Potassium and oxygen balance, but hydrogen does not. The hydrogen from water must go to two places, into H_2 and into KOH. Try two waters.

$$\text{Unbalanced:} \quad K + 2\ H_2O \longrightarrow H_2 + KOH$$

Now oxygen is unbalanced, with two on the left and one on the right.

$$\text{Unbalanced:} \quad K + 2\ H_2O \longrightarrow H_2 + 2\ KOH$$

Now oxygen is balanced, and in the process, hydrogen has also become balanced. Only potassium is unbalanced. Add one K.

$$\text{Balanced:} \quad \boxed{2\ K + 2\ H_2O \longrightarrow H_2 + 2\ KOH}$$

Recheck the equation. You will notice that there has been a lot of "juggling" of coefficients to reach the right answer.

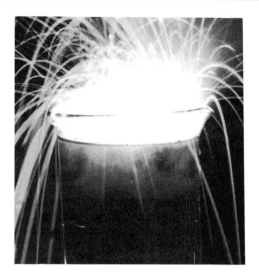

FIGURE 5–1 The reaction of potassium metal with water.

EXAMPLE 5c: Hydrogen burns in the presence of oxygen to give water. Write the equation. (See p. 4 to see how a passenger-carrying airship filled with hydrogen once burned disastrously.)

- -

ANSWER: The reactants are hydrogen and oxygen. What are the formulas? Both gases are diatomic, so we must use H_2 and O_2. (Remember the list of diatomic elements, H_2, N_2, O_2, and the halogens.)

$$\text{Unbalanced:}\quad H_2 + O_2 \longrightarrow H_2O$$

Oxygen is unbalanced. Try adding one water.

$$\text{Unbalanced:}\quad H_2 + O_2 \longrightarrow 2\ H_2O$$

Now hydrogen is unbalanced. Add one H_2.

$$\text{Balanced:}\quad \boxed{2\ H_2 + O_2 \longrightarrow 2\ H_2O}$$

Check the answer.

The process in Example 5c is called a *combination* reaction, where elements come together to make a compound.

EXAMPLE 5d: By passing a direct electrical current through water, we can decompose H_2O to its elements. Write the equation.

- -

ANSWER: The reactants are H_2O only. The products are O_2 and H_2. Therefore the balanced equation is the reverse of that in Example 5c:

$$\boxed{2\ H_2O \longrightarrow 2\ H_2 + O_2}$$

If we had not already done Example 5c, we would have gone through the steps shown there. (See Figure 1–3, p. 7, for a diagram of this process.)

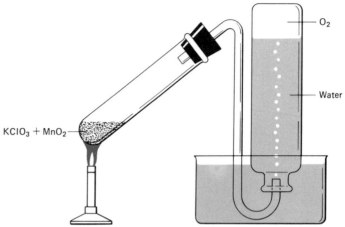

FIGURE 5–2   This mixture will produce O_2 gas when heated to about 200°C. The oxygen is usually collected and used in other experiments. (Example 5e.)

EXAMPLE 5e: A common freshman laboratory experiment involves heating potassium chlorate, $KClO_3$, solid in the presence of a small amount of manganese dioxide MnO_2 (Figure 5–2). The $KClO_3$ decomposes to oxygen and potassium chloride. Write the balanced equation.

- -

ANSWER: The reactants and products are given to you.

$$\text{Unbalanced:} \quad KClO_3 \longrightarrow KCl + O_2$$

Only oxygen is unbalanced. Try doubling the reactants.

$$\text{Unbalanced:} \quad 2\ KClO_3 \longrightarrow KCl + O_2$$

Now we must double the amount of potassium chloride.

$$\text{Unbalanced:} \quad 2\ KClO_3 \longrightarrow 2\ KCl + O_2$$

Finally we need to balance oxygen.

$$\text{Balanced:} \quad \boxed{2\ KClO_3 \longrightarrow 2\ KCl + 3\ O_2}$$

Why was MnO_2 needed in the test tube if it is not in the equation? It serves as a *catalyst,* something that speeds up the reaction without itself becoming used up. We will discuss catalysts further in Chapter 21. The enzymes required for all body reactions are also catalysts (Chapter 23).

Reminder: In Sections 5.2 and 5.3 be sure to answer each example yourself by working all the steps. Use a piece of paper or cardboard to cover parts you have not yet done. Write and balance the equation. Then check your answer against that given.

Writing nuclear equations

In Section 3.5 we discussed such nuclear changes as the emission of alpha or beta particles from natural radioactive atoms. These represent a third category of change, since they are not physical changes (in which chemical substances remain unchanged) or chemical changes (in which the formulas of substances change but the atoms of elements remain as they were). In a nuclear process, there is often a change in the isotope present, usually to a different number of protons and thus to a different element.

For example, when cobalt-60 is used to treat cancer it loses a beta particle (an electron). This can be written in equation form:

$$^{60}_{27}\text{Co} \longrightarrow ^{60}_{28}\text{Ni} + ^{0}_{-1}\text{e}$$

Like a conventional chemical equation, a **nuclear equation** shows the reactants (here $^{60}_{27}\text{Co}$) and the products (here, $^{60}_{28}\text{Ni}$ and an electron) with an arrow showing the direction of change. The superscripts giving the mass numbers must show that the Law of Conservation of Mass is obeyed, at least in broad totals. There are (approximately) 60 amu of mass in one atom of cobalt-60 and 60 amu of mass in total between nickel-60 and the beta particle. The subscripts showing the atomic number must reflect what happens to charge. Since the electron has a negative charge equal to the positive charge on a proton, it is shown with a -1 charge. Nickel has more protons than cobalt, since apparently one of the neutrons in cobalt-60 has converted to a proton plus an electron. That gives a net total of 27 positive charges on the two sides of the equation: $27 = 28 + (-1)$.

So long as you know the reactant in a natural radioactive decay process and know which particles are emitted, you can figure out the other products and write the nuclear equation.

EXAMPLE 5f: Write the nuclear equation for the emission of an alpha particle from radium-226, which is used to treat cancer.

- -

ANSWER: An alpha particle is a helium nucleus, ^4_2He. The helium nucleus contains four subparticles, two protons and two neutrons. We must therefore presume that the decay product atom has two fewer protons and two fewer neutrons than radium-226.

Radium-226 has 88 protons, and $(226 - 88) = 138$ neutrons. Taking away two protons and two neutrons would leave 86 protons and 136 neutrons. Since $Z = 86$ for the product, we have a radon (Rn) nucleus. Since the new mass number is $(86 + 136) = 222$, we have as a product $^{222}_{86}\text{Rn}$.

The nuclear equation is thus

$$\boxed{^{226}_{88}\text{Ra} \longrightarrow ^{4}_{2}\text{He} + ^{222}_{86}\text{Rn}}$$

The masses of the reactants and products in amu must be the same ($226 = 4 + 222$) and the positive charges must balance ($88 = 2 + 86$). The product isotope, radon-222, was discussed in Problem 3.89 as a noble gas that presents a natural source of radioactivity. It is found in some rocks used as building materials.

Similar nuclear equations are written to describe all types of radioactivity and nuclear changes, including those of fission and fusion (Section 3.5) and bombardment in nuclear laboratories.

SELF-CHECK

5.1)   Write a balanced equation for the formation of each of the following compounds from its elements. (Remember the diatomic gases.)
a)   KF   b)   CaO   c) NH_3 d) CH_4 e) N_2O_5 f) Al_2O_3
5.2)   You have already learned the names of the following compounds. Write the balanced equation for the formation of each from its elements.
a)   propane   c)   iron(III) fluoride (ferric fluoride)
b)   sodium oxide   d)   formaldehyde

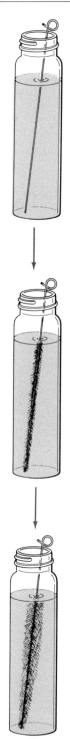

5.3)   Write the balanced equation for each of the following decomposition reactions, given the reactants and products.
a) $KClO_4$ (potassium perchlorate) gives KCl and oxygen gas
b) H_2SO_4 (sulfuric acid) gives water and sulfur trioxide, SO_3
c) HgO (mercury(II) oxide) decomposes to its elements
d) NH_4NO_2 (ammonium nitrite) gives water and nitrogen gas

5.2 SOME SIMPLE CHEMICAL REACTIONS

LEARNING GOAL 5C: Given the products and reactants in an aqueous solution reaction, write the chemical equation. Include the state of each reactant and product.

5D: Describe and recognize the difference between a conventional equation and an ionic equation for an aqueous reaction.

5E: Explain what is meant by reaction equilibrium.

5F: Given the formula of an organic compound containing carbon, hydrogen, and perhaps oxygen, write the balanced equation for its complete combustion.

There are many different kinds of inorganic chemical reactions, and we can only touch on a few here. The chemical industry, which has provided thousands of important products for modern living, uses many reactions between gases, liquids, and solids. The human body, however, provides a water-based environment for almost all of its chemistry. The reactants in a chemical process are brought together in the body by water, which we call an **aqueous** medium. Most of the chemistry of Chapters 17 to 28 takes place in water.

The manner in which water dissolves chemical substances will be discussed in Chapter 12. Water acts as a *solvent,* something that can draw chemical substances in between its own molecules and mix them thoroughly. Most inorganic substances, as well as many of the organic compounds of interest to us, dissolve in water.

States of reactants and products

Suppose we take a piece of copper metal (Cu) and place it in some solid silver nitrate ($AgNO_3$). Nothing will happen.

$$Cu + AgNO_3 \longrightarrow \text{no reaction}$$

However, if we dissolve the silver nitrate in water and *then* add a piece of copper, we will get a reaction (Figure 5–3):

$$Cu + 2\,AgNO_3 \longrightarrow Cu(NO_3)_2 + 2\,Ag$$

Now we have two chemical equations that seem to contradict each other. Does or does not copper react with silver nitrate?

Since water broke up the silver nitrate crystals and allowed the copper to react with silver ions (Ag^+), we should express that in some way. We can do so by indicating clearly for each reactant and product the **state** it is in:

FIGURE 5–3   Silver needles grow on copper wire in the reaction of copper with silver nitrate solution.

Solid state: (s)
Liquid state: (ℓ)

Gaseous state: (g)
Dissolved in water: (aq)

We can now rewrite the equation for Figure 5–3 showing states:

$$Cu_{(s)} + 2\ AgNO_{3(aq)} \longrightarrow Cu(NO_3)_{2(aq)} + 2\ Ag_{(s)}$$

We should read this as "one atom of copper metal reacts in water solution with two formula units of dissolved silver nitrate to give two atoms of silver metal plus one formula unit of dissolved copper(II) nitrate." Those particular metals do *not* dissolve in water, so both Cu and Ag are in their solid states. All nitrates do dissolve in water, so both silver nitrate and copper(II) nitrate are shown spread out (and mixed) into the water solution.

Make a habit of showing the states of all reactants and products (gaseous, liquid, solid, or in aqueous solution) whenever it might make a difference in the way a chemical reaction takes place.

Neutralization

A very important kind of reaction takes place between a compound that can *lose* H^+ (called an acid) and another that can *gain* H^+ (called a base). The reaction therefore involves the transfer of a proton from the acid to the base. There are many different kinds of acid-base reactions, some of which will be discussed in Chapter 13.

EXAMPLE 5g: Solid aluminum hydroxide is not very soluble in water. However, it is often used in antacids to treat "heartburn" and acid indigestion, since it will react with the dissolved HCl in stomach fluids. The products of a reaction between an acid and a *hydroxide* are an ionic salt and water. Write the balanced equation showing the states of all substances. $AlCl_3$ is soluble in water.

- -

ANSWER: The reactants are $Al(OH)_3$ solid and HCl solution. The products include a (different) ionic salt, which can only be aluminum chloride, $AlCl_3$. We are told that $AlCl_3$ is soluble in water. The other product is water, which is liquid. We can then write

Unbalanced: $Al(OH)_{3(s)} + HCl_{(aq)} \longrightarrow AlCl_{3(aq)} + H_2O_{(\ell)}$

Balance this in the usual fashion. There are three chlorines on the right.

Unbalanced: $Al(OH)_{3(s)} + 3\ HCl_{(aq)} \longrightarrow AlCl_{3(aq)} + H_2O_{(\ell)}$

Now only the number of water molecules needs to be adjusted.

Balanced: $\boxed{Al(OH)_{3(s)} + 3\ HCl_{(aq)} \longrightarrow AlCl_{3(aq)} + 3\ H_2O_{(\ell)}}$

EXAMPLE 5h: "Milk of magnesia" is a suspension of solid magnesium hydroxide in water. Vinegar is a solution of acetic acid, which we will write here $HC_2H_3O_2$. The acetate ion (from Table 4–2) is $C_2H_3O_2^-$. Magnesium acetate is soluble in water. Write the equation for the reaction of milk of magnesia with vinegar, showing all states.

- -

ANSWER: The reactants are $Mg(OH)_2$ solid and $HC_2H_3O_2$ solution. The products are water and the ionic salt $Mg(C_2H_3O_2)_2$ dissolved in water.

Unbalanced: $Mg(OH)_{2(s)} + HC_2H_3O_{2(aq)} \longrightarrow Mg(C_2H_3O_2)_{2(aq)} + H_2O_{(\ell)}$

Now balance acetates by doubling the number of acetic acid molecules.

Unbalanced: $Mg(OH)_{2(s)} + 2\ HC_2H_3O_{2(aq)} \longrightarrow Mg(C_2H_3O_2)_{2(aq)} + H_2O_{(\ell)}$

Hydrogen and oxygens still need balancing.

Balanced: $Mg(OH)_{2(s)} + 2\ HC_2H_3O_{2(aq)} \longrightarrow Mg(C_2H_3O_2)_{2(aq)} + 2\ H_2O_{(\ell)}$

You should notice from Examples 5g and 5h that the number of water molecules produced is equal to the number of OH^- ions neutralized.

Ionic equations

When a substance dissolves in water, it mixes completely so that each small amount of water contains the same amount of dissolved substance or *solute* (as described in Chapter 12). If the solute is covalently bonded, it will generally exist in *molecular* form as individual molecules dispersed (spread) through the water. This is true for table sugar, $C_{12}H_{22}O_{11}$, which in water solution still consists of sucrose molecules. We could write the dissolving of sugar crystals (or cubes)

$$C_{12}H_{22}O_{11(s)} \longrightarrow C_{12}H_{22}O_{11(aq)}$$

One of the properties of ionic salts is that they do not exist as molecules either in the solid state or in solution. The solid is held together by attraction between many cations and anions. In water, those cations and anions separate from each other. The dissolving of sodium chloride might be written

$$NaCl_{(s)} \longrightarrow NaCl_{(aq)}$$

but it would actually be more correct to write

$$NaCl_{(s)} \longrightarrow Na^+_{(aq)} + Cl^-_{(aq)}$$

The ionic solid breaks apart or *dissociates* into its ions. Each ion is surrounded by a group or cluster of water molecules, and the result is actually a chemical change, since ionic bonds between Na^+ and Cl^- are being broken.

Equations of the type in Examples 5a to 5h give a certain amount of information. In the case of dissolved ionic salts, even more accurate information is given by ionic equations.

While the equations in Examples 5g and 5h are correct for what they represent, the same processes could be written

5g: $Al(OH)_{3(s)} + 3\ H^+_{(aq)} \longrightarrow Al^{3+}_{(aq)} + 3\ H_2O_{(\ell)}$

5h: $Mg(OH)_{2(s)} + 2\ HC_2H_3O_{2(aq)} \longrightarrow Mg^{2+}_{(aq)} + 2\ C_2H_3O^-_{2(aq)} + 2\ H_2O_{(\ell)}$

You should recognize these as being **ionic equations**, since they show ions in aqueous solution. If your course requires you to be able to write such equations, the skill will be taught in Section 14.4. The HCl and $HC_2H_3O_2$ are treated differently in the above equations because one (HCl) is a *strong* acid and the other ($HC_2H_3O_2$) is a *weak* acid, as will be explained in Chapter 13.

Equilibrium

If you compare Example 5c with Example 5d, you will notice that one equation is simply the reverse of the other. Just about every chemical reaction is likely to happen both in the forward ($\rightarrow$) direction and also, to some extent, in the reverse ($\leftarrow$) direction. Sometimes this is significant; sometimes not. In the case of water and its elements, the two reactions shown go much in the direction shown by the arrows in each case.

Here is a different situation.

EXAMPLE 5i: Carbon dioxide gas (CO_2) will dissolve in water to give a solution called "club soda" or carbonated water. Under the conditions existing inside red blood cells, the dissolved CO_2 can be converted to H_2CO_3, carbonic acid, by reaction with water. Write the balanced equation, showing states.

- -

ANSWER: This is an easy combination equation.

$$CO_{2(aq)} + H_2O_{(\ell)} \longrightarrow H_2CO_{3(aq)}$$

EXAMPLE 5j: In the lungs, carbonic acid, H_2CO_3, dissolved in the fluid inside red blood cells will decompose to carbon dioxide and water. The carbon dioxide will then pass out of the blood and eventually be exhaled from the lungs. Write the equation, with states, for the decomposition of H_2CO_3.

- -

ANSWER: This is the reverse of Example 5i.

$$H_2CO_{3(aq)} \longrightarrow CO_{2(aq)} + H_2O_{(\ell)}$$

In the particular case of carbonic acid, like thousands of other biologically important reactions, both the forward reaction of Example 5i and the "reverse" reaction of Example 5j are happening *at the same time* to an important extent.

We call this situation **equilibrium.** We can write a chemical equation for an equilibrium situation, for example,

$$CO_{2(aq)} + H_2O_{(\ell)} \rightleftharpoons H_2CO_{3(aq)}$$

which indicates that, after some point in time, the number of H_2CO_3 molecules *decomposing* each second is equal to the number of H_2CO_3 molecules being *made* in that second. In other words, while both the forward and the reverse reactions are happening, the amount of each substance remains constant.

Vinegar, like lemon juice, has the characteristic tart taste of an acid. This taste is due to $H^+_{(aq)}$, a proton surrounded by water molecules, which is often instead written $H_3O^+_{(aq)}$ and called the *hydronium* ion. In the case of vinegar and lemon juice, there is an equilibrium between the acid and the $H^+_{(aq)}$ or H_3O^+ ions. For vinegar:

$$HC_2H_3O_{2(aq)} \rightleftharpoons H^+_{(aq)} + C_2H_3O_2{}^-{}_{(aq)}$$

This equilibrium will be discussed in Chapter 13. It is well to remember that almost all reactions do reach equilibrium at some stage.

SELF-CHECK

5.4)   Write balanced equations, showing the state of each reactant and product, for
a)   aluminum metal placed in iron(II) nitrate solution to give iron metal and a solution of aluminum nitrate

b) potassium oxide dissolved in water to give a solution of potassium hydroxide

c) sodium hydroxide solution added to solid oxalic acid, $H_2C_2O_4$, to give water and a solution of sodium oxalate, $Na_2C_2O_4$.

d) a solution of calcium hydroxide neutralized by sulfuric acid, H_2SO_4, solution to give a solution of calcium sulfate.

5.5) Describe and explain the differences in the following two ways of writing an equation for the neutralization of formic acid, HCOOH (found in ants), by sodium hydroxide solution.

a) $HCOOH_{(aq)} + NaOH_{(aq)} \longrightarrow HCOONa_{(aq)} + H_2O_{(\ell)}$

b) $HCOOH_{(aq)} + OH^-_{(aq)} \longrightarrow HCOO^-_{(aq)} + H_2O_{(\ell)}$

5.6) Inside red blood cells, there is an equilibrium set up between carbonic acid and bicarbonate ion:

$$H_2CO_{3(aq)} \rightleftharpoons HCO^-_{3(aq)} + H^+_{(aq)}$$

Explain exactly what we mean here by *equilibrium*.

Halogenation

In Section 4.4 we saw some simple organic molecules. The compounds methane, ethane, propane, and butane are all *alkanes,* which will be discussed in Section 7.1. An alkane may react with a halogen to produce an alkyl halide.

EXAMPLE 5k: Chloroethane, C_2H_5Cl, may be prepared by the reaction of ethane with chlorine gas. The other product is HCl gas. Write the balanced equation.

- -

ANSWER: The reactants are $C_2H_{6(g)}$ and $Cl_{2(g)}$. The products are HCl and C_2H_5Cl.

$$C_2H_6 + Cl_2 \longrightarrow C_2H_5Cl + HCl$$

The equation balances very easily.

EXAMPLE 5l: Chloroform, $CHCl_3$, is no longer used as an anesthetic but makes a good industrial solvent. It can be prepared by carefully controlled *chlorination* of methane. The equation?

- -

ANSWER: Reactants: CH_4 and Cl_2. Products: $CHCl_3$ and HCl.

Unbalanced: $CH_4 + Cl_2 \longrightarrow CHCl_3 + HCl$

We need as many chlorine molecules reacting as we have chlorines substituted on the methane. Try three chlorine molecules.

Unbalanced: $CH_4 + 3\ Cl_2 \longrightarrow CHCl_3 + HCl$

Now chlorines are unbalanced. Adjust the number of HCl molecules.

Balanced: $CH_4 + 3\ Cl_2 \longrightarrow CHCl_3 + 3\ HCl$

Combustion

Almost all organic compounds will burn in air. This is sometimes a disadvantage, often tragic, since billions of dollars worth of personal possessions and housing are lost each year to fires. On the other hand, the burning or **combustion** of organic fuels made of hydrocarbons allows us to drive our automobiles with *internal combustion* engines, ride in airplanes or motor boats, and heat our homes with oil and natural gas. Many people also obtain electricity from coal- or oil-burning power plants.

If there is plenty of air (containing 20% oxygen) available, the products of the combustion of an organic compound are generally carbon dioxide and water. We call this *complete* combustion.

EXAMPLE 5m: Write the equation for the complete combustion of methane. (Products: CO_2 and H_2O.)

- -

ANSWER: The reaction is with oxygen gas in the air.

Unbalanced: $CH_4 + O_2 \longrightarrow CO_2 + H_2O$

Balance hydrogen on both sides.

Unbalanced: $CH_4 + O_2 \longrightarrow CO_2 + 2\ H_2O$

Now balance oxygen atoms.

Balanced: $\boxed{CH_4 + 2\ O_2 \longrightarrow CO_2 + 2\ H_2O}$

The burning of natural gas consists largely of this reaction.

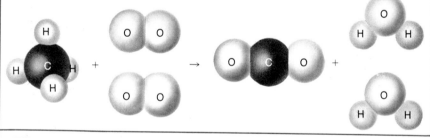

EXAMPLE 5n: Write the equation for the complete combustion of octane, C_8H_{18}, which is similar to the compounds in gasoline.

- -

ANSWER: Reactants: C_8H_{18} and O_2. Products: CO_2 and H_2O.

Unbalanced: $C_8H_{18} + O_2 \longrightarrow CO_2 + H_2O$

First balance carbon atoms, so that there are eight on each side.

Unbalanced: $C_8H_{18} + O_2 \longrightarrow 8\ CO_2 + H_2O$

Now balance hydrogen atoms so that there are 18 on each side.

Unbalanced: $C_8H_{18} + O_2 \longrightarrow 8\ CO_2 + 9\ H_2O$

Finally, balance oxygen atoms. We need $(8)(2) + 9 = 25$ atoms.

Balanced: $\boxed{C_8H_{18} + \dfrac{25}{2} O_2 \longrightarrow 8\ CO_2 + 9\ H_2O}$

Many chemists would leave the equation this way, even though we have a fractional coefficient of oxygen gas. Since we have asked you to consistently use whole number coefficients, multiply all coefficients by two.

Balanced: | $2 C_8H_{18} + 25 O_2 \longrightarrow 16 CO_2 + 18 H_2O$

A bit more complex this time, but the same rules apply. There are, to recheck, 16 carbon atoms, 36 hydrogen atoms, and 50 oxygen atoms on each side of the balanced equation.

Organic compounds containing oxygen will be discussed in detail in Chapter 9. You have already met several in earlier chapters, such as the alcohol used in drinks, C_2H_5OH, table sugar (sucrose), $C_{12}H_{22}O_{11}$, sodium benzoate, C_6H_5COONa, and calcium oxalate, CaC_2O_4.

Although you may not yet know the names and properties of all such compounds, you should be able to write equations for their complete combustion. The same steps apply as for the burning of hydrocarbons, except that you must remember, in counting *oxygen* atoms, to count those already inside the organic molecule.

EXAMPLE 5o: Many simple chemistry sets and field kits use alcohol lamps as a source of heat. Write the equation for the complete combustion of methyl alcohol.

- -

ANSWER: Reactants: CH_3OH and O_2. Products: CO_2 and H_2O.

Unbalanced: $CH_3OH + O_2 \longrightarrow CO_2 + H_2O$

Carbons are already balanced. Now balance hydrogens.

Unbalanced: $CH_3OH + O_2 \longrightarrow CO_2 + 2 H_2O$

Did you remember that CH_3OH has *four* hydrogens?
Finally balance oxygens, remembering the one inside CH_3OH.

Balanced: | $CH_3OH + \dfrac{3}{2} O_2 \longrightarrow CO_2 + 2 H_2O$

With whole number coefficients:

Balanced: | $2 CH_3OH + 3 O_2 \longrightarrow 2 CO_2 + 4 H_2O$

Since organic compounds will burn, fire is a particular hazard in organic and biochemical laboratories, where organic solvents like acetone, benzene, and ether are used. Smoking is very definitely OUT!

EXAMPLE 5p: Diethyl ether, $C_2H_5OC_2H_5$, is used both as a solvent and as an anesthetic for humans and for laboratory animals. What happens if you light a match around some ether?

- -

ANSWER: Reactants: $C_2H_5OC_2H_5$ and O_2. Products as usual.

Unbalanced: $C_2H_5OC_2H_5 + O_2 \longrightarrow CO_2 + H_2O$

Balance carbons first. There are *four* carbons in ether.

Unbalanced: $C_2H_5OC_2H_5 + O_2 \longrightarrow 4\ CO_2 + H_2O$

Now balance the *ten* hydrogens in ether.

Unbalanced: $C_2H_5OC_2H_5 + O_2 \longrightarrow 4\ CO_2 + 5\ H_2O$

Now balance oxygens, remembering the one in diethyl ether.

Balanced: $\boxed{C_2H_5OC_2H_5 + 6\ O_2 \longrightarrow 4\ CO_2 + 5\ H_2O}$

Many more organic reactions will be discussed in Chapters 7 to 9. Some of those reactions involve equilibrium, described in Section 5.2.

Equation shorthand

We have written balanced chemical equations showing all reactants and products. These equations are useful for keeping track of what is present in a chemical system and for developing weight relationships for the calculations of Section 5.4.

However, the organic chemist or biochemist is often interested in showing only the most important aspects of a chemical change. An arrow may be used in that case simply to show an organic reactant changing to an organic product, such as

$$CH_4 \xrightarrow{Cl_2} CHCl_3$$

This is *not* a chemical equation. It is a shorthand way for describing a chemical change. Be prepared to see many such diagrams in the chapters to come.

SELF-CHECK

5.7) Write balanced chemical equations for the complete combustion of
a) ethyl alcohol, which is occasionally used as an automobile fuel, especially in combination with gasoline as *gasohol*
b) propane, often used in stoves
c) the fuel acetylene, C_2H_2
d) glucose, a simple sugar (carbohydrate), $C_6H_{12}O_6$ (a similar process provides energy for living systems)

5.3 THE MOLE IN CHEMISTRY

LEARNING GOAL 5G: Given the number of grams of a substance whose formula is known, calculate the number of moles present; given the number of moles, calculate mass.

5H: Given the number of moles of a substance, use Avogadro's number to calculate the number of atoms, molecules, or formula units present.

You may someday wish to make up a solution for use in a hobby or profession or you may need to estimate how much heat will be produced by a given amount of fuel. Whenever in chemistry we have to answer the question "how much?" we must use mathematics.

There is no reason to be afraid of the kinds of arithmetic calculations we will be doing in the rest of this chapter or in the remainder of the course. Most chemists are not fond of higher mathematics. They rely on the *conversion-factor method* you learned in Chapter 2 to make their calculations simpler.

Avogadro's number

In Chapter 2 we discussed the atomic weight of an element, which is given in the periodic table and is measured in atomic mass units. In Section 4.5 we used those atomic weights to calculate the formula weight of a compound. Recall that

The formula weight of a substance is the sum of the atomic weights of all of the atoms that make up one formula unit or one molecule of that substance.

Since the atomic weight is the weighted average in amu of the masses of individual atoms, it, too, is measured in amu, and the formula weight has units of amu.

One atomic mass unit is equal to 1.66×10^{-24} grams, which can be written 0.000 000 000 000 000 000 000 001 66 grams. That's a pretty small weight. Also, 1 gram = 6.02×10^{23} amu = 602 000 000 000 000 000 000 000 amu. Since the mass of one gram was established hundreds of years ago and is in common use throughout the world, we must live with it. The mass of 1 amu is fixed by the actual masses of atomic nuclei. The relationship between them is called **Avogadro's number,** commemorating an important Italian scientist (see Section 10.4).

This number must be memorized: 6.02×10^{23}.

The mole

It is very difficult to work with individual atoms, molecules, and amu in the laboratory. Yet, much of our chemical information is in terms of what atoms and molecules do, and how much they weigh in amu. The chemist has saved much time and effort by inventing a unit of *amount,* the **mole,** such that

$$1 \text{ mole} = 6.02 \times 10^{23} \text{ objects}$$

One gram thus is the same as one mole of atomic mass units. We have a few other counting terms in common use, such as "a pair" or "a dozen." "A mole of" is simply the same kind of term. It is a very convenient amount of atoms, molecules, or formula units. For example, one mole of sodium chloride is a little less than $1/8$ of a pound. One cup of water is about 13 moles of water. A mole is an amount that can often be held, felt, and seen. The international symbol for mole is *mol,* as in "13 mol H_2O."

Mass of one mole

The wonderful advantage of having the mole as a chemical unit will quickly become apparent. One molecule of oxygen gas, which contains two atoms, has a formula weight of 32.0 amu. What is the mass of one mole of oxygen gas? Use conversion factors. We know that 1 mole of O_2 molecules $= 6.02 \times 10^{23}$ O_2 molecules and 1 mole of amu $= 6.02 \times 10^{23}$ amu $= 1$ g. Then we can calculate:

$$\frac{32.0 \text{ amu}}{1 \text{ molecule } O_2} \times \frac{1 \text{ g}}{6.02 \times 10^{23} \text{ amu}} \times \frac{6.02 \times 10^{23} \text{ } O_2 \text{ molecules}}{1 \text{ mole } O_2 \text{ molecules}} =$$

$$\frac{32.0 \text{ g}}{\text{mole } O_2 \text{ molecules}}$$

We get the *same number,* 32.0, although in different units.

One mole of atoms has the same mass *in grams* as the atomic weight written in the periodic table. One mole of carbon atoms has a mass of 12.0 grams. One mole of gold atoms has a mass of 197 grams, the same number as you find in the box for gold ($Z = 79$) in the periodic table (Figure 5–4).

One mole of formula units has the same mass *in grams* as the formula weight calculated from Section 4.5. Since one molecule of water has a mass of 18.0 amu, one mole of water has a mass of 18.0 grams. Since one formula unit of NaCl has a mass of 58.5 amu, one mole of NaCl has a mass of 58.5 grams.

We can summarize this by saying

The mass of one mole of atoms or formula units *in grams* **is the same as the atomic weight or formula weight in amu.**

The mole will be used for some very important calculations in Section 5.4, for gas calculations in Chapter 10, and for determining solution concentrations in Chapter 14. The pH scale used to describe acids and bases (Chapter 13) is based on the mole.

Some texts will call the weight of one mole of any substance the *molar weight* or *molar mass*. Others, especially older writings, distinguish between a *gram-atomic weight* (mass of one mole of atoms), a *gram-molecular weight* (mass of one mole of molecules), and a *gram-formula weight* (mass of one mole of formula units). Since they all mean "mass of one mole," you will understand these terms if you run across them.

Converting from grams to moles

The mass of one mole, given by the number of the atomic weight or formula weight, may be used as a conversion factor.

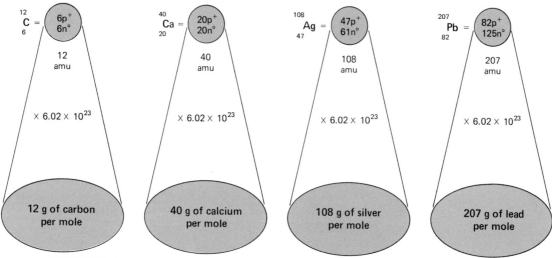

FIGURE 5–4 Avogadro's number (6.02×10^{23}) of atomic weights (in amu) will give the mass of one mole of atoms.

EXAMPLE 5q: How many moles
i) of iron atoms are there in 1 pound (454 grams) of iron metal?
ii) of hemoglobin molecules (formula weight 68 000 amu) are there in an average 150-pound person, who contains 900 grams of hemoglobin in the red blood cells?

ANSWER i) Use the conversion-factor method. The atomic weight or formula weight is always to be used as a conversion factor.

$$454 \text{ g Fe atoms} \times \frac{1 \text{ mole Fe atoms}}{55.85 \text{ g Fe atoms}} = \boxed{8.13 \text{ moles Fe atoms}}$$

ii)

$$900 \text{ g hemoglobin} \times \frac{1 \text{ mole hemoglobin}}{68\,000 \text{ g hemoglobin}} = \boxed{0.0132 \text{ mole hemoglobin}}$$

Converting from moles to grams

EXAMPLE 5r: What is the weight of
i) 1.50 moles of methane?
ii) 0.0788 mole of calcium chloride solid?
iii) 3.50 moles of carbon?

ANSWER i) You must calculate a formula weight for methane.
CH_4 has $(1 \text{ C})(12.0) + (4 \text{ H})(1.0) = 16.0$ amu/molecule
$= 16.0$ g/mole

Then

$$1.50 \text{ moles CH}_4 \times \frac{16.0 \text{ g CH}_4}{1 \text{ mole CH}_4} = \boxed{24.0 \text{ g CH}_4}$$

ii) Calculate a formula weight for $CaCl_2$.
$(1 \text{ Ca})(40.1) + (2 \text{ Cl})(35.5) = 111$ amu/formula unit $= 111$ g/mole

Then

$$0.0788 \text{ mole CaCl}_2 \times \frac{111 \text{ g CaCl}_2}{1 \text{ mole CaCl}_2} = \boxed{8.75 \text{ g CaCl}_2}$$

iii) The atomic weight of carbon from the periodic table is 12.0 amu, thus 12.0 g/mole.

$$3.50 \text{ moles C} \times \frac{12.0 \text{ g C}}{1 \text{ mole C}} = \boxed{42.0 \text{ g C}}$$

EXAMPLE 5s: What is the weight of 2.00 moles of oxygen?

ANSWER: ?
We don't know, because no formula has been given to us. Oxygen is an element. If what is meant is "2.00 moles of atoms of the element oxygen" then we can calculate:

$$2.00 \text{ moles O atoms} \times \frac{16.0 \text{ g O atoms}}{1 \text{ mole O atoms}} = \boxed{32.0 \text{ g O atoms}}$$

Oxygen also forms diatomic molecules. We usually mean, when we write "2.00 moles of oxygen," 2.00 moles of O_2 molecules.

$$2.00 \text{ moles } O_2 \times \frac{32.0 \text{ g } O_2}{1 \text{ mole } O_2} = \boxed{64.0 \text{ g } O_2 \text{ molecules}}$$

To choose between those two answers, we would need more information.

It is best, in doing this kind of problem, to look at each given quantity and decide which conversion factor will work best for it. Avoid trying to memorize "to go from grams to moles, we divide by the formula weight." It is much better to understand *how* to use conversion factors.

Converting between moles and atoms, molecules, or formula units

The conversion factor for going from the laboratory scale (grams, moles) to the atomic scale (atoms, molecules, formula units, and amu) is Avogadro's number.

EXAMPLE 5t: How many bromine *atoms* are in
  i) 8.56 moles of bromine atoms?
 ii) 0.0372 moles of Br_2 molecules?
iii) 1.67 moles of NaBr?
- -
ANSWER i)   The conversion factor is 6.02×10^{23} atoms/mole.

$$8.56 \text{ moles Br atoms} \times \frac{6.02 \times 10^{23} \text{ atoms Br}}{1 \text{ mole Br atoms}} = \boxed{5.15 \times 10^{24} \text{ Br atoms}}$$

ii)   We should first find the number of Br_2 molecules.

$$0.0372 \text{ moles } Br_2 \times \frac{6.02 \times 10^{23} \text{ molecules } Br_2}{1 \text{ mole } Br_2} = 2.24 \times 10^{22} \text{ } Br_2 \text{ molecules}$$

Now, realizing that there are two atoms of Br in one Br_2 molecule,

$$2.24 \times 10^{22} \text{ } Br_2 \text{ molecules} \times \frac{2 \text{ Br atoms}}{1 \text{ } Br_2 \text{ molecule}} = \boxed{4.48 \times 10^{22} \text{ Br atoms}}$$

iii)   Again, first find the number of NaBr formula units.

$$1.67 \text{ moles NaBr} \times \frac{6.02 \times 10^{23} \text{ NaBr units}}{1 \text{ mole NaBr}} = 1.01 \times 10^{24} \text{ NaBr units}$$

You know there is one atom of Br in each NaBr formula unit.

$$1.01 \times 10^{24} \text{ NaBr units} \times \frac{1 \text{ Br atom}}{1 \text{ NaBr unit}} = \boxed{1.01 \times 10^{24} \text{ Br atoms}}$$

5.8)   How many moles
a)   of fluorine atoms are in 190 grams of fluorine?
b)   of fluorine molecules in 190 grams of fluorine?
c)   of sodium fluoride units in 190 grams of NaF?
d)   of fluoromethane molecules in 190 grams of CH_3F?
5.9)   Calculate the mass in grams of
a)   17.5 moles of fluoromethane (see Question 5.8d)
b)   55.5 moles of water
c)   0.0125 mole of HCl
d)   1.27 moles of iodine atoms
5.10)   How many moles are contained in
a)   10 carbon atoms?
b) 6.02×10^{24} hydrogen molecules?
5.11)   How many
a)   oxygen molecules are in 0.890 moles?
b)   silver atoms in 18.5 moles?
c)   carbon atoms in 24.0 grams of carbon?
d)   carbon atoms in 3.50 grams of CH_4?

5.4 WEIGHT RELATIONSHIPS IN REACTIONS

LEARNING GOAL 5I: Interpret a chemical equation in terms of number of moles of reactants and products.
        5J: Given moles or grams of one reactant and assuming an excess of all other reactants, calculate the amount of product (in grams or moles) that could be formed.

In this section, we will answer the question "If I use so much reactant, how much product will I get?" We will use the conversion-factor method consistently to solve such problems, and the key is the use of *moles*.

Meaning of an equation (moles)

Let us look at the equation for the production of chloroform, which we saw in Example 5l:

$$CH_4 + 3 Cl_2 \longrightarrow CHCl_3 + 3 HCl$$

We could interpret this equation as meaning "one molecule of methane will react with three molecules of chlorine to give one molecule of chloroform and three molecules of hydrogen chloride."

Now, let us simply increase the number of molecules by a factor of Avogadro's number. Then "6.02×10^{23} molecules of methane react with 1.8×10^{24} molecules of chlorine to give 6.02×10^{23} molecules of chloroform and 1.8×10^{24} molecules of hydrogen chloride." That is the same as saying "one mole of methane reacts with three moles of chlorine to give one mole of chloroform and three moles of hydrogen chloride."

The coefficients in a balanced chemical equation give the mole ratios between the reactants and products.

Furthermore, since the coefficients give the mole ratios, we can obtain necessary *conversion factors* by looking at the balanced equation. Assuming that we are dealing with the above process, the following conversion factors (as examples) would come out of the equation:

$$\frac{1 \text{ mole } CH_4}{3 \text{ moles } Cl_2} \quad \frac{1 \text{ mole } CH_4}{1 \text{ mole } CHCl_3} \quad \frac{1 \text{ mole } CH_4}{3 \text{ moles } HCl} \quad \frac{3 \text{ moles } Cl_2}{3 \text{ moles } HCl}$$

Calculating amount of product

We can use the mole ratios gained from the coefficients of the balanced equation to relate the amount of reactant to the amount of product. To simplify matters, we will make the assumption that the conversion from reactant to product is 100% complete. In real life, this is not true, for reasons which include such factors as spillage and equilibrium situations. The **yield of products,** the amount obtained after a reaction is ''done,'' is always less than the theoretical amount, but knowing the theoretical yield is a start.

EXAMPLE 5u: Calculate the (theoretical) yield of chloroform in grams if 10.0 grams of methane react with an excess of chlorine.

- -

ANSWER: Looking at the balanced equation we have just written, one mole of CH_4 gives one mole of $CHCl_3$. Our problem can therefore be solved by

i)   changing grams of methane to moles of methane (using formula weight)

ii)   changing moles of methane to moles of chloroform (from the equation)

iii)   changing moles of chloroform to grams of chloroform (with formula weight)

Showing these three steps individually:

i) $\qquad 10.0 \text{ g } CH_4 \times \dfrac{1 \text{ mole } CH_4}{16.0 \text{ g } CH_4} = 0.625 \text{ mole } CH_4$

ii) $\qquad 0.625 \text{ mole } CH_4 \times \dfrac{1 \text{ mole } CHCl_3}{1 \text{ mole } CH_4} = 0.625 \text{ mole } CHCl_3$

iii)   Calculating a formula weight for $CHCl_3$ as 120 amu/molecule = 120 g/mole, we have

$$0.625 \text{ mole } CHCl_3 \times \frac{120 \text{ g } CHCl_3}{1 \text{ mole } CHCl_3} = \boxed{75.0 \text{ g } CHCl_3}$$

Or, we could use one long conversion factor set up as follows:

$$10.0 \text{ g } CH_4 \times \frac{1 \text{ mole } CH_4}{16.0 \text{ g } CH_4} \times \frac{1 \text{ mole } CHCl_3}{1 \text{ mole } CH_4} \times \frac{120 \text{ g } CHCl_3}{1 \text{ mole } CHCl_3} = \boxed{75.0 \text{ g } CHCl_3}$$

Given amount of reactant → moles of reactant → moles of product
→ mass of product

To summarize the steps involved in converting amount of reactant to amount of product (theoretical yield):

1) Change amount of reactant to moles (using formula weight as conversion factor)
2) Change moles of reactant to moles of product (using balanced equation)
3) Change moles of product to amount of product (using product formula weight)

The result will be the amount a "perfect chemist" would obtain if every atom of every element did exactly what it was "supposed to do" according to the chemical equation. In the real world, this never happens.

We will now try a situation where the mole ratio is *not* one to one. Remember to *cover the answers* and do your own work on each part of the example.

EXAMPLE 5v: Using the earlier equation,

$$CH_4 + 3\ Cl_2 \longrightarrow CHCl_3 + 3\ HCl,$$

i) if 9 molecules of Cl_2 react, how many molecules of $CHCl_3$ can be produced?

ii) if 5.0 moles of CH_4 are used up, how many moles of HCl can we obtain?

iii) if 71.0 grams of Cl_2 react, how many moles of HCl could result?

iv) if 25.0 grams of CH_4 are used up, how many grams of HCl could be produced?

- -

ANSWER:

i) $9 \text{ molecules } Cl_2 \times \dfrac{1 \text{ molecule } CHCl_3}{3 \text{ molecules } Cl_2} = \boxed{3 \text{ molecules } CHCl_3}$

ii) $5.0 \text{ moles } CH_4 \times \dfrac{3 \text{ moles HCl}}{1 \text{ mole } CH_4} = \boxed{15 \text{ moles HCl}}$

iii) $71.0 \text{ g } Cl_2 \times \dfrac{1 \text{ mole } Cl_2}{71.0 \text{ g } Cl_2} \times \dfrac{3 \text{ moles HCl}}{3 \text{ moles } Cl_2} = \boxed{1.00 \text{ mole HCl}}$

iv) $25.0 \text{ g } CH_4 \times \dfrac{1 \text{ mole } CH_4}{16.0 \text{ g } CH_4} \times \dfrac{3 \text{ moles HCl}}{1 \text{ mole } CH_4} \times \dfrac{36.5 \text{ g HCl}}{1 \text{ mole HCl}} = \boxed{171 \text{ g HCl}}$

Reactant-reactant relationships

Sometimes we wish to know how much of one reactant will be needed to react completely with a given amount of another reactant. The procedure is the same as for the previous examples.

EXAMPLE 5w: For the formation of water, $2\ H_2 + O_2 \longrightarrow 2\ H_2O$, how many grams of oxygen will be needed to react completely with:

i) 2.00 moles of hydrogen gas molecules?

ii) 12 grams of hydrogen gas?

- -

ANSWER:

i) $2.00 \text{ moles } H_2 \times \dfrac{1 \text{ mole } O_2}{2 \text{ moles } H_2} \times \dfrac{32.0 \text{ g } O_2}{1 \text{ mole } O_2} = \boxed{32.0 \text{ g } O_2}$

$$\text{ii)} \quad 12 \text{ g H}_2 \times \frac{1 \text{ mole H}_2}{2.0 \text{ g H}_2} \times \frac{1 \text{ mole O}_2}{2 \text{ moles H}_2} \times \frac{32.0 \text{ g O}_2}{1 \text{ mole O}_2} = \boxed{96 \text{ g O}_2}$$

If the amounts of the reactants are not equal, then one of them will be used up first. The other is in excess. We have to use the amount of the reactant that is used up first, the *limiting reactant*, to calculate the amount of product.

EXAMPLE 5x: For the reaction given in Example 5w, how many moles of water can be produced if we have as reactants
  i) 4.0 moles of H_2 and excess O_2?
 ii) 4.0 moles of H_2 and 2.0 moles of O_2?
iii) 4.0 moles of H_2 and 1.5 moles of O_2?

- -

ANSWER: i) Hydrogen will be used up first.

$$4.0 \text{ moles H}_2 \times \frac{2 \text{ moles H}_2\text{O}}{2 \text{ moles H}_2} = \boxed{4.0 \text{ moles H}_2\text{O}}$$

ii) How many moles of O_2 will react with 4.0 moles of H_2?

$$4.0 \text{ moles H}_2 \times \frac{1 \text{ mole O}_2}{2 \text{ moles H}_2} = 2.0 \text{ moles O}_2$$

Since we have exactly that much, both reactants will be used up at the same time. From above, we get 4.0 moles of H_2O. Or, using the amount of oxygen:

$$2.0 \text{ moles O}_2 \times \frac{2 \text{ moles H}_2\text{O}}{1 \text{ mole O}_2} = \boxed{4.0 \text{ moles H}_2\text{O}}$$

iii) How much O_2 is needed to react with all of the H_2? From before, we know that the amount needed is 2.0 moles of O_2. However, we do not have that much O_2. We have only 1.5 moles of O_2. Hydrogen is in excess, and the amount of water formed must be determined using the amount of the limiting reactant, O_2.

$$1.5 \text{ moles O}_2 \times \frac{2 \text{ moles H}_2\text{O}}{1 \text{ mole O}_2} = \boxed{3.0 \text{ moles H}_2\text{O}}$$

The general procedure to follow if you are given amounts of *two* reactants is to calculate the amount of product each reactant would give if it were all used up. That gives you two answers for the amount of product. Then choose the lower answer.

EXAMPLE 5y: In the Haber process for making ammonia, $3 H_2 + N_2 \longrightarrow 2 NH_3$, we mix 6.0 grams of H_2 with 8.0 grams of N_2. How many grams of NH_3 could result?

- -

ANSWER: First see what happens if all of the H_2 is used up.

$$6.0 \text{ g H}_2 \times \frac{1 \text{ mole H}_2}{2.0 \text{ g H}_2} \times \frac{2 \text{ moles NH}_3}{3 \text{ moles H}_2} \times \frac{17.0 \text{ g NH}_3}{1 \text{ mole NH}_3} = 34 \text{ g NH}_3$$

Now, what if all of the nitrogen were used up?

$$8.0 \text{ g N}_2 \times \frac{1 \text{ mole N}_2}{14.0 \text{ g N}_2} \times \frac{2 \text{ moles NH}_3}{1 \text{ mole N}_2} \times \frac{17.0 \text{ g NH}_3}{1 \text{ mole NH}_3} = 19 \text{ g NH}_3$$

It is clear that, in fact, all of the nitrogen *is* used up and hydrogen is present in excess. The theoretical yield is $\boxed{19 \text{ g } NH_3.}$

5.12)   A common antacid consists largely of chalk, $CaCO_3$, in a form that breaks apart quickly in the stomach. Its reaction with stomach acid is

$$CaCO_{3(s)} + 2 HCl_{(aq)} \longrightarrow CO_{2(g)} + H_2O_{(\ell)} + CaCl_{2(aq)}$$

State in words what is meant by this equation in terms of
a)   atoms, molecules, and formula units of reactants and products
b)   moles of reactants and products
5.13)   Using the equation of Question 5.12,
a)   how many moles of $CaCO_3$ will completely neutralize 1.0 mole of HCl?
b)   how many grams of $CaCO_3$ will completely neutralize 1.0 gram of HCl?
c)   how many grams of CO_2 gas (which is what makes you burp!) will be released by adding 1.0 gram of $CaCO_3$ to excess stomach acid?
d*)   how many grams of $CaCO_3$ will be needed to react completely with 1.5 liters of stomach acid with a concentration of 0.010 mole/liter?
e*)   if 5.0 grams of $CaCO_3$ are added to 0.080 mole of HCl in water solution, how many moles of CO_2 will be produced?

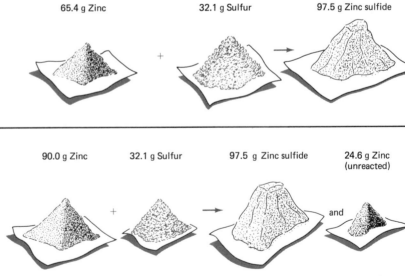

65.4 g Zinc   32.1 g Sulfur   97.5 g Zinc sulfide

90.0 g Zinc   32.1 g Sulfur   97.5 g Zinc sulfide   24.6 g Zinc (unreacted)

FIGURE 5–5   One reactant is almost always in excess in any real chemical reaction. By the law of conservation of mass, the amount in grams of ZnS produced by reaction of elemental zinc and sulfur must be the same as the amount of reactants lost. The reactants always react in the same mass ratio, as shown in the top drawing. If there is an excess of zinc, we find that excess left over at the end, unreacted, as in the bottom drawing.

CHAPTER FIVE IN REVIEW ■ Chemical Reactions and Equations

GLOSSARY FOR CHAPTER FIVE

aqueous Inside a water solution; pertaining to water; symbol "(aq)." (p. 130)

Avogadro's number The number of atoms, molecules, or formula units in a *mole*: 6.02×10^{23}; the number of atoms in exactly 12 grams of $^{12}_{6}C$. (p. 138)

chemical change A change in the elemental composition (chemical formula) of the substances present; bonds are broken and/or formed; *reactant* substances disappear and *product* substances are formed; represented by a *chemical equation*. (p. 124)

chemical equation A shorthand way of using chemical formulas to represent a chemical change, using equation coefficients to show the relative amounts of reactants and products. (p. 124)

combustion The reaction of a substance with oxygen to give oxides; particularly the complete reaction of an organic compound (in air) to give carbon dioxide and water; burning. (p. 135)

equation coefficient A number placed before a chemical formula in a *chemical equation* to indicate the relative number of units of that substance that participate in the reaction; also shows the relative number of *moles* of that substance. (p. 124)

equilibrium A condition in which a reverse reaction takes place at the same speed as a forward reaction so that there is no net change in the amounts of *reactants* or *products* over a period of time. (p. 133)

ionic equation A *chemical equation* that shows substances ionized in *aqueous* solution in the form of their ions. (p. 132)

mole The chemist's unit of amount of substance present; the amount containing *Avogadro's number* of formula units; the amount containing as many grams as the formula weight of the substance (the international symbol is "mol," but "mole" is still widely used). (p. 138)

nuclear equation A shorthand way of using nuclear symbols to represent a nuclear change, as in radioactivity. (p. 129)

physical change A change in the temperature, shape, or *state* of

matter without any change in the composition or formula unit of the substance. (p. 124)

products In a *chemical change,* the substances present after the change takes place which were not present earlier; the new substances formed. (p. 125)

reactants In a *chemical change,* the substances present at the start of the change which are not present in as great amounts later; the substances destroyed by the change. (p. 125)

state The physical form of a substance that indicates how tightly it is held in place by its neighbors; normally considered to include the solid (s), liquid (ℓ), and gaseous (g) states of a pure substance, as well as the *aqueous* (aq) state for a dissolved substance. (p. 130)

yield of products The amount of products obtained from a particular chemical change, especially in comparison with the amount (in moles) of reactants used up. (p. 143)

QUESTIONS AND PROBLEMS FOR CHAPTER FIVE ■
Chemical Reactions and Equations

SECTION 5.1 BALANCING A CHEMICAL EQUATION

5.14) Explain the meaning in terms of atoms, molecules, and formula units of
a) $2 \text{ KClO}_3 \longrightarrow 2 \text{ KCl} + 3 \text{ O}_2$
b) $2 \text{ CH}_3\text{OH} + 3 \text{ O}_2 \longrightarrow$
$$2 \text{ CO}_2 + 4 \text{ H}_2\text{O}$$

5.15) Write the balanced equation for the formation of each of the following compounds from its elements at room temperature:
a) calcium fluoride
b) carbon monoxide
c) sodium iodide
d) propane

5.16) Write the balanced equation for each decomposition reaction:
a) sodium chloride decomposes to its elements by electrolysis

5.34) Explain the meaning in terms of atoms, molecules, and formula units of
a) $\text{Na}_2\text{O} + \text{H}_2\text{O} \longrightarrow 2 \text{ NaOH}$
b) $(\text{C}_2\text{H}_5)_2\text{O} + 6 \text{ O}_2 \longrightarrow$
$$4 \text{ CO}_2 + 5 \text{ H}_2\text{O}$$

5.35) Write the balanced equation for the formation of each of the following compounds from its elements at room temperature:
a) potassium sulfide
b) ethyl alcohol
c) iron(II) oxide
d) butane

5.36) Write the balanced equation for each decomposition reaction:
a) hydrogen iodide, HI, decomposes to its elements by electrolysis

b) hydrogen sulfite, H_2SO_3, gives water and SO_2 gas

5.17*) Write the nuclear equation (refer to Table 3–5) for
a) the formation of technetium-99 by beta decay from another isotope
b) the decay of tritium
c) the decay of uranium-238 with emission of an alpha ray. ($Z = 92$.)

b) calcium hydroxide when heated gives calcium oxide and water

5.37*) Write the nuclear equation (refer to Table 3–5) for
a) the formation of radium-226 by alpha decay from another isotope
b) the decay of sulfur-35
c) the decay of uranium-235 with emission of an alpha ray. ($Z = 92$.)

SECTION 5.2 SOME SIMPLE CHEMICAL REACTIONS

5.18) Balance the following not-yet-balanced equations, in which correct chemical formulas are already written for reactants and products:
a) $P + O_2 \longrightarrow P_2O_3$
b) $P_2O_3 + H_2O \longrightarrow H_3PO_3$
c) $Al + Fe_2O_3 \longrightarrow Fe + Al_2O_3$
d) $NaBr + F_2 \longrightarrow NaF + Br_2$
e) $H_2O_2 \longrightarrow H_2O + O_2$
f) $MgCO_3 \longrightarrow MgO + CO_2$
g) $NH_4NO_2 \longrightarrow N_2 + H_2O$

5.38) Balance the following not-yet-balanced equations, in which correct chemical formulas are already written for reactants and products:
a) $P + O_2 \longrightarrow P_2O_5$
b) $P_2O_5 + H_2O \longrightarrow H_3PO_4$
c) $C + Fe_2O_3 \longrightarrow Fe + CO$
d) $KI + Cl_2 \longrightarrow I_2 + KCl$
e) $BaO_2 \longrightarrow BaO + O_2$
f) $Al_2(CO_3)_3 \longrightarrow Al_2O_3 + CO_2$
g) $K_4Fe(CN)_6 \longrightarrow KCN + Fe + C + N_2$

5.19) Balance the following:
a) $Na_{(s)} + H_2O_{(\ell)} \longrightarrow$
   $\qquad H_{2(g)} + NaOH_{(aq)}$
b) $Al_2O_{3(s)} + HCl_{(aq)} \longrightarrow$
   $\qquad AlCl_{3(aq)} + H_2O_{(\ell)}$
c) $H_{2(g)} + FeO_{(s)} \longrightarrow H_2O_{(\ell)} + Fe_{(s)}$
d) $Fe_2O_{3(s)} + CO_{(g)} \longrightarrow Fe_{(s)} + CO_{2(g)}$
e) $ZnCO_{3(s)} + HCl_{(aq)} \longrightarrow$
   $\qquad ZnCl_{2(aq)} + CO_{2(g)} + H_2O_{(\ell)}$
f) $FeS_{(s)} + HBr_{(aq)} \longrightarrow$
   $\qquad FeBr_{2(aq)} + H_2S_{(aq)}$
g) $AgNO_{3(aq)} + AlCl_{3(aq)}$
   $\qquad \longrightarrow AgCl_{(s)} + Al(NO_3)_{3(aq)}$

5.39) Balance the following:
a) $Ca_{(s)} + H_2O_{(\ell)} \longrightarrow$
   $\qquad H_{2(g)} + Ca(OH)_{2(aq)}$
b) $K_2O_{(s)} + HNO_{3(aq)} \longrightarrow$
   $\qquad KNO_{3(aq)} + H_2O_{(\ell)}$
c) $H_{2(g)} + Fe_2O_{3(s)} \longrightarrow H_2O_{(\ell)} + Fe_{(s)}$
d) $Al_{(s)} + AgNO_{3(aq)} \longrightarrow$
   $\qquad Al(NO_3)_{3(aq)} + Ag_{(s)}$
e) $Fe_2(CO_3)_{3(s)} + HNO_{3(aq)} \longrightarrow$
   $\qquad Fe(NO_3)_{3(aq)} + CO_{2(g)} + H_2O_{(\ell)}$
f) $Ca_3(PO_4)_{2(s)} + HCl_{(aq)} \longrightarrow$
   $\qquad CaCl_{2(aq)} + H_3PO_{4(aq)}$
g) $Ba(NO_3)_{2(aq)} + H_2SO_{4(aq)} \longrightarrow$
   $\qquad BaSO_{4(s)} + HNO_{3(aq)}$

5.20) Given the following acid and base reactants in a neutralization reaction, write the products (water and a dissolved ionic salt) and balance the equation. Show all states.
a) $NaOH_{(aq)}$ and $HNO_{3(aq)}$
b) $Ca(OH)_{2(s)}$ and $HI_{(aq)}$
c) $Ba(OH)_{2(aq)}$ and $H_2C_2O_{4(s)}$
d) solid magnesium hydroxide and hydrochloric acid, $HCl_{(aq)}$

5.40) Given the following acid and base reactants in a neutralization reaction, write the products (water and a dissolved ionic salt) and balance the equation. Show all states.
a) $KOH_{(aq)}$ and $H_2SO_{4(aq)}$
b) $Al(OH)_{3(s)}$ and $HF_{(aq)}$
c) $Cu(OH)_{2(s)}$ and $HC_2H_3O_{2(aq)}$
d) solid cobalt(II) hydroxide and nitrous acid, $HNO_{2(aq)}$

5.21) The reaction in Problem 5.20a may also be written in either of the following forms:

$Na^+_{(aq)} + OH^-_{(aq)} + H^+_{(aq)} + NO^-_{3(aq)}$
$\qquad \longrightarrow Na^+_{(aq)} + NO^-_{3(aq)} + H_2O_{(\ell)}$

5.41) The reaction in Problem 5.40b may also be written in the following form:

$Al(OH)_{3(s)} + 3\ HF_{(aq)} \longrightarrow$
$\qquad Al^{3+}_{(aq)} + 3\ F^-_{(aq)} + 3\ H_2O_{(\ell)}$

or

$$OH^-_{(aq)} + H^+_{(aq)} \longrightarrow H_2O_{(\ell)}$$

How do these ways of writing a neutralization equation differ from what you wrote in your earlier answer? What do we call these equations? What is their advantage?

5.22) Calcium ion can be added to or removed from bone, depending on the level of that ion in body fluids. Unwanted deposits of calcium and magnesium salt solids may occur in such organs as the kidneys and bladder. These deposits may block the tubules leading to the organs, causing severe pain; we call them stones or calculi. Part of the explanation for both of these facts lies in the equilibrium

$$Ca_3(PO_4)_{2(s)} \rightleftharpoons 3\ Ca^{2+}_{(aq)} + 2\ PO^{3-}_{4(aq)}$$

Explain the meaning of this equation.

5.23*) Balance the following ionic equations, making sure all charges and atoms balance:
a) $Ag^+_{(aq)} + SO^{2-}_{4(aq)} \longrightarrow Ag_2SO_{4(s)}$
b) $Cu^{2+}_{(aq)} + NH_{3(aq)} \longrightarrow Cu(NH_3)^{2+}_{4(aq)}$

5.24) Balance the following equations, for which the reactants and products are given:
a) making acetylene:

$$CaC_2 + H_2O \longrightarrow Ca(OH)_2 + C_2H_2$$

b) chlorinating methane:

$$CH_4 + Cl_2 \longrightarrow CH_3Cl + HCl$$

5.25) Write and balance the equations for the complete combustion (to CO_2 and water) of the following organic compounds:
a) ethene, C_2H_4
b) hexane, C_6H_{14}
c) butanol, C_4H_9OH
d) acetone, CH_3COCH_3
e) table sugar, $C_{12}H_{22}O_{11}$

SECTION 5.3 THE MOLE IN CHEMISTRY

5.26) How many grams of iron are in 0.25 moles of iron atoms?

How does this way of writing a neutralization equation differ from what you wrote in your earlier answer? What do we call this equation? What is its advantage?

5.42) The body needs a way to regulate the acidity of the urine. Two equilibrium *buffer* systems (Chapter 13) are involved, which can be represented by the equations

$$HPO^{2-}_{4(aq)} + H^+_{(aq)} \rightleftharpoons H_2PO^-_{4(aq)}$$

and

$$NH_{3(aq)} + H^+_{(aq)} \rightleftharpoons NH^+_{4(aq)}$$

Describe and explain what is meant by these two equations. (All of the substances should be familiar from previous chapters.)

5.43*) Balance the following ionic equations, making sure all charges and atoms balance:
a) $Ca^{2+}_{(aq)} + F^-_{(aq)} \longrightarrow CaF_{2(s)}$
b) $Zn(OH)_{2(s)} + OH^-_{(aq)} \longrightarrow$
$$Zn(OH)^{2-}_{4(aq)}$$

5.44) Balance the following equations, for which the reactants and products are given:
a) fermenting grape juice into wine:

$$C_6H_{12}O_6 \longrightarrow C_2H_5OH + CO_2$$

b) brominating ethane:

$$C_2H_6 + Br_2 \longrightarrow C_2Br_6 + HBr$$

5.45) Write and balance the equations for the complete combustion (to CO_2 and water) of the following organic compounds:
a) pentyne, C_5H_8
b) butane, C_4H_{10}
c) isopropyl alcohol, C_3H_7OH
d) acetaldehyde, CH_3CHO
e) cholesterol, $C_{27}H_{46}O$

5.46) How many grams of copper are in 0.33 mole of copper atoms?

5.27) How many moles of the substance indicated are in the masses given below?
a) 36.0 g of C atoms
b) 0.00471 g of Mg atoms
c) 4.04 g of H_2 molecules
d) 3.69×10^4 g of N atoms
e) 5.00 g of HF
f) 0.0593 g of NaCl
g) 17.6 g of $CHCl_3$

5.28) Calculate the mass in grams of the following amounts:
a) 0.0875 mole of K atoms
b) 3.75 moles of O_2 molecules
c) 31.4 moles of $CaCl_2$
d) 1.74 moles of octane, C_8H_{18}

5.29) The quantity 0.539 mole of methyl alcohol, CH_3OH, represents
a) what total mass?
b) how many CH_3OH molecules?
c) how many oxygen atoms?
d) how many hydrogen atoms?

5.30) Suppose we had 392 molecules of $C_{12}H_{22}O_{11}$, which is sucrose or table sugar. We would then have
a) how many hydrogen atoms?
b) how many moles of sucrose?
c) how many grams of sucrose?
d) how many moles of oxygen atoms?

5.47) How many moles of each substance indicated are in the masses given below?
a) 2.30 g of Na atoms
b) 0.0792 g of S atoms
c) 96.0 g of O_2 molecules
d) 1.82×10^7 g of Cl atoms
e) 5.00 g of HCl
f) 0.0391 g of CaS
g) 59.2 g of C_2H_5OH

5.48) Calculate the mass in grams of the following amounts:
a) 0.666 mole of Sn atoms
b) 17.6 moles of H_2 molecules
c) 217 moles of $Ca_3(PO_4)_2$
d) 8.63 moles of heptane, C_7H_{16}

5.49) A mass of 13.9 grams of ammonium nitrate, NH_4NO_3, represents
a) how many moles?
b) how many formula units of NH_4NO_3?
c) how many oxygen atoms?
d) how many nitrogen atoms?

5.50) Suppose we had 151 molecules of alanine, an amino acid shown in Figure 1–4, with formula $C_3H_7NO_2$. We would then have
a) how many hydrogen atoms?
b) how many moles of alanine?
c) how many grams of alanine?
d) how many moles of oxygen atoms?

SECTION 5.5 WEIGHT RELATIONSHIPS IN REACTIONS

5.31) Consider the breaking up of urea, H_2NCONH_2, in the body to give ammonia and carbon dioxide:

$$H_2NCONH_{2(aq)} + H_2O_{(\ell)} \longrightarrow$$
$$2\ NH_{3(aq)} + CO_{2(aq)}$$

a) Explain the meaning of this equation in terms of molecules.
b) Explain the meaning of this equation in terms of moles.
c) If 3.00 moles of urea react completely, how many moles of ammonia will be formed?
d*) How many moles of water are needed to react fully with 3.00 moles of urea?
e) If 10.0 g of H_2NCONH_2 react completely, how many grams of NH_3 are produced?

5.51) Methyl alcohol can be made commercially by the reaction

$$CO_{(g)} + 2\ H_{2(g)} \longrightarrow CH_3OH_{(g)}$$

a) Explain the meaning of this equation in terms of molecules.
b) Explain the meaning of this equation in terms of moles.
c) If 2.50 moles of H_2 gas react completely, how many moles of methyl alcohol will be formed?
d*) How many moles of carbon monoxide, CO, are needed to completely react with 0.568 mole of hydrogen molecules?
e) If 10.0 g of H_2 react completely, how many grams of CH_3OH will be formed?

5.32) Emergency oxygen masks contain potassium superoxide, KO_2, pellets. When the exhaled CO_2 from the lungs passes through the KO_2, we get the reaction

$$4 KO_{2(s)} + 2 CO_{2(g)} \longrightarrow 2 K_2CO_{3(s)} + 3 O_{2(g)}$$

The oxygen produced can then be breathed in, so no air from outside the mask is needed.
a) If 125 g of KO_2 are used up completely, how many grams of O_2 will be produced?
b*) How many grams of KO_2 are needed to completely react with 1.00 kg of CO_2? (Remember that 1 kg = 1000 g.)
c*) If we know that 5.00 moles of O_2 have been produced in a certain period of time, how many grams of KO_2 have been used up?
d*) If 150 g of KO_2 and 60.0 g of CO_2 react together, what is the maximum amount of O_2 (in grams) that can be formed?

5.33*) Baking cakes and pastries involves the production of CO_2 to make the batter "rise." For example, citric acid in lemon or orange juice can react with baking soda to give carbon dioxide gas:

$$H_3C_6H_5O_{7(aq)} + 3 NaHCO_{3(aq)} \longrightarrow$$
citric acid   baking soda
$$Na_3C_6H_5O_{7(aq)} + 3 CO_{2(g)} + 3 H_2O_{(\ell)}$$
sodium citrate

a) Suppose 6.00 g of citric acid react with 20.0 g of sodium hydrogen carbonate. Which reactant will be in excess? What is the maximum number of grams of CO_2 that can be formed?
b) One mole of CO_2 gas at the temperature of a baking oven (400°F = 204°C) occupies about 39.2 liters. How many liters of empty space do you thus expect for the cake made by the combination in Question 5.33a?
c) The actual size of the cake will be less than predicted, for various reasons. Can you think of any?

5.52) Spacecraft must carry adequate supplies of oxygen for the astronauts and must remove exhaled carbon dioxide. One method of removal is by the process

$$2 LiOH_{(s)} + CO_{2(g)} \longrightarrow Li_2CO_{3(s)} + H_2O_{(g)}$$

a) If 25.0 g of LiOH powder are completely used up, how many grams of water vapor will be produced?
b*) If one astronaut releases 1.00 kilogram of CO_2 each day, how many grams of LiOH will be needed per day for each member of the crew?
c*) If we know that 2.00 moles of water vapor have been produced in a certain period, how many grams of CO_2 were absorbed by the system in that period?
d*) If 50.0 g of LiOH and 50.0 g of CO_2 react together, what is the maximum amount of Li_2CO_3 (in grams) that can be formed?

5.53*) Photosynthesis is the most fundamental reaction of life, since it converts the sun's energy to energy for plants, and ultimately for animals. In green plants, the compound *chlorophyll* (Chapter 25) absorbs sunlight and makes the following reaction possible (oversimplified):

$$6 CO_{2(g)} + 6 H_2O_{(\ell)} \longrightarrow C_6H_{12}O_{6(s)} + 6 O_{2(g)}$$

a) Suppose 50.0 g of water react with 120 g of CO_2 in photosynthesis. Which reactant will be in excess? What is the maximum number of grams of the carbohydrate $C_6H_{12}O_6$ that can be formed?
b) One mole of O_2 gas at a normal summer air temperature of 68°F = 20°C occupies a volume of about 24.0 liters. How many liters of oxygen gas would you expect for the combination in Question 5.53a?
c) The actual yield of $C_6H_{12}O_6$ from this process may be less than predicted, for various reasons. Can you think of any?

Covalent Bonding 6

You received an introduction to ionic and covalent bonding in Chapter 4, at the same time you were learning how to write the formulas of some simple ionic and covalent compounds. At that point, we tried to keep away from "theory" so that you could concentrate on writing molecular and structural formulas.

In order to understand the properties of organic compounds, it is useful to know a little more about covalent bonding. Some covalent bonds are stronger than others; some are longer than others. Many covalent bonds are a bit "ionic," while *all* ionic bonds have some covalent character. The information in this chapter will help you to predict some of the physical properties of substances, such as the melting point and boiling point, which are mentioned in later chapters. When acids are discussed in Chapter 13, you will have a better understanding of why some are strong and some are weak. The unique properties of aromatic ring systems (Chapter 15) come from delocalized electrons, which will be discussed here. Finally, many of the bonds and attractions that hold together such biochemically important molecules as proteins will only make sense if you understand some of the differences between covalent bonds.

6.1 POLARITY OF COVALENT BONDS

LEARNING GOAL 6A: Describe the trends in electronegativity values for representative elements across and down the periodic table.

6B: Given a table of electronegativity values and given a particular bonding pair of atoms, predict whether the attraction between them should be considered an ionic bond, a polar covalent bond, or a nonpolar covalent bond.

6C: Given a polar covalent bond, state which side can be considered to have a partial positive charge and which a partial negative charge.

6D: Describe or predict the effect of bond polarity on the length and strength of covalent bonds.

Ionization energy trends

The trends in ionization energies for many of the representative elements were discussed briefly in Chapter 3.

1	2		3	4	5	6	7	8
							H 315	He 568
Li 126	Be 216		B 193	C 261	N 337	O 316	F 403	Ne 499
Na 120	Mg 178		Al 140	Si 189	P 244	S 240	Cl 302	Ar 365
K 102	Ca 142		Ga 140	Ge 184	As 228	Se 226	Br 274	Kr 324
Rb 98	Sr 133		In 135	Sn 171	Sb 201	Te 210	I 243	Xe 281
Cs 90	Ba 122		Tl 142	Pb 173	Bi 170	Po 196	At	Rn 249

FIGURE 6–1   Ionization energies of the representative elements in kilocalories per mole. The highest values are in the upper right-hand corner. The lowest values are for the metals in the lower left-hand corner.

Recall that an ionization energy is the "pull" required to remove an electron from an atom. Figure 3–9 graphed the ionization energies of the first 20 elements so that the periodic trends could be seen. Figure 6–1 lists the ionization energies for some elements. Note the trends in Figure 6–1.

Atomic size

The sizes of many atoms have been calculated from what we know about their spacing. Figure 6–2 shows the relative **atomic sizes** of different elements. The radius of an atom increases as one goes down a group of the periodic table because the outermost electrons are in higher principal energy levels, farther from the nucleus. The atoms get smaller from left to right across the table because nuclear charge is increasing.

The trends in atomic size are exactly opposite the trends in ionization energy. The same factors that make an outer (valence) electron difficult to remove from a nonmetal atom (high ionization energy) also bring it close to the nucleus.

Size of ions

When a metal atom loses an electron, the charge difference remaining (more protons than electrons) causes the outermost electrons to move closer to the nucleus, as shown in Figure 6–3. In terms of **ionic size,** then, a positive ion is smaller than its neutral atom. When an atom of a nonmetal gains electrons, it becomes larger for similar reasons; an anion is larger than its neutral atom.

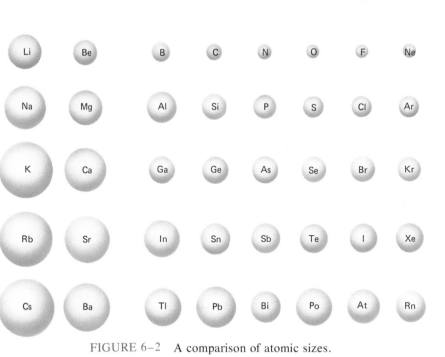

FIGURE 6–2   A comparison of atomic sizes.

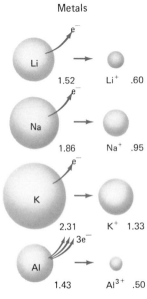

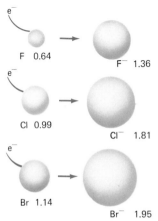

FIGURE 6–3   Relative size in Å. (1 Å = 10^{-8} cm) of some Group 1 and Group 7 atoms and ions.

The sizes of atoms and ions have a lot to do with the chemical bonds they form. The closer two nuclei come to each other, the more they repel (push away) each other. However, the closer a nucleus comes to an electron cloud of another atom, the more the two atoms will be attracted to each other (Figure 6–4). There is thus a balance of forces.

The sizes of the atoms involved in bonding also affect the physical properties of many compounds, especially organic substances containing oxygen and nitrogen, as will be seen when we discuss hydrogen-bonding in Chapter 11.

Electron affinity

A quantity that is difficult to measure but plays a role in chemical bonding is the tendency of a neutral atom to gain electrons. This tendency is clearly high (and important) for atoms that form 1 − ions, such as the halogens of Group 7. **Electron affinity** is the energy given off when a neutral gaseous atom adds one electron to become a 1 − ion. Some electron affinity values are, for second-period elements in kcal/mole, Li 14.3, Be −57, B 6, C 29, N 0, O 34, F 77, and Ne −7.

The values for ionization energies and electron affinities may be expressed in kilocalories per mole of atoms. The mole was defined in Chapter 5. A kilocalorie is perhaps most familiar as the common "Calorie" of food energy used in all nutrition discussions. Energy measurements and units will be discussed in more detail in Chapter 21.

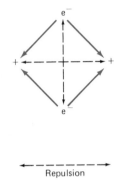

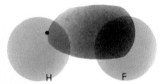

FIGURE 6–4   A bond is created if there is a balance of attractive and repulsive forces between two atoms.

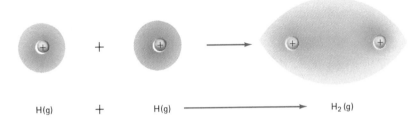

FIGURE 6–5   The electron density in the H—H bond of the H_2 molecule is evenly distributed between the two nuclei. Compare with Figure 4–2.

Electronegativity

Suppose we know that two atoms combine to form a covalent bond. We can show this process by a diagram like Figure 6–5, in which the electron "cloud" is represented by dots.

In the case shown in Figure 6–5, that of the hydrogen molecule, the bits of charge between the two hydrogen nuclei act like a kind of "glue" to bond the atoms together into a molecule. These charges are equally "shared" by the two nuclei. There is no particular reason for the electron cloud to be shifted toward one or the other nucleus.

Now compare the electron cloud in the HF molecule (Figure 6–6). There is clearly more cloud near the fluorine nucleus than near the hydrogen nucleus.

Our measure of the tendency to pull the electrons of a covalent bond over to one side is called **electronegativity** (EN). Figure 6–7 shows the electronegativities of the elements and relates the values to the metal (EN less than 2.0) and nonmetal (EN greater than 2.0) character of the elements.

Electronegativity is clearly related to ionization energy. If an electron is easily lost from a neutral atom, then that same electron is likely to be easily shifted *away* from a bonded atom. Elements with high ionization energies tend to have high electronegativities.

The electron affinity of a nonmetal is also relevant. If an atom tends to gain a whole electron to make a 1– ion, it tends also to shift a bonded electron close to it. High electron affinities thus go along with high electronegativities.

You should be able to predict which of two elements in the same group or period has the higher electronegativity.

FIGURE 6–6   The electron density in the polar F—H bond is shifted toward the fluorine because fluorine is more electronegative than hydrogen. Compare with Figure 4–3 on p. 100.

EXAMPLE 6a: Choose the member of each pair that should have the higher electronegativity.

i)   O or S   ii)   Si or C   iii)   Se or Br

- -

SOLUTION: i)   Oxygen is toward the *top* of the periodic table; it will have a higher electronegativity than sulfur, which is farther down. The reason? The oxygen nucleus is closer to its bonding electrons than the sulfur nucleus. Actual EN values are O 3.5 and S 2.5.

ii)   Carbon is toward the *top* of the table, thus has a higher electronegativity. Actual values are C 2.5 and Si 1.8. You should also remember that carbon is a nonmetal while silicon is a metalloid or semimetal.

iii)   Bromine is toward the *right* of the periodic table and has the higher electronegativity. Actual values are Br 2.8 and Se 2.4.

ELECTRONEGATIVITY INCREASES

ELECTRONEGATIVITY DECREASES

Most electronegative element

Most electropositive elements

H 2.1																	He —
Li 1.0	Be 1.5											B 2.0	C 2.5	N 3.0	O 3.5	F 4.0	Ne —
Na 0.9	Mg 1.2											Al 1.5	Si 1.8	P 2.1	S 2.5	Cl 3.0	Ar —
K 0.8	Ca 1.0	Sc 1.3	Ti 1.5	V 1.6	Cr 1.6	Mn 1.5	Fe 1.8	Co 1.8	Ni 1.8	Cu 1.9	Zn 1.6	Ga 1.6	Ge 1.8	As 2.0	Se 2.4	Br 2.8	Kr —
Rb 0.8	Sr 1.0	Y 1.2	Zr 1.4	Nb 1.6	Mo 1.8	Tc 1.9	Ru 2.2	Rh 2.2	Pd 2.2	Ag 1.9	Cd 1.7	In 1.7	Sn 1.8	Sb 1.9	Te 2.1	I 2.5	Xe —
Cs 0.7	Ba 0.9	La 1.1	Hf 1.3	Ta 1.5	W 1.7	Re 1.9	Os 2.2	Ir 2.2	Pt 2.2	Au 2.4	Hg 1.9	Tl 1.8	Pb 1.8	Bi 1.9	Po 2.0	At 2.2	Rn —
Fr 0.7	Ra 0.9	Ac 1.1	Ku —	Ha —	106 —												

Nonmetals   Metalloids

FIGURE 6–7   Electronegativity values for elements.

Bond polarity

Depending on the electronegativity difference between two elements, the electron cloud between their atoms may be essentially unshifted, shifted part way, or shifted almost all the way to one atom.

Figure 6–8 shows three typical cases of **bond polarity,** all involving the element fluorine. The F_2 molecule (left diagram) has an even distribution of electron density since the electronegativity difference, ΔEN, is $4.0 - 4.0 = 0$. We call F—F a nonpolar bond.

The middle diagram shows fluorine forming a *polar* bond with chlorine. The *density* of the electron charge is greater around the fluorine atom. This is shown in the picture by having more dots around fluorine. The fluorine thus has some extra negative charge, shown by the symbol δ^-, and the chlorine has a bit of net positive charge, shown by the symbol δ^+. The symbol δ, which is the lower-case Greek letter delta, stands for "part of an electron charge," or **partial charge.**

> A *polar* bond has one side more negatively charged than the other side. We then speak of the negative *pole* and the positive *pole,* just as a magnet has a north pole and a south pole.

The right diagram shows the meeting of two elements whose electronegativities are furthest apart, cesium ($Z = 55$) and fluorine ($Z = 9$). The difference in electronegativities, ΔEN, is $4.0 - 0.7 = 3.3$. Since a large electronegativity difference means an ionic bond, the charges shown are full cation (Cs^+) and anion (F^-) charges.

An ionic bond, as shown in Figure 6–8, still retains some covalent character. There is always some electron density shared between the two atoms. This is illustrated in Figure 6–9, which graphs "percent **ionic character**" (the degree to which the bond should be considered as that between two ions) against electronegativity difference. Even the cesium-fluorine bond does not have 100% ionic character. In fact, we consider a chemical bond to be ionic if it has greater than 50% ionic character, which corresponds to a ΔEN somewhere between 1.7 and 2.0. For ΔEN between 0.6 and 2.0, we usually consider a bond to be **polar covalent.** For ΔEN less than 0.6, the ionic character of the bond is so slight that we often consider the bond **nonpolar covalent.**

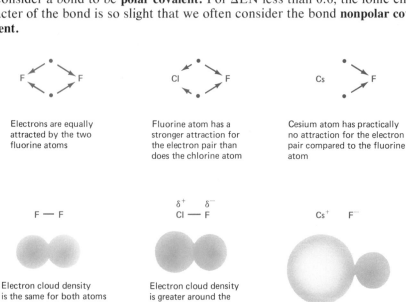

FIGURE 6–8   Bonds may be nonpolar or polar, depending on the difference in the electronegativity (ΔEN) of the two atoms.

FIGURE 6–9 The polarity of a bond may be expressed as "percent ionic character." No bond is 100% ionic.

(Graph: vertical axis "Percent Ionic Character" from 0 to 100; horizontal axis "Electronegativity Difference" from 0 to 3. Regions labeled "Primarily Ionic," "Polar Covalent," and "Nonpolar Covalent.")

Using a table of electronegativities (Figure 6–7), you should now be able to decide if a given bond is ionic, polar covalent, or nonpolar covalent. You should also be able to assign positive and negative charges or partial charges to the atoms.

EXAMPLE 6b: What kind of bond is formed between hydrogen and chlorine? Assign charges as appropriate. Find EN values in Figure 6–7.

- -

SOLUTION: Electronegativity values are H 2.1 and Cl 3.0, with a ΔEN = 0.9, which is greater than 0.6 and less than 1.7 units. This is a polar covalent bond. Since hydrogen has the lower electronegativity, it receives the partial positive (δ^+) charge. Figure 6–10 shows three ways to draw the H—Cl bond.

EXAMPLE 6c: What kind of bond is formed between nitrogen and
i) carbon? ii) sodium? iii) fluorine? Assign charges.

- -

SOLUTION: Electronegativities are N 3.0, C 2.5, Na 0.9, and F 4.0.
  i) ΔEN = 3.0 − 2.5 = 0.5. This is so small that we consider the bond essentially nonpolar.
  ii) ΔEN = 3.0 − 0.9 = 2.1. This is above the 50% ionic character level, so we consider this to be an ionic bond between a Na^+ ion and a negatively charged nitrogen (presumably N^{3-}).
  iii) ΔEN = 3.0 − 4.0 = − 1.0, thus a polar covalent bond with fluorine, not nitrogen, having the δ^- side.

Bond dipoles

A polar covalent bond can be considered as having two "poles" of electrical charge, one positive and one negative, in a manner similar to the way a bar magnet has two magnetic poles, one north and the other south. We thus say that a polar molecule has a charge *dipole*. The term *dipole* will be used again in Chapter 11, when we discuss the intermolecular forces that hold liquids and solids together.

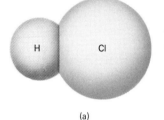

(a)

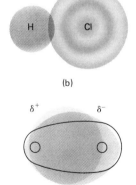

(b)

(c)

FIGURE 6–10 Three ways to draw the HCl molecule, which has a polar H—Cl bond: (a) a space-filling model; (b) an electron cloud picture of the atoms; (c) the electron cloud of the H—Cl bond, which is shifted toward the chlorine.

An alternative way to show the existence of a dipolar (polar) molecule, instead of using δ^+ and δ^- symbols, is to draw an arrow in the direction that runs from the center of positive charge to the center of negative charge, as shown at the bottom of Figure 6–10.

Bond strength and bond length

An ionic bond is usually considered to be stronger than a similar covalent bond. The separation of charges seems to increase **bond strength** to more than what would exist if there were no electronegativity difference. If the bond is stronger, it is harder to break. More energy must be supplied to break it.

It is a bit like using glue to fasten two pieces of wood together. Both polar and nonpolar bonds have the same "glue" of electron density between them; however, the polar bond has an additional *nail* of attraction between a positive charge center and a negative charge center, as shown in Figure 6–11.

The extra strength of a polar bond is also reflected in a shorter distance between the two nuclei. We call this the **bond length.** Thus, a polar bond has greater strength and shorter length than a similar but nonpolar bond.

SELF-CHECK

6.1) By looking at an ordinary periodic table, such as that inside the front cover of this text, predict which element in each of the following pairs should have the higher electronegativity.
a) I or Cl b) Ca or Mg c) Ca or Br d) S or Si
6.2–6.5) Using Figure 6–7, for each of the following bonds (a) decide whether it is nonpolar covalent, polar covalent, or ionic and (b) if polar or ionic, assign appropriate charges.
6.2) hydrogen-oxygen
6.3) potassium-chlorine
6.4) carbon-hydrogen
6.5) sulfur-oxygen
6.6) The silicon ($Z = 14$) and selenium ($Z = 34$) atoms are just about the same size. If no polarity were involved, the Si—F bond and the Se—F bond might be about the same strength and length. Based on electronegativity, which bond would you predict to be stronger? Which would you expect to be longer?

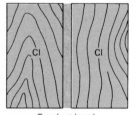

Covalent bond

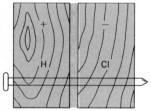

Polar
covalent
bond

FIGURE 6–11 If a covalent bond "glues" atoms together, then we can consider bond polarity as a "nail" of $+/-$ attraction that holds the atoms together even more tightly, and thus increases bond strength.

6.2 MULTIPLE BONDS

LEARNING GOAL 6E: Draw a Lewis electron-dot diagram for any molecule or polyatomic ion that obeys the octet rule, including a species that contains a double or triple bond.

6F: Describe and predict the effect of a double or triple bond on bond length and strength.

6G: Distinguish between a sigma (σ) bond and a pi (π) bond in a molecule. Explain what is meant by a molecular orbital.

6H: Describe the bonding in a molecule or polyatomic ion that requires a combination of several "resonance" diagrams to indicate its true electron distribution. Explain what is meant by a delocalized electron.

In Section 4.3 you began drawing some simple Lewis electron-dot diagrams. You are now familiar with the fact that most elements seek complete octets (noble-gas, ns^2np^6, electron configurations) and obtain them by gaining or losing electrons to form ions *or* by sharing electrons in covalent bonds.

In this section, we will deal with various situations in which there are not enough electrons in a compound or ion to allow each bonding pair to share only *two* electrons and still obey the octet rule.

The octet rule

This is a fancy name for something very simple that we started using early in Chapter 3. The **octet rule** states that a nonmetal atom generally completes its valence electron set by bringing it to *eight* electrons, through the transfer or sharing of electrons. Most organic molecules, as well as most inorganic ions and compounds, "obey" the octet rule. In a Lewis diagram of a compound that obeys the octet rule, each atom is written with eight dots around it.

Some molecules and ions do not "obey" the octet rule. For various reasons, a perfectly good electron configuration can result from a situation in which there is no octet of electrons around an atom.

Two examples should suffice. One of the stable compounds between nitrogen and oxygen is NO_2, nitrogen dioxide. The total number of valence electrons is 5 from nitrogen plus $2 \times 6 = 12$ from oxygen, or 17 in all. The octet rule only works if there is an even number of electrons.

Another relatively unusual molecule is PF_5. The phosphorus atom in the center of this molecule has ten electrons around it. Some of those electrons can use d atomic orbitals, while the octet rule assumes that only s and p orbitals will be used. A similar situation exists for the phosphate, PO_4^{3-}, ion and its derivatives, common in very important biochemicals such as ATP and DNA, discussed in Chapters 20 and 22. Unlike the nitrate ion, PO_4^{3-} acts somewhat as though it has ten electrons around the central atom.

However, most organic and biochemically important molecules follow the octet rule.

Counting valence electrons

The first skill to develop in writing more complicated Lewis diagrams is to count the total number of valence electrons provided by the atoms in a molecule or ion, as we did in Section 4.3.

For example, consider NH_4^+, the ammonium cation frequently seen in the health sciences. You must count the number of valence electrons brought by each atom. It doesn't matter *how* the atoms or electrons got there. We can count the valence electrons in NH_4^+ by saying "Nitrogen provides five, four hydrogens provide $4 \times 1 = 4$, that gives nine, but we have lost one electron in forming a cation. We are left with eight valence electrons, a complete octet around the nitrogen."

Or, we can assume we start with NH_3, which has eight valence electrons (five from N, three from the three H) and then combine it with a H^+ ion that has no valence electrons. The result is, again, eight.

Another example: How many valence electrons are there in C_2H_6? The carbon atoms bring four each, the hydrogens one each. The total is (2 carbons) $(4\ e^-/C)$ + (6 hydrogens) $(1\ e^-/H)$ = 14 electrons.

H	1
C, Si	4
N, P	5
O, S	6
F, Cl, Br, I	7

Table 6–1 lists the number of valence electrons for the elements you meet most commonly in Lewis diagrams.

To count valence electrons in a molecule or ion

1) Add up the number of valence electrons brought in by each individual atom, using Table 6–1 if necessary.
2) If you are working with a molecule, stop there! If you have an ion, add one electron for each negative charge on the ion or subtract one electron for each positive charge on the ion.

EXAMPLE 6d: Count the total number of valence electrons in
   i) CH_4 iv) $C_2H_5NH_2$
   ii) H_2O v) CN^-
   iii) C_4H_8 vi) $SO_4{}^{2-}$

- -

SOLUTION:

   i)   Valence electrons for C: 4, for H: 1; (1 C) (4) + (4 H) (1) = $\boxed{8 \text{ electrons}}$

   ii)   For H: 1, for O: 6; (2 H) (1) + (1 O) (6) = $\boxed{8 \text{ electrons}}$

   iii)   For C: 4, for H: 1; (4) (4) + (8) (1) = 16 + 8 = $\boxed{24 \text{ electrons}}$

   iv)   For C: 4, for N: 5, for H: 1; since there are two carbons, seven hydrogens, and one nitrogen, there are (2) (4) + (7) (1) + (1) (5) =

   8 + 7 + 5 = $\boxed{20 \text{ electrons}}$

   v)   For C: 4, for N: 5; 4 + 5 = 9. Subtract 1 since there is a 1 + charge on the ion: 9 − 1 = $\boxed{8 \text{ electrons}}$

   vi)   For S: 6, for O: 6; (1) (6) + (4) (6) = 6 + 24 = 30; now add two to account for the 2 − charge on the ion: 30 + 2 = $\boxed{32 \text{ electrons}}$

Rules for drawing Lewis diagrams

For most molecules and ions, we can use the following four-step procedure:

1) Count the number of valence electrons.
2) Connect all atoms bonded together with single bonds.
3) Add enough ''lone-pair'' electrons (those not involved in bonding) to give each atom an octet.
4) Count the number of dots you have drawn in the Lewis diagram. This number should agree with the number of available valence electrons from Step 1.

You may occasionally wonder which atom to put in the middle of a molecule or ion. The covalence numbers we have already used should solve that problem in most cases.

EXAMPLE 6e: Draw the Lewis electron-dot diagram for tetrachloromethane, CCl_4, commonly known as carbon tetrachloride.
- -

SOLUTION:
Step 1: Count 4e⁻ from carbon + (4) (7 e⁻) = 28 e⁻ from the four chlorines, for a total of 32 electrons.
Step 2: Putting carbon in the middle (since chlorine can only form one bond), connect single bonds.

$$\text{Cl} \atop \text{Cl} : \overset{..}{\underset{..}{\text{C}}} : \text{Cl} \atop \text{Cl}$$

Step 3: Carbon now has a complete octet. However, each chlorine has only two electrons. Eight are needed. Add six more lone-pair electrons (three pairs) around each chlorine.

$$: \overset{..}{\underset{..}{\text{Cl}}} :$$
$$: \overset{..}{\underset{..}{\text{Cl}}} : \overset{..}{\underset{..}{\text{C}}} : \overset{..}{\underset{..}{\text{Cl}}} :$$
$$: \overset{..}{\underset{..}{\text{Cl}}} :$$

Step 4: Count all the electron dots you have drawn. They add up to 32 electrons. Now compare with Step 1. There are indeed 32 valence electrons available.

EXAMPLE 6f: Draw the dot diagram for butane, C_4H_{10}.

SOLUTION: Follow the same procedure, so that you will become used to it.
Step 1: Count 4 e⁻ × 4 carbons = 16 e⁻ from carbon, plus 1 e⁻ × 10 hydrogens = 10 e⁻ from hydrogen. 10 + 16 = 26 e⁻.
Step 2: Draw the diagram.

$$\text{H H H H} \atop \text{H} : \overset{..}{\text{C}} : \overset{..}{\text{C}} : \overset{..}{\text{C}} : \overset{..}{\text{C}} : \text{H} \atop \text{H H H H}$$

Step 3: All carbons now have octets and each hydrogen has the two electrons needed to fill its valence level. The octet rule is already satisfied. No lone-pair electrons are needed.
Step 4: Count the number of electrons from Step 3. There are 26 electrons used. Check Step 1. We indeed have 26 valence electrons.

EXAMPLE 6g: Draw the Lewis diagram for diethyl ether, once commonly used as an anesthetic in hospitals. Its formula can be written $C_2H_5OC_2H_5$.

SOLUTION: Step 1: We have four carbon atoms, ten hydrogens, one oxygen. Count (4) (4 e⁻) + (10) (1 e⁻) + (1) (6 e⁻) = 32 electrons.
Step 2: Draw a singly bonded diagram.

$$\text{H H}\quad\text{H H} \atop \text{H} : \overset{..}{\text{C}} : \overset{..}{\text{C}} : \text{O} : \overset{..}{\text{C}} : \overset{..}{\text{C}} : \text{H} \atop \text{H H}\quad\text{H H}$$

Step 3: Does each atom have an octet (or, in the case of hydrogen, a duet) of electrons? All but oxygen are satisfied. Add four electrons to oxygen to give it an octet.

$$\text{H H}\quad\text{H H} \atop \text{H} : \overset{..}{\text{C}} : \overset{..}{\text{C}} : \overset{..}{\underset{..}{\text{O}}} : \overset{..}{\text{C}} : \overset{..}{\text{C}} : \text{H} \atop \text{H H}\quad\text{H H}$$

Step 4: Count the number of electrons in the diagram of Step 3. They add up to 32 electrons. Does this agree with Step 1? Yes.

Multiple bonds

Sooner or later we must run into a multiple bond. Let's see what happens when we do.

EXAMPLE 6h: Draw the Lewis diagram for ethene, C_2H_4, commonly known as ethylene.

– –

SOLUTION: Step 1: We have two carbons and four hydrogens. (2) (4 e⁻) + (4) (1 e⁻) = 12 electrons available.

Step 2:   Draw a singly bonded diagram.

$$\text{H} \quad \text{H}$$
$$\text{H}:\overset{..}{\text{C}}:\overset{..}{\text{C}}:\text{H}$$

Step 3:   Does each atom have an octet? No. Neither carbon has an octet. Add two electrons as lone pairs to each carbon, so that the octet rule is obeyed.

$$\text{H} \quad \text{H}$$
$$\text{H}:\overset{..}{\underset{..}{\text{C}}}:\overset{..}{\underset{..}{\text{C}}}:\text{H}$$

Step 4:   How many electrons do we now have in Step 3? There are 14 electrons. Does this agree with Step 1? No! Only 12 valence electrons are actually available. That's just as well, since the diagram in Step 3 looks rather strange!

We must now add a new step, Step 5. Remove the excess two electrons from the diagram. That leaves the proper number, 12 electrons, but one carbon now is lacking an octet.

$$\text{H} \quad \text{H}$$
$$\text{H}:\overset{..}{\text{C}}:\overset{..}{\underset{..}{\text{C}}}:\text{H}$$

Now move the lone-pair electrons to give a double bond, so that each carbon atom obeys the octet rule.

$$\boxed{\begin{array}{c}\text{H} \quad \text{H}\\ \text{H}:\overset{..}{\text{C}}::\overset{..}{\text{C}}:\text{H}\end{array}}$$

Check that everything is satisfied. You now see also that the covalences of carbon (4) and of hydrogen (1) are met by this final diagram.

We should now summarize Step 5.

Step 5:   If the number of electrons in the singly bonded structure of Step 3 is greater than the number of valence electrons available from Step 1, multiple bonding is involved. Reduce the number of dots to the proper total and make enough multiple bonds to insure that every atom obeys the octet rule.

Use the following guidelines:

If Step 4 creates no problems, there are only **single bonds.**

If Step 4 is two electrons high, there is one **double bond.**

If Step 4 is four electrons high, there are two double bonds or one **triple bond.**

If possible, always check that the final Lewis diagram agrees with what we know about the covalency of each element.

EXAMPLE 6i: Draw the Lewis diagram for acetylene (ethyne), C_2H_2.

- -

SOLUTION: Step 1:   Count valence electrons: $(2)(4\ e^-) + (2)(1\ e^-) =$ 10 electrons.
Step 2:   Make the necessary bonds.

$$H:C:C:H$$

Step 3:   Add electrons to make octets.

$$H:\overset{..}{C}:\overset{..}{C}:H$$

Step 4:   How many electrons have we used in Step 3? We wrote 14 electrons, but from Step 1, there are only 10 available. We are four over.
Step 5:   That means two double bonds or one triple bond. Hydrogen cannot be involved in a double bond. Thus, there must be a carbon-carbon triple bond. Write it

$$\boxed{H:C::C:H}$$

Now recheck that we have indeed used only ten electrons, that each atom obeys the octet rule, and that covalency numbers match.

Exactly the same procedures are used for ions. We will take a few short cuts to save space in the following examples. However, we are still using Step 1, Step 2, Step 3, Step 4, and, if necessary, Step 5.

EXAMPLE 6j: Draw the Lewis diagram for the hydroxide ion.

- -

SOLUTION: From Section 4.2, you should recall that this is OH^-.
Step 1:   Valence electrons $= (1)(6\ e^-) + (1)(1\ e^-)$ from the two atoms *plus* $1\ e^-$ because of the charge. Total is $8\ e^-$.
Step 2:

$$[O:H]^-$$

We use brackets and a minus sign to keep track of the fact that we are writing an anion.
Step 3:   Fill the oxygen octet.

$$\boxed{[:\overset{..}{\underset{..}{O}}:H]^-}$$

Step 4:   We have used eight electrons, which agrees with Step 1.

EXAMPLE 6k: Draw the Lewis diagram for the cyanide ion, CN^-.

- -

SOLUTION: Step 1: $(1)(4\ e^-) + (1)(5\ e^-) + 1\ e^-$ charge $= 10$ electrons.

Step 2: $[C:N]^-$

Step 3: $[:\overset{..}{C}:\overset{..}{N}:]^-$

Step 4: That requires 14 electrons. We only have ten.
Step 5: We are four short. There is one triple bond.

$[:C:::N:]^-$

That's correct. Each atom obeys the octet rule. In this particular ion, carbon is *not* forming four bonds, unless you wish to count the ionic bond that will be formed between CN^- and a metal cation. However, there's no way carbon can possibly form four bonds with *one* other atom. The limit is three.

EXAMPLE 6l: Write the Lewis diagram for acetone, CH_3COCH_3.

SOLUTION: Step 1: (3 C) ($4\ e^-$) + (6 H) ($1\ e^-$) + (1 O) ($6\ e^-$) = 24 electrons.

Step 2:

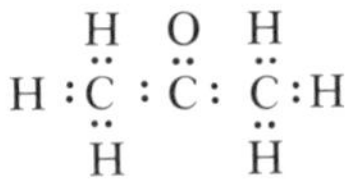

Step 3: Carbon needs one electron pair, oxygen three.

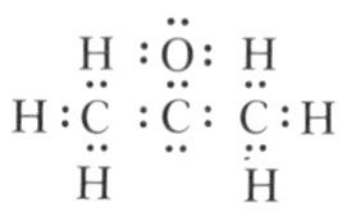

Step 4: The total count from Step 3 is 26 electrons. Wrong!
Step 5: We are two electrons over. There is one double bond.

If we try a carbon-carbon double bond, then one carbon atom would have five bonds, another only three. It must be a carbon-oxygen double bond.

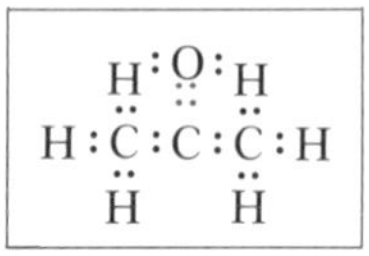

Recheck that only 24 electrons have been used in the final diagram.

Effects of double or triple bonds

A double bond is not twice as strong as a single bond. It is a bit stronger, however, because more electrons are helping "glue" the two atoms together. A triple bond is a bit stronger than a double bond for the same reason.

Conversely, a single bond is longer than a double bond, which in turn is longer than a triple bond. Table 6–2 lists some typical bond strengths and bond lengths of carbon-to-carbon single, double, and triple bonds.

TABLE 6–2 TYPICAL BOND LENGTHS AND STRENGTHS FOR SINGLE, DOUBLE, AND TRIPLE BONDS

–C—C– as in C_2H_6
length: 1.54 Å
strength: 83 kcal/mole
–C═C– as in C_2H_4
length: 1.33 Å
strength: 143 kcal/mole
–C≡C– as in C_2H_2
length: 1.20 Å
strength: 196 kcal/mole

Molecular orbitals

Whether electrons are in atoms or in molecules, we know as much (and as little) about them. We are still talking about electron clouds, rather than little flying particles. We can still only describe the *probability* of finding the electron in a region.

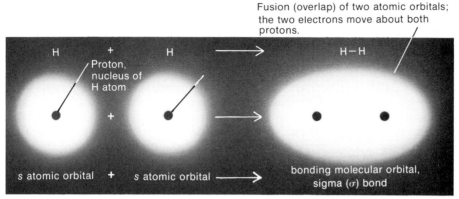

FIGURE 6–12   The combination of two atomic orbitals to make a bonding molecular orbital.

Therefore, the description of the electron in a molecule is still an orbital description, as vague and foggy as when we discussed atoms. However, the orbitals and energy levels are not those of individual atoms. The electrons, and particularly the electrons in a covalent bond, belong to the whole molecule. We therefore say they are in **molecular orbitals** and in molecular energy levels.

Sigma bonds

Chemists like to draw pictures. The picture of an electron in a molecular orbital can be drawn simply, as in Figure 6–10. However, we can also think of two atomic orbitals as *overlapping* or pushing into each other, as shown in Figure 6–12. The resulting molecular orbital is not like a ball; it is sort of oval. However, it is enough like a sphere to continue using an "s" to describe it. To distinguish between atomic orbitals (for electrons in isolated atoms) and molecular orbitals, we use Greek letters for molecules. Figure 6–12 shows how the mathematical treatment of electron clouds for 1s atomic orbitals of two hydrogens can be combined to give the cloud of the **sigma bond** (σ) molecular orbital for H_2.

Two electrons from atomic valence levels can enter a sigma bonding orbital to make an ordinary covalent bond. (Of course, the orbital may be empty, in which case there is no bond.) Each of the electrons spends most of its time somewhere between the atoms and only a small portion of its time close to one atom or the other.

Every covalent *single* bond is considered to be the result of having two electrons in a sigma-bonding molecular orbital. Not all of these orbitals are created as shown in Figure 6–12, but how they are made is of far more interest to physical chemists than to us. The most important thing about sigma bonds is that the electron "glue" is right between the two nuclei.

Pi bonds

Only when we consider double and triple bonds does the situation get somewhat more complex. When we show a double bond in a structural for-

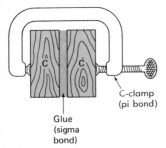

Glue
(sigma
bond)

In addition to the "glue" of Figure 6–11, a pi bond tends to "clamp" the two atoms in position.

mula or Lewis electron-dot diagram, we do not distinguish between bond #1 and bond #2. For ethene, C_2H_4, we write, as in Example 6h,

$$\underset{\displaystyle H}{\overset{\displaystyle H}{\text{H}-\text{C}}}=\underset{\displaystyle H}{\overset{\displaystyle H}{\text{C}-\text{H}}} \qquad \text{or} \qquad \overset{\displaystyle H}{\underset{}{\text{H}:\ddot{\text{C}}::\ddot{\text{C}}:\text{H}}}\overset{\displaystyle H}{}$$

However, in reality, the two parts of the double bond are different. They have in common *only* the fact that each involves two electrons in a bonding molecular orbital. The stronger of the two bonds is a sigma bond. The second bond is weaker and does not "glue" the two atoms together, but acts more like a C-shaped clamp. The second bond in the double bond is formed by overlap not of s (or similar) atomic orbitals but of p atomic orbitals.

The three 2p atomic orbital electron clouds are shown in Section 3.1 (p. 56). When similar p orbitals from two different atoms overlap, they do so above and below the two nuclei, as shown in Figure 6–13. They form a **pi bond** (π) molecular orbital. Or, the p orbitals of the atoms may overlap in front of and in back of the sigma bond.

The second bond in a double bond is the result of having two electrons in a pi-bonding molecular orbital. Such a pi bond is weaker than a sigma bond for two reasons: (a) the small amount of overlap between the p atomic orbitals creates a less dense electron cloud between the atoms (the two electrons spend more of their time with the individual atoms than they do in a sigma-bonding orbital, and less of their time holding the molecule together) and (b) the molecule is being held together rather indirectly, "from the side" instead of head-on.

A pi bond thus breaks much more easily than a sigma bond. This fact, as you will see in Chapter 7, is very important in organic chemistry.

A triple bond is made up of one sigma bond plus two pi bonds, one "above and below" and the other "in front and in back." The result is a cylinder-shaped charge cloud as shown in Figure 6–14, which shows not

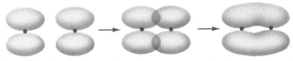

FIGURE 6–13   Side-by-side overlap of p atomic orbitals to give a pi bonding molecular orbital.

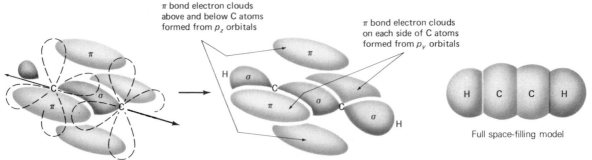

π bond electron clouds above and below C atoms formed from p_z orbitals

π bond electron clouds on each side of C atoms formed from p_y orbitals

Full space-filling model

FIGURE 6–14   The two pi bonds in acetylene, C_2H_2, surround the molecule with an electron charge cloud.

only how the one sigma bond and two pi bonds are made, but also a "space-filling model" for C_2H_2, the acetylene molecule discussed in Example 6i.

Delocalized electrons

All of our illustrations so far have been of electrons that "know their proper place." The electron in an atomic orbital is related to one particular atom. If the atomic orbital overlaps with one from a different atom to form a sigma- or pi-bonding molecular orbital, the electron will be found in that particular bond. All very neat and tidy, but not necessarily a complete description of nature.

There are electrons in molecular orbitals that are *not* confined to two atoms, but in fact are allowed to be anywhere in a large region of the molecule. The best known example is benzene (C_6H_6), in which the electron cloud looks like that shown in Figure 6–15, with the electrons spread above and below the ring of six carbon atoms. This explains many of the properties of aromatic compounds discussed in Chapter 15.

Many other substances, organic and inorganic, have **delocalized electrons.** How do we know when we come across one? We find that our traditional manner of drawing a single Lewis electron-dot diagram for a molecule or ion no longer works.

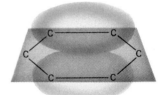

FIGURE 6–15 A delocalized electron cloud, shaped like a ring above and a ring below the plane of the carbon atoms, provides the pi bonding in benzene.

EXAMPLE 6m: Write the Lewis diagram for the carbonate ion.

SOLUTION: From Section 4.2 we know that this has the formula CO_3^{2-}.
Step 1:   Valence $e^- = (1\ C)\ (4) + (3\ O)\ (6) + 2\ e^- = 24$ electrons.
Step 2:   Carbon must be at the center.

$$\left[\begin{matrix} O \\ O:\ddot{C}:O \end{matrix} \right]^{2-}$$

Step 3:   Create octets.

$$\left[\begin{matrix} :\ddot{O}: \\ :\ddot{O}:\ddot{C}:\ddot{O}: \end{matrix} \right]^{2-}$$

Step 4:   Our diagram in Step 3 has 26 electrons. We only have 24 available.
Step 5:   We must therefore have one double bond. Where does it go? All three oxygens are equivalent; none can be different from the rest. We can thus draw three possibilities.

$$\left[\begin{matrix} \cdot\ddot{O}\cdot \\ :\ddot{O}:\ddot{C}:\ddot{O}: \end{matrix} \right]^{2-} \ \text{or} \ \left[\begin{matrix} :\ddot{O}: \\ :\ddot{O}::\ddot{C}:\ddot{O}: \end{matrix} \right]^{2-} \ \text{or} \ \left[\begin{matrix} :\ddot{O}: \\ :\ddot{O}:\ddot{C}::\ddot{O}\cdot \end{matrix} \right]^{2-}$$

Check these. They all obey the octet rule, and each uses 24 electrons. That still leaves us with three pictures for one anion.

It is tempting to think that perhaps the two electrons in the double bond jump back and forth between the carbon-oxygen bonds. The name for what we have just drawn, **resonance** structures, even tends to make you think that. However, the electrons do not move from place to place to make one of the diagrams correct, then another, then the third. There is only one correct description of the bonding in CO_3^{2-}, and this is shown in Figure 6–16. A delocalized pi molecular orbital is shown (with lines). It can hold two electrons, but those two electrons spend their time over all four atoms in the carbonate ion.

Delocalized electrons are also found in metals. A solid metal is simply a system of very large molecular orbitals, which extend over whole moles of atoms. An electron inserted at one end of a metal wire can thus push an electron out of the other end. That is how we get conduction of electricity.

SELF-CHECK

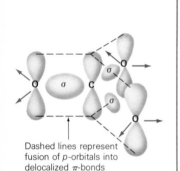

Dashed lines represent fusion of p-orbitals into delocalized π-bonds

FIGURE 6–16 The delocalized pi-electron bonds of the carbonate anion are spread over the four atoms.

6.7) Using the step-by-step process given in this chapter, draw a Lewis electron-dot diagram for each of the following.
a) ethyl alcohol
b) propane
c) propyne, C_3H_4
d) ethanal (acetaldehyde), CH_3CHO
e) phosphate ion, PO_4^{3-}
f) nitrite ion, NO_2^-
g) carbon monoxide, CO
h) octatriene, C_8H_{12}
i) sulfur trioxide gas, SO_3
j) prussic acid, HCN
6.8) Are delocalized electrons involved in the real electron distribution of any of the above molecules or ions? Explain.
6.9) The two molecules CH_3NH_2 and HCN both contain carbon-nitrogen bonding. In which of the two would you expect the C—N bond to be stronger? In which would the carbon nucleus be farther from the nitrogen nucleus? Explain.
6.10) Where will you find sigma bonds and where pi bonds in CH_3NH_2 and HCN?
6.11) How does a molecular orbital differ from an atomic orbital? Does a bonding molecular orbital *always* hold atoms together?
6.12*) As you draw more and more Lewis electron-dot diagrams, you find that certain numbers of valence electrons always turn up for diagrams in which there are only single bonds. What are these numbers?

6.3 THE SHAPES OF MOLECULES

LEARNING GOAL 6I: Recognize and draw a tetrahedron (the shape of methane and the basis for the shapes of most organic compounds).
         6J: Use electron-pair repulsion to predict the shape of a molecule (or ion) in which a central atom is surrounded by two, three, or four electron clouds.

You will see in later chapters that the biochemically important compounds of the human body tend to have rather large molecules. The shapes

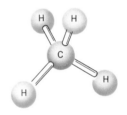

of those molecules are important to our functioning properly. If hemoglobin (the protein molecule in red blood cells that carries oxygen) takes on the wrong shape, it can't do its job. Shape is all important in transmission of hereditary information (Chapter 20). Our senses of smell and taste are also based on the shapes of molecules, as well as their charges.

The tetrahedron

We tend to diagram the simple hydrocarbon molecules as rectangles and squares, but the actual shapes of organic molecules tend to be different from these simple pictures. Angles of 90° are, in fact, not very common in chemistry and extremely uncommon in organic chemistry.

How is the shape of a molecule described? First of all, by a three-dimensional model that you can hold in your hand. If your class has molecular models available, try to use them. There is no better way to understand shape than to look at an object from different angles.

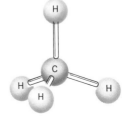

The second best way is to make a photograph or drawing of a molecular model. We will show you several such pictures, such as Figure 4–5 on p. 108. Less effective is a perspective drawing, which tries to show you in two dimensions what is going on in three-dimensional space. Lastly, we can use numbers, such as bond angles.

What does a methane molecule really look like? We showed you some pictures in Section 4.4. Several more are shown in Figure 6–17. The shape of CH_4 is **tetrahedral,** like a pyramid with a triangular base or a photographer's tripod with a camera on top. Does that give you the idea yet? It will grow on you. Every singly bonded carbon atom is at the center of a tetrahedron. Carbon chains, such as those of ethane, propane, and butane, are based on tetrahedra.

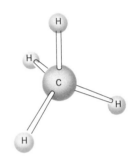

A **bond angle** is a measure of the angle made by two lines representing bonds. The bond angle in methane is roughly 109°, which represents how far apart four things can get from each other if they are all at the same distance from a central point.

Electron-pair repulsion

Why do the hydrogen atoms in methane get as far apart as they possibly can? Recall that opposite charges attract each other, but like charges repel each other. Each hydrogen atom in methane is surrounded by an electron cloud. One electron cloud repels all other electron clouds.

This gives us the **electron-pair repulsion** principle, which states that **the electron pairs surrounding an atom are located as far apart from each other as possible.**

To apply this principle, remember that an electron pair may be in a bond or may be a lone pair, as is the case for the two electron pairs in water, which are not involved in covalent (sigma) bonds to hydrogen.

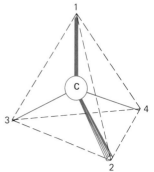

FIGURE 6–17   Four views of the tetrahedral molecule of methane, CH_4.

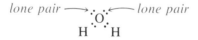

A third possibility is that the pair may be a group of electrons in a double or triple bond.

It takes three points to specify an angle. A bond angle may be described by listing the three atoms involved. For example, in methane, the 109° angle between one C—H bond and another C—H bond can be called an H—C—H bond angle.

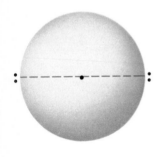

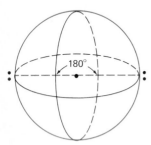

Minimum repulsion between two electron pairs around a central atom occurs when the pairs are at opposite ends of the diameter of a sphere.

Two pairs of electrons

Let us start with a molecule of beryllium chloride, $BeCl_2$,

$$:\ddot{Cl}:Be:\ddot{Cl}:$$

There are two electron pairs around the beryllium atom, so those pairs (and the bonds they form) get as far apart as possible. If you and a friend wanted to get as far apart on the earth as you could, you would be on opposite sides. Similarly, the chlorine atoms will be found on opposite sides of the beryllium atom. The angle made by one Cl—Be bond with the other Be—Cl bond is 180°, since the three atoms are in a straight line.

We call such a straight-line geometry a **linear** geometry. Another molecule with similar geometry is acetylene,

$$H:C:::C:H$$

Each carbon atom has two electron clouds around it, one larger than the other (Figure 6–14), and all four atoms are in a straight line.*

The geometry around any triple bond is linear. For example, the HCN molecule, with Lewis diagram

$$H:C:::N:$$

has the three atoms in a straight line.

Three pairs of electrons

Our inorganic example here is boron trichloride, BCl_3. The Lewis diagram is

$$:\ddot{Cl}:B:\ddot{Cl}:$$
$$:\ddot{Cl}:$$

However, in actual fact, the two "upper" chlorines are positioned so that the three chlorines form a triangle around the boron atom (Figure 6–18).

An interesting aspect of this molecule is that all four nuclei (including that of central boron) are in the same plane.

Many organic compounds have their shapes determined by this kind of relationship. For example, formaldehyde has the Lewis diagram

$$H:C::\ddot{O}:$$
$$\ddot{H}$$

The carbon atom has three electron clouds around it, which get as far apart as possible. The carbon atom, the oxygen atom, and both hydrogen atoms are all in the same plane. The angle between one H—C bond and the other C—H bond is 120°, the same as every other bond angle in the molecule.

Because a triangle is formed and all atoms lie in the same plane, we call this a **triangular planar** arrangement. It is always found around an atom with one double bond.

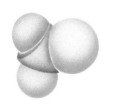

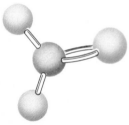

The geometry of formaldehyde, H_2CO, is triangular planar with a 120° H—C—H bond angle.

---

* There are cases when the Lewis electron-dot diagram (structural formula) may have the same shape as the actual molecule. This is only possible for molecules that lie in a straight line or in a plane. Organic molecules with double or triple bonds may qualify, and the Lewis diagram may be shown with 120° or 180° bond angles. Organic molecules with only single bonds have tetrahedral geometry around each carbon atom. The actual shape of such molecules does not resemble the Lewis diagrams

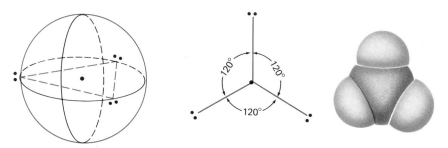

FIGURE 6–18 Minimum repulsion among three electron pairs around a central atom occurs when the pairs are 120° apart.

The triangular planar geometry also applies when there are three electron pairs but one of them is a lone pair. The compound stannous fluoride, used in toothpastes to prevent tooth decay has a Lewis diagram

$$:\ddot{F}:\ddot{Sn}:\ddot{F}:$$

Since there are three electron pairs around the central tin atom, we expect the fluorines to be in a bent arrangement, so the angle between one F—Sn bond and the other Sn—F bond is approximately 120°.

Four pairs of electrons

We already know that four pairs of electrons get as far apart as they can if they go to the corners of a tetrahedron. Figure 6–19 summarizes the cases of a central atom surrounded by two, three, and four bonds.

A very interesting aspect of the fact that four electron pairs around a central atom form a tetrahedron is its prediction for the shape of two of the most important molecules in chemistry, water and ammonia. As you see in Figure 6–20, CH_4, NH_3, and H_2O have essentially the same geometry of electron pairs. Nitrogen has four electron pairs (an octet), although only three bond with hydrogen in ammonia. The oxygen in water also has four electron pairs, two of which bond with hydrogen and two of which are lone pairs.

If a central atom obeys the octet rule, and if there are no double or triple bonds to it, the geometry of the electron pairs about it will be tetrahedral.

The molecular geometry is limited to the shapes of the molecules themselves. On this basis, the ammonia molecule is a pyramid and the water molecule is bent, as shown in Figure 6–20. You should not assume that the bond angles in various molecules will be exactly 120° or 109°, because some electron clouds are more effective than others at repulsion.

Hybridization

To a physical chemist, there is a theoretical gap in what we have said so far. The atomic orbitals we drew in Section 3.1 are at angles of 90° to each other. We said in Section 6.2 that bonding molecular orbitals are created by overlap of atomic orbitals. That should imply bond angles of 90°, but each molecule we have discussed in Section 6.3 has bond angles of 180°, 120°, or 109° (more or less).

Of course, the atom and its electrons don't know that we are having problems with our mathematics. They just go on doing what they do. Chemists must therefore

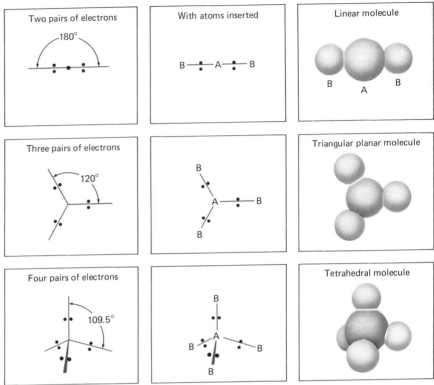

FIGURE 6–19 The geometry that results from electron-pair repulsion of two, three, or four pairs of electrons around a central atom.

adjust their mathematical answers to agree with the real world. The result of this adjustment is to say that an atomic orbital that overlaps to make a bonding molecular orbital may be s, p, d (which we have seen before) or *some combination of these* that gives the required geometry.

The most popular arrangements are to combine an s and a p orbital if we have a bond angle of 180°, an s and two p orbitals if we want 120°, and an s and three p orbitals if we want a tetrahedron. We can therefore calculate the effect of having two sp, three sp², or four sp³ atomic orbitals.

Although many texts provide these "hybrid" or mixed atomic orbitals as something to learn, you frankly can't do much more with them than you can with

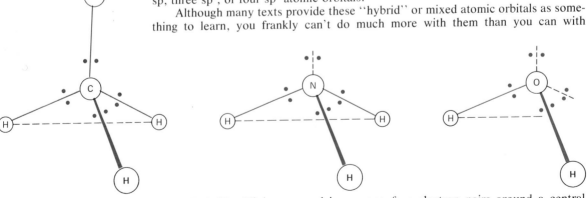

FIGURE 6–20 Minimum repulsion among *four* electron pairs around a central atom occurs when the pairs are arranged in a tetrahedral configuration with angles of about 109°. The three bonds in NH_3 form a pyramid, while the two bonds in H_2O make it a bent molecule.

the electron-pair repulsion principle. For this reason, we have de-emphasized "hybrid" atomic orbitals in this text.

6.13) Draw the tetrahedral carbon tetrachloride, CCl_4, molecule.

6.14) Draw a Lewis electron-dot diagram and predict the shape and bond angles for each of the following molecules and ions.

a) ClCCH   d) PH_3
b) H_2S e) NO_3^-
c) H_2CCH_2

6.15*) Explain why it is not possible to *completely* show the shape of ethane on a piece of paper, but it is possible to show the shape of H_2CO and HCCH correctly in simple drawings.

6.4 POLARITY OF MOLECULES

LEARNING GOAL 6K: Given the shape of a molecule and given a table of electronegativities, estimate the polarity of the molecule.

You may have thought we were done discussing polarity after Section 6.1, but a simple illustration will show why we are not. Can you choose a side of the CO_2 molecule that is positive and a side that is negative?

The Lewis diagram for CO_2 is

$$:\overset{..}{O}::C::\overset{..}{O}:$$

By the electron-pair repulsion principle, this will be a *linear* molecule, like HCCH or HCN. The electronegativity difference between oxygen (3.5) and carbon (2.5) is certainly enough to make polar bonds. We can label those bonds with partial charges as follows:

$$\overset{\delta^-}{:\overset{..}{O}}::\overset{\delta^+}{C}::\overset{\delta^-}{\overset{..}{O}}:$$

What we find is that, although each bond is polar, the polarities cancel out. The CO_2 molecule *as a whole* is nonpolar.

Consider the $BeCl_2$ and BCl_3 molecules we looked at in Section 6.3. Each of these has polar bonds. However, the bond polarities cancel out. Figure 6–21 shows that the polar bonds in CCl_4 cancel each other out, while $CHCl_3$ is polar because of molecular shape.

Water would not be polar (and would not have many of its amazing properties) if it were linear like $BeCl_2$ or BeF_2. The approach to determining whether a **molecule** is **polar** or not is

1) Compare electronegativities to see if there are any polar bonds (remember that an electronegativity difference of less than 0.6 units is often considered essentially nonpolar).

2) Look at the molecule as a whole to see if any polarities from the bonds cancel out.

EXAMPLE 6n: Check each of the following molecules and ions to see if it is polar.

i) NH_3 ii) SO_2 iii) the nitrate ion, NO_3^-

SELF-CHECK

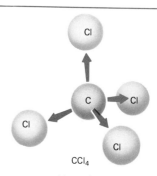

CCl_4

Nonpolar

(Dipoles from polar bonds cancel due to symmetry)

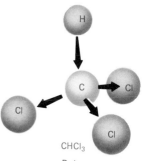

$CHCl_3$

Polar

(Dipoles from polar bonds do not cancel)

FIGURE 6–21 A polar molecule has a positive side and a negative side; a nonpolar molecule does not. If a molecule contains polar bonds, it may be helpful to decide which atoms carry plus charges and which atoms carry minus charges. Find the center of the atoms with plus charges (the plus pole) and the center of the atoms with minus charges (the minus pole). If the two centers are at the same spot, you have a nonpolar molecule. In this drawing of CCl_4, the center of the four (negative) chlorines is at the same point as the center of the (positive) carbon atom

---

SOLUTION: Draw a Lewis diagram for each substance. Determine if the bonds are polar. Then look for canceling.

$$H:\ddot{N}:H$$
$$\ddot{H}$$

i) NH_3 has $\Delta EN = 3.0 - 2.1 = 0.9$, so the three bonds are polar. The shape is pyramidal, not planar. The bond dipoles do not cancel. Ammonia is a polar molecule.

ii) SO_2 has 18 valence electrons. Its Lewis diagram is $:\ddot{O}::\ddot{S}:\ddot{O}:$

(with two possibilities, thus a delocalized pi-electron situation). The central sulfur atom effectively has three electron clouds around it, thus the angle between one O—S bond and the other S—O bond is more like 120° than 180°. The $\Delta EN = 3.5 - 2.5 = 1.0$, so the bonds are polar. The bond dipoles do not cancel out, so SO_2 is a polar molecule.

iii) The Lewis diagram for the nitrate ion is, with 24 valence electrons,

$$:\ddot{O}::N:\ddot{O}:,$$
$$\phantom{:\ddot{O}::N}:\ddot{O}:$$

with two additional "resonance" forms. There are effectively three electron pairs around the central nitrogen, each of which is a bond to oxygen. The $\Delta EN = 3.5 - 3.0 = 0.5$. The bond dipole is close to zero. In addition, the ion is symmetric, so even if there were a bond dipole, the three bonds would cancel each other. Thus, the NO_3^- ion is nonpolar.

Note: the fact that the NO_3^- ion as a whole is charged does not affect whether one end of the molecule is more positive or negative than the other.

In Chapter 11 we will be looking very carefully at the polarity of a molecule *as a whole* when we examine intermolecular forces that hold together liquids and solids.

SELF-CHECK

6.16) Decide whether each of the following molecules is polar or nonpolar.
a) H_2CO c) HCCH   e) HCCF   g) PH_3 i) CH_3I
b) C_4H_{10} d) H_2O f) CF_4 h) $C_8H_{17}O$ j) BeH_2
6.17*) Is the CH_2F_2 molecule polar or nonpolar? Draw a good picture.

CHAPTER SIX IN REVIEW ■ Covalent Bonding

6A: Describe the trends in electronegativity values for representative elements across and down the periodic table.

6B: Given a table of electronegativity values and given a particular bonding pair of atoms, predict whether the attraction between them should be considered an ionic bond, a polar covalent bond, or a nonpolar covalent bond.

6C: Given a polar covalent bond, state which side can be considered to have a partial positive charge and which a partial negative charge.

GLOSSARY FOR CHAPTER SIX

atomic size   The size of an atom when it is covalently bonded to other similar atoms; half of the distance between two neighboring nuclei in the pure element (called the *atomic radius*); depends on the number of protons pulling on the electron cloud and on the distance of the valence electron cloud from the nucleus. (page 154)

bond angle   The angle formed between two straight lines that meet at a common central atom and represent bonds between atoms, such as the 109° angle between any two C–H bonds in methane; in organic chemistry, a 120° angle is found in a situation involving one double bond, while a 180° angle is typical of one triple bond. (p. 171)

bond length   The distance between the two nuclei of atoms that are bonded together, typically one to several angstrom units; the effect of *ionic character* is to shorten the bond length; the effect of *pi bonding* is to shorten the bond length. (p. 160)

bond polarity   The degree to which the electron cloud between two bonded atoms is not shared equally; the extent of *ionic character;* represented by showing *partial charges* on the atoms. (p. 158)

bond strength   The degree of attraction between two bonded atoms; the energy required to break the bond and move the atoms away from each other (also known as *bond energy); ionic character* and *pi bonding* both have the effect of increasing bond strength. (p. 160)

delocalized electron   An electron that contributes to bonding in a chemical compound but is not found specifically between two distinct atoms; part of an electron cloud that is spread among three or more atoms, as in metals and some inorganic and organic compounds; cannot be represented by a single Lewis diagram and thus requires a series of *resonance* diagrams to show the delocalization. (p. 169)

double bond The sharing of four electrons (two electron pairs) by two atoms; a *sigma bond* plus a *pi bond*, as seen in ethylene, $H_2C=CH_2$. (p. 164)

electron affinity A measure of the tendency of an atom or ion to accept an additional electron; the energy given off when a neutral atom becomes a 1– anion; high for Groups 6 and 7. (p. 155)

electronegativity A measure of the relative tendency of the atoms of an element to attract the electrons in a bond and thus to become the negative side of a *polar bond*; high for elements with high *electron affinity* and high ionization energy; low for metals. (p. 156)

electron-pair repulsion The principle that the electron pairs around an atom will repel each other because of the negative charges on each and will thus get as far away from each other as possible; used to predict the shapes and bond angles of molecules. (p. 171)

ionic character The degree to which a bond between two atoms is actually between a cation and an anion; the degree to which the electron cloud of a bond is related to only one of the two atoms; depends on the *electronegativity* difference (ΔEN) between the two elements; may vary from zero in a completely *nonpolar* covalent bond to over 90% for the Cs—F bond; the degree of *bond polarity*. (p. 158)

ionic size The size of a cation or anion when it is ionically bonded; the ionic radius; a negative ion is larger than the corresponding neutral atom, and a positive ion is smaller. (p. 154)

linear The shape of a molecule (or ion) that has three or more atoms in a straight line; a single straight line passes through all of the nuclei; the *bond angles* are all 180°; seen in acetylene HC $\equiv$ CH, $BeCl_2$; a *triple bond* creates linear geometry around each atom involved. (p. 172)

molecular orbital The region of space around a molecule in which an electron has a comparatively high chance of being found; a mathematical description similar to an atomic orbital; holds 0, 1, or 2 electrons; electrons in certain molecular orbitals can form *sigma* or *pi* bonds. (p. 167)

nonpolar covalent bond A bond in which the valence electron cloud between the atoms is evenly shared; there are no partial charges; the *bond polarity* is extremely low; the *ionic character* is close to zero; strictly true of bonds in pure elements, such as O_2 and F_2; considered also to be approximately true in bonds with ΔEN less than 0.6, as in N—Cl or H—C. (p. 158)

octet rule The principle that a bonded atom of a nonmetal tends to obtain or have a share in *eight* valence electrons; an aid to writing Lewis diagrams. (p. 161)

partial charge In a polar covalent bond, the indication by use of the Greek letter delta (δ^+ and δ^-) that one nucleus has more of the electron cloud near it, and thus has some extra negative charge (but not a "whole" electron's worth) and the other nucleus has an equal but opposite partial positive charge; shows the degree of bond polarity. (p. 158)

pi (π) bond Two electrons in a bonding *molecular orbital* in which the two-electron cloud is above and below (or in front of and in back of) the line joining the two nuclei; since there is no direct sharing of electrons between the atoms, the pi bond is weaker than a *sigma bond*; a double bond consists of one pi bond and one sigma bond; a triple bond has two pi bonds and one sigma bond; *delocalized electrons* are in pi bonds. (p. 168)

polar covalent bond A bond with *polarity* or *ionic character*; a bond for which *partial charges* may be written; may be considered as corresponding to a ΔEN of between 0.6 and 1.7–1.9 units; differences greater than this produce *ionic* bonds; a bond with a dipole of electrical charge. (p. 158)

polar molecule A molecule for which one side has a partial negative charge, the other side a partial positive charge; the centers of positive and negative partial charge are not at the same point, and so the bond polarities do not cancel out; the molecule as a whole has a charge dipole; a molecule containing only nonpolar bonds cannot be polar; a molecule with polar bonds may or may not be a polar molecule. (p. 175)

resonance A situation in which the real electron distribution cannot be adequately described by a single Lewis electron-dot diagram, owing to delocalized electrons; several dot diagrams are drawn, each of which is helpful in understanding the overall molecule (each such diagram is a contributing or resonance form). (p. 169)

sigma (σ) bond A covalent bond created by the direct sharing of two electrons between atoms; two electrons in a bonding *molecular orbital* centered between the nuclei; present in *single* bonds as well as in *double* and *triple* bonds. (p. 167)

single bond A covalent bond created by the sharing of two electrons in a *sigma bond;* to be distinguished from a multiple (double or triple) bond. (p. 164)

tetrahedral A shape in which four atoms are placed at the corners of a regular tetrahedron; the *angle* between any two bonds is about 109°, as in all organic compounds with single bonds; the four bonds around a central atom are as far apart as they can get because of *electron-pair repulsion*. (p. 171)

triangular planar A shape in which four atoms are arranged with one in the center, the other three forming an equilateral triangle around it, with all four nuclei in the same plane; the bond angles are all 120°; associated with one *double bond* on the central atom, as in $H_2C=CH_2$ or $H_2C=O$; the three bonds around a central atom are as far apart as they can get because of *electron-pair repulsion*. (p. 172)

triple bond A combination of one sigma bond and two pi bonds between two atoms; produces a linear geometry, as in $HC\equiv CH$ or $H-C\equiv N$; shorter and stronger, in general, than the corresponding double and single bonds. (p. 164)

QUESTIONS AND PROBLEMS FOR CHAPTER SIX ■ Covalent Bonding

SECTION 6.1 POLARITY OF COVALENT BONDS

6.18) Choose the element from each pair that should have the *higher* electronegativity.
a) C or N c) Ba or I
b) K or Na

6.19) Use Figure 6–7 to decide whether each of the following bonds is nonpolar, polar covalent, or ionic. If polar or ionic, assign appropriate charges.
a) Na—F c) H—S
b) C—F

6.20*) The unstable molecule C_2 has a bond length of 1.24 Å, while the O_2 molecule has a bond length of 1.21 Å. Considering *only* the polarity of

6.43) Choose the element from each pair that should have the *higher* electronegativity:
a) P or S c) Be or F
b) Br or I

6.44) Use Figure 6–7 to decide whether each of the following bonds is nonpolar, polar covalent, or ionic. If polar or ionic, assign appropriate charges.
a) Si—O c) Cl—Br
b) K—Cl

6.45*) The N_2 molecule has a bond length of 1.09 Å and the F_2 molecule has a bond length of 1.41 Å. Considering *only* the polarity of the N—F

the C—O bond, would you expect it to have a length greater than, less than, or equal to 1.225 Å? Explain.

6.21) Do you expect the electronegativity of a metal to be relatively high or low?

6.22*) If element A has a lower ionization energy than element Z, what would you predict about the relative (a) atomic sizes? (b) electronegativities?

6.23*) Rank the following in order of increasing radius.

K	Ca^{2+}
Ca	Ca^+

6.24*) What is the meaning of the partial charge assigned to an atom in a polar bond?

6.25*) Separate these formulas into two groups, using Figure 6–7: (a) compounds with predominantly ionic bonds and (b) compounds with predominantly covalent bonds.

Rb_2O	XeF_4
ClF	GeH_4
SO_2	K_2S
CO_2	CsF

6.26*) Not every compound has only ionic or covalent bonds; some have both kinds. From Chapter 4, you should be able to write the formulas of the following ionic salts. In each case, show the anion and cation, and then list the covalent bonds to be found in the formula unit.
a) ammonium nitrate
b) copper(II) monohydrogen phosphate
c) aluminum acetate. The acetate anion is

$$CH_3\overset{\|}{\underset{O}{C}}-O^-$$

SECTION 6.2 MULTIPLE BONDS

6.27) Draw an octet-rule Lewis diagram or structural formula for each of the following molecules. In some cases, the skeleton of atoms is shown to help you.

bond, would you expect it to have a length greater than, less than, or equal to 1.25 Å? Explain.

6.46) Do you expect the electronegativity of a halogen to be relatively high or low?

6.47*) If element D has a greater atomic radius than element X, what would you predict about the relative (a) electronegativities? (b) ionization energies?

6.48*) Rank the following in order of increasing radius.

S^-	S
Cl	S^{2-}

6.49*) With which element should bromine form a bond in order for Br to have the greatest value of δ^+? With which element to have the greatest possible value of δ^-?

6.50*) Separate these formulas into two groups, using Figure 6–7: (a) compounds with predominantly ionic bonds and (b) compounds with predominantly covalent bonds.

NO	IF_7
KI	BeO
SiF_4	RbBr
P_2S_3	KH

6.51*) Follow the instructions for Question 6.26, using the compounds listed below.
a) ammonium cyanide
b) calcium dihydrogen phosphate
c) sodium oxalate. The oxalate anion is

$$^-O-\overset{\|}{\underset{O}{C}}-\overset{\|}{\underset{O}{C}}-O^-$$

6.52) Draw an octet-rule Lewis diagram or structural formula for each of the following molecules. In some cases, the skeleton of atoms is shown to help you.

a) N_2 (nitrogen gas)
b) ClO^- (hypochlorite ion)
c) $HOPO_3^{2-}$ (monohydrogen phosphate ion)
d) SiO_2 (sand)
e) ONONO (dinitrogen trioxide)
f) C_3H_8
g) C_3H_4
h) $C_2H_5COCH_3$

a) O_2 (oxygen gas)
b) ClO_4^- (perchlorate ion)
c) $HOPO_2OH^-$ (dihydrogen phosphate ion)
d) CO_2 (carbon dioxide)
e) NNO (dinitrogen oxide)
f) C_5H_{12}
g) C_5H_8
h) C_3H_7CHO

6.28) Which do you expect to have a longer C—C bond, ethane (C_2H_6) or ethene (C_2H_4)? Explain, using structural formulas.

6.29) Given two atoms, how many sigma bonds may be formed between them? How many pi bonds? Explain your answer.

6.30) How do molecular orbital descriptions of electron behavior resemble those of atomic orbitals?

6.31) Delocalized electrons cannot possibly be described fully by atomic orbital descriptions. Why?

6.32) A typical triple bond is made up of how many σ- and how many π-bonds?

6.33) Draw all the resonance Lewis diagrams for sulfur dioxide, OSO, a poisonous gas. How would you describe an S—O bond in this molecule?

6.34*) Draw a Lewis diagram for a polyatomic anion that has the same number of atoms and electrons as sulfur dioxide.

6.35*) A metal is held together by delocalized electrons. Can you use this fact to explain why a metal can be easily drawn out into a wire but a salt crystal cannot be?

6.53) Which do you expect to have a shorter C—O bond, carbon monoxide (CO) or carbon dioxide (CO_2)? Explain, using Lewis diagrams.

6.54) Describe the difference in position and in strength between a sigma bond and a pi bond formed by the same two atoms.

6.55) How many electrons must be in a bonding molecular orbital before a covalent bond can exist?

6.56) Do the electrons in a series of contributing resonance diagrams shift back and forth between the bonds shown? Explain.

6.57) A typical double bond is made of how many σ- and how many π-bonds?

6.58) Draw all the resonance Lewis diagrams for the hydrogen carbonate ion, $HOCO_2^-$. How would you describe a C—O bond in this anion?

6.59*) Draw a Lewis diagram for a polyatomic anion that has the same number of atoms and electrons as carbon dioxide, OCO.

6.60*) A metal is held together by delocalized electrons. Can you use this fact to explain why a metal conducts electricity but solid salt crystals do not?

SECTION 6.3 THE SHAPES OF MOLECULES

6.36) Which of the following drawings represents methane in its correct three-dimensional shape?

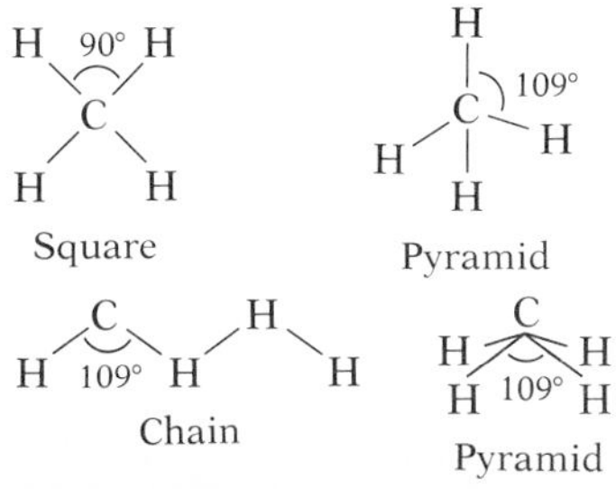

6.61) Draw a recognizable tetrahedron to show the shape of the CF_4 molecule.

H   90° H
C
H   H
Square

H
|
C 109°
H—|—H
H
Pyramid

C
H 109° H   H
H
Chain

C
H   H
H 109° H
Pyramid

6.37) For each of the following, draw a Lewis diagram and then predict the shape and bond angles.
a) SF_2
b) $CHBr_3$
c) CaH_2
d) H_2CNH
e) sulfate ion
f) F_2CO
g) BF_3
h) NSF

6.38*) Explain why methane, water, and ammonia all have relatively similar bond angles, even though the number of atoms differs.

6.39*) The following bond angles have been observed experimentally. Compare them with what you would predict from electron-pair repulsion as described in this chapter.
a) In chlorine dioxide, ClO_2, the O—Cl—O bond angle is 118.5°.
b) In difluorodiazine, FNNF, each F—N—N bond angle is about 115°.
c) In bromomethane, CH_3Br, each H—C—H bond angle is 111°.

6.62) For each of the following, draw a Lewis diagram and then predict the shape and bond angles.
a) IO_2^-
b) H_2CCBr_2
c) $AlCl_3$
d) H_3CCN
e) nitrate ion
f) CH_3F
g) BeF_2
h) OCS

6.63*) Explain why HCN and HCCH have the same bond angles, even though the number of atoms differs in the two cases.

6.64*) The following bond angles have been observed experimentally. Compare them with what you would predict from electron-pair repulsion as described in this chapter.
a) In hydrogen peroxide, HOOH, each H—O—O bond angle is 100°.
b) In nitrosyl bromide, ONBr, the O—N—Br bond angle is about 117°.
c) In formaldehyde, H_2CO, the H—C—H bond angle is about 126°.

SECTION 6.4 POLARITY OF MOLECULES

6.40) Using Figure 6–7, determine for each species in Problem 6.37 whether it is completely nonpolar or has some net polarity (charge dipole).

6.41*) Determine the shape and overall charge dipole (if any) of each of the following.
a) NCO^- (cyanate ion)
b) HNNN (hydrazoic acid)
c) $(NC)_2CC(CN)_2$ (tetracyanoethylene)

6.42*) In general, the geometry of a molecule with an unpaired electron is the same as though the unpaired electron were *not* present in the molecule. From this, predict the shape of the fragment $CH_3 \cdot$ (methyl).

6.65) Using Figure 6–7, determine for each species in Problem 6.62 whether it is completely nonpolar or has some net polarity (charge dipole).

6.66*) Determine the shape and polarity or overall charge dipole (if any) of each of the following.
a) CNO^- (fulminate ion)
b) $(CH_3)_2SO$ (dimethyl sulfoxide)
c) HCCCCH (diacetylene)

6.67*) The ethylene molecule, H_2CCH_2, is very important in modern organic chemistry. It is used in thousands of daily applications, including the making of polyethylene plastics. Only one of the following ways that chemists have used to depict ethylene (since Dalton) is *entirely* incorrect. Which one?

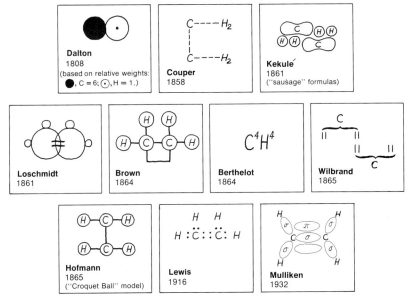

Some historical drawings of the ethylene molecule.

7 Hydrocarbons

In Chapter 1 we discussed some of the differences between *inorganic* and *organic* compounds. Organic compounds always involve carbon and generally contain chains of carbon atoms connected by covalent bonds. In Section 4.4, we discussed some simple organic compounds, such as methane, ethyl alcohol, formaldehyde, and chloroform. We will now review in a systematic fashion the naming of hydrocarbons and some of their reactions.

For the past several thousand years, people have been using organic compounds for dyes, beverages (ethyl alcohol), medicines, and soaps. Many useful compounds were known to ancient civilizations, but it was only at the beginning of the 18th century that scholars began to investigate the chemical nature of such substances.

By the early 1800's, it began to be possible to divide chemical compounds into two groups: those that came from minerals and would not burn (inorganic compounds) and those that came from living animals or plants and would burn (organic compounds). As we have learned more about the chemistry of these substances, our understanding of the nature and reactions of organic compounds has grown tremendously. Today, there are over *three million* known organic compounds. The study of such a vast number of substances would be impossibly difficult if we couldn't group them together in logical ways.

In Chapter 4 you learned to write structural formulas for methane, ethane, propane, and butane. These four compounds have something in common, which will be discussed in Section 7.1. As organic molecules become more complicated, it becomes more difficult to transmit information about them unless we understand the system used by scientists to name organic compounds. Therefore, this naming method will be introduced in Section 7.1.

7.1 ALKANES

LEARNING GOAL 7A: Given the name of any continuous-chain alkane with from one to ten carbon atoms, write its structural formula.

7B: Given the structural formula of a branched-chain alkane, write its IUPAC name.

7C: Given a series of structural formulas for alkanes, state which formulas show isomers and which depict identical molecules.

An **alkane** is a hydrocarbon (Chapter 4) in which all of the carbon atoms have *single* covalent bonds. Among the examples we saw in Section 4.4 are methane (CH_4), ethane (C_2H_6), propane (C_3H_8), and butane (C_4H_{10}). We also briefly discussed pentane (C_5H_{12}), hexane (C_6H_{14}), and octane (C_8H_{18}).

Hydrocarbons such as the alkanes are important as fuels for our modern technological society. We find them in deposits several thousand feet under the surface of the earth in the form of natural gas, oil, and coal—the remains of plants buried millions of years ago. These are nonrenewable resources, which cannot be replaced when they run out. Hydrocarbons are also very important raw materials for the chemical industry. Because the alkanes are the simplest hydrocarbons, the system for assigning names to the millions of known organic compounds, called the **IUPAC** system (after the *I*nternational *U*nion of *P*ure and *A*pplied *C*hemistry), is based on the names of the alkanes.

The continuous-chain alkanes with from one to ten atoms are summarized in Table 7–1. You already know most of them from Chapter 4, so this table should be largely review. Remember that the shape of each molecule is not as shown in the structural formula since the bonds are arranged in a *tetrahedral* fashion (Section 6.3) around each carbon atom.

The word "continuous" means that we can count the carbon atoms from one end of the molecule to the other. Molecules with side-chains or *branching* will be discussed shortly.

Alkane word stems

Since the names of most organic molecules are derived from the names of the alkanes, you must learn the names in Table 7–1. Then, part of each alkane name (the *stem*), formed by removing the ending *-ane,* is used in organic chemistry to show a specific number of carbon atoms. **Learn these stems.**

meth- means *one* carbon
eth- means *two* carbons
prop- means *three* carbons
but- means *four* carbons
pent- means *five* carbons

hex- means *six* carbons
hept- means *seven* carbons
oct- means *eight* carbons
non- means *nine* carbons
dec- means *ten* carbons

Some of these stems should be familiar, since we have already used them (Section 4.4) to name inorganic covalently bonded compounds, such as Si_2F_6, disilicon *hex*afluoride. Once we know the stems, we can work back to the names of the alkanes by adding the characteristic ending -ane.

EXAMPLE 7a: Give the name of
i) a hydrocarbon with seven carbons in a continuous chain and no multiple bonds

ii)   the molecule

$$H-\overset{\displaystyle H}{\underset{\displaystyle H}{C}}-\overset{\displaystyle H}{\underset{\displaystyle H}{C}}-\overset{\displaystyle H}{\underset{\displaystyle H}{C}}-\overset{\displaystyle H}{\underset{\displaystyle H}{C}}-\overset{\displaystyle H}{\underset{\displaystyle H}{C}}-\overset{\displaystyle H}{\underset{\displaystyle H}{C}}-\overset{\displaystyle H}{\underset{\displaystyle H}{C}}-\overset{\displaystyle H}{\underset{\displaystyle H}{C}}-\overset{\displaystyle H}{\underset{\displaystyle H}{C}}-H$$

SOLUTION: Count the number of carbon atoms in the chain. Then apply the proper stem plus the ending -ane:

i)   with seven carbons, we have hept- plus -ane = heptane

ii)   with nine carbons, we have non- plus -ane = nonane

TABLE 7–1   THE FIRST TEN CONTINUOUS-CHAIN
ALKANE HYDROCARBONS

Name	Formula	Structural Formula
Methane	CH_4	$H-\overset{\displaystyle H}{\underset{\displaystyle H}{C}}-H$
Ethane	C_2H_6	$H-\overset{H}{\underset{H}{C}}-\overset{H}{\underset{H}{C}}-H$
Propane	C_3H_8	$H-\overset{H}{\underset{H}{C}}-\overset{H}{\underset{H}{C}}-\overset{H}{\underset{H}{C}}-H$
Butane	C_4H_{10}	$H-\overset{H}{\underset{H}{C}}-\overset{H}{\underset{H}{C}}-\overset{H}{\underset{H}{C}}-\overset{H}{\underset{H}{C}}-H$
Pentane	C_5H_{12}	$H-\overset{H}{\underset{H}{C}}-\overset{H}{\underset{H}{C}}-\overset{H}{\underset{H}{C}}-\overset{H}{\underset{H}{C}}-\overset{H}{\underset{H}{C}}-H$
Hexane	C_6H_{14}	$H-\overset{H}{\underset{H}{C}}-\overset{H}{\underset{H}{C}}-\overset{H}{\underset{H}{C}}-\overset{H}{\underset{H}{C}}-\overset{H}{\underset{H}{C}}-\overset{H}{\underset{H}{C}}-H$
Heptane	C_7H_{16}	$H-\overset{H}{\underset{H}{C}}-\overset{H}{\underset{H}{C}}-\overset{H}{\underset{H}{C}}-\overset{H}{\underset{H}{C}}-\overset{H}{\underset{H}{C}}-\overset{H}{\underset{H}{C}}-\overset{H}{\underset{H}{C}}-H$
Octane	C_8H_{18}	$H-\overset{H}{\underset{H}{C}}-\overset{H}{\underset{H}{C}}-\overset{H}{\underset{H}{C}}-\overset{H}{\underset{H}{C}}-\overset{H}{\underset{H}{C}}-\overset{H}{\underset{H}{C}}-\overset{H}{\underset{H}{C}}-\overset{H}{\underset{H}{C}}-H$
Nonane	C_9H_{20}	$H-\overset{H}{\underset{H}{C}}-\overset{H}{\underset{H}{C}}-\overset{H}{\underset{H}{C}}-\overset{H}{\underset{H}{C}}-\overset{H}{\underset{H}{C}}-\overset{H}{\underset{H}{C}}-\overset{H}{\underset{H}{C}}-\overset{H}{\underset{H}{C}}-\overset{H}{\underset{H}{C}}-H$
Decane	$C_{10}H_{22}$	$H-\overset{H}{\underset{H}{C}}-\overset{H}{\underset{H}{C}}-\overset{H}{\underset{H}{C}}-\overset{H}{\underset{H}{C}}-\overset{H}{\underset{H}{C}}-\overset{H}{\underset{H}{C}}-\overset{H}{\underset{H}{C}}-\overset{H}{\underset{H}{C}}-\overset{H}{\underset{H}{C}}-\overset{H}{\underset{H}{C}}-H$

The alkane series

The alkanes are not limited to the ten compounds shown in Table 7–1. For one thing, we can have more than ten carbons in the continuous chain, as in $C_{12}H_{26}$ or $C_{15}H_{32}$. All of the continuous-chain alkanes, however, fit the very general formula C_nH_{2n+2}, where n is the number of carbon atoms in the molecule. Heptane, with seven carbons, has the molecular formula C_7H_{16}.

Octane, with eight carbons, is C_8H_{18}. Each higher member in this series differs from the previous one by a $-CH_2-$ unit. A series of compounds that differ in this systematic way is called a *homologous* series. We will meet other such series in Section 7.2.

The alkane series shown in Table 7–1 is sometimes called the *paraffins* because some of the higher members of the series are found in candles and other kinds of wax.

Alkyl groups

When we discuss the naming of branched chain compounds, and also when we make other organic compounds (*derivatives*) from the alkanes, we often find ourselves referring to a molecular fragment, a part of an alkane that has lost one hydrogen atom. We discussed the methyl fragment, CH_3-, and the ethyl fragment, C_2H_5-, in Section 4.4. In the real world, such fragments quickly react to form new substances, such as methyl alcohol, CH_3OH. As you can see, the term *methyl* means CH_3- bonded to something else. Methyl chloride is CH_3Cl.

The term used to represent the molecular fragment is obtained by adding the ending *-yl* to the alkane stem.

CH_3- is *methyl* C_3H_7- is *propyl*
C_2H_5- is *ethyl* C_4H_9- is *butyl*

Table 7–2 shows the **alkyl** groups (where *alk-* comes from the word *alkane* and stands for any of the stems we are using) derived from the first three alkanes. Organic chemists often use the letter R to stand for an alkyl group. An alkane is then "R—H."

TABLE 7–2 SOME ALKYL GROUPS

Alkane (R—H)		Alkyl Group (R—)	
H | H—C—H | H Methane	CH_4	H | H—C— | H Methyl group	CH_3-
H H | | H—C—C—H | | H H Ethane	CH_3CH_3	H H | | H—C—C— | | H H Ethyl group	CH_3CH_2-
H H H | | | H—C—C—C—H | | | H H H Propane	$CH_3CH_2CH_3$	H H H | | | H—C—C—C— | | | H H H Propyl group	$CH_3—CH_2—CH_2-$

EXAMPLE 7b:
i) Write the name of the alkyl group C_5H_{11}—.
ii) What is the chemical formula of the *octyl* group?

- -

SOLUTION: i)   There are five carbon atoms, thus pent- plus -yl = $\boxed{\text{pentyl}}$

ii)   We have oct- meaning eight carbons, plus -yl so the formula is $\boxed{C_8H_{17}-}$

Branched-chain compounds

You have learned that the compound C_4H_{10} with four carbon atoms in a continuous chain is *butane*. Butane is shown in Figure 7–1, along with another molecule that also has the formula C_4H_{10}. These two molecules are **isomers.**

Two different molecules are isomers if they have the same molecular formula (thus the same number of atoms of each element in one molecule of the compound) but different chemical and physical properties. We saw one such situation in Example 4f (p. 102), where two different compounds had the overall molecular formula C_2H_6O. We will encounter many more isomers as we look at other kinds of organic compounds.

How can we describe the two isomers with formula C_4H_{10} shown in Figure 7–1? If the left-hand isomer is called *butane,* what about the one on the right? You should notice that the right-hand molecule has three carbons in a continuous chain (propane) with a methyl group (—CH_3) sticking out from the propane like a branch of a tree. We thus call this molecule a **branched-chain compound,** and its name is *methylpropane.*

There are only two different compounds with the molecular formula C_4H_{10}, and they are both shown in Figure 7–1. However, as the number of carbon atoms increases, we have much greater difficulty distinguishing between isomers. There are 3 isomeric forms of pentane, 5 of hexane, 9 of heptane, 75 of decane, and over 300 000 for $C_{20}H_{42}$.

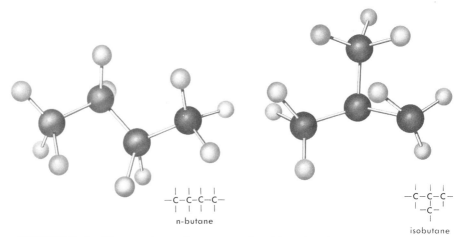

FIGURE 7–1   The two isomeric compounds with molecular formula C_4H_{10}. Left: *butane*, a continuous-chain alkane. Right: methylpropane (or *isobutane*), a branched-chain alkane.

Naming hydrocarbons by the IUPAC system

To distinguish between these molecules, we use the following system.

Step 1: Find the *longest* continuous carbon chain in the molecule. Count the number of carbon atoms in that chain and use that number to choose the stem. We consider this stem to come from the parent compound. If there are no double or triple bonds, the parent compound is an alkane.

The chains of carbon atoms may have to be counted in various ways to find the longest chain in the molecule.

EXAMPLE 7c: Name the parent compounds of

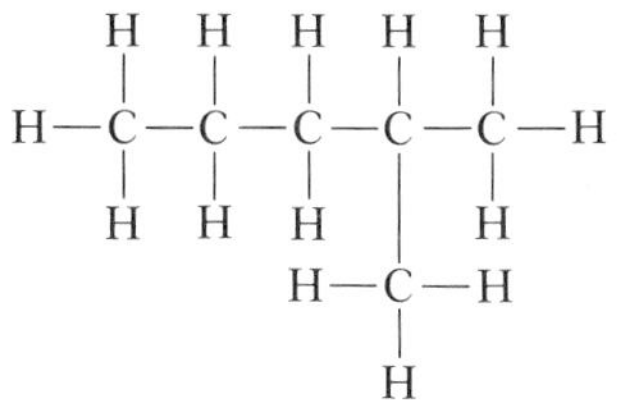

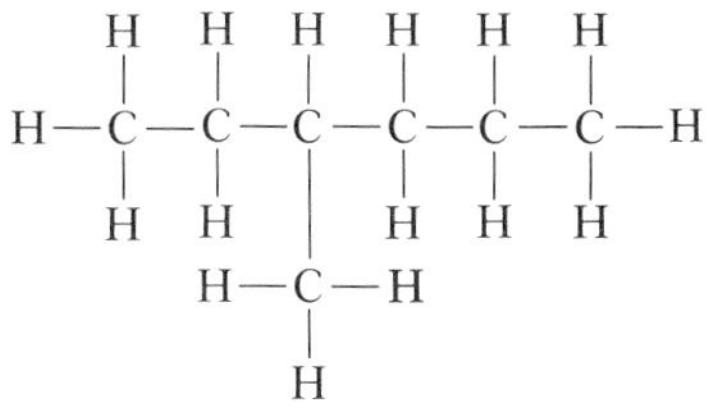

SOLUTION: Count the number of carbons in the longest continuous chain.

i)   *five* carbon atoms, so the parent compound is pentane

ii)   *six* carbon atoms (you will also find a five-carbon chain and a four-carbon chain), so the parent compound is hexane

---

Step 2: Locate any branches in the molecule. Once you have found the carbon atoms that form the longest chain, see if there are any other carbon atoms in the molecule. Each branch must replace a hydrogen in the parent compound with an alkyl group. Number the longest continuous carbon chain, choosing the direction of numbering so that the branches are attached to the carbon atoms with the *lowest* numbers. In other words, start numbering at the end of the chain closest to a branch.

EXAMPLE 7d: Number each of the following chains of carbon atoms, and state to which carbon atom each branch is attached.

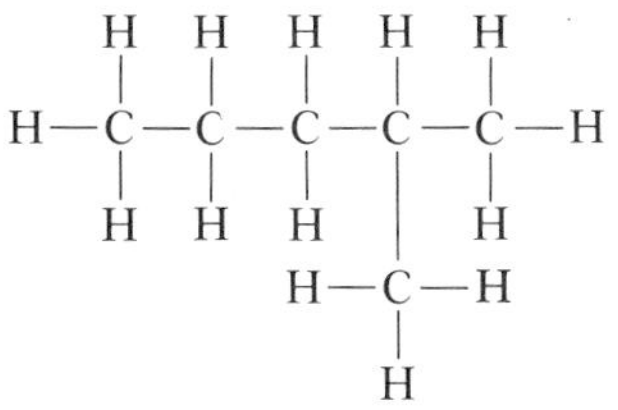

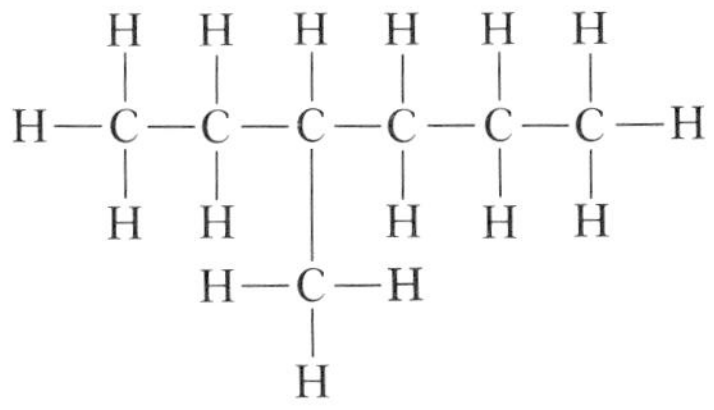

SOLUTION: Start numbering from the chain end closest to the branch.

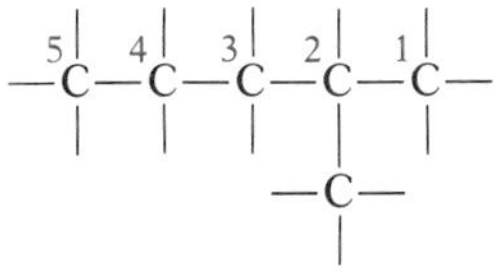

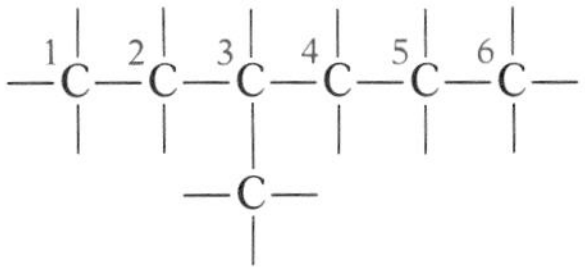

The CH_3— (methyl) branch is on carbon 2 of the pentane chain.

The CH_3— (methyl) branch is on carbon 3 of the hexane chain.

The molecule in Example 7di also has a different five-carbon chain, but with no effect on its name. In the compound shown in Example 7dii, there is also a four-carbon chain and a five-carbon chain; do not use these in naming the molecule because neither one is the longest chain in the molecule.

Step 3: Name each branch according to the alkyl group involved. This will usually be methyl (CH_3—) or ethyl (C_2H_5—).

Step 4: Identify the position of each alkyl branch by giving the number of the carbon atom to which it is attached. Place this number, separated by a hyphen, and the name of the alkyl branch in front of the name of the parent compound.

EXAMPLE 7e: Write the IUPAC name for

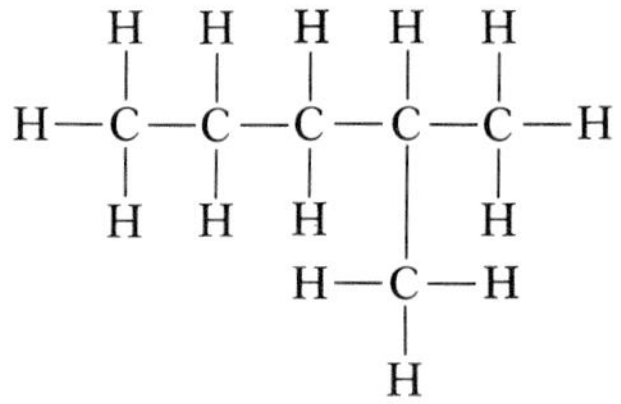

SOLUTION: First number the carbons:

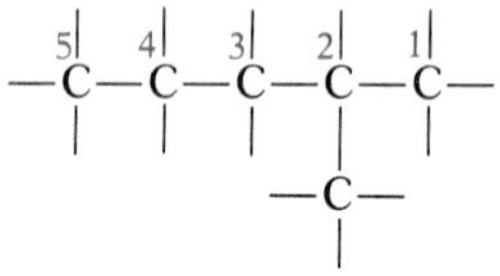

The methyl branch is bonded to carbon 2 of the parent chain. (If you used carbon 4, you started numbering from the wrong end.) The name of the compound is 2-methylpentane .

Step 5: If the same branch occurs two or more times, indicate the number of appearances by the Greek prefixes *di-* (2), *tri-* (3), *tetra-* (4), and *penta-* (5), as in Section 4.4. Place this prefix before the name of the branch and show each position, separating numbers by commas.

EXAMPLE 7f: Write the IUPAC name of the following isomer of pentane.

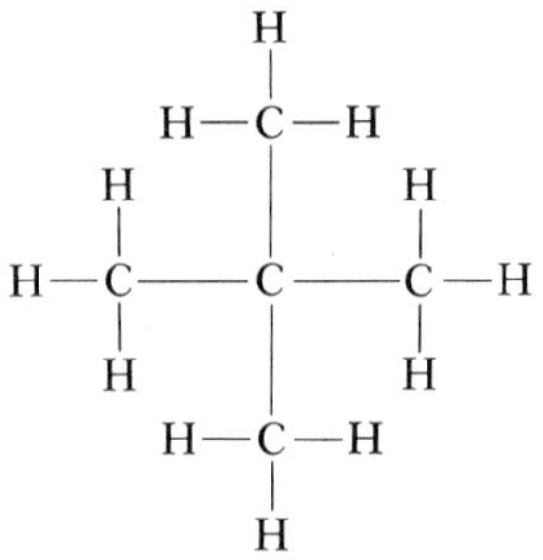

SOLUTION: The parent compound is propane, since there is no continuous chain with more than three carbons, no matter how you count. There are two methyl branches on the central carbon, which must be carbon 2, again no matter which way you count the atoms. The name of this molecule in the IUPAC system is 2,2-dimethylpropane .

Remember that the name cannot be 2-dimethylpropane or 2,2-methylpropane. Each part of the IUPAC name is important.

EXAMPLE 7g: Write the IUPAC name of the following isomer of octane.

SOLUTION: There are three methyl branches on the parent pentane (five-carbon) chain. The <u>lowest numbering is 2,2,4</u> (rather than 2,4,4), so this molecule is named ┃ 2,2,4-trimethylpentane ┃ .

Step 6: If different kinds of alkyl branches are involved, their naming follows the alphabetical order of the group names. For example, ethyl before methyl before propyl.

EXAMPLE 7h: Write the IUPAC name of the following isomer of decane.

SOLUTION: The parent compound is heptane (seven carbons). (Don't make the mistake of taking a side-branch and ending up with six carbons.) The numbering is

The branches are methyl (on carbon 3) and ethyl (on carbon 4), and ethyl goes before methyl alphabetically. The name of this compound in the IUPAC system is ┃ 4-ethyl-3-methylheptane ┃ .

We are omitting hydrogen atoms so you can see the carbon chain more clearly.

There is a way to check that all these steps have been applied correctly. Remember that part of the IUPAC name gives the number of carbon atoms in the longest continuous chain (*hept*ane shows seven carbons in Example 7h). Another part, the naming of branches, gives us the remaining carbon atoms. Add the numbers of carbon atoms indicated by the parent compound name and by all the branch names. Then the total number of carbon atoms in the molecule is obtained. This number must be identical to the number of carbon atoms in the molecular formula if it has been named correctly. This is a good way to check that no carbon atoms have been omitted in naming the molecule.

EXAMPLE 7i: What is the IUPAC name of

$$H-\overset{\displaystyle H}{\underset{\displaystyle H}{C}}-\overset{\displaystyle H}{\underset{\displaystyle H}{C}}-\overset{\displaystyle H-\overset{\displaystyle H}{\underset{\displaystyle }{C}}-H}{\underset{\displaystyle H-\overset{\displaystyle }{\underset{\displaystyle H}{C}}-H}{C}}-\overset{\displaystyle H}{\underset{\displaystyle H}{C}}-H$$

- -

SOLUTION:

Step 1: The longest continuous carbon chain has four carbons. The parent compound is butane.

$$\overset{1}{C}-\overset{2}{C}-\overset{3}{\underset{\displaystyle C}{C}}-\overset{4}{C} \quad \text{or} \quad \overset{2}{C}-\overset{3}{\underset{\displaystyle {}^{1}C}{C}}-C \quad {}^{4}C$$

Although there are eight possible ways to number this molecule, they all lead to the same name.

Step 2: Branches are attached at carbon 2 and carbon 3.
Step 3: Each branch is a methyl group.
Step 4: One methyl branch is at carbon 2, the other is at carbon 3.
Step 5: Since there are two identical branches, the prefix *di-* is used. Each methyl group is also assigned a number to locate its position on the chain.

Not **dimethylbutane or 2,3-methylbutane.**

The IUPAC name is $\boxed{\text{2,3-dimethylbutane}}$.

EXAMPLE 7j: What is the IUPAC name for

$$H-\overset{H}{\underset{H}{C}}-\overset{H}{\underset{\underset{\displaystyle H}{|}}{C}}-\overset{H}{\underset{H}{C}}-\overset{H}{\underset{\underset{\displaystyle H-C-H}{|}}{C}}-\overset{H}{\underset{H}{C}}-\overset{H}{\underset{H}{C}}-H$$

- -

SOLUTION:

Step 1: The longest continuous chain has six carbons. The parent compound is hexane.

$$\overset{1}{C}-\overset{2}{\underset{\displaystyle C}{C}}-\overset{3}{C}-\overset{4}{\underset{\underset{\displaystyle C}{\displaystyle C}}{C}}-\overset{5}{C}-\overset{6}{C} \quad [A] \quad \text{or} \quad \overset{6}{C}-\overset{5}{\underset{\displaystyle C}{C}}-\overset{4}{C}-\overset{3}{\underset{\underset{\displaystyle C}{\displaystyle C}}{C}}-\overset{2}{C}-\overset{1}{C} \quad [B]$$

Other combinations of numbering give either one of the above or a shorter parent chain.

Step 2: Branches occur at carbon 2 and carbon 4 in [A]. Branches occur at carbon 3 and carbon 5 in [B]. So, to give the branches the lowest numbers, we must use [A].

Step 3: One branch is methyl and the other branch is ethyl.

Step 4: The methyl branch is attached at carbon 2 in [A]; the ethyl branch is attached at carbon 4 in [A].

Step 6: Alphabetically, ethyl comes before methyl, so the IUPAC name is 4-ethyl-2-methylhexane .

Step 5 of the IUPAC system is not needed here since each type of branch appears only once.

Not **3-ethyl-5-methylhexane**, because the numbers used (3 + 5) add up to eight, while the numbers used in the answer (4 + 2) add up to six.

Distinguishing between structural isomers

In Figure 7–1 we showed the two different structures having the alkane molecular formula C_4H_{10}. You now understand why the two compounds are named *butane* and *methylpropane*. By far the best way to distinguish between two different organic compounds is to name each molecule. If the names (done correctly by the IUPAC method) are different, then the compounds are different.

Consider the alkanes with molecular formula C_5H_{12}. There are three different ways to position the carbon atoms, and thus three isomeric forms:

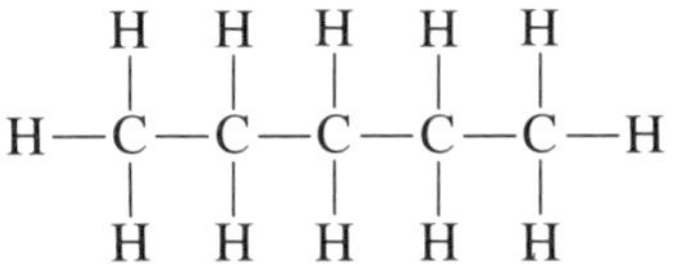

pentane 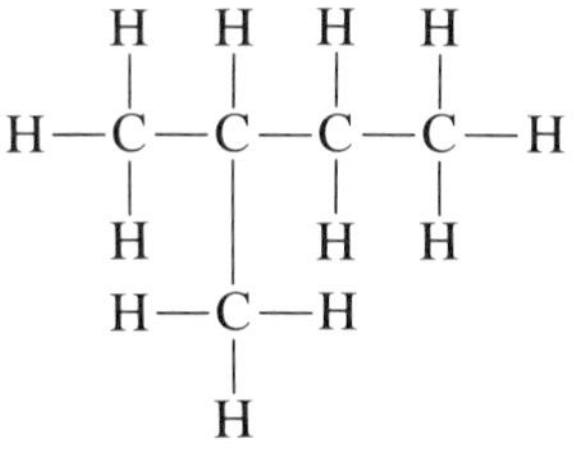   2-methylbutane 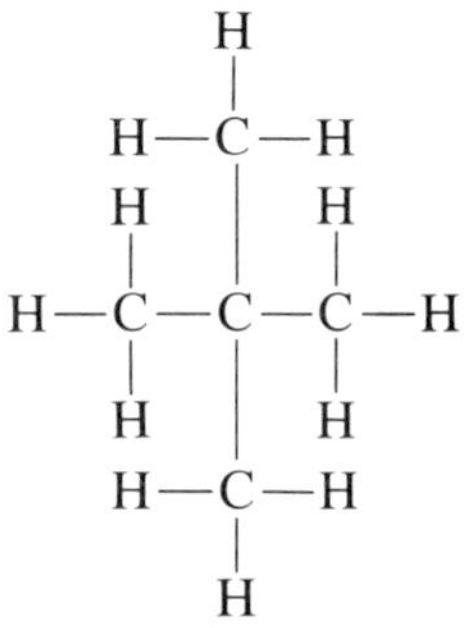   2,2-dimethylpropane

When we reach C_6H_{14}, there are five possible isomers:

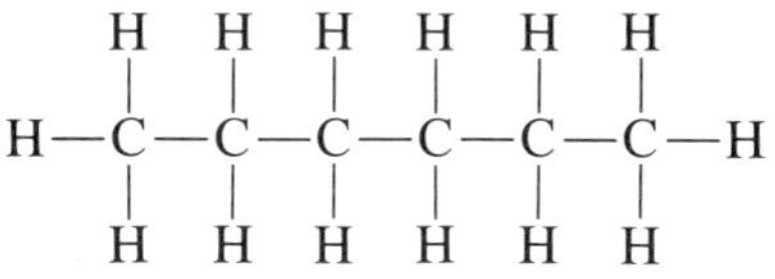

hexane 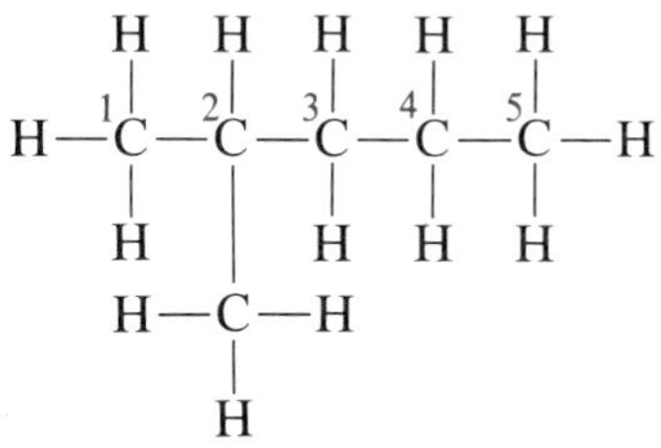   2-methylpentane

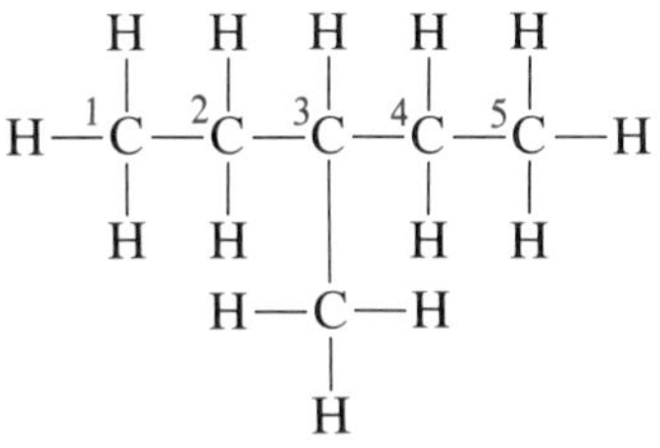

3-methylpentane

$$
\begin{array}{c}
\text{H} \\
\text{H}-\text{C}-\text{H} \\
\text{H}\text{H}\text{H} \\
\overset{1}{|}\overset{2}{|}\overset{3}{|}\overset{4}{|} \\
\text{H}-\text{C}-\text{C}-\text{C}-\text{C}-\text{H} \\
\text{H}\text{H}\text{H} \\
\text{H}-\text{C}-\text{H} \\
\text{H}
\end{array}
$$

2,3-dimethylbutane

$$
\begin{array}{c}
\text{H} \\
\text{H}-\text{C}-\text{H} \\
\text{H}\text{H}\text{H} \\
\overset{1}{|}\overset{2}{|}\overset{3}{|}\overset{4}{|} \\
\text{H}-\text{C}-\text{C}-\text{C}-\text{C}-\text{H} \\
\text{H}\text{H}\text{H} \\
\text{H}-\text{C}-\text{H} \\
\text{H}
\end{array}
$$

2,2-dimethylbutane

Figure 7–2 shows space-filling molecular models of all five molecules with the formula C_6H_{14}. You can see from these models that the three-dimensional geometry around each carbon atom is tetrahedral, rather than rectangular as shown in the structural formula.

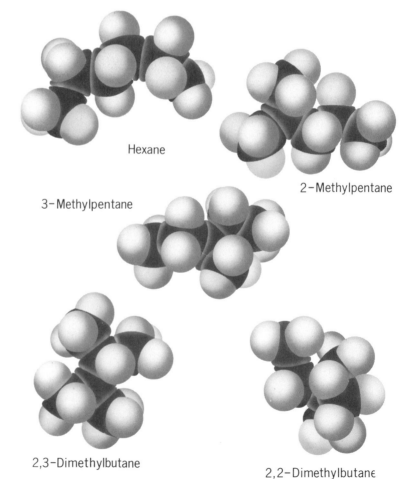

Hexane

2–Methylpentane

3–Methylpentane

2,3–Dimethylbutane

2,2–Dimethylbutane

FIGURE 7–2 Space-filling models of the five isomers with the molecular formula C_6H_{14}.

The types of isomers we have been drawing are called **structural isomers** because they differ in the bonding arrangements in the carbon chains. There are other kinds of isomers, which will be considered later.

In attempting to draw all the possible structures for a collection of carbon atoms, it's usually easiest to start with the longest continuous carbon chain. Then, shorten the chain by one carbon, and again by one, and so forth, drawing all possible structures each time the chain is shortened by one until all combinations are exhausted. When drawing these structures, it is important to distinguish true structural isomers from a mere rearrangement of atoms that only gives the same molecule drawn in different ways. If no chemical bonds are broken or no atoms are moved to new positions, no new structural isomer has been formed. For example,

> Structural isomers are like different constructions made by a child using a single set of building blocks.

$$CH_3—CH_2—CH_2—CH_2 \quad CH_3—CH_2—CH_2—CH_2—CH_3$$

pentane CH_3 pentane

$$\begin{array}{c} CH_3 \\ | \\ CH_2—CH_2—CH_2 \end{array}$$

pentane CH_3

All are the same molecule, pentane. Similarly,

$$\begin{array}{c} CH_3 \\ | \\ CH_3—C—CH_3 \\ | \\ CH_2—CH—CH_3 \\ | \\ CH_2—CH_2—CH_2—CH_3 \end{array}$$

is the same as

$$\begin{array}{c} CH_3 \qquad CH_3 \\ | \qquad\quad | \\ CH_3—C—CH_2—CH—CH_2—CH_2—CH_2—CH_3 \\ | \\ CH_3 \end{array}$$

These two apparently different structures are really the same molecule (trace the longest carbon chain) called 2,2,4-trimethyloctane. Each of the carbon atoms, with the atoms bonded to it, is free to rotate (turn around) and is in constant motion. At one instant, the molecule may be stretched out, at another time it may be curled around, just as a snake or worm may assume many different shapes by arranging its body in various ways. We can likewise write the same structural formula in a variety of ways and still be showing only one single compound.

Because of the many different arrangements that may be used to write a structural formula, it's very easy to become confused when drawing structural isomers. How do you know that you have not drawn the same isomer more than once in a different arrangement? With experience, you will be able to pick out the identical compounds by visual inspection, but, obviously, that isn't foolproof! The best method to spot identical molecules drawn in different arrangements is to *name each structural isomer* that you have sketched. Then, if you follow the IUPAC rules for naming the isomers, *any isomers that differ only in arrangement will have the same IUPAC name.*

EXAMPLE 7k: Some possible structural formulas of C_7H_{16} are

$$\begin{array}{c} CH_3—CH—CH_2—CH—CH_3 \\ | \qquad\quad | \\ CH_3 \qquad CH_3 \end{array} \qquad \begin{array}{c} CH_3 \\ | \\ CH_3—CH—CH_2—CH \\ | \qquad\qquad | \\ CH_3 \qquad CH_3 \end{array}$$

[A]   [B]

$$[C] \quad \begin{array}{c} CH_3 \\ | \\ CH-CH_2-CH_2-CH_2-CH_3 \\ | \\ CH_3 \end{array} \qquad [D] \quad \begin{array}{c} CH_3 \\ | \\ CH_3-CH-CH_2-CH_2 \\ | \\ CH_2-CH_3 \end{array}$$

$$[E] \quad \begin{array}{c} CH_3 \\ | \\ CH_3-CH-CH-CH_2-CH_3 \\ | \\ CH_3 \end{array}$$

Which of these molecules are structural isomers and which are simply different arrangements of the same molecule?

- -

SOLUTION:
If we apply the six steps we learned to name the molecules, their names are
[A] 2,4-dimethylpentane
[B] 2,4-dimethylpentane
[C] 2-methylhexane
[D] 2-methylhexane
[E] 2,3-dimethylpentane
Thus, [A], [C], and [E] are structural isomers. [A] and [B] are identical, and [C] and [D] are identical.

Condensed structural formulas

In order to save space, organic chemists often write the structural formula of a compound so that it all fits on a single printed line. While such formulas provide the same information as the complete diagram, they can be somewhat confusing. You should be particularly aware that

1) A series of singly bonded carbon atoms with attached hydrogens can be condensed using parentheses. **Example:** For octane, the full formula is

$$\begin{array}{c} H \quad H \quad H \quad H \quad H \quad H \quad H \quad H \\ | \quad | \quad | \quad | \quad | \quad | \quad | \quad | \\ H-C-C-C-C-C-C-C-C-H \\ | \quad | \quad | \quad | \quad | \quad | \quad | \quad | \\ H \quad H \quad H \quad H \quad H \quad H \quad H \quad H \end{array}$$

The condensed structural formula can be either $CH_3(CH_2)_6CH_3$ or
$$CH_3CH_2CH_2CH_2CH_2CH_2CH_2CH_3$$

(Do not make the mistake of thinking hydrogens are bonded between the carbon atoms. The carbons are bonded to each other so that each carbon forms four bonds and each hydrogen forms one bond.)

2) Two or more groups on an end carbon may be collected in a condensed structural formula. **Example:** 2,4-dimethylpentane

$$\begin{array}{c} H \quad H \quad H \quad H \quad H \\ | \quad | \quad | \quad | \quad | \\ H-C-C-C-C-C-H \\ | \quad | \quad | \quad | \quad | \\ H \quad | \quad H \quad | \quad H \\ \quad H-C-H \quad | \\ \quad | \qquad H-C-H \\ \quad H \quad H \qquad | \\ \qquad\qquad\qquad H \end{array}$$

can be written $(CH_3)_2CHCH_2CH(CH_3)_2$.

3) Side-chains can be shown in parentheses *after* the carbon to which they are bonded. **Example:** 3-ethyl-2,2,3-trimethylhexane

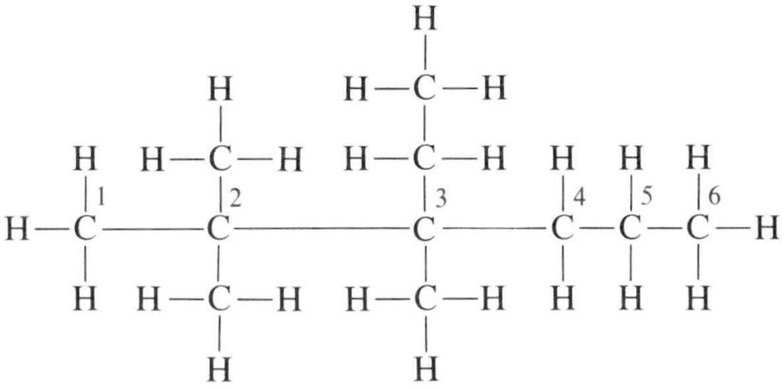

can be written $H_3CC(CH_3)_2C(CH_3CH_2)(CH_3)CH_2CH_2CH_3$.

7.1)   Write the structural formula for
a) heptane   b) decane   c) 3-ethyl-4,4-dimethyloctane
Write the correct IUPAC name for

d) 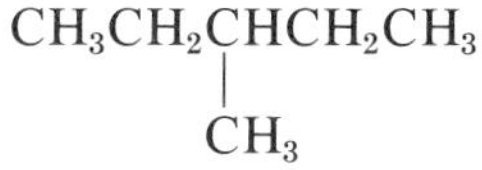 $CH_3CH_2CHCH_2CH_3$
$\qquad\qquad |$
$\qquad\qquad CH_3$

$\qquad\qquad CH_3$
$\qquad\qquad\ \ |$
e) 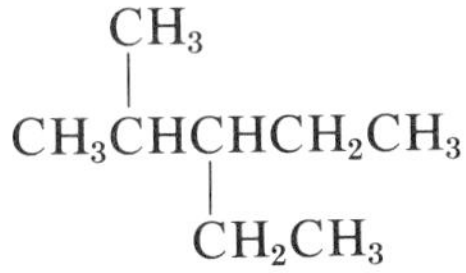 $CH_3CHCHCH_2CH_3$
$\qquad\qquad |$
$\qquad\qquad CH_2CH_3$

f) $CH_3CH_2CHCH_2CH_2CH_2CH_3$
$\qquad\qquad\ \ |$
$\qquad\qquad CH_2CH_2CH_3$

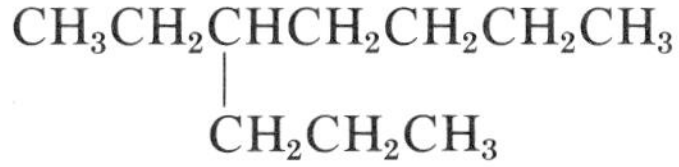

7.2)   Which of the following structural formulas are identical and which are structural isomers? Name each compound.

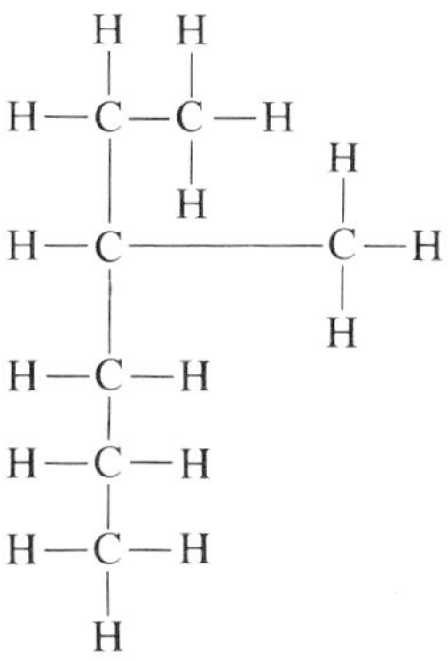

a) 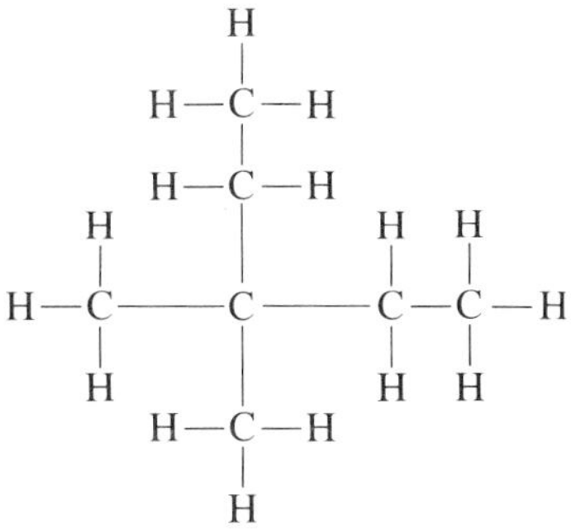   b) 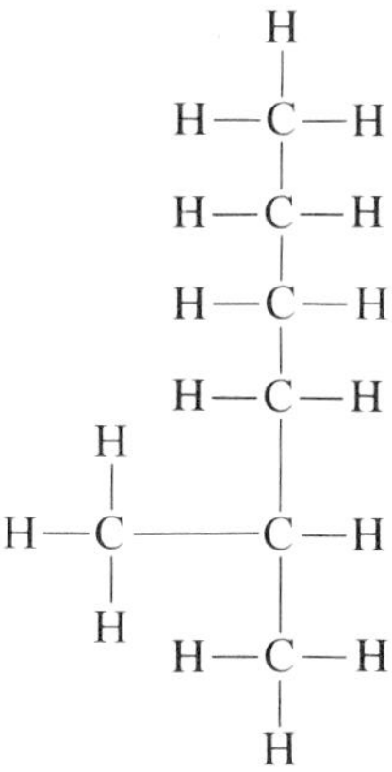   c)

d)

$$H-\overset{\overset{\displaystyle H}{|}}{\underset{\underset{\displaystyle H}{|}}{C}}-\overset{\overset{\displaystyle H-\overset{\displaystyle H}{\overset{|}{C}}-H}{|}}{\underset{\underset{\displaystyle H-\overset{\displaystyle H}{\overset{|}{C}}-H}{|}}{C}}-\overset{\overset{\displaystyle H}{|}}{\underset{\underset{\displaystyle H-\overset{\displaystyle H}{\overset{|}{C}}-H}{|}}{C}}-\overset{\overset{\displaystyle H}{|}}{\underset{\underset{\displaystyle H}{|}}{C}}-H$$

7.2 ALKENES AND ALKYNES

LEARNING GOAL 7D: Write the IUPAC name for an alkene or alkyne, given the structural formula.

7E: Distinguish between structural isomers of a given alkene or alkyne.

7F: Distinguish between and name cis *and* trans *isomers of a given alkene.*

7G: Write a chemical equation for the conversion of an alkane to an alkene (oxidation) and one for the hydrogenation of an alkene (reduction).

7H: Write a chemical equation for an addition to an alkene to produce a given alkyl halide. Apply Markownikoff's rule.

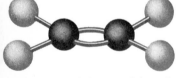

Ball-and-stick model of ethene.

In Chapter 6, you learned that two carbon atoms may be bonded to each other by a single covalent bond, by two covalent bonds (a double bond) or by three covalent bonds (a triple bond). A hydrocarbon that contains only single bonds is an alkane. Since each carbon atom in an alkane is bonded to four other atoms (the maximum possible number), an alkane is often referred to as a *saturated* hydrocarbon.

A hydrocarbon containing a carbon-to-carbon double bond is an *alkene*. One with a triple bond between neighboring carbon atoms is an *alkyne*.

$$H-\overset{\overset{\displaystyle H}{|}}{\underset{\underset{\displaystyle H}{|}}{C}}-\overset{\overset{\displaystyle H}{|}}{\underset{\underset{\displaystyle H}{|}}{C}}-H \qquad H-\overset{\overset{\displaystyle H}{|}}{C}=\overset{\overset{\displaystyle H}{|}}{C}-H \qquad H-C\equiv C-H$$

an alkane (ethane)   an alkene (ethene)   an alkyne (ethyne)

Alkenes and alkynes contain fewer hydrogen atoms than the corresponding alkanes. We shall soon see that it is possible to *add* hydrogen to such compounds under certain conditions. Since alkenes and alkynes do not contain as much hydrogen as alkanes, we consider them to be *unsaturated* hydrocarbons, not yet containing the maximum amount of hydrogen. The terms saturated and unsaturated are also applied to other molecules containing long carbon chains which may include multiple bonds. Of particular interest are the fats and fatty acids (Chapter 18) with and without double bonds.

Alkenes form a homologous series with the formula C_nH_{2n}, where n is the number of carbon atoms (two or more). Alkynes form a similar series with group formula C_nH_{2n-2}.

A structural formula does not show the difference between the sigma and pi parts of a double or triple bond, as discussed in Section 6.2. However, the presence of pi bonding makes alkenes and alkynes react chemically in a fashion quite different from that of alkanes, and also makes them slightly more difficult to name.

Naming alkenes and alkynes

The IUPAC rules for naming alkenes and alkynes are very similar to those you learned for alkanes. The main differences are (a) the longest continuous carbon chain must contain the double bond or triple bond and (b) in many cases the position of the double bond or triple bond in the longest chain must be identified by a number.

Let's see how this system applies.

Step 1: Select the longest continuous carbon chain that includes the double or triple bond. The alkane having this number of carbon atoms is considered to be the parent compound and provides the basic name. For an alkene, the *-ane* ending of the parent compound name is changed to *-ene*. For an alkyne, the *-ane* ending is changed to *-yne*.

EXAMPLE 7l: What is the IUPAC name for

$$\begin{array}{ccc} H & & H \\ \diagdown & & \diagup \\ & C{=}C & \\ \diagup & & \diagdown \\ H & & CH_3 \end{array}$$

- -

SOLUTION: The longest continuous carbon chain has three carbon atoms, so the parent compound is propane. If we drop the *-ane* ending and add *-ene*, propane becomes ⎡propene⎤ .

EXAMPLE 7m: What is the IUPAC name for $CH_3{-}C{\equiv}C{-}H$?

- -

SOLUTION: The longest continuous carbon chain has three carbon atoms, so the parent compound is again propane. This time, drop the *-ane* ending and add *-yne,* so that propane becomes ⎡propyne⎤ .

Step 2: When the multiple bond may be located at more than one position in the molecule, the position of the first carbon atom of the multiple bond is indicated by a number placed immediately in front of the longest chain name. This number is separated from the chain name by a hyphen. The molecule is always numbered from the end nearest the multiple bond, so that the first carbon of the multiple bond has the lowest possible number.

EXAMPLE 7n: What is the IUPAC name for

$$\begin{array}{ccccccc} & H & & H & H & H & \\ & | & 1 & 2\,| & 3\,| & 4\,| & \\ H{-} & C & {-}\!\!-\!\!- & C{=} & C{-} & C & {-}H \\ & | & & & & | & \\ & H & & & & H & \end{array}$$

SOLUTION: Because the longest chain has four carbons, the name is butene. The double bond is located between carbon 2 and carbon 3 so its lower number is 2 and therefore the name of this compound is $\boxed{\text{2-butene}}$.

EXAMPLE 7o: What is the IUPAC name for

$$H-\overset{\overset{\displaystyle H}{|}}{\underset{\underset{\displaystyle H}{|}}{C}}\overset{1}{-}\overset{\overset{\displaystyle H}{|}}{\underset{\underset{\displaystyle H}{|}}{C}}\overset{2}{-}\overset{3}{C}\equiv\overset{4}{C}-\overset{\overset{\displaystyle H}{|}}{\underset{\underset{\displaystyle H}{|}}{C}}\overset{5}{-}\overset{\overset{\displaystyle H}{|}}{\underset{\underset{\displaystyle H}{|}}{C}}\overset{6}{-}\overset{\overset{\displaystyle H}{|}}{\underset{\underset{\displaystyle H}{|}}{C}}\overset{7}{-}H$$

Not **4-heptyne; start counting from the end nearest the triple bond.**

SOLUTION: The longest chain has seven carbons, and its name is heptyne. The triple bond is located between carbon 3 and carbon 4; therefore the name of the compound is $\boxed{\text{3-heptyne}}$.

An alkene or alkyne can also have branches on the longest continuous carbon chain. Since the multiple bond must be assigned the lowest possible number, the positions of the branches are automatically fixed once we assign the position of the multiple bond. Thus, for a branched-chained alkene or alkyne, we first apply Steps 1 and 2. Then

Step 3: Name the alkyl branches and identify their positions on the longest carbon chain by the appropriate numbers. Place these numbers (separated by a hyphen) in front of the name of the alkyl group.

Step 4: Indicate a repeat of any alkyl branch by the appropriate prefix (*di-, tri-*, etc.)

Step 5: Arrange all the alkyl branches in alphabetical order. Place the numbers and alkyl branch names in front of the entire parent name, with hyphens separating any numbers from the word parts of the name.

EXAMPLE 7p: What is the IUPAC name for

$$H-\overset{5}{\underset{\underset{\displaystyle H}{|}}{\overset{\overset{\displaystyle H}{|}}{C}}}-\overset{4}{\underset{\underset{\displaystyle H}{|}}{\overset{\overset{\displaystyle H}{|}}{C}}}-\overset{3}{\underset{\underset{\displaystyle |}{|}}{\overset{\overset{\displaystyle H}{|}}{C}}}-\overset{2}{\overset{\overset{\displaystyle H}{|}}{C}}=\overset{1}{\overset{\overset{\displaystyle H}{|}}{C}}-H$$

$$H-\overset{\overset{\displaystyle }{}}{\underset{\underset{\displaystyle H}{|}}{C}}-H$$

SOLUTION: The longest continuous carbon chain has five carbons, so the name of the parent compound is pentane, which becomes pentene because of the double bond.

Since the double bond is between the first and second carbons, this isomer is 1-pentene. A methyl ($-CH_3$) branch located at carbon 3 on the longest continuous chain makes the name of this compound $\boxed{\text{3-methyl-1-pentene}}$.

EXAMPLE 7q: What is the IUPAC name for

$$H-\overset{\overset{\displaystyle H}{|}}{\underset{\underset{\displaystyle H}{|}}{C}}\overset{1}{}-\overset{2}{C}\equiv\overset{3}{C}-\overset{\overset{\displaystyle H}{|}}{\underset{\underset{\displaystyle H}{|}}{C}}\overset{4}{}-\overset{\overset{\displaystyle H}{|}}{\underset{\underset{\displaystyle H}{|}}{C}}\overset{5}{}-\overset{\overset{\displaystyle H}{|}}{\underset{\underset{\displaystyle H}{|}}{C}}\overset{6}{}-H$$

SOLUTION: The parent chain name is hexyne. Because the position of the first carbon of the triple bond is 2, this isomer is 2-hexyne. A methyl branch located at carbon 5 leads to the name 5-methyl-2-hexyne .

Not **2-methyl-4-hexyne**, even though the numbers add up to less than the answer given, because we start counting from the end nearest the multiple bond.

Earlier in this chapter, you learned that the alkane C_4H_{10} had two possible arrangements of the carbon atoms. The two structural isomers were butane and methylpropane. Through branching of the carbon chain, alkenes and alkynes show similar structural isomerism. For example, 1-butene and 2-methylpropene are structural isomers of the hydrocarbon C_4H_8:

$$H_2C=CHCH_2CH_3 \qquad H_2C=C\overset{\displaystyle CH_3}{\underset{\displaystyle CH_3}{<}}$$

1-butene   2-methylpropene

Similarly, 1-pentyne and 3-methyl-1-butyne are structural isomers of the hydrocarbon C_5H_8:

$$HC\equiv CCH_2CH_2CH_3 \qquad HC\equiv C\underset{\underset{\displaystyle CH_3}{|}}{C}HCH_3$$

1-pentyne   3-methyl-1-butyne

In all the examples so far, we have rearranged the carbon atoms to draw the structural isomers. However, with alkenes and alkynes, structural isomers are also possible simply by changing the position of the multiple bond in the carbon chain, *without* changing the position of any of the carbon atoms in the molecule. For example, in the alkene C_4H_8 we may write the four carbon atoms in a continuous chain. The double bond can be then located between carbon 1 and carbon 2 to give 1-butene. However, we could just as well put the double bond between carbon 2 and carbon 3 to give another isomer, 2-butene. By branching the chain, we get 2-methylpropene:

$$H_2C=CHCH_2CH_3 \qquad CH_3CH=CHCH_3 \qquad H_2C=C\overset{\displaystyle CH_3}{\underset{\displaystyle CH_3}{<}}$$

1-butene   2-butene   2-methylpropene

Thus, structural isomers of alkenes and alkynes are possible either by rearranging the carbon atoms in the molecule or by changing the position of the multiple bond.

EXAMPLE 7r: What are the structural isomers of the hydrocarbon C_5H_8 that contain a triple bond?

– –

SOLUTION: The carbon atoms may be drawn in a continuous chain or they may be branched from a shorter carbon chain.

$HC\equiv CCH_2CH_2CH_3$ 1-pentyne

$CH_3C\equiv CCH_2CH_3$ 2-pentyne

$CH_3CHC\equiv CH$ 3-methyl-1-butyne
$\quad|$
CH_3

Any other arrangement of the carbon atoms or position of the triple bond gives one of these molecules. Thus, there are three structural isomers of the alkyne C_5H_8.

Cis-trans isomers

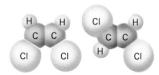

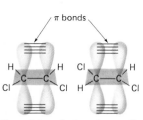

π bonds

The pi bond that forms the second bond in a carbon-carbon double bond prevents the molecule from rotating. This creates two different isomers, as shown for the molecular formula $ClHC\equiv CHCl$. The top diagram shows space-filling models. The bottom diagram shows that the six atoms all lie in the same plane, with the pi bonds above and below that plane. These molecules follow the same naming system described for alkenes.

In Section 7.1 we referred to the many different shapes that may be assumed by a long-chain alkane molecule owing to the ability of every carbon atom to *rotate* around each bond which links it to its neighbors. An alkane thus does not have a fixed three-dimensional geometry. We can be sure that bonds are arranged tetrahedrally around each carbon, but we cannot predict the overall size or shape of an alkane molecule with three or more carbon atoms.

The situation is different if there is a multiple bond in the carbon chain. For example, the double bond in ethene, $H_2C\equiv CH_2$, presents a barrier to rotation of either carbon atom since a pi bond restricts rotation of the two carbon atoms it connects. Rotation can only occur if the pi bond is broken. The amount of energy required to break a pi bond is about 68 kcal/mole, a relatively large amount of energy. Most molecules don't have this much extra energy available to them. Thus, the groups attached to pi-bonded carbon atoms are generally *fixed in space relative to one another.*

This **restricted rotation** of double bonds in alkenes has some interesting structural consequences that depend on the number of different groups attached to the double bond. By ''group,'' we mean any atom or group of atoms bonded to the carbon. Each double-bonded carbon atom has two such groups. One of the structural isomers is 2-butene. A detailed study of 2-butene has shown that there are really two different molecules that have a four-carbon chain with a double bond between carbon 2 and carbon 3 and with the remaining bonds to carbon occupied by hydrogens. These two molecules have the planar structures

$$H_3C \diagdown \qquad \diagup H$$
$$C=C$$
$$H \diagup \qquad \diagdown CH_3$$
[A]
trans-2-butene

$$H_3C \diagdown \qquad \diagup CH_3$$
$$C=C$$
$$H \diagup \qquad \diagdown H$$
[B]
cis-2-butene

In [A] the two methyl groups are located *across* the double bond from each other, as are the two hydrogen atoms. This situation is called **trans,** meaning "across," as in a *trans* continental (across the continent) trip. In [B] the two methyl groups are located on the same side of the double bond, as are the two hydrogen atoms. This situation is called **cis,** meaning "on the same side." To indicate which molecule is being named, the prefix *trans* or *cis* is included in the name. This prefix is placed in front of the number that indicates the position of the double bond and is separated from this number by a hyphen. Thus, the 2-butene isomers are *trans*-2-butene and *cis*-2-butene. Overall, there are four structural isomers of the alkene C_4H_8.

The *trans* and *cis* isomers of 2-butene differ only with respect to the arrangement in space of the atoms or groups of atoms in the molecule. Both isomers contain the double bond, the same number of carbon atoms, and the same number of hydrogen atoms. However, they are not identical and are called **geometrical isomers.**

Geometrical isomers are compounds that have the same molecular formula but different arrangements of the atoms because of the presence of restricted rotation in the molecule. For now, we will only discuss alkenes. In Section 7.3, you will see examples of restricted rotation in compounds that do *not* contain a double bond.

Now that you have seen that 2-butene exists in two isomeric forms, what about 1-butene? Does it also have two geometrical isomers? Chemical evidence says no! There is only one 1-butene. The presence of a double bond in the molecule does not automatically signal the presence of *cis-trans* (geometrical) isomers. There are two requirements for a molecule to exist in *cis-trans* isomeric forms:

1) Restricted rotation of some kind must be present in the molecule.
2) Each carbon atom involved in the double bond (or any other situation of restricted rotation) must carry two different groups.

So, 1-butene meets the first requirement. It has restricted rotation (the double bond). However, 1-butene does not meet the second requirement, since one of the carbon atoms has two identical atoms (the hydrogens) bonded to it.

Similarly, the other C_4H_8 structural isomer, 2-methylpropene, does not exist as *cis-trans* isomers. It has two identical groups on each carbon of the double bond. A molecule must fulfill *both* requirements in order for *cis-trans* isomerism to be present.

You may be asking yourself why we are bothering to point out these geometrical isomers. Such isomers are of great importance in living cells. They may exhibit widely different chemical and physical properties, as well as different responses in the body.

cis-isomer

trans-isomer

The sex-attractant of the female housefly. Only the *cis* isomer is effective.

For example, two unsaturated organic acids, maleic acid and fumaric acid, are geometrical isomers. Fumaric acid is an important intermediate in metabolic processes, whereas maleic acid is poisonous to living organisms.

maleic acid

fumaric acid

A long-chain alkene (23 carbons) is secreted by the female housefly. This secretion contains the *cis* isomer and is the attractant perfume for the male housefly. The *trans* isomer does not attract him, and so geometrical isomers are very important to houseflies!

Geometrical isomers also play an important role in human vision. One of the important chemical compounds involved in vision is *retinal*. When light strikes the retina of the eye, it causes the conversion of a *cis* double bond in retinal to a *trans* double bond.

cis-retinal

light

trans-retinal

Bright light temporarily destroys our ability to see in dim light because it takes time for the formation of a new supply of *cis*-retinal. When less light hits the eye, the conversion of *trans*-retinal back to the necessary *cis*-retinal is slowed and we find it more difficult to see.

You may be wondering why we have focused all our attention on alkene examples of *cis-trans* isomers. What about alkynes—do they also show geometrical isomerism? Chemical evidence says no! An alkyne is a linear molecule, and the two groups attached to the triple bond lie in a straight line with the triple bond. No geometrical isomerism is possible.

Oxidation-reduction of hydrocarbons

Organic compounds take part in many chemical reactions that can be viewed as the addition or loss of hydrogen atoms. Such reactions are important in many processes of living cells. In this section, we will introduce you to the concept of oxidation and reduction as applied to organic molecules. In Chapter 8, we will expand our discussion of these ideas to include more general definitions of oxidation and reduction.

When hydrogens are lost by organic molecules, *oxidation* has occurred. In the United States, alkenes are made commercially by heating (cracking) petroleum alkanes at very high temperatures. Carbon-hydrogen bonds are broken under these conditions, and alkenes are formed:

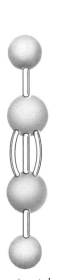

Ethyne (acetylene).

$$CH_3CH_2CH_2CH_3 \xrightarrow{700°C} H_2C{=}CHCH_2CH_3 \text{ and } CH_3CH{=}CHCH_3 + H_2$$
butane 1-butene 2-butene

The butane has lost hydrogen atoms in this chemical reaction. *Oxidation* of butane has occurred, or, in other words, butane has been *oxidized*.

When hydrogen atoms are gained by an organic molecule, *reduction* has occurred. Alkenes react readily with hydrogen (H_2) gas when nickel or platinum is used as a catalyst:

$$CH_3\underset{\;}{C}H{=}CH_2 + H{-}H \xrightarrow{\text{Ni}} CH_3CH_2CH_3$$
$$\quad\text{propene}\qquad\qquad\qquad\qquad\text{propane}$$

The hydrogen atoms add across the double bond of propene to give propane as the product of this chemical reaction. *Reduction* of propene has occurred, that is, the propene has been *reduced*.

Alkynes can also be reduced with hydrogen gas and a catalyst. An alkene or alkane may be formed, depending on the number of molecules of hydrogen gas added.

$$CH_3\underset{\;}{C}{\equiv}CH + H{-}H \xrightarrow{\text{Pt}} CH_3CH{=}CH_2 \xrightarrow[\text{Pt}]{H_2} CH_3CH_2CH_3$$
$$\quad\text{propyne}\qquad\qquad\qquad\text{propene}\qquad\qquad\text{propane}$$

Catalytic hydrogenation is also an important commercial process. Vegetable oils contain long-chain unsaturated organic molecules, each of which contains one or more carbon-carbon double bonds. Margarine and cooking shortenings are prepared by hydrogenation of these polyunsaturated vegetable oils. By controlling the amount of hydrogenation (that is, the number of double bonds reduced) the degree of polyunsaturation can be controlled. Commercial shortenings such as Crisco or Spry contain about 20 to 25 per cent saturated and 75 to 80 per cent unsaturated carbon chains.

Thus, one simple way to look at some organic chemical reactions is in terms of oxidation and reduction. Focus your attention on the product of the chemical reaction. If it has lost hydrogen atoms (relative to the reactant), oxidation has occurred; if it has gained hydrogen atoms (relative to the reactant), reduction has occurred. The rules are:

1) Oxidation has occurred if the number of carbon-hydrogen bonds *decreases* from reactant to product.
2) Reduction has occurred if the number of carbon-hydrogen bonds *increases* from reactant to product.

Addition of hydrogen halides to alkenes

We have just considered the addition of hydrogen to a double bond. The adding agent (the H_2 molecule) splits and one part of it adds to each carbon of the multiple bond. When the reaction is complete, each carbon of the multiple bond has bonded with another atom. This type of reaction, called an *addition reaction,* is the most common chemical reaction of alkenes:

$$\underset{X{-}Y}{\overset{\diagdown}{C}{=}\overset{\diagup}{C}} \longrightarrow -\overset{|}{\underset{X}{C}}-\overset{|}{\underset{Y}{C}}-$$

product of an addition to an alkene

The addition of H_2 gas in the presence of a metal catalyst is *catalytic hydrogenation.*

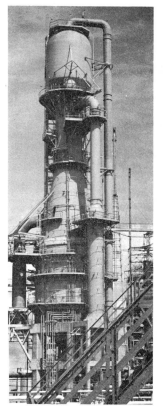

Catalytic cracking unit at Humble Oil and Refining Co.

You will see these rules again in Chapter 8.

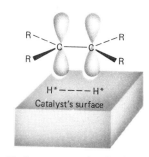

Hydrogen gas adsorbed onto the surface of the metal catalyst leads to catalytic hydrogenation.

Hydrogen halides (HF, HCl, HBr, HI) readily add to a double bond. The product of the reaction is an alkyl halide (Section 4.4):

$$H_2C{=}CH_2 + H{-}Cl \longrightarrow CH_3CH_2Cl$$

ethene   hydrogen   chloroethane
chloride

At first glance, this addition reaction may seem to be exactly like the addition of hydrogen to alkenes. However, hydrogen is a symmetrical molecule (both ends are the same), and it does not make any difference how the molecule splits and adds to the double bond.

The hydrogen halides are unsymmetrical reagents. Both ends are not alike. For most alkenes, there are two possible ways to add the hydrogen halide, for example:

$$CH_3CH{=}CH_2 + H{-}Cl \longrightarrow \underset{\underset{Cl}{|}}{CH_3CHCH_3}$$

propene   hydrogen   2-chloropropane
chloride

or

$$CH_3CH{=}CH_2 + H{-}Cl \longrightarrow CH_3CH_2CH_2Cl$$

propane   hydrogen   1-chloropropane
chloride

Thus, two products, 1-chloropropane and 2-chloropropane, are possible. But what really happens in this reaction? Do we get mainly 1-chloropropane, mainly 2-chloropropane, or a mixture of the two? The actual product is mainly 2-chloropropane, with very little 1-chloropropane being formed. We therefore say that the reagent (HCl) adds *selectively*.

From a study of many reactions of this type, chemists have found that unsymmetrical reagents generally add to a double bond in only one way. The Russian chemist Vladimir Markownikoff proposed a rule that allows you to predict the product to be expected in this type of addition reaction. **Markownikoff's Rule** is

When an unsymmetrical reagent adds to an alkene, the hydrogen of the reagent adds to the carbon atom of the double bond with the greater number of hydrogens.

In the addition of HCl to propene, the hydrogen of the HCl added to the carbon atom that already had two hydrogens. The other carbon of the double bond only had one hydrogen. Another way to remember Markownikoff's Rule is to remember the old saying that "the rich get richer."

EXAMPLE 7s: What is the product of the addition of HI to 1-butene?

SOLUTION:

$$\underset{CH_3CH_2CH{=}CH_2}{\overset{4\quad 3\quad 2\quad 1}{}} \xrightarrow{HI} \begin{cases} CH_3CH_2CH_2CH_2I & [A] \\ \\ CH_3CH_2CHICH_3 & [B] \end{cases}$$

Addition of the hydrogen from HI to carbon 1 leads to compound [B], 2-iodobutane. Addition of the hydrogen to carbon 2 leads to [A], 1-iodobutane. Carbon 1 already has two hydrogens bonded to it, and carbon 2 has one hydrogen bonded to it. Markownikoff's Rule predicts addition of hydrogen to carbon 1, and so the product of this reaction is [B].

EXAMPLE 7t: What is the product of the addition of HCl to 2-methyl-2-butene?

- -

SOLUTION:

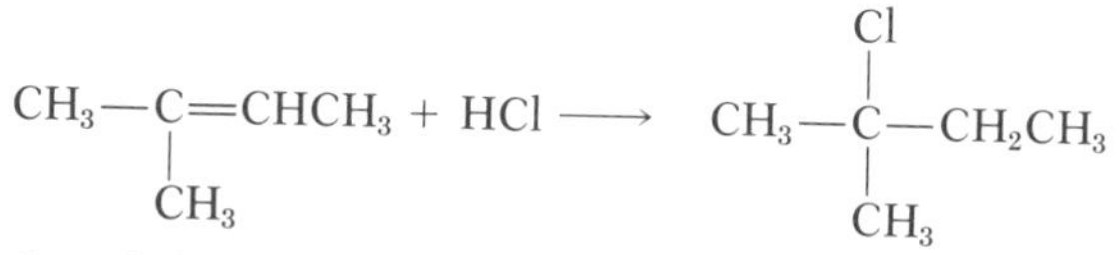

$$
\underset{\substack{|\\ CH_3}}{CH_3-C}=CHCH_3 + HCl \longrightarrow \underset{\substack{|\\ CH_3}}{\overset{\overset{\displaystyle Cl}{|}}{CH_3-C}}-CH_2CH_3
$$

2-methyl-2-butene   2-chloro-2-methylbutane

Addition follows Markownikoff's Rule and the hydrogen from the HCl adds to the carbon already having the greater number of hydrogens.

7.3) Write the IUPAC name for each of the following alkenes and alkynes.
a) $CH_3CH_2CH_2CH_2CH=CH_2$
b) $(CH_3)_2CHCH_2CH=CH_2$

c) 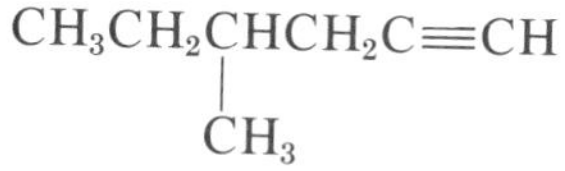 $CH_3CH_2\underset{\substack{|\\ CH_3}}{CH}CH_2C\equiv CH$

d) $CH_3CH_2CH_2CH_2C\equiv CCH_2CH_2CH_3$
7.4) Write the IUPAC names for
a) all structural isomers of the alkene C_5H_{10}
b) the compound

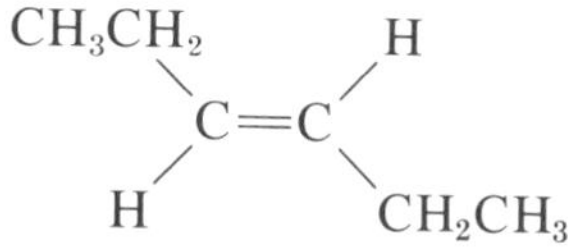

$$
\underset{H}{\overset{CH_3CH_2}{\diagdown}}C=C\underset{CH_2CH_3}{\overset{H}{\diagup}}
$$

7.5) Which of the following compounds would exhibit geometrical isomerism?
a) $(CH_3)_2C=CHCH_3$
b) $CH_3CH=CHCH_2CH(CH_3)_2$

c) 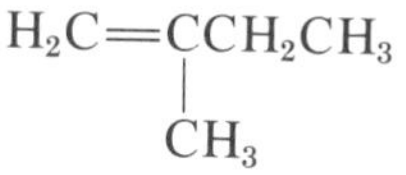 $H_2C=\underset{\substack{|\\ CH_3}}{C}CH_2CH_3$

7.6) Using Markownikoff's Rule, predict the product of each of the following reactions.
a) $(CH_3)_2CHCH=CH_2 + HF \longrightarrow$
b) $(CH_3)_2C=CHCH_2CH_3 + HCl \longrightarrow$
c) $H_2C=CHCl + HCl \longrightarrow$

SELF-CHECK

7.3 SIMPLE ORGANIC RING SYSTEMS

> *LEARNING GOAL 7I: Name and identify* cis *and* trans *isomers of cyclo-alkanes and their simple derivatives.*

Thus far, we have mainly discussed compounds in which the carbon atoms are attached to one another to form continuous or branched chains. Other carbon compounds exist that have closed chains and are classified as *cyclic* ("circle") *compounds.* Some of these compounds, which occur in nature and may have one or more rings, are cholesterol, nicotine, DNA, RNA, and THC (from marijuana). In later chapters, you will see these and many other important cyclic chemicals of life.

Cycloalkanes

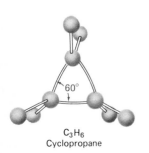

C_3H_6
Cyclopropane

The simplest cyclic compounds are the **cycloalkanes,** which contain only carbon and hydrogen. A cycloalkane can be viewed as being formed by the removal of one hydrogen atom from each of the end carbons of a continuous-chain alkane. These two carbons are then joined together. Cycloalkanes are not really formed this way, but it is an easy way for the mind to get the idea of cyclic ring formation.

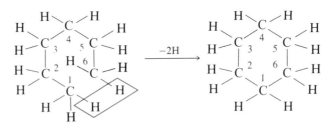

Chemists usually use a shorthand method for drawing cyclic structures. For example, a *triangle* is used to represent a three-membered ring, a *square* is used for a four-membered ring, a *pentagon* (like that in Washington, D.C.) for a five-membered ring, and a *hexagon* for a six-membered ring:

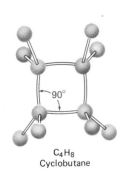

C_4H_8
Cyclobutane

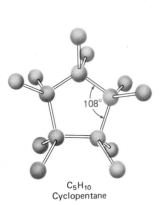

C_5H_{10}
Cyclopentane

$$H_2C\!-\!CH_2$$
$$\diagdown\;\diagup$$
$$C$$
$$H_2$$
cyclopropane
C_3H_6

$$H_2C\!-\!CH_2$$
$$|\qquad\;\;|$$
$$H_2C\!-\!CH_2$$
cyclobutane
C_4H_8

$$H_2C\!-\!CH_2$$
$$H_2C\qquad CH_2$$
$$C$$
$$H_2$$
cyclopentane
C_5H_{10}

$$H_2$$
$$C$$
$$H_2C\qquad CH_2$$
$$H_2C\qquad CH_2$$
$$C$$
$$H_2$$
cyclohexane
C_6H_{12}

In polygon ("many-sided") structures, each corner represents a singly bonded carbon atom along with its two hydrogens. The sides of the polygon represent the covalent single bonds joining the carbon atoms.

The simplest cycloalkanes are named by adding the prefix *cyclo-* to the name of the corresponding alkane. Substituted cycloalkanes are named and numbered in the same way as alkanes. Each branch is again given the lowest possible number.

EXAMPLE 7u: What is the IUPAC name for the cycloalkane , a seven-membered ring?

- -

SOLUTION: The cycloalkane contains seven carbon atoms. Hence, it is the cyclic version of heptane. To indicate it is a cycloalkane, we place the prefix cyclo- in front of the alkane name. The name of this compound is cycloheptane .

EXAMPLE 7v: What is the IUPAC name for

- -

SOLUTION: The ring structure is a cyclopentane. It has two branches (both methyl) attached to it. We must name each branch, indicate identical branches by a suitable prefix (di- in this case), and indicate the position of each branch on the ring by the lowest number.
The name is   1,1-dimethylcyclopentane .

When the ends of an alkane chain are joined together to form a cycloalkane, the carbon atoms of the ring are "locked" into place. No free rotation of the carbon atoms of the ring structure is possible without breaking the ring. Cycloalkanes may thus potentially show geometrical isomerism like the alkenes. You might want to review the requirements for geometrical isomerism in Section 7.2.

EXAMPLE 7w: Does 1,1-dimethylcyclohexane show geometrical isomerism?

- -

SOLUTION:

1,1-dimethylcyclohexane

The molecule has restricted rotation because it contains a ring.
Both carbon 1 and carbon 2 contain identical groups, and so no geometrical isomerism is possible. Only one form of this compound exists.

EXAMPLE 7x: Does 1,2-dimethylcyclohexane show geometrical isomerism?

- -

SOLUTION:

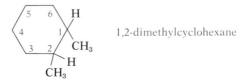

1,2-dimethylcyclohexane

The molecule has restricted rotation because it contains a ring. Neither carbon 1 nor carbon 2 bears identical groups, so this molecule does show geometrical isomerism and can exist as either the *cis* or the *trans* isomer. The two geometrical isomers are

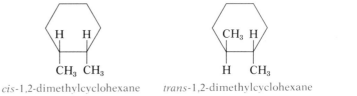

cis-1,2-dimethylcyclohexane   *trans*-1,2-dimethylcyclohexane

Note that, as for alkenes, the prefix *cis* or *trans* is incorporated into the name of the compound to indicate the relative position of identical groups in the molecule.

Ring strain

Only the three- and four-membered cycloalkanes exhibit much chemical reactivity. To account for this, a German chemist by the name of Adolf Baeyer proposed in 1885 a "ring strain" theory. He assumed that all the cycloalkanes were *planar* and that the carbon atoms of the ring were most "comfortable" if they had normal tetrahedral bond angles (109°). In cyclopropane, the bond angle is 60°; in cyclobutane it is 90°; in cyclopentane 108°.

60°   90°   108°

He proposed that the more the bond angle differed from 109°, the more stress or strain the molecule would be subjected to. Thus, he subtracted the bond angles of each cycloalkane from 109° to obtain the "degree of strain." The larger this difference, the more strain in the cycloalkane and the higher the chemical reactivity.

This idea worked quite well for the three-, four-, and five-carbon cycloalkanes. The amount of strain decreased in the order cyclopropane is more strained than cyclobutane, which is more strained than cyclopentane. Correspondingly, the chemical reactivity decreased in the order cyclopropane is more reactive than cyclobutane, which is more reactive than cyclopentane, as predicted by Baeyer's theory.

When the cycloalkanes are six-membered rings or larger, Baeyer also predicted a lot of strain, since if these larger rings were planar the bond angles would be larger than 109°:

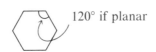 120° if planar

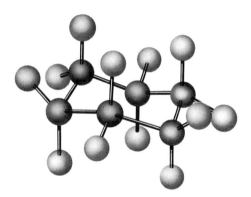

FIGURE 7–3   The puckered form of
cyclohexane, C_6H_{12}.

However, chemical evidence shows that these larger cycloalkane rings are similar to
cyclopentane and have low chemical reactivity. Baeyer's strain theory fails for these
larger rings because they are not planar, as he assumed. We now know that they are
puckered (bent) so that each carbon atom of the ring attains the tetrahedral (109°)
bond angle. By assuming this puckered shape, the molecule has no strain and is quite
"comfortable" and relatively unreactive. Figure 7–3 shows the shape of the cyclohexane ring.

   Although Baeyer's strain theory did not survive the test of time, it did stimulate
chemists to determine the bond angles of many cycloalkanes. Thus, it did help advance our understanding of cycloalkanes and the shapes of ring structures.

7.7)   Which of the following cycloalkanes would show geometrical
isomerism?
a)   1,1,3-trimethylcyclohexane
b)   1,2-diethylcyclopropane
c)   1,1,2-trimethylcyclobutane

SELF-CHECK

CHAPTER SEVEN IN REVIEW ■ Hydrocarbons

7.1 ALKANES   Page 184
   *7A: Given the name of any continuous-chain alkane with from
one to ten carbon atoms, write its structural formula.*
   *7B: Given the structural formula of a branched-chain alkane,
write its IUPAC name.*
   *7C: Given a series of structural formulas for alkanes, state which
formulas show isomers and which depict identical molecules.*
7.2 ALKENES AND ALKYNES   Page 198
   *7D: Write the IUPAC name for an alkene or alkyne, given the
structural formula.*
   *7E: Distinguish between structural isomers of a given alkene or
alkyne.*
   7F: Distinguish between and name cis *and* trans *isomers of a
given alkene.*
   7G: Write a chemical equation for the conversion of an alkane to

an alkene (oxidation) and one for the hydrogenation of an alkene (reduction).

7H: Write a chemical equation for an addition to an alkene to produce a given alkyl halide. Apply Markownikoff's Rule.

7.3 SIMPLE ORGANIC RING SYSTEMS   **Page 208**

7I: Name and identify cis *and* trans *isomers of cycloalkanes and their simple derivatives.*

GLOSSARY FOR CHAPTER SEVEN

alkane A hydrocarbon in which the carbon atoms are connected by only single bonds; group formula C_nH_{2n+2}; carbon chain may be continuous or branched. (p. 185)

alkyl An alkane with one hydrogen atom removed; a group of atoms that is often found as a substituent on a hydrocarbon chain or connected to another group, such as CH_3OH, methyl alcohol, in which CH_3— is the alkyl fragment called *methyl.* (p. 187)

branched-chain compound An organic compound in which not all the carbon atoms are arranged in a single continuous chain. (p. 188)

cis A prefix indicating the geometrical isomer that contains two identical groups on the same side of a double bond. (p. 203)

cycloalkane A hydrocarbon that includes at least one ring of carbon atoms joined only by single bonds. (p. 208)

geometrical isomers Isomers that have different arrangements of their atoms in space because of the presence of restricted rotation in the molecule. (p. 203)

isomers Different compounds that have the same molecular formula. (p. 188)

IUPAC International Union of Pure and Applied Chemistry, the body that devises official systems for naming chemical compounds. (p. 185)

Markownikoff's Rule A rule for predicting the product of the addition of an unsymmetrical reagent to a multiple bond. (p. 206)

restricted rotation An energy barrier in a molecule that fixes the groups of the molecule in space relative to one another. (p. 202)

structural isomers Compounds that have the same molecular formula but with the atoms bonded in different ways. (p. 195)

trans A prefix indicating the geometrical isomer that contains two identical groups on opposite sides of a double bond. (p. 203)

QUESTIONS AND PROBLEMS FOR CHAPTER SEVEN ■ Hydrocarbons

SECTION 7.1 ALKANES

7.8) Write the correct IUPAC name for

a) $CH_3CH_2CH_2CH_2CH_2CH_2CH_3$

b) the fragment CH_3CH_2—

c) $(CH_3)_2CHCH_2CH_2CH_2CH_3$

d) $CH_3CH(CH_3)CH_2CH(CH_3)CH_2CH_3$

e) $(CH_3)_3CCH_2CH_3$

f) $(CH_3CH_2)_3CH$

7.9) Write a correct structural formula for

a) nonane

b) butyl-

7.21) Write the correct IUPAC name for

a) $CH_3CH_2CH_2CH_2CH_2CH_3$

b) the fragment CH_3—

c) $CH_3CH(CH_3)CH_2CH_2CH_2CH_3$

d) $(CH_3)_2CHCH_2CH_2CH(CH_3)CH_2CH_3$

e) $CH_3C(CH_3)_2CH_2CH(CH_3)CH_3$

f) $CH_3CH_2CH_2C(CH_2CH_3)_3$

7.22) Write a correct structural formula for

a) octane

b) propyl-

c) methylpropane
d) 3-ethyloctane
e) 2,3,3-trimethylpentane

7.10) Do the following sets of structural formulas show different structural isomers or identical compounds?

a) $CH_3CH_2CH_2$
           |
           CH_2CH_3

     and

CH_3CH_2
  |
CH_2CH_2
    |
    CH_3

b) $CH_3CH(CH_3)CH_2CH_2CH_3$
    and
$CH_3CH_2CH_2CH(CH_3)CH_3$

7.11*) Draw the structural formula for the alkane 4-ethyl-3-methylheptane. Does this molecule obey the octet rule? Write the molecular formula of this compound and calculate the weight of one mole.

c) ethylpentane
d) 4-methylheptane
e) 2-methyl-3-ethylhexane

7.23) Do the following sets of structural formulas show different structural isomers or identical compounds?

a) CH_3 H
           | |
CH_3-C-H and CH_3CCH_3
        | |
    CH_2CH_2 CH_2CH_2
        | |
      CH_2CH_3 CH_2
                             |
                             CH_3

b) $(CH_3)_2CHCH_2CH(CH_3)CH_2CH_3$
    and
$CH_3CH(CH_3)CH_2CH_2CH(CH_3)_2$

7.24*) Draw the structural formula for 2,3,4-trimethyl-4-propylheptane. Does this molecule obey the octet rule? Do the covalence numbers of Chapter 4 apply? Calculate the weight of one mole of this compound.

SECTION 7.2 ALKENES AND ALKYNES

7.12) Write the IUPAC name for
a) $CH_3(CH_2)_3CH=CH_2$
b) $(CH_3CH_2)_2C=CHCH_2CH_3$
c) $CH_3CH_2C≡CCH_2CH_3$

7.13) Draw the structural formula for
a) 4,4-dimethyl-2-pentyne
b) *trans*-2-pentene

7.14) Draw the geometrical isomers of the alkene
$CH_3(CH_2)_3CH=CHCH_2CH_3$
and give the IUPAC name for each isomer.

7.15) Draw the structural formula for the product obtained through the catalytic hydrogenation of 1-octene. Write the IUPAC name of the product.

7.16) Write the structural formula of the product from
a) the reaction of 1-pentene and HBr
b) the reaction of 2-methylpropene and HF

7.25) Write the IUPAC name for
a) $CH_3(CH_2)_5CH=CH_2$
b) $(CH_3)_2C=CHCH(CH_3)_2$
c) $CH_3(CH_2)_4C≡CCH_3$

7.26) Draw the structural formula for
a) *cis*-3-hexene
b) 2,5-dimethyl-3-hexyne

7.27) Draw the geometrical isomers of the alkene
$CH_3(CH_2)_2CH=CH(CH_2)_2CH_3$
and give the IUPAC name for each isomer.

7.28) Draw the structural formula for the product obtained through the catalytic hydrogenation of 2-octene. Write the IUPAC name of the product.

7.29) Write the structural formula of the product from
a) the reaction of 1-octene and HI
b) the reaction of 3-ethyl-2-pentene and HCl

c) the reaction of 2-methyl-2-butene and HBr

c) the reaction of 2-methyl-1-butene and HCl

SECTION 7.3 SIMPLE ORGANIC RING SYSTEMS

7.17) Draw the structural formula of

a) methylcyclopentane

b) 1,1-dimethylcyclopropane

7.18) Write the IUPAC name of

a)  —CH$_2$CH$_3$

b)

        H
    H
        CH$_3$
    CH$_3$

7.19) Draw the structural formula of *trans*-1,2-dimethylcyclopentane.

7.20*) Draw *all* the geometrical isomers of a cyclobutane that has two methyl branches. Give the IUPAC name of each isomer.

7.30) Draw the structural formula of

a) ethylcyclohexane

b) 1,1,2-trimethylcyclobutane.

7.31) Write the IUPAC name of

a)   CH$_2$CH$_3$

    H$_3$C   CH$_3$

b)   H CH$_3$

  H$_3$C H

7.32) Draw the structural formula of *cis*-1,2-diethylcyclobutane.

7.33*) Draw *all* the geometrical isomers of a cyclohexane that has two methyl branches. Give the IUPAC name of each isomer.

Oxidation and Reduction

In the last chapter we defined oxidation and reduction on the basis of the loss or gain of hydrogen atoms by alkanes, alkenes, and alkynes. This simple definition, however, does not include atoms, ions, and oxygen-containing organic molecules, which also take part in oxidation-reduction or **redox reactions.** In this chapter we will consider redox reactions of various types and expand the definition of oxidation and reduction.

Redox is an abbreviated term for *oxidation-reduction.*

8.1 ELECTRON TRANSFER REACTIONS

LEARNING GOAL 8A: Given the formula of a chemical species (atom, molecule, or ion), determine the oxidation state of each of its elements.

8B: Given a chemical equation, decide from oxidation states whether or not it represents a redox reaction. If it does, list the oxidation state changes and determine the element oxidized and the element reduced.

Oxidation

The process of oxidation was once considered to be simply a "combining with oxygen." For example, the chemical equation for what happens when iron rusts is

$$4 \text{ Fe}_{(s)} + 3 \text{ O}_{2(g)} \longrightarrow 2 \text{ Fe}_2\text{O}_{3(s)}$$

Iron(III) oxide is a reddish-brown ionic compound. Since it contains only ions, we could have written the same equation as

$$4 \text{ Fe}_{(s)} + 3 \text{ O}_{2(g)} \longrightarrow (4 \text{ Fe}^{3+} + 6 \text{ O}^{2-})_{(s)}$$

There are actually two processes happening here:

$$4 \text{ Fe}_{(s)} \longrightarrow 4 \text{ Fe}^{3+}, \textit{ losing } (4)(3) = 12 \text{ electrons}$$

$$3 \text{ O}_{2(g)} \longrightarrow 6 \text{ O}^{2-}, \textit{ gaining } (6)(2) = 12 \text{ electrons}$$

The iron has become oxidized (combined with oxygen) but at the same time has *lost electrons* to oxygen. **Oxidation** means the *loss of electrons.*

Remember, oxidation state numbers have signs *and* magnitudes.

Oxygen forms *oxides* when it combines with other elements, and it then has an oxidation state of -2, as described in Section 3.4. We thus consider each oxygen to have *gained two electrons* when it went from O_2 gas in the air to the oxygen in the iron(III) oxide. The oxygen has been reduced. **Reduction** means the *gain of electrons*.

As another example, let's look at what happens when we burn hydrogen:

$$2\ H_{2(g)} + O_{2(g)} \longrightarrow 2\ H_2O_{(g)}$$

For bookkeeping purposes (since there are no ionic bonds in the water molecule, only covalent bonds), we pretend that all of the transferred electrons have gone to the oxygen atoms of the water molecule. Each water molecule contains eight valence electrons, one from each of the two hydrogens and six from the oxygen. If all eight are on the oxygen to make an octet, each hydrogen has *lost an electron* and has become oxidized to the $+1$ oxidation state. The burning or combustion of hydrogen is also the oxidation of hydrogen gas, using both meanings of oxidation: (a) a combining with oxygen and (b) a loss of electrons. Hydrogen goes from a lower oxidation state (0 in H_2 gas) to a higher oxidation state ($+1$ in water).

Each oxygen atom in the O_2 gas has *gained two electrons* and has been reduced from a higher oxidation state (0 in the O_2 gas) to a lower oxidation state (-2 in water).

Another typical example of oxidation-reduction is the combustion of methane in natural gas to heat homes:

$$CH_{4(g)} + 2\ O_{2(g)} \longrightarrow CO_{2(g)} + 2\ H_2O_{(g)}$$

Again, since carbon dioxide contains only covalent bonds, we say, only for bookkeeping purposes, that the oxygen has gained all the available electrons to reach a -2 oxidation state. If each oxygen has gone from a 0 oxidation state in O_2 to a -2 oxidation state in CO_2, then the four oxygen atoms have gained a total of eight electrons. The source of those eight electrons is the methane molecule. Methane is *oxidized* to carbon dioxide and water when it burns. (We will return to this example later to account for the change in the oxidation state of carbon in this combustion reaction.)

Electrons are neither made nor destroyed in redox reactions. They are merely transferred, usually from an element with a low electronegativity (such as a metal) to an element with a higher electronegativity (such as oxygen).

We can summarize our definition of oxidation and reduction as electron transfer:

Oxidation occurs when electrons are *lost* by a species (molecule or ion). This loss of electrons may result from combining with oxygen or a loss of hydrogen, or through other processes.

Reduction occurs when electrons are *gained* by a species (molecule or ion). This gain of electrons may result from combining with hydrogen or through other processes.

Oxidation states in compounds

After the burning of methane, each oxygen atom in the CO_2 molecule has an oxidation state of -2. The oxidation states of all the atoms in a molecule or ion must add up to the net charge. Since the CO_2 molecule is neutral (no net charge), the oxidation state of carbon plus the sum of the two oxygen oxidation numbers must add up to zero. Then $(x) + 2(-2) = 0$, so the oxidation state of carbon must be $+4$. Since there is a net change of eight electrons gained by the four oxygen atoms in the combustion equa-

TABLE 8–1   RULES FOR DETERMINING OXIDATION STATES OF ELEMENTS

1. The oxidation state of any elemental substance is zero, e.g., sodium in Na, oxygen in O_2, and hydrogen in H_2 all have zero oxidation states.
2. The oxidation state of a monatomic ion is equal to the charge on that ion, e.g., iron in Fe^{2+} has an oxidation state of $+2$, iodine in I^- has an oxidation state of -1.
3. The oxidation state of oxygen in a compound is generally -2.
4. The oxidation state of hydrogen in an organic compound is $+1$.
5. The oxidation states of all the atoms in a molecule must add up to zero.
6. The oxidation states of all the atoms in a polyatomic ion must add up to the charge on that ion.

tion, these electrons must have come from the carbon atom in the methane molecule. Thus, the carbon atom in CH_4 must have an oxidation state of -4, since the change from -4 to $+4$ gives a net loss of the eight electrons gained by the oxygen atoms. If carbon in CH_4 has an oxidation state of -4, the hydrogens in this neutral molecule must each have an oxidation state of $+1$. Thus, we have determined the oxidation state of each element in each molecule, and we can do the same thing for any other molecule or ion.

Oxidation state numbers are calculated rather than measured experimentally.

There is a way of determining oxidation states by following a simple set of rules. Some of them you already know from Section 3.3. They are summarized in Table 8.1.

Rules 5 and 6 permit us to calculate the various oxidation states of elements that have different oxidation states in different compounds and ions. Let's see how these rules are applied.

EXAMPLE 8a: Calculate the oxidation state of nitrogen in each of the following.
i) N_2
ii) NO_2
iii) NH_3
iv) $Ca(NO_3)_2$
v)   NO
vi) N_2O
vii) NF_3

- - - - - - - - - - - - - - - - - - - -

SOLUTION: Apply the rules listed in Table 8–1.

i)   0 in N_2: The first rule applies. You may also use Rule 5 to get the same result: The oxidation states of the two nitrogen atoms must add up to zero; since they are identical, each must be $\boxed{\text{zero}}$.

ii) $+4$ in NO_2: Each oxygen atom is -2 (Rule 3), so two oxygens make -4. The nitrogen oxidation state added to -4 must give zero (Rule 5). Therefore, N is in the $\boxed{+4 \text{ state}}$.

iii) -3 in NH_3: Each hydrogen is $+1$ (Rule 4), so the three hydrogens add up to $+3$. The nitrogen must then be $\boxed{-3}$ (Rule 5). The ammonium ion, NH_4^+, and the amide ion, NH_2^-, also involve nitrogen in the -3 oxidation state and are formed from ammonia, NH_3, by the gain or loss of a proton, H^+.)

iv) $+5$ in $Ca(NO_3)_2$: This is an ionic compound with Ca^{2+}; thus calcium has a $+2$ state. In the nitrate ion, NO_3^-, each oxygen is -2, and there are three oxygens. If we let x be the state of each nitrogen, $x + (3)(-2) = -1$ (Rule 6) and $x = \boxed{+5}$.

v) $+2$ in NO: Oxygen is -2, so N must be $\boxed{+2}$ (Rule 5) so that the two of them add up to zero.

vi) $+1$ in N_2O: By the same reasoning, $2x + (-2) = 0$, so $x = \boxed{+1}$.

vii) $+3$ in NF_3: You should remember that fluorine is the most negative element in the periodic table; since it forms a $1-$ ion to obtain a noble-gas electron configuration, it will always have a -1 oxidation state in its compounds. Then $x + (3)(-1) = 0$ and $x = \boxed{+3}$.

Note the change in sign when you solve these algebraic expressions.

> **EXAMPLE 8b:** When iron rusts, Fe_2O_3 is formed. What is the oxidation state of iron in Fe_2O_3?
>
> -
>
> *SOLUTION:* Oxygen has an oxidation state of -2 (Rule 3), and there are three oxygens. If we let x be the state of each iron, $2x + (3)(-2) = 0$, so $2x = +6$ and $x = \boxed{+3}$ as described in Section 3.3.

> **EXAMPLE 8c:** What is the oxidation state of manganese (Mn) in the permanganate ion, MnO_4^-?
>
> -
>
> *SOLUTION:* Oxygen has an oxidation state of -2 (Rule 3), and there are four oxygen atoms in this $1-$ anion. If we let x be the state of the manganese, $x + (4)(-2) = -1$, so $x = \boxed{+7}$.

Within a polyatomic ion, the atoms are covalently bonded to each other.

> **EXAMPLE 8d:** Calculate the oxidation state of sulfur in
> i) SO_2 ii) SO_4^{2-}
>
> -
>
> *SOLUTION:* i) $+4$ in SO_2: Oxygen has an oxidation state of -2. Thus, $x + (2)(-2) = 0$, so $x = \boxed{+4}$.
>
> ii) $+6$ in SO_4^{2-}: Oxygen has an oxidation state of -2. If we let x be the state of sulfur in this $2-$ anion, then $x + (4)(-2) = -2$, and $x = \boxed{+6}$.

> **EXAMPLE 8e:** What is the oxidation state of chromium (Cr) in the dichromate anion of $K_2Cr_2O_7$?
>
> -
>
> *SOLUTION:* The potassium ion (K^+) has an oxidation state of $+1$. Since the compound is neutral, the dichromate ion must have a net charge of -2, to give $Cr_2O_7^{2-}$. Since each oxygen atom has an oxidation state of -2, if we let x be the state of each chromium, $2x + (7)(-2) = -2$, so $2x = 14 - 2 = +12$, and $x = \boxed{+6}$.

Carbon oxidation states

In its inorganic compounds, carbon is usually found in the $+4$ oxidation state.

> **EXAMPLE 8f:** Calculate the oxidation state of carbon in sodium bicarbonate, $NaHCO_3$.
>
> -
>
> *SOLUTION:* The oxidation state of the sodium ion is $+1$. Thus, the bicarbonate anion, HCO_3^-, has a net charge of -1. Hydrogen has an oxidation state of $+1$, and that of oxygen is -2. If we let x be the oxidation state of carbon, then $x + (+1) + (3)(-2) = -1$, and $x = +6 - 2 = \boxed{+4}$.

Similar exercises with Na_2CO_3 and carbon dioxide also give a $+4$ oxidation state for carbon.

However, in organic compounds it is more difficult to use the oxidation state number system for bookkeeping. The main reason is that carbon and hydrogen attract electrons almost equally, so that the main assumption we have been making (that all electrons in a bond go to the more negative atom) is more difficult to apply. We may not be sure whether carbon or hydrogen is more negative in a given situation.

We can, if we wish, apply the above rules of bookkeeping to determine at least if carbon gets oxidized or reduced in a chemical reaction. We simply assume that hydrogen is $+1$ and oxygen is -2, as usual, and solve for the oxidation state of carbon.

EXAMPLE 8g: Calculate the change of oxidation state for carbon in the burning of methane:

$$CH_{4(g)} + 2\ O_{2(g)} \longrightarrow CO_{2(g)} + 2H_2O_{(g)}$$

- -

SOLUTION: Applying the rules to methane, we get $x + (4)(+1) = 0$, and $x = -4$ for the oxidation state of carbon in CH_4.

For CO_2, $x + 2(-2) = 0$, and $x = +4$ for the oxidation state of carbon in CO_2.

Thus, we calculate a loss of eight electrons for each carbon atom, from the -4 oxidation state in methane to the $+4$ oxidation state in carbon dioxide. Whether or not carbon itself actually loses all of these electrons (hydrogen doubtless plays some part), the number of electrons (eight) agrees with the number gained by two O_2 molecules going to oxides.

We can now add something new and useful to our definition of oxidation: **Oxidation occurs when the oxidation state of a species becomes more positive.**

In Chapter 7 we saw that butane is oxidized when it loses hydrogens to form the butene isomers. Let us check the oxidation states for the carbon atoms in this chemical change.

EXAMPLE 8h:

$$2\ CH_3CH_2CH_2CH_3 \xrightarrow{700°C} H_2C{=}CHCH_2CH_3 + CH_3CH{=}CHCH_3 + 2\ H_2$$

What are the oxidation states for the carbon atoms in butane and the butenes?

- -

SOLUTION: Applying the rules, we get

butane: $4x + (10)(+1) = 0$, so $x = \boxed{-2^1/_2}$

1-butene: $4x + (8)(+1) = 0$, so $x = \boxed{-2}$

2-butene: $4x + (8)(+1) = 0$, so $x = \boxed{-2}$

Carbon has indeed gone to a more positive (less negative) oxidation state, from $-2^1/_2$ to -2. Carbon has lost electrons and has been oxidized. Since there are four carbons, two electrons have been given up: $(4)(2^1/_2 - 2) = 2$. Where did these two electrons go? To hydrogen to make H_2.

Let us see what happens if we reverse this process.

EXAMPLE 8i: Calculate the oxidation states for carbon in the catalytic hydrogenation of propene to propane:

$$CH_3CH{=}CH_2 + H_2 \xrightarrow{Ni} CH_3CH_2CH_3$$

- -

SOLUTION: Applying the rules to calculate the oxidation state of carbon, we get $CH_3CH_2CH_3$: $3x + 8(+1) = 0$, so $x = \boxed{-8/3}$

$CH_3CH{=}CH_2$: $3x + 6(+1) = 0$, so $x = \boxed{-2}$

"Less positive" is the same as "more negative."

Carbon has gone to a more negative (less positive) oxidation state, from -2 to $-8/3$. Carbon has gained electrons and has been reduced.

Reduction occurs when the oxidation number of a species becomes less positive and is "reduced."

Admittedly, this is only a method of bookkeeping. However, by using this system, you should be able to define oxidation and reduction in terms of electron loss or gain and also in terms of oxidation state changes. You should also be able to determine the oxidation state of each element in a molecule or ion by applying the rules listed in Table 8–1.

You are now in a position to look at a chemical equation and decide (from oxidation state changes) whether or not the equation represents a redox reaction. If it does, you should be able to list the oxidation state changes and determine the element oxidized and the element reduced.

In this section, we will examine some simple redox reactions of inorganic compounds. In the next section, we will look at redox reactions of organic compounds.

EXAMPLE 8j: The reaction of copper with aqueous silver nitrate was considered in Chapter 5 (p. 130). The net reaction is

$$\underset{0}{Cu_{(s)}} + \underset{+1}{2\,Ag^+_{(aq)}} \longrightarrow \underset{+2}{Cu^{2+}_{(aq)}} + \underset{0}{2\,Ag_{(s)}}$$

Is this reaction a redox process? If so, what element is oxidized and what element is reduced?

SOLUTION: The copper metal, $Cu_{(s)}$, has *lost* two electrons to become $Cu^{2+}_{(aq)}$. Each $Ag^+_{(aq)}$ has *gained* one electron to become $Ag_{(s)}$.

Electrons have been lost and gained in this chemical reaction, so it is a redox process.

The oxidation and reduction reactions occur at the same time.

The $Cu_{(s)}$ has lost electrons, and the oxidation state of $Cu_{(s)}$ has become more positive. Therefore, $Cu_{(s)}$ has been oxidized. The $Ag^+_{(aq)}$ has gained electrons, and its oxidation state has become less positive. Therefore, $Ag^+_{(aq)}$ has been reduced. Since there are two $Ag^+_{(aq)}$ ions involved, two electrons are gained. These are the two electrons lost by the $Cu_{(s)}$.

EXAMPLE 8k: If we put solid zinc metal into a solution containing Fe^{2+} cations, the zinc metal will dissolve to become Zn^{2+} cations and the Fe^{2+} will become iron metal. The equation can be written

$$Zn_{(s)} + Fe^{2+}_{(aq)} \longrightarrow Zn^{2+}_{(aq)} + Fe_{(s)}$$

Which element is oxidized and which reduced?

SOLUTION: Zinc metal, $Zn_{(s)}$, has *lost* two electrons to become the zinc cation, and the oxidation state of zinc has become more positive. Thus, zinc has been oxidized. The $Fe^{2+}_{(aq)}$ cation has *gained* two electrons to become iron metal. The oxidation state of iron has become less positive. Iron has been reduced.

Oxidizing and reducing agents

Let us examine the equation in Example 8k more closely. The zinc metal is losing its electrons to the $Fe^{2+}_{(aq)}$ cations. The $Fe^{2+}_{(aq)}$ cations are accepting electrons from the zinc metal. In a redox process, one element acts as an acceptor of electrons and another element acts as a donor of electrons. These two reactants in a redox process are given special names to indicate the parts they play. The species that brings about oxidation by accepting (gaining) electrons is called the **oxidizing agent;** the species that donates (loses) the electrons so that reduction may occur is called the **reducing agent.**

In the above example, the $Fe^{2+}_{(aq)}$ cation has accepted electrons from zinc metal—it has oxidized Zn to $Zn^{2+}_{(aq)}$—and is therefore the oxidizing agent. Conversely, zinc metal has donated electrons to $Fe^{2+}_{(aq)}$ cations—it has reduced the $Fe^{2+}_{(aq)}$ to iron metal—and is therefore the reducing agent.

Notice that oxidizing agents are themselves reduced and reducing agents are oxidized: $Fe^{2+}_{(aq)}$ is the oxidizing agent and is reduced to $Fe_{(s)}$, and $Zn_{(s)}$ is the reducing agent and is oxidized to $Zn^{2+}_{(aq)}$.
To summarize:

An *oxidizing agent* accepts electrons from some other atom, molecule, or ion and is, in turn, reduced.

A *reducing agent* donates electrons to some other atom, molecule, or ion and is, in turn, oxidized.

A practical example of a redox process is the lead storage battery in an automobile or truck.

EXAMPLE 8l: Which element is oxidized and which is reduced in a lead storage battery? The equation is

$$Pb_{(s)} + PbO_{2(s)} + 4\ H^+_{(aq)} + 2\ SO^{2-}_{4(aq)} \longrightarrow 2\ PbSO_{4(s)} + 2\ H_2O_{(\ell)}$$

- -

SOLUTION: Assign oxidation states to as many elements as necessary until you come up with a pair that has changed. Then identify the oxidation and reduction changes. Apply the rules listed in Table 8–1, so that hydrogen, sulfur, and oxygen do not change oxidation state.

The $Pb_{(s)}$ changes to Pb^{2+} in $PbSO_4$. The Pb in $PbO_{2(s)}$, changes to Pb^{2+} in $PbSO_4$. Thus, lead is both *oxidized* (0 in $Pb_{(s)}$ to $+ 2$ in $PbSO_4$) and *reduced* ($+4$ in PbO_2 to $+ 2$ in $PbSO_4$). $Pb_{(s)}$ donates electrons, so it is the reducing agent. $PbO_{2(s)}$ accepts electrons, so it is the oxidizing agent.

Batteries

There are two ways in which redox reactions may be used in everyday life. One is to use the electrons lost by the substance being oxidized as an electric current to do work, while the same current provides electrons to enter the substance being reduced. This is what happens in an electrochemical cell or *battery,* such as the one shown for silver and zinc in Figure 8–1.

Silver cations from the Ag^+ solution are being reduced at the *cathode.* (The word *cat*ion is related, in fact, to the word *cat*hode, while the word *an*ion comes from the opposite electrode or piece of metal, the *an*ode.) The electrons to reduce the silver come out of the wire. They have passed through the light bulb filament, heating it enough to light it up. The ammeter shows that an electric current is flowing in the

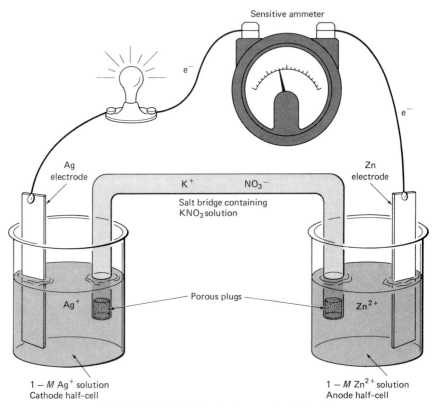

FIGURE 8-1   A simple electrochemical cell.

wire. Electrons came originally from the zinc electrode, the *anode*, where zinc metal is oxidized and dissolves in the solution as Zn^{2+} ions.

There has to be a "return path" of electric current so that the amount of negative charge that left the zinc and went into the wire eventually comes back to the Zn^{2+} solution to keep it electrically neutral. In the simple battery shown, the potassium and nitrate ions, K^+ and NO_3^-, in the salt bridge solution move about to keep each solution neutral without allowing the Zn^{2+} and Ag^+ solutions to mix.

The voltage for the battery shown could be as high as 1.5 volts. There are other battery designs, such as the flashlight (dry cell) battery shown in Figure 8-2. This type also can produce 1.5 volts. Other common cells are the lead storage battery used in automobiles (Figure 8-3), the alkaline cell, and the nickel-cadmium cell. Several of these may be recharged. This is necessary because as any battery delivers electricity, it uses up the chemical reactants that are producing the redox reaction. Today, mercury cells are used in miniature batteries to supply energy for transistor radios, hearing aids, and heart pacemakers.

Electrolysis

The reactions we have been discussing involve redox processes that go all by themselves, once you put the reactants together. We don't have to do anything to an auto battery to get it to work. The cell shown in Figure 8-3 will give out a voltage or current until most of the lead metal and PbO_2 are used up.

What if we change the wiring of the lead storage battery and instead put in a *source* of electrons so that the electrons go *into* the $Pb_{(s)}$ and *out of* the $PbO_{2(s)}$, in

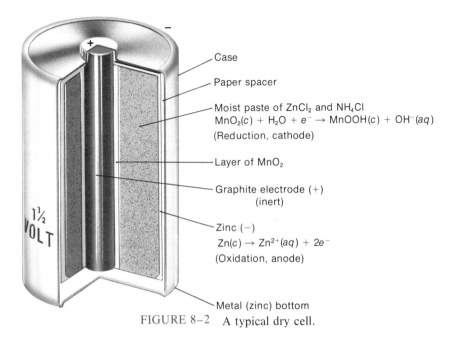

Case

Paper spacer

Moist paste of $ZnCl_2$ and NH_4Cl
$MnO_2(c) + H_2O + e^- \rightarrow MnOOH(c) + OH^-(aq)$
(Reduction, cathode)

Layer of MnO_2

Graphite electrode (+)
(inert)

Zinc (−)
$Zn(c) \rightarrow Zn^{2+}(aq) + 2e^-$
(Oxidation, anode)

Metal (zinc) bottom

FIGURE 8–2   A typical dry cell.

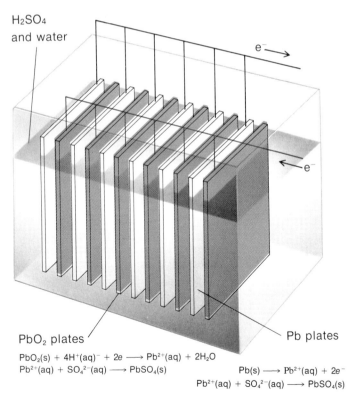

H_2SO_4 and water

$e^- \longrightarrow$

e^-

PbO_2 plates

Pb plates

$PbO_2(s) + 4H^+(aq)^- + 2e \longrightarrow Pb^{2+}(aq) + 2H_2O$
$Pb^{2+}(aq) + SO_4{}^{2-}(aq) \longrightarrow PbSO_4(s)$

$Pb(s) \longrightarrow Pb^{2+}(aq) + 2e^-$
$Pb^{2+}(aq) + SO_4{}^{2-}(aq) \longrightarrow PbSO_4(s)$

FIGURE 8–3   A lead storage battery. A battery like this has a voltage of 2 volts per cell and can deliver a large amount of electrical energy for a short time. Another advantage of this battery is that it can be recharged. A disadvantage is that it is very heavy.

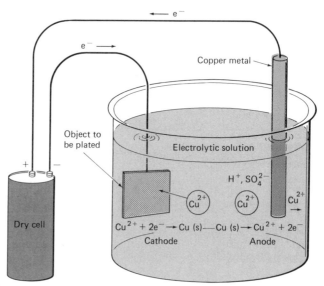

FIGURE 8–4   An electrolytic cell used for electroplating copper. The object to be plated is connected to the negative terminal of the electrochemical cell, which serves as the source of electrons. The copper anode of the electrolytic cell is connected to the positive terminal of the electrochemical cell.

the reverse direction of that shown in Figure 8–3? In that case, we can force lead metal to be produced from $PbSO_4$ and also force $PbSO_4$ to change to PbO_2. We will essentially put a thin layer of lead, an electroplate, on the $Pb_{(s)}$ electrode. This process is called *electrolysis* and is how an automobile battery is recharged.

This principle can be illustrated well by a system that involves only copper (Figure 8–4). We can make the Cu^{2+} ions from the solution reduce (plate) onto the object we want to coat with copper by pumping electrons into that object, which acts as the cathode. At the other end of the wire, electrons are being pulled out of copper atoms, which then dissolve as Cu^{2+}.

The commercial method for making chlorine similarly uses electrolysis to convert melted sodium chloride to sodium metal and chlorine gas. You may have had the experience in an earlier science course of seeing water *electrolyzed* to hydrogen and oxygen (Figure 1–3, p. 7).

The redox reaction is thus something that can work both ways. Left to itself, it will go one way, possibly in a manner we can harness to make a battery. Given a source of electrons from outside, a "pump" such as a large battery, we can make the redox reaction go in the reverse direction, or recharge a run-down battery.

SELF-CHECK

8.1)   Calculate the oxidation state of each element in the following species.

a) MnO_2 d) CO_3^{2-} g) SO_3^{2-} i) ClO_3^-
b) $Fe_2(SO_4)_3$ e) ClO^- h) $H_2PO_4^-$ j) ClO_4^-
c) PbO_2 f) PO_3^{3-}

8.2)   A reaction that is sometimes used in the chemical laboratory to prepare chlorine gas from hydrochloric acid is

$$MnO_{2(s)} + 4H^+_{(aq)} + 2Cl^-_{(aq)} \longrightarrow Mn^{2+}_{(aq)} + Cl_{2(g)} + 2H_2O_{(\ell)}$$

Assign oxidation state numbers to the elements that have changed oxidation states. What element is oxidized and what element is reduced? What species is the oxidizing agent? What species is the reducing agent?

8.2 ORGANIC REDOX REACTIONS

LEARNING GOAL 8C: Given an organic process, decide from the number of oxygen and hydrogen atoms in each molecule whether or not a redox reaction has occurred. If so, determine the oxidized form and the reduced form.
8D: List at least three common oxidizers (oxidizing agents) and three common reducers (reducing agents) useful in organic synthesis.
8E: Describe the products formed in step-by-step oxidation of a hydrocarbon, through alcohols, aldehydes, and carboxylic acids, to CO_2 and H_2O.

One of the primary concerns of the organic chemist is how a compound can be made or *synthesized*. Organic compounds are usually made by changing a small reactive part of the molecule called a *functional group*. The rest of the organic molecule remains unchanged. For example, the following change can be carried out under the proper conditions. The reactive part of the molecule (—CH₂OH part) is changed to —C=O.

A functional group is an atom or group of atoms that can take the place of a hydrogen in an alkane (Section 9.1).

ethanol ⟶ ethanal

The —OH group is the functional group in the alcohol. The aldehyde group, will be discussed in Section 9.3.

The organic chemist calls this type of change "the synthesis of ethanal from ethanol." Note that the methyl group portion of the molecule does not change. The success of such a synthesis depends on many things, such as the type of chemical reagent used to effect the change, the temperature of the reaction, the solvent used, and, in some cases, the pressure of the reactants. The ability of the organic chemist to synthesize new molecules is directly related to his or her skill in choosing the reagents, solvents, temperature, and pressure to carry out an organic reaction.

Throughout this text you will encounter many different reagents that will change one functional group into another. Oxidizing and reducing agents are common types of reagents for carrying out this kind of change. Each time the oxidation state of the carbon atom is changed, a new functional group results. In this section, we will briefly examine some of the simple redox reactions of organic molecules. We will formulate simple rules to recognize both an organic redox process and each form in the redox reaction.

Let's look more closely at the ethanol-to-ethanal conversion. The oxidation states of carbon in ethanol and ethanal are

$$
\begin{array}{c}
\text{H} \quad \text{H} \\
| \quad | \\
\text{H}-\text{C}-\text{C}-\text{OH:} \quad 2x + 6(+1) + (1)(-2) = 0 \\
| \quad | \\
\text{H} \quad \text{H}
\end{array}
$$

$$x = -2$$

$$
\begin{array}{c}
\text{H} \quad \text{H} \\
| \quad | \\
\text{H}-\text{C}-\text{C}=\text{O:} \quad 2x + 4(+1) + (1)(-2) = 0 \\
| \\
\text{H}
\end{array}
$$

$$x = -1$$

The oxidation state of carbon changes as the functional group changes.

The oxidation state of the carbon atoms becomes more positive (from -2 to -1) in this reaction. The ethanol has been oxidized. Closer inspection reveals some other differences between these two molecules. Ethanol has five carbon-hydrogen bonds, and ethanal has four. Thus, the number of carbon-hydrogen bonds has decreased from reactant to product. This is consistent with our earlier definition of oxidation of organic molecules (p. 205). Notice also that the ethanal contains two carbon-oxygen bonds, while the ethanol contains only one carbon-oxygen bond. Even though the number of oxygen atoms (one) has stayed the same, the number of carbon-oxygen bonds has increased (from one to two) from reactant to product. Organic chemists find it easier to decide quickly whether oxidation or reduction has occurred by counting the number of carbon-oxygen bonds or carbon-hydrogen bonds in the reactants and the products. The rules they use are

1) Oxidation has occurred if the number of carbon-oxygen bonds *increases* or if the number of carbon-hydrogen bonds *decreases* from reactant to product.
2) Reduction has occurred if the number of carbon-oxygen bonds *decreases* or if the number of carbon-hydrogen bonds *increases* from reactant to product.

Using these rules for organic redox processes gives exactly the same results as using oxidation states. However, these rules are usually easier and faster to apply to complex organic molecules. Some examples will demonstrate their usefulness.

EXAMPLE 8m: Ethanal can be easily converted to ethanoic acid:

$$
\begin{array}{ccc}
\text{H} & & \text{O} \\
| & & \| \\
\text{CH}_3-\text{C}=\text{O} & \longrightarrow & \text{CH}_3-\text{C}-\text{OH} \\
\text{ethanal} & & \text{ethanoic acid}
\end{array}
$$

The oxidized form in an organic redox process is the molecule with the greater number of carbon-oxygen bonds.

The reduced form in an organic redox process is the molecule with the lower number of carbon-oxygen bonds.

Is this process an oxidation or a reduction? What are the oxidized form and the reduced form?

SOLUTION: In ethanal, there are two carbon-oxygen bonds and four carbon-hydrogen bonds. In ethanoic acid, there are three carbon-oxygen bonds and three carbon-hydrogen bonds. Thus, from reactant to product, the number of carbon-oxygen bonds has increased and the number of carbon-hydrogen bonds has decreased. This is an oxidation process. The oxidized form is ethanoic acid, and the reduced form is ethanal.

EXAMPLE 8n: Ethylene oxide (a cyclic compound) can be converted to ethanol under the proper conditions:

$$H_2C{-}CH_2 \xrightarrow[\text{catalyst}]{H_2} H{-}\overset{\displaystyle H}{\underset{\displaystyle H}{C}}{-}\overset{\displaystyle H}{\underset{\displaystyle H}{C}}{-}OH$$

$$\underset{O}{\diagdown\diagup}$$

ethylene oxide   ethanol

Is this process an oxidation or a reduction? What are the oxidized form and the reduced form?

- -

SOLUTION: In ethylene oxide, there are two carbon-oxygen bonds and four carbon-hydrogen bonds. In ethanol, there are one carbon-oxygen bond and five carbon-hydrogen bonds. The number of carbon-oxygen bonds has decreased and the number of carbon-hydrogen bonds has increased from reactant to product. This is a reduction process. The oxidized form is the ethylene oxide, and the reduced form is the ethanol.

Organic redox reactions are also important in a wide variety of body processes. For example, when your body uses glycogen for energy (Chapter 25), the conversion of pyruvic acid to lactic acid is one of the important steps.

EXAMPLE 8o: Is the conversion of pyruvic acid to lactic acid an oxidation or a reduction?

$$CH_3{-}\overset{\displaystyle O}{\overset{\|}{C}}{-}\overset{\displaystyle O}{\overset{\|}{C}}{-}OH \longrightarrow CH_3{-}\overset{\displaystyle OH}{\underset{\displaystyle H}{C}}{-}\overset{}{\underset{\displaystyle O}{\overset{\|}{C}}}{-}OH$$

pyruvic acid   lactic acid

- -

SOLUTION: The pyruvic acid contains five carbon-oxygen bonds and three carbon-hydrogen bonds. The lactic acid contains four carbon-oxygen bonds and four carbon-hydrogen bonds. The number of carbon-oxygen bonds has decreased and the number of carbon-hydrogen bonds has increased from reactant to product. This is a reduction process. The oxidized form is pyruvic acid, and the reduced form is lactic acid.

A more complex example of a biochemical redox process is the conversion of six-carbon sugars to ethanol and carbon dioxide.

EXAMPLE 8p: The fermentation of glucose in the enzyme mixture called zymase can be represented

$$\xrightarrow{\text{zymase}} 2\ CH_3CH_2OH + 2\ CO_2$$

glucose

ethanol   carbon dioxide

Is the fermentation of glucose an oxidation or reduction process?

- -

SOLUTION: In glucose, there are seven carbon-oxygen bonds and seven carbon-hydrogen bonds. In ethanol, there are one carbon-oxygen bond and five carbon-hydrogen bonds. In carbon dioxide, there are four carbon-oxygen bonds and no carbon-hydrogen bonds.

Reactant:	7 C—H bonds, 7 C—O bonds	
Products:	ethanol	(2)(1) C—O bonds
		(2)(5) C—H bonds
	CO_2	(2)(4) C—O bonds
		no C—H bonds
	(Products:	10 C—O bonds
		10 C—H bonds)

The number of carbon-oxygen bonds has increased and the number of carbon-hydrogen bonds has increased from reactant to products! The carbons in the sugar have been both oxidized (to carbon dioxide) and reduced (to ethanol). Compare this redox process with that in the lead storage battery (p. 223).

The above example looks more complex than some of the earlier ones. However, application of the rules for counting carbon-oxygen and carbon-hydrogen bonds easily lets you decide what type of redox process has occurred. Apply these rules to all the organic reactions you encounter in later chapters.

Oxidizers and reducers in organic synthesis

Something that gives up electrons easily is a good reducer (reducing agent) because to reduce something you have to give it electrons. Most metals (such as the alkali metals, the alkaline earth metals, iron, and zinc) and hydrogen gas are good reducers and can be used for organic and inorganic reduction processes.

Something that oxidizes must take up electrons. You may think of a good oxidizer (oxidizing agent) as something like an electron "vacuum cleaner" (and a reducer as an electron "pump"). A metal cannot be an oxidizer since it cannot take in electrons; if it did it would become a negative ion, and metals do not form anions. The best oxidizers in organic chemistry are oxygen gas or complex oxygen-containing anions. Since the oxidizing agent is taking electrons from another substance, it is itself undergoing an increase of electrons, a reduction process. Since the reducing agent is giving away electrons, it must itself be losing them and undergoing oxidation. This is an area of frequent confusion among students, so be sure you have these definitions straight: An oxidizing agent is an electron acceptor; a reducing agent is an electron donor.

Oxidizers

In organic redox processes, some of the common oxidizers are oxygen gas, potassium permanganate, chromic oxide, and potassium dichromate.

Let's first look at the O_2 molecule. Air oxidation is what gave us the word *oxidation* in the first place. Hydrocarbons react with O_2 gas in several ways. When burned with sufficient oxygen, an alkane is oxidized to CO_2 and H_2O (Section 5.2):

$$CH_4 + 2\ O_2 \xrightarrow{\text{flame}} CO_2 + 2\ H_2O + heat$$
methane   as in a gas heater

$$CH_3CH_2CH_3 + 5\ O_2 \xrightarrow{\text{flame}} 3\ CO_2 + 4\ H_2O + heat$$
propane   as in a propane camp stove

$$2\ CH_3(CH_2)_6CH_3 + 25\ O_2 \xrightarrow{\text{flame}} 16\ CO_2 + 18\ H_2O + heat$$
octane   as in an automobile engine

The heat given off is used to heat homes (CH_4 and C_3H_8) or to power cars (C_8H_{18}). If there is insufficient oxygen present when the alkane is burned, the toxic gas carbon monoxide (CO) is formed.

Notice that in all the above combustion reactions, the number of carbon-oxygen bonds increases and the number of carbon-hydrogen bonds decreases from reactants to products. The alkane is oxidized, and the O_2 gas is reduced. The O_2 gas is the oxidizer, and the alkane is the reducer.

Earlier, we saw the conversion of an organic compound called ethylene oxide to ethanol. Ethylene oxide is produced industrially by the reaction of ethene with O_2 gas in the presence of a silver oxide catalyst at high temperatures:

$$2\ H_2C{=}CH_2 + O_2 \xrightarrow[\text{heat}]{Ag_2O} 2\ H_2C\!\!\overset{\displaystyle}{\diagdown}\underset{O}{}\overset{}{\diagup}\!\!CH_2$$
ethene   ethylene oxide

The O_2 gas is the oxidizer, and the ethene is the reducer. As an exercise for yourself, count the increase or decrease in the carbon-oxygen and carbon-hydrogen bonds from reactants to product.

In the presence of copper at 300°C, methanol can be oxidized by air (O_2) to a compound called methanal, which contains a carbon-oxygen double bond. The oxygen in the air is the oxidizer; the alcohol is the reducer.

$$2\ CH_3OH + O_2 \xrightarrow[\text{Cu}]{300°C} 2\ H_2C{=}O + 2\ H_2O$$
methanol   methanal

Oxygen gas is a weak oxidizer and reacts only slowly with most organic compounds at room temperature. Higher temperatures or catalysts are needed to speed up the oxidation process. Thus, for many oxidations, the organic chemist prefers a stronger oxidizer that can be used under relatively mild conditions, such as potassium permanganate ($KMnO_4$), chromic oxide (CrO_3), and potassium dichromate ($K_2Cr_2O_7$). These may be used in acid solution (the two chromium compounds) or in neutral or basic solution ($KMnO_4$) and will oxidize a wide variety of organic molecules.

Permanganate ion, MnO_4^-, contains manganese in its +7 oxidation state. Reduction in neutral or basic solution gives the +4 oxidation state in the form of manganese dioxide, MnO_2. The MnO_4^- ion is dark purple and the MnO_2 solid is brown, so there is a way of keeping track of the

When the oxidation state of an element changes, its properties change.

process by watching color changes. The reaction of an alkene with $KMnO_4$ may be represented by the following equation:

$$3\ CH_3CH{=}CH_2 + 2\ KMnO_4 + 4\ H_2O \longrightarrow 3\ CH_3CH{-}CH_2 + 2\ MnO_{2(s)} + 2\ KOH$$

$$\underset{OH\ \ \ OH}{\big|\ \ \ \big|}$$

| propene | (purple) oxidizer | a diol | brown insoluble solid |

The MnO_4^- is the oxidizer, and propene is reducer. How many carbon-oxygen bonds and carbon-hydrogen bonds are there in the organic reactants? in the organic products?

Ethanol is quickly oxidized by potassium dichromate in acidic solution (H_2SO_4) to ethanal:

$$3\ CH_3CH_2OH + K_2Cr_2O_7 + 4\ H_2SO_4 \longrightarrow 3\ CH_3\overset{\overset{\textstyle H}{\big|}}{C}{=}O + Cr_2(SO_4)_3 + K_2SO_4 + 7\ H_2O$$

| ethanol | (orange oxidizer) | ethanal | green product |

The dichromate ion, $Cr_2O_7^{2-}$, is bright orange and contains chromium in its $+6$ oxidation state, while the product, Cr^{3+} ion, is green. The $Cr_2O_7^{2-}$ ion is the oxidizer, and the alcohol is the reducer. These color changes are the basis for the use of dichromate solutions in "breathalyzer" testing kits. If a certain concentration of alcohol (from alcoholic beverages) is on your breath, as you exhale into a dichromate solution, the color changes from orange-red to green.

Similar oxidations of alcohols occur with CrO_3 in acidic solution. Much recent research has been devoted to this reagent, and it is now more commonly used than the older oxidation procedure with $K_2Cr_2O_7$.

$$3\ CH_3\overset{\overset{\textstyle OH}{\big|}}{C}HCH_3 + 2\ CrO_3 + 3\ H_2SO_4 \longrightarrow 3\ CH_3{-}\overset{\overset{\textstyle O}{\|}}{C}{-}CH_3 + 2\ Cr_2(SO_4)_3 + 6\ H_2O$$

| 2-propanol | | propanone | |

Oxidizing agents as antiseptics

The purpose of an antiseptic or disinfectant is to kill bacteria. Several strong oxidizing agents are commonly used in hospitals, including $KMnO_4$ in the form of a dilute solution (to treat infections of the bladder and urethra), as well as $NaOCl$ and H_2O_2 solutions. Potassium chlorate ($KClO_3$) solution was once widely used for sore throats, but is now considered too irritating. Chlorine (Cl_2) is widely used to disinfect drinking water, although ozone (O_3) is replacing it for some purposes. Iodine solutions (I_2) were once widely used to prevent infection of cuts and bruises. Since I_2 will also oxidize the damaged skin, it is now recommended for other antibacterial purposes and for the purification of small amounts of drinking water.

Nearly any oxidizing agent will also serve as a bleach; solutions of $NaOCl$ (javel water, laundry bleach) and hydrogen peroxide are widely used. Some oxidizing agents are also very useful in removing stains from fabrics.

Reducers

Some common reducers for organic compounds are hydrogen gas; inorganic reagents, such as sodium borohydride ($NaBH_4$) and lithium aluminum hydride ($LiAlH_4$); and active metals, such as lithium or zinc.

We have already seen hydrogen gas in a reduction process (p. 205). A catalyst, Ni or Pt, for example, is required with this reducer. Multiple bonds of many types are reduced with hydrogen and a catalyst, in a process called *catalytic hydrogenation*. They do not have to be carbon-carbon multiple bonds. Some examples are

A catalyst speeds up a reaction so that it will provide useful amounts of products in a reasonable time period. Enzymes are catalysts (Chapters 21 and 23).

$$CH_3CH_2CH{=}CH_2 + H_{2(g)} \xrightarrow{Pt} CH_3CH_2CH_2CH_3$$
$$\text{1-butene} \qquad\qquad\qquad \text{butane}$$

$$CH_3{-}\overset{\overset{\displaystyle H}{|}}{C}{=}O + H_{2(g)} \xrightarrow{Pt} CH_3CH_2OH$$
$$\text{ethanal} \qquad\qquad\qquad \text{ethanol}$$

$$CH_3{-}\overset{\overset{\displaystyle O}{\|}}{C}{-}CH_3 + H_{2(g)} \xrightarrow{Ni} CH_3{-}\underset{\underset{\displaystyle H}{|}}{\overset{\overset{\displaystyle OH}{|}}{C}}{-}CH_3$$
$$\text{propanone} \qquad\qquad\qquad \text{2-propanol}$$

Has the number of carbon-oxygen bonds and carbon-hydrogen bonds increased or decreased in these reactions?

Catalytic hydrogenation is not a selective process and will reduce any multiple bond in the molecule. Sometimes more selective reagents are needed. The two most common reducers for organic compounds that contain a carbon-oxygen double bond are sodium borohydride and lithium aluminum hydride. In aqueous solution, sodium borohydride reacts with a carbon-oxygen double bond to form an alcohol:

$$4\ CH_3\overset{\overset{\displaystyle H}{|}}{C}{=}O + NaBH_4 + 4\ H_2O \longrightarrow 4\ CH_3CH_2OH + NaB(OH)_4$$
$$\text{ethanal} \qquad\qquad\qquad\qquad \text{ethanol}$$

Lithium aluminum hydride is a more reactive reducer. However, it reacts violently with water or alcohols, generating hydrogen gas:

$$LiAlH_4 + 4\ H_2O \longrightarrow LiOH + Al(OH)_3 + 4\ H_2$$

For this reason, it is generally dissolved in dry ether, and the reduction processes are conducted in this solvent. The reagents $NaBH_4$ and $LiAlH_4$ do not generally reduce carbon-carbon double bonds. They selectively reduce the $-C{=}O$ group. Note that these reactions allow the chemist to reverse the oxidation of alcohols.

Some metals, such as lithium or zinc, will reduce an alkyl halide to a hydrocarbon. These reactions are actually more complex than shown in the following equation, which summarizes the results of several steps.

$$CH_3CH_2CH_2Br + 2\ Li + H_2O \longrightarrow CH_3CH_2CH_3 + LiBr + LiOH$$
$$\text{1-bromopropane} \qquad\qquad\qquad \text{propane}$$

Note that the number of carbon-hydrogen bonds increases from reactant to product, hence this is a reduction process. The Li is the reducer, and the alkyl halide is the oxidizer.

The oxidizers and reducers introduced here will be used in the next section and in subsequent chapters. You will, however, probably see redox equations written in a more condensed form. Detailed balanced equations like those you have seen in this section are not usually used by organic chemists. Everything is simplified until *only the change* in the organic molecule is shown. Thus, some of the equations seen earlier can be rewritten as unbalanced expressions, rather than balanced equations:

$$CH_3CH_2OH \xrightarrow[H_2SO_4]{K_2Cr_2O_7} CH_3-\overset{\displaystyle H}{\underset{}{C}}=O$$

$$CH_3\overset{\displaystyle H}{\underset{}{C}}=O \xrightarrow[2)\ H_2O]{1)\ NaBH_4} CH_3CH_2OH$$

The necessary inorganic reagents are written above and below the arrow, and the inorganic by-products are ignored. In this way, all attention is focused on the organic reactant and product and less time is spent balancing complicated equations. This type of organic shorthand will be used in later chapters to illustrate many organic and biochemical reactions.

Oxidation levels of organic compounds

As we have seen, organic chemists define oxidation and reduction in terms of the gain or loss of oxygen or hydrogen. When considering organic compounds, it is often helpful to assess the **oxidation level** of any molecule or group by referring to the successive steps of the oxidation of methane.

Starting from methane, we can form a series of methane derivatives by successive changes in the number of carbon-oxygen bonds, as shown in Table 8–2. In each successive step across this series of compounds, the

[O] is commonly used to represent an oxidizing agent such as KMnO$_4$ or CrO$_3$.

TABLE 8–2   OXIDATION LEVELS FOR THE METHANE SERIES

$$H-\overset{\displaystyle H}{\underset{\displaystyle H}{C}}-H \xrightarrow{[O]} H-\overset{\displaystyle H}{\underset{\displaystyle H}{C}}-OH \xrightarrow{[O]} H-\overset{\displaystyle H}{\underset{}{C}}=O \xrightarrow{[O]} H-\overset{\displaystyle O}{\underset{}{C}}-OH \xrightarrow{[O]} O=C=O$$

	methane (alkane)	methanol (alcohol)	methanal (aldehyde)	methanoic acid (carboxylic acid)	carbon dioxide
Number of C—O bonds	0	1	2	3	4
Oxidation state of carbon	−4	−2	0	+2	+4

Increasing oxidation state of C $\longrightarrow$

Increasing oxidation level

number of carbon-oxygen bonds increases by one and the oxidation state of carbon becomes more positive.

In theory, any of the compounds in this series can be oxidized (to a compound at a higher oxidation level) by reaction with the appropriate oxidizer. Alcohols may be oxidized to aldehydes or carboxylic acids. Further oxidation gives carbon dioxide. The organic molecule loses one carbon atom. Some of these types of oxidation were seen earlier in this section.

Depending on the structure of the alcohol, the next higher oxidation level may be a *ketone* rather than an aldehyde.

Ketones, which have

$$-\overset{\displaystyle O}{\underset{\displaystyle \|}{C}}-$$

as their functional group, will be studied in Section 9.3.

$$CH_3-\underset{\underset{\displaystyle H}{|}}{\overset{\overset{\displaystyle OH}{|}}{C}}-CH_3 \xrightarrow{[O]} CH_3-\overset{\overset{\displaystyle O}{\|}}{C}-CH_3$$

2-propanol   propanone
(alcohol)   (ketone)

Oxidations are widely used in the organic chemical laboratory and in industry, and they also occur in many biological systems. For example, when you drink a beverage that contains alcohol (ethanol), the alcohol you take in is first oxidized in the liver with the aid of an enzyme called alcohol dehydrogenase. The aldehyde (ethanal) formed is further oxidized to the acetate anion, CH_3COO^-, which then reacts with a sulfur-containing enzyme called coenzyme A (abbreviated HSCoA).

$$CH_3CH_2OH \xrightarrow[\text{dehydrogenase}]{\text{alcohol}} CH_3-\overset{\overset{\displaystyle H}{|}}{C}{=}O \xrightarrow{[O]} CH_3-\overset{\overset{\displaystyle O}{\|}}{C}-O^-$$

ethanol
(from alcoholic
beverages)   ethanal

$$\downarrow \text{HSCoA}$$

$$CH_3-\overset{\overset{\displaystyle O}{\|}}{C}-SCoA$$

$$CO_2 + H_2O$$

Eventually the alcohol is converted to CO_2 and H_2O after this series of oxidations. The important point here is not to try to memorize the details but to recognize that biological oxidations and chemical oxidations involve the same kinds of steps and changes in oxidation level. The only difference between these two types of oxidation is the kind of oxidizer.

If we look at this same series of reactions in the *opposite* direction, the number of carbon-oxygen bonds decreases and the oxidation number of carbon decreases. This is then a reduction series. If we chose the appropriate reducer, a carboxylic acid could be reduced to an aldehyde, an aldehyde could be reduced to an alcohol, and an alcohol could be reduced to an alkane.

An example of an important industrial reduction process is the synthesis of the alcohol *glucitol* (sorbitol) from glucose:

$$HOCH_2CH(OH)CH(OH)CH(OH)CH(OH)\overset{\overset{\displaystyle H}{|}}{C}{=}O \xrightarrow{\underset{\text{Ni}}{H_2}} HOCH_2CH(OH)CH(OH)CH(OH)CH(OH)CH_2OH$$

glucose   glucitol

Natural glucitol can be isolated from such fruits as cherries, plums, apples, and pears. The synthetic glucitol, produced by reduction of glucose, is used as an artificial sweetener.

SELF-CHECK

SELF-CHECK

8.3)   The alcohol 1-butanol ($CH_3CH_2CH_2CH_2OH$) is converted to the aldehyde $CH_3CH_2CH_2CHO$ using a copper catalyst at high temperatures. Is this reaction a redox process? If so, identify the oxidized form and the reduced form of the organic molecule.

8.4)   The alcohol menthol is found in mint and is used to flavor cigarettes and throat lozenges. It reacts readily with CrO_3 in acid solution to give the ketone menthone:

Remember that a hexagon represents a cyclohexane ring (p. 208).

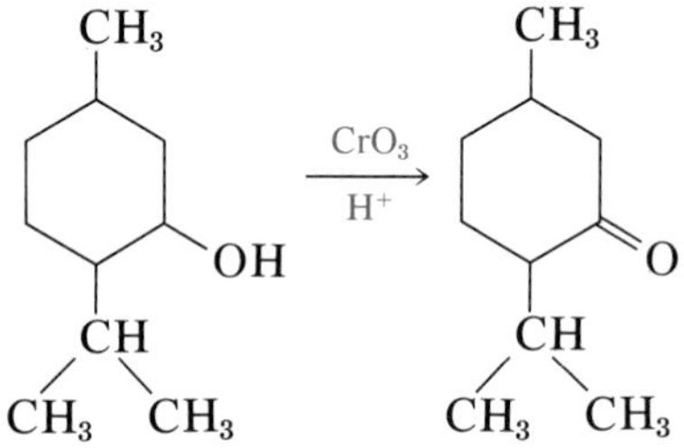

menthol   menthone

Is this reaction a redox process? If so, name the oxidizer and reducer. What is the oxidized form of the organic molecule? the reduced form? Has the oxidation level been increased or decreased in this transformation?

8.5)   The reaction of 2-butanone with aqueous $NaBH_4$ gives 2-butanol:

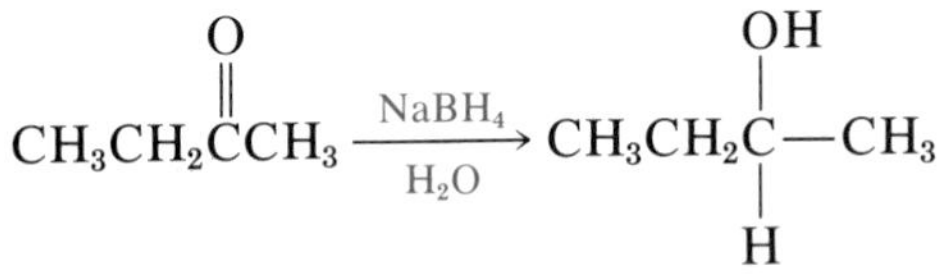

2-butanone   2-butanol

Is this reaction a redox process? If so, name the oxidizer and reducer. What is the oxidized form of the organic molecule? the reduced form? Has the oxidation level been increased or decreased in this reaction?

CHAPTER EIGHT IN REVIEW ■ Oxidation and Reduction

8.1 ELECTRON TRANSFER REACTIONS   Page 215

8A: Given the formula of a chemical species (atom, molecule, or ion), determine the oxidation state of each of its elements.

8B: Given a chemical equation, decide from oxidation states whether or not it represents a redox reaction. If it does, list the oxidation state changes and determine the element oxidized and the element reduced.

8.2 ORGANIC REDOX REACTIONS   Page 225

8C: Given an organic process, decide from the number of oxygen and hydrogen atoms in each molecule whether or not a redox reaction has occurred. If so, determine the oxidized form and the reduced form.

8D: List at least three common oxidizers (oxidizing agents) and three common reducers (reducing agents) useful in organic synthesis.

8E: Describe the products formed in step-by-step oxidation of a hydrocarbon, through alcohols, aldehydes, and carboxylic acids, to CO_2 and H_2O.

GLOSSARY FOR CHAPTER EIGHT

oxidation A reaction that results in (a) a loss of electrons, (b) an increase in the oxidation number of an element, (c) an increase in the number of carbon-oxygen bonds, or (d) a decrease in the number of carbon-hydrogen bonds in a molecule. (p. 215)

oxidation level A term that relates the oxidation state of carbon in an organic molecule to the successive steps in the oxidation of methane. (p. 232)

oxidizer, oxidizing agent A species that accepts electrons and brings about oxidation, such as O_2 or MnO_4^-. (p. 221)

redox reaction A reaction in which oxidation and reduction take place. (p. 215)

reducer, reducing agent A species that donates electrons to bring about reduction, such as H_2 or some metals. (p. 221)

reduction A reaction that results in (a) a gain of electrons, (b) a decrease in the oxidation number of an element, (c) a decrease in the number of carbon-oxygen bonds, or (d) an increase in the number of carbon-hydrogen bonds in a molecule. (p. 216)

QUESTIONS AND PROBLEMS FOR CHAPTER EIGHT ▪ Oxidation and Reduction

SECTION 8.1 ELECTRON TRANSFER REACTIONS

8.6) A sulfur atom gains two electrons to form a S^{2-} ion. Is this process an oxidation or a reduction?

8.7) The copper in CuO becomes copper metal. Is this process an oxidation or a reduction?

8.8) The oxidation state of chlorine changes from + 3 to + 1. Is this an oxidation or a reduction?

8.9) An alkane is burned and produces CO_2 and water. Is this process an oxidation or a reduction of the alkane?

8.10*) Explain why oxidation-reduction reactions are often called "electron transfer" processes.

8.11*) Define reduction in terms of electrons gained or lost.

8.12) When oxygen from the air is added to an organic molecule, has oxidation or reduction occurred?

8.33) A copper atom loses two electrons to become a Cu^{2+} ion. Is this process an oxidation or a reduction?

8.34) The sulfur in SO_2 goes to SO_3. Is this process an oxidation or a reduction?

8.35) The oxidation state of nitrogen changes from +3 to +5. Is this an oxidation or a reduction?

8.36) The phosphorus in P_2O_5 becomes the pure element. Is this change an oxidation or a reduction?

8.37*) Can you have an oxidation process without a reduction? Explain.

8.38*) Define oxidation in terms of electrons gained or lost.

8.39) When hydrogen from H_2 gas is added to an organic molecule, has oxidation or reduction occurred?

8.13) What is the oxidation state of chlorine in
a) $AlCl_3$?   c) $HClO_4$?
b) Cl^-?

8.14) Does oxidation or reduction occur to any of the elements involved when $NaCl$ becomes $NaClO_2$? Explain.

8.15) What is the oxidation state of nitrogen in N_2O_3?

8.16) In the reaction

$$16 H^+_{(aq)} + 2 MnO^-_{4(aq)} + 10 Cl^-_{(aq)} \longrightarrow$$
$$2 Mn^{2+}_{(aq)} + 8 H_2O_{(\ell)} + 5 Cl_{2(g)},$$

identify the element oxidized and the element reduced.

8.17*) Define oxidation in terms of change in oxidation state.

8.40) What is the oxidation state of sulfur in
a) SO_2?   c) S_8?
b) H_2S?

8.41) Does oxidation or reduction occur to any of the elements involved when liquid Br_2 is produced from Br^- in sea water? Explain.

8.42) What is the oxidation state of manganese in MnO_4^{2-}?

8.43) In the reaction

$$8 H^+_{(aq)} + SO^{2-}_{4(aq)} + 6 I^-_{(aq)} \longrightarrow$$
$$S_{(s)} + 4 H_2O_{(\ell)} + 3 I_{2(s)},$$

identify the element oxidized and the element reduced.

8.44*) Define reduction in terms of change in oxidation state.

SECTION 8.2 ORGANIC REDOX REACTIONS

8.18) When $CH_3CH_2CH_2OH$ is changed to CH_3CH_2CHO, has oxidation or reduction occurred?

8.19) When formaldehyde is changed to methyl alcohol, has oxidation or reduction occurred?

8.20) Define oxidation and reduction of organic compounds in terms of the number of carbon-oxygen bonds gained or lost by the organic molecule.

8.21) 2-Butanone reacts with H_2 to give 2-butanol:

$$\underset{\substack{|| \\ CH_3CH_2CCH_3}}{O} \xrightarrow[Ni]{H_2} \underset{\substack{| \\ CH_3CH_2CHCH_3}}{OH}$$

Is this change an oxidation or a reduction? What are the oxidized and reduced forms?

8.45) When
$$\underset{\substack{| \\ CH_3CH_2C=O}}{H} \text{ is}$$
changed to
$$\underset{\substack{|| \\ CH_3CH_2C-OH,}}{O} \text{ has oxi-}$$
dation or reduction occurred?

8.46) When
$$\underset{\substack{|| \\ CH_3CH_2C-OH}}{O} \text{ is}$$
changed to $CH_3CH_2CH_2OH$, has oxidation or reduction occurred?

8.47) Define oxidation and reduction of organic compounds in terms of the number of carbon-hydrogen bonds gained or lost by the organic molecule.

8.48)
$$\underset{\substack{| \\ CH_3CH_2CH_2CH_2C=O}}{H} \text{ reacts with}$$

H_2 to give $CH_3CH_2CH_2CH_2CH_2OH$. Is this change an oxidation or a reduction? What are the oxidized and reduced forms?

8.22) List three common oxidizers of organic molecules.

8.23) Define oxidizer.

8.24*) In the redox reaction

$$CH_3CH_2\overset{H}{\underset{}{C}}=O \xrightarrow[H^+]{CrO_3} CH_3CH_2\overset{O}{\underset{}{C}}-OH,$$

identify the oxidizer and the reducer.

8.25*) In the reduction reaction

$$(CH_3)_2CH-\overset{O}{\underset{}{C}}-CH_3 \xrightarrow[H_2O]{NaBH_4} (CH_3)_2CH-\overset{OH}{\underset{H}{C}}-CH_3,$$

identify the reducer.

8.26*) What is the oxidizer when propane is burned in air and produces CO_2 and H_2O?

8.27*) What is the reducer when 1-pentene reacts with H_2 to give pentane:

$$CH_3(CH_2)_2CH=CH_2 \xrightarrow[Ni]{H_2} CH_3(CH_2)_3CH_3?$$

8.28*) Using what you've learned about the oxidation levels of organic compounds, would you expect an alcohol to be oxidized to an alkane? Explain.

8.29) What type of compound would you expect if an aldehyde

$$(\overset{O}{\underset{}{-C}}-H)$$ is oxidized to the next higher oxidation level?

8.30) What type of compound would you expect if an alkane is oxidized to the next higher oxidation level?

8.31*) Would you predict that an alcohol could be oxidized by the appropriate reagent to a carboxylic acid? Explain.

8.49) List three common reducers of organic molecules.

8.50) Define reducer.

8.51*) In the redox reaction

$$CH_3CH_2CH_2OH \xrightarrow[OH^-]{KMnO_4} CH_3CH_2\overset{H}{\underset{}{C}}=O,$$

identify the oxidizer and the reducer.

8.52*) In the oxidation reaction

$$CH_3\overset{OH}{\underset{H}{C}}-CH(CH_3)_2 \xrightarrow[H^+]{K_2Cr_2O_7} CH_3\overset{O}{\underset{}{C}}CH(CH_3)_2,$$

identify the oxidizer.

8.53*) What is the oxidizer when methanal is converted to methanoic acid by $KMnO_4$:

$$H_2C=O \xrightarrow[OH^-]{KMnO_4} H-\overset{O}{\underset{}{C}}-O-H?$$

8.54*) What is the reducer when iodobutane is reacted with Zn and H^+ to give butane:

$$CH_3(CH_2)_2CH_2I \xrightarrow[H^+]{Zn} CH_3(CH_2)_2CH_3?$$

8.55*) Using what you've learned about the oxidation levels of organic compounds, would you expect an aldehyde to be reduced to a carboxylic acid? Explain.

8.56*) What type of compound would you expect if a ketone $$(\overset{O}{\underset{}{-C}}-)$$ is reduced to the next lower oxidation level?

8.57*) What type of compound would you expect if a carboxylic acid

$$(\overset{O}{\underset{}{-C}}-OH)$$ is reduced to the next lower oxidation level?

8.58*) Would you predict that a ketone could be reduced by the appropriate reagent to an alkane? Explain.

8.32*) The following reaction has been observed:

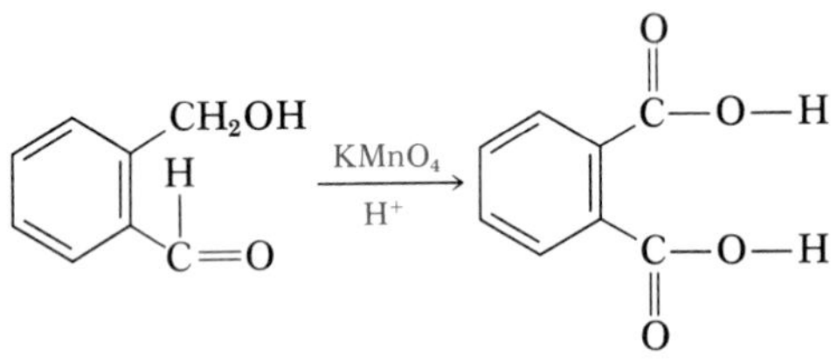

Is this an oxidation or a reduction? What is the oxidizer or reducer? By how many oxidation levels has each group involved in the redox process changed?

8.59*) The following reaction has been observed:

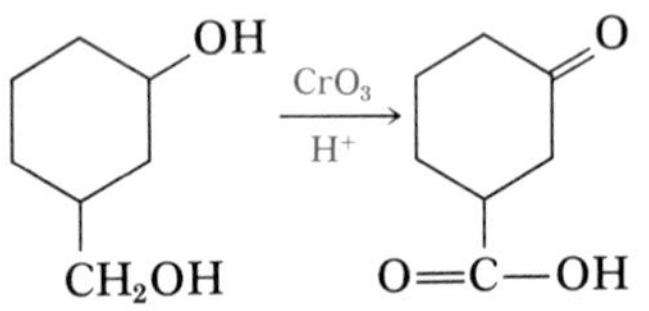

Is this a redox reaction? If so, what is the oxidizer or reducer? By how many oxidation levels has each group involved in the redox process changed?

Oxygen-Containing Organic Compounds

In Chapter 8 the redox reactions of organic compounds were examined in detail. The systematic oxidation of an alkane yields first an alcohol, then an aldehyde, then a carboxylic acid. Our emphasis in that chapter was on keeping track of any changes in the number of carbon-oxygen bonds in the organic molecules so that we could classify each process as an oxidation or a reduction reaction. Little attention was devoted to the oxidized or reduced products.

In this chapter we will take a closer look at these products. You will learn to name these organic derivatives, to distinguish the different types of oxygen-containing functional groups, and to write some basic reactions of these groups. Many molecules essential to life contain these functional groups, and you will see many examples of such compounds in later chapters devoted to biochemistry. Don't be frightened by the complexity of a biologically important chemical of life. Learn to split up the complex molecule into its functional groups. Then you will be able to recognize the various redox processes that occur and relate these reactions to the principles that you learned in Chapter 8.

A functional group is an atom or group of atoms that give certain properties to an organic compound. Carbon-carbon double bonds and triple bonds are functional groups, as are the —OH, —CHO, and —COOH groups we have seen.

9.1 FUNCTIONAL GROUPS

LEARNING GOAL 9A: List several pairs of functional groups that form isomers.

9B: List the functional groups in a molecule, given its structural formula.

In Chapter 7 we saw examples of alkanes, alkenes, and alkynes that are *structural isomers*. They have the same molecular formula, the same number and kinds of atoms, but the atoms are bonded in different ways. Butane and 2-methylpropane, 1-butene and 2-butene, 1-butyne and 2-butyne are examples of structural isomers. In these hydrocarbons, isomers are formed either by branching the carbon chain or by moving the position of the double or triple bond in the carbon chain. However, the type of functional group does not change. Both 1-butene and 2-butene contain the double bond; both 1-butyne and 2-butyne contain the triple bond.

In this chapter we will examine another type of structural isomer. These isomers will have the same molecular formula, the same number and kinds of atoms, but the atoms will be bonded in different ways to give different functional groups. The functional group is generally the reactive part of an organic molecule, and it defines the type of chemical reactions that the molecule takes part in. Thus, depending upon how the atoms are arranged, a different functional group can result, and hence the chemical and physical properties of the molecule will be affected.

The functional group is the site (place) of most chemical reactions in an organic molecule.

How can we arrange the atoms in a molecule that has the molecular formula C_3H_6? From our previous experience, drawing structural diagrams so that carbon always has four bonds, we can bond these atoms in only two ways to give either propene or cyclopropane:

cyclopropane   propene

The functional groups are the double bond and the three-carbon ring.

Thus, an alkene and the corresponding cycloalkane are a pair of structural isomers that have different functional groups.

The following examples will illustrate other pairs of structural isomers that have different functional groups. Learn how to draw pairs of structural isomers of this type and to recognize the kinds of functional group.

EXAMPLE 9a: Draw the structural formulas for the two compounds with the molecular formula C_2H_6O.

– –

SOLUTION: Since carbon forms four covalent bonds, oxygen two covalent bonds, and hydrogen one covalent bond, we can draw

ethanol, C_2H_6O dimethyl ether, C_2H_6O

Ethers are named by naming the two alkyl groups joined to the oxygen followed by the word *ether*. If the two groups are identical, the prefix *di-* is used.

Any other arrangements will not satisfy the bonding requirements of the atoms involved. Note that the ethanol contains the —OH group. This group is the *alcohol* functional group. The dimethyl ether contains an oxygen atom covalently bonded to two other carbon atoms (C—O—C). This arrangement of atoms is called an **ether** functional group.

Most ethers will easily ignite and burn, and caution must be used when working with them, as noted on p. 136.

CH_3CH_2—O—CH_2CH_3 is diethyl ether, the one commonly used in hospitals.

Chemically, ethers and alcohols are as different as night and day (dimethyl ether is a gas at room temperature, while ethanol is a liquid). Ethers, in general, are some of the most chemically unreactive molecules. They do not react with the strong oxidizers or strong reducers we saw in Chapter 8. In contrast, as we also saw in Chapter 8, alcohols are easily oxidized by strong oxidizers to aldehydes. Thus, alcohols and ethers make up a pair of structural isomers with different functional groups and widely different physical and chemical properties.

EXAMPLE 9b: Draw structural formulas containing carbon-oxygen double bonds for two compounds with the molecular formula C_3H_6O.

- -

SOLUTION: Using the bonding requirements for C, H, and O as before, two possible arrangements of the atoms are

$$
\begin{array}{ccc}
& H & O & H \\
& | & \| & | \\
H - & C - & C - & C - H \\
& | & & | \\
& H & & H \\
\end{array}
\qquad
\begin{array}{ccc}
& H & H & H \\
& | & | & | \\
H - & C - & C - & C = O \\
& | & | & \\
& H & H & \\
\end{array}
$$

propanone, C_3H_6O propanal, C_3H_6O

Propanal is an **aldehyde** and, like all aldehydes, contains the $-\overset{\overset{\displaystyle H}{|}}{C}=O$

The aldehyde functional group is often written —CHO.

functional group. Propanone is a **ketone** and contains the $C-\overset{\overset{\displaystyle O}{\|}}{C}-C$ group.

Note that both of these isomers contain $\overset{\diagdown}{\underset{\diagup}{C}}=O$, the **carbonyl** group. In the aldehyde the carbonyl group is bonded to one other carbon atom and to one hydrogen atom. In the ketone, the carbonyl group is bonded to two other carbon atoms. In many of their reactions, aldehydes and ketones behave similarly. They do, however, show some differences in chemical reactivity. Aldehydes are easily oxidized by strong oxidizers to carboxylic acids, whereas ketones are not easily oxidized. Thus, aldehydes and ketones make up a pair of structural isomers that contain different functional groups.

Perhaps, in trying to draw the structural formulas in Example 9b, you arrived at some diagrams that were different from those shown. For example, $H_2C=CHCH_2OH$ fits the molecular formula C_3H_6O. This molecule, also a structural isomer of propanone and propanal, contains the alkene functional group ($C=C$) and the alcohol functional group ($-OH$). As you can see, the number of structural isomers possible for a molecular formula increases rapidly as the number of carbon atoms increases. In some cases, the molecule can be multi-functional (contain more than one functional group).

Thus, the molecular formula C_3H_6O has three possible arrangements of the atoms. Our main concern here is simple pairs of structural isomers containing different functional groups. Keep in mind that multi-functional compounds may allow additional structural formulas that fit the molecular formula.

Recognition of functional groups

In our discussion thus far in this chapter, you have learned that structural isomers can be created by (a) branching the carbon chain, (b) moving the position of the functional group, (c) changing the type of functional group, or (d) putting in more than one functional group. In order to understand organic chemistry and biochemistry, it is important that you be able to easily recognize the parts of the molecule that change during a chemical reaction (for example, in a redox process). You should be capable of identifying what **functional groups** are present in a structural formula of a molecule. Let's summarize the kinds of functional groups you have seen.

Functional group	Identifying feature

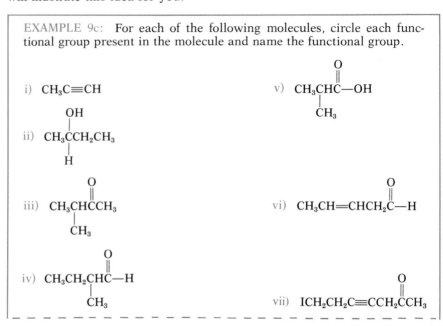

Alkene

Alkyne

Alcohol

Aldehyde (carbonyl)

Ketone (carbonyl)

Carboxylic acid

Ether

Alkyl halide

The carboxylic acid functional group is often written —COOH or —CO₂H.

When you see the structural formula of an organic molecule, learn to pick out the types of functional groups present in the molecule. Some examples will illustrate this idea for you.

EXAMPLE 9c: For each of the following molecules, circle each functional group present in the molecule and name the functional group.

i) $CH_3C\equiv CH$

ii) $CH_3\overset{\displaystyle OH}{\underset{\displaystyle H}{C}}CH_2CH_3$

iii) $CH_3\overset{\displaystyle O}{\underset{\displaystyle CH_3}{CH}}CCH_3$

iv) $CH_3CH_2\overset{\displaystyle O}{\underset{\displaystyle CH_3}{CH}}C-H$

v) $CH_3\overset{\displaystyle O}{\underset{\displaystyle CH_3}{CH}}C-OH$

vi) $CH_3CH=CHCH_2\overset{\displaystyle O}{C}-H$

vii) $ICH_2CH_2C\equiv CCH_2\overset{\displaystyle O}{C}CH_3$

SOLUTION:

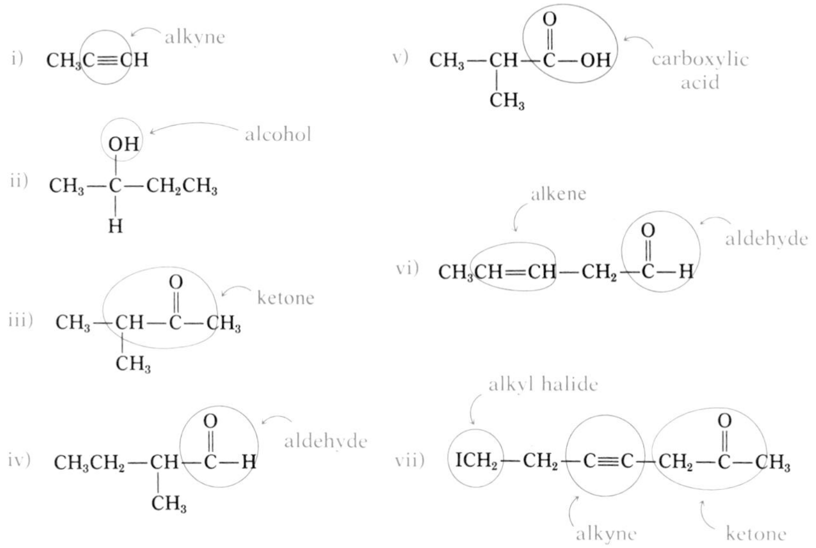

i) $CH_3C\equiv CH$ alkyne

ii) $CH_3-\overset{\overset{\displaystyle OH}{|}}{\underset{\underset{\displaystyle H}{|}}{C}}-CH_2CH_3$ alcohol

iii) $CH_3-CH-\overset{\overset{\displaystyle O}{\|}}{C}-CH_3$ ketone
$\underset{\displaystyle CH_3}{|}$

iv) $CH_3CH_2-CH-\overset{\overset{\displaystyle O}{\|}}{C}-H$ aldehyde
$\underset{\displaystyle CH_3}{|}$

v) $CH_3-CH-\overset{\overset{\displaystyle O}{\|}}{C}-OH$ carboxylic acid
$\underset{\displaystyle CH_3}{|}$

vi) $CH_3CH=CH-CH_2-\overset{\overset{\displaystyle O}{\|}}{C}-H$ alkene aldehyde

vii) $ICH_2-CH_2-C\equiv C-CH_2-\overset{\overset{\displaystyle O}{\|}}{C}-CH_3$ alkyl halide alkyne ketone

No matter how complex the molecule, you should be able to split it up into its functional groups.

9.1) For each of the following molecular formulas, draw the structural formulas for a pair of isomers containing different functional groups.
a) $C_4H_{10}O$ b) C_3H_8O c) $C_2H_4O_2$
9.2) Draw the structural formula for an isomer of $CH_3C\equiv CCH_3$ that does not contain a triple bond.
9.3) For each of the following compounds, circle the functional group and name the type of functional group.

a) $CH_3CH_2\overset{\overset{\displaystyle H}{|}}{C}=O$

b) $CH_2=CHCH_2\overset{\overset{\displaystyle O}{\|}}{C}-OH$

c) $CH_3-O-CH_2CH_2Br$

d) $(CH_3)_2CHC\overset{\overset{\displaystyle O}{\|}}{}CH_2\overset{\overset{\displaystyle O}{\|}}{C}-H$

e) $CH_3C\equiv CCH_2\overset{\overset{\displaystyle OH}{|}}{\underset{\underset{\displaystyle H}{|}}{C}}CH_2\overset{\overset{\displaystyle O}{\|}}{C}-OH$

f) 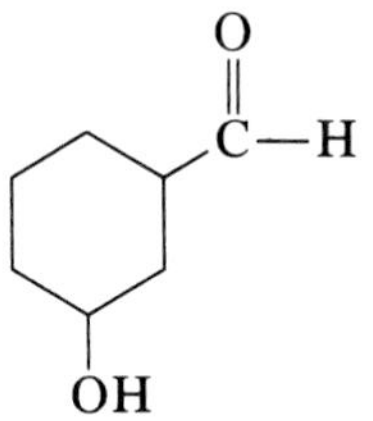 a cyclohexane ring with a $\overset{\overset{\displaystyle O}{\|}}{C}-H$ group and an OH group

9.2 ALCOHOLS

LEARNING GOAL 9C: Write the IUPAC name for an alcohol, given the structural formula.
                9D: Describe a reaction that produces a given alcohol from
   an alkyl halide or from an alkene.
                9E: Predict the oxidation product of a given primary or
   secondary alcohol.

Names

In Chapter 7, the IUPAC rules for naming alkanes and alkenes were introduced. Proper application of these rules allows you to write an unam-
biguous name for any type of hydrocarbon. When naming alkanes, the main
concern is to find the longest continuous carbon chain. In naming alkenes,
we saw that the longest chain *must* contain the carbon-carbon double bond.
Indeed, the rules that you learned to name alkenes can be applied to any
organic molecule containing a functional group. These rules are summarized
below in a general form. In this section, we will see how they apply to alcohols. In later sections of this chapter, we will use them to name aldehydes,
ketones, and carboxylic acids.

Rules for Naming Organic Compounds Containing Functional Groups
1)   Find the longest continuous carbon chain that contains the functional
   group. Give the name of the corresponding alkane with the same number
   of carbon atoms. This is the parent compound.
2)   Replace the -e ending of the alkane with the characteristic ending of the
   functional group contained in the longest carbon chain.
3)   Indicate the position of the functional group by the lowest possible
   number.
4)   Name any branches on the longest chain and identify their positions on
   the chain by the appropriate numbers. Place each number (separated by a
   hyphen) in front of the name of the branch.
5)   Indicate the number of similar branches by use of the appropriate prefix
   (di-, tri-, tetra-, etc.).
6)   Arrange the branches in alphabetical order. Place the numbers and
   branch names in front of the parent compound name, with hyphens separating any numbers from the word parts of the name.

The terms *hydroxy* and
hydroxyl are both used to
refer to the alcohol functional
group.

Let's see how these rules apply to alcohols. The characteristic ending
that indicates the presence of a **hydroxyl (alcohol)** functional group in a molecule is -*ol*.

EXAMPLE 9d: What is the IUPAC name for $CH_3CH_2CH_2CH_2OH$?

SOLUTION:

$$H-\underset{\underset{H}{|}}{\overset{\overset{H}{|}}{\underset{4}{C}}}-\underset{\underset{H}{|}}{\overset{\overset{H}{|}}{\underset{3}{C}}}-\underset{\underset{H}{|}}{\overset{\overset{H}{|}}{\underset{2}{C}}}-\underset{\underset{H}{|}}{\overset{\overset{H}{|}}{\underset{1}{C}}}-OH$$

1)   The longest carbon chain has four carbons. The parent alkane is *butane*.

2)   Replace -e of the alkane with -ol to obtain *butanol*.
3)   The lowest number of the carbon attached to the —OH group is 1. The
name is 1-butanol .

Not simply "butanol."

EXAMPLE 9e: What is the IUPAC name for $CH_3CHOHCH_3$?

SOLUTION:

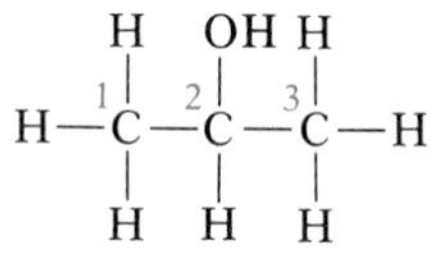

$$\begin{array}{ccccc} & H & OH & H \\ & | & | & | \\ H - & \underset{1}{C} - & \underset{2}{C} - & \underset{3}{C} - H \\ & | & | & | \\ & H & H & H \end{array}$$

1)   The longest carbon chain has three carbons. The parent alkane is *pro-pane*.
2)   Replace -e ending of the alkane with -ol to obtain *propanol*.
3)   Carbon 2 contains the alcohol functional group. The name is

2-propanol .

EXAMPLE 9f: What is the IUPAC name for $(CH_3)_3COH$?

SOLUTION:

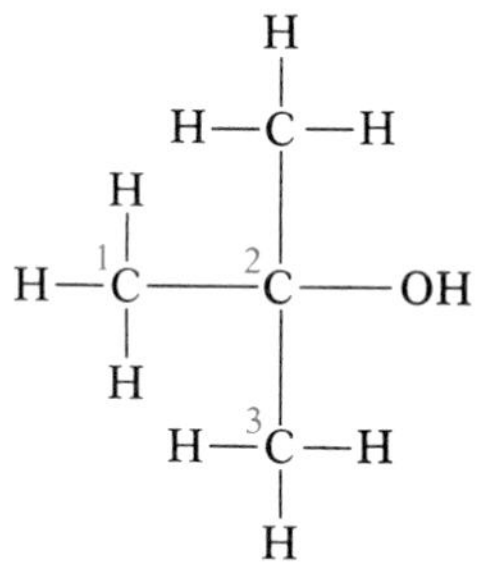

$$\begin{array}{c} H \\ | \\ H - C - H \\ H \quad\quad | \\ | \quad\quad\quad \\ H - \underset{1}{C} - \underset{2}{C} - OH \\ | \quad\quad | \\ H \quad\quad H - \underset{3}{C} - H \\ | \\ H \end{array}$$

1)   The longest continuous carbon chain has three carbons. The parent al-kane is *propane*.
2)   Replace -e with -ol to obtain *propanol*.
3)   Carbon 2 is attached to the alcohol functional group, so this com-pound is a derivative of *2-propanol*.
4)   A methyl branch is also located at carbon 2. The name is

2-methyl-2-propanol .

Not "2-methyl-propanol"
or "methyl-2-propanol."

EXAMPLE 9g: What is the IUPAC name for
$(CH_3CH_2)_2CHCH_2C(CH_3)_2CH(OH)CH_2CH_3$?

SOLUTION:

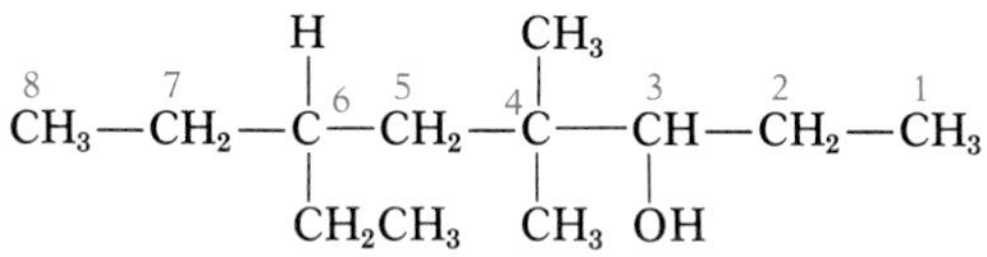

$$\begin{array}{c} H \quad\quad CH_3 \\ | \quad\quad\quad | \\ \underset{8}{CH_3} - \underset{7}{CH_2} - \underset{6}{C} - \underset{5}{CH_2} - \underset{4}{C} - \underset{3}{CH} - \underset{2}{CH_2} - \underset{1}{CH_3} \\ | \quad\quad | \quad | \\ CH_2CH_3 \quad CH_3 \; OH \end{array}$$

1)   The longest continuous carbon chain has eight carbons. The parent al-kane is *octane*.
2)   Drop the -e of the alkane name and replace with -ol to give *octanol*.
3)   The lowest possible number for the alcohol functional group is three, so this is a *3-octanol*.

4) An ethyl branch is located at carbon 6 and two methyl branches at carbon 4.

5) The prefix di- is used to indicate two identical branches on the same carbon.

6) Arrange ethyl and methyl alphabetically to give the name

6-ethyl-4,4-dimethyl-3-octanol .

Not "3-ethyl-5,5-dimethyl-6-octanol" or "6-ethyl-4-methyl-3-octanol."

Synthesis of alcohols

Since alcohols are important compounds, a wide variety of methods have been developed to synthesize them from other organic molecules. Our purpose here is not to overburden you with a long list of such methods but to illustrate two general methods that an organic chemist might use in trying to change one functional group to another. Indeed, the art of organic synthesis is how to selectively change one functional group to another *without* affecting any other part of the molecule.

A common way to accomplish a functional group change is to carry out a **displacement reaction.** To make alcohols, the halogen of an alkyl halide can be displaced by the hydroxyl (—OH) group. Such a displacement process is accomplished by heating an alkyl halide with aqueous sodium hydroxide:

$$CH_3CH_2Br + NaOH \xrightarrow[water]{heat} CH_3CH_2OH + NaBr$$

bromoethane   ethanol

The attacking species is the hydroxide ion (OH⁻). This ion approaches the carbon to which the halogen is attached from the side opposite the halogen (Figure 9–1). The hydroxide ion forms a new bond with this carbon atom. At the same time, the bond between this carbon atom and the bromine atom is broken. Thus, bromide ion is *displaced* by hydroxide ion, and the alcohol product is formed.

Displacement processes are quite common in organic synthesis. By changing the attacking species, many different types of functional groups may be introduced into organic molecules.

Although alkyl halides are usually not found in living organisms, other groups that are, such as phosphate, can be ejected in similar types of displacement reactions. These types of reactions will be observed frequently when you study the chemistry of carbohydrates and amino acids in later chapters. For example, the nucleoside thymidine (Section 20.2) is formed by the displacement of phosphate by thymine:

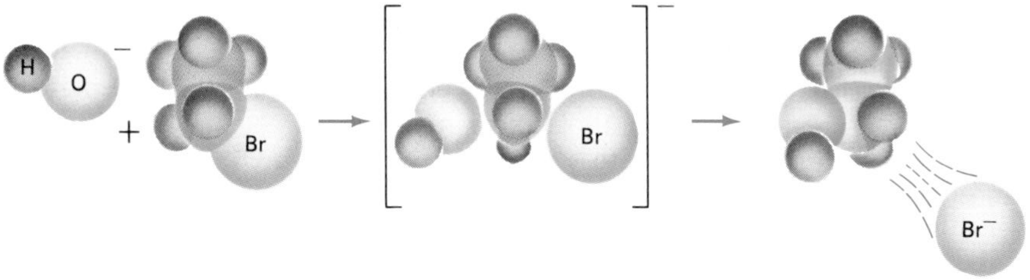

FIGURE 9–1   The displacement of bromide ion from bromoethane by hydroxide ion.

Note that the phosphate group leaves from one side of the ring and the thymine group attaches to the opposite side.

Alcohols can also be made by an addition reaction. In the presence of an acid catalyst, a water molecule will add across the carbon-carbon double bond of an alkene. The addition reaction follows Markownikoff's Rule (p. 206):

$$CH_3CH{=}CH_2 + H{-}OH \xrightarrow{\ H^+\ } CH_3CHCH_3$$
$$\overset{\displaystyle |}{OH}$$

propene   2-propanol

$$CH_3CH{=}C(CH_3)_2 + H{-}OH \xrightarrow{\ H^+\ } CH_3CH_2C(CH_3)_2$$
$$\overset{\displaystyle |}{OH}$$

2-methyl-2-butene   2-methyl-2-butanol

We do not obtain $CH_3CH_2CH_2OH$ and $CH_3CHOHCH(CH_3)_2$, since these addition products do not obey Markownikoff's Rule.

Subclasses of alcohols

It is convenient (for discussion purposes) to call alcohols *primary, secondary,* and *tertiary,* according to the condition of the carbon atom holding the —OH group. If the carbon joined to the —OH group has just one other carbon directly attached to it, the alcohol is a **primary alcohol.** If there are two other carbons bonded directly to the carbon atom carrying the —OH group, the alcohol is a **secondary alcohol.** If there are three other carbon atoms bonded directly to the carbon bearing the —OH group, the alcohol is a **tertiary alcohol.** Almost all alcohols can be classified by this scheme. Thus, when the symbol R is used for any alkyl group, we have

Methanol, CH_3OH, can't be classified under this scheme since its carbon is attached to no other carbon atoms.

$$\overset{\displaystyle H}{\underset{\displaystyle H}{R{-}\overset{|}{\underset{|}{C}}{-}OH}} \qquad \overset{\displaystyle H}{\underset{\displaystyle R}{R{-}\overset{|}{\underset{|}{C}}{-}OH}} \qquad \overset{\displaystyle R}{\underset{\displaystyle R}{R{-}\overset{|}{\underset{|}{C}}{-}OH}}$$

primary alcohol   secondary alcohol   tertiary alcohol

Look again at the alcohols already seen in this section. Ethanol and 1-butanol are examples of primary alcohols. The 2-propanol and 6-ethyl-4,4-dimethyl-3-octanol are examples of secondary alcohols. The 2-methyl-2-propanol and 2-methyl-2-butanol are examples of tertiary alcohols.

Primary alcohols react with strong oxidizers ($KMnO_4$, CrO_3, $K_2Cr_2O_7$) under the proper conditions to give aldehydes:

Such redox processes were discussed in Chapter 8.

$$CH_3CH_2CH_2OH \xrightarrow{CrO_3} CH_3CH_2\overset{\displaystyle H}{\underset{}{C}}=O$$

1-propanol   propanal

Aldehydes themselves are also easily oxidized (Section 9.3) to carboxylic acids, so when carrying out this reaction special precautions must be taken to prevent aldehyde oxidation. The general rule is

Oxidation of a primary alcohol under controlled conditions gives an aldehyde.

A secondary alcohol, on the other hand, is oxidized by strong oxidizers to a ketone:

$$CH_3-\overset{\displaystyle OH}{\underset{\displaystyle H}{C}}-CH_3 \xrightarrow[H^+]{K_2Cr_2O_7} CH_3-\overset{\displaystyle O}{C}-CH_3$$

2-propanol   propanone

$$CH_3CH_2CHCH_2-\overset{\displaystyle CH_3}{\underset{\displaystyle CH_2CH_3}{C}}-\underset{\displaystyle OH}{CHCH_2CH_3} \xrightarrow{KMnO_4} CH_3CH_2CHCH_2-\overset{\displaystyle CH_3}{\underset{\displaystyle CH_2CH_3}{C}}-\overset{\displaystyle O}{C}CH_2CH_3$$

6-ethyl-4,4-dimethyl-3-octanol   6-ethyl-4,4-dimethyl-3-octanone

In contrast to aldehydes, ketones are comparatively inert to further oxidation. No special precautions are needed to obtain high yields of ketones from secondary alcohols. Here, the general rule is

Ketones will burn (oxidize) in air to give CO_2 and H_2O.

Oxidation of secondary alcohols gives ketones.

Tertiary alcohols generally do not react with strong oxidizers.

SELF-CHECK

9.4) Give the IUPAC name for each of the following alcohols.

a) $CH_3\overset{\displaystyle OH}{\underset{\displaystyle CH_2CH_3}{CHCHCH_3}}$ b) $CH_3CH_2\underset{\displaystyle CH_3}{CHCH_2CH_2OH}$ c) $(CH_3)_2\underset{\displaystyle OH}{CCH_2CH_2CH_3}$

9.5) Classify the alcohols in Self-Check 9.4 as primary, secondary, or tertiary.

9.6) Which of the alcohols in Self-Check 9.4 would you expect to react with strong oxidizers? Draw the structural formula of each oxidized product and name the functional group present.

9.7) Draw the structural formula of the product expected from each of the following chemical reactions.

a) $CH_3CH_2CH_2CH_2I + NaOH_{(aq)} \xrightarrow{heat}$

b) $(CH_3)_2C{=}CH_2 + H_2O \xrightarrow{H^+}$

c) $(CH_3)_3CCH_2OH \xrightarrow{CrO_3}$

d) $(CH_3CH_2)_2CHOH \xrightarrow{KMnO_4}$

9.3 ALDEHYDES AND KETONES

LEARNING GOAL 9F: Write the IUPAC name for an aldehyde or ketone, given its structural formula.
> *9G: Describe a reaction that produces a given aldehyde or ketone by oxidation of an alcohol.*
> *9H: Describe the role of a Grignard reagent in organic synthesis.*

Names

The rules for naming organic compounds containing a functional group that we used to name alcohols (Section 9.2) may also be applied to aldehydes and ketones. The characteristic ending for an **aldehyde** is *-al.* (Be careful not to confuse this ending with that used for alcohols, *-ol.*) Thus, in naming an aldehyde, the *-e* ending of the parent alkane name is replaced by *-al.* The carbon atom of the aldehyde group is *always* given the lowest number (1) in the longest continuous carbon chain when numbering substituent positions.

EXAMPLE 9h: What is the IUPAC name for $(CH_3)_2CHCH_2CHO$?

SOLUTION:

$$\overset{4}{C}H_3 - \overset{\overset{\displaystyle H}{|}}{\underset{\underset{\displaystyle CH_3}{|}}{\overset{3}{C}}} - \overset{2}{C}H_2 - \overset{\overset{\displaystyle O}{||}}{\overset{1}{C}} - H$$

1)   The longest continuous carbon chain has four carbons. The parent alkane is *butane.*
2)   Drop the *-e* of the alkane name and replace it with *-al* to give *butanal.*
3)   The aldehyde carbon atom is given the lowest number (which, since it is the number 1, is understood and not placed in front of the name).
4)   A methyl branch is located at carbon 3, so the name is

> 3-methylbutanal .

EXAMPLE 9i: What is the IUPAC name for
$(CH_3CH_2)_2CHCH_2CH(CH_3)CHO$?

Numbering the chain

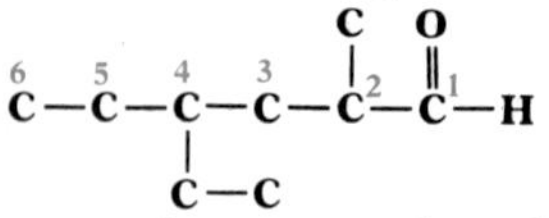

$$\overset{6}{C}-\overset{5}{C}-\overset{4}{\underset{|}{C}}-\overset{3}{C}-\overset{2}{\overset{||}{C}}-\overset{1}{C}-H$$
$$\underset{C-C}{}$$

with the C at position 4 bearing a C—C branch and position 2 bearing a C and O (ketone/carbonyl)

gives the same result as that shown in Example 9i.

SOLUTION:

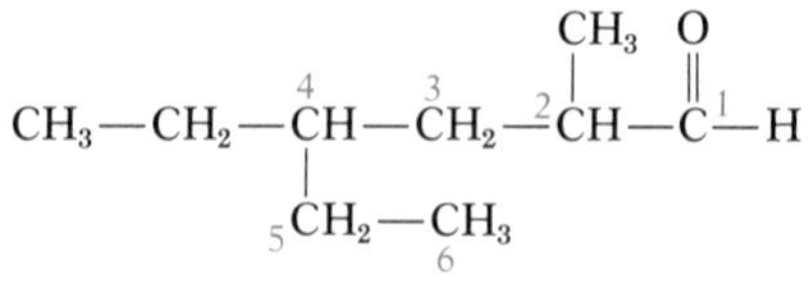

$$CH_3-CH_2-\overset{4}{CH}-\overset{3}{CH_2}-\overset{2}{\underset{\underset{5}{CH_2-CH_3}}{CH}}-\overset{\overset{O}{||}}{\underset{}{C}}-\overset{1}{H}$$

with CH_3 branch on carbon 2 and $\overset{5}{CH_2}-\overset{6}{CH_3}$ branch on carbon 4

1) The longest continuous carbon chain has six carbons. The parent alkane is *hexane*.
2) Replace the *-e* of hexane with *-al* to obtain *hexanal*.
3) Assign the aldehyde carbon the lowest number. (Again, the 1 is understood and does not appear in the name.)
4) A methyl branch is located at carbon 2 and an ethyl branch at carbon 4.
5) Arrange branch names alphabetically, and the name is

    | 4-ethyl-2-methylhexanal | .

For **ketones,** the characteristic ending is *-one*. For ketones that contain more than three carbon atoms, the location of the carbon atom of the ketone functional group *must* be given by a (lowest possible) number.

EXAMPLE 9j: What is the IUPAC name for

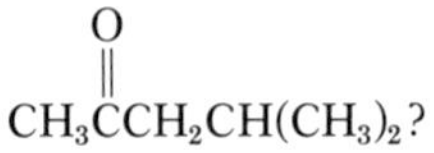

$$\overset{O}{\underset{||}{CH_3CCH_2CH(CH_3)_2}} ?$$

– –

SOLUTION:

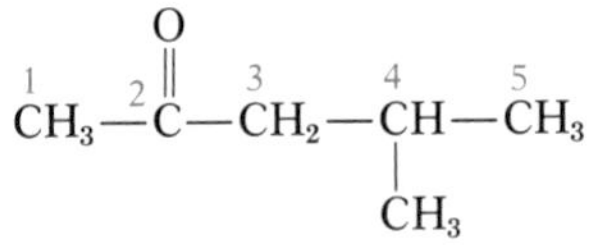

$$\overset{1}{CH_3}-\overset{2}{\overset{\overset{O}{||}}{C}}-\overset{3}{CH_2}-\overset{4}{\underset{\underset{CH_3}{|}}{CH}}-\overset{5}{CH_3}$$

1) The longest continuous carbon chain has five carbons. The parent alkane is *pentane*.
2) Replace the *-e* of pentane with *-one* to obtain *pentanone*.
3) The lowest possible number for the carbon atom of the ketone group is 2; thus this is a *2-pentanone*.
4) A methyl branch is located at carbon 4, and the name is

    | 4-methyl-2-pentanone | .

Synthesis of aldehydes and ketones

In Section 9.2 we looked at the controlled oxidation of primary and secondary alcohols. Many aldehydes and ketones are synthesized by this type of reaction:

Both aldehydes and ketones can be made by the controlled oxidation of alcohols. If we just burned the alcohols in air (uncontrolled oxidation), the products would be CO_2 and H_2O.

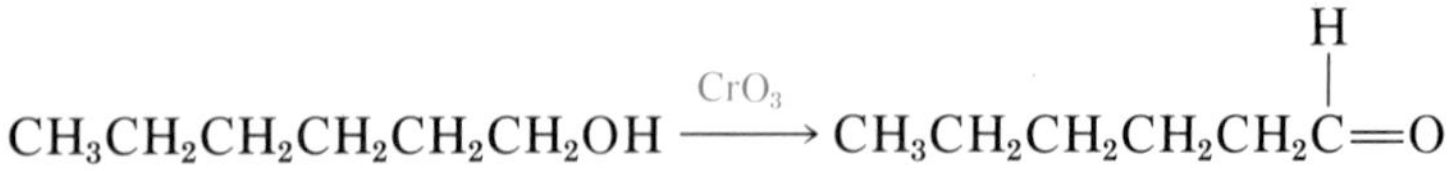

$$CH_3CH_2CH_2CH_2CH_2CH_2OH \xrightarrow{CrO_3} CH_3CH_2CH_2CH_2CH_2\overset{\overset{H}{|}}{C}{=}O$$
$$\text{1-hexanol} \qquad\qquad\qquad\qquad \text{hexanal}$$

In the oxidized molecule (hexanal), the number of carbon-oxygen bonds has increased (from 1 to 2), the number of carbon-hydrogen bonds has decreased (from 14 to 12), and the oxidation state number of carbon in the product is more positive ($-1\frac{2}{3}$) than that of carbon in the reactant (-2).

The metabolism of the ethyl alcohol from alcoholic drinks is accomplished by a series of complex oxidation steps (p. 233). When the amount of aldehyde in the blood goes up, your blood pressure goes down, your face flushes red, your heart beats faster, and you feel uncomfortable. This feeling is caused by an "acetaldehyde syndrome" (more commonly known as a hangover!).

The sulfur-containing compound disulfiram blocks the further oxidation of acetaldehyde. Thus, the acetaldehyde builds up in the blood, and the symptoms of the syndrome are felt. This has led to an interesting medical

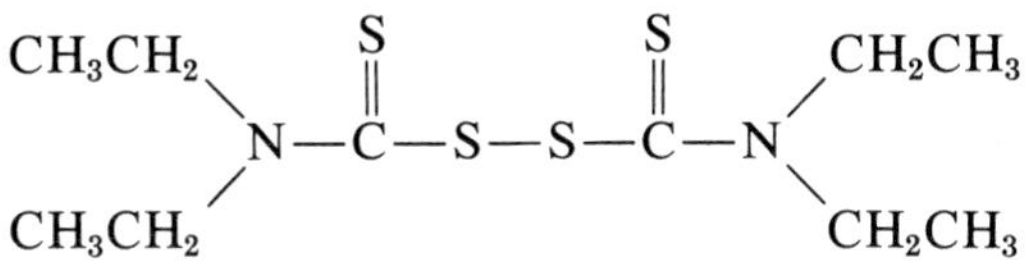

$$
\begin{array}{c}
CH_3CH_2 \\
\diagdown \\
N-\overset{\overset{\displaystyle S}{\|}}{C}-S-S-\overset{\overset{\displaystyle S}{\|}}{C}-N \\
\diagup \\
CH_3CH_2
\end{array}
\begin{array}{c}
CH_2CH_3 \\
\diagup \\
 \\
\diagdown \\
CH_2CH_3
\end{array}
\qquad \text{disulfiram}
$$

treatment for alcoholism. If given disulfiram, an alcoholic will feel uncomfortable even after only one drink, and will probably refuse any more. Eventually the alcoholic, accustomed to "refusing more," may become less dependent on drinking. What is needed to combat alcoholism is not only a desire not to drink but also the self-confidence in one's ability to refuse a drink. Disulfiram might help the "problem drinker" build up this confidence and overcome the problem.

A reaction of industrial importance is the oxidation of methanol by air (O_2). The methanol and air are passed over hot copper, and oxygen is used to convert the hydrogen (that is lost in the oxidation) to water:

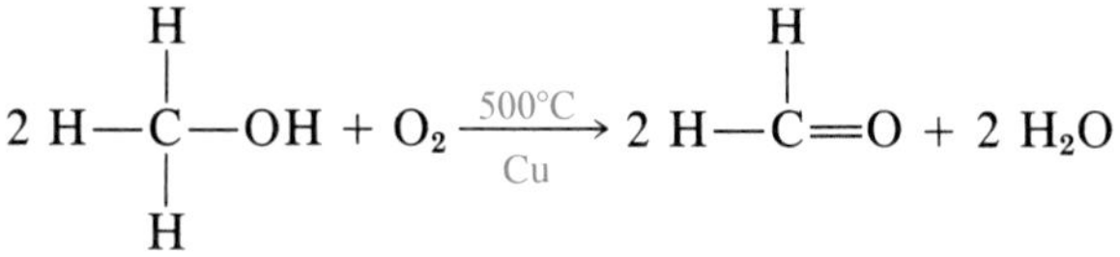

$$
2\ \overset{\overset{\displaystyle H}{|}}{\underset{\underset{\displaystyle H}{|}}{H-C-OH}} + O_2 \xrightarrow[\text{Cu}]{500°C} 2\ \overset{\overset{\displaystyle H}{|}}{H-C{=}O} + 2\ H_2O
$$

$$\text{methanol} \qquad\qquad\qquad \text{methanal}$$

The oxidation of secondary alcohols gives ketones:

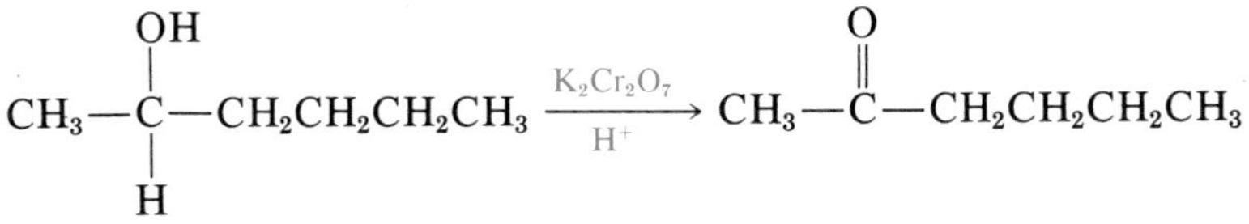

$$
\overset{\overset{\displaystyle OH}{|}}{\underset{\underset{\displaystyle H}{|}}{CH_3-C-CH_2CH_2CH_2CH_3}} \xrightarrow[\text{H}^+]{K_2Cr_2O_7} \overset{\overset{\displaystyle O}{\|}}{CH_3-C-CH_2CH_2CH_2CH_3}
$$

$$\text{2-hexanol} \qquad\qquad\qquad \text{2-hexanone}$$

Since ketones are not easily oxidized further by strong oxidizers, this type of reaction is widely used to make ketones in the laboratory. Many secondary alcohols can be made by the addition of water to alkenes (p. 247). Thus, ketones can be made in a two-step process from an alkene, as illustrated here for the synthesis of 2-butanone:

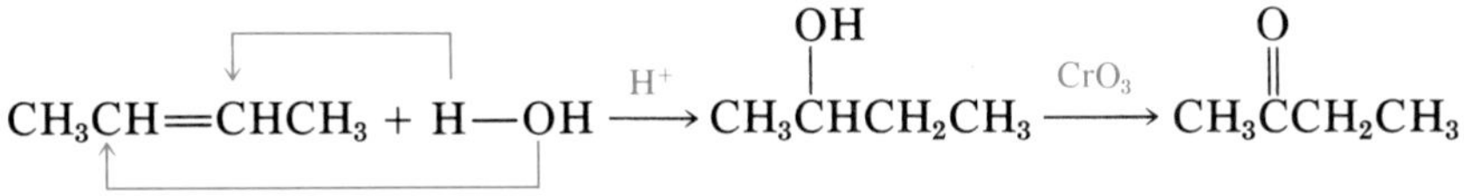

$$
CH_3CH{=}CHCH_3 + H-OH \xrightarrow{H^+} \overset{\overset{\displaystyle OH}{|}}{CH_3CHCH_2CH_3} \xrightarrow{CrO_3} \overset{\overset{\displaystyle O}{\|}}{CH_3CCH_2CH_3}
$$

$$\text{2-butene} \qquad\qquad\qquad \text{2-butanol} \qquad\qquad \text{2-butanone}$$

Grignard reagents

We have seen that hydrogen readily adds across the carbonyl group of aldehydes and ketones (p. 231). One of the most useful reagents in organic chemistry is the **Grignard reagent,** which is prepared by direct reaction between an alkyl halide and magnesium (Mg) metal in dry ether:

$$\text{R—X} + \text{Mg} \xrightarrow{\text{ether}} \text{R—Mg—X}$$

R = alkyl group
X = halogen (Cl, Br, I)

Grignard reagent
(alkyl magnesium halide)

This reagent can react with an aldehyde or ketone:

$$\underset{\text{R}'-\overset{\displaystyle O}{\overset{\|}{C}}-\text{H}}{} + \text{R—MgX} \longrightarrow \text{R}'-\overset{\text{O—MgX}}{\underset{\text{R}}{\overset{|}{C}}}-\text{H} \xrightarrow[\text{H}_2\text{O}]{\text{H}^+} \text{R}'-\overset{\text{OH}}{\underset{\text{R}}{\overset{|}{C}}}-\text{H} + \text{Mg(OH)X}$$

The alkyl portion of the Grignard reagent adds to the carbon atom of the carbonyl group, and the —MgX portion adds to the oxygen atom of the carbonyl group. If an acid solution is used ("acid hydrolysis"), an alcohol product is produced.

EXAMPLE 9k: What alcohol is formed by addition of ethyl magnesium bromide to 2-butanone?

- -

SOLUTION:

$$\text{CH}_3\text{CH}_2-\overset{\displaystyle O}{\overset{\|}{C}}-\text{CH}_3 + \text{CH}_3\text{CH}_2-\text{MgBr} \longrightarrow$$

2-butanone   ethyl magnesium bromide

$$\text{CH}_3\text{CH}_2-\overset{\text{O—MgBr}}{\underset{\text{CH}_2\text{CH}_3}{\overset{|}{C}}}-\text{CH}_3 \xrightarrow[\text{H}_2\text{O}]{\text{H}^+} \text{CH}_3\text{CH}_2-\overset{\text{OH}}{\underset{\text{CH}_2\text{CH}_3}{\overset{|}{C}}}-\text{CH}_3$$

3-methyl-3-pentanol

The addition of a Grignard reagent to an aldehyde or ketone provides a way of making an alcohol of any class. By choosing the appropriate carbonyl reactant, we can synthesize a primary alcohol (from methanal), a secondary alcohol (from aldehydes other than methanal), or a tertiary alcohol (from a ketone). This type of reaction is one of the organic chemist's most versatile methods for making alcohols. For the discovery of this reagent, Victor Grignard received the Nobel prize in 1912.

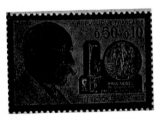

SELF-CHECK

9.8) Give the IUPAC names for the following aldehydes and ketones.

a) $\text{CH}_3\text{CH}_2\text{CHCH}_2\text{CHCH}_2\text{CHO}$
$|\phantom{\text{CH}_2\text{CH}}|$
$\text{CH}_3\ \ \ \text{CH}_2\text{CH}_3$

b) $(\text{CH}_3)_2\text{CHCH}_2\overset{\displaystyle O}{\overset{\|}{\text{C}}}\text{CH}_2\text{CH}_2\text{CH}(\text{CH}_3)_2$

9.9) Draw the structural formula of the CrO_3 oxidation product of each of the following alcohols.

a) $(CH_3)_2CHCH_2CH_2OH$ b) $CH_3CH(OH)CH_2C(CH_3)_3$ c) $CH_3CHCH(CH_3)_2$
                                                                                $|$
                                                                              CH_2OH

9.10) Draw the structural formula of the alcohol formed (after acid hydrolysis) from methyl magnesium bromide and methanal.

9.4 CARBOXYLIC ACIDS

LEARNING GOAL 9I: Write the IUPAC name for a carboxylic acid, given its structural formula.
9J: Write the common name for a continuous-chain alcohol, aldehyde, ketone, or carboxylic acid with one, two, or three carbon atoms, given the structural formula.
9K: Write an equation that represents the neutralization of a given carboxylic acid with aqueous NaOH or KOH to produce a salt.

As we noted earlier (p. 248), special precautions must be taken in the oxidation of primary alcohols to aldehydes. Otherwise, the aldehyde is further oxidized to a **carboxylic acid:**

$$R-CH_2OH \xrightarrow{[O]} R-\underset{H}{\overset{H}{C}}=O \xrightarrow{[O]} R-\underset{}{\overset{O}{C}}-O-H$$

Names

The functional group in carboxylic acids is the **carboxyl** group (—COOH). The carbon atom bonded to this functional group is as usual assigned the lowest number. As with the aldehydes, this will always be carbon 1, and this number will not appear in the name. The characteristic ending for carboxylic acids in the IUPAC system is *-oic acid*. The rest of the naming rules are applied as before.

EXAMPLE 9l: What is the IUPAC name for the carboxylic acid CH_3COOH?

- -

SOLUTION:

$$H-\overset{2}{\underset{H}{\overset{H}{C}}}-\overset{1}{\overset{O}{C}}-OH$$

1)   The longest continuous carbon chain has two carbons. The parent alkane is *ethane*.
2)   Replace the *-e* of ethane by *-oic acid* to obtain *ethanoic acid*.

EXAMPLE 9m: What is the IUPAC name for the carboxylic acid $(CH_3)_2CHCH(CH_3)CH_2COOH$?

- -

SOLUTION:

$$\overset{5}{CH_3}-\overset{4}{CH}-\overset{\overset{\displaystyle CH_3}{|}}{\underset{|}{\overset{3}{CH}}}-\overset{2}{CH_2}-\overset{\overset{\displaystyle O}{\|}}{\overset{1}{C}}-OH$$
$$CH_3$$

1) The longest continuous carbon chain has five carbons. The parent alkane is *pentane.*
2) Replace the *-e* of pentane with *-oic acid* to obtain *pentanoic acid.*
3) The carbon of the carboxyl group is assigned the lowest number (1). The rest of the chain is then numbered accordingly.
4) Methyl branches are located on carbon 3 and carbon 4.
5) Since there are two identical branches, use the prefix *di-*.
6) The name is ⌐3,4-dimethylpentanoic acid⌐ .

Nonsystematic (common) names

The IUPAC system of naming organic molecules was introduced after chemists had been working with organic compounds for many years and had already given common names to many substances. We still use some of these common names today, and many of them are probably more familiar to you than the systematic IUPAC names. Thus far in this text, we have avoided such common names and have tried to show you how organic compounds can be named by a logical set of rules. However, in your practical work with organic chemicals, you will likely hear many of these common names, and you should at least know some of the more widely used ones.

Carboxylic acids were among the earliest known organic compounds. The common names given to them generally reflect natural sources of the acids. Table 9–1 gives the common names of a few carboxylic acids. Formic acid adds sting to the bite of an ant. Acetic acid is present in vinegar. Butyric acid gives rancid butter its typical smell.

The common name of an aldehyde is derived from the common name of the carboxylic acid with the same number of carbon atoms by replacing the

TABLE 9–1   COMMON NAMES OF SOME
CARBOXYLIC ACIDS

Compound	Common Name	Source of the Name
$H-\overset{\overset{\displaystyle O}{\|}}{C}-OH$	Formic acid	Latin, *formica,* ant
$CH_3-\overset{\overset{\displaystyle O}{\|}}{C}-OH$	Acetic acid	Latin, *acetum,* vinegar
$CH_3CH_2-\overset{\overset{\displaystyle O}{\|}}{C}-OH$	Propionic acid	Greek, *proto* (first), + *pion* (fat)
$CH_3CH_2CH_2-\overset{\overset{\displaystyle O}{\|}}{C}-OH$	Butyric acid	Latin, *butyrum,* butter

-ic acid ending of the acid name with the ending *-aldehyde*. The common names of the first four continuous-chain aldehydes are given in Table 9–2.

For alcohols, the common name is formed by adding the word alcohol *after* the name of the alkyl group to which the —OH group is joined. Some examples are

$$H_3C \!\!-\!\!|\!\!-\!\! OH \qquad \text{methyl alcohol}$$

$$CH_3CH_2 \!\!-\!\!|\!\!-\!\! OH \qquad \text{ethyl alcohol}$$

$$CH_3CH_2CH_2 \!\!-\!\!|\!\!-\!\! OH \qquad \text{propyl alcohol}$$

The simplest ketone (CH_3CCH_3) has the common name *acetone*. All other common names of ketones are formed by naming the two alkyl groups joined to the carbonyl group followed by the word "ketone." As an example, $CH_3—\overset{\overset{\displaystyle O}{\|}}{C}—CH_2CH_3$ is called methyl ethyl ketone (or ethyl methyl ketone).

Salt formation

All carboxylic acids will react with aqueous solutions of bases, such as sodium or potassium hydroxide, to form salts:

$$R—\overset{\overset{\displaystyle O}{\|}}{C}—O\boxed{—H \quad + \quad Na}\,OH \longrightarrow RCO_2Na \ + \ H_2O$$

$$\text{acid} \qquad\qquad \text{base} \qquad\qquad \text{salt} \qquad \text{water}$$

The acid is said to be *neutralized* by the base (Section 13.1). The carboxyl group donates a proton (H^+) to the hydroxide ion (OH^-) of the base to form water and an ionic salt of the acid.

The salts of the long-chain **fatty acids** (C_{12} to C_{20}) are called soaps:

$$CH_3(CH_2)_{16}COOH \ + \ NaOH \longrightarrow CH_3(CH_2)_{16}CO_2Na \ + \ H_2O$$

$$\text{stearic acid} \qquad\qquad\qquad \text{sodium stearate}$$
$$\text{(a soap)}$$

Ordinary **soap** is a mixture of the sodium salts of long-chain fatty acids. Soaps may vary in composition and method of processing. If soap is made from olive oil, it is a *castile* soap; if it is filled with air it will float; perfumes and dyes can be added to provide fragrance or to match the home "decor." If a potassium (instead of a sodium) salt is used, it is a *soft soap*. Chemically, however, all the soaps are pretty much the same and work in the same way. Ivory soap is sodium stearate. Palmolive soap is sodium palmitate. In Chapter 12, we will look in more detail at soaps and detergents.

The name of a salt of a carboxylic acid is composed of two words. First, the cation (from the base used) is named. This is followed by the name of the anion **(carboxylate ion),** which is formed by changing the *-ic* ending of the acid (either the IUPAC or common name) to *-ate*.

($CH_3)_2CH$— is the isopropyl group. Rubbing alcohol is isopropyl alcohol or isopropanol, $(CH_3)_2CHOH$.

TABLE 9–2   **COMMON NAMES OF ALDEHYDES**

Compound and Name
$H—\overset{\overset{\displaystyle O}{\|}}{C}—H$
Formaldehyde
$CH_3—\overset{\overset{\displaystyle O}{\|}}{C}—H$
Acetaldehyde
$CH_3CH_2—\overset{\overset{\displaystyle O}{\|}}{C}—H$
Propionaldehyde
$CH_3CH_2CH_2—\overset{\overset{\displaystyle O}{\|}}{C}—H$
Butyraldehyde

The formation of ionic salts was discussed in Section 4.1. Table 4–2 (p. 97) includes the acetate and stearate (carboxylate) ions. The acidity of carboxylic acids is discussed in Section 13.2, and neutralization reactions in Section 13.3.

Palmitic acid, $CH_3(CH_2)_{14}COOH$, is found in coconut oil.

The anion $RCOO^-$ is a *carboxylate ion.*

The common name of CH_3CO_2Na is sodium acetate (Section 4.1).

The sodium and calcium salts of propionic acid—sodium propionate, $CH_3CH_2CO_2Na$, and calcium propionate, $(CH_3CH_2CO_2)_2Ca$—are widely used in baked goods and cheese to prevent the formation of mold.

EXAMPLE 9n: What is the IUPAC name of the salt formed in the neutralization of ethanoic acid by sodium hydroxide?

SOLUTION:

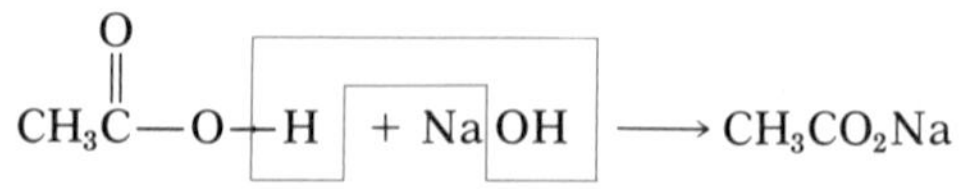

$$CH_3\overset{\displaystyle O}{\overset{\displaystyle \|}{C}}-O-H \;+\; Na\,OH \longrightarrow CH_3CO_2Na$$

1) The cation (from the base) is *sodium.*
2) Drop *-ic* of ethanoic acid and add *-ate* to obtain *ethanoate.*
3) The name of the salt is sodium ethanoate .

SELF-CHECK

9.11) Give the IUPAC name for each of the following.
a) $(CH_3)_2CHCH_2COOH$
b) $CH_3CH_2CH(CH_3)COOH$
c) $(CH_3)_3CCH_2CH_2COOH$
9.12) Draw the structural formula for
a) sodium formate   b) propionaldehyde   c) ethyl alcohol

9.5 ESTERS

LEARNING GOAL 9L: Write the IUPAC name for an ester, given its structural formula.
9M: Write an equation for the hydrolysis of a given ester.

The product of the reaction between an alcohol and a carboxylic acid is called an **ester,** and the overall reaction process is called *esterification:*

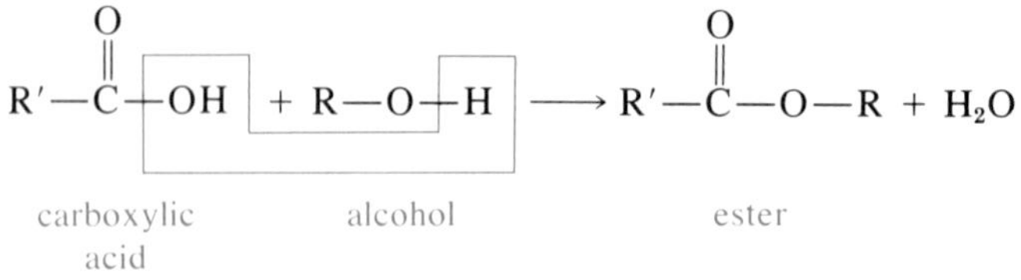

$$R'-\overset{\displaystyle O}{\overset{\displaystyle \|}{C}}-OH \;+\; R-O-H \longrightarrow R'-\overset{\displaystyle O}{\overset{\displaystyle \|}{C}}-O-R \;+\; H_2O$$

carboxylic   alcohol   ester
acid

Close examination of the above equation shows that the —OH group of the acid has been replaced with the —OR group of the alcohol. Esters are sometimes written $R'CO_2R$, where R and R' are alkyl groups.

Names

Esters are easy to name. First, remember that an ester has been made from an acid and an alcohol by the loss of water:

In naming an ester, the alcohol portion of the name comes first, then the acid portion.

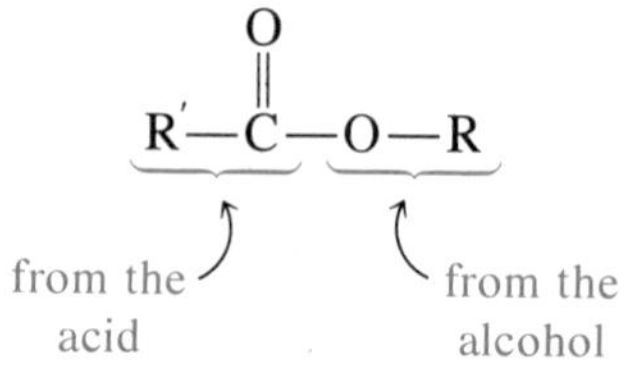

$$R'-\overset{\displaystyle O}{\overset{\displaystyle \|}{C}}-O-R$$

from the   from the
acid   alcohol

Name the alkyl group from the alcohol (designated R in the general formula). Then, name the part derived from the acid with the *-ic* part of the acid name replaced by *-ate* (as in the names of salts).

EXAMPLE 9o: What is the IUPAC name of the ester with the structural

formula $CH_3\overset{\displaystyle O}{\overset{\|}{C}}-O-CH_3$?

- -

SOLUTION:
1)   The CH_3— of the —OCH_3 comes from the alcohol. It is the methyl group.

$$CH_3\overset{\displaystyle O}{\overset{\|}{C}}\overset{\vdots}{-}OCH_3$$
$$\text{acid} \quad \text{alcohol}$$
$$\text{part} \quad \text{part}$$

2)   The acid part (CH_3CO—) comes from ethanoic acid. Drop *-ic* and replace this suffix by *-ate* to obtain *ethanoate*.
3)   The name of this ester is ⟦ methyl ethanoate ⟧.

Many simple esters also have common names. The common name of the ester is formed as described above from the common name of the acid.

EXAMPLE 9p: Write the common name of the ester $CH_3\overset{\displaystyle O}{\overset{\|}{C}}-OCH_2CH_3$.

- -

SOLUTION:
1)   The CH_3CH_2— comes from the alcohol. It is the ethyl group.
2)   The common name of the acid CH_3CO— part is *acetic*. Drop *-ic* and add *-ate* to obtain *acetate*.
3)   The common name is ⟦ ethyl acetate ⟧. See Figure 9–2.

Ethyl acetate is an excellent solvent. It is a common constituent of many brands of paint remover and fingernail polish remover. It has a characteristic odor.

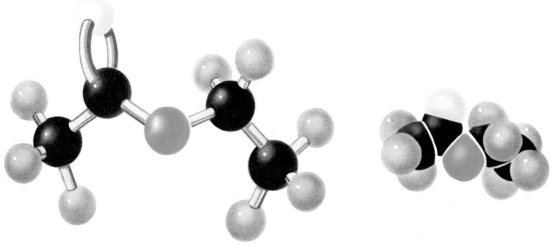

FIGURE 9–2   Two molecular models of ethyl acetate.

Esters are common in the biological world. The most important esters found in animals are fats, which are triesters with glycerol of fatty acids (Chapter 18). Fats have several biochemical functions, the most important of which is the storage of energy. When the body has taken in more food than it needs for immediate use, the excess is converted to fat and stored until it is needed (Chapter 26).

Acids other than carboxylic acids also form esters. For example, phosphate esters, which are of extreme importance in biochemistry, can be formed by esterification of alcohols with phosphoric acid:

$$\underset{\text{phosphoric acid}}{\text{HO}-\overset{\displaystyle O}{\overset{\|}{\underset{\underset{\text{OH}}{|}}{P}}}-\text{OH}} + \text{R}-\text{O}-\text{H} \longrightarrow \underset{\substack{\text{phosphate}\\\text{ester}}}{\text{HO}-\overset{\displaystyle O}{\overset{\|}{\underset{\underset{\text{OH}}{|}}{P}}}-\text{OR}} + H_2O$$

In biochemical systems, a more complex phosphoric acid derivative is used to form the phosphate ester.

Ester hydrolysis

An ester can be broken apart by the addition of water to reform the carboxylic acid and alcohol from which the ester was originally made. This reaction is called **hydrolysis** of an ester. It is catalyzed by either acid or base:

$$\underset{\text{ethyl ethanoate}}{CH_3-\overset{\displaystyle O}{\overset{\|}{C}}-OCH_2CH_3} + \text{H}-\text{OH} \xrightarrow{\text{acid}} \underset{\substack{\text{ethanoic}\\\text{acid}}}{CH_3-\overset{\displaystyle O}{\overset{\|}{C}}-OH} + \underset{\text{ethanol}}{CH_3CH_2OH}$$

Hydrolysis in basic (OH^-) solution is called **saponification** and was once a widely used reaction for making soaps from animal fats.

$$\begin{matrix}
CH_3(CH_2)_{16}-\overset{\displaystyle O}{\overset{\|}{C}}-O-CH_2 \\
\\
CH_3(CH_2)_{16}-\overset{\displaystyle O}{\overset{\|}{C}}-O-CH \\
\\
CH_3(CH_2)_{16}-\overset{\displaystyle O}{\overset{\|}{C}}-O-CH_2
\end{matrix} + H_2O \xrightarrow{\text{NaOH}} 3\ CH_3(CH_2)_{16}CO_2Na + \underset{\substack{\quad|\quad\ \ |\quad\ \ |\\\ \ OH\ \ OH\ \ OH}}{CH_2-CH-CH_2}$$

ester of stearic   sodium stearate   glycerol
acid and glycerol   (soap)
(from animal fat)

Saponification of the fat gives glycerol and the salt of the fatty acid (soap). Early civilizations made their soaps this way.

9.13) Give the IUPAC names for the following esters.

$$
\begin{array}{cc}
\quad\quad\overset{\displaystyle O}{\underset{\displaystyle \parallel}{}} & \quad\quad\overset{\displaystyle O}{\underset{\displaystyle \parallel}{}} \\
a)\ \ CH_3CH_2C\!-\!OCH_3 & b)\ \ CH_3CH_2C\!-\!OCH_2CH_3
\end{array}
$$

9.14) What are the hydrolysis products from the saponification of
a) ethyl ethanoate?   b) methyl methanoate?

9.6 SOME IMPORTANT OXYGEN-CONTAINING COMPOUNDS

Many oxygen-containing organic compounds are common materials in our daily life or important molecules in biological functions. In this section, we will briefly review some of the more common compounds. In later chapters, other members of these classes will be introduced to you.

Methanol is sometimes called wood alcohol because it was once made by heating wood in the absence of oxygen (Figure 9–3). Today, methanol is prepared mainly by the catalytic hydrogenation of carbon monoxide. Methanol is a colorless liquid with a characteristic odor. It is used as an antifreeze

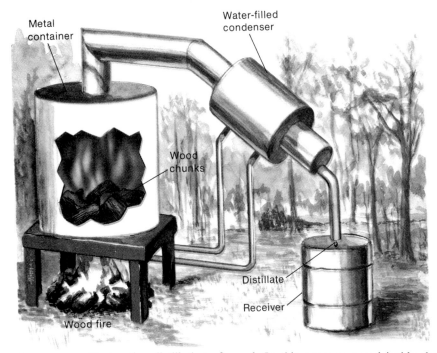

FIGURE 9–3 Destructive distillation of wood. In this process, wood inside the container on the left is heated, probably by a wood fire, in the absence of air. The distillate is mainly water but contains a significant amount of methyl alcohol. The latter can be recovered by a second distillation. The apparatus is crude and could be assembled in a lumber yard or out in the woods. Charcoal is the other product.

for automobile radiators and as a raw material for the synthesis of other organic compounds, such as formaldehyde.

When taken internally, methanol is poisonous. Small doses produce blindness through the breakdown of the optic nerve. Large doses are fatal. During the prohibition era in the United States, many people were blinded and many died after drinking ethanol *denatured* with methanol.

Ethanol is commonly known as "alcohol" or as grain alcohol, since it has been obtained for thousands of years through the fermentation of grains (corn, rye, rice), potatoes, or molasses. Yeast can change complex sugars into simple sugars (Chapter 17) and then into alcohol and CO_2:

$$C_{12}H_{22}O_{11} + H_2O \xrightarrow{\text{yeast}} 2\ C_6H_{12}O_6 \xrightarrow{\text{yeast}} 4\ CH_3CH_2OH + 4\ CO_2$$

sucrose, a complex sugar   glucose, a simple sugar   ethanol   carbon dioxide

Ethanol is a colorless liquid with a rather faint, sharp odor. It is the "active" ingredient of alcoholic drinks and is used in the preparation of medicines, flavoring extracts, and perfumes. Ethanol also is a mild antiseptic (germ-killer) and so is often used to clean the skin before an injection.

When ethanol is consumed in a drink, it is rapidly absorbed and oxidized in the body. It may therefore be used as a source of energy (Chapter 21) and is often used to overcome shock or collapse. If large amounts of alcohol are taken, there is a depression of the nerve centers in the uppermost level of the brain. This results in mental confusion, lack of muscle coordination, lowering of normal inhibitions, and eventually unconsciousness. Alcohol abuse constitutes a major drug problem in many countries.

Some alcohols contain more than one hydroxyl group per molecule. Sugars are good examples of such compounds and will be studied in Chapter 17. The simplest di-alcohol (diol), $HOCH_2CH_2OH$, is called *ethylene glycol*. It is a liquid that doesn't boil away easily. This property makes it an excellent antifreeze for automobile radiators. Preparations such as Prestone consist of ethylene glycol plus a small amount of dye.

The most important triol (three alcohol groups) is glycerol ($CH_2OHCHOHCH_2OH$), also called glycerin. It is a sweet, syrupy liquid, safe to take internally, that mixes in all proportions with water and alcohol. It is used to prepare liquid medicines and sometimes as a lubricant. Since glycerol can take up moisture from the air, it tends to keep the skin soft and moist. It is thus commonly used in cosmetics and hand lotions. More important, it is the alcohol that combines with fatty acids to form *fats* (Chapter 18).

An important aldehyde is methanal (formaldehyde), a gas that readily dissolves in water. A solution of 37% methanal and 7 to 15% methanol in water is called *formalin*. Formalin acts as a disinfectant and is used as embalming fluid and to preserve biological specimens. It combines readily with proteins, killing microorganisms and hardening tissues.

The aldehyde CCl_3CHO readily adds water to give $CCl_3CH(OH)_2$. This compound, called *chloral hydrate,* is a solid used as a sedative (sleep producer). It is the principal ingredient of "knock-out drops" and has received some fame as the "Mickey Finn" of mystery stories.

Propanone or acetone (Figure 9–4) is the most important ketone and is made industrially by the oxidation of 2-propanol. It is one of the most important industrial solvents. It not only dissolves many organic substances but also mixes with water in all proportions. It is used to dissolve varnishes, lacquers, resins, and plastics.

An individual who was blinded temporarily after drinking a small amount of methanol was said to be "blind drunk."

When ethanol is made unfit to drink (by adding an obnoxious substance) without reducing its usefulness for other purposes, it is said to be *denatured*.

The automobile fuel *gasohol* contains about 10 per cent ethanol and 90 per cent gasoline.

The concentration of alcohol in bottled "spirits" and other beverages is usually expressed as per cent or "proof." In the United States, proof is double the per cent alcohol. Thus, 100-proof whiskey is 50 per cent alcohol by volume. Standard laboratory 95-per cent alcohol is 190 proof. See Section 14.1 for the effect of various concentrations of alcohol in the blood stream.

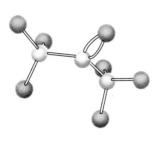

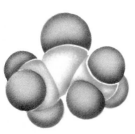

FIGURE 9–4   Acetone.

The most important carboxylic acid is ethanoic (acetic) acid. This acid has been known for thousands of years as an essential component of vinegar. Cider vinegar from the fermentation of fruit juices contains about 4% of this acid, in addition to flavoring and coloring agents from the fruit. White vinegar is made by diluting ethanoic acid with water. Commercial ethanoic acid is about 99.5% pure and is called "glacial acetic acid," since at temperatures below 17°C it freezes to an ice-like solid.

Acetic acid is also used in making cellulose acetate, commonly known as rayon.

Most esters formed from the first several organic acids and alcohols are nontoxic liquids with good properties for use as lacquer solvents. For example, butyl ethanoate serves as the solvent for fingernail polishes. Many esters have pleasant odors and are widely found in nature. The fragrance and flavor of a flower or fruit is often due to an ester. Artificial fruit flavors are often mixtures of esters (Table 9–3).

Polyesters are large synthetic molecules containing many repeating units of the ester functional group arranged in long, unbranched chains. They will be discussed in Chapter 16.

Dacron is a polyester.

TABLE 9–3   SOME TYPICAL ESTERS

Ester	Flavor
$\overset{\displaystyle O}{\overset{\|}{H-C}}-O-CH_2CH_3$	Rum
$\overset{\displaystyle O}{\overset{\|}{H-C}}-O-CH_2CH(CH_3)_2$	Raspberries
$\overset{\displaystyle O}{\overset{\|}{CH_3C}}-O-(CH_2)_4CH_3$	Banana
$\overset{\displaystyle O}{\overset{\|}{CH_3C}}-O-(CH_2)_7CH_3$	Orange
$CH_3CH_2CH_2\overset{\displaystyle O}{\overset{\|}{C}}-O-CH_2CH_3$	Pineapple
$CH_3CH_2CH_2\overset{\displaystyle O}{\overset{\|}{C}}-O-(CH_2)_4CH_3$	Apricot
$(CH_3)_2CHCH_2CH_2\overset{\displaystyle O}{\overset{\|}{C}}-O$ $(CH_3)_2CHCH_2-CH_2$	Apple

CHAPTER NINE IN REVIEW ■ Oxygen-Containing Organic Compounds

9.1 FUNCTIONAL GROUPS   Page 239

9A: *List several pairs of functional groups that form isomers.*
9B: *List the functional groups in a molecule, given its structural formula.*

9.2 ALCOHOLS — Page 244

9C: Write the IUPAC name for an alcohol, given the structural formula.

9D: Describe a reaction that produces a given alcohol from an alkyl halide or from an alkene.

9E: Predict the oxidation product of a given primary or secondary alcohol.

9.3 ALDEHYDES AND KETONES — Page 249

9F: Write the IUPAC name for an aldehyde or ketone, given its structural formula.

9G: Describe a reaction that produces a given aldehyde or ketone by oxidation of an alcohol.

9H: Describe the role of a Grignard reagent in organic synthesis.

9.4 CARBOXYLIC ACIDS — Page 253

9I: Write the IUPAC name for a carboxylic acid, given its structural formula.

9J: Write the common name for a continuous-chain alcohol, aldehyde, ketone, or carboxylic acid with one, two, or three carbon atoms, given the structural formula.

9K: Write an equation that represents the neutralization of a given carboxylic acid with aqueous NaOH or KOH to produce a salt.

9.5 ESTERS — Page 256

9L: Write the IUPAC name for an ester, given its structural formula.

9M: Write an equation for the hydrolysis of a given ester.

9.6 IMPORTANT OXYGEN-CONTAINING COMPOUNDS — Page 259

GLOSSARY FOR CHAPTER NINE

alcohol An organic compound in which the —OH functional group is attached to a carbon atom that has only single bonds. (p. 244)

aldehyde An organic compound in which the $-\overset{\displaystyle O}{\overset{\|}{C}}-H$ group is attached to either a hydrogen atom or a carbon atom. (p. 241)

carbonyl The functional group $-\overset{|}{C}=O$, found in aldehydes and ketones. (p. 241)

carboxyl The functional group $-\overset{\displaystyle O}{\overset{\|}{C}}-OH$ found in carboxylic acids. (p. 253)

carboxylate ion An anion formed by the removal of H^+ from a carboxylic acid through neutralization by a base; carboxylate ions found in Table 4–2 are acetate (CH_3COO^-), benzoate ($C_6H_5COO^-$), and stearate ($C_{17}H_{35}COO^-$). (p. 255)

carboxylic acid An organic compound containing the carboxyl group. (p. 253)

displacement reaction A reaction in which an anion bonds with a carbon atom of an organic molecule and displaces the functional group attached to that carbon to form an anion. (p. 246)

ester An organic compound containing the $-\overset{\displaystyle O}{\overset{\|}{C}}-OR$ group. (p. 256)

ether An organic compound of the form R—O—R′, which contains the functional group $-\underset{|}{\overset{|}{C}}-O-\underset{|}{\overset{|}{C}}-$, such as the common anesthetic diethyl ether, $CH_3CH_2OCH_2CH_3$. (p. 240)

fatty acid   A carboxylic acid with up to 20 carbon atoms. (p. 255)

functional group   A group of atoms bonded together to give characteristic properties of a distinct type of organic compound, such as the hydroxyl, carbonyl, or alkene functional groups. (p. 241)

Grignard reagent   An important reactant prepared from an alkyl halide and magnesium metal; represented by RMgX. (p. 252)

hydrolysis   A reaction with water which results in the splitting of a molecule into two parts, one of which bonds with the H— of water, the other with the —OH from water; acid hydrolysis of an ester gives the carboxylic acid and alcohol; biochemical hydrolysis reactions break down larger molecules into smaller ones. (p. 258)

hydroxyl   The functional group —OH, found in alcohols and also typical of many carbohydrates (Chapter 17). (p. 244)

ketone   An organic compound in which the
$$\overset{O}{\underset{\|}{-C-}}$$
(carbonyl) group is attached to two other carbon atoms. (p. 241)

primary alcohol   An alcohol in which the carbon atom attached to the —OH functional group is also attached directly to only one other carbon atom. (p. 247)

saponification   The breaking apart of an ester (basic hydrolysis) by sodium hydroxide solution to form a sodium salt, a *soap*. (p. 258)

secondary alcohol   An alcohol in which the carbon atom attached to the —OH functional group is also attached directly to two other carbon atoms. (p. 247)

soap   A salt of a long-chain (fatty) carboxylic acid. (p. 255)

tertiary alcohol   An alcohol in which the carbon atom attached to the —OH functional group is also bonded directly to three other carbon atoms. (p. 247)

QUESTIONS AND PROBLEMS FOR CHAPTER NINE ■
Oxygen-Containing Organic Compounds

SECTION 9.1 FUNCTIONAL GROUPS

9.15)   Draw the structural formulas of two alcohols isomeric with $CH_3CH_2OCH_3$.

9.16)   Draw the structural formula for the cycloalkane isomeric with 1-butene.

9.17)   Draw the structural formulas for the alkynes isomeric with $H_2C{=}CH{-}CH{=}CH_2$.

9.18)   Name the functional groups in the molecule $CH_3CH{=}CHCH_2CHO$.

9.19*)   Draw the structural formulas of the isomers with the molecular formula $C_5H_{10}O$. Name the functional groups in each isomer.

9.42)   Draw the structural formulas of three ethers isomeric with $CH_3CH_2CH_2CH_2OH$.

9.43)   Draw the structural formulas for the alkenes isomeric with cyclopentane.

9.44)   Draw the structural formula for an aldehyde isomeric with
$$\overset{O}{\underset{\|}{CH_3CCH_2CH_3}}.$$

9.45)   Name the functional groups in the molecule

9.46*)   Draw the structural formulas of ten isomers with the molecular formula $C_5H_8O_3$. Name the functional groups in each isomer.

SECTION 9.2 ALCOHOLS

9.20) Write the IUPAC name for the alcohol

$$(CH_3)_2CHCH_2CH_2CHCH_3 .$$
$$| \atop OH$$

9.21) Draw the structural formula for 2-hexanol.

9.22) Write the IUPAC name for the alcohol

$$OH \atop |$$
$$(CH_3CH_2)_2CHCHCH_2CH_3 .$$

9.23) Classify the alcohols in Questions 9.20 and 9.22 as primary, secondary, or tertiary.

9.24) Draw the structural formula for the product of the reaction between propyl bromide and aqueous sodium hydroxide.

9.25) Draw the structural formula for the alcohol formed by addition of water to 1-butene.

9.26*) Draw the structural formulas of the alcohols with the molecular formula $C_4H_{10}O$. Give the IUPAC name of each alcohol and classify each as primary, secondary, or tertiary.

9.27) Draw the structural formula of the product of the CrO_3 oxidation of 2-butanol.

9.28) Is 2-methyl-1-octanol oxidized to an aldehyde or ketone by CrO_3?

9.47) Write the IUPAC name for the alcohol $CH_3CH_2CH(CH_3)CH_2CH_2OH$.

9.48) Draw the structural formula for 2,3,4-trimethyl-2-pentanol.

9.49) Write the IUPAC name for the alcohol

$$OH \atop |$$
$$(CH_3)_2CHCH_2CHCH_2CH(CH_3)_2 .$$

9.50) Classify the alcohols in Questions 9.47 and 9.49 as primary, secondary, or tertiary.

9.51) Draw the structural formula for the product of the reaction between 2-bromohexane and aqueous sodium hydroxide.

9.52) Draw the structural formula of the alcohol formed by addition of water to 2-methyl-1-butene.

9.53*) Draw the structural formulas of the alcohols with the molecular formula $C_5H_{12}O$. Give the IUPAC name of each alcohol and classify each as primary, secondary, or tertiary.

9.54) Draw the structural formula of the product of the $K_2Cr_2O_7$ oxidation of 2,6-dimethyl-4-heptanol.

9.55) Is 4-ethyl-3-hexanol oxidized to an aldehyde or ketone by $KMnO_4$?

SECTION 9.3 ALDEHYDES AND KETONES

9.29) Write the IUPAC name of the

$$O \atop ||$$
compound $CH_3CH_2CCH_2CH_2CH_3 .$

9.30) Write the IUPAC name of the

$$O \atop ||$$
aldehyde $CH_3CH_2CH_2CH{-}C{-}H .$
$$| \atop CH_3$$

9.31) What alcohol can be oxidized to 2-methylpropanal?

9.32) Draw the structural formula for the alcohol formed (after acid hydrolysis) from the reaction of ethyl magnesium bromide with propanal.

9.56) Write the IUPAC name of the compound,

$$H \atop |$$
$$CH_3CH_2CH(CH_3)CH_2CH_2C{=}O .$$

9.57) Write the IUPAC name of the ketone,

$$O \atop ||$$
$$CH_3CH_2CH_2CC(CH_3)_3 .$$

9.58) What alcohol can be oxidized to 3-methyl-2-pentanone?

9.59) Draw the structural formula of the alcohol formed (after acid hydrolysis) from the reaction of methyl magnesium iodide with propanone.

9.33*) Devise a synthesis for 2-methyl-2-butanol starting with 2-butene. (More than one step is required.)

SECTION 9.4 CARBOXYLIC ACIDS

9.34) Write the IUPAC name for the carboxylic acid $CH_3CH_2CH_2CH_2COOH$.

9.35) Draw the structural formulas of
a) ethyl alcohol
b) acetic acid
c) formaldehyde
d) acetone

9.36) Draw the structural formula of the salt formed by neutralization of ethanoic acid with aqueous sodium hydroxide.

9.37*) Give the IUPAC name of the salt formed in Question 9.36.

SECTION 9.5 ESTERS

9.38) Write the IUPAC name of the ester $CH_3CH_2CH_2\overset{\overset{\displaystyle O}{\displaystyle \|}}{C}-OCH_3$.

9.39) Draw the structural formula for methyl formate.

9.40) Draw the structural formulas of the products from the saponification of methyl propanoate with NaOH.

SECTION 9.6 SOME IMPORTANT OXYGEN-CONTAINING COMPOUNDS

9.41*) List two important alcohols and their uses.

9.60*) Devise a synthesis for 2-methyl-2-butanol starting from propene. (More than one step is required.)

9.61) Write the IUPAC name for the carboxylic acid $CH_3CH_2C(CH_3)_2CH_2COOH$.

9.62) Draw the structural formulas of
a) methyl alcohol
b) formic acid
c) acetaldehyde
d) diethyl ketone

9.63) Draw the structural formula of the salt formed by neutralization of propanoic acid with aqueous potassium hydroxide.

9.64*) Give the IUPAC name of the salt formed in Question 9.63.

9.65) Write the IUPAC name of the ester $CH_3CH_2\overset{\overset{\displaystyle O}{\displaystyle \|}}{C}OCH_3$.

9.66) Draw the structural formula for ethyl butyrate.

9.67) Draw the structural formulas of the products from the acid hydrolysis of ethyl methanoate.

9.68*) List two important carbonyl-containing compounds and their uses.

Gases

The air that surrounds us is a mixture of invisible gases called the atmosphere. Our bodies contain several gases. Some gases are used as fuels for stoves and furnaces. Of the three states of matter—solid, liquid, and gas—the simplest to study is the gas state.

All atoms of matter are in constant motion. In the gas state, this motion determines the physical properties we will describe in this chapter. In liquids and solids, the attraction between particles is so strong that the molecular motion is very limited. For this reason, the physical properties of liquids and solids, to be described in Chapter 11, are more difficult to explain than those of gases because they depend on chemical composition. Since gases can be converted to liquids and solids, our ideas about gases can often be used to better understand the nature of the other two states.

10.1 THE NATURE OF GASES

LEARNING GOAL 10A: List the four most important measurable properties of a gas.

10B: Summarize the kinetic molecular theory of an ideal gas.

10C: Given a gas property, explain it in terms of the kinetic molecular theory.

We are all familiar with some of the properties of gases. We can smell perfume, feel the wind, and pump up a bicycle tire because of these properties.

For example, we have all observed that a gas generally has a very low density. It is mostly empty space. Because of the empty space, we can push together or *compress* a gas, as with a tire pump. We can also mix gases together as we wish, since there is always "room for more." Anesthetics used in surgery are commonly gas mixtures (Section 10.5). We may also note that, because gas molecules move quickly into the empty space available to them, gases expand to fill up a whole container. These properties of gases will be discussed further in Section 10.2.

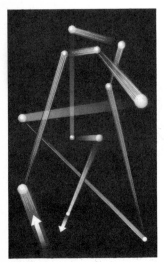
The molecules of a gas are in constant random motion.

Gas measurements

In order to describe a gas exactly, we have to specify four measurements. If we carry out an experiment or reaction involving gases, we can measure or calculate the amount (n), volume (V), temperature (T), and pressure (P) of the gases.

Amount. The quantity or amount of gas might be measured as its mass in grams. The number of moles (n) or formula units can then be calculated by the methods of Section 5.4.

Volume. If we wish to measure a property of a gas, or allow it to react, we must first confine it in a container. The capacity of the closed container is the **volume** of the gas. The inner surface of the container we refer to as the *walls*, and the gas molecules hit these walls in their travels.

Volume measurements were discussed in Section 2.1. The same volume units that we use for liquids (liters, milliliters, cubic centimeters) are applied to gases. Recall from Table 2–2 that $1 \text{ L} = 1000 \text{ mL} = 1000 \text{ cm}^3 = 0.001 \text{ m}^3$.

The container of a gas may be a closed flask or box, a rubber balloon, a spray can, etc. The easiest way to find the volume of a rigid container like a flask is to fill it with water. Since a gas expands to fill the space available to it, the volume of the water must be the same as the volume of any gas confined in the closed flask.

Temperature. The temperature of a gas sample is generally measured with a thermometer, as discussed in Section 10.2. A special *absolute temperature scale* is used with gases.

Pressure. The pressure, as described in Section 10.3, is a measure of the collision force of gas particles against a unit area of the container wall. A common scientific unit of pressure is the standard atmosphere (atm).

The kinetic molecular theory

It is easiest to understand and explain the physical properties of a gas if you can visualize a **model**, a mental picture of a gas molecule. A model airplane looks very much like the "real thing," but scaled down in size and simplified. A well-prepared model airplane can be used to compare the relative dimensions of a real airplane, and sometimes even to see how the wings function in flight. A model of the human body can show the relative positions of the organs. Models are idealized in order to be of maximum use. They do not contain all of the complexities of the real world.

Similarly, our model for a gas is *ideal*. It makes certain assumptions, which are more or less true for the gases we encounter in our daily lives. The assumptions are less true for gases that have been compressed to high density, or that have been cooled to a very low temperature, since such gases behave somewhat like liquids.

The **kinetic molecular theory** for an ideal gas was developed in the last half of the 19th century and is based on a simple model of a gas particle for which the following assumptions are true.

Assumption 1: An ideal gas consists of individual molecules or atoms that are far apart from each other in comparison to their size.

When we walk through air, we do not have to make an effort to "push away" many particles. When we pump up an automobile tire, we find that

To find the volume of a closed container such as a flask, we first weigh the empty container. We then fill it with water and weigh it again. The difference in weights gives the mass of water that exactly fills the flask. Knowing the density of water at that temperature (Section 2.3), we can calculate the volume occupied by the water.

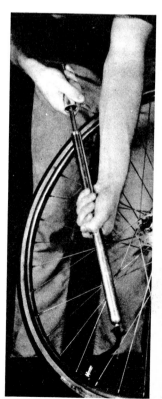

In a tire pump, we *compress* air in order to force it into the tire.

Attractions between real molecules depend very strongly on the distance between them. In assuming that ideal gas molecules are far apart, we are at the same time assuming that they do not attract each other at all.

we can add a considerable amount of air without changing the volume of the tire greatly. A gas molecule is typically one to several angstrom units (1 Å = 10^{-8} cm) in length. Air molecules are perhaps 30 Å apart on the average, and only about 1/1000 of the total volume of air is occupied by the molecules themselves.

Assumption 2: An ideal gas particle is moving very fast in a series of straight-line paths.

Figure 10–1 shows that if only a few gas molecules are present, then each molecule collides only with the walls of the container. If many molecules are present, then there are collisions with other gas molecules as well as with the walls. This assumption is in agreement with the fact that a gas quickly expands to fill its container. It also explains why perfume (or other odors) released in one part of a room can after a short while be smelled anywhere in the room.

The speed of sound is related to the high speeds of gas molecules. The device making the sound creates a chain of collisions, gas molecule against gas molecule, at a rate of about 770 miles/hour at room temperature. The speed at which the sound wave travels across the room is almost as great as the average speed of an individual molecule.

Assumption 3: Gas particles bounce off each other, and off the container walls, with no loss of energy. The pressure of a gas results from collisions with the walls of the container.

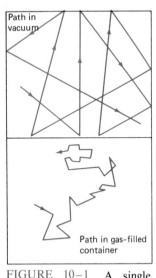

FIGURE 10–1 A single gas molecule in a container would follow the type of path shown in the top drawing. In a gas-filled container, the molecule is involved in many collisions, and its path is like that shown in the bottom illustration.

In everyday life, a rubber ball does not keep bouncing forever. It loses energy and stops. Gas molecules are forever moving. We thus say that gas collisions are completely *elastic* and no energy is lost as heat to the walls.

Each collision between a gas molecule and a wall creates a small "push" against the wall. The total of all pushes, measured as the total force against a unit area (such as a square inch or square meter) of wall, is the gas **pressure.**

Let us summarize the three assumptions of the ideal gas model: **Gases consist of very small particles moving quickly in straight-line paths. These particles move through empty space, occasionally colliding with each other and with the container walls, creating pressure. No energy is lost from the gas through these collisions.**

These assumptions allowed the development of the kinetic molecular theory, which is used to explain a large number of observed gas laws and properties. You may have noticed that we have not yet discussed any particular gases, such as CO_2, O_2, or CH_4. One advantage of the **ideal gas** model is that **ideal gas molecules, regardless of chemical composition, all "look" the same to each other and to the walls.**

We are disregarding any attractions between gas particles. Because we are assuming that all ideal gas molecules are very small compared with the space between them, we can make no distinction between a very small gas molecule, such as H_2, and a much larger one, such as C_4H_{10}. In real life, no gas is really 100% "ideal." Nonideal behavior occurs at high pressures and at low temperatures, when molecular size and attraction become important. If these factors are significant enough, the gas becomes a liquid or a solid.

In the next several sections, we will examine the properties of an ideal gas.

10.1)   Some of the following are important measurable properties of a gas, while others are physical properties that may or may not be directly measurable. Which are the four most important ones?

color   temperature   compressability
volume   particle size   amount of substance
pressure   average speed   density

10.2)   State in your own words the three assumptions of the kinetic molecular theory.

10.3)   What do we mean by the "walls" with which gas molecules collide?

10.4)   What causes gas pressure against the walls?

10.5)   Does the ideal gas model make any distinction between an O_2 molecule and a CH_4 molecule?

10.6)   Explain in terms of the kinetic molecular theory why it is possible to compress a gas.

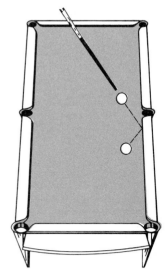

Gas collisions with the walls (and between molecules) are elastic, somewhat like the motion of billiard balls.

10.2 TEMPERATURE

LEARNING GOAL 10D: Relate temperature to energy of motion.
            10E: Convert a temperature expressed in °F, °C, or K to any of the other scales.
            10F: Given the initial volume and the initial and final temperatures of a fixed amount of ideal gas at constant pressure, use Charles' Law to calculate the final volume.

Temperature and heat flow

We are all familiar with the meaning of "hot" and "cold." When you touch a hot stove, energy in the form of heat passes from the stove into your fingers, causing cell damage. The heat flows from the object at a higher temperature (the stove) into the object at a lower temperature (your finger).

Similarly, frostbite occurs when body tissues freeze because they have lost heat to a cold (lower temperature) object. We can describe temperature in terms of heat flow:

Heat flows from a hot (higher temperature) body to a cold (lower temperature) body.

Heat is a form of energy of motion (**kinetic energy**). If you add heat to water, as when you plug in an electric coffeepot, the water temperature goes up. If the pot is plugged in for one minute, the water will gain a certain amount of heat. If you have used a lot of water, you are spreading the added heat over many molecules (as discussed in Chapter 21) and the temperature only goes up by a small amount. If you use only a little bit of water, the temperature shoots up quickly to boiling.

We may consider heat to be *total* energy of motion, so that the more substance you have, the more heat it contains. **Temperature,** on the other hand, does not depend on the amount of substance:

Temperature is a measure of the *average* energy of motion of the particles in a sample of a substance.

To raise the temperature of a substance, we add heat. This added heat, distributed among all the molecules, raises the average energy of motion (the temperature). As the substance cools, it loses heat and the temperature is lowered (by lowering the average energy of motion). This interpretation of temperature is good for all substances: gases, liquids, and solids. The difference between these three states is mainly in the *kinds* of motion contributing to the average kinetic energy. Gases travel through space in straight-line paths. Liquids have some motion from place to place, plus a back-and-forth movement called *vibration*. Solids can only vibrate, since the atoms cannot change their relative positions in space.

The average kinetic energy of the units in a solid—for example, a windowpane—becomes the same as the average kinetic energy of the air molecules hitting that solid. If the air molecules have a higher average energy of motion (higher temperature), they transfer heat to the windowpane and its temperature increases. As the air becomes colder, the air molecules hitting the pane remove heat until the temperatures of the air and windowpane are again equal.

The molecules in a gas do not all have the same energy or the same speed. Some molecules are moving so slowly that they may, if intermolecular forces are present, form a liquid, as discussed in Chapter 11. Other gas molecules are moving at very high speeds.

Thermometers

Temperature-measuring devices or **thermometers** work just like the windowpane. They gain or lose heat until the average kinetic energy inside the thermometer is the same as that of the substance being measured. Because a mercury column expands considerably as its temperature increases and contracts as its temperature decreases, it is commonly used in thermometers. Thermometers may also be made in other ways, but all must come to *thermal equilibrium* with the environment so that heat is neither lost nor gained. That's why a clinical thermometer must be kept in place for several minutes to obtain a correct reading.

A clinical thermometer that reads body temperature in °F. Modern hospitals often use similar thermometers that read in °C.

Absolute temperatures

You might conclude from the preceding discussion that as the temperature goes down, molecules move more and more slowly until they finally stop. If substances remained as ideal gases at low temperatures, this would be true. The average speed of the gas molecules would have to be zero at zero temperature. We call the temperature at which all ideal gas motion stops the **absolute zero** of temperature.

The International System of Units (SI) uses the **Kelvin scale,** with the symbol K, which is understood to mean ''degrees Kelvin.'' The degree symbol (°) is not used. Absolute zero of temperature is 0 K. The normal freezing point of water is 273.15 K. The Kelvin scale must be used when calculating gas properties.

However, the daily weather report would sound a bit strange if it read ''We predict a high tomorrow of a sweltering 304 K, followed by a low of 295

The word *normal* here has a particular technical meaning: the atmospheric pressure must be exactly one standard atmosphere. At sea level on earth, this represents a typical air pressure.

K and a range Monday of 290 to 296 K." To avoid the use of high temperature values, a different scale, Celsius, has been adopted by scientists and for everyday use in almost all nations.

Celsius temperatures

The **Celsius scale,** with the symbol °C, was chosen so that the normal freezing point of pure water is exactly 0°C and the normal boiling point exactly 100°C. Absolute zero is −273.15°C.

The size of one degree on the Celsius scale is *exactly* the same as the size of one degree on the Kelvin scale. The strange weather report we quoted above may sound more familar with "a high of 31°C, a low of 22°C, and a Monday range of 17°C to 23°C." The day is no hotter or colder than previously described, since 31°C = 304 K. The °C numbers are just more convenient to use.

Celsius temperatures become negative below 0°C, the freezing point of water.

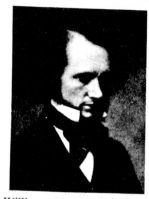

William Thomson (1824–1907), Baron Kelvin, the British physicist after whom the absolute temperature scale is named.

Fahrenheit temperatures

The earliest temperature scale, still used for most public purposes in the United States, is the Fahrenheit scale, marked in °F. Figure 10–2 shows the three scales, °F, °C, and K (absolute), side by side so that you may compare their values. You see that water freezes at 32°F and boils at 212°F.

Temperature conversions

You should be able to convert between the three temperature scales, since different scales are used (in the United States, at least) for different purposes.

Conversion between Kelvin and Celsius is easiest. They are alike except for the zero point:

Celsius to Kelvin: $T_K = T_{°C} + 273$
Kelvin to Celsius: $T_{°C} = T_K - 273$

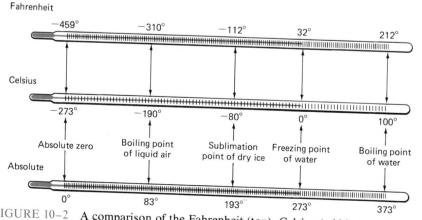

FIGURE 10–2   A comparison of the Fahrenheit (top). Celsius (middle), and Kelvin (bottom) temperature scales.

EXAMPLE 10a: Give the Celsius temperature corresponding to
  i)   the boiling point of liquid nitrogen (used to treat warts and other skin problems), 77 K
  ii)   the boiling point of the common solvent acetone, 329 K
  iii)   a typical room temperature, 293 K

SOLUTION: Subtract 273 from each of the Kelvin temperatures to get °C.

  i)   77 K − 273 = $\boxed{-196°C}$ for the boiling point of liquid nitrogen

  ii)   329 K − 273 = $\boxed{56°C}$ for the boiling point of acetone

  iii)   293 K − 273 = $\boxed{20°C}$ for a typical room temperature

EXAMPLE 10b: Determine the Kelvin temperature corresponding to
  i)   the melting point of iron, 1535°C
  ii)   the temperature of commercial dry ice (solid CO_2), −80°C
  iii)   the boiling point of liquid helium, −269°C

SOLUTION: Add 273 to each Celsius temperature to get Kelvin temperature.

  i)   1535°C + 273 = $\boxed{1808\ K}$ for the melting point of iron metal

  ii)   −80°C + 273 = $\boxed{193\ K}$ for dry-ice temperature

  iii)   −269°C + 273 = $\boxed{4\ K}$ for the boiling point of liquid helium

Note that a *change* in temperature is the same on both the Celsius and Kelvin scales.

EXAMPLE 10c: The air temperature dropped 30 Celsius degrees in a few hours at a remote Arctic post. What was the temperature change in Kelvins?

SOLUTION: The two scales have the same size unit, so the temperature drop must be the same, $\boxed{30\ K}$

Both Celsius and Fahrenheit temperature readings are commonly given in weather reports from radio and TV stations that are near the border between the United States and Canada or Mexico, since the United States is in the process of metric conversion, while people in all other countries are familiar with °C.

For converting between Fahrenheit and Celsius temperatures, you must realize that a change of nine Fahrenheit degrees is the same as a change of five Celsius degrees. Also, the zero points of the two scales are different: 0°C = 32°F.

The most common equations for converting between °F and °C are

$$\text{Fahrenheit to Celsius:}\quad T_{°C} = \frac{5}{9}(T_{°F} - 32)$$

$$\text{Celsius to Fahrenheit:}\quad T_{°F} = \left(\frac{9}{5}T_{°C}\right) + 32$$

EXAMPLE 10d: What is the Celsius temperature corresponding to
  i)   the world's highest recorded shade temperature, 136.4°F, in Libya?

ii)   the world's lowest screened temperature, − 126.9°F, at Vostok Research Station, Antarctica?
iii) the average normal body temperature, 98.6°F?
iv)   a room temperature of 70.0°F?
v)   the famous "book-burning" temperature of Fahrenheit 451?
vi)   the recommended temperature for a home hot-water supply, 140°F?

SOLUTION: Use the first equation above, $T_{°C} = \dfrac{5}{9}(T_{°F} − 32)$.

i) $(^5/_9)(136.4°F − 32) = (^5/_9)(104.4) = \boxed{58.0°C}$ severe desert heat

ii) $(^5/_9)(− 126.9°F − 32) = (^5/_9)(− 158.9) = \boxed{− 88.3°C}$ the worst chill

iii) $(^5/_9)(98.6°F − 32) = (^5/_9)(66.6) = \boxed{37.0°C}$ for normal bodies

iv) $(^5/_9)(70.0°F − 32) = (^5/_9)(38.0) = \boxed{21.1°C}$ in a classroom

v) $(^5/_9)(451°F − 32) = (^5/_9)(419) = \boxed{233°C}$ for burning paper

vi) $(^5/_9)(140°F − 32) = (^5/_9)(108) = \boxed{60.0°C}$ hot water

---

EXAMPLE 10e: Calculate the Fahrenheit temperature corresponding to
i)   the freezing point of liquid mercury, − 39°C
ii) absolute zero of temperature, − 273.15°C
iii) the temperature for fast pasteurization of milk, 72°C
iv) the temperature at the center of the sun, 15 000 000°C
v)   the boiling point of liquid air, − 190°C

SOLUTION: Use the second equation given, $T_{°F} = \left(\dfrac{9}{5}T_{°C}\right) + 32$.

i) $(^9/_5)(− 39°C) + 32 = − 70.2 + 32 = \boxed{− 38.2°F}$ mercury freezes

ii) $(^9/_5)(− 273.15°C) + 32 = − 491.67 + 32 = \boxed{− 459.67°F}$ absolute zero

iii) $(^9/_5)(72°C) + 32 = 130 + 32 = \boxed{162°F}$ to pasteurize milk

iv) $(^9/_5)(1.5 \times 10^7°C) + 32 = (2.7 \times 10^7) + 32 = \boxed{2.7 \times 10^7°F}$ inside the sun

v) $(^9/_5)(− 190°C) + 32 = − 342 + 32 = \boxed{− 310°F}$ for liquid air

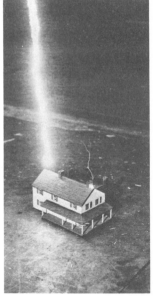

A lightning bolt can heat the air in its path to nearly 35 000 °C, hotter than the surface of the sun. About 600 flashes of lightning happen every second somewhere on earth. Lightning provides the energy for some very important chemical reactions that happen in the atmosphere.

Since liquid mercury freezes at − 39°C (− 38°F), a mercury thermometer cannot be used at very low temperatures, such as might be found in a polar research station.

If a temperature *difference* is to be calculated, remember that nine Fahrenheit degrees is the same temperature change as five Celsius degrees.

EXAMPLE 10f: A freak temperature rise occurred at Spearfish, South Dakota, on January 22, 1943. In two minutes, the temperature went from − 4°F all the way up to 49°F. What is this rise in Celsius degrees?

SOLUTION: Celsius degrees = $^5/_9$ Fahrenheit degrees

$\dfrac{5}{9}[49°F − (− 4°F)] = \dfrac{5}{9}(53$ F degrees$) = \boxed{29.4 \text{ Celsius degrees}}$

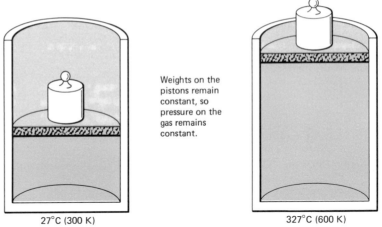

Weights on the pistons remain constant, so pressure on the gas remains constant.

27°C (300 K)   327°C (600 K)

FIGURE 10–3 Illustration of Charles' Law. If the Kelvin temperature is doubled, then the volume of a gas is doubled if pressure and amount of gas remain constant.

Charles' Law

We will consider several relationships between the measurable properties of a gas: amount, volume, temperature, and pressure. First let's look at the dependence of volume on temperature.

Let us assume that a gas is inside a closed container, such as the piston shown in Figure 10–3. The pressure on the gas is constant. We find that doubling the Kelvin temperature, from 300 K to 600 K, doubles the volume.

Many experiments of this kind have been performed, and they always lead to the same result. At constant pressure, and with a constant amount of gas, we have **Charles' Law:**

The volume of a gas is directly proportional to the Kelvin temperature.

This relationship may be used to solve numerical problems. Suppose, in a situation like that of Figure 10–3, the initial volume is 1.5 liters at 300 K. What will be the final volume at 600 K?

If we recognize that volume is directly proportional to temperature, we can set up this problem using a conversion factor that will take the first volume, V_1, and change it to the second volume, V_2:

$$\text{initial volume } (V_1) \times \text{factor} = \text{final volume } (V_2)$$

There are only two numbers available, 300 K and 600 K. From these, there are two possible factors: $\dfrac{300 \text{ K}}{600 \text{ K}}$ or $\dfrac{600 \text{ K}}{300 \text{ K}}$. Which one do we choose? Don't try to memorize anything. Instead, use logic. Volume and temperature are directly proportional to each other. The temperature is going up. Then the volume must also increase. We need a factor that will *increase* the volume.

Only $\dfrac{600 \text{ K}}{300 \text{ K}}$ will do this:

$$V_1 \times \frac{600 \text{ K}}{300 \text{ K}} = V_2$$

$$1.5 \text{ L} \times 2 = V_2 = 3.0 \text{ L}$$

We will call this approach the **proportionality factor method.** It is recommended as a good way to solve problems.

EXAMPLE 10g: The most common situation in which we have constant pressure, and thus may use Charles' Law, is with a balloon, such as that shown in Figure 10–4. Suppose the balloon of Monsieur Charles had a volume of 200 m³ (2×10^5 L) when it was filled with hot air at a temperature of 500°C. What volume would it occupy if it were sealed and then cooled to 27°C?

- -

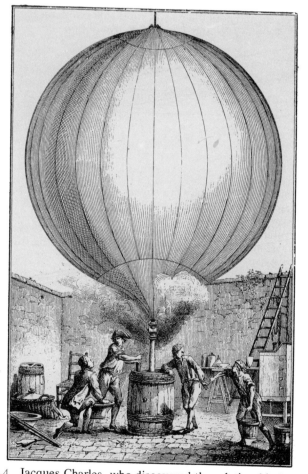

FIGURE 10–4   Jacques Charles, who discovered the relationship between the volume of a gas and its temperature, was really more interested in balloons. In 1783, he rose to a height of more than five miles in this hot-air balloon. (*Bettmann Archives.*)

SOLUTION: The possible conversion factors use the two temperatures, 500°C = 773 K and 27°C = 300 K. Do we use $\dfrac{773 \text{ K}}{300 \text{ K}}$ or $\dfrac{300 \text{ K}}{773 \text{ K}}$? The initial volume is 200 m³. The balloon cools down. Since volume is directly proportional to temperature, the volume must decrease. We need the factor that is less than one:

$$200 \text{ m}^3 \times \frac{300 \text{ K}}{773 \text{ K}} = \boxed{77.6 \text{ m}^3}$$

Once the balloon is cooled, it occupies only about one third the original volume.

Students who enjoy algebra will notice that if volume is proportional to temperature, then V = kT, where k is some constant. Then if V_1 and V_2 are the initial and final volumes and T_1 and T_2 are the initial and final temperatures, we can solve for k:

$$k = \frac{V}{T} = \frac{V_1}{T_1} = \frac{V_2}{T_2}$$

This gives us a second possible way to solve this problem. By substituting V_1 = 200 m³, T_1 = 773 K, and T_2 = 300 K, we obtain

$$\frac{V_1}{T_1} = \frac{200 \text{ m}^3}{773 \text{ K}} = \frac{V_2}{T_2} = \frac{V_2}{300 \text{ K}}$$

This can be solved to give V_2 = $\boxed{77.6 \text{ m}^3}$.

Graham's Law of Diffusion

We know that all gas molecules are moving fast. However, at a given temperature, some are moving faster than others. We can find the relative speeds of molecules by noting that the average kinetic energy of the molecules of two different gases at the *same* temperature must be the same. Let A and B be the two gases. The kinetic energy of any single molecule is $KE = \frac{1}{2} mv^2$, where m is the mass of the molecule and v is its velocity (speed).

Then for an *average* molecule of A:

$$KE_A = \frac{1}{2} m_A v_A^2$$

Similarly, for an average B molecule:

$$KE_B = \frac{1}{2} m_B v_B^2 = KE_A$$

Then

$$\frac{1}{2} m_A v_A^2 = \frac{1}{2} m_B v_B^2$$

which can be simplified to

$$\frac{v_A}{v_B} = \sqrt{\frac{m_B}{m_A}}$$

This equation expresses Graham's Law of Diffusion, which states that at a given temperature, gas particles with smaller mass tend to travel faster than gas particles with larger mass.

EXAMPLE 10h: At room temperature, an average H_2 molecule travels at a speed of 1700 m/sec (about 3800 miles/hr). What is the speed of an average O_2 molecule?

- -

SOLUTION: The masses are H_2, 2.0 amu, and O_2, 32.0 amu. Oxygen has a molecular mass 16 times greater than hydrogen. The ratio of speeds is inversely proportional to the *square root* of the mass ratio. The square root of 16 is 4. Hydrogen has an average speed four times that of oxygen. The speed for oxygen is thus

$$\frac{1}{4} \times 1700 \text{ m/sec} = \boxed{425 \text{ m/sec}}$$

SELF-CHECK

10.7) A sick person has a temperature of 105.0°F. What is that in °C?

10.8) The best temperature for brewing coffee is said to be 82°C. What is that temperature in °F? in K? Should you boil coffee?

10.9) While freezing is dangerous to body tissue, *hypothermia* (the lowering of body temperature) has one possibly beneficial aspect: it slows down body processes, and the brain can last longer without oxygen. A person rescued from drowning who has been without air for five minutes in warm weather may suffer severe brain damage; if the water is very cold, however, recovery without brain damage is possible even if the rescued person has been underwater for more than 20 minutes. A young patient once survived a body temperature of 293.5 K. Calculate that temperature in °C and °F, and compare it with the average normal body temperature.

10.10) What is the relationship between temperature and molecular motion? Is it possible to measure a meaningful temperature for a region of interstellar space in which there are very few atoms? Explain.

10.11) A child's balloon is filled with helium at 20°C to a volume of 2.00 liters. The child, as you would expect, lets go of the string, and the balloon floats up to a cloud layer where the temperature is 0°C. Assuming constant pressure, what is the new balloon volume? Remember to use Kelvin degrees!

10.3 PRESSURE

LEARNING GOAL 10G: Convert a gas pressure between atmospheres and torr (mm Hg).*

10H: Given the initial pressure and the initial and final temperatures of a fixed amount of ideal gas in a container of constant volume, use Gay-Lussac's Law to calculate the final pressure.

---

* Your instructor may ask you to be able to convert gas pressures to and from other units that are particularly important for your type of course.

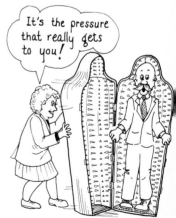

It's the pressure that really gets to you!

A small force applied to a very small area can produce great pressure. A knife blade cuts well for exactly that reason.

10I: *Apply Dalton's Law of Partial Pressures to a gas mixture.*

10J: *Given the initial pressure and volume and the final pressure (or volume) of a fixed amount of ideal gas at constant temperature, use Boyle's Law to calculate the final volume (or pressure).*

How do you feel a breeze? The force of the wind on you is the result of a gigantic number of air molecules hitting you and bouncing back. The force of the wind can be used to turn windmills and generate electricity. Extremely high winds, as in hurricanes and tornados, can do tremendous damage.

Pressure is simply a continuous and uniform "wind" that hits against all of the walls confining a gas. It is measured in force per unit area of wall, as shown in Figure 10–5. Because the gas molecules are moving in all directions, the pressure is applied equally to all surfaces. If an ant were to find itself anywhere inside the box shown in Figure 10–5, it would be subjected to the same gas pressure as the walls.

A small force applied to a small area will create a higher pressure than the same force applied to a larger area. An increase in the volume of a gas gives the molecules a greater wall surface area to strike and thus lowers the pressure. We can calculate this effect using Boyle's Law, as we shall see shortly.

If we double the force on a given area, we double the pressure. If we replace the 10-gram weight in Figure 10–5 by a 20-gram weight, we double the pressure. An increase in pressure thus results if we increase the amount of gas (usually expressed as n, the number of moles), since this leads to a greater number of collisions with the walls. Increasing the temperature leads to more frequent and more energetic collisions, and thus also to greater pressure.

Atmospheric pressure

We live at the bottom of a sea of air, the atmosphere. The effect of having a column of air above our bodies is similar to the effect shown in Figure 10–5. Since air molecules have mass, we are "supporting" a stack of molecules many miles high. At the earth's surface, this stack weighs 14.7 pounds for each square inch of area. Your hand thus supports about 300 pounds of air.

Air exerts pressure in all directions, so there is also a 300 pound "push up" on the bottom of your hand. The net effect is zero, so you can move your hand through the air. There are situations in which air pressure creates problems for the body, however. Your eardrum, which separates the inner ear from the atmosphere, will feel comfortable (and function well) if the internal pressure is equal to that of the atmosphere. As you go up in an airplane, the two forces on the drum equalize at a lower pressure than on the ground. Then when you come down, the atmospheric pressure is higher than that in the middle ear and you feel uncomfortable until the ear "pops."

If pressures are unequal on the two sides of a surface, the surface will be pushed by the region of higher pressure. A piece of tissue paper floating in air has equal pressure above it and below it. What if you catch it with the nozzle of a vacuum cleaner? The force on the room side of the tissue is still very high. Since a vacuum is a lack of gas molecules, the force from inside

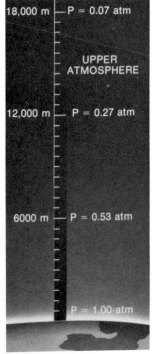

The air pressure above the surface of the earth is produced by the weight of the air column that is over that spot. As you move up into the atmosphere, the air pressure drops because there is less air above you. For comparison, Mount Everest is 29 028 feet or 8848 meters high, about halfway up the diagram.

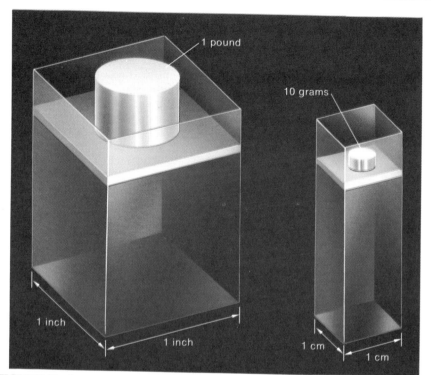

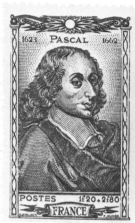

Blaise Pascal (1623–1662) was a great French philosopher and mathematician who helped explain how a barometer measures pressure.

FIGURE 10–5 Gas pressure is equal to force divided by area. A mass of one pound resting on one square inch of area exerts a downward pressure (because of gravity) of 1 lb/in.² (1 psi). Ten grams on a surface of one square centimeter exerts a pressure of 0.1 N/cm², about one kilopascal.

the vacuum is much lower. The result is that the atmosphere *pushes* the tissue paper into the vacuum cleaner. We often say that a vacuum cleaner "sucks up" dirt, but that's not true at all. The pressure of the atmosphere pushes dirt into the machine. A vacuum is not a "pulling" force, it is the absence of a push, caused by a low pressure. You discover this when you try to open a pressure cooker or vacuum jar before first equalizing the pressures.

Units of pressure

The SI unit of pressure is the **pascal** (Pa), a rather small unit defined as a force of one newton applied over an area of 1 m². The force applied by a 10-g weight on an area of 1 cm² (Figure 10–5) is about 1000 pascals.

Canadian weather reports give air pressure in kilopascals, kPa, which use the metric prefix *kilo-* that you learned in Chapter 2 (1 kPa = 1000 Pa). One standard **atmosphere** (atm) of pressure is 101.3 kPa. A low-pressure region usually brings wet and stormy weather. Inside a cyclone or hurricane, the pressure can fall to as low as 0.866 atm, or 87.7 kPa. A high-pressure weather region usually brings good weather. The highest recorded sea-level pressure was 1.070 atm, or 108.3 kPa.

Traditional British and U.S. pressure-measuring devices record pounds per square inch (psi). A standard atmosphere is 14.7 psi. Tire pressures are stated in psi *above* atmospheric pressure. If the pressure inside a flat tire

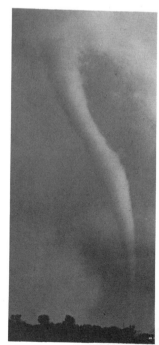

The air pressure inside a tornado is rather low.

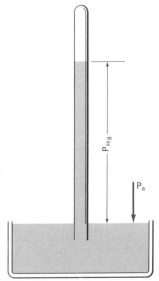

FIGURE 10–6 A mercury barometer. The atmospheric pressure (P_a) must be equal to the height of the mercury column (P_{Hg}).

TABLE 10–1 PRESSURES EQUAL TO ONE STANDARD ATMOSPHERE

760 torr or 760 mm Hg
101.325 kPa (kilopascals, the SI unit)
14.696 psi (pounds/square inch)
29.92 inches of mercury
1013.25 millibars (used in U.S. weather reports)

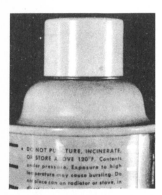

A spray can warning about the effects of Gay-Lussac's Law.

reads zero on a tire gauge, the pressures inside and outside the tire are equal. The same is true for pressure gauges on tanks of compressed gases.

All other pressure units are based on observed readings from a **barometer,** a device first designed by Torricelli in the 1600's. The principle of a mercury barometer (Figure 10–6) is that the height of the column of mercury (shown as P_{Hg}) is directly proportional to the atmospheric pressure (P_a). A standard atmosphere will support a mercury column 76.0 cm (760 mm) high. Scientists long ago began using millimeters of mercury height in a barometer (mm Hg) as a pressure unit. Because of Torricelli's contribution, this unit is now known as a **torr,** and 1 atm = 760 torr. If a mercury barometer is calibrated in inches, you will obtain numbers near 30 inches of mercury for atmospheric pressures.

Table 10–1 shows the value of one standard atmosphere in various units so that conversion factors may be used to solve various types of problems.

EXAMPLE 10i: One common type of home pressure cooker can be set to cook food at 5, 10, or 15 psi above atmospheric pressure. Convert 15.0 psi to torr, to atm, and to kPa.

- -

SOLUTION: Using the factors in Table 10–1:

$$15.0 \text{ psi} \times \frac{760 \text{ torr}}{14.70 \text{ psi}} = \boxed{776 \text{ torr}}$$

$$15.0 \text{ psi} \times \frac{1 \text{ atm}}{14.70 \text{ psi}} = \boxed{1.02 \text{ atm}}$$

$$15.0 \text{ psi} \times \frac{101.325 \text{ kPa}}{14.70 \text{ psi}} = \boxed{103 \text{ kPa}}$$

Gay-Lussac's Law

In the previous section you studied Charles' Law: if the amount of gas and the pressure are fixed, the volume is directly proportional to the temperature.

A similar relationship exists if the amount of gas and the volume are kept constant, as in a metal can or glass bottle, and the temperature is changed. In such a situation, we have **Gay-Lussac's Law:**

The pressure inside a fixed volume is proportional to the Kelvin temperature.

Consider a spray can of the type commonly used for deodorants, oven cleaners, and paints. One of the warnings on such cans is *"Do not place in hot water or near radiators or stoves. Do not incinerate, even when empty. Do not store at temperatures above 120°F."*

Such a can is built to withstand a certain inside pressure. Beyond that pressure, the can bursts or explodes. But why is there a caution against incinerating an *empty* can? If the extra pressure is all gone (when you press the button, nothing happens), isn't the can safe?

EXAMPLE 10j: The contents of a spray can are all used up, and the can thus contains gas at a pressure of 1.00 atm. The can is removed from the bathroom cupboard (T = 27°C = 300 K) and thrown into a fire, where its temperature quickly rises to 900 K (627°C). Why does the can explode?

- -

SOLUTION: Use the proportionality factor method, just as for Charles' Law in Example 10g. The two possible factors are $\dfrac{300\ K}{900\ K}$ and $\dfrac{900\ K}{300\ K}$. We are increasing the temperature, which should result, by Gay-Lussac's Law, in increasing the pressure. The correct factor is greater than one:

$$1.00\ atm \times \frac{900\ K}{300\ K} = \boxed{3.00\ atm}$$

This pressure is more than enough to break the can, since the internal pressure is now 2.00 atm greater than the outside pressure.
  Alternatively, you could use algebra to solve the problem:

$$P \propto T^* \quad so \quad \frac{P_1}{T_1} = \frac{P_2}{T_2} \quad and \quad \frac{1.00\ atm}{300\ K} = \frac{P_2}{900\ K} \quad so\ P_2 = \boxed{3.00\ atm}$$

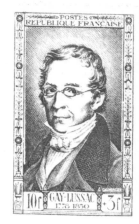

Joseph Louis Gay-Lussac (1778–1850).

The same principle is used in a pressure cooker or in an autoclave to sterilize medical instruments. When you heat a sealed metal container (constant volume, constant amount of gas), the pressure increases. Water boils at a higher temperature at high pressure (as you will see in Chapter 11), so the food is cooked or the instruments are sterilized more quickly.

EXAMPLE 10k: A pressure cooker (or autoclave) is closed at 20°C. To what temperature must the gas be heated in order to create an internal pressure of 2.00 atm?

- -

SOLUTION: The original pressure is 1.00 atm. The two possible conversion factors are $\dfrac{1.00\ atm}{2.00\ atm}$ and $\dfrac{2.00\ atm}{1.00\ atm}$. From the problem and from Gay-Lussac's Law, you know that the temperature increases. The correct factor must be the second one. The original temperature is 20°C = 293 K:

$$293\ K \times \frac{2.00\ atm}{1.00\ atm} = \boxed{586\ K = 313°C}$$

Or, using algebra:

$$\frac{P_1}{T_1} = \frac{P_2}{T_2}, \quad so \quad \frac{1.00\ atm}{293\ K} = \frac{2.00\ atm}{T_2} \quad and\ T_2 = \boxed{586\ K}$$

At an internal pressure of 2.00 atm, the boiling point of water is raised higher than at 1.00 atm, and the temperature of the steam is 120°C, rather than the normal 100°C.

Another practical example of Gay-Lussac's Law is related to automobile safety. It is important to keep tires at the proper inflation pressure. Tires build up heat while they roll, because of flexing and friction with the road. Under-inflated tires become hotter than properly inflated tires. Higher gas

---

* The symbol ∝ means ''is proportional to.''

temperature inside the tire naturally increases the pressure, which may cause a blowout and an accident.

Relationship of pressure and amount of gas

The number of molecules is proportional to n, the number of moles. If n increases, the number of gas molecules increases.

The amount of gas can be measured in grams or calculated in number of moles (n) or molecules. More gas molecules inside a container (at fixed V, T) must result in more collisions with the walls, and thus greater pressure.

For example, when you pump air into a tire, the volume stays just about constant, as does the temperature. The added air goes almost entirely into an increased pressure. At constant V and T,

Pressure is proportional to the amount of an ideal gas.

Dalton's Law of Partial Pressures

In the preceding paragraph, we did not say that the gas had to consist of only one element or compound. Recall that in the kinetic molecular theory, we cannot distinguish between different kinds of gas particles. Thus, two gas molecules of *different* substances contribute to the gas pressure in exactly the same manner as do two molecules of the same substance. In each case, the two molecules have the same average kinetic energy, since the temperature is the same for both.

A very important general rule is

The pressure of an ideal gas depends on the number of molecules present, rather than on the type of molecule.

With a gas mixture, the number of particles is what counts. If the mixture of particles consists of a certain number (N_A) of particles of gas A, and a different number of particles (N_B) of gas B, then the A molecules will contribute to the total pressure as if B were not present, and the B molecules will collide with the walls as if A were not present.

The pressure exerted by a given amount of an ideal gas in a container of fixed volume is the same whether that gas is alone in the container or mixed with other gases.

This is illustrated by Figure 10–7. At a fixed temperature, gas A is occupying a box of volume V and exerts pressure P_A. Gas B is doing the same, exerting pressure P_B. When the gases are mixed, the total pressure is $P_A + P_B$. We may now write **Dalton's Law of Partial Pressures:**

The total pressure of a mixture of ideal gases is the sum of the partial pressures of the individual gases in the mixture.

Consider the oxygen collected from the decomposition of KClO$_3$, shown in Figure 5–2. Since the oxygen is collected over water, there will be a mixture of O$_2$ molecules and H$_2$O vapor molecules in the collection bottle.

The **partial pressure** of any gas is the pressure that results *only* from the molecules of that particular gas. It is equal to the pressure that would result if that gas were *alone* in the container. We may write this law algebraically:

$$P_{total} = P_A + P_B + P_C + P_D + ...$$

where P_A is the partial pressure of gas A, etc. The concept of partial pressures is important in human biochemistry because we breathe not pure ox-

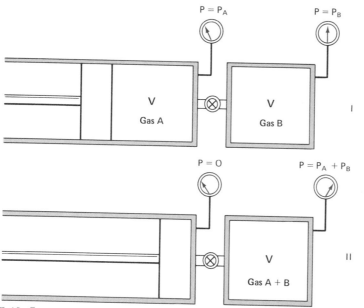

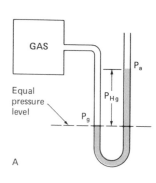

FIGURE 10–7   An experimental apparatus to demonstrate Dalton's Law of Partial Pressures.

ygen but air, a mixture of gases. The total atmospheric pressure is thus the sum of several partial pressures:

$$P_{air} = P_{N_2} + P_{O_2} + P_{CO_2} + P_{H_2O} + P_{Ar} + \ldots$$

In Section 10.5 we will discuss the partial pressures of oxygen and carbon dioxide in the human body. You should be able to solve problems using Dalton's Law of Partial Pressures.

Pressure measurements on confined gases are made with a **manometer** (Figure 10–8).

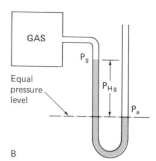

FIGURE 10–8   An open-end manometer, which works on the same principle as a barometer, is used to determine the gas pressure in a closed vessel. *Barometer* is from the Greek word for measuring weight, in this case the weight of the atmosphere. *Manometer* is from the Greek word for measuring something very thin or rare. If the gas pressure P_g is greater than atmospheric pressure P_a, we have case A. The pressure P_{Hg} is the difference in pressure. If the pressure of the gas in the container is less than atmospheric pressure, we have case B.

EXAMPLE 10l: A mixture of gases in a 3.00-liter flask consists of N_2 at a partial pressure of 100 torr and O_2 at a partial pressure of 300 torr. i) What is the volume of each gas? ii) Calculate the total pressure in the flask.

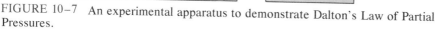

SOLUTION: i)   The volume available to a gas is the overall volume of its container. The presence of another gas has no effect, since every gas expands to fill its container. Each gas thus has V = $\boxed{3.00 \text{ liters}}$.
ii)   By Dalton's Law of Partial Pressures, the total pressure in the flask is obtained by adding together the partial pressures of the contents:

$$P_{total} = P_{N_2} + P_{O_2} = 100 \text{ torr} + 300 \text{ torr} = \boxed{400 \text{ torr}}$$

EXAMPLE 10m: Air has relatively constant proportions of nitrogen (78.1% of the molecules), oxygen (21.0%), argon (0.9%), and CO_2 (0.03%). The partial pressure of each gas in normal dry air at sea level is proportional to the number of molecules: N_2, 0.781 atm; O_2, 0.210 atm; Ar, 0.009 atm; CO_2, 0.0003 atm.

We are thus accustomed to breathing air with an oxygen partial pressure of 0.210 atm. When we go to a high-altitude mountaintop or city, the total air pressure is lower. Oxygen still makes up the same 21.0% of air. Calculate the oxygen partial pressure if the total pressure is 0.316 atm, as it is at the top of Mount Everest.

- -

SOLUTION: Since 21.0% of the molecules of air are oxygen molecules, oxygen makes up 21.0% of the pressure.

$$(0.210)(0.316 \text{ atm}) = \boxed{0.0664 \text{ atm O}_2} ,$$

less than one third of the O_2 pressure we are accustomed to at sea level.

Boyle's Law

So far, we have discussed only the relationships between the important measurable gas quantities (T,V,P,n) that are *direct* proportionalities:

$$V \propto T \text{ (at fixed P,n)} \qquad P \propto T \text{ (at fixed V,n)} \qquad P \propto n \text{ (at fixed V,T)}$$

where n is the number of moles of ideal gas.

As you might expect, nature is not always so simple. We must learn one *inverse* relationship.

Imagine squeezing a child's balloon between your hands. You are *decreasing the volume* of the balloon. What happens? The balloon pushes back (or bursts) from the *increased* pressure.

Expand your lungs. You are *increasing the volume* of your lungs, thus *decreasing* the pressure inside the air passages. This creates a partial "vacuum," which causes air to rush into your body. At fixed temperature and amount of ideal gas:

If volume goes up, pressure goes down. $P \propto \dfrac{1}{V}$ $P_1V_1 = P_2V_2$
If volume goes down, pressure goes up.

This is the law of Robert Boyle:

The pressure of an ideal gas is inversely proportional to the volume at constant temperature and constant amount of gas.

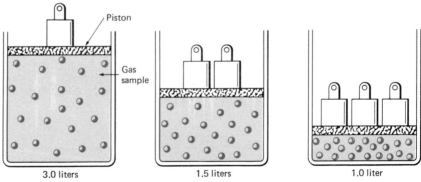

FIGURE 10–9 Boyle's Law. If the pressure on a fixed amount of gas at constant temperature is increased, the volume decreases. The product of pressure and volume is constant.

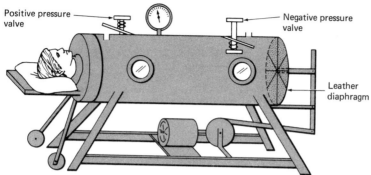

FIGURE 10–10   A hospital application of Boyle's Law, the emergency respirator. Smaller versions are now available for portable use.

Boyle's Law is shown in Figure 10–9, which could be considered to show the *compression* stroke inside a cylinder of an automobile engine. As the gas is compressed to higher pressure, the volume decreases. When the compressed gas is ignited and explodes, it creates a very high pressure (in a small volume). This high pressure is then relieved by increasing the volume (pushing the piston *up*), which provides power to the wheels of the car.

Medical respirators

Boyle's Law is the principle behind the devices used in hospitals to aid patients' breathing. One such device is called an *iron lung* (Figure 10–10). A slight increase of respirator volume causes a lower-than-normal pressure on the patient's body. The air in the lungs (at 1 atm pressure) pushes out against this lower pressure, expanding the lungs and causing air to flow in. A higher pressure inside the respirator then compresses the lungs, forcing its gases out. The pressure usually alternates between 760 torr and 751 torr. A similar, smaller device that fits just over the chest of the patient can permit some movement.

The Heimlich maneuver

Another important application of Boyle's Law can help remove food stuck in the trachea (windpipe) of a choking person. The traditional "backslap" advocated in some first-aid manuals has often been ineffective and has sometimes worsened the situation. The Heimlich maneuver, which works on the principle of Boyle's Law, consists of a kind of "bear hug," using vigorous upward pushes on the abdomen. The result is an increased pressure inside the lungs, which generally expels the obstruction in the same way a cork pops out of a champagne bottle (Figure 10–11).

Posting of signs in restaurants showing how to use this technique is required by law in some cities, such as New York and Cincinnati. Recent evidence shows that the maneuver is also useful in removing water from the lungs of drowning victims, before starting mouth-to-mouth resuscitation.

The syringe

Boyle's Law also permits medical personnel to give injections using a syringe. When the plunger is drawn back, the increase in volume inside the syringe creates a low pressure (vacuum) that draws the liquid from a vial into the chamber.

When you suck up a liquid through a straw, you do essentially the same thing, using your lungs as the chamber that increases in volume. Similarly, a water pump

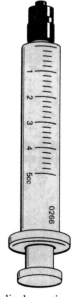

A medical syringe uses Boyle's Law.

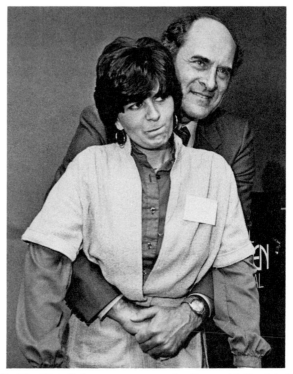

FIGURE 10–11 The Heimlich maneuver—saving lives with Boyle's Law. Choking on food can cause death or irreversible brain damage in four minutes. The procedure demonstrated in this photograph by Dr. Henry Heimlich has already saved many lives. (Montreal *Gazette* photo by Richard Arless, Jr.)

works by increasing a volume (creating a vacuum), causing the water under normal atmospheric pressure in the well to flow into the pipe.

EXAMPLE 10n: Suppose a syringe plunger is pushed all the way in, so that (counting the needle) the syringe contains 0.10 mL of air at 1.00 atm. The plunger is now pulled back quickly so that the total volume changes to 3.00 mL. Calculate the momentary pressure before any liquid comes into the syringe.

SOLUTION: The initial pressure is 1.00 atm. There are two possible conversion factors: $\dfrac{0.10 \text{ mL}}{3.00 \text{ mL}}$ and $\dfrac{3.00 \text{ mL}}{0.10 \text{ mL}}$. Which do we choose? Since we are increasing the volume, we expect the gas pressure to *decrease*. That also makes sense if we want to draw liquid into the syringe. Thus we want the conversion factor that is less than one:

$$1.00 \text{ atm} \times \frac{0.10 \text{ mL}}{3.00 \text{ mL}} = \boxed{0.033 \text{ atm}}$$

Or, we may use algebra:

$$P_1V_1 = P_2V_2 \qquad (1.00 \text{ atm})(0.10 \text{ mL}) = P_2 (3.00 \text{ mL})$$

$$P_2 = \boxed{0.033 \text{ atm}}$$

EXAMPLE 10o: A small child carrying an inflated balloon with a volume of 2.00 liters gets on an airplane in New York at P = 760 torr. What will be the volume of the balloon on arrival in Mexico City, which is 7347 feet above sea level and thus has an average atmospheric pressure of 600 torr?

- -

SOLUTION: Of two possible conversion factors, $\dfrac{760 \text{ torr}}{600 \text{ torr}}$ and $\dfrac{600 \text{ torr}}{760 \text{ torr}}$, which do we use? The pressure is going down, so the volume must go *up*. We need the conversion factor greater than one:

$$2.00 \text{ liters} \times \frac{760 \text{ torr}}{600 \text{ torr}} = \boxed{2.53 \text{ liters}}$$

Or, using algebra:

$$P_1V_1 = P_2V_2 \qquad (760 \text{ torr})(2.00 \text{ liters}) = V_2 (600 \text{ torr})$$

$$V_2 = \boxed{2.53 \text{ liters}}$$

The Ideal Gas Law

We have developed four relationships between the most important measurable properties of an ideal gas:

Charles' Law: $V \propto T$ at constant n,P
Gay-Lussac's Law: $P \propto T$ at constant n,V
Unnamed law: $P \propto n$ at constant V,T
Boyle's Law: $P \propto \dfrac{1}{V}$ at constant n,T

These laws can be combined into one grand equation called the *equation of state* for an ideal gas:

$$PV = nRT$$

The *R* is a *gas constant* that relates the units of pressure and volume to the units of moles and temperature. If, as is quite common, P is in atmospheres and V is in liters, then R = 0.0821 $\dfrac{\text{L-atm}}{\text{mole-K}}$. If P is in torr (mm Hg) and V is again in liters, the value of R is 62.4 $\dfrac{\text{L-torr}}{\text{mole-K}}$.

The product of pressure and volume has the units of work or energy.

The ideal gas equation of state can be used to solve almost any gas problem.

EXAMPLE 10p: A steam autoclave is used to sterilize hospital instruments. Suppose an autoclave with a volume of 15.0 liters contains pure steam (H_2O) at a temperature of 121°C and a pressure of 1550 torr. How many grams of water does it contain?

- -

SOLUTION: First convert the Celsius temperature to Kelvin: 121°C + 273 = 394 K. Now we can substitute in the ideal gas equation

$$PV = nRT$$

$$(1550 \text{ torr})(15.0 \text{ L}) = n \left(62.4 \frac{\text{L-torr}}{\text{mole-K}}\right)(394 \text{ K})$$

$$n = \frac{(1550)(15.0)}{(62.4)(394)} \text{ moles } H_2O = 0.946 \text{ mole } H_2O$$

For water, one mole has a mass of 18.0 grams:

$$0.946 \text{ mole } H_2O \times \frac{18.0 \text{ g } H_2O}{1 \text{ mole } H_2O} = \boxed{17.0 \text{ grams } H_2O}$$

Remember to use the value of R that corresponds to the units in the problem.

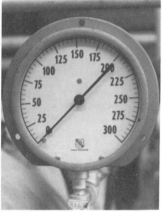

The pressure gauge on a compressed gas cylinder reads the *extra* gas pressure above atmospheric pressure. An empty cylinder will have zero gauge reading and will have the same pressure inside and outside. Many such gauges are calibrated in the United States in psi.

EXAMPLE 10q: A hospital uses an oxygen gas cylinder containing 3.50 kg of O_2 gas in a volume of 20.0 liters and at a temperature of 24°C. What is the pressure in atm in the cylinder? What pressure would the gauge at the top of the cylinder read?

SOLUTION: Convert to Kelvin: 24°C + 273 = 297 K. Convert the amount of oxygen to moles:

$$3.50 \text{ kg } O_2 \times \frac{1000 \text{ g } O_2}{1 \text{ kg } O_2} \times \frac{1 \text{ mole } O_2}{32.0 \text{ g } O_2} = 109 \text{ moles } O_2$$

Now you are ready to substitute into the ideal gas equation. Since we are asked for pressure in atmospheres, we use the corresponding value of R:

$$PV = nRT$$

$$P (20.0 \text{ L}) = (109 \text{ moles})(0.0821 \frac{\text{L-atm}}{\text{mole-K}})(297 \text{ K})$$

$$P = \frac{(109)(0.0821)(297)}{(20.0)} \text{ atm} = \boxed{133 \text{ atm}}$$

The gauge at the top of the cylinder reads the *difference* between atmospheric pressure and the pressure inside the cylinder, so if the tank is empty (gauge reads zero), the inside pressure will be equal to that outside, 1 atm. The gauge thus reads 133 atm (inside) − 1 atm (outside) = $\boxed{132 \text{ atm}}$

SELF-CHECK

10.12)   The inside of ordinary incandescent light bulbs is filled with an inert gas such as argon, since if the bulbs contained air, the wire filament would burn up. The argon may be at a reduced pressure of 2.00 torr. What is this in atmospheres?

10.13)   During a storm, the air pressure goes down because water vapor (mass, 18 g/mole) mixes with the air (mass, 29 g/mole) and lowers its density somewhat. If the mercury in a barometer had a height of 736 mm, what would be the air pressure in atm?

10.14)   A nurse inflates the rubber cuff of an apparatus for measuring blood pressure (a sphygmomanometer) until the patient's pulse can no longer be felt. That takes a pressure of 0.151 atm. What is the equivalent reading in mm Hg?

10.15)   A steel tank contains N_2O anesthetic gas at a pressure of 16.0 atm. The temperature is 20°C. The safety valve on the tank will pop open at a pressure of 25.0 atm. To what temperature would we need to heat the gas in the tank to create enough pressure to open the valve? (Gay-Lussac's Law.)

10.16)   The partial pressure of the oxygen you exhale averages about 115 torr. What must be the total of the partial pressures of all other gases (CO_2, N_2, H_2O) expelled from the lungs? (Dalton's Law of Partial Pressures.)

10.17)   A diver working deep underwater is under very great external pressure. If the diver emits a gas bubble with a volume of 2.50 mL at a pressure of 5.00 atm, what is the volume of the gas bubble when it reaches the water surface, where the pressure is 1.00 atm? This diver is about 120 feet below the surface. (Boyle's Law.)

10.18)   A weather balloon has a volume of 1000 m³ at sea level (P = 1.00 atm) at a temperature of 0°C. It rises into an atmospheric layer where the temperature is again 0°C, but the balloon volume is now 3500 m³. What is the atmospheric pressure at this level? (Boyle's Law.)

10.19*)   One of the standard ways to find the mass of one mole of an unknown liquid is to put a small amount into a flask and vaporize it (Figure 10–12) until it fills the flask with its gas vapor and no liquid is left. In one such experiment, 1.67 grams of an unknown organic gas fills a 0.250-liter flask at a temperature of 125°C and a pressure of 749 torr. What is the mass of one mole of that gas, using the ideal gas equation?

10.20*)   In designing a lunar landing vehicle for astronauts, we wish to be able to check that the cabin air pressure is maintained properly so any leak will be noticed. Should we include a mercury barometer on the vehicle for this purpose? Explain.

10.21*)   Would it make any difference in the use of a tire on a bicycle if the tire were blown up with freon gas instead of air? Ignore any possible chemical reactions.

10.22*)   Explain, using the kinetic molecular theory, why you have to push hard on a bicycle pump in order to add air to a tire.

10.23*)   Compressing a gas, such as in a bicycle pump, raises the temperature of the gas in the pump, so it becomes hot to the touch. Can you give some reasons for this?

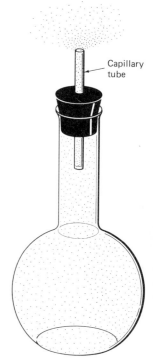

Capillary tube

FIGURE 10–12 The vapor density method for finding the mass of one mole of gas. Molecules escape through the capillary tube until the pressure of the unknown gas inside the flask equals the air pressure outside the flask, and all liquid is *just* evaporated to vapor. The flask is then cooled and weighed, and its volume is determined as in Self-Check 10.19.

10.4 GAS REACTIONS

LEARNING GOAL 10K: *Apply Avogadro's Principle, which relates gas volume to number of molecules.*
        10L: *Use the molar volume of an ideal gas, especially at STP, to relate number of moles to number of liters.*

Avogadro's Principle

    We stressed earlier that different kinds of ideal gas molecules function identically with respect to the ideal gas laws. That led us to Dalton's Law of

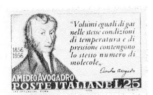

Amedeo Avogadro, Count of Quaregna (1776–1856), made the famous statement "Equal volumes of gas at fixed temperature and pressure contain equal numbers of molecules." We honor him by naming the important number "6.02 × 10²³ molecules in a mole" (Section 5.3) "Avogadro's number."

Partial Pressures. Another statement of this fact, **Avogadro's Principle,** was largely developed by Amedeo Avogadro:

Equal volumes of ideal gases (measured at the same temperature and pressure) contain the same numbers of molecules.

This principle is illustrated in Figure 10–13, which shows that eight molecules of each of three different gases will occupy the same volume at a given temperature and pressure. What is true for eight molecules will also be true for 6.02×10^{23} molecules. Avogadro's Principle holds true for moles as well as for molecules.

We may also derive Avogadro's Principle if we know the ideal gas equation. At fixed temperature and pressure, the ratio n/V (moles/liters) will be the same for every different kind of gas, since we can derive from $PV = nRT$ the equivalent equation $\dfrac{n}{V} = \dfrac{P}{RT}$ = constant at fixed P, T. If we know n, the number of moles, we therefore know V.

Avogadro's Principle gives us a convenient "handle" on the amounts of gas involved in chemical reactions.

EXAMPLE 10r: The reaction $N_{2(g)} + 3\,H_{2(g)} \rightarrow 2\,NH_{3(g)}$ is of great importance since it is used to "fix" nitrogen from the air to make ammonia fertilizer. Interpret this equation in terms of liters of pure gas at a known temperature and pressure.

– –

SOLUTION: The equation indicates that one molecule of N_2 gas reacts with three molecules of H_2 gas to give two molecules of NH_3 (ammonia); it also indicates that one mole of N_2 reacts with three moles of H_2 to give two moles of NH_3. From Avogadro's Principle, we can extend this to say that **one liter of nitrogen gas reacts with three liters of hydrogen gas to give two liters of ammonia gas, if all three substances are measured at the same temperature and pressure.**

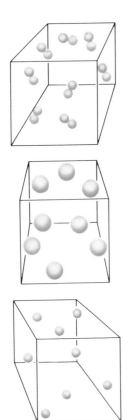

Same volume, temperature, and pressure

FIGURE 10–13 Avogadro's Principle: Equal volumes of gases, measured at the same temperature and pressure, contain the same number of molecules.

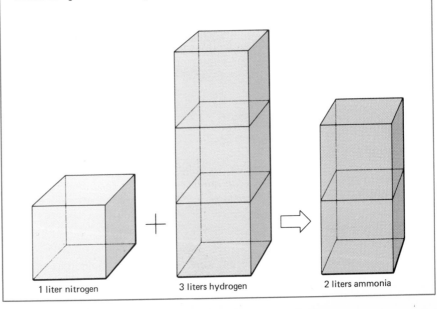

1 liter nitrogen   3 liters hydrogen   2 liters ammonia

Molar volume

It is sometimes very convenient to have a factor that relates moles of an ideal gas to volume. In a different situation, we may wish to relate grams of a pure substance to liters. There is a convenient conversion factor that has the units $\frac{\text{liters}}{\text{moles}}$ and is called the **molar volume,** or volume of one mole.

At a pressure of *1.00 atm,*

The volume in liters for one mole of an ideal gas = (0.0821)(T)

where T is (as usual) in Kelvins. At room temperature (25°C) and 1.00 atm, one mole of ideal gas occupies (0.0821)(298 K) = 24.5 liters. At human body temperature (37°C), one mole occupies (0.0821)(310 K) = 25.4 liters. At the boiling point of water (100°C), the same one mole will occupy (0.0821) (373 K) = 30.6 liters.

We can use this information to solve problems at 1.00 atm pressure.

EXAMPLE 10s: We wish to fill a 5.00-liter box with steam at 100°C in such a way that its pressure will be 1.00 atm. No other gas will be in the box. How many grams of liquid water must we evaporate?

- -

SOLUTION: The condition is met that P = 1.00 atm, and we know the temperature to be 100°C. From the previous paragraph, then, the volume of one mole is 30.6 liters under these conditions:

$$5.00 \text{ liters} \times \frac{1 \text{ mole H}_2\text{O at } 1.00 \text{ atm}, 100°\text{C}}{30.6 \text{ liters}} = 0.163 \text{ mole H}_2\text{O}$$

$$0.163 \text{ mole H}_2\text{O} \times \frac{18.0 \text{ g H}_2\text{O}}{1 \text{ mole H}_2\text{O}} = \boxed{2.93 \text{ grams H}_2\text{O}}$$

Molar volume at STP

To make calculations even simpler, chemists have defined a **standard temperature and pressure** (STP) to which gas measurements can be referred. The standard pressure is 1.00 atm. The standard temperature is the freezing point of water, 0.00°C = 273.15 K. Under these conditions, one mole of ideal gas occupies (0.0821)(273) = 22.4 L. Remember that this STP value is only good for an ideal gas. It cannot be used for liquids or solids. Figure 10–14 shows a cube of solid CO_2 (dry ice) for comparison. It occupies not 22.4 liters but 0.0282 liters.

If you ever need to convert to or from STP, you can use the proportionality factor method that we applied to Charles' Law and Boyle's Law.

Standard temperature and pressure is 0°C and 1.00 atm.

EXAMPLE 10t: We wish to prepare 3.50 kg of ammonia by the Haber process described in Example 10r: $N_2 + 3 H_2 \rightarrow 2 NH_3$. Commercially, this is carried out at 500°C and at a pressure of 350 atm. How many liters of ammonia will we obtain?

- -

28.2 ml
6.02×10^{23}
molecules
44.0 g

22.4 liters (STP)
6.02×10^{23} molecules
44.0 g

22.4 liters (STP)
6.02×10^{23} molecules
2.02 g

22.4 liters (STP)
6.02×10^{23} molecules
222 g

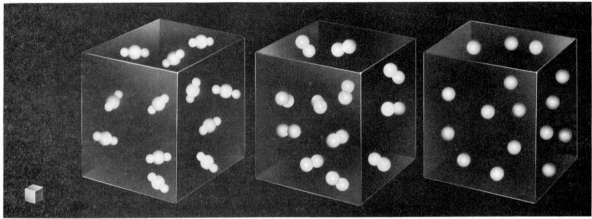

1 mole of
solid CO_2

1 mole CO_2
A triatomic* gas
Triatomic molecules

1 mole H_2
A diatomic* gas
Diatomic molecules

1 mole Rn**
A monatomic* gas
Monatomic molecules

*From *tri, di,* and *monos,* the Greek words for
three, two, and one.

**Rn, radon, a radioactive gas, consists of
individual atoms.

FIGURE 10–14 The molar
volume at standard temperature (0°C) and pressure (1
atm) is 22.4 liters for all ideal
gases. The molar volumes of
solids and liquids are much
smaller; one mole of solid
CO_2 occupies 28 *milli*liters.

SOLUTION: There are many ways to approach this problem, several
using molar volume. First of all, we must convert the amount of ammonia
to moles:

$$3.50 \text{ kg } NH_3 \times \frac{1000 \text{ g } NH_3}{\text{kg } NH_3} \times \frac{1 \text{ mole } NH_3}{17.0 \text{ g } NH_3} = 206 \text{ moles } NH_3$$

At STP, what would be the volume of 206 moles of ideal gas?

$$206 \text{ moles } NH_3 \times \frac{22.4 \text{ L } NH_3 \text{ at STP}}{1 \text{ mole } NH_3} = 4.61 \times 10^3 \text{ liters } NH_3 \text{ at STP}$$

Now convert to the higher temperature. Volume is directly proportional
to temperature, so the conversion factor is $\frac{500°C + 273}{0°C + 273} = \frac{773 \text{ K}}{273 \text{ K}}$:

$$4.61 \times 10^3 \text{ liters } NH_3 \text{ at STP} \times \frac{773 \text{ K}}{273 \text{ K}} = 1.31 \times 10^4 \text{ liters at 500°C, 1 atm}$$

Now correct for the pressure. As pressure goes up, volume goes down. The
correct conversion factor is $\frac{1 \text{ atm}}{350 \text{ atm}}$:

$$1.31 \times 10^4 \text{ liters at } \begin{smallmatrix}500°C\\1 \text{ atm}\end{smallmatrix} \times \frac{1 \text{ atm}}{350 \text{ atm}} = \boxed{37.3 \text{ liters } NH_3} \text{ at 500°C, 350 atm}$$

Calculations using gas equations

We can now apply all of the skills learned in Section 5.4, but now also add the ability to use liters of gas.

EXAMPLE 10u: How many liters of hydrogen gas will be used up to make the 37.3 liters of ammonia in Example 10t?

SOLUTION: Assuming that both gases are at the same temperature (500°C) and the same pressure (350 atm), we can apply Avogadro's Principle to note that

$$N_{2(g)} + 3\ H_{2(g)} \longrightarrow 2\ NH_{3(g)}$$

1 mole + 3 moles $\longrightarrow$ 2 moles

1 liter + 3 liters $\longrightarrow$ 2 liters

$$37.3 \text{ liters NH}_3 \times \frac{3 \text{ liters H}_2}{2 \text{ liters NH}_3} = \boxed{56.0 \text{ liters H}_2}$$

Always make conversions to and from *moles*.

SELF-CHECK

10.24) A 0.100-liter container holds 3.1×10^{21} molecules of O_2 gas at a fixed temperature and pressure.
a) At the same temperature and pressure, how many molecules of SO_2 (twice as massive as O_2) and how many gaseous atoms of He (one eighth as massive as O_2) would be contained in the same flask?
b*) If the pressure is 1.00 atm, find the temperature.
10.25) How many liters of gas at STP will be produced by
a) 0.335 moles of Cl_2?
b) 100 grams of CO_2?
c) 10.0 grams of liquid water? (Careful!)
d*) mixing 4.00 liters of N_2 gas and 2.00 liters of H_2 gas at STP, assuming complete reaction, to give ammonia?

10.5 THE BREATH OF LIFE

LEARNING GOAL 10M: Describe the chemical composition of air, giving approximate partial pressures at sea level for O_2 and N_2.
        10N: Name three major air pollutants, and indicate one source of each.
        10O: Describe the process by which O_2 from the atmosphere enters the blood stream.

We have already discussed the important role of the lungs in connection with Boyle's Law (Section 10.3). With every breath, an average adult takes in at least 500 mL of dry air, containing about 10^{22} molecules. The composition of such air is shown in Table 10–2.

TABLE 10–2 COMPOSITION OF CLEAN, DRY AIR NEAR SEA LEVEL

in parts per million (μg per gram of air)

Nitrogen (N_2)	780 900
Oxygen (O_2)	209 400
Argon (Ar)	9 300
Carbon dioxide (CO_2)	318
Neon (Ne)	18
Helium (He)	5.2
Methane (CH_4)	1.5
Krypton (Kr)	1.0
Hydrogen (H_2)	0.5
Dinitrogen oxide (N_2O)	0.25
Carbon monoxide (CO)	0.10
Xenon (Xe)	0.08
Ozone (O_3)	0.02
Ammonia (NH_3)	0.01

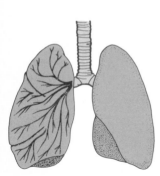

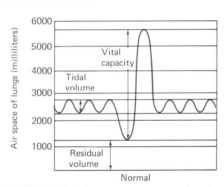

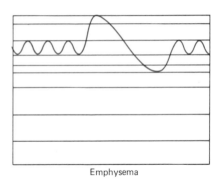

FIGURE 10–15 Changes in lung air volume during breathing. It is never possible to empty the lungs completely; about 1.2 liters of air remain behind as the *residual volume*. Normal lung capacity is shown on the left, that of a patient with emphysema on the right.

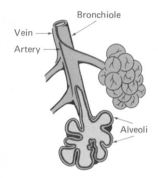

The lungs

Inhaled air enters the lungs, where it encounters a gigantic area of tissue that allows the exchange of gas in the lungs with gas in the blood. If the lung is damaged, the alveoli walls may be destroyed (causing emphysema) or scar tissue may form in the bronchioles (causing chronic bronchitis).

Figure 10–15 shows in graphic form the changes in lung air content during breathing. The *tidal volume* (about 500 mL) is what an average man takes in and breathes out while at rest. His *vital capacity* (maximum ability of the lungs to take in or exhale gases) is much greater—about five liters. The corresponding values for an average adult woman are somewhat lower.

In the **alveoli,** inhaled oxygen normally comes into contact with an area of tissue as large as a tennis court. Here, about 25% of the inhaled oxygen molecules are absorbed into red blood cells and carried to the rest of the body. As mentioned in Self-Check 5.7d of Section 5.2, the overall process by

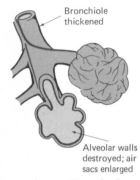

Human lungs. Top: the lung on the left is shown in cross-section so the branching bronchial tubes may be seen. Middle: enlarged view of section of normal lung. Bottom: view of lung with chronic bronchitis and emphysema.

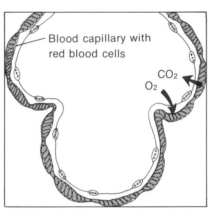

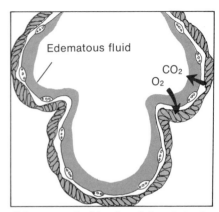

FIGURE 10–16 Gas exchange in the alveoli between the blood and the air in the lungs. Left: a normal lung has only a thin layer of cells separating the air from the red blood cells. Right: accumulation of fluid (*edema*) partially blocks exchange. Substances passing from areas of high concentration to low concentration are *diffusing*.

which the body gains energy is similar to the combustion of sugar, which of course requires oxygen. At the same time, CO_2 gas is coming out of the blood and going into the lungs (as mentioned in Example 5j, p. 133). This exchange process is shown in Figure 10–16. Normal breathing results in about 12 breaths (approximately 6 liters) per minute at rest. The maximum breathing capacity of a young male adult is 125 to 170 L/min. We have considerable ability to increase the amount of air exchanged.

A gas passes across cell *membranes* (Chapter 18) from a region of higher partial pressure to one of lower partial pressure. Oxygen diffuses from the alveoli ($P_{O_2} \approx 105$ torr) to the red blood cells ($P_{O_2} \approx 40$ torr); eventually it passes from red blood cells ($P_{O_2} \approx 105$ torr) to tissue cells ($P_{O_2} < 40$ torr). In one minute, roughly 200 mL of O_2 go from the lungs into the blood stream, and similarly from the blood stream into the cells. An equal and opposite process normally brings CO_2 from the cells into the lungs to be exhaled. This process will be discussed in more detail in Chapter 24 on body fluids.

Effect of high altitude

As seen in Example 10m, the total air pressure decreases with altitude and the oxygen partial pressure, 21% of the total pressure, decreases correspondingly. The oxygen masks demonstrated at the beginning of each airplane flight are provided in case the cabin loses its extra pressure and takes the same total pressure as the air outside. Since most jet planes fly somewhat higher than Mount Everest on long trips, the oxygen partial pressure available outside the plane would be less than one third that at sea level.

Effects vary, but individuals who climb rapidly to heights above 10 000 feet usually suffer some degree of "mountain sickness," including a lowered ability to see and think clearly. If one remains at high altitude, the body gradually adjusts by increasing the breathing rate (*hyperventilation*) and by other means. Some villagers in the Andes Mountains work permanently at an elevation of 18 000 feet and function quite normally. However, pregnant women from these villages come to lower altitudes in order to protect the fetus.

Air pollution and health

Damage to the lungs may be caused by various factors, including recurrent infections, severe asthma, smoking, and air pollution (Figure 10–17).

Certain air pollutants have a direct effect on the ability of the body to transport oxygen. Lead poisoning, for example, interferes with the body's ability to manufacture *hemoglobin* (which carries oxygen in the red blood cells), producing severe chronic anemia.

Carbon monoxide replaces oxygen on hemoglobin molecules and thus reduces the efficiency with which the blood transfers oxygen to the cells. The first effects of CO poisoning are headache and nausea. Breathing an atmosphere containing 0.1% carbon monoxide for four hours can cause death, as can shorter exposure time at a higher concentration (Figure 10–18). Smokers suffer chronically from the effects of carbon monoxide poisoning, as do many workers in automobile garages. The effects happen without warning because CO is a colorless, odorless gas.

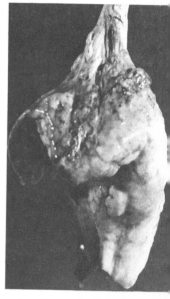

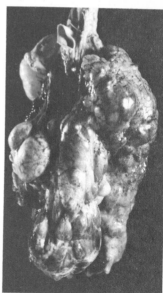

FIGURE 10–17 Photographs of actual human lungs. Top: a normal lung. Bottom: a lung with emphysema, such as is commonly caused by cigarette smoking, is enlarged and misshapen. (Photo by Glen Cuerden, Cuerden Advertising Design.)

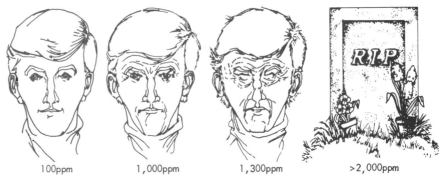

FIGURE 10–18 The effects of carbon monoxide on health. A healthy adult can tolerate 100 ppm of CO in air (about 0.0001 gram of CO in a liter of air) without any ill effects. A one-hour exposure to 1000 ppm causes a mild headache. One hour at 1300 ppm turns the skin cherry red, and causes a throbbing headache to develop. One hour at greater than 2000 ppm probably would be fatal. (From Meyer, E., *Chemistry of Hazardous Materials,* Prentice-Hall, 1977.)

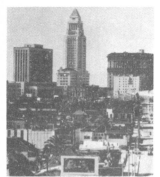

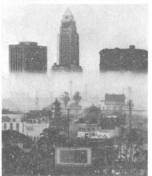

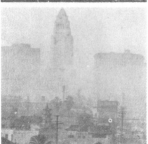

FIGURE 10–19 Three views of the same part of downtown Los Angeles, California. Top: on a clear day. Middle: pollution trapped beneath an inversion layer at a height of 75 meters. Bottom: pollution under an inversion layer at 450 meters. (Photos from Los Angeles Air Pollution Control District.)

Some other toxic gases often found in the smog of cities as a result of industrial pollution are the oxides of sulfur and nitrogen, and ozone (O_3). Figure 10–19 shows the smog of Los Angeles; the content of that smog is described in Table 10–3. Some of the pollutants are made from air and smokestack fumes, as well as from the hydrocarbons of automobile exhausts, by the action of sunlight. Nitrogen and sulfur oxides form very strong acids when they dissolve in the water of lung membranes:

$$SO_{3(g)} + H_2O \longrightarrow H_2SO_{4(aq)} \quad \text{(sulfuric acid)}$$

$$4\,NO_{2(g)} + 2\,H_2O + O_2 \longrightarrow 4\,HNO_{3(aq)} \quad \text{(nitric acid)}$$

These gases thus cause damage to the bronchial tubes and alveoli.

The *suspended particles* in air pollution (soot, dust, and smoke) present a different sort of problem. They collect on the walls of the bronchial tubes and interfere with the ability of the lungs to get rid of irritants. The lungs of city dwellers, and particularly of smokers, thus accumulate many different kinds of small particles, some of which simply interfere with gas exchange.

TABLE 10–3 APPROXIMATE CONCENTRATIONS OF POLLUTANTS IN LOS ANGELES ON A CLEAR DAY (VISIBILITY 7 MILES) AND ON A SMOGGY DAY (VISIBILITY 1 MILE)

	Concentration (ppm)		
Pollutant	*Clear Day*	*Smoggy Day*	*Increase*
Carbon monoxide	3.5	23.0	×6.5
Hydrocarbons	0.2	1.1	×5.5
Peroxides	0.1	0.5	×5.0
Oxides of nitrogen	0.08	0.4	×5.0
Lower aldehydes	0.07	0.4	×6.0
Ozone	0.06	0.3	×5.0
Sulfur dioxide	0.05	0.3	×6.0

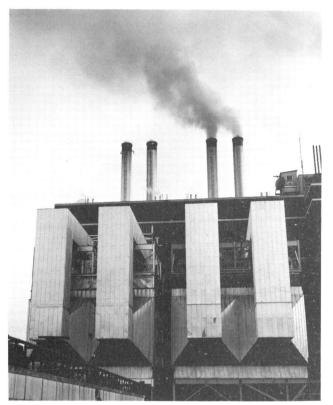

An electrostatic precipitator greatly reduces the soot and ash released into the air by smokestacks. The two chimneys to the left are equipped with pollution-control devices, while the two to the right are not.

Other particles have the ability to cause cancer, particularly asbestos fibers (and some other industrial fibers) and some hydrocarbons.

Cigarette smoke contains a particularly dangerous hydrocarbon, 1,2-benzopyrene (BaP), which is probably responsible for many cases of lung cancer. Marihuana cigarettes contain greater amounts of this pollutant than tobacco and are even more likely than regular cigarettes to have their smoke inhaled deeply. In addition, large amounts of this hydrocarbon are released into the air from burning coal, oil, and gas, garbage incinerators, industrial emissions, and automobiles. British research has shown ten times greater amounts of BaP in city air than in rural air, which parallels a lung cancer rate which is nine times greater in cities than in the countryside. Coal smoke presents a particular problem in this respect.

However, we must not assume that all air pollution is the result of human technology. Nitrogen oxides (0.5 ppm N_2O and 0.02 ppm NO_2) are produced in air by the sun's rays and by lightning, as is ozone (0.02 ppm). Carbon monoxide and soot particles are generated by forest fires. The 1980 eruption of Mount St. Helens demonstrated that nature can put as much energy into an explosion and provide as much particle pollution as can human beings. The total of particles entering the atmosphere each year from all sources amounts to about 10^{18} grams, of which only about 10^{15} grams, or about 0.1%, come from human efforts.

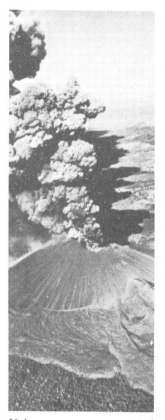

Volcanos are natural sources of air pollution, as many residents of Oregon and Washington can testify. The Cerro Negro Volcano in Nicaragua (shown in this photo) blanketed the countryside with ash for 45 days in 1968. (Reprinted with permission of *Science & Public Affairs,* the Bulletin of the Atomic Scientists.)

The amount of dissolved O_2 or CO_2 in a given volume of body fluid is usually expressed in terms of the partial pressure of gas right above the solution that would result in such a concentration. This measure is often called the *tension* of O_2 or CO_2 in the body fluid involved, and is generally expressed in torr (or mm Hg).

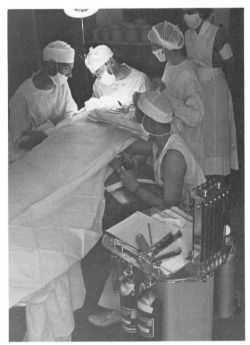

An anesthesia unit containing dinitrogen oxide, N_2O, is shown in an operating room. (Courtesy of S. C. Cullen, University of Iowa Hospitals.)

Inhalation therapy

Medical facilities are often called upon to treat cases of lung damage or poisoning. In these cases, the ability of the patient to transport oxygen to the cells must be increased. An *inhalation therapist* is specially trained to administer gases and operate respirators in emergency situations, as well as to assist with the administration of gaseous anesthetics and to handle gases involved in other kinds of treatment.

If a patient is having difficulty breathing, the rate and volume of oxygen being passed through the lungs may be increased by use of a respirator (Figure 10–10). It may help to give the patient a higher partial pressure of O_2 to breathe than the 159 torr (0.21 atm) contained in air at normal pressures. The extra oxygen may be provided by a nasal tube, mask, face tent, or—in the case of a newborn infant—an incubator.

The word hyperbaric comes from *hyper* (over) plus *baric*, as in *bar*ometer, meaning pressure. A system under partial vacuum would be *hypo*baric. Wherever the partial pressure of oxygen is high, precautions must be taken to prevent all sparks or fire, since objects burn very quickly in an excess of oxygen gas.

The patient may be placed in a *hyperbaric* chamber that supplies normal air at a pressure higher than 1.00 atm. The effect is to increase the partial pressure of oxygen. Such chambers are also useful in the treatment of gangrene (caused by bacteria that are very sensitive to oxygen), as well as in the treatment of underwater divers who have returned to the surface too fast. A special kind of cancer therapy uses such a chamber because cancer cells are more likely to be destroyed by x-rays if under high oxygen partial pressure, while the vulnerability of normal cells does not change.

Part of inhalation therapy is the maintenance of proper humidity in the lungs. We breathe out a lot of water vapor, since the air in the alveoli is surrounded by water-covered membranes. When the air you breathe is too dry, your throat feels parched and you're thirsty. Gases administered by an inhalation therapist are generally accompanied by water vapor for this reason. Home humidifying units are often recommended in situations where the amount of water vapor in the air (the "relative humidity") is low. Many people also find a "cool mist" vaporizer of help in relieving a cough, since the lungs and throat work best if they are kept humid.

Special atmospheres for divers and astronauts

People often adventure in places where there is not a good air supply and so the air must be piped in or carried along on the trip. Himalayan mountain climbers need oxygen (Example 10n) to supplement their air. Astronauts must take along their entire supply. Too high an oxygen partial pressure is dangerous to breathe, so other gases must be mixed with the oxygen.

Deep-sea divers have a different kind of hazard. The pressure of liquid water depends on depth, so that the total pressure on the outside of a diver's body increases by one atmosphere for every 30 feet below the surface of the water. A diver at a depth of 90 feet thus has an external pressure of four atmospheres to contend with. If air is pumped from above, it must be at four atmospheres to keep the rubber hoses open. Scuba divers have the same problem. This extra air pressure causes nitrogen gas to dissolve in the blood. If a diver comes up to the surface too quickly, the nitrogen gas will form bubbles in the blood, which can lead to death.

One solution to this problem is to use an artificial atmosphere that contains the normal 159 torr of oxygen partial pressure, but uses other gases (such as helium) to replace nitrogen. In this way, both deep-sea divers and astronauts may function at their best, with a normal partial pressure of oxygen available to the lungs.

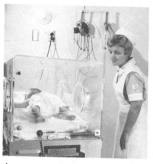

An oxygen tent connected to the oxygen supply of the hospital helps an infant breathe.

SELF-CHECK

10.26)   No matter what the total pressure of artificial atmospheres fed to astronauts or divers, the partial pressure of oxygen should come close to that of normal air. What is the O_2 partial pressure *in atmospheres* in normal air at sea level?

10.27)   Besides oxygen, what are the two substances present in the greatest quantities in normal air? How does the body react to these two substances? (Hint: both are elements.)

10.28)   Name three major air pollutant substances, and indicate one source of each.

10.29*)   Name three air pollutant compounds that strongly affect the efficiency of the lungs, and describe the health effect of each.

10.30)   Describe in simple terms the progress of an O_2 molecule from the air outside your body into your blood stream. Does every O_2 molecule you breathe in actually enter your blood?

10.31*)   Explain in terms of the structure of the lungs why the Heimlich maneuver works.

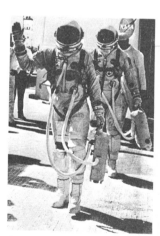

An astronaut carries along the entire air supply for a trip into space.

CHAPTER TEN IN REVIEW ■ Gases

10.1 THE NATURE OF GASES

Page 266

10A: *List the four most important measurable properties of a gas.*

10B: *Summarize the kinetic molecular theory of an ideal gas.*

10C: *Given a gas property, explain it in terms of the kinetic molecular theory.*

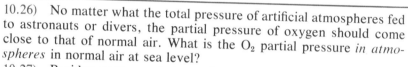

10.2 TEMPERATURE

10D: Relate temperature to energy of motion.
10E: Convert a temperature expressed in °F, °C, or K to any of the other scales.
10F: Given the initial volume and the initial and final temperatures of a fixed amount of ideal gas at constant pressure, use Charles' Law to calculate the final volume.

10.3 PRESSURE

10G: Convert a gas pressure between atmospheres and torr (mm Hg).
10H: Given the initial pressure and the initial and final temperatures of a fixed amount of ideal gas in a container of constant volume, use Gay-Lussac's Law to calculate the final pressure.
10I: Apply Dalton's Law of Partial Pressures to a gas mixture.
10J: Given the initial pressure and volume and the final pressure (or volume) of a fixed amount of ideal gas at constant temperature, use Boyle's Law to calculate the final volume (or pressure).

10.4 GAS REACTIONS

10K: Apply Avogadro's Principle, which relates gas volume to number of molecules.
10L: Use the molar volume of an ideal gas, especially at STP, to relate number of moles to number of liters.

10.5 THE BREATH OF LIFE

10M: Describe the chemical composition of air, giving approximate partial pressures at sea level for O_2 and N_2.
10N: Name three major air pollutants, and indicate one source of each.
10O: Describe the process by which O_2 from the atmosphere enters the blood stream.

GLOSSARY FOR CHAPTER TEN

absolute zero The temperature at which an ideal gas would have no energy of motion; the lowest possible temperature; 0 K; −273.15°C; a temperature scale based on absolute zero (like the Kelvin scale) is an absolute temperature scale since it cannot have a negative reading. (p. 270)

alveoli Small air sacs in the lungs through which O_2 passes from the lungs into the bloodstream and CO_2 passes from the bloodstream into the lungs. (p. 294)

atmosphere A unit of pressure, equal to exactly 760 torr; symbol *atm*; roughly the same as the average air pressure at sea level; also, the layer of air that surrounds all objects at the surface of the earth. (p. 279)

Avogadro's Principle The observation that at a constant temperature and pressure, equal volumes of two different ideal gases contain the same number of molecules (or moles). (p. 290)

barometer A device for measuring atmospheric *pressure*; read in *torr* (mm Hg) or, occasionally, in inches of mercury. (p. 280)

Boyle's Law The pressure and volume of a fixed amount of ideal gas at constant temperature are inversely proportional to each other; $P_1V_1 = P_2V_2$; when the pressure goes up, the volume goes down. (p. 285)

Celsius scale A temperature scale based on the normal freezing point of water being zero (0°C) and the normal boiling point of water being 100°C; once called "centigrade"; Celsius degree intervals are the same as Kelvin degree intervals. (p. 271)

Charles' Law The volume of a fixed amount of ideal gas at constant pressure is directly proportional to the Kelvin temperature; $V_1/T_1 = V_2/T_2$. (p. 274)

Dalton's Law of Partial Pressures The total pressure of a mixture of ideal gases is the sum of the partial pressures of the individual gases. (p. 282)

Gay-Lussac's Law The pressure of a fixed amount of ideal gas in a constant volume is proportional to the Kelvin temperature; $P_1/T_1 = P_2/T_2$. (p. 280)

ideal gas A gas for which the kinetic molecular theory is valid; a gas in which the particles do not attract each other and have negligible sizes. (p. 268)

Kelvin scale An absolute scale of temperature based on the same degree intervals as the Celsius scale; absolute zero is 0 K; 0°C = 273.15 K; the temperature scale used for all ideal gas calculations. (p. 270)

kinetic energy Energy of motion; for straight-line motion, kinetic energy equals $\frac{1}{2}mv^2$, where m is mass and v is velocity; temperature measures the average kinetic energy of a group of particles; heat flow is a transfer of kinetic energy. (p. 269)

kinetic molecular theory A set of assumptions about the behavior of gas particles that leads to the ideal gas model. (p. 267)

manometer A device for measuring gas pressure. (p. 283)

model A mental picture, usually simplified, that helps explain the behavior of something we cannot adequately measure; used in the scientific method, usually as part of a theory. (p. 267)

molar volume The volume of one mole, particularly of an ideal gas, where the molar volume in liters is equal at one atmosphere pressure to 0.0821T; at STP, the molar gas volume is 22.4 liters. (p. 291)

partial pressure The pressure that one gas in a mixture of gases would exert if it alone occupied the same container at the same temperature; the pressure of one particular gas in a mixture; used in Dalton's Law of Partial Pressures; often referred to as *gas tension* in medical applications in which a gas is dissolved in a body fluid in an amount corresponding to a particular partial pressure right above that liquid. (p. 282)

pascal A unit of pressure in SI; 1 atm = 101.325 kPa. (p. 279)

pressure The force of molecules hitting a surface, per unit area of that surface; may be measured in pascals, atmospheres, or torr (mm Hg). (p. 268)

proportionality factor method The use of the ratio of an initial to final (or final to initial) measurement as a conversion factor in a calculation involving a gas law. (p. 275)

standard temperature and pressure The conditions of exactly 1.00 atm and 0°C, at which the molar volume of an ideal gas will be 22.4 liters. (p. 291)

temperature A property that determines the direction of heat flow; a measure of the average kinetic energy of a group of particles; measured by a thermometer; normally expressed in scientific work in the Celsius scale; for ideal gas calculations, measured in the Kelvin scale. (p. 269)

thermometer A device for measuring temperature. (p. 270)

torr A unit of pressure, exactly equal to the pressure of a column of mercury (in a barometer) that is 1 mm high, thus equal to the older unit of "mm Hg"; 1/760 of a standard atmosphere. (p. 280)

volume The space available to gas molecules inside a container; the capacity of the container; usually measured in liters or mL. (p. 267).

QUESTIONS AND PROBLEMS FOR CHAPTER TEN ■ Gases

SECTION 10.1 THE NATURE OF GASES

10.32) According to the kinetic molecular theory of an ideal gas,
a) what do we assume about the size of gas particles?
b) why doesn't friction slow down the gas particles and cause them to stop moving?
c) why can gases be easily compressed to a smaller volume?

10.33) Which of the following physical properties of a gas can be measured directly?

density   molecule speed
volume   pressure

10.34*) If cigarette smoke is observed under a microscope, the solid particles can be seen bouncing around in a random fashion, moving continuously. Explain this effect, called *Brownian motion*.

SECTION 10.2 TEMPERATURE

10.35) The following are record high temperatures for U.S. cities. Convert each value to the scale indicated.
a)   115°F to °C (Phoenix, AZ)
b)   30°C to °F (Seattle, WA)
c)   311 K to °F (Washington, DC)

10.36) A hospital patient's temperature went up by 2.5 Celsius degrees. What was the increase in Fahrenheit degrees?

10.37*) British and U.S. engineers invented an absolute temperature scale based on Fahrenheit degrees. What is the boiling point of water on this *Rankine* scale?

10.63) According to the kinetic molecular theory of an ideal gas,
a) what do we assume about the speed of gas particles?
b) what causes pressure on the walls of a container of gas?
c) why do gases quickly diffuse throughout a room?

10.64) Which of the following physical properties of a gas can be measured directly?

particle size   temperature
color   mass

10.65*) Does gravity ever have an effect on gas properties? in a small room? in the earth's atmosphere?

10.66) The following are record low temperatures for U.S. cities. Convert each value to the scale indicated.
a)   2°C to °F (Los Angeles, CA)
b)   −32°F to °C (Caribou, ME)
c)   277 K to °C (Miami, FL)

10.67) A sick child had a temperature 5 Fahrenheit degrees above normal temperature. How many Celsius degrees above normal is this?

10.68*) On which of the three major scales will you find negative temperatures? Explain.

All of the following problems are at constant pressure.

10.38) A circus vendor blew up balloons at 10:00 A.M., when T = 15°C. Each balloon had a volume of 4.00 liters. The balloons started popping at 2:00 P.M., when T = 30°C on this hot summer day. Calculate the 2:00 P.M. volume of each balloon.

10.69) A weather balloon had a volume of 2000 liters on the ground, where T = 20°C. Going aloft, it hit a very cold air layer where T = −5°C, but the pressure was still one atmosphere. What was the volume of the balloon in this cold air layer?

10.39) Hot air rises and cold air falls; that is the basis of much of our weather and is also the reason warm-air heating registers are placed low in a room. Explain why warm air is less dense than cold air.

10.40*) When a rubber balloon is blown up with air, it gets smaller after a few days. When the same balloon is filled with helium, it shrinks overnight. Explain, using Graham's Law.

SECTION 10.3 PRESSURE

10.41) Figure 10–20a shows a karate chop. Explain why the board breaks in half and doesn't just fall off the table.

10.70) On a cold January day, some students in a college dormitory blew up a basketball indoors. When they took the ball outside, it seemed to have "lost its bounce" and had flat spots. Explain.

10.71*) You wish to impress a member of the opposite sex by your perfume or eau de Cologne. Would it be wisest to select a substance that has a *high* or *low* formula weight to make a quick impression? Explain, using Graham's Law.

10.72) Figure 10–20b shows that if you attach a vacuum pump to a tin can, the can will collapse. Explain.

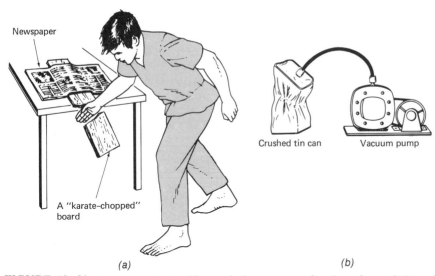

Newspaper

A "karate-chopped" board

(a)

Crushed tin can   Vacuum pump

(b)

FIGURE 10–20 Some practical effects of air pressure, for Questions 10.41 and 10.72.

10.42) Convert each of the following pressures to the units indicated. Use Table 10–1.
a) 78.9 torr to atm
b) 30 psi to torr
c) 145 mm Hg to kPa

10.43*) What is the difficulty in using a mercury barometer to measure pressures at the South Pole? (Hint: see Example 10e)

10.73) Convert each of the following pressures to the units indicated. Use Table 10–1.
a) 0.459 atm to mm Hg
b) 1500 psi to atm
c) 76.9 kPa to torr

10.74*) Explain with a diagram how a mercury barometer measures atmospheric pressure.

10.44*) Special kinds of reaction flasks can withstand a high inside vacuum without bursting. Could such flasks equally tolerate having a pressure of 1.00 atm inside and a vacuum outside?

10.45) An automobile tire contains 43 psi (total) when it is filled on a winter day at 0°C. Calculate its pressure when the temperature falls to $-25°C$ overnight? Assume constant volume.

10.46*) A small cylinder of oxygen gas has a pressure of 10.0 atm. Some of the O_2 molecules react to form ozone:

$$3\ O_{2(g)} \longrightarrow 2\ O_{3(g)}$$

Assuming constant volume and temperature, how will this reaction affect the *total* pressure in the container?

10.47) Use the kinetic molecular theory to explain Gay-Lussac's Law.

10.48) One kind of hospital anesthetic is a mixture of 20% dinitrogen oxide, N_2O, and 80% oxygen, O_2. If the total pressure is 3.00 atm, calculate the partial pressure in mm Hg of each gas.

10.49*) Explain, using Boyle's Law,
a) why a gas cylinder whose valve is broken off is propelled like a rocket across the room
b) why yawning opens up some of the alveoli that are normally closed to air, thus allowing more gas exchange with the blood
c) how we create the suction that allows us to drink through straws.

10.50) An adult woman has a lung volume of 3.0 L after exhaling. She expands her lungs to create an internal pressure of 0.90 atm. What will be the total volume of the air that then fills her lungs and brings them back to 1.00 atm?

10.75*) Suppose we know that a flask is able to withstand a vacuum inside it of 10^{-2} torr. What are its chances of withstanding the best vacuum we can get in a modern laboratory, 10^{-10} torr? Explain.

10.76) A hospital tank of oxygen gas is filled to a pressure of 150 atm (total) at 25°C. The tank may burst at a pressure higher than 408 atm. At what temperature would the inside gas reach this danger point?

10.77*) A small cylinder contains pure H_2O_2 gas at a pressure of 0.20 atm. Some of the molecules dissociate as follows:

$$2\ H_2O_{2(g)} \longrightarrow 2\ H_2O_{(g)} + O_{2(g)}$$

Assuming constant volume and temperature, how will this reaction affect the *total* pressure in the container?

10.78) Use the kinetic molecular theory to explain Dalton's Law of Partial Pressures.

10.79) A mixture of cyclopropane, C_3H_6, and O_2 gas has been used as an anesthetic for surgery. If the partial pressure of C_3H_6 is 150 torr and that of O_2 is 550 torr,
a) calculate the total pressure
b) calculate the per cent of molecules of each kind of gas

10.80*) Explain, using Boyle's Law,
a) why the air in a spaceship will be lost if there is a leak to outer space
b) how a medicine dropper works
c) how the Heimlich maneuver works

10.81) An adult man had a total lung volume of 4.6 L filled with air at 1.00 atm. He became frightened, and quickly exhaled. What was the throat pressure at the moment he began to breathe out, assuming his lungs were compressed to 3.7 L at that point?

10.51*) Why is it forbidden to carry a butane cigarette lighter aboard an airplane and into the cabin?

10.52*) If an Apollo spacecraft had a volume of 3×10^4 L at a temperature of 20°C and contained only pure oxygen at a pressure of 0.25 atm, how many grams of O_2 would be needed to fill the cabin? (Hint: use the ideal gas equation)

SECTION 10.4 GAS REACTIONS

10.53) At 1.00 atm and 25°C, a 3.00-L balloon contains 7.4×10^{22} air molecules. A second balloon contains helium at a volume of 9.00 L under the same conditions. How many He atoms does it contain?

10.82*) A mountain climber was surprised to find his bag of potato chips popped open when he reached the peak. Why did it break?

10.83*) The gases in some white dwarf stars are incredibly dense. A volume of 1.00 cm³ contains 1.0×10^5 moles of gas (H_2 and He) at a temperature of 10 000 K. What would be the ideal gas pressure in atm? Would this gas behave ideally? (Use the ideal gas equation.)

10.84) A weather balloon has a volume of 1.0×10^5 L. It contains 2.7×10^{26} H_2 molecules. How many atoms of He are contained in a helium-filled balloon that occupies 4.0×10^4 L under the same conditions?

Assume constant temperature and pressure as well as ideal gas behavior for the following problems.

10.54) Ethene burns to give carbon dioxide and water:

$$C_2H_4 + 3\ O_2 \longrightarrow 2\ CO_2 + 2\ H_2O$$

How many liters of oxygen are needed to react fully with 3.7 liters of ethene? If the reaction is complete, how many liters of CO_2 will be formed?

10.55*) Stomach acid is neutralized by sodium bicarbonate:

$$NaHCO_{3(s)} + HCl_{(aq)} \longrightarrow$$
$$NaCl_{(aq)} + CO_{2(g)} + H_2O_{(\ell)}$$

Suppose 8.00 grams of sodium hydrogen carbonate react with excess stomach acid (HCl). How many liters (maximum) of CO_2 at 37°C and 1.00 atm will be "burped"?

10.85) Methanol is made commercially by combining carbon monoxide and hydrogen:

$$CO_{(g)} + 2\ H_{2(g)} \longrightarrow CH_3OH_{(g)}$$

How many liters of hydrogen gas are required to react completely with 173 liters of carbon monoxide? If the reaction is complete, how many liters of methanol will be formed?

10.86*) An untuned automobile engine can be a major source of air pollution. The poisonous gas carbon monoxide, CO, is produced by reactions such as:

$$2\ C_8H_{18(\ell)} + 17\ O_{2(g)} \longrightarrow$$
$$16\ CO_{(g)} + 18\ H_2O_{(g)}.$$

Suppose one U.S. gallon of gasoline has a mass of 2.60 kg and consists 20% of octane that burns according to the above equation to give CO gas at 30°C and 1.00 atm. How many liters of CO will be produced? If the CO is released into a sealed garage of dimensions 8 m by 3 m by 4 m, what will be the CO level in ppm? Would this be enough to kill a person after one hour? Use Figure 10– 18.

10.56) How many liters at STP are occupied by 10.0 grams of propane, C_3H_8?

SECTION 10.5 THE BREATH OF LIFE

10.57) Which of the following gases are present in air in large amounts?

H_2 NH_3 N_2 Cl_2 O_2

10.58) Give a major source for each of the following pollutants.

a) ozone

b) sulfur dioxide

c) soot (carbon particles)

10.59*) How does breathing SO_3 gas damage the lungs?

10.60) What is the function of the bronchioles in the lungs? What is the effect of having the bronchioles constrict (tighten), as in bronchial asthma?

10.61*) Name a situation in which an emergency room patient in a hospital might be placed in a hyperbaric chamber.

10.62*) The hemoglobin of red blood cells carries oxygen to the body by reacting with O_2. One mole of hemoglobin (68 000 grams) can react with up to four moles of O_2 to form oxyhemoglobin. There are 900 grams of hemoglobin in the red blood cells of a 150-pound adult. How many liters of O_2 at STP are needed to change all of this hemoglobin to oxyhemoglobin?

10.87) How many liters at STP are occupied by 10.0 grams of cyclopropane, C_3H_6?

10.88) Describe the chemical composition of air by naming the two most important gases and their approximate partial pressures at sea level.

10.89) Give a major source for each of the following pollutants.

a) carbon monoxide

b) nitrogen dioxide

c*) lead

10.90*) How does breathing smoke (as from tobacco or marihuana) containing 1,2-benzopyrene damage the lungs?

10.91) What is the function of the alveoli in the lungs? What is the effect of having the alveoli cell walls break apart, as in emphysema?

10.92*) Name a situation in which an emergency room patient in a hospital might be given pure oxygen to breathe through a mask.

10.93*) From data given in this chapter, estimate the number of grams of oxygen that are absorbed into the body of a resting adult in a single day.

Liquids and Solids

In Chapter 10, we discussed the properties of a relatively simple type of substance, the ideal gas. Chemistry would be easier to learn if all substances behaved as ideal gases. We would then be able to use the kinetic molecular theory to explain all physical properties. On the other hand, we would not be here!

Liquids and solids, which make up most of our bodies, are not described by the kinetic molecular theory. Most real substances, in fact, have particles that attract each other quite strongly. As a result, the particles cluster together to form the liquids and solids described in this chapter. With liquids and solids, the volume of each molecule is not negligible in comparison to the space between molecules. The density of matter in a *condensed state* is generally between 0.50 and 20 g/cm³, compared with roughly 1 g/liter for gases. A liquid or solid is thus roughly 1000 times as dense as a common ideal gas. This extra density makes such a substance difficult to compress, but easier to push, pour, chew, kick, and move about.

See Table 2–4 for the densities of some common solids and liquids.

11.1 THE LIQUID STATE

LEARNING GOAL 11A: *Describe the major differences in the physical properties of a liquid and a gas.*
         11B: Describe how the viscosity, surface tension, and normal boiling point of a liquid are affected by the strength of intermolecular forces.

Intermolecular forces

No gas behaves *exactly* in the manner predicted by the ideal gas model. Nothing is truly "ideal." The gas laws of Chapter 10 are approximations that work best at low pressure and high temperature. If we lower the temperature or increase the pressure, a gas may behave differently (Table 11–1).

As the pressure of a gas increases, the actual volume occupied by the molecules themselves becomes significant. As the temperature decreases and the molecules move more slowly, attractions between them have more effect. The equations that account for the differences in the physical properties of ideal gases and real gases were first developed by the Dutch scientist

TABLE 11–1   BEHAVIOR OF ONE MOLE OF
GASEOUS METHANE AT 0°C AND
VARIOUS PRESSURES

Pressure (atm)	Volume (L)	Product P × V	Behavior	Density (g/L)
0.100	224	22.4	ideal	0.071
1.00	22.4	22.4	ideal	0.714
50.0	0.374	18.7	nonideal	42.8
100	0.169	16.9	nonideal	94.7
600	0.0420	25.2	nonideal	381

Johannes van der Waals in 1873. In honor of his work, the intermolecular attractive forces that create liquids and solids are often called **van der Waals forces.**

There are several different kinds of van der Waals forces, and we will discuss the differences in Sections 11.3 and 11.4. Right now, we will be concerned only with the relative strength of the forces.

You know that when you heat a beaker containing an ice cube (Figure 11–1), you get liquid water, and if you continue heating, you will eventually obtain *steam,* water in its gaseous form. The reverse process, called **condensation,** is also familiar. Water vapor in the air (gas) *condenses* on cold surfaces to form liquid water. The liquid can freeze, at temperatures below 0°C, to form solid ice. The three conditions in which we find matter under normal circumstances—solid, liquid, or gas—are known as *states*. Changes of state will be discussed further in Section 11.5.

> Condensation is observed when dew forms on the (cold) grass and automobile windshields in the early morning.

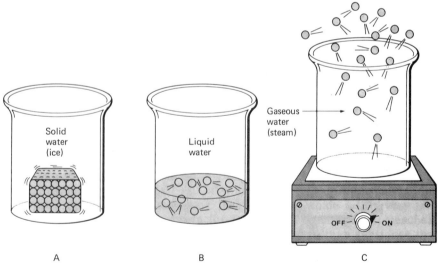

FIGURE 11–1   The three states of matter, illustrated by water. A: Solid water (ice) has a definite volume and shape. Particles vibrate in place, holding fixed positions relative to each other. B: Liquid water has a definite volume, but takes the shape of the bottom of its container to the depth necessary to hold that volume. Molecules are free to move relative to each other within that volume. C: Gaseous water (steam) has neither definite volume nor shape, but expands to fill the container if the container is closed and escape from it if the container is open. Particles move in random fashion, completely independent of each other.

Formation of a liquid

If a gas is at high temperature, most molecules are moving about at high speed. Even if there are attractions between molecules, the collisions are not "sticky" enough to result in the formation of a liquid. The high kinetic energy tends to break the molecules apart.

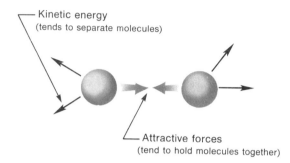

Kinetic energy
(tends to separate molecules)

Attractive forces
(tend to hold molecules together)

As the temperature goes down, the kinetic energy has less effect, and the attractive forces can sometimes keep the molecules together. Some of the gas molecules are moving more slowly than others. If two slow molecules collide, they might stick together.

The effect of gravity on a pair of molecules stuck together is greater than on a single fast-moving molecule. If even more molecules collide with the pair and stick together, a **liquid** drop is formed. Eventually, if the temperature is low enough, most of the gas molecules will stick to the growing liquid surface and become "caught" in the liquid phase. They cannot travel throughout the container. They can only roll about in the liquid, which settles to the bottom of the container.

A few molecules, moving very quickly and thus with high kinetic energy, will remain in the gas state even at low temperature. Some fast-moving liquid molecules will escape from the surface of the liquid to join the gas phase. Some of the slower gas molecules will hit the liquid and join it.

Viscosity

It is easy to transfer a liquid from one container to another. You simply pour it. You can't pour a gas, however, since it will fill the room as well as the other container!

Of course, some liquids are more difficult to pour than others. Liquid water flows very easily. It is much more difficult to pour petroleum jelly and catsup; they resist flow. Diethyl ether and acetone flow more easily than water.

Resistance to flow is called **viscosity.** Gases have extremely low viscosity. The closer a liquid is to acting like a gas (low attractions between molecules), the less viscous it is. You may think of viscosity as "stick-togetherness." Viscosity measures how freely the molecules move about within the liquid. A solid generally has extremely high viscosity.

If we compare the viscosities of two liquid substances at the same temperature, we find that

A liquid with strong intermolecular attractions is generally more viscous than a liquid with weak attractions.

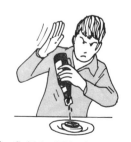

If a fluid is difficult to pour, it has a high viscosity. A fluid is any substance that will flow and therefore includes both gases and liquids.

Since increased kinetic energy tends to break the attractions between particles, a liquid tends to be *less* viscous at *higher* temperature. Warm molasses flows more easily than cold.

Surface tension

Some small insects can walk on the surface of water. Yet, they are not floating. The force holding them up is called **surface tension.** As shown in Figure 11–2, the molecules at the surface of a liquid are attracted unevenly and are pulled inward. If you have seen a drop of mercury on a table, you may have noticed that the liquid does not spread out over the table, but instead stays in a drop. Mercury has a very high surface tension. This surface tension creates a mercury **meniscus** in a barometer or thermometer (Figure 11–3).

Because of surface tension, you may obtain two distinct layers when you pour two liquids together. The liquid with the higher density goes to the bottom, and the liquid with the lower density goes to the top, as, for example, oil on water. Each of the two distinct groups of molecules is called a **phase.**

High surface tension means high resistance to breakage or stretching of the liquid surface. In general,

A liquid with high intermolecular attractions will have higher surface tension than a liquid with weak attractions.

Like viscosity, surface tension should decrease with increasing temperature. The surface tension of a pure liquid may also be decreased by certain "wetting agents," which may be dissolved in it. A detergent is one such wetting agent. When detergents are used to clean up oil spills in bodies of water, one unfortunate side effect is to reduce the surface tension in the oils that coat the feathers of water birds. The birds may then become "waterlogged" and drown.

The same effect is useful in killing bacteria, however. Antiseptics and disinfectant solutions tend to have lower surface tension than water. They

One health effect of surface tension is a leading cause of death among small or premature babies. Respiratory distress syndrome (RDS) results if the cells in the linings of the lungs have abnormally high surface tension. The air passageways do not expand as they should, and not enough air reaches the alveoli (Section 10.5).

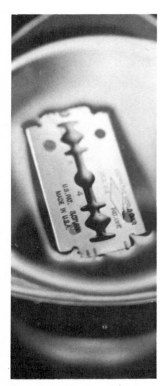

A solid object, such as a razor blade, will be held up on the surface of the water by the forces we call *surface tension.*

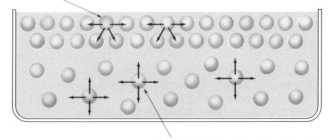

Molecules on surface are attracted only by molecules below and beside them; there are practically no molecules above.

Molecules in body of liquid are attracted equally on all sides by surrounding molecules.

FIGURE 11–2 The cause of surface tension. The molecules at the surface of a liquid are attracted unevenly and tend to be pulled inward. The strength of surface tension is directly related to the strength of intermolecular attractions.

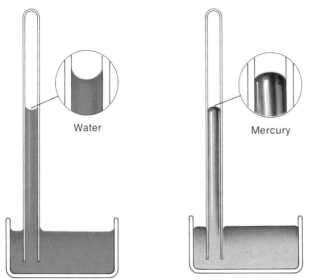

Water   Mercury

FIGURE 11–3   The combined effects of surface tension and the attraction between the liquid and the glass create a *meniscus* or curved surface for water and mercury. In reading a buret (Section 14.5), you must read the *bottom* of the water meniscus. When you read the pressure on a mercury barometer (Section 10.3), you read the *top* of the mercury column.

TABLE 11–2   SOME
SURFACE TENSION
VALUES AT 20°C

mercury	436
water	73
glycerol	63
acetone	24
ethanol	23
diethyl ether	17
normal urine	66
urine in jaundice	55

Values are in dynes/cm.

spread out over a microorganism and lower the surface tension at the cell membrane. This may speed the disintegration of the cell.

Normal urine has a higher surface tension than the urine of a person with jaundice, a liver disease that causes bile to accumulate in the urine. If powdered sulfur is sprinkled on the surface of normal urine, it stays on the top; on the urine of someone with jaundice, the sulfur sinks because of the lower surface tension. Table 11–2 lists the relative surface tensions of several liquids.

Normal boiling point

A liquid always contains molecules that are evaporating into the gas (**vapor**) phase, since there are always some fast-moving molecules that will escape the surface tension. At some temperature, and given additional heat energy, all of the liquid molecules can be converted (in a process called **vaporization**) to gas. We call the lowest such temperature the **boiling point** of that liquid.

The boiling point of a liquid is dependent on air pressure, as discussed in Section 11.5. To avoid this complication, we usually compare the boiling points of liquids at 1.00 atm pressure. This is the *normal boiling point* of a liquid. For water, the normal boiling point is exactly 100°C. Substances that are gases at room temperature, such as H_2, Cl_2, NH_3, and N_2O, must have normal boiling points lower than 20°C (average room temperature). Table 11–3 gives some normal boiling points.

A pure substance will boil away at a constant temperature. Thus, the normal boiling point is often used to identify an unknown organic liquid. If a liquid boils over a wide temperature range, it is not a pure substance.

TABLE 11–3   BOILING
POINTS OF SOME
PURE SUBSTANCES
(at 1 atm pressure)

Solids at room temperature	
C (diamond)	4827°C
Fe (iron)	2750°C
SiO_2 (quartz)	2230°C
NaCl (table salt)	1413°C
S (sulfur)	445°C
I_2 (iodine)	184°C

Liquids at room temperature	
Hg (mercury)	357°C
H_2O (water)	100°C
C_6H_6 (benzene)	80°C
C_2H_5OH (ethanol)	78°C
CH_3COCH_3 (acetone)	56°C
C_5H_{12} (pentane)	36°C

Gases at room temperature	
C_4H_{10} (butane)	0°C
HCHO (formaldehyde)	−21°C
NH_3 (ammonia)	−33°C
CH_4 (methane)	−164°C
N_2 (nitrogen)	−196°C
He (helium)	−269°C

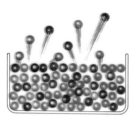
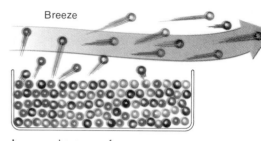

Breeze

a   **b**   Larger surface area

FIGURE 11–4   Evaporation of a liquid. The "hottest" molecules (those with the highest kinetic energy) on the surface of the liquid escape into the gas (a). Heating, increasing the surface area (b), and providing a breeze all increase the rate of evaporation.

The higher the attraction between molecules in a liquid, the more difficult it is for heat to break a molecule out of the liquid into the gas. Thus, as a general rule

A liquid with high intermolecular attractions will have a higher normal boiling point than a liquid with weak attractions.

Even at temperatures below the boiling point, a liquid will evaporate, that is, become a gas. If you leave a glass of water on a table, the liquid level will get lower and lower as some fast-moving molecules vaporize, escape into the gas phase, and disperse around the room (Figure 11–4).

A **volatile** liquid is one that evaporates easily. It has relatively low attractive forces between molecules and thus a relatively low normal boiling point, viscosity, and surface tension. You can usually smell the gas molecules that evaporate from such a liquid. The *vapor pressure* of a volatile liquid is higher than that of a liquid with stronger attractive forces, as will be discussed in Section 11.5.

In summary, a liquid with strong intermolecular forces will have a relatively high viscosity, high surface tension, high normal boiling point, and low evaporation rate.

SELF-CHECK

11.1)   List the major characteristics of an ideal gas. Do liquids share these characteristics? Why not?

11.2)   In each of the following pairs of substances, which one would you expect to have the stronger intermolecular forces at 25°C? Explain.
a)   liquid vegetable oil or white solid hydrogenated shortening
b)   a gelatin dessert or pure water
c)   water or ethanol

11.3)   Which would you expect to have a
a)   higher viscosity: water at 10°C or water at 90°C?
b)   higher surface tension: water or gelatin dessert?
c)   higher normal boiling point: perfume or liquid soap?

11.2 BLOOD PRESSURE

> *LEARNING GOAL 11C:* Describe the major factors affecting the blood pressure in a vein or artery.

Hydrostatic pressure

In Section 10.3 we discussed gas pressure as a *force per unit area* of surface in contact with the gas. This force is a result of collisions between the gas molecules and the surface. On p. 278 it was noted that the gas pressure is applied equally to *all* surfaces inside the container.

The same is true if a container holds a liquid. In any small section of the container, the pressure caused by the liquid molecules is constant and is transmitted in all directions. We call this pressure *hydrostatic* if the liquid is water or an aqueous solution such as blood.

We live at the bottom of a "sea" of air. The gas pressure on our bodies actually represents the weight (a result of gravity) of a column of air molecules many miles high. This pressure is exerted equally on eardrums, chest, hands, and feet.

Some living organisms must survive at the bottom of the ocean. The pressure on their bodies represents the weight of the column of air on the top of the ocean (one atmosphere) *plus* the weight of the column of water above them. A fish living one mile down in the ocean is under a total pressure (on all of its membranes and surfaces) of about 160 atmospheres!

Our blood must keep our bodies at a pressure of one atmosphere. That deep-sea fish must have body fluids that push out against the sea water at 160 atm. If that fish is brought to the surface, the internal pressure may cause it to burst.

Liquid pressure is thus dependent upon depth. This is the principle behind use of a mercury column in a barometer or manometer (Section 10.3).

A sea laboratory is shown in Figure 11–5. The air pressure at a point inside the research vessel must be about two atmospheres. In spite of what is implied in James Bond films, underwater diving is a dangerous sport because of the high pressures. Coming up from high pressures can cause nitrogen bubbles to form in the blood and can cause particular problems for people with colds, sinus congestion, or ear difficulties. A diver generally cannot go below 150 feet because the pressure at that depth, six atmospheres, is the limit for air to be pumped to a diver. Imagine the difficulty scientists had in exploring the Marianas trench in the Pacific Ocean, where the pressure is over 1000 atm!

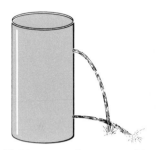

Fluid pressure increases with depth. When two holes are punched in the side of a can, water will flow faster from the hole nearer the bottom.

The amount of dissolved oxygen and nitrogen in the blood under an air pressure of two atm is double that at sea level (*Henry's Law*, Section 12.2). If return to the surface is too rapid, there is not enough time for the extra dissolved nitrogen to be excreted through the lungs. Bubbles of nitrogen forming in the blood stream then block the capillaries, causing the painful condition known as "the bends." Brain damage and death may quickly follow from nitrogen bubbles in brain capillaries, which cause *air embolism*. The only emergency solution is to *recompress* the diver to an external pressure of two atm and then very slowly allow decompression back to one atm. Some hospitals now use hyperbaric chambers (Section 10.5) for this purpose.

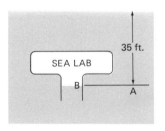

FIGURE 11–5 The air pressure inside a sea laboratory (point B) must be equal to the water pressure outside (point A). That water pressure is made up of the weight of the atmosphere on the surface of the water (1.0 atm) plus the weight of the water above point A (equivalent to 1.0 atm).

The extra fluid pressure in the legs may cause some of the blood plasma to pass out of the capillaries into the cells through *osmosis* (Section 12.5). That is why airplane passengers on long trips tend to suffer from swollen ankles.

Increase in pressure with depth has a more direct effect on the human body. If blood pressure were due simply to gravity, it would be highest in the feet and lowest in the head. The body must compensate for this. Varicose veins in the legs are a result of the inability of the blood vessel walls to withstand this pressure without swelling. Fortunately, gravity is not a major factor in providing blood pressure. If it were, astronauts could not possibly function in the weightlessness of space.

Hydraulic pressure

If you apply pressure to a gas, you can compress it and reduce the volume. However, the volume of a liquid is almost completely taken up by the electron clouds of the molecules. There is very little empty space.

Pressure exerted on a liquid (*hydraulic pressure*) is thus transmitted to all parts of the liquid with very little loss. If you squeeze the bottom of a tube of toothpaste, the pressure causes the paste to come out the hole at the top. Since pressure is force per unit area, a small force on a small unit area can be magnified into a large force on a large unit area, as shown in Figure 11–6. In this way, the pressure of a driver's foot on the brake pedal of a car becomes a large force to stop the car, or a small compressed-air pump can be used in an automobile garage to lift a large truck far off the ground.

A great deal of force is required to push the blood through the many vessels of your body. Even though the heart is a fairly small organ, it uses the same hydraulic principle to maintain pressure throughout the body.

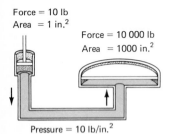

FIGURE 11–6 The hydraulic press. A small push at the left-hand end results in a very large force in the right-hand platform. In theory, the multiplying factor for the force exerted (here, 10 pounds of force lifts 10 000 pounds of weight, a mechanical advantage of 1000) is equal to the ratio of the piston areas.

Measuring blood pressure

There are actually two different **blood pressures.** One, **systolic blood pressure,** is caused by a heart beat (contraction of the left ventricle). The second, **diastolic pressure,** is the pressure in the system while the heart is recovering for its next beat. The systolic pressure in a young person is typically between 110 and 140 torr, and the diastolic pressure between 70 and 90

Blood is carried from the heart to body tissues by *arteries*, is distributed to the cells by very narrow *capillaries*, and returns to the heart through *veins*, as shown in Section 24.2.

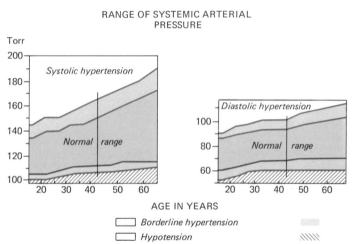

Blood pressure as a function of age. Normal and abnormal ranges are shown.

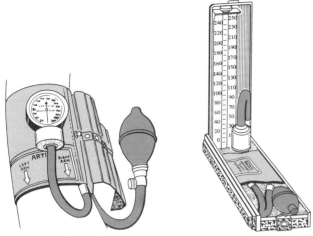

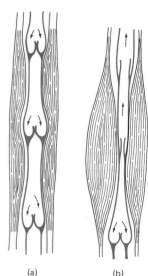

A sphygmomanometer is used to measure both systolic and diastolic blood pressures.

Veins contain one-way valves with pockets (a) that fill with blood and close the valve when blood tends to back up. When the muscles contract (b), the valves open and the blood is moved toward the heart.

torr. The blood pressure reading is reported as systolic/diastolic; for example, a reading might be 120/75.

Modern blood pressure readings are taken on the upper arm because its artery is close to the heart. As the blood gets farther from the heart, the pressure decreases until it is about 32 torr at the artery end of a small capillary. Veins have even less pressure, so the body has a system of valves to return the blood to the heart from the veins. The arterial circulation of the four to six liters of blood in a typical adult is accomplished partly by the pumping action of the heart and partly by the muscle action of the walls of the arteries.

High blood pressure (**hypertension**) may be caused by an increase in resistance of the blood vessels to the passage of blood or by a loss of muscle action in arteries ("hardening of the arteries"). One type of hypertension is due to a narrowing of the arteries because of a buildup of fat deposits (atherosclerosis).

Glaucoma

Another important medical application of the concepts of liquid pressure is in glaucoma, a common cause of blindness. This condition arises from an increase in the fluid pressure inside the eyeball, caused by a blockage of the pores that allow the aqueous humor to drain into the blood stream. The retina is very sensitive to such increased pressure. Early diagnosis of glaucoma using a *tonometer* is becoming an important part of eye examinations, especially for older people.

SELF-CHECK

11.4)   Explain what is meant by systolic blood pressure.

11.5)   The blood pressure in a vein leading into the heart is almost zero. How does the blood then get into the heart?

11.6*)   Some sudden strokes causing loss of brain function are due to the tearing of an artery wall. Explain why a weak point in an artery wall can lead to death, while weakness in the wall of a vein is much less serious.

11.7*) Nervous tension may lead to constriction (tightening) of arteries leading to the brain. The resulting lack of oxygen leads to dizziness or fainting. This is often treated by lowering the patient's head. Why?

11.3 INTERMOLECULAR FORCES

LEARNING GOAL 11D: Explain the origin of dipole forces and of dispersion forces between molecules.

11E: Given structural formulas for two pure liquids, predict which is likely to have the stronger intermolecular attractions and the higher viscosity or normal boiling point.

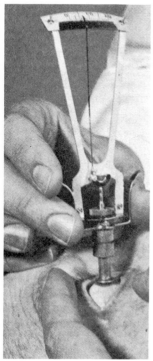

A tonometer, placed on the cornea, measures fluid pressure in the eye. An excess of pressure may destroy the retina and cause blindness through *glaucoma*. (Photo by John P. Goeller)

In a real gas, the collisions between molecules are "sticky" because of intermolecular attraction. In a liquid, the molecules roll over each other because they are attracted to each other. Since these are neutral molecules, the attraction cannot be that of a cation for an anion, as is the case in ionic bonding.

The forces are, indeed, electrostatic attractions between positive and negative centers of charge. However, they are between *partial charges*, such as those discussed in Section 6.4, rather than between ions. Intermolecular attractions are generally weaker than bonds, either covalent or ionic. There are two major categories of such forces between molecules: permanent *dipole* forces and the *dispersion* forces created by temporary dipoles. Dipole forces occur between polar molecules (discussed in Section 6.4), while dispersion forces are present in all types of molecules.

Dipole forces

If the electronegativity difference between two elements is substantial, the bond formed between atoms of those elements will be a polar bond (Section 6.1). For example, the bond between carbon (EN = 2.5) and hydrogen (EN = 2.1) is only very slightly polar, but that between carbon and fluorine (EN = 4.0) is highly polar. For each carbon-fluorine bond, we may indicate partial charges as

$$\overset{\delta^+}{C} - \overset{\delta^-}{F}$$

This indicates that the electron pair that forms the carbon-fluorine bond is shifted towards the fluorine atom, making the fluorine somewhat negatively charged with respect to the carbon atom.

In Section 6.4 we discussed the fact that a molecule with polar bonds may or may not actually have a *net* polarity or dipole. The bond polarities may cancel out.

Note that you cannot always predict the polarity of a molecule from its structural formula. We could write CH_2F_2

$$\overset{\delta^+}{H} - \underset{\underset{F_{\delta^-}}{|}}{\overset{\overset{F^{\delta^-}}{|}}{C}} - \overset{\delta^+}{H}$$

Here, the C—F dipoles seem to cancel out. However, this diagram is not a true picture of the molecule; it is simply a way of showing what is bonded to what. We must know the molecular geometry (Section 6.3) before we can predict dipole forces.

In fact, the molecule CH_2F_2 is polar, as you can see if we draw it as follows:

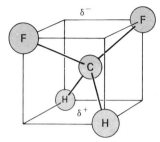

A useful test you may apply to see if a molecule is polar or not is to try to *slice* the molecule into two halves, one of which is more positively charged, the other more negatively charged. If you can do so with one clean slice, the molecule is polar.

A polar molecule has a charge *dipole*. Two polar molecules can line up in such a way that the δ^+ charge of one molecule attracts the δ^- charge on a second molecule (Figure 11–7). The force of attraction in this case is called a **dipole force.**

The difference between a covalent *bond* and an intermolecular dipole *force* of attraction is shown in Figure 11–8. A large amount of work (256 kcal/mole) is needed to break the covalent bond between carbon and oxygen in carbon monoxide. In contrast, only a small amount of energy (1.4 kcal/mole) is needed to pull the negative (oxygen) side of one CO molecule away from the positive (carbon) side of a second CO molecule to break the liquid apart into a gas.

The electronegativities of the elements are shown in Figure 6–7 (p. 157). For your convenience, the values for eight elements frequently encountered in organic molecules are listed again in Table 11–4. An element with electronegativity greater than 3.0 is more negative than carbon and thus will tend to form a polar bond with carbon. This means that, in an organic molecule, you can expect nitrogen, chlorine, and particularly oxygen and fluorine atoms to have partial negative charges.

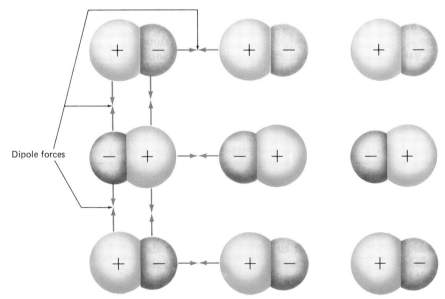

Dipole forces

FIGURE 11–7   Dipole forces between molecules result from attraction between the δ^+ side of one molecule and the δ^- side of a neighboring molecule. In a solid held together by dipole forces, such as ICl, the molecules are in a regular pattern. However, in a polar liquid, such as water, the molecules will not be in any kind of straight-line pattern.

TABLE 11–4 ELECTRO-NEGATIVITY VALUES OF SOME COMMON ELEMENTS

H (hydrogen)	2.1
P (phosphorus)	2.1
C (carbon)	2.5
S (sulfur)	2.5
N (nitrogen)	3.0
Cl (chlorine)	3.0
O (oxygen)	3.5
F (fluorine)	4.0

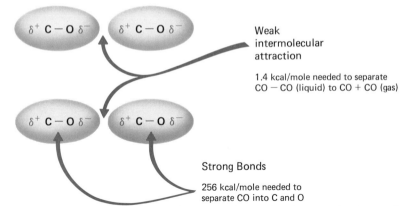

Weak intermolecular attraction

1.4 kcal/mole needed to separate CO — CO (liquid) to CO + CO (gas)

Strong Bonds

256 kcal/mole needed to separate CO into C and O

FIGURE 11–8 The attraction holding two polar molecules together in the liquid state is much weaker than the covalent bonds between the atoms in the molecule. When we boil carbon monoxide, we obtain CO gas, not C atoms and O atoms.

If none of these elements are present in an organic molecule, the molecule is likely to be nonpolar.

The effect of molecular polarity in a series of compounds is shown in Table 11–5. The increase in boiling point shown in each case is mainly because one type of molecule is polar and the other is not.

Dipole forces are relatively easy to understand because the partial charges are *always* present in the molecule.

Dispersion forces

There is another type of force, called a London force or **dispersion force,** that causes attractions in *all* substances. This force is a consequence of the fact that an electron cloud does not stay rigidly fixed in place. As an electron cloud moves, it comes closer to the electron cloud of a second molecule. The two clouds will repel each other because both have negative charge. This effect, shown in Figure 11–9, creates an *induced* dipole in the second mole-

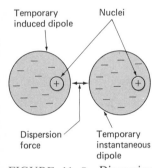

Temporary induced dipole   Nuclei

Dispersion force   Temporary instantaneous dipole

FIGURE 11–9 Dispersion (London) forces. A change in position of the electron cloud of the right-hand molecule makes that particle polar for an instant. At that moment, the electron cloud of the left-hand molecule is repelled, making that particle temporarily polar. The two temporary dipoles attract each other for a moment.

TABLE 11–5   EFFECT OF DIPOLE FORCES ON SOME NORMAL BOILING POINTS

No Dipole Present	Normal BP	Polar Molecule	Normal BP
H_2	−253°C	HF	20°C*
F_2	−188°C		
O_2	−183°C	NO	−152°C
N_2	−196°C		
trans-1,2-dichloroethene	48°C	*cis*-1,2-dichloroethene	60°C

* The astoundingly high effect of polarity in HF is called *hydrogen-bonding* and will be discussed in the next section.

cule. Each of the two molecules is momentarily polar. During that moment, there is an attraction.

The same thing happens if two neutral atoms, such as those of helium, come together. A momentary shift in the electron cloud of one atom will *polarize* (make polar) the second atom, and there will be a temporary attraction. For this reason, even helium (which forms no chemical bonds) can be made into a liquid, although at the extraordinarily low temperature of 4 K (−269°C).

Although temporary dipoles exist for only a small fraction of a second, that is enough to make some collisions between molecules "sticky." Weak dispersion forces account for our ability to turn air into a liquid. Much stronger dispersion forces account for the fact that bromine, Br_2 (nonpolar), is a liquid at room temperature.

Because electron clouds are constantly shifting, dispersion forces exist between all kinds of molecules and atoms. For large polar molecules, the dispersion forces are generally more important than the dipole forces.

The relative strength of dispersion forces depends on the number of electrons forming the electron clouds of the molecule and on the overall size of the molecule. In compounds with only a few electrons and small size, dispersion forces tend to be quite weak. As the size and number of electrons go up, dispersion forces become more important (Table 11–6).

A common rule of thumb is that, among *similar* compounds, the strength of dispersion forces increases with increasing molecular weight. Since the molecular weight (in amu) is usually about twice the number of electrons in the molecule, and since heavier molecules of the same type are generally larger molecules, this is a useful indirect way of predicting physical properties. However, among different kinds of compounds with similar molecular weights, the intermolecular forces can vary widely.

TABLE 11–6   NORMAL BOILING POINTS OF SOME CONTINUOUS-CHAIN ALKANES

CH_4	−162°C
C_2H_6	−89°C
C_3H_8	−42°C
C_4H_{10}	0°C
C_5H_{12}	36°C
C_6H_{14}	69°C
C_7H_{16}	98°C
C_8H_{18}	126°C
C_9H_{20}	151°C
$C_{10}H_{22}$	174°C
$C_{15}H_{32}$	268°C
$C_{20}H_{42}$	343°C

SELF-CHECK

11.8)   In what kinds of liquids will we find dipole attractions?
11.9)   What causes dispersion forces in H_2 gas?
11.10)   Which of the following liquids would you predict to have the higher viscosity (at a given temperature)? Explain.
a) CF_4 or CHF_3
b)   ethane   or   octane
c)   diethyl ether, $C_2H_5OC_2H_5$, or butanal, C_3H_7CHO
d) N_2 or   NO

11.4 WATER AND HYDROGEN-BONDING

> *LEARNING GOAL 11F: Given the structural formula for a pure liquid, predict whether hydrogen-bonding will play an important role in determining its properties.*

Water is an amazing compound. From its molecular formula, H_2O, you might expect it to be very similar to hydrogen sulfide, H_2S, a poisonous gas at room temperature. Yet, water remains a liquid up to 100°C and thus provides the basis for life on earth. Water dissolves many chemical substances and allows many aqueous-solution processes to take place in the body.

Water is highly stable. It provides excellent heat storage, gaining or losing heat very slowly with respect to many other pure liquids, and so allows bodies of water (as well as our own bodies) to maintain a fairly constant temperature.

Many of these properties of water, as well as some of the unique aspects of ice, the solid form of water, are due to a particularly strong form of dipole attraction between the hydrogen atoms (δ^+) and oxygen atoms (δ^-) in different molecules.

Hydrogen-bonding

Figure 11–10 compares the normal boiling points of some *hydrides*, compounds formed by hydrogen with the elements in a particular group of the periodic table. The boiling points increase for the hydrogen compounds of the Group 4 elements in the order CH_4, SiH_4, GeH_4, and SnH_4 (just as we would expect). The heavier hydrides have greater dispersion forces. All are nonpolar, since each has a tetrahedral shape. The boiling points are all quite low and follow a regular pattern.

Group 5 gives us the first surprise. We know that NH_3 is polar (Example 6n) while CH_4 is nonpolar. The boiling point of ammonia should thus be somewhat higher than that of methane. However, the intermolecular forces

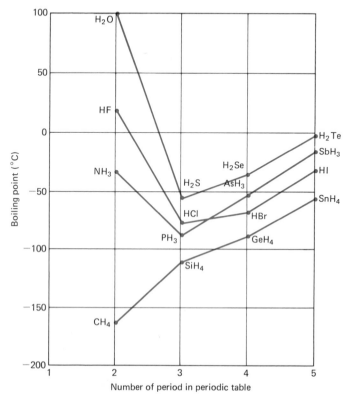

FIGURE 11–10 The effect of hydrogen-bonding. The three molecules H_2O, HF, and NH_3 have unusually high normal boiling points when compared with similar compounds.

in ammonia are *very* strong and give it a boiling point more than 100 Celsius degrees higher than that of methane.

The same happens with water. Again, only the first compound in the series is "out of step" with the rest, and even more sharply than ammonia. Finally, for Group 7, the boiling point of HF is much higher than would be expected from the trend in HCl, HBr, and HI.

We are thus dealing with an extraordinary kind of dipole attraction, which only occurs between a very *small* hydrogen atom carrying a *partial positive charge* and one of the following very small atoms carrying a *partial negative charge:*

N nitrogen   O oxygen   F fluorine

as in

NH₃   H₂O   HF

Chemists have (somewhat unfortunately) given the name "hydrogen bond" to this very strong dipole attraction. In this text, we will use a hyphen to distinguish the intermolecular force of a "hydrogen-bond" from a covalent bond formed between hydrogen and another atom.

Figure 11–11 shows how **hydrogen-bonding** can cause H₂O and HF to form chains of molecules that are attracted to each other. Moreover, HF dissolved in water can form *intermolecular* hydrogen-bonds:

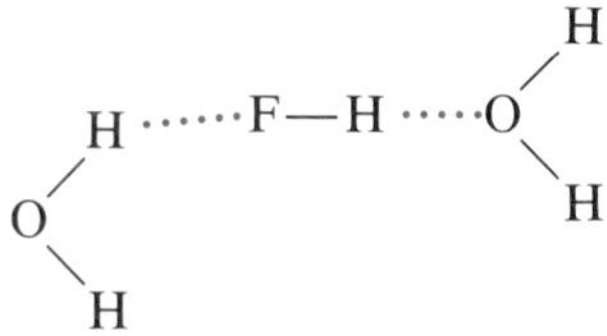

These dipole attractions make aqueous HF solutions behave quite differently from solutions of HCl, HBr, and HI.

To summarize:

A hydrogen-bond is a very strong dipole attraction between a hydrogen acting as the δ⁺ side of a polar molecule and a fluorine, oxygen, or nitrogen acting as the δ⁻ side of a polar molecule.

You will not find hydrogen-bonds in a hydrocarbon. Carbon is not sufficiently electronegative to either create a strong enough δ⁺ on the hydrogen of a C—H bond or to create a δ⁻ on the carbon atom. The hydrogen atom must itself generally be bonded to a N, O, or F to have hydrogen-bonding.

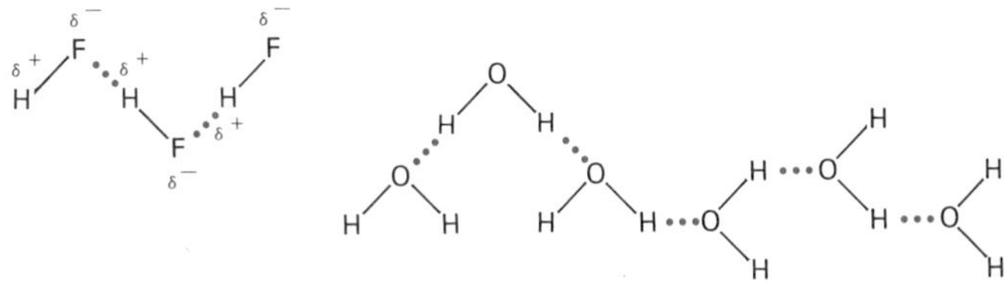

For hydrogen-bonding to result, the hydrogen atom must carry a δ⁺ charge in its molecule, and so the atom must itself be bonded to a highly electronegative element such as N, O, or F. It is then attracted by the δ⁻ lone pair on a highly electronegative atom (N, O, F, or possibly Cl) of a neighboring molecule. The closer these two partial charges can come to each other, the stronger the dipole force will be. The strength of the hydrogen-bond force is therefore mostly due to the fact that both the hydrogen atom and the electronegative (N, O, F) atom are quite small.

Do not confuse covalent bonds, such as the O—H bond in water, with hydrogen-bonding forces, such as the

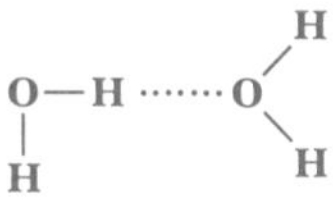

attraction in liquid water.

FIGURE 11–11 Hydrogen-bonding in HF and H₂O gives these substances very high normal boiling points.

C_2H_6O	
CH_3OCH_3 (dimethyl ether)	−23°C
CH_3CH_2OH (ethanol)	78°C
four carbons	
$CH_3CH_2CH_2CH_3$ (butane)	0°C
$CH_3CH_2OCH_2CH_3$ (diethyl ether)	35°C
$CH_3CH_2CH_2CHO$ (butanal)	76°C
$CH_3CH_2CH_2CH_2OH$ (1-butanol)	117°C
$HOCH_2CH_2CH_2CH_2OH$ (1,4-butanediol)	235°C

On the other hand, it is possible for a long molecule to hydrogen-bond to itself. It is not actually necessary for the molecule as a whole to be polar, so long as in a local region of the molecule there is a charge separation giving a δ^+ and a δ^-.

Hydrogen-bonding in alcohols

An alcohol, with its —OH functional group, fulfills the requirement for hydrogen-bonding, no matter where the —OH group is on the molecule. Table 11–7 compares the normal boiling points of some organic compounds with and without hydroxyl groups. As a general rule, a compound with hydrogen-bonding will boil at a high temperature.

The strength of the hydrogen-bonding increases with the number of —OH groups, as you may have noticed if you have used isopropyl alcohol (not very viscous, C_3H_7OH) to treat a cut and glycerol (very viscous, $C_3H_5(OH)_3$) to lubricate a piece of glass tubing.

On the other hand, a hydroxyl group on an end carbon forms more effective hydrogen-bonding attractions than if the —OH group is "hidden" in the middle of the molecule. 1-hexanol boils at 158°C, 2-hexanol at 140°C, and 3-hexanol at 135°C. The longer the carbon chain, the more an alcohol begins to resemble its parent alkane, and the less important is hydrogen-bonding. While short-chain alcohols dissolve easily in water through formation of hydrogen bonds, hexanol is only slightly soluble, and decanol ($C_{10}H_{21}OH$) is insoluble in water.

Ice

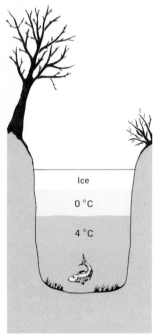

Ice

0 °C

4 °C

Freezing of water in a lake

The three-dimensional structure of ice is shown in Figure 11–12. To a great extent, this is also the structure of liquid water. Each water molecule can be hydrogen-bonded to *four* other water molecules. Such attractions are completed in solid ice, which keeps the structure rigid. In liquid water, the hydrogen-bonding creates clusters of ice-like groups of molecules.

Notice that the ice structure has a good deal of empty space. In fact, ice is less dense than liquid water and thus floats on the top of a lake or ocean. This is fortunate for life on earth. If ice, like most solids, were more dense than its liquid state, the polar ice caps would sink into the sea, to be covered by more and more ice. Sea life would be impossible in winter anywhere except near the equator because of the accumulation of ice. Actually, ice forming on the surface of arctic seas protects the water from the very cold air and helps sustain the sea life below.

SELF-CHECK

11.11)   In which of the following liquids do you expect to find hydrogen-bonding?
a) H_2NNH_2 hydrazine (a rocket fuel)
b)   HF   hydrogen fluoride
c) $CH_3CH_2OCH_2CH_3$ diethyl ether
d) H_2NCONH_2 urea
e) CH_3OH methanol
f) CH_3F fluoromethane

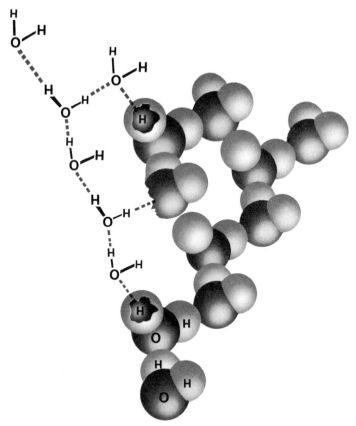

FIGURE 11–12 Hydrogen-bonding in ice, compared with the intermolecular attractions in liquid water. In the liquid, there is less hydrogen-bonding than in the solid. As a result, the solid structure is more open and less dense; ice floats on liquid water.

g)   HOOH   hydrogen peroxide
h*) NH_4NO_3 ammonium nitrate
11.12*) Predict which of the following liquids will have the highest surface tension (all at the same temperature).
a) $CH_3CH_2CH_2CH_2CH_2CH_3$ hexane
b) $CH_3CH_2CH_2CH_2CH_2CH_2OH$ 1-hexanol
c) $CH_3CH_2CHOHCH_2CH_2CH_3$ 3-hexanol
d) $CH_2OHCHOHCHOHCHOHCHOHCH_2OH$ glucose
11.13) Explain why ethanol, CH_3CH_2OH, easily dissolves in water to give a variety of alcoholic beverages.

11.5 CHANGES OF PHASE

LEARNING GOAL 11G: Explain why a particular phase change is endothermic or exothermic.

A pure substance may exist in at least three different phases at different temperatures. At low temperatures, we generally find the *solid* phase. As we add heat to the solid, its temperature rises until we reach the **melting point,** the temperature at which the solid enters the *liquid* phase.

As we add more heat to the liquid, its temperature goes up until we reach the boiling point, the temperature at which the liquid enters the *gas* phase. Any additional heat will then raise the temperature of the gas.

This whole process may be shown on a heating curve (Figure 11–13). Note that while a pure substance is melting (changing from a solid to a liquid), the temperature remains constant at the melting point. Similarly, when the liquid boils and becomes vapor, the temperature is constant at the boiling point until all the liquid is converted to gas.

Endothermic processes

The steps shown in Figure 11–13 all require heat. A process that requires heat is **endothermic:**

Increasing the temperature of a substance is endothermic.

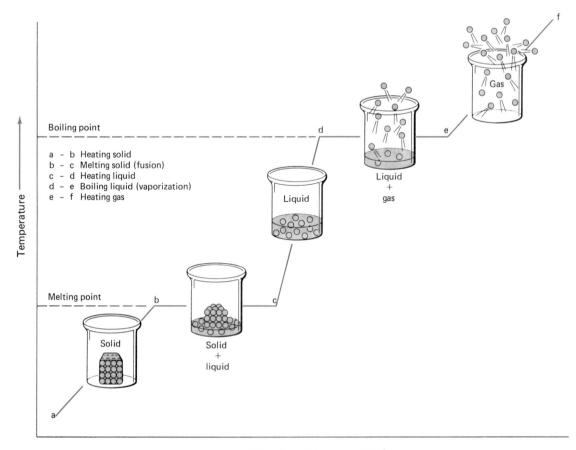

Boiling point

a – b Heating solid
b – c Melting solid (fusion)
c – d Heating liquid
d – e Boiling liquid (vaporization)
e – f Heating gas

Gas

Liquid + gas

Liquid

Melting point

Solid + liquid

Solid

Temperature

Time (or heat energy added) ⟶

FIGURE 11–13   A heating curve for a pure substance, showing changes in temperature and state (solid, liquid, gas).

Melting a solid to a liquid is endothermic.
Vaporizing a liquid to a gas is endothermic.

The reasons should not be difficult to understand if you apply the kinetic molecular theory. Temperature is proportional to the average kinetic energy of the molecules (Section 10.2). If we are to raise the temperature, we must add kinetic energy (heat) to the molecules of the substance.

The difference between a liquid and a solid is largely in degree of movement. A liquid molecule moves about, while a solid molecule is locked pretty well into one position. To convert from a solid to a liquid, we must break some of the intermolecular forces of the solid. This takes energy.

To go from a liquid to a gas, we must break all of the remaining intermolecular forces (dipole, dispersion, hydrogen-bonding) so that the molecules are free to fill their container. Breaking intermolecular attractions requires energy, in the form of heat. This heat may come from a stove, which we use to boil water, or from your hand if you use it to melt an ice cube. An endothermic process simply cannot happen unless there is heat available.

Exothermic processes

A process that gives off heat is **exothermic.** We may reverse our steps in Figure 11–13, going from right to left, if we take a gas and cool it. In cooling the gas, we are removing heat:

Decreasing the temperature of a substance is exothermic.
Condensing a gas into a liquid is exothermic.
Freezing a liquid into a solid is exothermic.

In each of these cases, we must remove heat. Heat is transferred from the object to its environment. A refrigerator or freezer removes heat from food (and transfers it to the surrounding room), an exothermic change.

Most chemical reactions that happen "by themselves" are exothermic, that is, they give off heat. An explosion is an exothermic process.

Phase equilibrium

We have already discussed equilibrium in terms of the reactants and products of a chemical reaction (p. 133). Another type of equilibrium may take place at the melting point of a solid. As shown in Figure 11–13, both solid and liquid are present along line b-c. While solid is changing to liquid, some liquid is changing back to solid. If the system is kept exactly at the melting point and no heat is added or removed, we will eventually reach a situation in which the number of solid molecules melting in one minute is exactly equal to the number of liquid molecules freezing in the same amount of time. We are in a situation of **phase equilibrium:**

$$\text{solid} \underset{\text{at melting point}}{\rightleftharpoons} \text{liquid}$$

We can now define equilibrium in terms that apply both to phase changes and to chemical reactions:

Equilibrium is a situation in which two opposing reactions or processes are taking place at the same rate, so there is no net change in the amount of each substance present.

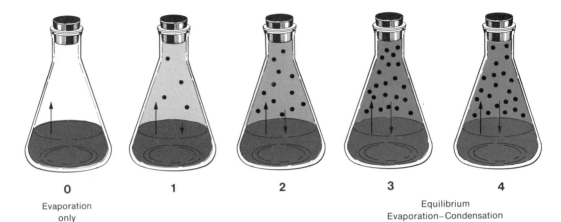

FIGURE 11–14 The development of liquid-vapor equilibrium. The partial pressure of the vapor (black dots) in equilibrium with the liquid in flasks 3 and 4 is called the *vapor pressure* of the liquid at the particular temperature being used.

TABLE 11–8 WATER VAPOR PRESSURE

Temperature (°C)	Vapor Pressure (mm Hg or torr)
0	4.6
5	6.5
10	9.2
15	12.8
16	13.6
17	14.5
18	15.5
19	16.5
20	17.5
21	18.6
22	19.8
23	21.1
24	22.4
25	23.8
26	25.2
27	26.7
28	28.3
29	30.0
30	31.8
31	33.7
32	35.7
33	37.7
34	40.0
35	42.2
40	55.3
45	71.9
50	92.5
60	149.4
70	233.7
80	355.1
90	525.8
100	760.0

Let us suppose we have a cloudy day in winter, with the air temperature at exactly 0°C. Some of the snow on a driveway will begin melting, and some of the water in contact with that snow will freeze. Eventually, we will have equilibrium:

$$H_2O_{(s)} \rightleftharpoons H_2O_{(\ell)}$$

If the day gets warmer, this equilibrium will be shifted to the right. Heat will be absorbed by the solid. The ice may all melt. If the day gets colder than 0°C, the air will absorb heat from the liquid. All of the liquid may freeze to solid.

At equilibrium, the amount of solid and amount of liquid stay constant. However, the situation is *dynamic* and always moving. Ice is changing to liquid water and liquid water is changing to ice all the time.

At the boiling point of a liquid, we may have a similar situation, with the vapor (gas) in equilibrium with the liquid. However, there are other situations in which the liquid and vapor are in equilibrium.

Vapor pressure

Since liquid molecules (unlike those in solids) are in constant motion through space, rolling over one another, there will be a range of kinetic energies. Some liquid molecules will be moving rather fast. If these molecules are at the outer surface of the liquid, they may escape and become gas molecules. If the liquid surface is open to the air of a room, the vapor will become dispersed throughout the room, and eventually all of the liquid will evaporate. This happens at *any* temperature, although the *rate* of evaporation clearly depends on temperature.

If instead of an open room we keep the liquid inside a sealed flask, then there is a limit to the number of molecules of liquid that can evaporate. As soon as the vapor begins forming, some of the slow-moving gas molecules are trapped by intermolecular forces on the surface of the liquid. Eventually, there are as many vapor molecules condensing into liquid (like dew on cool morning grass) as there are liquid molecules evaporating, and an equilibrium is set up:

liquid $\rightleftharpoons$ vapor

The partial pressure of the vapor under these conditions is known as the **vapor pressure** of that particular liquid (Figure 11–14). It is a constant that depends only on temperature, not on the volume of the container.

The vapor pressure of a liquid is also a measure of the evaporation rate. It goes up with temperature, as you might expect. Some values of the vapor pressure of water are given in Table 11–8.

So long as a sealed flask contains liquid water at a given temperature (say 25°C), it will develop a concentration of water vapor that will exert a pressure equal to the vapor pressure at that temperature (in this case, 24 torr). To the limited extent that we may consider the human lungs to be a ''closed'' vessel, we would expect a water vapor level corresponding to the vapor pressure at 37.0°C, or about 47 torr.

We sometimes say that the air is then *saturated* with water vapor.

When the weather report says that the humidity is 100%, what is meant is that the partial pressure of water vapor (steam) in the air is equal to the vapor pressure of water at that temperature. In summer, this makes us uncomfortable because the amount of steam condensing on the skin is equal to the amount of sweat evaporating. Therefore, we cannot use the endothermic process of evaporation to draw heat from our bodies. In a cold climate, even ''100% humidity'' may represent very dry air.

One important use of vapor pressure is related to the fact that

A liquid will boil at a temperature at which its vapor pressure is equal to the atmospheric pressure around it.

If the air is at 1.00 atm pressure, then water will boil at 100°C, because that is the temperature (Table 11–8) at which its vapor pressure is 760 torr. If the air is at 634 torr in a mountain resort, water will boil much earlier, at 95°C. Eggs will cook much more slowly at 95°C than they will at 100°C. For similar reasons, the pressure cooker and autoclave discussed in Examples 10k and 10p increase the temperature at which water boils by increasing the pressure.

When gases are collected over water, the vapor pressure of water must be taken into account when calculating the amount of gas. This process is relevant to an important medical test, the measurement of basal metabolism, which determines how much oxygen is being used by the body each minute (Figure 21–4).

Sublimation

While many solids do not convert very easily to gases, some solids (often the ones you can smell!) are undergoing continual loss of molecules directly to the gas phase. This process is called *sublimation*. There is a vapor pressure of a solid associated with sublimation, which can be appreciated if you work with dry ice (solid CO_2), mothballs (naphthalene), or camphor ice. For this reason, snow and ice on the ground will very slowly evaporate, even at temperatures below 0°C. The vapor pressure of ice is about 1 torr at −17°C, rising to 4.6 torr at 0°C.

Phase changes and intermolecular forces

All of the processes discussed in this section are related to the intermolecular forces (dipole, dispersion, and hydrogen-bonding) of Sections 11.3 and 11.4. A substance with a relatively high attractive force between molecules may be expected to have a

1) relatively high melting point and boiling point
2) relatively high heat of fusion (heat required to melt the solid)
3) relatively high heat of vaporization (heat required to evaporate the liquid)

and

4) relatively low vapor pressure of the liquid at a given temperature

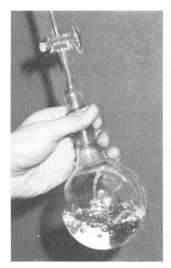

In the photograph, water is boiling at room temperature. The flask was attached to a vacuum pump, which lowered the pressure below the vapor pressure of the water. No heat was needed. Actually, the temperature of the water fell as the boiling proceeded. Can you suggest why?

11.14)   Is each of the following processes exothermic or endothermic? Explain why in each case.
a)   evaporation of diethyl ether
b)   freezing of water to make ice cubes
c)   condensation of water vapor on a cold windowpane
d)   warming your hands in front of a fire
11.15*)   Under what conditions do we expect to find phase equilibrium between liquid and gas?

11.6 SOLIDS

LEARNING GOAL 11H: Distinguish between molecular and ionic solids.
         11I: Describe a hydrated crystal.
         11J: Explain how a precipitate can result from the mixing of two solutions.

In a liquid, the molecules stick to one another, but move around. When the motion of a molecule in space slows down enough for it to be "locked" into one average position, the solid state results. The solid has a definite shape and volume. While each atom or molecule has a given "spot," it doesn't stay exactly fixed but vibrates back and forth around that position. We know by now that electron clouds "blur" the positions of atoms and molecules somewhat. The nuclei also vibrate somewhat, but in a manner that we can ignore in this discussion.

Amorphous solids

Some kinds of solids are simply "frozen liquids." The molecules are arranged haphazardly, as they are in the liquid, but their motion through space has been stopped. Such a solid, with no long-range order, is an **amorphous solid.** Window glass is one example; most plastics, rubber, and coal also fit into this category. Amorphous solids tend to break irregularly or stretch, and do not have sharp melting points.

Crystals

Most solids are **crystals.** They form three-dimensional patterns that repeat themselves, so that atoms and molecules are lined up very regularly, in a fashion similar to the way a wallpaper pattern repeats itself. The fixed pattern is called the *crystal lattice*. It is often cubic, like the pattern of girders used to construct a skyscraper. Figure 11–15 shows some of the differences between amorphous and crystalline solids.

Much of the beauty of diamonds and other carefully cut gemstones is due to a pleasing external shape. Such smooth faces and sharp corners can only result from a crystal with considerable order at the molecular level. Crystals of table salt are cubic in a way that corresponds to the way the Na^+ and Cl^- ions are "packed" in the lattice. Remember, however, that it takes many, many ions to make up a crystal large enough to be seen. The beautiful

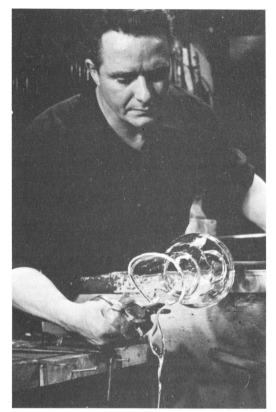

A craftsman working with molten glass, an amorphous solid when it cools. (Courtesy of Corning Glass)

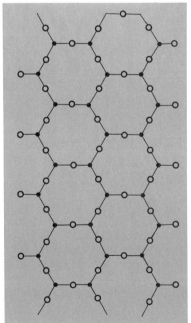

Crystalline

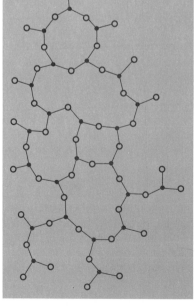

Amorphous

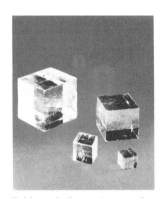

Table salt is made up of a regular pattern of Na$^+$ and Cl$^-$ ions, which form a cube. The external appearance of a large crystal, made up of 10^{22} Na$^+$ and 10^{22} Cl$^-$ ions, also shows the shape of a cube. However, crystals with cubic atomic patterns do not always have the overall shape of a cube.

FIGURE 11–15   A crystalline solid has a regular pattern of molecules or atoms as its structural unit. An amorphous solid has no regular pattern.

colors of some gems are due to very slight amounts of metal cation impurities.

Molecular crystals

Molecular (covalently bonded) substances form crystals in which the molecules are held in position by intermolecular forces. Ice (Figure 11–12) is one example of a **molecular crystal.** Such crystals are generally rather soft and melt at low temperatures. Organic compounds, of course, tend to form molecular crystals. The melting point of an organic solid is often used as a means of identification, since it is low enough to be determined easily in the laboratory.

Ionic crystals

The forces holding **ionic crystals** together are very strong since they are ionic bonds. Sodium ion is ionically bonded to six chloride ions in the lattice of table salt. Each chloride anion is similarly bonded to six sodium cations.

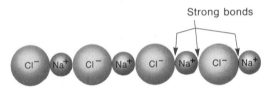

Strong bonds

183 kcal/mole are needed to separate a collection of bonded Na$^+$Cl$^-$ ions into individual Na$^+$ and Cl$^-$ ions

FIGURE 11–16 Sodium chloride, an ionic solid. Model shows how Na$^+$ and Cl$^-$ ions pack in a cubic crystal.

The melting point of NaCl is 1413°C, which is higher than ordinary laboratory ovens can go. Ionic crystals tend to be very hard and brittle. They often dissolve in water, for reasons to be discussed in Chapter 12. All ionic compounds form ionic crystals (Figure 11–16).

Macromolecular crystals

A few substances form crystal lattices that are held together not by ionic bonds (as in ionic salts) or by weak intermolecular forces (as in molecular compounds) but instead by a network of *covalent bonds* that extends throughout the lattice. One good example is diamond, which is extremely hard with a very high melting point (over 3550°C). There is essentially one huge covalently bonded molecule making up the entire crystal. Another example of a *macromolecular crystal* is quartz, found in sand and in many kinds of rock. It is a network of SiO$_2$ units and melts at 1710°C.

Metal crystals

As mentioned briefly at the end of Section 6.2, a metal is held together by a large cloud of delocalized electrons. The metal cations are fixed in position in regular rows, and the electrons are free to move while acting as a kind of "glue" holding the metal nuclei in place. Because the electrons are so free to move, metals are good conductors of electricity. They are also very good conductors of heat.

Because of their structure, it is fairly easy to draw metals into wires, roll them into sheets and foils, and press them into useful shapes (Figure 11–17). The more electrons there are in the valence-electron "sea" surrounding the cations, the stronger and higher-melting the metal is likely to be.

TABLE 11-9   COMPOSITION AND PROPERTIES OF SOME
COMMON ALLOYS

	Composition (Mass %)*	Properties
Alnico	Fe(51), Co(14), Ni(14), Al(8), Cu(3)	Magnetic (electromagnets)
Brass	Cu(70), Zn(30)	Easily machined
Bronze	Cu(88), Sn(8), Zn(4)	Hard, brittle
Coinage metal	Cu(70), Ni(30)	Cheaper than silver
Gold, 18 karat	Au(75), Cu(25)	Harder than pure gold (24 karat)
Monel metal	Ni(72), Cu(25), Fe(3)	Resists corrosion
Nichrome	Ni(80), Cr(20)	High electrical resistance
Pewter	Sn(85), Pb(15)	Inexpensive, malleable
Silver, sterling	Ag(92.5), Cu(7.5)	Harder than pure silver
Solder, soft	Pb(62), Sn(38)	Low melting point
Steel	Fe(99), C(1)	Stronger than pure iron
Steel, stainless	Fe(76), Cr(15), Ni(8), C(1)	Resists corrosion
Wood's metal	Bi(50), Pb(25), Cd(12.5), Sn(12.5)	Melts at 70°C

* Several of the compositions are approximate.

Impurities in metals often give them useful properties. A combination of metals called an *alloy* (Table 11–9) may give us a material with better properties than pure elements. Iron is often alloyed with carbon and other metals to make steel. Copper is found in brass (with zinc), bronze (with tin), sterling silver, and 14-karat gold. Most surgical instruments and metal implants intended for use inside the human body are made of stainless steel, an alloy of iron, chromium, nickel, and sometimes other metals.

Hydrated crystals

We have discussed ionic crystals as though they contain only metal cations and nonmetal anions. This is largely true for sodium chloride. However, most other ionic salts form crystal lattices that include a certain fixed amount of water.

For example, washing soda is a crystalline form of sodium carbonate, Na_2CO_3. However, its true formula is $Na_2CO_3 \cdot 10\ H_2O$, since ten water molecules accompany every Na_2CO_3 formula unit in the crystal lattice. The name of this substance is *sodium carbonate decahydrate*, with a Greek prefix (as in Chapter 4) used to give the number of waters.

Table 11-10 lists some **hydrates** and their uses. You should remember that most rocks contain hydrated salts. It is not always easy to obtain an ionic compound in *anhydrous* (without water of hydration) powder form.

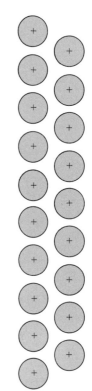

FIGURE 11–17 A metallic crystal. Unlike an ionic crystal, a metal can be "worked" into thin sheets or drawn into wires. This is because the positively charged atomic kernels can be moved within the "sea" of electrons without fundamentally altering their environment.

TABLE 11-10   SOME HYDRATED IONIC SALTS
AND THEIR FORMULAS

aluminum sulfate	$Al_2(SO_4)_3 \cdot 9H_2O$	papermaker's alum
calcium chloride	$CaCl_2 \cdot 2\ H_2O$	melting ice on roads, drying compound
calcium sulfate	$CaSO_4 \cdot \frac{1}{2}\ H_2O$	plaster of Paris
	$CaSO_4 \cdot 2\ H_2O$	gypsum, plaster casts
cobalt(II) chloride	$CoCl_2 \cdot 6\ H_2O$	humidity indicator, turns from red to blue
copper(II) acetate	$Cu(C_2H_3O_2)_2 \cdot H_2O$	paint pigment
copper(II) sulfate	$CuSO_4 \cdot 5\ H_2O$	insect poison, called "blue vitriol"
potassium sodium tartrate	$KNaC_4H_4O_6 \cdot 4\ H_2O$	Rochelle salt
sodium borate	$Na_2B_4O_7 \cdot 10\ H_2O$	borax for washing
sodium carbonate	$Na_2CO_3 \cdot 10\ H_2O$	washing soda
sodium hyposulfite	$Na_2S_2O_3 \cdot 5\ H_2O$	photography

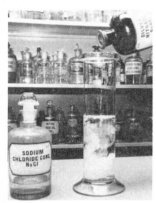

Formation of a precipitate by mixing two clear solutions to obtain a solid. The formation of a white AgCl precipitate is sometimes used as a test for the presence of Cl⁻ ions in a mixture.

We will here be writing ionic equations of the type first described in Section 5.2. The skill of writing such equations for precipitation reactions is included in Section 14.4.

One of the most important hydrated salts in medicine is calcium sulfate, used for making plaster casts to keep broken bones and torn ligaments in place. A bandage containing plaster of Paris powder (hydrated calcium sulfate) is dipped in water and wrapped around the limb. As the plaster sets, it absorbs water and turns into a very hard hydrated salt called gypsum:

$$2\ CaSO_4 \cdot \tfrac{1}{2}\ H_2O + 3\ H_2O \longrightarrow 2\ CaSO_4 \cdot 2\ H_2O$$
plaster of Paris + water gives   gypsum

As hydrated salts are heated, they tend to release their water of hydration. Gypsum may thus be heated to 128°C to convert it to plaster of Paris. Plaster of Paris will itself lose its water of hydration at 163°C to become anhydrous calcium sulfate, $CaSO_4$.

Precipitates

When ionic salts dissolve in water, they dissociate and the ions are quickly surrounded by clusters of water molecules called *hydration spheres*. The anions and cations, with their accompanying waters, then move about separately.

It is possible for a hydrated anion, such as $SO_{4(aq)}^{2-}$, to collide with a hydrated cation, such as $Ba_{(aq)}^{2+}$, to form an ionically bonded pair. If such bonding is strong enough, more ions will add to the growing crystal nucleus and a solid will form in the water solution. We call such a solid a **precipitate.**

Suppose, for some unknown reason, someone had swallowed some crystals of barium nitrate, $Ba(NO_3)_2$. This salt is very soluble in water (Section 12.3), so the following reaction occurs in the stomach:

$$Ba(NO_3)_{2(s)} \rightleftharpoons Ba_{(aq)}^{2+} + 2\ NO_{3(aq)}^{-}$$

The Ba^{2+} ion is very poisonous. We need an *antidote* to remove it from circulation. Fortunately, we can easily give the person a drink of sodium sulfate solution, which contains dissolved Na_2SO_4 in the form of hydrated Na^+ and SO_4^{2-} ions. The sulfate ions collide with the barium ions, forming solid crystals of barium sulfate precipitate:

$$SO_{4(aq)}^{2-} + Ba_{(aq)}^{2+} \rightleftharpoons BaSO_{4(s)}$$

While there is some equilibrium here, it is shifted far toward the (insoluble) solid barium sulfate, as shown by the relative lengths of the arrows. Solid $BaSO_4$ is harmless to the body and, in fact, is widely used to outline body organs in x-rays of the gastrointestinal tract.

As shown by the previous equations, there is an equilibrium between an ionic salt placed in water and its dissolved ions. If a salt is very soluble, there will be no solid apparent until an upper limit of ion concentrations in solution is reached, at which point a precipitate forms.

Although NaCl is a soluble salt, it will precipitate (or remain undissolved) if there are more than 370 grams of sodium chloride per liter of water. In that case, the solution is *saturated* (Section 12.2). In small pools along the seashore, salt water accumulates at high tide and then evaporates, leaving solid salt, which is collected and purified for our use.

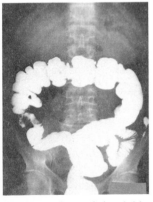

A suspension of insoluble $BaSO_4$ makes the colon block x-rays and permits detection of a cancer visible on the left side of this x-ray photo.

Calcium phosphate, $Ca_3(PO_4)_2$, is a constituent of bone, teeth, and kidney stones. This ionic salt is only very slightly soluble (0.020 grams per liter in cold water). An excess of calcium ions and phosphate ions in body fluids may thus lead to an unwanted precipitate:

$$3\ Ca^{2+}_{(aq)} + 2\ PO^{3-}_{4(aq)} \rightleftharpoons Ca_3(PO_4)_{2(s)}$$

Calcium ions in river water will react with carbonate ions (created by dissolved CO_2 from the atmosphere) to form limestone.

Calcium fluoride is insoluble in water. This plays an important part in the use of fluoride to prevent tooth decay in children, since F^- ions are incorporated into tooth solids and replace OH^- ions. The bacteria that cause tooth decay liberate acid that can react with the OH^- ions but not with the F^- ion.

Some rules to help you determine which ionic solids are soluble in water and which are not will be provided in Section 14.4.

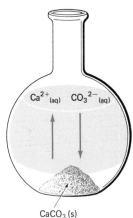

$CaCO_3$ (s)

In a saturated calcium carbonate solution, solid $CaCO_3$ is at equilibrium with the $Ca^{2+}_{(aq)}$ and the $CO^{2-}_{3(aq)}$ ions. Addition of solid $CaCO_3$ does not change the concentration of the ions.

SELF-CHECK

11.16) What kinds of particles occupy the lattice positions in a molecular solid? in an ionic solid?

11.17) Why is a molecular solid generally softer than an ionic solid?

11.18*) Is each of the following an amorphous or crystalline solid?
a) table salt   b) sugar   c) glass

11.19) Cobalt chloride occurs in two hydrated forms, a blue $CoCl_2 \cdot 2\ H_2O$ and a red $CoCl_2 \cdot 6\ H_2O$. Describe each crystal. Some "weather predictors" sold in novelty shops contain cobalt chloride crystals. What color would you expect when the humidity is very high and it is about to rain?

11.20*) Explain why water of hydration is often incorporated into a solid crystal when it precipitates.

11.21) Silver bromide, $AgBr$, is an insoluble ionic salt, while both silver nitrate and sodium bromide are soluble. Explain, using a chemical equation, how we may mix two solutions to obtain the silver bromide crystals used on photographic film.

CHAPTER ELEVEN IN REVIEW ■ Liquids and Solids

11.1 THE LIQUID STATE   Page 307

11A: Describe the major differences in the physical properties of a liquid and a gas.

11B: Describe how the viscosity, surface tension, and normal boiling point of a liquid are affected by the strength of intermolecular forces.

GLOSSARY FOR CHAPTER ELEVEN

amorphous solid A solid in which the particles are randomly ordered, such as glass; not crystalline; does not have a sharp melting point. (p. 328)

blood pressure The liquid pressure inside blood vessels that helps move blood through the circulatory system; more strictly, the *systolic* and *diastolic* pressures of an artery close to the heart. (p. 314)

boiling point The temperature at which liquid and vapor are in equilibrium in an open vessel; vapor bubbles are formed inside the liquid phase; the *vapor pressure* is equal to the external gas pressure; the *normal boiling point* is the boiling point under an atmospheric pressure of 1.00 atm. (p. 311)

condensation Change of state from a gas to a liquid (or solid); often occurs on a cold surface in humid weather, where water vapor condenses to liquid water or ice; a *condensed state* is a liquid or solid. (p. 308)

crystal A solid in which the particles are arranged in a very orderly pattern; the relationship between a few particles repeats itself throughout the crystal; may be *ionic*, *molecular*, or *macromolecular*; the structure is called a crystal *lattice*; a solid that forms crystals is *crystalline*. (p. 328)

diastolic pressure The blood pressure when the heart is resting between beats; the lower blood pressure resulting from muscle action in the arteries. See *systolic* pressure. (p. 314)

dipole force An intermolecular force in a real gas, liquid, or solid resulting from the attraction of a δ^+ side of one polar molecule for the δ^- side of another polar molecule; a hydrogen-bond is an especially strong case of a dipole force. (p. 317)

dispersion force An intermolecular force in a real gas, liquid, or solid caused by the attraction of a temporary dipole on one particle (caused by a shift in the electron cloud) for an induced temporary dipole on a second particle; the London force; present in all substances, but strongest in long molecules with many electrons. (p. 318)

endothermic Absorbs heat; the reactants gain energy to go to products; examples are melting and boiling. (p. 324)

exothermic Gives off heat; the reactants lose energy to go to products; examples are condensing, freezing, and combustion. (p. 325)

hydrate A particle surrounded by water molecules; a solid crystal that includes *water of hydration* within its orderly structure, as in gypsum, $CaSO_4 \cdot 2H_2O$; all substances dissolved in water solution are *hydrated*. (p. 331)

hydrogen-bonding An intermolecular force in a real gas, liquid, or solid caused by the attraction of a partially positively charged hydrogen to a partially negatively charged atom such as fluorine, oxygen, or nitrogen; a particularly strong kind of dipole attraction found in water, alcohols, ammonia, HF, etc. (p. 321)

hypertension A blood pressure that is significantly higher than normal; for example, a systolic pressure greater than 170 torr; in connection with disease of the arteries, hypertension can be very dangerous. (p. 315)

ionic crystal A crystalline solid composed of anions and cations held together by ionic bonds; often has a very high melting point. (p. 330)

liquid A state of matter in which the particles attract each other substantially; the molecules are touching but can move about and take the shape of the container; a liquid does not expand (like a gas) to fill its container; it may vaporize to a gas or freeze to a solid. (p. 309)

melting point The temperature at which the solid and liquid phases of a pure substance are in equilibrium; 0°C for water at 1 atm pressure; the melting point of a solid substance is the same as the freezing point of the liquid. (p. 324)

meniscus The curved surface of a liquid in a container; the curved surface at the top of a column of mercury or water in a tube such as a barometer or buret. (p. 310)

molecular crystal A crystalline solid made up of individual molecules held together by intermolecular forces (dipole or dispersion forces or *hydrogen-bonding*); generally has a low melting point. (p. 330)

phase One of two or more distinct portions of matter separated from each other by visible surfaces; examples are the solid, gas, and liquid phases in a glass of water containing an ice cube, or the two liquid phases when oil is floating on water. (p. 310)

phase equilibrium A situation in which two different states of a pure substance are present in phases touching each other, and in which the rate of conversion in both directions is the same; examples are ice and liquid water at 0°C and liquid water and steam at 100°C and 1 atm. (p. 325)

precipitate A solid formed from a reaction in a liquid or solution. (p. 332)

surface tension The resistance of particles at the surface of a liquid to the breaking or stretching of that surface; caused by *van der Waals forces*. (p. 310)

systolic pressure The maximum blood pressure caused by a pumping action of the heart in an artery near the heart; high systolic blood pressure is *hypertension*. See *diastolic* pressure. (p. 314)

van der Waals forces Intermolecular attractive forces that hold liquids and molecular crystals together and cause real gases to show nonideal behavior; includes dipole, dispersion, and hydrogen-bonding attractions; high van der Waals forces lead to high viscosity, high surface tension, and a high boiling point. (p. 308)

vapor The gas state of a substance when found in connection with the liquid phase, as in water vapor in the air, which comes from the vaporization of liquid in seas and lakes. (p. 311)

vaporization Change of state from liquid to gas; evaporation; the higher the *van der Waals forces*, the more difficult it is to vaporize a liquid. (p. 311)

vapor pressure A measure of the ease of vaporization of a liquid (a high vapor pressure means low intermolecular forces); specifically, the partial pressure of the vapor in equilibrium with a liquid. (p. 327)

viscosity Resistance of a substance to flow; a viscous liquid is hard to pour and seems "thick"; it will not pass quickly through a tube; viscosity depends on *van der Waals forces.* (p. 309)

volatile Easy to vaporize; if you can smell the vapor from a liquid, the vapor pressure must be high and the intermolecular forces must be low. (p. 312)

QUESTIONS AND PROBLEMS FOR CHAPTER ELEVEN ■ Liquids and Solids

SECTION 11.1 THE LIQUID STATE

11.22) One gram of steam occupies 1700 mL at 100°C, while one gram of liquid water occupies only 1.04 mL at the same temperature. Explain.

11.23) In a container of fixed volume, when we increase the temperature on a gas, we increase the pressure. If we increase the temperature of a liquid under the same conditions, the liquid pressure remains relatively constant. Explain.

11.24) How is the surface tension of a liquid related to the strength of intermolecular attractions?

11.25) A saline (NaCl) solution for use in intravenous injections has a viscosity lower than that of water. Will it pass through a needle more or less easily than water?

SECTION 11.2 BLOOD PRESSURE

11.26) A person with hypertension may have a systolic pressure as high as 300 mm Hg. What is that in atmospheres?

11.27) A blood clot in a brain artery can quickly cause death. A similar clot in a vein is less dangerous. Why?

11.55) Two different gases will mix with each other much more quickly than will two different liquids. Why?

11.56) At constant temperature, if we compress a gas (by increasing the pressure), we decrease its volume. If we try to compress a liquid, we find that we cannot make much of a change in its volume. Explain.

11.57) How is the viscosity of a liquid related to the strength of intermolecular attractions?

11.58) If the body temperature drops (as sometimes it does when a person is in shock), the blood becomes more viscous. How do you think this will affect the rate at which gases are exchanged in the alveoli of the lungs?

11.59) Normal systolic blood pressure is about 120 mm Hg for a young adult. What is this in atmospheres?

11.60) The blood pressure in the veins of the legs is less than that required to lift the blood (against gravity) to the heart. How does the blood return to the heart while we are walking or standing?

11.28) Why is diastolic blood pressure lower than systolic pressure?

11.29*) Lying on a normal bed, weight is concentrated in certain spots. Severely burned people suffer less pain if they use water beds. Why?

11.30*) Many boxers have died from brain damage caused by severe blows to the head. However, the damage usually results not at the front of the head (where the punch landed) but on the *opposite* side of the skull. Explain.

11.61) What is meant by a blood pressure reading of 125/80?

11.62*) If a pregnant woman engages in sports activities, the fetus might not be injured by a fall or bump. How does the amniotic fluid inside the uterus protect it from such shocks?

11.63*) When a blood transfusion is being given intravenously, the fluid should not be suspended too far above the patient, or pain will result. Why?

SECTION 11.3 INTERMOLECULAR FORCES

11.31) Explain where dispersion forces come from.

11.32) In what kind of compound do you expect dispersion forces to be most important?

11.33) At a given temperature, which of the following liquids do you expect to have the greater viscosity? Explain.
a) propane or heptane
b) $H_2C=CHF$ or $H_2C=CH_2$
c) boron nitride, BN, or nitrogen gas, N_2
d) 2,2-dimethylpropane or pentane

11.34) Which has the higher boiling point, Kr ($Z = 36$) or Ar ($Z = 18$)? Why?

11.64) Explain where dipole forces come from.

11.65) In what kind of compound do you expect dipole forces to be most important?

11.66) At a given temperature, which of the following liquids do you expect to have the higher surface tension? Explain.
a) NO or O_2
b) nonane or 3,3-diethylpentane
c) ethene or 2-pentene
d) methylamine, CH_3NH_2, or ethane

11.67) Which has the higher boiling point, Cl_2 or Br_2? Why?

SECTION 11.4 WATER AND HYDROGEN-BONDING

11.35) What chemical substance do you get when you boil NH_3 liquid?

11.36) For which of the following substances would hydrogen-bonding be important in determining liquid properties?
a) 2-propanol, $CH_3CHOHCH_3$
b) PH_3
c) $H_2C=CH_2$
d) $(CH_3)_2NH$

11.37) Compare the strength of intermolecular forces in H_2O with the forces in H_2S. Explain any differences.

11.68) What chemical substance do you get when you boil H_2O liquid?

11.69) For which of the following substances would hydrogen-bonding be important in determining liquid properties?
a) NF_3
b) $HONH_2$
c) 1,2-propanediol,
$CH_2OHCHOHCH_3$
d) CH_3CH_2F

11.70) Compare the strength of intermolecular forces in NH_3 liquid with the forces in PH_3. Explain any differences.

11.38) Compare the strength of the hydrogen-bonding in liquid NH_3 with the strength of the N—H bond in NH_3.

11.39*) When formic acid (HCOOH) vaporizes, we find that the gas consists not of individual molecules but of *dimers* made up of two HCOOH units each. Explain.

11.40*) Both alcohols and ethers can have a molecular formula C_3H_8O. Which, if any, have hydrogen-bonding?

11.41*) Hydrogen-bonding is quite important in providing some of the forces that affect proteins. What is the maximum number of hydrogen-bonds that can be formed by one molecule of the amino acid asparagine, shown below.

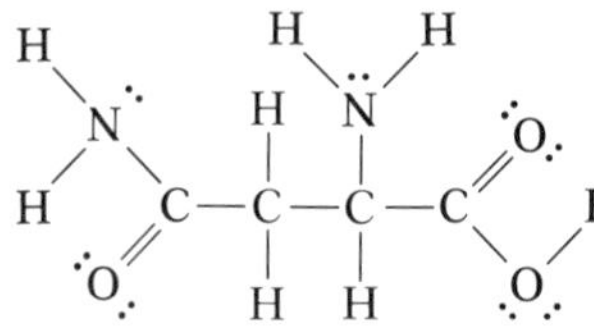

11.42*) In cold climates, water seeps into cracks in roadways and home foundations during winter thaws and then freezes. The result is cracks and potholes. Why?

11.71) Compare the strength of the hydrogen-bonding in liquid H_2O with the strength of the O—H bond in H_2O.

11.72*) In a concentrated ("glacial") solution of acetic acid, CH_3COOH, we find that many individual acetic acid molecules have joined together in *dimers*, each made of two CH_3COOH units. Explain.

11.73*) Many different kinds of compounds could have the molecular formula C_3H_6O. Draw structural formulas of at least three such compounds that have hydrogen-bonding.

11.74*) Hydrogen-bonding is very important in biological systems. Draw dotted lines representing any hydrogen-bonds that can form between the protein fragment shown below (left) and the enzyme portion (right).

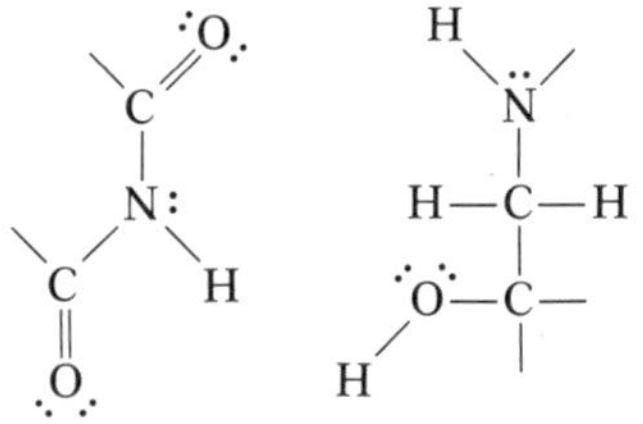

11.75*) Some people hope we can freeze the bodies of cancer victims so that at some future time when a cure is available they can be revived and cured. However, currently known ways of freezing bodies tend to destroy the membranes of brain cells, making revival highly unlikely. Why does freezing destroy cell membranes?

SECTION 11.5 CHANGES OF PHASE

11.43) Why is melting of ice endothermic? How does the air temperature affect the amount of snow that melts in winter?

11.44*) Camphor is a ketone with the molecular formula $C_{10}H_{16}O$. It has many uses in over-the-counter drugs. When camphor "ice" is left on a table, it changes directly from solid

11.76) Why is condensation of dew on grass exothermic? How would formation of dew be affected by the temperature of the air?

11.77*) On a very hot, humid summer day, you may notice the cold water pipes in the basement of a home dripping with water ("sweating"). The same does not happen to gas. What is this process called? Is it endothermic or exothermic?

11.45*) Do you expect water at the bottom of a deep well to boil at a higher or lower temperature than water at the surface? Explain.

SECTION 11.6 SOLIDS

11.46) How does a solid differ from a liquid?

11.47*) Charcoal is amorphous, and diamond is a crystal. Which properties of charcoal are due to the fact it is amorphous?

11.48) Arsenic trichloride, $AsCl_3$, forms needlelike crystals that melt at $-8.5°C$. Do you expect these crystals to be ionic or molecular? Explain.

11.49*) Two solids have the properties described below. Classify each as ionic, molecular, macromolecular, or metallic.
a) melts at 1050°C; dissolves easily in water; forms hard, colorless crystals
b) melts at 2000°C; does not dissolve in water; forms very hard, colorless crystals

11.50*) If you were choosing an alloy to use in making an artificial heart valve, what properties would you seek?

11.51*) Glauber's salt is sodium sulfate decahydrate. It has been used as a cathartic (laxative) and diuretic. However, it may find a more important use as a material that can store heat during the day for release at night and thus save heating fuel. Write the formula of this salt.

11.52*) The compound $FeCl_3·6H_2O$ may be dissolved to give a solution used in a medical test for phenylketonuria. How would you name this crystal? What is its formula weight?

with hot water pipes. Explain what is going on.

11.78*) At what temperature will water boil for yak soup at the top of Mount Everest, where the average air pressure is 0.316 atm? Use Table 11–8.

11.79) How does a molecular solid differ from an ionic solid?

11.80*) Silicon dioxide, SiO_2, may be found in amorphous solids like glass, as well as in quartz crystals. Compare the melting process for a quartz crystal with that for a glass.

11.81) Bismuth trifluoride, BiF_3, forms gray cubic crystals that melt at 727°C. Do you expect these crystals to be ionic or molecular? Explain any differences between BiF_3 and $AsCl_3$ (Problem 11.48).

11.82*) Two solids have the properties described below. Classify each as ionic, molecular, macromolecular, or metallic.
a) melts at 1450°C; conducts electricity very well; does not dissolve in water; may be drawn into a fine wire easily
b) forms a very soft powder that melts at 150°C; does not dissolve easily in water

11.83*) What properties does a dentist seek in an alloy to make a dental bridge between molar teeth? Would pure gold ever be used? Explain.

11.84*) Epsom salt is magnesium sulfate heptahydrate. It has been used as a cathartic and muscle relaxant in medicine, as well as in many industrial applications. Write the formula for Epsom salt.

11.85*) The compound
$$Cu(NO_3)_2·3H_2O$$
may be used to give a blue color to ceramics and as a catalyst. What is the name of this crystal? What is its formula weight?

Write a chemical equation to show that

solutions of hydrochloric acid and silver nitrate may be mixed to give a precipitate of silver chloride

solutions of magnesium iodide and sodium hydroxide may be mixed to give a precipitate of magnesium hydroxide

Explain how a solution containing F^- ions and a solution containing Ca^{2+} ions might be mixed together and have *no* precipitate of CaF_2 formed.

11.86) Write a chemical equation to show that

a) solutions of aluminum nitrate and sodium carbonate may be mixed to give a precipitate of aluminum carbonate

b) solutions of potassium sulfide and zinc acetate may be mixed to give a precipitate that is the same as the zinc sulfide solid used as a phosphor on some television screens

11.87*) Write a chemical equation to show how a crystal of $Ca(OH)_2$ solid can dissolve in a solution of HF, hydrofluoric acid, to give a stable crystal of CaF_2. Explain how this type of process can be used to help strengthen tooth enamel, with reference to Questions 4.26 and 4.51 on page 120.

Solutions abound in nature and are involved in our daily living. The oceans are a water solution of sodium chloride and other dissolved compounds. Even drinking water is a solution, although we may think of it as "pure." Natural "hard" water contains enough calcium and magnesium cations to form solid salt deposits in water pipes. Some other familiar solutions are gasoline, household ammonia, air, and steel.

A solution is one type of mixture, combining at least two different pure substances. Depending on the size of each particle of one substance mixed with a second substance, we may obtain either a mixture with the properties of a colloid or suspension or a mixture with the properties of a true solution.

In this chapter, we will discuss which mixtures are likely to form solutions. We will briefly explore the difficult problems of water pollution and its control. Finally, we will discuss one process that carries water into and out of cells, a process called osmosis.

LEARNING GOAL 12A: Distinguish on the basis of particle size between a solution, a colloid, and a suspension.

12B: Give one example of an aerosol, a sol, a gel, an emulsion, and a foam.

If you drop some nuts into cake batter and bake the result, you will get a nut cake. You can pick out the individual nuts; they have been mixed with the cake batter, but they have not dissolved in it. On the other hand, as you add sugar to a cake batter, it dissolves. You can taste it in the cake, but you cannot pick out individual sugar crystals from the baked product.

The nut cake gives us an example of a **heterogeneous mixture.** If you can pick out individual particles of one substance from those of a different substance, you have such a mixture.

If the substance present in a heterogeneous mixture in the greatest amount (called the *medium*) is not a solid but a liquid or gas, we may have a

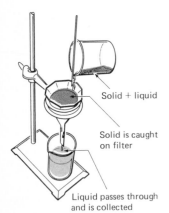

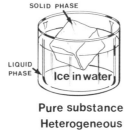

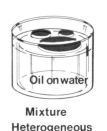

FIGURE 12–2 Two examples of heterogeneous mixtures. Note the different phases (layers) in each case.

FIGURE 12–1 Filtration of a suspension or precipitate.

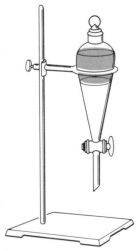

FIGURE 12–3 A separatory funnel may be used to separate a heterogeneous mixture of two liquids.

Remember that 1 cm = 10^8 Å;

$$1 \text{ Å} = \frac{1}{100\,000\,000} \text{ cm} = 10^{-8} \text{ cm}$$

suspension. Smoke is a suspension of solid particles in a gas (air). Muddy water is a suspension of solid particles in a liquid (water). The substances in a suspension can often be separated by *filtration,* as shown in Figure 12–1. Air conditioners filter the air, removing large soot particles and grains of pollen, by passing the air through small spaces in paper or metal screening.

A heterogeneous mixture of a solid in a liquid, such as ice and water, or of two liquids, such as oil and water, will often divide into two pure phases (Figure 12–2).

Heterogeneous mixtures of two liquids can often be separated by *decanting* (pouring off) the top liquid, as you might skim the cream from the top of a bottle of milk fresh from the farm, or by use of a device called a *separatory funnel* to drain off the bottom liquid (Figure 12–3).

A suspension contains particles larger than 1000 Å (10^{-5} cm), which is just below the size visible through an ordinary (light) microscope. In general, a suspension is something that will block light; it is *opaque.* You cannot see through a bottle of milk because the particles are big enough to reflect the light. A thick smoke acts in the same way; you cannot see through it.

Colloids

A *solution* contains very small particles of the "mixed" substance. The particles are so small that the mixing is complete, as when you add sugar to cake batter. The particle size is that of individual, single molecules—usually less than 10 Å in diameter. We will look at the properties of solutions in Section 12.2.

What about dispersions (mixtures) of particles with sizes ranging from 10 Å to about 1000 Å in a gas or liquid medium? These are called **colloids.** Some common colloids are skim milk, fog, gelatin dessert, whipped cream, rain clouds, mayonnaise, and beer.

The particles in colloids are not large enough to settle out of the medium, but they are too small to be filtered. They are not visible to the naked eye, but they are large enough to scatter light more than the extremely small particles in a true solution. When a light beam is passed through colloidal particles in a gas or liquid, the beam of light is often visible from the side (as a beam of sunlight entering a room is visible because it is reflected by the dust particles in the air). This is the **Tyndall effect** (Figure 12–4). It is an accepted way of deciding whether a particular mixture is a colloid or a solution. If it scatters light so that you can see the light beam, it is a colloid.

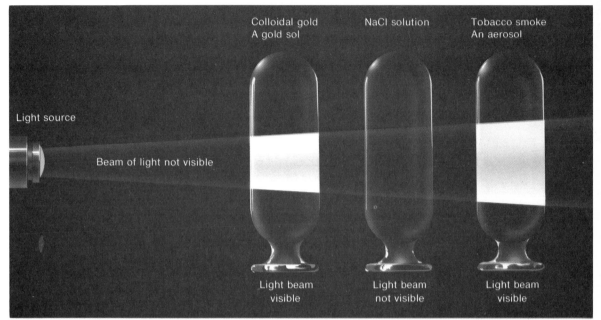

FIGURE 12–4 The presence of colloidal particles is easily detected with the aid of a light beam.

Types of colloids

A colloid may be an aerosol, a sol, a gel, an emulsion, or a foam. For an **aerosol,** the dispersing medium is a gas. The dispersed particles are solid (as in smoke) or liquid (as in fog).

The most common gas medium is air. Mists, fogs, and clouds are aerosols of tiny water droplets in air. A dust cloud may be created when small particles are swept up from the soil to form an aerosol. Such dust clouds may be blown hundreds of miles before the particles are brought down by rain.

An aerosol containing particles that burn can be very dangerous. Air contains more than enough oxygen to support the combustion of such an aerosol. Thus, coal dust in a mine may be easily ignited by a spark; an explosion may result. Similarly, flour mills and grain elevators can be blown apart by such dust explosions.

An electrostatic precipitator can clean particles from a stream of gas (p. 297). Such a device may be used in homes to help persons suffering from pollen allergies by clearing some of the pollen out of the air.

Sols and gels

A **sol** consists of a solid dispersed in a liquid, usually water. Fountain-pen ink and some kinds of paints are sols. Proteins in water (Chapter 19) form a sol of interest to biochemists. Figure 12–5 shows how protein molecules may be separated from ions in a solution by a process called *dialysis*.

Because of the Tyndall effect, automobile drivers should avoid driving in foggy conditions with their "high-beam" headlights on, since the beam will be reflected back into their eyes.

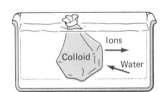

FIGURE 12–5 Dialysis of a protein in water. The special parchment bag has very small holes that permit small ions to pass through but block larger colloidal particles. The ions move through until equal numbers are on both sides of the bag, which reduces the number inside. A series of such processes purifies the protein inside the bag.

Quicksand is a gel of water and sand. It "flows" when someone steps on it.

A **gel** consists of the reverse situation: liquid droplets dispersed in a solid. The familiar gelatin desserts and fruit jellies provide examples. The liquid phase is water. The solid phase is open like a honeycomb in a beehive, so the liquid becomes trapped inside the three-dimensional solid structure and is not free to move. Nondrip paint is a gel that flows when brushed or shaken.

Emulsions and foams

An **emulsion** consists of one liquid dispersed in a second liquid, generally involving a substance that will not dissolve in water and thus forms droplets in water. Milk contains both a sol (proteins in water) and an emulsion (droplets of butterfat in water). Mayonnaise and cream hair oils are emulsions of oils in water. Cold cream is an emulsion of water dispersed in an oil. After application the water evaporates, leaving an oil layer on the skin.

Emulsions will often separate into their original substances if left for a time. They are often stabilized with **emulsifying agents,** which prevent separate layers from forming. Mayonnaise is stabilized by egg yolk and milk by proteins.

A soap molecule (p. 258) has one end that will dissolve in and bond with oil or grease and one end that will dissolve in water. When soap is used for cleaning, the oil connected to one end of the soap molecule is emulsified to make it something that can be washed away. Detergents work the same way. Figure 12–6 shows how detergents act to wash cloth.

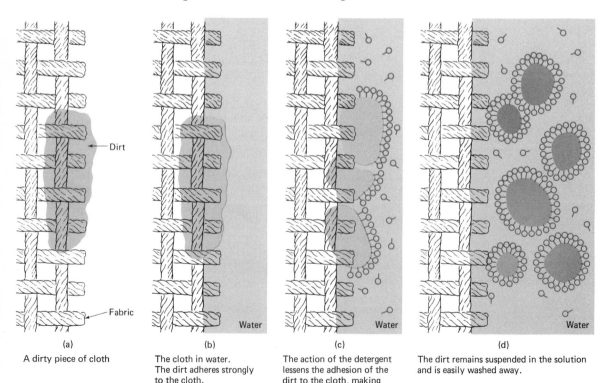

(a)	(b)	(c)	(d)
A dirty piece of cloth	The cloth in water. The dirt adheres strongly to the cloth.	The action of the detergent lessens the adhesion of the dirt to the cloth, making it easier to detach the dirt from the fabric.	The dirt remains suspended in the solution and is easily washed away.

FIGURE 12–6 The action of a detergent in removing dirt from a piece of cloth.

Foams are familiar as soapsuds, shaving cream, whipped cream, meringue, and similar dispersions of *gases* in *solids* or *liquids*.

12.1) Several solids are dispersed in water. Would you classify the dispersion as a solution, colloid, or suspension if the average diameter of the solid particles is
a) 4 Å   b) 155 Å   c) 10^{-6} cm   d) 1 mm
12.2) Classify each of the following dispersions as an aerosol, sol, gel, emulsion, or foam.
a) the head on a glass of beer
b) extremely small pollen grains carried in air
c) dishwater

12.2 SOLUTIONS AND SOLUBILITY

LEARNING GOAL 12C: *Given a common solution, identify the solute and the solvent.*

12D: *Describe how you would prepare an aqueous solution of any common ionic solid that is saturated, unsaturated, or supersaturated.*

12E: *Use Henry's Law to predict how the solubility of a gas in water is affected by a change in the partial pressure of that gas over the solution.*

A **solution** is a special kind of mixture. Earlier, we defined a solution as one in which the average diameter of the dispersed particles is less than 10 Å. The particles of the dispersing medium, such as water, are also roughly of that size. Thus, in a solution, the particles of the substance present in smaller amounts, called the **solute,** can move freely between the particles of the dispersing medium, called the **solvent** (Figure 12–7). Since this mixing process takes place very quickly and thoroughly, the solution has the same composition throughout; it is a **homogeneous mixture.** No matter from where in the solution we take a sample, or how large or small the sample is, it will have the same per cent composition of each element and will have the same color, density, taste, smell, boiling point, and other physical properties.

Homogeneous is from the Greek *homos*, the same.

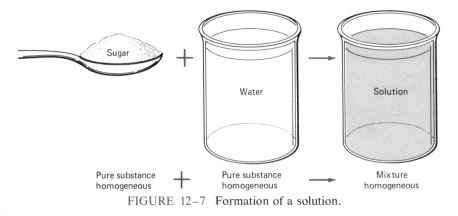

FIGURE 12–7 Formation of a solution.

Unlike a heterogeneous mixture, a solution cannot be divided into its solute and its solvent by any type of filtration or settling process. The properties of a solution are so uniform that you might almost think of it as a pure substance—except for one factor: The relative amounts of solute and solvent can be controlled almost at will. We can thus make a "salt-water" solution that has 1% by weight of NaCl, that is, 1 gram of NaCl in 100 grams of solution. Or we can make it 2%, or 9.5%, or 25%. Each of these amounts of solute per 100 grams of solution will have different physical properties. Each is considered to be at a different **concentration.**

The concentration of solute in a solution is a measure of the amount of solute present in a given amount of solvent or of total solution.

The many different ways of expressing concentration of solute will be discussed in Chapter 14. In this chapter, we will avoid arithmetic as much as possible and concentrate on *why* and *how* solutions have the properties they do.

Nonaqueous solutions

When we speak of a solution, it is usually understood that the solvent is water. Such solutions are inside us (blood, lymph, urine, etc., as described in Chapter 24) and outside us (rain, ocean, juice, and so many others). Most of our discussion will concern these *aqueous* (water) solutions.

However, there are other homogeneous mixtures that must also be considered solutions. First of all, the solvent need not be water, or even a liquid. Any mixture of *gases* is a solution, since all of the particles can move freely among each other and all are already of molecular size. The air we breathe is thus a solution.

The solvent may be a *solid*. The alloys (steel, brass, bronze) that we discussed in Section 11.6 are solutions.

The solvent may be a *liquid other than water*. Many of the common organic compounds we have studied, such as acetone, ether, and hexane, may be used as solvents to dissolve other organic compounds to create *nonaqueous* solutions. In our own bodies, the fats (lipids) discussed in Chapter 18 will dissolve certain organic substances that may be only slightly soluble in the water-based body fluids.

Aqueous solutions

We now turn our attention to solutions in which water is the solvent, which will occupy us for several chapters. Some of these solutions are very familiar to us. For example:

Gases in water. Carbonated water (club soda, "seltzer"), which is the basis of soft drinks, is a solution of CO_2 in water. Fish can survive because sea water and fresh water are solutions of O_2 in water. Household ammonia is a solution of NH_3 gas in water. Chlorine bleach is partially a solution of Cl_2 gas in water.

Liquids in water. Vinegar is a solution of acetic acid in water. Alcoholic beverages are solutions of ethyl alcohol in water. Most types of antifreeze are solutions of ethylene glycol in water.

Ionic solids in water. "Salt water" from the ocean and brine for pickling cucumbers are solutions of NaCl in water. Many drug and medical solutions contain ionic solids dissolved in water.

Covalently bonded solids in water. Solutions of sugar, as an example, contain covalent molecules dissolved in water.

As a general rule, we consider water to be the *solvent* in such solutions and the dissolved gas, liquid, or solid to be the *solute*.

This choice of terms is in line with the way we usually think about solutions. We view CO_2 or NaCl as "dissolving in water," rather than the reverse.

Solubility

The **solubility** of a solute in water is a measure of how much solute we can add to a given amount of water before no more solute will dissolve. The solution is then at equilibrium with undissolved solute. We usually measure solubility in grams of solute dissolved in 100 mL of water at a known temperature.

Near the solubility limit, there are three possibilities. Suppose we add sodium chloride to a glass of water at room temperature (Figure 12–8). As we continue to add NaCl crystals, the concentration of dissolved salt increases. Eventually, we reach a point where, even with stirring, no additional salt will dissolve.* At this stage, we have a **saturated solution** of NaCl. It cannot hold any more solute. The concentration is constant. The amount of NaCl contained in 100 mL of water under these conditions is the measured *solubility* of NaCl in water at room temperature.

---

* In reality, some of the extra crystals will dissolve while some of the dissolved solute will crystallize (precipitate) to form a solid. The total amount of solid remains constant in this *dynamic equilibrium* situation.

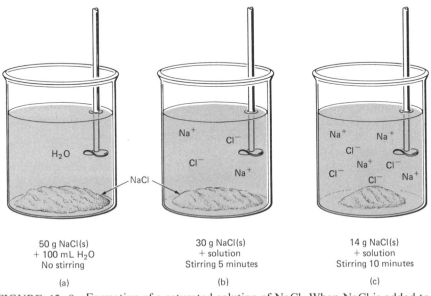

50 g NaCl(s)	30 g NaCl(s)	14 g NaCl(s)	14 g NaCl(s)
+ 100 mL H$_2$O	+ solution	+ solution	+ solution
No stirring	Stirring 5 minutes	Stirring 10 minutes	Stirring 1 hour
(a)	(b)	(c)	(d)

FIGURE 12–8   Formation of a saturated solution of NaCl. When NaCl is added to water, most of the solid goes to the bottom. On stirring, the solid slowly dissolves. After a period of time, the amount in solution becomes constant, and the solution is said to be saturated.

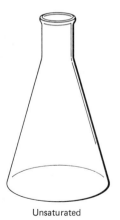

Unsaturated

Any solution that contains less NaCl than the solubility limit is an *unsaturated* solution. An unsaturated solution can accept more solid crystals and will dissolve them.

Under special conditions, usually by cooling a hot saturated solution, we may obtain a solution that contains more dissolved solute than the solubility limit at a given temperature. This is a **supersaturated solution.** It will not remain in that state, because if a speck of dust or a small seed crystal is added, crystallization (formation of solid) occurs until the amount of dissolved solute is down to that of a *saturated* solution.

Two other terms commonly used to indicate in a rough manner the concentration of a solution are *dilute* and *concentrated*. The meanings of these terms for some common laboratory stock reagents will be discussed in Section 13.1.

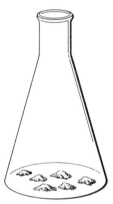

Saturated

You may have noticed that, in a home aquarium, air is continuously bubbled into the water. This maintains the level of oxygen dissolved in the water so that the fish may absorb it through their gills; otherwise, the fish would die.

Solutions of gases in water may be saturated or unsaturated and are easily prepared by bubbling the gas through the water. The solubility or *saturation limit* depends very strongly on two factors:

Temperature. Gases become less soluble in water as the temperature increases. Fish may die if their water supply is warmed up by more than a few degrees (as by the wastewater outlet from a plant producing electricity) because the warmer water contains a lower concentration of dissolved oxygen. An open bottle of beer or soda loses its fizz quickly if it becomes warm.

Partial pressure. The solubility of the gas is partially determined by the partial pressure of the dissolved gas *over* the solution in which it is being dissolved. Figure 12–9 shows how *Henry's Law* applies to gases dissolved in a liquid. A practical effect of this law is that when a soft drink is bottled, some CO_2 escapes from the liquid and fills the space at the top of the bottle. When the bottle is opened, you lose that CO_2 partial pressure over the solution and some CO_2 bubbles out of solution to replace it. If the bottle is left open, eventually all of the CO_2 will bubble out and the drink will go flat. Pressurized containers for shaving cream and whipped cream operate on the same princi-

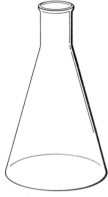

Supersaturated

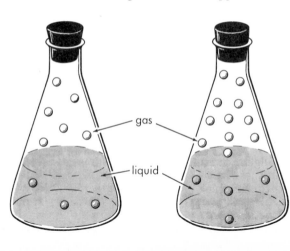

Henry's Law. The effect of the partial pressure of a gas on its solubility in a liquid. The concentration of solute vapor, and therefore its partial pressure, is lower in the flask on the left than in that on the right. Thus, the solution concentration of dissolved gas is lower in the flask on the left.

ple. When the valve is opened, some of the dissolved gas comes out of solution, carrying the liquid with it as a *foam*.

Biochemical oxygen demand

Oxygen from the air dissolves in rivers, lakes, and streams because the constant flow of water brings it into contact with the air. For each million molecules of water, about six molecules of oxygen are dissolved. This comes to roughly 10 grams of oxygen per million grams of water or 10 ppm (parts per million by weight). Ocean water contains only about seven ppm of O_2 because oxygen is less soluble in salt water. Aquatic animals and plants depend on this oxygen supply for life just as we depend on the air we breathe. If the oxygen content is too low, the life forms may not be able to survive.

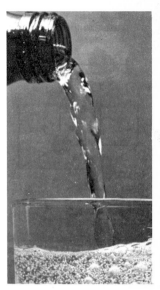

Bubbles of CO_2 come out of a solution of soda water when the pressure drops. (Fredrik D. Bodin/Stock Boston)

Modern industrial processes in the pulp and paper, food, chemical, and other industries have added large amounts of organic waste materials to our lakes and streams. Water-borne bacteria use oxygen to convert this organic material to simple molecules and ions such as carbon dioxide, nitrate ion, and sulfate ion. That's fine for breaking down the wastes! However, in this process the bacteria use up some of the dissolved oxygen. If they use up too much, the oxygen supply is depleted and the organisms dependent on the oxygen will die.

The amount of oxygen needed by the bacteria to convert the waste organic material is measured as the **biochemical oxygen demand,** or **BOD.** The more organic wastes we dump, the greater the BOD. Drinking water has a BOD of 0 to 3. Sewage, containing organic wastes from humans, typically has a BOD of 100 to 400. Some industrial wastes have BOD values in the thousands, which causes severe environmental problems.

Brine is a solution of NaCl and water. Which is the solvent and which is the solute?

The solubility of sodium fluorosilicate, Na_2SiF_6 (often used in water supplies for fluoridation to prevent tooth decay), in 100 mL of water is 2.46 grams in boiling water (100°C) and 0.65 grams in cold water (12°C). Describe how you would prepare a solution of sodium fluorosilicate, using one liter of water, that is

a)   unsaturated   b)   saturated   c)   supersaturated

Fish are swimming in an aquarium with air being bubbled through. Would their oxygen intake be affected if

a)   the nitrogen in the air were replaced by helium, as is sometimes done for air pumped to deep-sea divers?

b)   the air in the tube were at a total pressure of two atm, instead of the (usual) one atm?

c)   the tube were removed and the water became still?

LEARNING GOAL 12F: Given the formula of a solute, predict whether it will be more soluble in water or in a nonpolar organic solvent.

12G: Given a solute that dissolves in water, describe an experiment that will tell you if that solute is a strong electrolyte, a weak electrolyte, or a nonelectrolyte.

Sometimes water is described as the "universal solvent." While water does dissolve many chemical substances, it does not dissolve *everything*. Rainwater does not dissolve a roof, brickwork, an automobile, or a cotton sweater. Wooden boats do not dissolve in the ocean. Common metals, such as aluminum, tin, lead, and the transition metals, do not dissolve in water, although the presence of water often speeds up rusting and corrosion. Most simple organic molecules, such as alkanes, are not soluble in water.

Yet, ionic salts like $NaCl$, alcohols like CH_3OH, carbohydrates like $C_6H_{12}O_6$, and simple organic acids like CH_3COOH do dissolve in water. Why are some compounds soluble in water while others are not?

Solutions of liquids in water

When ethyl alcohol and water are mixed in *any* proportions, they form a homogeneous mixture, a solution. They never form two layers and never form a saturated solution. They are mutually soluble, regardless of the amounts mixed. They are said to be **miscible with** each other.

Miscible is from the Latin **miscere**, *to mix, and thus means* mixable.

Some other liquid pairs, such as diethyl ether and water, are soluble in each other but only in limited amounts. Such liquid pairs are said to be *partially miscible*. They usually form two layers.

If two liquids are insoluble in each other, which in practical terms means that the solubilities are so small that we cannot measure them, we say they are *immiscible*. Oil and water, mercury and water, and carbon tetrachloride and water are three examples of pairs of immiscible liquids that form heterogeneous mixtures as shown in Figure 12–2.

Separation of miscible liquids

If two liquids are mutually soluble and form a homogeneous solution, they may be separated by *fractional distillation*. The separation is based on the difference in boiling point of the two liquids, as shown in Fig. 12–10. The

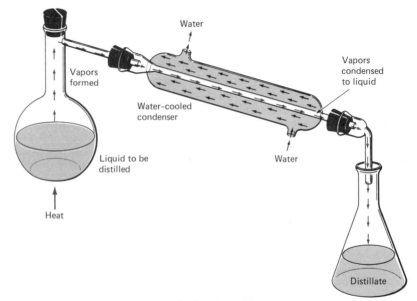

FIGURE 12–10 A simple distillation apparatus.

lower-boiling liquid vaporizes more rapidly. Thus, at the beginning of the distillation, the gases (vapors) coming into the condenser contain more of this component than of the other, higher-boiling, liquid. When the vapors are cooled by the cold water running through the condenser, they turn to a liquid (the *distillate*) that is "enriched" in the lower-boiling liquid. Repeated distillations of this type lead to almost complete separation of the two liquids.

Immiscible liquids form two layers on standing. The complete separation of the two layers is accomplished by a simple piece of laboratory apparatus called a separatory funnel (Figure 12–3).

Fractional distillation on a large scale is used to separate the various hydrocarbons in crude oil to make gasoline and other petroleum products.

Intermolecular attractions and solubility

We noted earlier that alcohol and water are miscible, while carbon tetrachloride and water are immiscible. Why do some organic molecules dissolve in water, while others do not?

In Sections 11.3 and 11.4, you learned that liquids are held together by three major kinds of intermolecular forces: dipole forces (for polar molecules), dispersion (London) forces, and the special kind of dipole attractions called hydrogen-bonding.

Look for a moment at the process of dissolving ethanol in water. To remove an ethanol molecule from the rest of the ethanol liquid, we must break the forces inside the ethanol liquid (largely hydrogen-bonding). To force that molecule into the water, we must push apart the water molecules. We must therefore also break apart the water-to-water forces (very strong hydrogen-bonds) to allow the ethanol molecule in.

These two steps both involve putting energy into the breaking of intermolecular attractions. When the ethanol molecule is finally inside the water, it forms new hydrogen-bonding attractions with the water molecules that surround it. These new attractions *give off* energy and thus make the ethanol molecule more stable in its water environment.

The attraction between solute molecules and water is mainly of two types: ordinary dipole forces and hydrogen-bonding. In practice, the dipole attraction of water for a polar organic solute molecule depends on the number of carbon atoms in the molecule. Only the first few members (one, two, three carbons) of a group of polar organic compounds will be highly soluble. Solubility drops off with increasing number of carbon atoms, so—in the absence of any special features—an organic molecule with more than six carbon atoms is generally insoluble (or immiscible) in water. What kind of "special features" in an organic molecule would increase its water solubility?

Let us consider more closely some compounds that form familiar water solutions. Commercial alcoholic beverages contain ethanol, C_2H_5OH. Automobile antifreeze contains ethylene glycol, $HOCH_2CH_2OH$. Glycerol, $HOCH_2CHOHCH_2OH$, is used in many cosmetics. Vinegar contains acetic acid, CH_3COOH. What do all of these compounds have in common? Inspection of these molecules shows that each contains one or more hydroxyl (—OH) groups. Thus, each of them can hydrogen-bond to water.

Water molecules form hydrogen-bonds among themselves. Organic substances with —OH groups can exchange place with H—OH molecules and form similar attractions, as shown in Figure 12–11. The number of hydroxyl groups has an influence on solubility. Sucrose (table sugar, $C_{12}H_{22}O_{11}$) has eight —OH groups to help it dissolve in water and sweeten desserts.

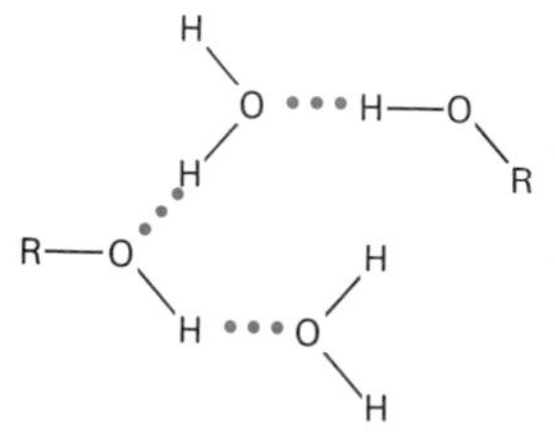

Alcohol in water

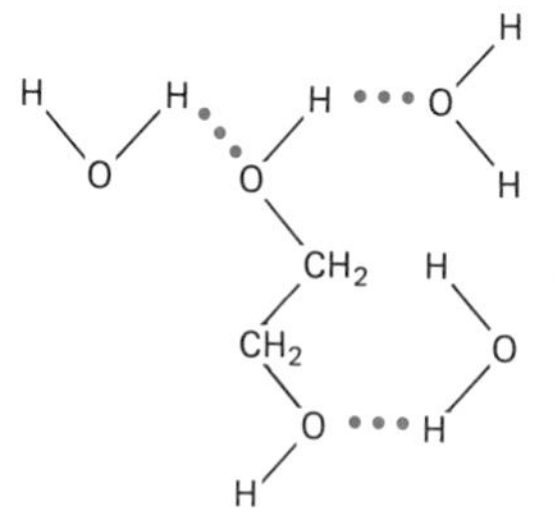

Ethylene glycol in water

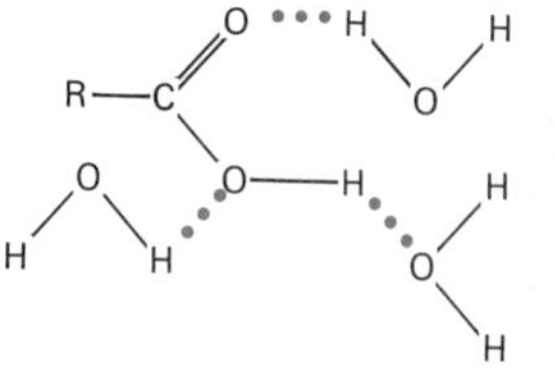

Carboxylic acid in water

FIGURE 12–11   Hydrogen-bonding is the major factor in water solubility of an organic compound.

Nonpolar solvents

Carbon tetrachloride, CCl_4, is immiscible with water. Why? Because it is not polar, so there is very little attraction between it and water. On the other hand, the dispersion forces between two molecules of CCl_4, although relatively strong, are quite similar to the dispersion forces between other nonpolar organic molecules, and between the CCl_4 molecule and molecules of a nonpolar solvent surrounding it. Thus, if CCl_4 is placed in the nonpolar solvent octane, C_8H_{18}, it will dissolve.

As a general rule,

Nonpolar compounds will dissolve only in nonpolar solvents.

Another way of saying the same thing is "Like dissolves like."

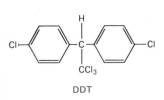

DDT

The very damaging biological effects of the insecticide DDT are due largely to its ability to dissolve in (nonpolar) fats but not in water. Once DDT is deposited in the soil, perhaps as part of a mosquito spraying program to prevent malaria, it is washed (undissolved) into rivers, lakes, and streams. There, it contaminates the food eaten by birds, fish, and other forms of life. Since it is soluble in lipids (nonpolar fats), it is stored in fatty tissue and nerve tissues and may interfere with metabolism or reproductive processes.

Even if lower animals are relatively unaffected by the DDT, birds and mammals eating them will concentrate the DDT in their own tissues. One result has been bird eggs with shells too thin to survive. As some of these animals become part of the food chain, DDT is consumed by humans and may pose long-term health problems. Furthermore, DDT is not **biodegradable,** that is, it stays as DDT for many years. For these reasons, DDT use is banned in the United States, although it is still used in many parts of the world where malaria and rats pose immediate health threats.

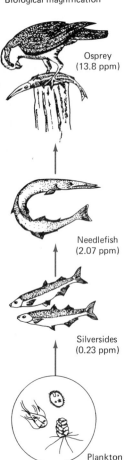

Biological magnification

Osprey
(13.8 ppm)

Needlefish
(2.07 ppm)

Silversides
(0.23 ppm)

Plankton
(0.04 ppm)

DDT in a food chain

Aqueous solutions of ionic solids

The vast majority of everyday compounds that are soluble in water are inorganic ionic salts. Let us examine the detailed process of dissolving an ionic solid and see how we can make predictions about which salts will dissolve and which will not.

What happens when a crystal of sodium chloride dissolves in water? You see only the solid disappearing and a clear solution afterwards. What really happened to the very small units? Did they form smaller and smaller NaCl crystals, or did they dissolve as Na^+ cations and Cl^- anions?

Three things actually happen when NaCl dissolves in water. The NaCl crystal consists entirely of Na^+ ions and Cl^- ions. The positively charged Na^+ ions at the surface of the crystal are attracted by the partial negative charge on the oxygen atoms of the water molecules, as shown in Figure 12–12. The Cl^- ions in the crystal are attracted to the hydrogen atoms of the water. A "tug of war" results between the water molecule pulling ions "out" and the other ions in the crystal trying to keep the ions "in."

We earlier referred to three forces that must balance if we are to dissolve an organic liquid molecule in water. A similar set of three forces operates for the dissolving of an ionic crystal in water. The forces holding ions in a crystal are *much stronger* than those holding C_2H_5OH in the liquid, as you can tell from the melting points (1413°C for NaCl, −117°C for ethanol). The ionic bonds tend to keep an ionic salt from dissolving.

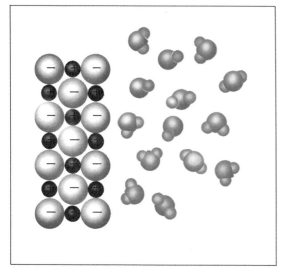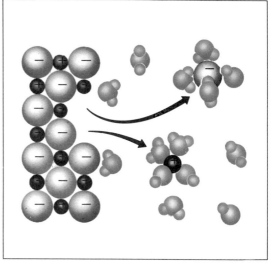

FIGURE 12–12. The process of dissolving an ionic solid in water.

When an ion dissolves in water by separating from the surface of the crystal, it is surrounded by water molecules, as shown in Figure 12–13. If the ion is a cation, such as K^+, each water molecule has its oxygen atom closest to the ion. If it is an anion, such as Cl^- or S^{2-}, then the hydrogen atoms point towards the ion to obtain the maximum attractive force. This process is called **hydration.** It gives off tremendous amounts of energy.

The dissolving process is reversible. If we have a saturated solution, the number of ions forming solid crystals in any period of time will be equal to the number dissolving in the solvent. We have a situation of dynamic equilibrium. Figure 12–14 shows how the amount of solid in solution builds up to the saturation point, after which the system is in equilibrium.

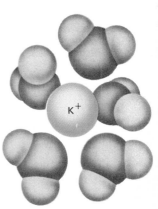

FIGURE 12–13 Water molecules surround K^+ ions in solution.

If water is not the solvent, this process is called by its general name, *solvation*. Hydration is also discussed in Section 11.6 on solids.

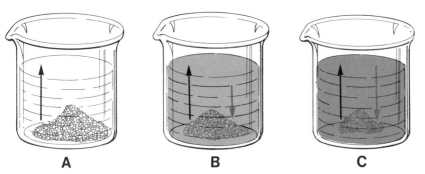

A   **B**   **C**

FIGURE 12–14 Development of equilibrium in producing a saturated solution. The solute dissolves at a constant rate, shown by the black arrows. In A, when dissolving has just begun, the solute concentration in the solvent is zero, so no crystallization can occur. In B, the solute concentration has risen to yield a crystallization rate indicated by the colored arrow—still less than the dissolving rate. Eventually, in C, the concentration has increased to the point where the dissolving and crystallization rates are equal. Equilibrium has been reached, and the solution is saturated.

Pressure has almost no effect on the solubility of solids and liquids in water.

Temperature plays an important role in the solubility of most ionic salts, for reasons which will be clearer after you read Chapter 21. Generally, solubility goes up with increasing temperature, but there are exceptions.

Solubility rules for ionic solutes

Since the dissolving of an ionic solute requires that we break the ions out of the crystal lattice, the forces holding the lattice together become very important. The attraction between a 1+ charge and a 1− charge is less than that between a 1+ charge and a 2− charge, which in turn is less than the force between 2+ and 2−. A practical result is that almost all compounds containing cations with 1+ charge (Li^+, Na^+, K^+, and NH_4^+, in particular) are soluble, and almost all compounds containing anions with 1− charge (NO_3^-, Cl^-, Br^-, I^-, CH_3COO^-, CN^-, etc.) are soluble. There are many exceptions to these general ideas; for example, compounds of the silver ion, Ag^+, the hydroxide ion, OH^-, and the fluoride ion, F^-, are largely insoluble.

As you can see, it is not easy to predict solubility because several factors are involved. Table 12–1 gives some general rules that, although there are a number of exceptions, will serve to predict the properties of most of the compounds you are likely to meet in everyday chemistry.

TABLE 12–1 SOME SIMPLE SOLUBILITY RULES FOR IONIC SOLUTES

With rare exceptions, an ionic salt is soluble in water if it contains

Na^+	Cl^-
K^+	Br^-
NH_4^+	I^-
NO_3^-	CH_3COO^-

and insoluble (will not dissolve) if it contains

Ag^+	Pb^{2+}

If none of the above ions are in the compound, then the following ions tend to make an ionic salt *insoluble:*

CO_3^{2-}	PO_4^{3-}
F^-	S^{2-}
OH^-	

Electrolytes

When we dissolve an ionic salt in water, we create a solution that contains hydrated cations and anions. These ions can, with their accompanying water molecules, move freely through the solution. Such a solution will conduct an electric current, as shown in Figure 12–15(a). A solid solute whose

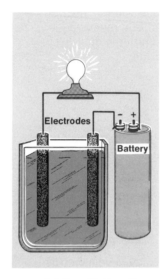
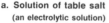

a. Solution of table salt
(an electrolytic solution)

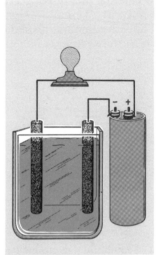

b. Solution of table sugar
(a nonelectrolytic solution)

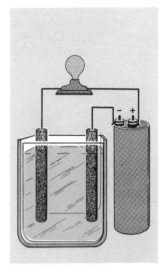

c. Pure water
(a nonelectrolyte)

FIGURE 12–15 Electrolytes and nonelectrolytes. (a) NaCl solution conducts electricity, as shown by the glowing light bulb. NaCl is an electrolyte. (b) Sugar solution does not conduct electricity, so the bulb does not glow. Sugar is a nonelectrolyte. (c) Pure water does not conduct electricity; it is a nonelectrolyte. Therefore the light bulb does not glow.

aqueous solution is a good conductor of electricity is called a **strong electrolyte.** The crystals of a strong electrolyte break up completely into ions when dissolved in water.

Some solutes when dissolved in water form few cations and anions, remaining mostly in molecular form. These solutes are *weak electrolytes*. Their aqueous solutions will conduct electricity, but to a far lesser extent than a strong electrolyte. The light bulb shown in Figure 12–15 would light up for a solution of vinegar (acetic acid, CH_3COOH), but only dimly.

Pure water does not conduct electricity, according to our test for conductivity using a light bulb. That makes it a *nonelectrolyte,* a substance that does not ionize appreciably, as shown in Figure 12–15(c). When table sugar is added to water, it dissolves, but the bulb does not light up, as shown in Figure 12–15(b). This organic compound, like most organic compounds, is a *nonelectrolyte.* Solutions of nonelectrolytes contain molecules of both solute and solvent, but few if any ions.

In summary: An *electrolyte* is a solute that when dissolved conducts electricity by means of its cations and anions. The terms *strong* and *weak* refer to high and low degrees of ionization. Solutions of nonelectrolytes consist of neutral molecules.

Body fluids contain cations, mostly Na^+, K^+, Ca^{2+}, and Mg^{2+}, and anions, such as HCO_3^-, Cl^-, HPO_4^{2-}, $H_2PO_4^-$, SO_4^{2-}, carboxylate anions, and protein. These electrolytes maintain a delicate balance in the blood plasma and other body fluids. It is important to maintain this *electrolyte balance* in the body because serious health problems may result if various concentrations are changed beyond narrow limits.

> The term *electrolyte* is also used occasionally to refer to a *solution* that conducts electricity, that is, a solution of a strong electrolyte.

> Pure water does ionize, but only to the extent of one part in ten million, as discussed in Section 13.1.

SELF-CHECK

12.6)   For each of the following solutes, predict if its solubility will be higher in water or in hexane. Give a brief explanation for your answer in each case.

a) KBr   b) CH_4 c) HF   d) Cl_2
e) NF_3 f) CH_3OCH_3 g) $CH_3(CH_2)_8CH_2OH$
h) CH_3CHO i) C_2Cl_6

12.7)   You are given three white powders, any of which may be dissolved in water. One is a strong electrolyte, one is a weak electrolyte, and one is a nonelectrolyte. What apparatus would you need and how would you use it to match each powder with its correct category of electrolyte?

12.4 WATER POLLUTION AND PURIFICATION

> *LEARNING GOAL 12H: List three major sources of water pollution.*
>   *12I: Describe briefly how a water treatment plant might remove a pollutant from water used for drinking.*
>   *12J: Describe one method for softening hard water.*
>   *12K: Describe a way to obtain drinking water from sea water.*

Water is the most abundant compound in our environment. It is more widely distributed on the surface of the earth and in the tissues of living orga-

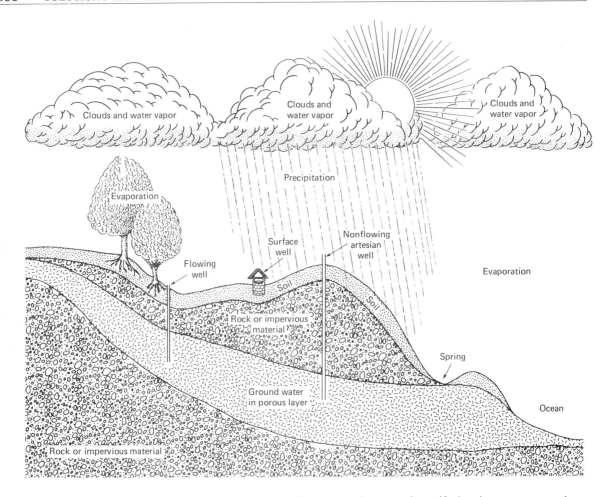

In nature's water cycle, water is purified as it evaporates and returns to earth. Exposure of flowing water to air helps remove organic liquids and gases. Solid material settles to the bottom of waterways or is filtered out as the water passes through layers of sand and rock. Oxidation by bacteria removes some organic material. Before people came along to overwhelm this purification system, it worked very well.

nisms than any other chemical substance. Water is a natural resource that is constantly being renewed by the *water cycle* (Figure 12–16). This cycle moves water to various parts of the earth and also purifies the water by evaporating it into the air and separating it from any solute impurities.

The rainwater that falls to earth is thus very pure unless it is mixed with pollutants (smoke, soot, etc.) in the air. Various natural purification processes also clean the water of springs, streams, and rivers. Thus, before extensive contamination by people, natural cleansing processes provided water pure enough to safeguard the environment for different life forms.

CLASSES OF WATER POLLUTANTS AND SOME EXAMPLES

1. Oxygen-demanding wastes	Plant and animal material
2. Infectious agents	Bacteria and viruses
3. Plant nutrients	Fertilizers, such as nitrates and phosphates
4. Organic chemicals	Pesticides, such as DDT, and detergent molecules
5. Other minerals and chemicals	Acids from coal mine drainage; inorganic chemicals, such as iron from steel plants
6. Sediment from land erosion	Clay silt (on stream bed may reduce or even destroy life forms living there)
7. Radioactive substances	Waste products from mining and processing of radioactive material; radioactive isotopes after use
8. Heat from industry	Cooling water used in steam generation of electricity

In recent years, increases in the human population and in the industrial waste of our technology-based society have strained the natural purification system to and beyond its limits. Fish kills resulting from "acid rain" (p. 376) have been reported hundreds of miles from the smokestacks that produced the SO_2 pollutants responsible. Oil slicks and pesticides have damaged water life. Heat pollution and oxygen depletion are also to blame. Contamination with heavy metals, such as mercury, has injured humans as well as wildlife.

All sources of contamination to our water supply are *pollutants*. A pollutant is a substance that makes water unfit for drinking, unfit to support aquatic life, or unfit for any other specific purpose. Table 12-2 lists some types of water pollutants.

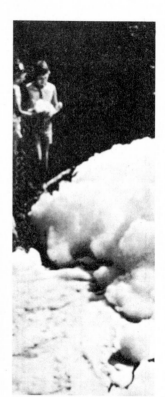

To eliminate the soap scum caused by the reaction of soap with Ca^{2+} and Mg^{2+} ions in hard water, a new type of cleaner was developed, a detergent, which is a branched-chain sulfonic acid derivative:

$$CH_3-CH-CH_2-CH-CH_2-CH-CH_2-CH \underset{}{\bigcirc} -SO_3^{\ominus} Na^{\oplus}$$
$$\quad\ \ |\qquad\quad |\qquad\quad |\qquad\quad |$$
$$\quad CH_3\quad\ \ CH_3\quad\ \ CH_3\quad\ \ CH_3$$

This type of detergent is not biodegradable. It cannot be broken down into simpler soluble molecules by the bacteria in rivers and streams. The result is buildup of foam in natural waters. Chemists have found that continuous-chain detergent molecules eliminate the foam since they can be attacked by bacteria:

$$CH_3CH_2CH_2CH_2CH_2CH_2CH_2CH_2CH_2CH_2CH_2CH_2OSO_3^-Na^+$$

In addition to sulfonic acid derivatives, modern laundry and dishwasher detergents often contain large amounts of a sodium phosphate, $Na_5P_3O_{10}$, to improve washing action and to bleach and brighten dishes or clothes. More than a quarter of a million tons of phosphorus is dumped yearly into U.S. waterways in the form of phosphates. This poses a special pollution problem because green plant life, algae, grow rapidly in solutions containing phosphate and can "choke off" a waterway.

Foam in natural waters. A high concentration of detergent materials dissolved in water causes foam because of the lowered surface tension of the water. If the water is badly polluted, the foam may exist miles from the pollution source. (From Singer, S.F., "Federal interest in estuarine zones builds," *Environmental Science and Technology*, Vol. 3, p. 2, 1969.)

Fertilizers

Fertilizers contain large amounts of phosphate, which is carried off the fields and into rivers to add to the problem just discussed. They also contain nitrates, which may add to the algae growth.

Nitrates in drinking water present an additional hazard. The nitrate ion, NO_3^-, is reduced in the human body to nitrite ion, NO_2^-. Nitrite destroys the ability of hemoglobin to transport oxygen to the cells. High nitrate concentrations in drinking water are thus particularly dangerous to small infants. Unfortunately, the usual procedures used to purify city water supplies do not remove nitrates, so attention must be paid to the lowering of nitrate levels in runoff from fields.

Heavy metals and industrial waste

Many industries produce large amounts of highly poisonous waste products that include cyanide ions, acids, bases, heavy metal ions, oils, dyes, and organic solvents.

Heavy metal ions, such as those of mercury, lead, arsenic, cadmium, chromium, copper, and zinc, are found in varying amounts as waste products of industrial processes. In more than trace amounts, these metal ions are toxic (Table 12-3).

The major source of lead pollution in waterways has been lead tetraethyl, $Pb(C_2H_5)_4$, added to gasoline and emitted by automobiles into the atmosphere. This has, of course, been in addition to the lead ion pollution from industrial sources, such as some pigments for paints.

Arsenic is a poison famous from murder mysteries. The recent use of a lead arsenate, $Pb_3(AsO_4)_2$, spray to kill insects has managed to contaminate natural waters with both lead ion and arsenic in one blow.

Mercury

Of all types of heavy metal ion pollution, that of mercury has received the most attention. Yet, we know that mercury is not always poisonous; you probably have some mercury in your mouth as part of dental fillings. The

TABLE 12–3   TOXIC TRACE ELEMENTS IN THE ENVIRONMENT

Element	Major Sources	Effects on Humans
Arsenic	Coal burning, impurity in phosphates, processing of sulfide ores	Large doses cause gastrointestinal disorders; even small quantities may be carcinogenic
Beryllium	Coal burning, nuclear fuel processing, some rocket fuels	Long exposure even at low levels causes lung damage, often fatal
Cadmium	Electroplating wastes, impurity in all products containing Zn	Low levels (0.2 mg/day) cause hypertension; degenerative bone disease at high levels
Lead	Leaded gasolines, paints	Nausea, irritability at low levels; large doses cause brain damage
Mercury	Electrochemical industry, certain fungicides	Large doses of organic Hg compounds cause brain damage, often fatal

mercury liquid used in thermometers is not very harmful if swallowed, as might happen if an oral thermometer broke. For a long time there was very little concern about mercury pollution.

Of 10 000 tons of mercury mined each year, half is somehow released into the environment after industrial use, largely in factories that produce chlorine gas. The major problem is not the emission of liquid mercury, but a product that is synthesized by the bacteria in the mud of river bottoms. They convert the Hg to the very poisonous substance dimethylmercury, $Hg(CH_3)_2$ (similar to lead tetraethyl), and to methylchloromercury, $HgCH_3Cl$.

The dimethylmercury is concentrated by the food chain. It may end up in humans in several ways, but most obviously by eating fish which are contaminated, as discussed on p. 70.

Water treatment

Let us briefly consider how a municipal water treatment plant purifies the water that comes to homes. Figure 12–17 outlines the operation of such a plant. The water intake from a lake, river, or reservoir is pumped into a *sedimentation* tank where suspended solids settle out. Colloidal particles do not settle out. They are removed by adding aluminum sulfate, $Al_2(SO_4)_3$, which reacts with the water to produce a gel-type solid that traps the colloidal particles and pulls them down.

The water from the settling tanks is then *filtered*, often by letting the water trickle through a sand layer, to remove any remaining particles. Then the water is *aerated* by spraying it into the air. This helps oxidize any dissolved organic matter, since bacteria in the aeration tank can degrade fats, proteins, and sugars.

After aeration, the water is still loaded with bacteria. Chlorine gas (or, in a few cases, ozone gas) is added to kill the bacteria so that the water is fit to drink.

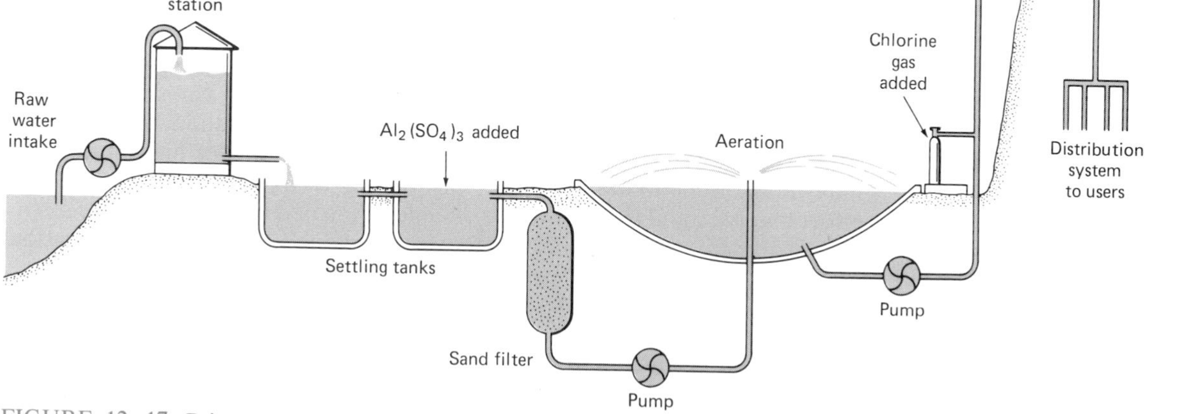

FIGURE 12–17 Primary water purification removes particles that will settle or can be filtered, usually by sand-bed filters. Aeration adds oxygen and gets rid of gases, and chlorination kills microbes.

Fluoridation

In Section 3.4, you learned that a small concentration of F^- ion in drinking water can make teeth more resistant to decay. Thus, many communities add small levels of NaF or Na_2SiF_6 to drinking water in order to improve the dental health of local children. The level of the F^- ion used in the water is important, however, because excessive levels can cause discoloring and brittleness in the tooth enamel. There is no scientific evidence that, in the levels used for water treatment, fluoridation presents any hazard to public health.

Hard and soft water

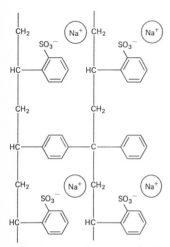

Structure of a synthetic cation exchange resin. The Na^+ ions readily change places with Ca^{2+} or Mg^{2+} ions when hard water is passed through the resin. The resin is manufactured as small beads packed in a tube.

Ordinary water treatment does not remove dissolved inorganic substances, particularly salts of Ca^{2+} and Mg^{2+}. If these two ions are present in large concentrations, we have **hard water.** Such water is perfectly safe to drink and to use for almost any purpose. However, it is annoying because it forms precipitates with soap. In addition, when hard water is boiled, it forms *scale* as salts such as limestone, $CaCO_3$, deposit on the sides of coffee pots, pipes, and water boilers. This not only wastes fuel but also eventually corrodes the metal.

The principal home method of removing Ca^{2+} and Mg^{2+} ions from hard water is to use a cation *exchange resin* (water softener). The Ca^{2+} and Mg^{2+} ions are trapped in the resin, which keeps them in preference to Na^+ ions, which are released into the water. The overall process is

$$2\,Na^+ \cdot resin^-_{(s)} + Ca^{2+}_{(aq)} \longrightarrow Ca^{2+} \cdot (resin^-)_{2(s)} + 2\,Na^+_{(aq)}$$

After the resin, usually a mineral called *zeolite,* has been used for some time, the ''holes'' become filled with Ca^{2+} ions and no further ''softening'' of water will occur. The column can be regenerated by flushing it with salt water brine. The reaction in the above equation is reversed, and the resin is ready to use again.

Fresh water from ocean water

In some very dry parts of the world and in sea research stations, the most economical way to obtain fresh water is to purify salt water. Removal of dissolved NaCl, called **desalination,** is generally very expensive and is used where there is no freshwater spring or stream and very little rain.

College laboratories often use an ion-exchange method similar to that described for water-softening to obtain **deionized water** of high purity. The major limitations to the use of deionization on a large scale are the time and effort involved and the cost of the chemicals needed to regenerate the resins. This process is only useful for water that contains very small concentrations of NaCl.

Electrodialysis involves attracting cations to a negatively charged plate and anions to a positively charged plate, using thin walls or *membranes* between compartments to make sure that the ions do not mix easily with the purified water in the middle. For this purpose, semipermeable membranes are chosen that will pass only selected solute particles. Such *dialyzing* membranes are also used for artificial kidneys (Figure 12–23). Electrodialysis may be used on a small scale to make pure water from salt water. However,

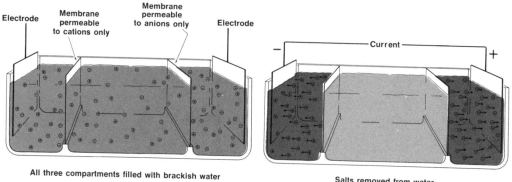

Electrodialysis. All three compartments are filled with salt water. Putting charges on the electrodes causes cations to move to the left, attracted by the negative electrode, and anions to move to the positive electrode. The salt is thus removed from the center area.

this method does not remove dissolved organic substances and is not practical for solving drinking water problems.

Reverse osmosis

A more promising method for large-scale water purification is **reverse osmosis**, using a **semipermeable membrane.**

Such a membrane is a thin wall of material such as cellophane or a piece of parchment paper that allows water molecules to pass through it. The holes or pores in the osmotic membrane are small enough to block *all* solute particles from crossing over (Figure 12–18), unlike a dialyzing membrane which allows some solute particles through but not others.

Osmosis, to be discussed in Section 12.5, works by allowing water to flow from the side of a semipermeable membrane with lower solute concentration to the side with the greater level of solute. Reverse osmosis applies pressure to a concentrated solution, such as sea water, to force pure water through the pores in the membrane and into a collection area, as shown in Figure 12–19. The Na^+ and Cl^- ions (as well as other dissolved matter) of sea water cannot pass through the pores and thus remain in the original compartment.

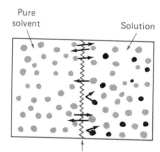

Rigid membrane, permeable to solvent molecules, ⬤ but impermeable to solute particles, ●

FIGURE 12–18 A semipermeable membrane allows solvent to pass in both directions, but acts as a wall that prevents solute (black dots) from passing through.

12.8)   How do exhaust emissions from automobiles using leaded gasolines contribute to heavy metal pollution of our lakes and rivers?

12.9)   Why does a water treatment plant spray the water into the air before it is allowed to come into contact with the bacteria that degrade organic wastes?

12.10)   How does a home water softener work?

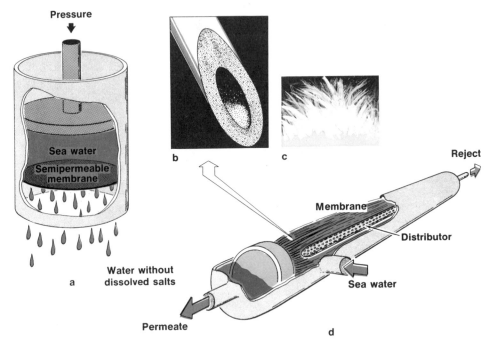

FIGURE 12–19 Reverse osmosis. (a) Mechanical pressure forces water against osmotic pressure to region of pure water. (b) Enlargement of individual membrane. (c) Mass of many membranes. (d) Industrial unit; feed water (salt) that passes through membranes collects at left end (permeate). The more concentrated salt solution flows out to the right as the reject.

12.5 OSMOSIS AND LIVING CELLS

> *LEARNING GOAL 12L: Describe two situations in which osmosis is important to biological systems.*
>
> *12M: Describe the effect on a living cell of immersion in an isotonic solution, a hypertonic solution, and a hypotonic solution.*

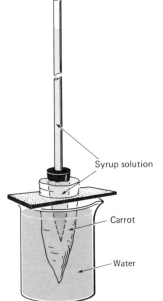

FIGURE 12–20 A simple osmosis experiment involving a carrot and maple syrup.

Osmosis is of vital importance to many plant and animal life processes. It explains how trees take in water through their roots, how cucumbers can be "pickled," how ham can be protected from bacteria by curing it in salt or sugar, and how we sense our own thirst.

Cell membranes in our bodies (Section 18.3) form selective walls, which allow some substances through but not others. Osmosis is the flow of solvent through a semipermeable membrane, such as a cell membrane, from a dilute solution to one that is more concentrated.

Let us consider a very simple experiment, one that you might even be able to do in your home. A carrot is hollowed out and filled with maple syrup, as shown in Figure 12–20. The hole at the top of the carrot is plugged tightly with a stopper containing a clear straw or glass tube. The carrot is then placed in a jar of water.

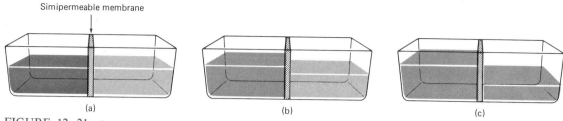

FIGURE 12–21 Osmosis. In (a) the solution on the left has a concentration twice that of the solution on the right. In (b) the solvent flows from right to left, and in (c) the concentrations are equal.

As time passes, the syrup *rises* into the straw so that you can see it. The water level in the glass jar drops. Water has passed through the carrot into the maple syrup, and the syrup has risen against the force of gravity!

A very simple laboratory picture of osmosis is shown in Figure 12–21. Again you will note that the level rises where the solution is more concentrated in solute, indicating that water has passed through the semipermeable membrane. There seems to be some force that makes water enter and *dilute* the more concentrated solution until the hydrostatic pressure simply keeps the water out.

At the point at which equilibrium is reached, the hydrostatic pressure of the maple syrup in the straw in Figure 12–20 or the extra height of solution on the left side of Figure 12–21(c) keeps more water from passing through the membrane.* This pressure, the pressure that *prevents* further osmosis, is defined as the **osmotic pressure** of the original concentrated solution.

From repeated experimentation, we know that the osmotic pressure does not depend on the kind of solute but only on the number of solute particles in the given amount of solution. This will be discussed in greater detail in Section 14.2.

The osmotic pressure of a maple syrup solution will depend on the number of sugar molecules. However, the osmotic pressure of a saline solution, NaCl in water, will depend on the total number of particles, including both Na^+ cations and Cl^- anions. Thus, if we dissolve 10^{-3} moles of NaCl in water, we will have almost twice the osmotic pressure as with 10^{-3} moles of sugar dissolved in the same amount of water.

When osmosis occurs, the flow of water is from a region of low solute concentration (greater water concentration) to one of high solute concentration (less water). The osmotic pressures of two solutions can be related to each other in three possible ways:

Isotonic. The solutions are **isotonic** if they have equal osmotic pressures, thus equal concentrations of particles.

Hypertonic. Suppose we are interested in the effect of putting a body cell (containing its own fluid) into a solution. If the osmotic pressure of the solution is *greater than* that of the cell fluid, the solution is **hypertonic** with respect to the cell fluid. Water will drain out of the cell in order to dilute the outside solution.

Hypotonic. If, on the other hand, the outside solution has an osmotic pressure *less than* that of the cell fluid, then the solution is **hypotonic** with

Isotonic comes from the Greek *isos*, which means equal. Other uses are *iso*tope, *iso*mer, and *iso*electronic. Hypertonic is from the Greek *hyper*, over or above, as in *hyper*active, *hyper*thyroid, *hyper*ventilate. Hypotonic is from the Greek *hypo*, under, as in *hypo*dermic (under the skin) and *hypo*ventilate. It generally means the opposite of *hyper*.

---

* More accurately, since a dynamic equilibrium has been reached, water is passing through the membrane in *both* directions at the *same* rate.

H$_2$O

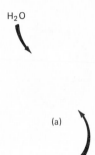

(a)

(b)

H$_2$O

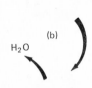

(c)

In a hypotonic solution (a), a cell swells and contents become more dilute. In an isotonic solution (b), the cell stays the same size. In a hypertonic solution (c), the cell loses its water and shrinks.

respect to the cell fluid. In that case, water will flow from the solution into the cell.

These three terms are illustrated in Figure 12–22. The cell shown could represent a sea urchin suddenly placed in water with a different concentration of NaCl (as in fresh water), or more relevant to the chapters you will be reading soon on human biochemistry, the cell could be a red blood cell.

If red blood cells are put into water, they begin to swell. Water passes through the cell wall (membrane) to dilute the more concentrated cell fluid, so the cell gets larger. When the walls finally reach their stretching limit, the cell bursts. When red blood cells break in a *hypotonic* solution such as pure water, the process is called *hemolysis*.

In contrast, if red blood cells are placed in a concentrated brine (NaCl) solution, water flows out of the cell into the solution and the cell gets smaller. This process of shrinking and eventually shriveling up in a *hypertonic* environment is called *crenation*.

In many clinical situations, fluids and nutrients are added to the body by intravenous injection. It is extremely important that each injected fluid be *isotonic* with the blood plasma and the red blood cells. Otherwise, hemolysis or crenation could occur and possibly cause serious harm to the patient.

A special NaCl solution that is isotonic with blood is generally used to replace body fluids. It is called *physiological saline* solution and contains about 0.9% NaCl. To prevent shock after operations, a 5.5% glucose solution is usually fed into a vein; this, too, is isotonic with blood.

Osmotic pressure is also important in the plant world, since all living cell walls serve as semipermeable membranes. Trees take up water from the ground by the osmotic flow of water through root cells into the concentrated sap solution. Flowers should be put in fresh water if they are to last. If they are put into salt water, they will wilt as the water is lost from their cells.

The food industry contains many interesting applications of osmosis. Pickles shrivel as they are kept in brine because they lose water to the hypertonic environment; the skin of your fingers may similarly wrinkle if you take a long swim in salt water. Dehydrated fruit, such as prunes, will swell and become plump if placed in water, since the water flows through the skin to dilute the solution inside the prune. For similar reasons, salt-water and fresh-water fish are generally limited to their own waterways.

In the human body, water sometimes tends to flow from the bloodstream into cells and tissues, creating edema, or pass by osmosis in the opposite direction, creating dehydration. The role of the kidneys is to regulate this *water balance* by retaining or excreting urine. The kidneys also contain semipermeable membranes that remove waste organic products from the bloodstream through dialysis. When the kidneys do not function, the blood must be cleansed by a process called *hemodialysis*, as shown in Figure 12–23. The detailed role of the kidneys is described in Section 24.3.

In some clinical situations, a doctor might prescribe that a patient drink a lot of water. Explain why this is done, in terms of osmotic pressure.

When a fresh-water fish is placed in salt water, its body will shrivel and wrinkle and it will (with a few exceptions) die of dehydration. Explain.

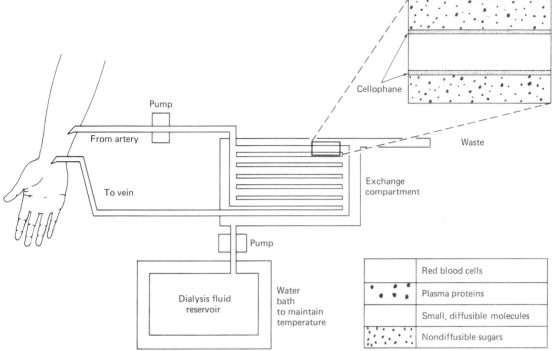

Diagram of an artificial kidney machine. Blood flows between sheets of cellophane (supported on plastic, not shown here). Dialysis fluid, warmed to body temperature, contains normal blood nutrients plus nondiffusible table sugar. The latter helps draw excess water from the blood. Na^+, urea, ammonia, H^+, and other wastes diffuse from blood to dialysis fluid.

LEARNING GOAL 12N: Describe the effect on the boiling or freezing point of water if an ionic or covalent solid is dissolved in it to form a solution.

In Section 12.5 it was noted that the osmotic pressure of a solution depends only on the number of particles contained in a given amount of solution and not on the particular substance used as solute. Several other properties of liquid solutions show a similar dependence on the number of particles present. We call these the **colligative properties** of a solution.

Although we will only discuss aqueous solutions here, these characteristics hold for any solvent.

A pure liquid has certain physical properties, as described in Chapter 11, such as vapor pressure at a given temperature, boiling point at 1 atm pressure, and freezing (melting) point. Adding solute molecules affects these properties in a way that depends only on how many particles are added. We wish to predict the kind of effect the solute will have in a water solution.

Boiling point

The boiling point of a solvent in an open container is the temperature at which its vapor pressure is equal to atmospheric pressure, as described on p. 327. At that point, the liquid will (given enough heat) continue to boil until it has all been converted to vapor. Below that temperature, some of the liquid will evaporate, but it will not boil (form vapor bubbles throughout the liquid).

When solute particles are dissolved in water, some of the dissolved particles are at the surface of the liquid. They prevent some of the water molecules from leaving the surface by blocking the way; they may also (through solute-solvent forces described in Section 12.2) attract water molecules which otherwise would leave the liquid. Either way, they reduce the vapor pressure of the liquid.

Figure 12-24 shows the effect of added solute on the vapor pressure, and thus on the boiling point. As soon as solute is added to water at 100°C, the vapor pressure is lowered below 1.00 atm, and the water will no longer boil. That's why adding salt to boiling water will temporarily stop the boiling; it's not because the salt is so cold you are cooling the water!

If you continue heating the water, eventually it *will* boil, but at a higher temperature. The difference between the normal boiling point of water (100.0°C) and the boiling point of the solution (in Figure 12-24, 100.5°C) is the *boiling point elevation* caused by the added solute.

In dilute solution, the boiling point goes up approximately 0.5 Celsius degrees for *each mole of particles* present in a liter of water.

One practical effect of boiling point elevation is that the oceans evaporate less as salt solutions than they would if they contained pure water. In another situation, antifreeze should be used in an automobile radiator all year round, not just in the winter, since it helps keep the car from boiling over in summer.

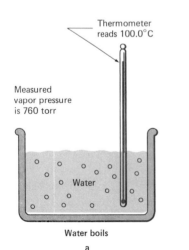
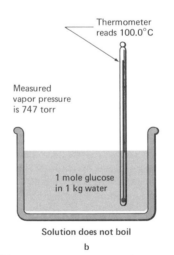
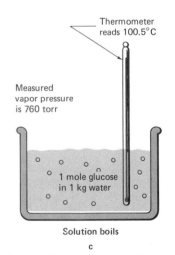

FIGURE 12-24 Boiling point elevation. (a) A solution of pure water boils at 100.0°C at 760 torr (1 atm) pressure because its vapor pressure is 760 torr. (b) When glucose is added to the water, the solution will not boil at 100.0°C and 760 torr because its vapor pressure has been reduced by the glucose molecules in solution. (c) If the glucose solution is heated to 100.5°C, it will finally begin to boil because the vapor pressure has been brought back to 760 torr.

Freezing point

Just as solute particles keep the liquid water molecules from being completely free to evaporate, they also keep some of the water molecules from lining up properly to form the crystal lattice of the solid (ice) at 0°C. If one mole of glucose (or 0.5 mole of NaCl) is dissolved in 1 kg of water, the observed freezing point is not 0.0°C, but −1.9°C. There is a *freezing point depression* or lowering.

There are many practical uses of the freezing point depression, especially in northern climates where snow and ice cause problems. Antifreeze lowers the freezing point of automobile coolant water to as low as −40°C, depending on how much is used. A similar fluid is used in the windshield washer system to avoid having the cleaning liquid freeze as soon as it hits the glass. Road ice is often melted by pouring water-soluble compounds on it. The most popular is rock salt (NaCl), which is also the most corrosive to automobile bodies, unfortunately, and can cause rusting out in only a few years. More expensive, but safer for plants and not much worse for car bodies, is calcium chloride, $CaCl_2$. Best for the environment is urea, H_2NCONH_2, which melts ice and acts as a fertilizer, too!

SELF-CHECK

12.13) Will human blood freeze at 0°C? Explain.

12.14) Mole for mole, which will be more effective in lowering the freezing point of water, NaCl or $CaCl_2$?

12.15) Which will cause the higher elevation in the boiling point of a given amount of water, one mole of NaCl or one mole of glucose?

CHAPTER TWELVE IN REVIEW ■ Solutions and Colloids

12.1 SUSPENSIONS AND COLLOIDS **Page 341**

12A: Distinguish on the basis of particle size between a solution, a colloid, and a suspension.

12B: Give one example of an aerosol, a sol, a gel, an emulsion, and a foam.

12.2 SOLUTIONS AND SOLUBILITY **Page 345**

12C: Given a common solution, identify the solute and the solvent.

12D: Describe how you would prepare an aqueous solution of any common ionic solid that is saturated, unsaturated, or supersaturated.

12E: Use Henry's Law to predict how the solubility of a gas in water is affected by a change in the partial pressure of that gas over the solution.

12.3 AQUEOUS SOLUTIONS **Page 349**

12F: Given the formula of a solute, predict whether it will be more soluble in water or in a nonpolar organic solvent.

12G: Given a solute that dissolves in water, describe an experiment that will tell you if that solute is a strong electrolyte, a weak electrolyte, or a nonelectrolyte.

GLOSSARY FOR CHAPTER TWELVE

aerosol A colloidal dispersion of a solid or liquid in a gas. (p. 343)

biochemical oxygen demand (BOD) A measure of the amount of oxygen required by aquatic bacteria to break down organic substances into simple molecules, thus reducing their environmental impact. (p. 349)

biodegradable Capable of being broken down by bacteria into simpler substances. (p. 352)

colligative property A physical property of a liquid solution, such as vapor pressure, melting point, boiling point, or osmotic pressure, that depends only on the number of dissolved particles and not on their kind. (p. 365)

colloid A heterogeneous mixture that contains particles of a dispersed substance of average size between 10 Å and 1000 Å. (p. 342)

concentration A measure of the amount of solute present in a given amount of solvent or of total solution. (p. 346)

deionized water Water that has had all cations and anions removed by ion exchange resins. (p. 360)

desalination Conversion of ocean water to fresh water by removal of dissolved $NaCl$. (p. 360)

electrolyte, strong A solute, usually an ionic solid, that dissolves in water to give a solution that conducts electricity well; a *weak electrolyte* dissolves in water to give a solution that ionizes only partially, and thus conducts only weakly; a solution of a *nonelectrolyte* does not conduct electricity. (p. 355)

emulsifying agent A substance added to an emulsion to prevent separation of the two liquids into different layers. (p. 344)

emulsion A colloidal dispersion of one liquid in another liquid. (p. 344)

foam A colloidal dispersion of a gas in a liquid or solid. (p. 345)

gel A colloidal dispersion of a liquid in a solid. (p. 344)

hard water Water that contains high concentrations of Ca^{2+} and Mg^{2+} cations. (p. 360)

heterogeneous mixture A mixture of two pure substances in which the dispersed particles have average sizes much larger than those of the medium; includes *colloids* and *suspensions*. (p. 341)

homogeneous mixture A solution; the solute particles have average sizes similar to those of the solvent molecules; the properties of the mixture are uniform, unlike those of a *heterogeneous mixture*. (p. 345)

hydration The surrounding of a dissolved molecule or ion by a group of water molecules which are attracted to it. (p. 353)

hypertonic Describing a solution that has an osmotic pressure higher than that of a given fluid. (p. 363)

hypotonic Describing a solution that has an osmotic pressure lower than that of a given fluid. (p. 363)

isotonic Describing a solution that has an osmotic pressure the same as that of a given fluid. (p. 363)

miscible with For a liquid, soluble in another liquid; if only partly soluble, the term *partially miscible* is used; if insoluble, the two liquids are *immiscible*. (p. 350)

osmosis Flow of solvent (usually water) through a semipermeable membrane from a solution of lower concentration to a solution of higher concentration. (p. 362)

osmotic pressure A measure of the number of particles dissolved in a solution; the mechanical pressure that must be applied to prevent osmosis. (p. 363)

reverse osmosis A method of desalinating sea water by forcing it to flow through a semipermeable membrane. (p. 361)

saturated solution A solution that contains dissolved solute in equilibrium with undissolved solute; the limit to how much solute may be dissolved by direct addition to a solvent; any solution that (at the same temperature) contains less than this amount of solute is an *unsaturated solution*. (p. 347)

semipermeable membrane A thin wall of cellophane, parchment, plant tissue, etc., that permits water to pass through but acts as a barrier to colloids and to some or all dissolved solutes. (p. 361)

sol A colloidal dispersion of a solid in a liquid. (p. 343)

solubility The amount of solute in a given amount of solvent in a saturated solution; depends on temperature. (p. 347)

solute In a solution, the pure substance present in lesser amounts than the solvent. (p. 345)

solution A homogeneous mixture containing a dispersed solute with average particle diameter less than 10 Å. (p. 345)

solvent The dispersing medium for a solution; the substance present in greater amounts than the solute; usually water. (p. 345)

supersaturated solution A solution containing an amount of dissolved solid greater than the solubility limit because no crystals have yet formed; an unstable condition. (p. 348)

suspension A heterogeneous mixture that contains dispersed particles of diameter greater than 1000 Å (10^{-5} cm); can usually be filtered or allowed to settle to separate the two substances. (p. 342)

Tyndall effect A test for dispersed particle size; in a colloid, a beam of light shining through the dispersion will be reflected; neither a suspension nor a solution will make the beam visible. (p. 342)

QUESTIONS AND PROBLEMS FOR CHAPTER TWELVE ■

Solutions and Colloids

SECTION 12.1 SUSPENSIONS AND COLLOIDS

12.16) Colloidal gold particles are sometimes used in medicine. Within what range do you expect to find the size of an average piece of gold in this dispersion?

12.17) Give an example of a sol.

12.18) Give an example of a foam.

12.44) When sucrose (table sugar) dissolves in water, within what range do you expect to find the size of an average particle of sucrose?

12.45) Give an example of a gel.

12.46) Give an example of an emulsion.

12.19*) When volcanos give off lava, melted rock, it may form a very porous stone known as *pumice*. Would you classify pumice as an *aerosol* or a *foam*? Why?

SECTION 12.2 SOLUTIONS AND SOLUBILITY

12.20) Vinegar is a solution containing two liquids, water and acetic acid, CH_3COOH. From what you know about vinegar, state which is the *solute* and which is the *solvent*.

12.21) Air is mostly a solution of oxygen and nitrogen. If it is 21% oxygen, which gas could be considered the solute?

12.22) Potassium iodide, KI, has a solubility of 128 grams in 100 mL of water at 20°C. How would you prepare a saturated solution of KI?

12.23) Calcium iodide, CaI_2, has a solubility in 100 mL of water of 426 grams at 100°C and 209 grams at 20°C. How would you prepare a supersaturated solution of CaI_2?

12.24) Hyperventilation, or breathing very quickly, raises the partial pressure of O_2 in the lungs. What effect does this have on the concentration of O_2 in the blood? Why?

SECTION 12.3 AQUEOUS SOLUTIONS

12.25) Which of the following solutes do you expect to be more soluble in water than in cyclohexane? Explain.
a) formic acid, HCOOH
b) benzene, C_6H_6
c) hydrazine, H_2NNH_2
d) tetrafluoromethane, CF_4

12.26) Acetic acid, CH_3COOH, when dissolved in water to make vinegar, conducts electricity only weakly. What kind of electrolyte is

12.47*) Proteins may be studied when they form a kind of colloid in water. Is this colloid a *sol* or a *gel*? How may the protein be separated from the remaining ions in the solution?

12.48) Wine is a solution of two liquids, water and from 10% to 20% ethanol. Which is the *solute* and which is the *solvent*?

12.49) Red brass contains 85% copper and 15% zinc in an alloy, a solution of a solid in a solid. Which metal is the solvent?

12.50) Sodium fluoride has a solubility of 4.22 grams in 100 mL of water at 18°C. Is fluoridated water (10^{-4} grams/100 mL) saturated or unsaturated? Explain.

12.51) Silver acetate, CH_3COOAg, has a solubility in 100 mL of water of 2.52 grams at 80°C and 1.02 grams at 20°C. How would you prepare a supersaturated solution of CH_3COOAg?

12.52) An automobile mechanic who has breathed in too much carbon monoxide gas should be taken outside and told to breathe deeply. Why? How will this reduce the amount of CO in the bloodstream?

12.53) Which of the following solutes do you expect to be more soluble in cyclohexane than in water? Explain.
a) diethyl ether, $(C_2H_5)_2O$
b) decane, $C_{10}H_{22}$
c) tetrachloroethene, $Cl_2C=CCl_2$
d) hydrogen fluoride, HF

12.54) Perchloric acid, $HClO_4$, when dissolved in water conducts electricity very well. What kind of electrolyte is it? What would you

it? What would you predict about the degree to which this acid ionizes to form H^+ and CH_3COO^- ions?

12.27*) List the forces that must be overcome when liquid diethyl ether, $(C_2H_5)_2O$, dissolves in water. What new forces are created that allow the solution to form?

12.28*) If we wish a drug to dissolve in the fatty membranes of the body, what properties should the drug molecules have?

12.29*) Describe a way of separating two immiscible liquids.

predict about the degree to which this acid ionizes to form H^+ and ClO_4^- ions in water?

12.55*) List the forces that must be overcome when solid NaF crystals dissolve in water. What new forces are created that allow the solution to form?

12.56*) Explain why DDT is dangerous to wildlife that eat the fatty parts of fish, but is less dangerous to birds that eat seeds and other plants.

12.57*) Describe a way to separate two miscible liquids.

12.4 WATER POLLUTION AND PURIFICATION

12.30) Give a source of organic solvent pollution in rivers.

12.31*) Which pollutant is often associated with detergents?

12.32*) How might cyanide ion, CN^-, find its way into lakes?

12.33) What is the purpose of the sedimentation (settling) step in water purification?

12.34) How might an ion-exchange resin remove Ca^{2+} ions from hard water?

12.35*) How does water get from the surface of the earth into the atmosphere? Does this process clean polluted water?

12.36*) How might fertilizers be modified to produce less pollution?

12.37*) In what form is mercury most hazardous to living organisms?

12.38*) Why is fluoride added to the water supply of most U.S. cities?

12.58) Give a source of phosphate ion pollution in rivers.

12.59*) Name a major source of nitrate ion pollution in streams.

12.60*) How might a compound of arsenic find its way into lakes?

12.61) What is the purpose of adding Cl_2 gas in the purification of drinking water for cities?

12.62) What ions are *substituted for* Ca^{2+} and Mg^{2+} ions in any process to soften hard water?

12.63*) How does water get from the atmosphere to the surface of the earth? Can this water ever come down already polluted? How?

12.64*) How were early detergents modified to make them biodegradable?

12.65*) Describe the process by which industrial mercury waste could eventually damage the health of a trapper in the wilderness.

12.66*) How might solar energy be used to make *reverse osmosis* an economical way to desalinate water?

12.5 OSMOSIS AND LIVING CELLS

12.39) Why are nurses instructed *never* to inject pure water into a patient's vein?

12.40) What happens to a red blood cell when it is immersed in sea water?

12.67) What is the function of physiological saline solution?

12.68) What happens to a red blood cell when it is immersed in pure water?

12.6 SOME COLLIGATIVE PROPERTIES OF AQUEOUS SOLUTIONS

12.41) How does dissolving an ionic salt in water affect the freezing point of the solution?

12.69) How does dissolving an ionic salt in water affect the boiling point of the solution?

12.42) Does maple sap boil at a higher or lower temperature than pure water?

12.70) Does beer freeze at a higher or lower temperature than pure water?

12.43*) Some insects living in arctic regions must withstand outside temperatures as low as −50°C. Unlike warm-blooded mammals, their bodies must continue to function without freezing solid at the same temperature as the outside air. How do you suppose they manage?

Acids and Bases

13

Although we may not think about them very much, acids and bases are very important to us. If the proper balance between acid and base were not maintained in the blood stream, our body functions would slow down. The *enzymes* that help biochemical reactions along by speeding them up (Chapter 23) are very sensitive to this acid-base balance. Our body has several systems that *buffer* and control the amount of acidity in body fluids. These will be discussed in Section 13.5.

Hydrochloric acid in our stomachs helps to digest proteins and convert them to amino acids, which are then used by the body to build new proteins. We break down dietary fats into fatty acids, which also provide building blocks for the construction of new molecules in the body. Some other acids, such as citric and lactic, play important roles in the metabolic reactions that produce energy for the body (Chapter 22).

Some common acids and bases.

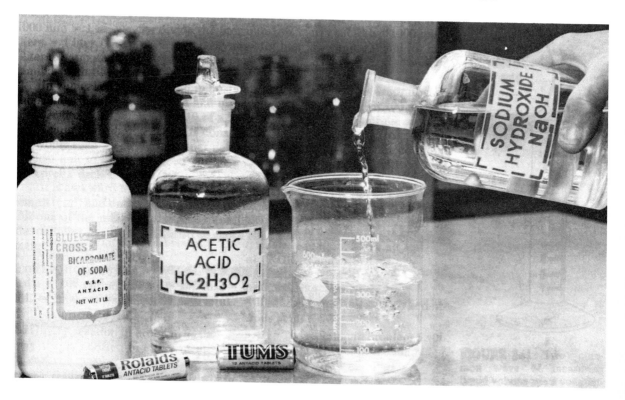

The food you eat and the liquids you drink may occasionally taste sour. The tart taste of sauerkraut, spinach, vinegar, rhubarb, buttermilk, and citrus fruits is due to acid content. Any water solution that feels "soapy" and slippery probably contains a *base* (or *alkali*), such as sodium hydroxide, sodium carbonate (washing soda), sodium bicarbonate (baking soda), or ammonia. Most bases taste somewhat bitter. You may have noticed this with caffeine (in coffee and tea), which is an *alkaloid*, one of a class of organic bases that includes nicotine and morphine. Many different kinds of drugs are organic bases containing *amine groups* (Section 13.4).

In this chapter, we will look at the nonmathematical aspects of acids and bases. If your course requires you to perform calculations for pH, buffer concentrations, titration problems, or other practical aspects of aqueous acid and base solutions, see these skills in Chapter 14.

13.1 STRONG ACIDS AND BASES

> *LEARNING GOAL 13A: Write the chemical equations for dissociation (in aqueous solution) of three common strong acids and one strong base.*
>
> *13B: Write a balanced equation for the neutralization of a strong acid by a strong base.*
>
> *13C: Given the pH of a solution, describe it as acidic, basic, or neutral; given pH values for two solutions, state which is more acidic.*

Proton donors

In water solution, we consider an **acid** to be a substance that can lose H^+ protons and donate them to water molecules. For example, HNO_3, nitric acid, reacts as follows:

$$HNO_{3(aq)} + H_2O_{(\ell)} \longrightarrow NO^-_{3(aq)} + H_3O^+_{(aq)}$$

The water molecule that has added a proton (H^+) becomes a *hydronium ion,* H_3O^+. However, this equation showing the formation of H_3O^+ doesn't really tell you much more than that nitric acid has lost a H^+ ion. You already know that everything in water solution is *hydrated,* that is, surrounded by H_2O molecules. Although the above equation is correct, the following equation says the *same* thing:

$$HNO_{3(aq)} \longrightarrow NO^-_{3(aq)} + H^+_{(aq)}$$

We therefore say that HNO_3 *dissociates* (breaks apart) into a nitrate ion and an aqueous H^+ ion.

The idea that an acid is a substance that dissociates to give H^+ ions was first proposed (in his Ph.D. thesis of 1884) by Svante Arrhenius at Uppsala University in Sweden. The idea was so strange that his professors only grudgingly gave Arrhenius his degree. Yet his concepts about the formation of ions in water solution laid the foundation for much of modern-day chemistry.

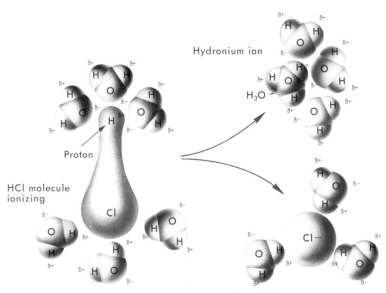

Hydronium ion

$H_3O \rightarrow$

Proton

HCl molecule
ionizing

Hydrated chloride ion

FIGURE 13–1   Proton transfer between dissolved HCl and water molecules leads
to an acid solution.

If you have ever experienced "heartburn" or acid indigestion, you may
have been feeling the effects of aqueous hydrochloric acid in your gastric
fluids. Remembering that all of the particles in an aqueous solution are hydrated (Figure 13–1), we can write the equation for dissociation of HCl:

$$HCl_{(aq)} \longrightarrow H^+_{(aq)} + Cl^-_{(aq)}$$

Hydrochloric acid, like nitric acid, is a source of hydrated protons. The
typical reactions of acids always involve the giving away or donating of such
$H^+_{(aq)}$ ions to other particles.

An acid is a proton donor in water solution.

Strong acids

You may feel that a strong acid is one that is very dangerous if it touches
your skin. The chemist has a different definition of strong. A **strong acid** is a
substance that almost completely dissociates or ionizes in water solution to
give $H^+_{(aq)}$ ions. The arrows in the equations for dissociation of nitric and
hydrochloric acids point only to the right, indicating that we generally do not
find many HNO_3 or HCl molecules in such solutions. When we write chemical equations or do calculations with such strong acids, we assume them to
be completely broken up.

The third common strong acid is sulfuric acid, H_2SO_4:

$$H_2SO_{4(aq)} \longrightarrow H^+_{(aq)} + HSO^-_{4(aq)}$$

While the first proton leaves H_2SO_4 very easily, the second proton, the one
on the HSO_4^- hydrogen sulfate ion, is only partly lost in water solution. We
will see in Section 13.2 that the HSO_4^- ion may be classified by chemists as a
weak acid, since it is not fully dissociated in typical solutions.

We have some contact with these three strong acids every day. Both nitric and sulfuric acids are formed when pollutant gases in the atmosphere react with oxygen and water to form *acid rain:*

$$4 \ NO_{2(g)} + 2 \ H_2O_{(\ell)} + O_{2(g)} \longrightarrow 4 \ HNO_{3(aq)}$$

$$SO_{3(g)} + H_2O_{(\ell)} \longrightarrow H_2SO_{4(aq)}$$

Oxides of both nitrogen and sulfur are naturally present in the atmosphere as a result of the action of lightning and volcanos. However, smokestack and automobile pollution has considerably increased the amounts of these gases, which can be carried long distances before they fall in rain. The result has been destruction of the fish populations of some wilderness areas.

All three of the common strong acids are widely used industrially and also find many applications in organic chemistry. A special solution that combines HCl and HNO$_3$, called *aqua regia,* is the only solvent that will dissolve gold. The other strong acids in aqueous solution are HBr, HI, and HClO$_4$.

Properties of acid solutions

An acid solution has a surplus of hydrated protons, which are available to add to a species that accepts protons (called a *base*). Water itself contains a very small amount of H$_{(aq)}^+$, as we will discuss shortly. We refer to an acid solution only when we mean a solution that has an amount of H$_{(aq)}^+$ considerably greater than that provided by the water itself.

Highly acidic solutions have some useful properties:

1) Acids can *oxidize* certain metals to give hydrogen gas and a solution of an ionic salt. For example:

$$Zn_{(s)} + 2 \ HCl_{(aq)} \longrightarrow H_{2(g)} + ZnCl_{2(aq)}$$

This is a common way of preparing hydrogen gas in the laboratory.

2) Acids can *dissolve* metal oxides and hydroxides that are insoluble in pure water:

$$FeO_{(s)} + 2 \ HCl_{(aq)} \longrightarrow FeCl_{2(aq)} + H_2O_{(\ell)}$$

$$Al(OH)_{3(s)} + 3 \ HCl_{(aq)} \longrightarrow AlCl_{3(aq)} + 3 \ H_2O_{(\ell)}$$

3) Acids can *neutralize* basic solutions to give ionic salt solutions:

$$KOH_{(aq)} + HCl_{(aq)} \longrightarrow KCl_{(aq)} + H_2O_{(\ell)}$$

$$NH_{3(aq)} + HCl_{(aq)} \longrightarrow NH_4Cl_{(aq)}$$

4) As a special case of neutralization: If a very small amount of a particular kind of colored organic base is placed in an acid solution, the base will be neutralized to an acid form that has a different color. Such a substance, called an acid-base *indicator,* can be used to test for acidity. One such indicator you may have seen is *litmus,* which is red in acid solution and blue in base:

$$blue \ litmus + H_{(aq)}^+ \longrightarrow red \ litmus$$

5) Acids can destroy protein molecules and thus cause cell damage (Chapter 19). This accounts for the use of acids, as in Compound W, to treat warts on the skin. It also explains why spilling concentrated acid solution on the skin can cause serious injury.

6) Acids will react with carbonates (containing CO_3^{2-} ion) to liberate CO_2 gas. The acid-base equilibrium involving bicarbonate ions (HCO_3^-) in the blood stream and the release of CO_2 to the lungs is extremely important in human biochemistry.

Strong bases

Arrhenius considered a **base** to be a substance that dissociates in water to give hydroxide ions, $OH_{(aq)}^-$. This is still our definition of a **strong base** or **alkali.** Those metal hydroxides that dissolve in water are considered to ionize completely to the metal ion and OH^-:

$$\text{(lye)} \qquad NaOH_{(aq)} \longrightarrow Na_{(aq)}^+ + OH_{(aq)}^-$$

$$\text{(limewater)} \quad Ca(OH)_{2(aq)} \longrightarrow Ca_{(aq)}^{2+} + 2\ OH_{(aq)}^-$$

The strong bases are all hydroxides of Group 1 and Group 2 metals. Other metal hydroxides, such as $Al(OH)_3$, are insoluble in pure water. Other substances classified as bases do not themselves contain OH^- ions, but will produce such ions on reaction with water. We call all such substances *weak bases* (Section 13.3).

Properties of basic solutions

Some highly basic solutions feel slippery because the OH^- can react with skin oils to make soap. If a strong base remains on the skin, it will react with the fats in the cell membrane and cause serious damage.

The other properties of bases are related to those of acids; for example, a base will neutralize an acid. A basic solution will react with red litmus, turning it blue:

$$\text{red litmus} + OH_{(aq)}^- \longrightarrow \text{blue litmus}$$

An equation describing the **neutralization** of a strong acid by a strong base is

$$HNO_{3(aq)} + NaOH_{(aq)} \longrightarrow H_2O_{(\ell)} + NaNO_{3(aq)}$$

However, you know from the definitions of strong acid and strong base that both are ionized in aqueous solution. Sodium nitrate solution is also completely dissociated. The actual reaction is

$$H_{(aq)}^+ + OH_{(aq)}^- \longrightarrow H_2O_{(\ell)}$$

This same *ionic* equation describes every possible strong acid/strong base neutralization.

Since most metal hydroxides are insoluble, one common reaction of a strong base is the *precipitation* of a hydroxide:

$$Ni_{(aq)}^{2+} + 2\ OH_{(aq)}^- \longrightarrow Ni(OH)_{2(s)}$$

Molarity and acid-base concentration

The chemist generally uses the units of moles per liter to measure the amount of solute in an aqueous solution. For example, gastric fluids typically contain about 0.05 moles of HCl in each liter of fluid. We then say that the concentration of HCl is 0.05 moles/liter. The term **molarity** is used to describe a concentration in moles/liter, using the symbol M or brackets around the formula, as in [HCl].

Molarity is concentration in moles/liter.

Chapter 14 will discuss the ways of preparing a solution of a given molarity and how molarity can be used in other types of calculations. Meanwhile, comparing the molarities of $H^+_{(aq)}$ in different solutions will give us a way of comparing the acidities.

Chemists often describe the commercial *stock* solutions normally stored on laboratory shelves as **concentrated** solutions. Table 13–1 gives the strengths of some stock acids and bases.

A **dilute** solution may mean several different things. A commercial dilute solution may be 6 M, which is still extremely dangerous if spilled on the eyes or skin. A laboratory dilute solution may be 3 M, or 1 M, or even less concentrated, depending on need. Most of the solutions you will encounter, and which we will call "dilute," have concentrations of under 1 M.

A *concentrated* solution of a substance has a relatively higher concentration of solute than a *dilute* solution.

If we are dealing with a strong acid, such as HCl, we assume that the reaction

$$HCl_{(aq)} \longrightarrow H^+_{(aq)} + Cl^-_{(aq)}$$

goes to completion in dilute solution. The $H^+_{(aq)}$ concentration in moles/liter, or [H^+], should be equal to the theoretical concentration we would get if we divided the number of moles of HCl by the number of liters of solution. Gastric fluid is typically around 0.05 M in HCl. However, *actually* present in that fluid would be 0.05 moles/liter of H^+ and 0.05 moles/liter of Cl^-.

TABLE 13–1 CONCENTRATIONS OF SOME CONCENTRATED COMMERCIAL STOCK SOLUTIONS

Strong acids	
HCl	11.6 M
HNO$_3$	16.0 M
H$_2$SO$_4$	18.0 M
HBr	8.9 M
HI	7.6 M
Weak acids	
H$_3$PO$_4$	14.6 M
CH$_3$COOH	17.4 M
Strong bases	
NaOH	19.1 M
KOH	13.5 M
(not commonly used)	
Weak base	
NH$_{3(aq)}$	14.8 M

Acid-base properties of water

An acid solution contains a large number of available $H^+_{(aq)}$ ions, and a basic solution a large number of available $OH^-_{(aq)}$ ions. We know that if both kinds of ions are present, they neutralize each other to give water. A solution cannot be both acidic and basic at the same time.

On the other hand, pure water dissociates very slightly, so slightly, in fact, that the concentration of H^+ and of OH^- in pure water is only about 10^{-7} moles/liter (10^{-7} M):

$$H_2O_{(\ell)} \rightleftharpoons H^+_{(aq)} + OH^-_{(aq)}$$

There are so few ions in pure water, in fact, that it is an insulator, that is, it does not conduct electricity. This comes as a surprise to many people who have been warned not to use any electrical appliances near the bathtub. Tap water contains many dissolved ions and so is an electrolyte. Pure water, free of the impurities, is a nonelectrolyte.

In pure water, the small number of H^+ ions produced by the dissociation of H_2O molecules is the same as the small number of OH^- ions produced. If we add H^+ ions to the pure water, it is more difficult for OH^- ions to be present because the few that are produced are almost all "gobbled up" by H^+ ions to form water. One definition of an acidic solution, then, is that it is a solution that has an OH^- concentration lower than that of water (10^{-7} M). In other words, the OH^- concentration in an acidic solution is less than 10^{-7} M.

If we add OH^- ions to pure water, some react with the H^+ ions present. The result is a lowering of the H^+ concentration to below 10^{-7} M.

Since water is in *equilibrium* with its ions, we can represent the balance between H^+ and OH^- ions by an equilibrium expression:

$$K_w = [OH^-][H^+] = 1 \times 10^{-14} \qquad \text{(at 25°C)}$$

The symbol K_w is called the *ion product constant* for water. It depends only on temperature. It is equal to the hydrogen ion concentration in *any* water solution multiplied by the hydroxide ion concentration. In pure water,

$$[H^+] = [OH^-] = \sqrt{K_w} = 1 \times 10^{-7} \text{ at 25°C}$$

In any water solution, we can turn the K_w expression around:

$$[H^+] = \frac{1 \times 10^{-14}}{[OH^-]} \qquad [OH^-] = \frac{1 \times 10^{-14}}{[H^+]}$$

A solution that is 10^{-2} M in H^+ will have a hydroxide concentration of 10^{-12} M. The two numbers multiplied together give 10^{-14}.

You have probably noticed that it would be much easier if we simply looked at the powers of ten. The powers of ten of the two molarities must add up to -14. This is the basis of the *pH scale*.

The pH scale of acidity

We use the fact that the powers of ten of $[H^+]$ and $[OH^-]$ are related to provide a simple way of expressing the acidity (or basicity) of an aqueous solution. We let the symbol **pH** represent the **p**ower of ten of the **H**$^+$ concentration, and for convenience we change all minus signs to plus signs.

If $[H^+]$ is 0.1 $M = 1 \times 10^{-1}$ M, the pH = 1.0.
If $[H^+]$ is 0.000 000 1 $M = 1 \times 10^{-7}$ M, the pH = 7.0.
If $[H^+]$ is 0.000 000 000 01 $M = 1 \times 10^{-11}$ M, the pH = 11.0.

This relationship is shown in Figure 13–2.

In mathematical terms, pH $= -\log_{10}\left(\dfrac{\text{moles } H^+ \text{ ion}}{\text{liter of solution}}\right)$. We have so far used only whole-number pH values, which do not require any knowledge of logarithms. If you need to calculate pH to one decimal place from H^+ concentrations, this skill is included in Section 14.3.

An increase in acidity by one pH unit, say from pH = 5.0 to pH = 4.0, represents ten times as many H^+ ions in solution. Remember that

A low pH value means *acidic*.
A high pH value means *basic*.
A neutral solution, neither acid nor base, has a pH of 7.0.

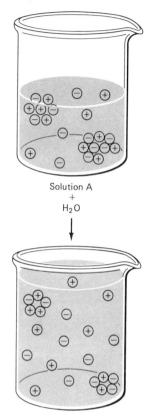

Solution A
+
H_2O

Solution B

Dissociation of a strong acid depends on concentration. A 1.0 M HCl solution is only about 90% dissociated because there are clusters of oppositely charged ions (Solution A). Diluted with water to 0.010 M, the HCl becomes almost 100% dissociated (Solution B).

A similar definition exists for pOH, which measures the basic strength of a solution containing OH^- ion. If $[OH^-] = 10^{-3}$ M, then pOH = 3. The pH and the pOH always add together to make 14.00. Later in this chapter, we will use pK_a, where K_a is an acid equilibrium constant. If $K_a = 1 \times 10^{-8}$, then $pK_a = 8.0$.

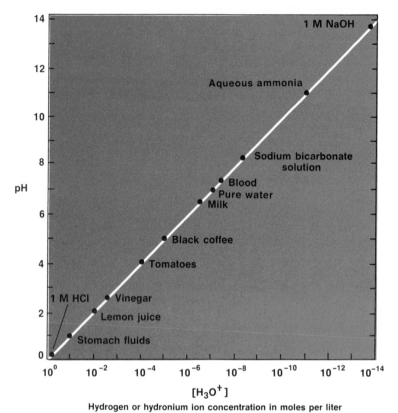

FIGURE 13–2 The relationship between pH and [H⁺]. The pH *increases* as the acidity *decreases*. The pH values of some common solutions are given for reference.

TABLE 13–2 RELATIONSHIPS OF THE pH SCALE

Description	pH	[H⁺]	[OH⁻]
Strongly acidic	0	$10^0 \, M = 1 \, M$	$10^{-14} \, M$
	1	$10^{-1} \, M = 0.1 \, M$	$10^{-13} \, M$
	2	$10^{-2} \, M = 0.01 \, M$	$10^{-12} \, M$
	3	$10^{-3} \, M = 0.001 \, M$	$10^{-11} \, M$
Weakly	4	$10^{-4} \, M = 0.000 \, 1 \, M$	$10^{-10} \, M$
acidic	5	$10^{-5} \, M = 0.000 \, 01 \, M$	$10^{-9} \, M$
Slightly acidic	6	$10^{-6} \, M = 0.000 \, 001 \, M$	$10^{-8} \, M = 0.000 \, 000 \, 01 \, M$
Neutral	7	$10^{-7} \, M = 0.000 \, 000 \, 1 \, M$	$10^{-7} \, M = 0.000 \, 000 \, 1 \, M$
Slightly basic	8	$10^{-8} \, M = 0.000 \, 000 \, 01 \, M$	$10^{-6} \, M = 0.000 \, 001 \, M$
Weakly	9	$10^{-9} \, M$	$10^{-5} \, M = 0.000 \, 01 \, M$
basic	10	$10^{-10} \, M$	$10^{-4} \, M = 0.000 \, 1 \, M$
Strongly basic	11	$10^{-11} \, M$	$10^{-3} \, M = 0.001 \, M$
	12	$10^{-12} \, M$	$10^{-2} \, M = 0.01 \, M$
	13	$10^{-13} \, M$	$10^{-1} \, M = 0.1 \, M$
	14	$10^{-14} \, M$	$10^{-0} \, M = 1 \, M$

Table 13–2 summarizes what we know about the pH unit. Remember, however, that the terms "weakly acidic" and "strongly acidic" (and the corresponding terms for basic solutions) are relative. For one purpose, a solution with pH = 3 might be sufficiently acidic to do a job; for another purpose, it might be too weak. Pure water has a pH of 7.0, but the tap water we use for various purposes has a range of pH values because of various impurities and is often around pH = 6.

You should be able to apply this knowledge.

EXAMPLE 13a: Three bottles of liquids in a home were tested for pH. The grape juice tested at pH = 4.0, the liquid soap at pH = 11.0, and some lime juice at pH = 2.0.
 i)   Which of the liquids were acidic, which were basic?
 ii) List them in order of increasing acidity.
 iii) Calculate the molarity of $H^+_{(aq)}$ in each solution.
 iv) Calculate the molarity of $OH^-_{(aq)}$ in each solution.

ANSWER:
 i)   The pH values under 7.0 are acidic; thus the grape juice and lime juice are acids. A pH value greater than 7.0 is that of a basic solution; the soap is basic.
 ii) Increasing acidity means *decreasing* value of pH:
soap (pH = 11.0)   grape juice (pH = 4.0)   lime juice (pH = 2.0)
 iii) The pH is the negative of the power of ten of the H^+ molarity:

Therefore, $[H^+] = \boxed{1 \times 10^{-11}}$ for soap (pH = 11.0)

$= \boxed{1 \times 10^{-4}}$ for grape juice (pH = 4.0)

$= \boxed{1 \times 10^{-2}}$ for lime juice (pH = 2.0)

 iv) You may use the equation given earlier: $[OH^-] = \dfrac{1 \times 10^{-14}}{[H^+]}$

$[OH^-] = \dfrac{1 \times 10^{-14}}{1 \times 10^{-11}} = \boxed{1 \times 10^{-3}}$ for soap

$= \dfrac{1 \times 10^{-14}}{1 \times 10^{-4}} = \boxed{1 \times 10^{-10}}$ for grape juice

$= \dfrac{1 \times 10^{-14}}{1 \times 10^{-2}} = \boxed{1 \times 10^{-12}}$ for lime juice

The most basic solution is soap. Lime juice is least basic.

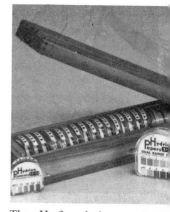

The pH of a solution may be estimated by dipping in a piece of pH paper. The paper contains dyes that change color depending on the acidity of the solution. By comparing the paper color with a standard chart, the pH of the solution may be determined.

Almost all foods are acidic. An exception is egg white (pH = 7.8). Human body fluids (Chapter 24) tend to have very slightly basic pH values, in the range 7.0 to 7.6. For example, human milk has a pH of 7.1, while cow's milk has a pH of 6.5.

Antacids for stomach distress

While persons with stomach ulcers may require medication to neutralize excessive stomach acid, the volume of sales of various antacid preparations, such as

Alka-Seltzer, Tums, and Rolaids, suggests that many healthy people also use antacids. They are presumably taking these drugs to relieve "heartburn," acid indigestion, and "sour stomach."

However, it is most likely that these symptoms are occurring with no excess stomach acid present. They may be the result of stress, diet, or eating habits rather than excess production of HCl. One of the most frequent causes of gastritis, an inflammation of the stomach lining that causes severe pain, is consumption of alcohol.

About two liters of HCl solution are secreted each day by cells in the stomach walls, mostly after a meal. The proteins in food, and certain drugs such as caffeine and alcohol, stimulate production of HCl. Emotions play a part also. If the pH of the stomach rises to a neutral level, this causes secretion of more acid, a gastric "rebound." If there is excess HCl production, it averages only about 0.010 moles greater than normal at any particular time. An ideal antacid should neutralize just this amount of HCl.

The normal acid content of the stomach serves several purposes. HCl breaks up some protein and connective tissue in food, thus speeding up digestion. It also kills almost all of the bacteria that enter the body with food. A third function is to create a pH in the stomach that is favorable to the work of certain protein-digesting enzymes known as pepsin. Pepsin works well in the pH range from 1.5 to 2.0 and is useless if the pH rises above 4.5.

TABLE 13–3   THE CHEMISTRY OF SOME ANTACIDS

Aluminum hydroxide $Al(OH)_{3(s)} + 3\ H^+_{(aq)} \longrightarrow Al^{3+}_{(aq)} + 3\ H_2O_{(\ell)}$
Found by a panel of the U.S. Food and Drug Administration to be effective and nonhazardous. No dosage restriction, but may cause constipation. Found alone in Amphojel, but usually combined with magnesium compounds in brands such as Aludrox, Gelusil, Maalox, Di-Gel, Mylanta, and in a generic form, Magnesium-Aluminum Hydroxide Gel USP. Generally most recommended.

Magnesium hydroxide $Mg(OH)_{2(s)} + 2\ H^+_{(aq)} \longrightarrow Mg^{2+}_{(aq)} + 2\ H_2O_{(\ell)}$
Found effective by FDA. Small dosages are antacid, but larger dosages are laxative. Dose must be limited for patients with kidney disease. May be purchased as Milk of Magnesia (USP or Phillips) or in combination with $Al(OH)_3$ above.

Dihydroxyaluminum sodium carbonate
$NaAl(OH)_2CO_{3(s)} + 4\ H^+_{(aq)} \longrightarrow Na^+_{(aq)} + Al^{3+}_{(aq)} + 3\ H_2O_{(\ell)} + CO_{2(g)}$
Effective, but poses danger in long-term use because of high sodium content. FDA recommends no more than 0.115 grams of sodium per day for persons on low-sodium diets. *Rolaids,* which contains this antacid, has 0.053 grams of sodium per tablet. Individuals may have high blood pressure without realizing it and worsen the problem with excessive sodium intake. Kidney disorders also require low-sodium diets.

Sodium bicarbonate $NaHCO_{3(aq)} + H^+_{(aq)} \longrightarrow Na^+_{(aq)} + H_2O_{(\ell)} + CO_{2(g)}$
Ordinary baking soda or in products such as Alka-Seltzer, Bromo Seltzer, Eno, and Brioschi. Fast and effective for short-term use. Dangerous for regular or frequent use for reasons given for Rolaids, as well as because of its ability to cause an increase in the pH of body fluids. Prolonged use may lead to kidney stones and possibly contribute to recurrent urinary tract infections. Two tablets of Alka-Seltzer contain more than one gram of sodium.

Calcium carbonate $CaCO_{3(s)} + 2\ H^+_{(aq)} \longrightarrow Ca^{2+}_{(aq)} + H_2O_{(\ell)} + CO_{2(g)}$
Purified limestone (chalk), found in Tums, Pepto-Bismol tablets, and many other products. Once highly recommended, but causes constipation and may cause "acid rebound." Prolonged use presents more serious problems, since high blood calcium levels can cause kidney stones and damage, especially in people who drink large amounts of milk. FDA panel recommends no more than 8 grams (16 Tums tablets) per day, and for not more than 2 weeks.

(Information and value judgments from Chapter 7 of *The Medicine Show,* 5th edition, published by Consumers Union, Mount Vernon, N.Y., 1980.)

The enzymes in the small intestine are adequate for digesting proteins, even if pepsin does not do its job in the stomach. However, it has been suggested that pepsin plays a more important role in the stomach: it breaks up proteins so that the liberated amino acids will stimulate production of enzymes from the pancreas.* An ideal antacid, then, would keep the pH of stomach contents below 4.0 and one dosage unit would not neutralize more than 0.010 moles of HCl.

Do any of the popular brands of antacids meet these criteria? Products such as Tums and Alka-2, which use only precipitated chalk, $CaCO_3$, and such as Milk of Magnesia, which is $Mg(OH)_2$, neutralize only slightly more than 0.010 moles of HCl but raise the stomach pH well above 5.0. Products that contain mixtures of $Al(OH)_3$, $Mg(OH)_2$, and other substances, such as Maalox, DiGel, and Gelusil, neutralize more HCl (0.012 to 0.014 moles per tablet) but maintain the pH of the stomach at 4.5. The only tested product that met both criteria was Rolaids, which contains a mixed salt of aluminum hydroxide and sodium bicarbonate. Several antacid products are listed in Table 13–3.

It is important to realize that these data represent the action of only *one* tablet of each product. Many people chew and swallow antacid tablets like candy mints. Such a practice will raise the stomach pH and perhaps hinder digestion.

The effect of an antacid is not simply a matter of neutralizing hydrochloric acid, however. Each substance added to the body has its own effect and may disturb the balance of ions in the body fluids. In particular, any product with high levels of sodium is inadvisable. Many antacid products are also laxatives and may produce unwanted side effects along with relief from stomach acidity. The long-term use of any antacid should be the subject of medical supervision.

SELF-CHECK

13.1)   Write the chemical equations for the dissociation in water of
a)   a strong acid that contains nitrogen
b)   a strong base that contains potassium
13.2)   Write the balanced equation for the neutralization reaction that occurs when limewater, $Ca(OH)_{2(aq)}$, is swallowed and mixes with the HCl in stomach fluid.
13.3*)   It is extremely dangerous to drink concentrated solutions of lye (NaOH) or caustic potash (KOH), but not nearly so harmful to drink suspensions of the strong bases $Mg(OH)_2$ (milk of magnesia) or $Ca(OH)_2$ (limewater). Explain.
13.4*)   Why is zinc hydroxide not considered a "strong base"?
13.5*)   Write a balanced equation for the reaction of sulfuric acid with zinc metal to give hydrogen gas.
13.6)   Classify each of the following solutions as acidic, basic, or neutral. The pH of each is a typical average value.
a)   sea water, pH = 8.1
b)   human spinal fluid, pH = 7.4
c)   plum juice, pH = 2.9
d)   human saliva, pH = 7.0
e)   rainwater, pH = 6.2
f)   beer, pH = 4.5
g)   black coffee, pH = 5.0
13.7)   Rank the seven solutions of Self-Check 13.6 in order of *increasing* acidity.

---

* See W. B. Batson and P. H. Laswick, "Pepsin and Antacid Therapy: A Dilemma," *J. Chem. Educ.* **56**, 485 (July 1979).

13.2 WEAK ACIDS

LEARNING GOAL 13D: *Given the formula of a weak acid, write the equilibrium equation for its partial dissociation.*
13E: *Given pK$_a$ values for two different weak acids, decide which of them will form a more acidic aqueous solution if both are at the same concentration.*
13F: *Given the formula of a weak acid, identify its conjugate base.*

Chemists often use simple one-letter symbols to represent a variety of formulas. The symbol "R" in Chapter 9 represented an alkyl group in an organic compound. Similarly, "A" here means an *anion* such as Cl^-, NO_3^-, or CH_3COO^-. It is also possible for "A" to represent a neutral basic molecule, such as NH_3, in which case "HA" stands for the basic molecule with H$^+$ added: NH_4^+.

We assume *strong* acids to be completely dissociated in aqueous solution. However, most acids do *not* ionize to any great extent in water. If we represent a typical weak acid by HA, where "A" represents not a strange element but a symbol for "some anion," then the ionization process is

$$HA_{(aq)} \rightleftharpoons H^+_{(aq)} + A^-_{(aq)}$$

For example, the dissociation of acetic acid can be written

$$HC_2H_3O_{2(aq)} \rightleftharpoons H^+_{(aq)} + C_2H_3O^-_{2(aq)}$$

or

$$CH_3COOH_{(aq)} \rightleftharpoons H^+_{(aq)} + CH_3COO^-_{(aq)}$$

The dissociation process shown in Figure 13–1 is followed in each case. Some acid molecules are "pulled apart" by water more easily than others. A hydrogen that can be pulled off to form $H^+_{(aq)}$ must be the δ^+ side of a polar molecule, which means it must be bonded to an electronegative atom. Carbon is not sufficiently electronegative to create such a dipole. The three hydrogens bonded to carbon in CH_3COOH are therefore not acidic.

The second way of writing the formula for acetic acid is preferred in this course, since we will be dealing frequently with carboxylic acids and anions. Either way, we are showing that the acetic acid molecule dissolved in water dissociates slightly to give one hydrated proton and one acetate anion.

Weak acids vary considerably in the acidity of their water solutions. For example, oxalic acid (found in spinach and rhubarb) is a relatively strong "weak acid," as is the hydrogen sulfate anion, HSO_4^-. Unlike strong acids, however, they are found primarily in their *associated* form (except in very dilute solution). We expect to find substantial concentrations of the parent acid molecule ($H_2C_2O_4$ for oxalic acid, HSO_4^- for hydrogen sulfate ion) in typical solutions of these substances.

EXAMPLE 13b: Write equations to show the dissociation of the following acids.
  i)   hydrofluoric acid, HF (used to etch glass)
  ii)   carbonic acid, H_2CO_3 (important in red blood cells)
  iii)   phosphoric acid, H_3PO_4 (whose anions are very important in the human body)

- -

ANSWER: The only strong acids known were mentioned in Section 13.1. These three acids are therefore weak acids. We must write equilibrium equations.

i) $$HF_{(aq)} \rightleftharpoons H^+_{(aq)} + F^-_{(aq)}$$

ii) $$H_2CO_{3(aq)} \rightleftharpoons H^+_{(aq)} + HCO^-_{3(aq)}$$

The bicarbonate ion, HCO_3^-, is basic and is one of the most important ions in the human body.

iii) $$H_3PO_{4(aq)} \rightleftharpoons H^+_{(aq)} + H_2PO^-_{4(aq)}$$

A **weak acid** is thus a substance that, when dissolved in water, provides substantial amounts of both the molecular acid and hydrated protons.

Polyprotic acids

If you look at Table 4–2 on p. 97, you will find some anions which themselves contain ionizable hydrogens. These include HCO_3^-, HSO_4^-, $H_2PO_4^-$, and HPO_4^{2-}. Although each of these anions comes from dissociation of an acid, each has the capability of dissociating again.

EXAMPLE 13c: Write equilibrium equations for the ionization of the three hydrogens of phosphoric acid.

- -

ANSWER: We already have one such equation from Example 13b. We must continue with two more:

phosphoric acid $H_3PO_{4(aq)} \rightleftharpoons H^+_{(aq)} + H_2PO^-_{4(aq)}$

dihydrogen
phosphate ion $H_2PO^-_{4(aq)} \rightleftharpoons H^+_{(aq)} + HPO^{2-}_{4(aq)}$

monohydrogen
phosphate ion $HPO^{2-}_{4(aq)} \rightleftharpoons H^+_{(aq)} + PO^{3-}_{4(aq)}$

The final product of full ionization of all three protons is the phosphate ion.

A molecule that can give up more than one proton is a **polyprotic** acid. One organic example is $H_2C_2O_4$, oxalic acid. From the name of *mono*sodium glutamate (a flavor enhancer used for many centuries in the Far East), you should be able to infer that glutamic acid is polyprotic and that it is possible to create *di*sodium glutamate. Another such acid, found in citrus fruits and in many other foods, is citric acid. In the human body, this acid is important enough to have a metabolic process named after it, the citric acid cycle (Chapter 22).

In all cases of polyprotic acids, the second H^+ comes off with more difficulty than the first, and the third with more difficulty than the second. We usually treat the dissociation steps of a polyprotic acid as if they were completely independent of each other.

$H_2N-CHCOOH$
|
CH_2CH_2COONa
monosodium
glutamate

CH_2COOH
|
$HO-C-COOH$
|
CH_2COOH
3-hydroxy-3-carboxy-
pentanedioic acid
(citric acid)

Conjugate acid-base pairs

The Arrhenius theory limited acids to those substances that could provide H^+ to water. It also limited bases to those substances that could provide OH^- ion, which would mean that only soluble metal hydroxides qualified as bases. It turns out that all of the strong acids and bases fit this theory.

In 1923, two scientists, Bronsted and Lowry, independently proposed that acid-base reactions involve *proton transfer* from a proton donor (an acid) to a proton acceptor (a base).

The Bronsted–Lowry picture adds an important feature to our understanding of acids and bases. When any acid actually loses its proton, it becomes a particle that can accept back the same proton. In other words, it becomes a base. For example, acetic acid, CH_3COOH, loses a proton to become the acetate ion, CH_3COO^-. The acetate ion must be a base, since it is capable of accepting a proton to become acetic acid.

Similarly, ammonia, NH_3, is a base. When it accepts a proton we get the ammonium ion, NH_4^+, which is capable of giving back that proton and thus is an acid.

Each acid is paired with a particle that contains one fewer H^+. CH_3COOH is paired with CH_3COO^-. NH_4^+ is paired with NH_3. HCl is paired with Cl^-. H_2CO_3 is paired with HCO_3^-. We call the acid and the base resulting from the loss of one proton a **conjugate acid-base pair.**

The word conjugate *means "joined" or "married."*

Acid constants and pK_a

Each weak acid has its own ionization characteristics. We should have a way to compare such substances so that we know which are more likely than others to lose $H_{(aq)}^+$. For simplicity in this chapter, we will use a constant called the **pK_a**. Each weak acid has its own particular value of pK_a such that, in the same way that low pH means *highly* acidic and high pH means *less* acidic,

An acid with a lower pK_a results in a more acidic solution than an acid with a higher pK_a.

This rule assumes that both acids are present in the same concentration in an aqueous solution.

The pK_a now gives us a way to compare acid strengths. Table 13–4 lists some inorganic and organic weak acids in order of decreasing acid strength, that is, in order of *increasing* pK_a. In this listing, the conjugate bases will be found in order from strongest at the bottom to weakest at the top.

Some of the acids in Table 13–4 may be unfamiliar to you. Ascorbic acid is Vitamin C (Chapter 23). The conjugate bases of lactic and pyruvic

TABLE 13–4   IONIZATION PROPERTIES OF SOME WEAK ACIDS AT 25°C IN SOLUTION

Name of Acid	pK_a	Ionization Equation		Name of Conjugate Base
Oxalic acid	1.2	HOOCCOOH	$\rightleftarrows H^+ + HOOCCOO^-$	Hydrogen oxalate ion
Sulfurous acid	1.9	H_2SO_3	$\rightleftarrows H^+ + HSO_3^-$	Hydrogen sulfite ion
Hydrogen sulfate ion	1.9	HSO_4^-	$\rightleftarrows H^+ + SO_4^{2-}$	Sulfate ion
Phosphoric acid	2.1	H_3PO_4	$\rightleftarrows H^+ + H_2PO_4^-$	Dihydrogen phosphate ion
Pyruvic acid	2.5	$CH_3COCOOH$	$\rightleftarrows H^+ + CH_3COCOO^-$	Pyruvate ion
Salicylic acid	3.0	HOC_6H_4COOH	$\rightleftarrows H^+ + HOC_6H_4COO^-$	Salicylate ion
Citric acid	3.1	$H_3C_6H_5O_6$	$\rightleftarrows H^+ + H_2C_6H_5O_6^-$	Dihydrogen citrate ion
Hydrofluoric acid	3.2	HF	$\rightleftarrows H^+ + F^-$	Fluoride ion
Nitrous acid	3.3	HNO_2	$\rightleftarrows H^+ + NO_2^-$	Nitrite ion
Formic acid	3.7	HCOOH	$\rightleftarrows H^+ + HCOO^-$	Formate ion
Lactic acid	3.9	$CH_3CHOHCOOH$	$\rightleftarrows H^+ + CH_3CHOHCOO^-$	Lactate ion
Ascorbic acid	4.1	$HC_6H_7O_6$	$\rightleftarrows H^+ + C_6H_7O_6^-$	Ascorbate ion
Benzoic acid	4.2	C_6H_5COOH	$\rightleftarrows H^+ + C_6H_5COO^-$	Benzoate ion
Acetic acid	4.7	CH_3COOH	$\rightleftarrows H^+ + CH_3COO^-$	Acetate ion
Carbonic acid	6.4	H_2CO_3	$\rightleftarrows H^+ + HCO_3^-$	Hydrogen carbonate ion
Dihydrogen phosphate ion	7.2	$H_2PO_4^-$	$\rightleftarrows H^+ + HPO_4^{2-}$	Monohyd. phosphate ion
Ammonium ion	9.3	NH_4^+	$\rightleftarrows H^+ + NH_3$	Ammonia (aqueous)
Phenol	9.9	C_6H_5OH	$\rightleftarrows H^+ + C_6H_5O^-$	Phenolate ion
Hydrogen carbonate ion	10.2	HCO_3^-	$\rightleftarrows H^+ + CO_3^{2-}$	Carbonate ion
Monohyd. phosphate ion	12.0	HPO_4^{2-}	$\rightleftarrows H^+ + PO_4^{3-}$	Phosphate ion
Water	14.0	H_2O	$\rightleftarrows H^+ + OH^-$	Hydroxide ion

LOWEST — ↑ — LOW — ↑ — ↑ — ↑ — (ACID STRENGTH) — ↑ — ↑ — HIGHER

LOWER — ↓ — ↓ — (BASE STRENGTH) — ↓ — ↓ — HIGHEST

acids are keys to the biochemical cycles to be discussed in Chapter 22. Several of the other acids and anions will be touched upon later.

You should be able to use Table 13–4 to make some predictions about chemical behavior.

EXAMPLE 13d: Two solutions are standing side by side. One contains 0.10 *M* HNO_2, nit*rous* acid (not to be confused with its much stronger cousin, nitric acid, HNO_3). The other is 0.10 *M* lactic acid, found in milk and in all muscle tissue. Which has the *lower* pH? Use Table 13–4.

– –

ANSWER: The compound with the lower pK_a is the stronger acid and will have the more highly acidic solution, thus the lower pH. The pK_a for nitrous acid is 3.3, for lactic acid 3.9. The nitrous acid solution will have the lower pH.

Table 13–4 can also show you the direction in which a reaction will go if a weak acid is used to neutralize one of the listed conjugate bases. The rule is that the *stronger* acid and base react to form the *weaker* acid and base.

EXAMPLE 13e: What will be present in the greatest concentrations if the following solutions (all 0.10 *M*) are mixed at 25°C?
i) pyruvic acid and sodium benzoate
ii) ascorbic acid and sodium salicylate

– –

ANSWER: Compare the weak acids in each case.
i) Pyruvic acid (pK_a = 2.5, from Table 13–4) is stronger than benzoic acid (pK_a = 4.2). The reaction will go from strong to weak. Also, the benzoate ion is a stronger base than the pyruvate ion, and again we go from strong to weak. Therefore the products are benzoic acid and sodium pyruvate.
ii) Ascorbic acid (pK_a = 4.1) is weaker than salicylic acid (pK_a = 3.0), and so the salicylate ion is a weaker base than the ascorbate ion. Since we already have the weaker acid and base present, there is very little reaction. The substances left at the end are mostly what we started with, ascorbic acid and sodium salicylate.

You may notice that a *stronger* acid has a *weaker* conjugate base, and vice versa. The conjugate bases of the common strong acids (NO_3^- from nitric acid, Cl^- from hydrochloric acid, HSO_4^- from sulfuric acid) have almost no ability to accept protons. They are not basic at all. Similarly, the conjugate acids of the strong bases, such as the hydrated Na^+ cation from NaOH or the hydrated Ca^{2+} cation from $Ca(OH)_2$ do not act as acids in aqueous solution. We will return briefly to this point in Section 13.3.

Acid equilibrium constants

In Sections 5.2 and 11.5, we discussed equilibrium without trying to assign numbers to the relative amounts of reactants and products. However, to properly describe what is present in a solution of a weak acid, we must solve some very simple algebraic expressions.

We have already seen one equilibrium expression, that for water:

$$K_w = [H^+][OH^-] = 1 \times 10^{-14} \text{ at } 25°C$$

There are many different kinds of **equilibrium constants** (K's), since there are many processes that do not go to completion. In the case of a weak acid, which only partly dissociates,

$$HA \rightleftharpoons H^+ + A^- \text{ (all in aqueous solution)}$$

the equilibrium constant, K_a, depends only on temperature and is

$$K_a = \frac{[H^+][A^-]}{[HA]}$$

In words, "the acid dissociation constant is equal to the molarity of hydrated protons in the solution $[H^+]$, times the molarity of the conjugate base $[A^-]$, divided by the molarity of the conjugate acid form $[HA]$."

If we are simply dissolving a weak acid in water, the number of moles of H^+ produced is equal to the number of moles of A^-, and $[H^+] = [A^-]$. In that particular case,

In this type of calculation, we ignore the amount of H^+ that would come from the dissociation of water molecules.

$$K_a = \frac{[H^+][A^-]}{[HA]} = \frac{[H^+]^2}{[HA]}$$

$$[H^+] = \sqrt{K_a[HA]}$$

The **pK_a** values in Table 13–4 are simply the negative powers of ten of the K_a values. If $K_a = 1 \times 10^{-4}$, then p$K_a = 4.0$. In the very special case of an acid that dissociates only slightly and has an overall concentration of about 1.0 mole/liter, $[HA] = 1.0$. In this unusual situation, the expression is even simpler:

$$[H^+] = \sqrt{K_a[HA]} = \sqrt{K_a(1.0)} = \sqrt{K_a}$$

$$-\log[H^+] = pH = \frac{1}{2}pK_a = -\log\sqrt{K_a}$$

In other words, the pH of the solution is directly proportional to the pK_a. In fact, at *any* acid concentration, and assuming only slight dissociation of the acid, since $[H^+] \simeq \sqrt{K_a[HA]}$ we can use the expression pH $\simeq \frac{1}{2}pK_a - \frac{1}{2}\log_{10}[HA]$ for a pure weak acid dissolved in water.

EXAMPLE 13f: Barbituric acid, the "parent" acid of several kinds of sleeping pills, has a p$K_a = 4.0$ at 25°C. What is the pH of a 0.010 M solution of barbituric acid in water?

- -

ANSWER: The $\log_{10}$ of 0.010 is -2.0, so $\frac{1}{2}\log_{10}[HA] \approx +1.0$. Then pH $= \frac{1}{2}pK_a - \frac{1}{2}\log_{10}[HA] \approx 2.0 + 1.0 = \boxed{3.0}$. This means that in this solution, $[H^+] \approx 1 \times 10^{-3} M$, and the acid is roughly 10% dissociated.

In other situations, the acid and its conjugate base may come from two different sources. For example, in the human blood stream, the concentrations of bicarbonate ion (hydrogen carbonate ion), HCO_3^-, and of H_2CO_3 from dissolved carbon dioxide are quite independent of each other. In such a case, we obtain a very important equation for *buffer solutions*. We already know that

$$K_a = \frac{[H^+][A^-]}{[HA]} = [H^+]\frac{[A^-]}{[HA]}$$

Turning this around we get

$$[H^+] = K_a\frac{[HA]}{[A^-]}$$

$$pH = pK_a - \log_{10}\frac{[HA]}{[A^-]}$$

This is the Henderson–Hasselbalch equation. We will refer back to this equation when we study buffer solutions in Section 13.5.

Relative acidity of carboxylic acids

Except for the extremely weak acids called phenols (Chapter 15), with pK_a around 10.0, all of the organic compounds that are acidic in aqueous solution are carboxylic acids, with the functional group

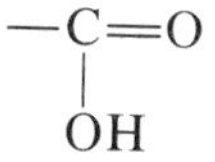

$$-\overset{\displaystyle |}{\underset{\displaystyle OH}{C}}=O$$

The presence of the doubly bonded oxygen in the $-C=O$ part of the molecule helps pull electrons away from the hydrogen:

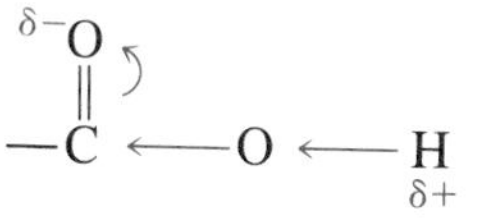

$$-\overset{\overset{\displaystyle \delta^- O}{\|}}{C} \longleftarrow O \longleftarrow \underset{\delta+}{H}$$

After the hydrogen is lost, the two oxygen atoms become equivalent. The second bond (pi bond) of the $C=O$ bond becomes *delocalized* (p. 170) over the three atoms. This makes it slightly more difficult for the H^+ to return, since neither oxygen is more attractive than the other:

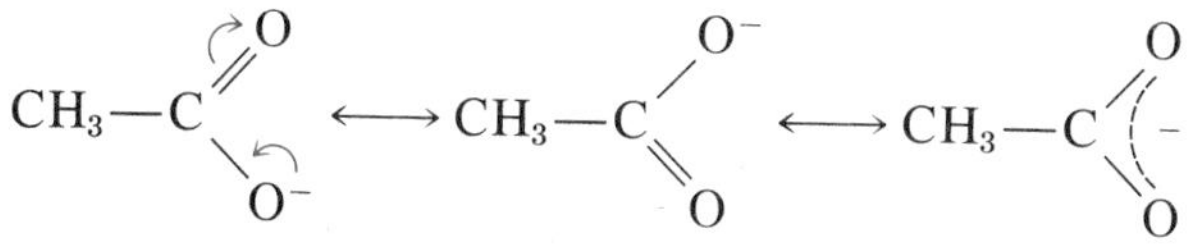

A nearby electron-pulling (highly electronegative) atom will also increase the acidity of a carboxylic acid. For example, look at the effect of a neighboring hydroxyl or carbonyl group:

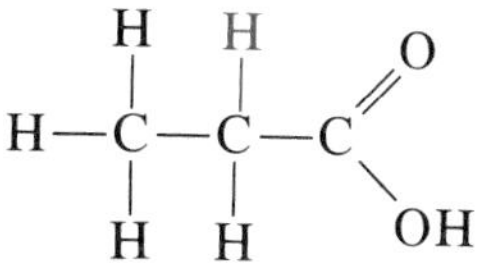

propanoic acid
$pK_a = 4.9$

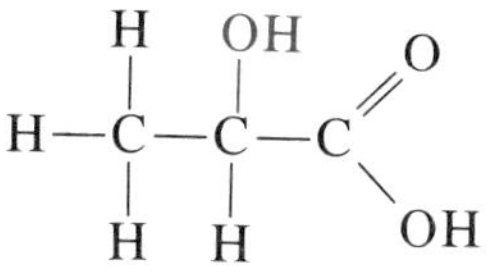

lactic acid
$pK_a = 3.9$

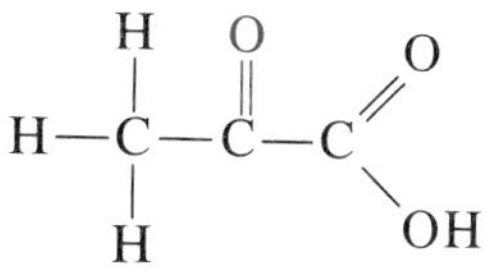

pyruvic acid
$pK_a = 2.5$

The hydrogen bonded to oxygen in an alcohol, such as CH_3OH, is not acidic in water solution. It takes the extra oxygen of a $-COOH$ group, or an aromatic ring (Chapter 15), to make the hydrogen easier to release as $H^+_{(aq)}$.

Chlorine is also highly electronegative, so we might expect chlorinated compounds to be more acidic than the simple hydrocarbon acids:

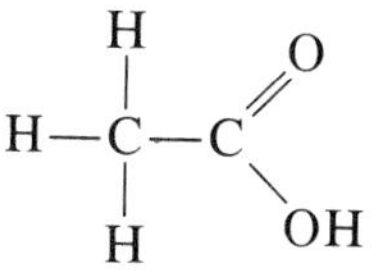

acetic acid
$pK_a = 4.7$

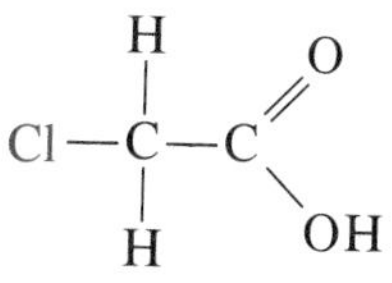

chloroacetic
acid
$pK_a = 2.9$

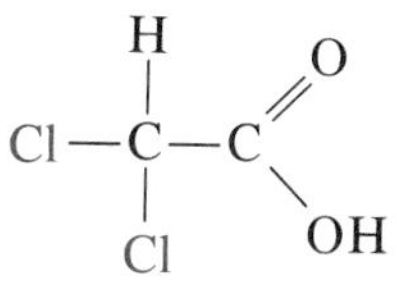

dichloroacetic
acid
$pK_a = 1.5$

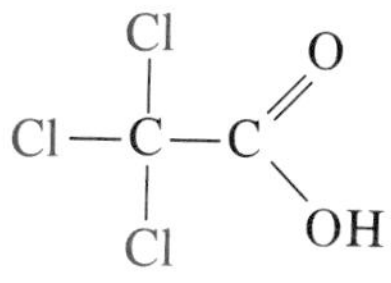

trichloroacetic
acid
$pK_a = 0.7$

In fact, trichloroacetic is one of the strongest organic acids; a 0.10 M solution has a pH $= 1.14$ and is over 70% dissociated. It is thus very close to being a *strong* acid like HCl.

SELF-CHECK

13.8) Write the equilibrium equation for the partial dissociation of
a) acetic acid, CH_3COOH, $pK_a = 4.7$
b) succinic acid, $HOOCCH_2CH_2COOH$, $pK_a = 4.2$
c) sulfurous acid, H_2SO_3, $pK_a = 1.9$
d) the ammonium ion, NH_4^+, $pK_a = 9.3$
e) nicotinic acid (niacin), a B-vitamin, C_5NH_4COOH

13.9) For the conjugate base of each of the acids in Self-Check 13.8,
a) write the formula
b*) write the common name

13.10) Rank the four acids in Self-Check 13.8 whose pK_a values are given in order of *decreasing acidity* of a 0.10 M solution.

13.11*) Determine whether each of the following is a polyprotic acid in water:
a) H_3PO_3 b) fumaric acid, $HOOCCH{=}CHCOOH$
c) acetoacetic acid, CH_3COCH_2COOH d) NH_4^+

13.12*) Determine what substances will be present in the greatest concentrations if equal amounts of 0.10 M solutions of the following are mixed at 25°C. Use Table 13–4.
a) HF and sodium ascorbate
b) phenol and potassium formate
c) sulfuric acid and sodium carbonate

13.13*) The pK_a values for several organic substances at 25°C are given below. Which are aqueous acids, that is, stronger acids than water in solution?
a) butyric acid (found in sweat, rancid butter) with $pK_a = 4.81$
b) glycerol (a viscous liquid) with $pK_a = 14.15$
c) saccharin (a sugar substitute) with $pK_a = 11.7$

13.14*) In each of the following pairs of acids, which would you expect to have the *lower* pK_a (greater acidity) based on the discussion of this section?
a) 2-chloropropanoic acid or propanoic acid
b) iodoacetic acid or chloroacetic acid
c) $HClO_4$ or $HClO$

13.3 WEAK BASES

LEARNING GOAL 13G: Given the formula of a basic molecule or anion, write the equilibrium equation for its reaction with water.
13H: Given formulas of any acid and any base, write the neutralization equation.
13I: Given the pK_a of a weak acid, calculate the pK_b of its conjugate base.

You have already seen a number of weak bases in Table 13-4. Every conjugate base of a weak acid has the ability to increase the $OH^-_{(aq)}$ concentration of a water solution:

$$A^-_{(aq)} + H_2O_{(\ell)} \rightleftharpoons HA_{(aq)} + OH^-_{(aq)}$$

A **weak base** is thus a substance that does not contain OH^- ion but reacts

TABLE 13–5   REACTIONS AND pK_b OF SELECTED BASES AT 25°C

Name of Base	Reaction with Water (hydrolysis) to Produce a Weak Acid		pK_b of Base = $14.0 - pK_a$ of Weak Acid
Phosphate ion	PO_4^{3-}	$+ H_2O \rightleftharpoons OH^- + HPO_4^{2-}$	2.0
Methylamine	CH_3NH_2	$+ H_2O \rightleftharpoons OH^- + CH_3NH_3^+$	3.3
Carbonate ion	CO_3^{2-}	$+ H_2O \rightleftharpoons OH^- + HCO_3^-$	3.8
Phenolate ion	$C_6H_5O^-$	$+ H_2O \rightleftharpoons OH^- + C_6H_5OH$	4.1
Ammonia	NH_3	$+ H_2O \rightleftharpoons OH^- + NH_4^+$	4.7
Monohydrogen phosphate ion	HPO_4^{2-}	$+ H_2O \rightleftharpoons OH^- + H_2PO_4^-$	6.8
Hydrogen carbonate (bicarbonate) ion	HCO_3^-	$+ H_2O \rightleftharpoons OH^- + H_2CO_3$	7.6*
Acetate ion	CH_3COO^-	$+ H_2O \rightleftharpoons OH^- + CH_3COOH$	9.3
Aniline	$C_6H_5NH_2$	$+ H_2O \rightleftharpoons OH^- + C_6H_5NH_3^+$	9.4
Benzoate ion	$C_6H_5COO^-$	$+ H_2O \rightleftharpoons OH^- + C_6H_5COOH$	9.8
Fluoride ion	F^-	$+ H_2O \rightleftharpoons OH^- + HF$	10.8

* The pK_b of bicarbonate ion in the blood stream is about 7.9, since it is then not at 25°C but at body temperature, 37°C. In the body, the weak acid involved is largely H_2CO_3, *carbonic acid*. In water solutions outside the body, such as cake batters and Alka-Seltzer, very little H_2CO_3 exists and most of the reaction involves $CO_{2(aq)}$, carbon dioxide gas dissolved in water.

with water to gain a proton and release OH^- from the water. This process is sometimes called *hydrolysis*, which literally means "the breaking apart of water."

Table 13-5 shows the reactions of a number of bases with water. In most cases, these reactions are the reverse of what you saw in Table 13-4.

Just as the pK_a is used to measure the relative ability of a weak acid to *lose* its H^+, a **pK_b** is used to measure the relative ability of a weak base to *gain* H^+ and become its conjugate acid. The calculation of pK_b for the conjugate base of any acid in Table 13-4 is simplified by the fact that

The pK_a of a weak acid + the pK_b of its conjugate base = 14.0 at 25°C

To find the pK_b, we simply subtract the pK_a of the conjugate acid from 14.0. For example, the pK_a of the ammonium ion is 9.3. Then the pK_b of NH_3 must be $(14.0 - 9.3) = 4.7$.

Our list of useful bases is somewhat short. Carboxylate ions are generally less basic than their parent carboxylic acids are acidic. The pK_a values are generally around 3.0 to 5.0, leading to pK_b values of the anions between 9.0 and 11.0. That is one reason foods tend to be acidic rather than basic. On the other hand, many of these carboxylate anions are found in useful food additives, such as citrates, sodium benzoate, and calcium propionate.

Sodium bicarbonate (baking soda) is useful in making cakes rise; it also seems to be very effective in absorbing odors in the air. Ammonia is a valuable cleaning agent.

Two of the strongest bases in Table 13-5 are commonly used in very strong detergents. Trisodium phosphate, Na_3PO_4, and washing soda, Na_2CO_3, are so basic that they will severely damage the esophagus if swallowed. For this reason, dishwasher detergents should always be kept out of the reach of small children.

You have now developed skills that should permit you to answer questions like the following.

Hydrolysis was defined in Section 9.5 in a situation in which water breaks up an ester, the H— from water making the carboxylic acid and the —OH from water making the original alcohol. The same word is used in a similar sense here. In both cases, water is "breaking up" into H— and —OH.

Do not refer to aqueous ammonia as "ammonium hydroxide," NH_4OH, as occasionally seen on reagent bottles. Such a formula would imply the existence of the ionic salt NH_4OH, which would be a *strong* base if it truly existed.

EXAMPLE 13g: Write the equilibrium equation for the reaction with water of each of the following bases.
i) the sulfite ion, SO_3^{2-}
ii) the acetate ion, CH_3COO^-

- -

ANSWER: The reaction must involve gaining one $H_{(aq)}^+$ from water.
i) $SO_{3(aq)}^{2-} + H_2O_{(\ell)} \rightleftharpoons HSO_{3(aq)}^- + OH_{(aq)}^-$
ii) $CH_3COO_{(aq)}^- + H_2O_{(\ell)} \rightleftharpoons CH_3COOH_{(aq)} + OH_{(aq)}^-$

You should be able to apply the equation $pK_b = 14.0 - pK_a$.

EXAMPLE 13h: Rank the following bases in order of *decreasing* OH^- concentration of their 0.10 M solutions, by calculating the pK_b for each base. Use Table 13–4 as needed.
i) monohydrogen phosphate ion, HPO_4^{2-}
ii) carbonate ion, CO_3^{2-}
iii) sulfide ion, S^{2-} (pK_a for $HS_{(aq)}^-$ is 12.0)
iv) picrate ion, $C_6H_2N_3O_7^-$ (pK_a for picric acid is 0.4)
v) propanoate (propionate) ion (pK_a for propanoic acid is 4.9)

- -

ANSWERS:
i) $H_2PO_4^-$ has $pK_a = 7.2$; thus pK_b of HPO_4^{2-} is $14.0 - 7.2 = \boxed{6.8}$.
ii) HCO_3^- has $pK_a = 10.2$, thus pK_b of CO_3^{2-} is $14.0 - 10.2 = \boxed{3.8}$.
(These two values can also be checked in Table 13–5.)
iii) pK_b for S^{2-} is $14.0 - 12.0 = \boxed{2.0}$.
iv) pK_b for $C_6H_2N_3O_7^-$ is $14.0 - 0.4 = \boxed{13.6}$.
v) pK_b for $CH_3CH_2COO^-$ ion is $14.0 - 4.9 = \boxed{9.1}$.
Putting the bases in order, strongest base first, we obtain

Base:	S^{2-}	HCO_3^-	HPO_4^{2-}	$CH_3CH_2COO^-$	$C_6H_2N_3O_7^-$
pK_b:	2.0	3.8	6.8	9.1	13.6

Solutions of ionic salts

If we wish to determine whether a solution of an ionic salt dissolved in water is acidic or basic, we might consult Tables 13–4 and 13–5. For example, three ions are very definitely acidic: HSO_4^-, $H_2PO_4^-$, and NH_4^+. If any one of these is in combination with an ion that is neither acidic nor basic, such as Na^+, Ca^{2+}, Cl^- or NO_3^-, then the resulting solution will be acidic.

Many ions are basic, such as F^-, HCO_3^-, PO_3^{3-}, or OH^-. If any of these is in combination with a Group 1 or 2 metal ion, the resulting solution will be basic.

The only doubtful salt would be one that combines an acidic cation (such as NH_4^+ or an ammonium salt such as those described in Section 13.4) with a basic anion. In that case, the pK_a of the acid must be compared with the pK_b of the base to see which is stronger.

EXAMPLE 13i: Is a 0.10 M solution of each of the following ionic salts acidic, basic, or neutral?
i) NaF ii) $CaCl_2$ iii) NH_4NO_3 iv) $KHCO_3$ v) CH_3COONH_4

- -

ANSWER:
i) Na^+ is neither acidic nor basic, F^- is basic. A solution of NaF would be $\boxed{basic}$.

ii) Ca^{2+} is neither acidic nor basic; Cl^- is neither. A solution of $CaCl_2$ would be neutral .

iii) NH_4^+ is acidic; NO_3^- is neither acidic nor basic. A solution of NH_4NO_3 would be acidic .

iv) K^+ is neither acidic nor basic; HCO_3^- is basic. A solution of $KHCO_3$ would be basic .

v) CH_3COO^- is basic; NH_4^+ is acidic. We must compare pK's. The $pK_a = 9.3$ for NH_4^+; the $pK_b = 9.3$ for CH_3COO^-. Since the acidity of ammonium is equal to the basicity of the acetate ion, the resulting solution should be neutral .

Finally, you should be able to write any chemical equation that involves neutralization.

EXAMPLE 13j: Write the chemical equation for the reaction between the following substances in aqueous solution, showing the products as ions.
  i) hydrochloric acid and aniline (see Table 13–5)
  ii) acetic acid and monohydrogen phosphate ion
  iii) benzoic acid and sodium hydroxide
  iv) pyruvic acid (see Table 13-4) and phosphate ion
  v) tartaric acid, HOOCCHOHCHOHCOOH, and hydrazine, H_2NNH_2

- -

ANSWER:
  i) $HCl + C_6H_5NH_2 \longrightarrow C_6H_5NH_3^+ + Cl^-$
  ii) $CH_3COOH + HPO_4^{2-} \longrightarrow CH_3COO^- + H_2PO_4^-$
  iii) $C_6H_5COOH + NaOH \longrightarrow C_6H_5COO^- + Na^+ + H_2O$
  iv) $CH_3COCOOH + PO_4^{3-} \longrightarrow CH_3COCOO^- + HPO_4^{2-}$
  v) $HOOCCHOHCHOHCOOH + H_2NNH_2 \longrightarrow$
                      $HOOCCHOHCHOHCOO^- + H_2NNH_3^+$

SELF-CHECK

13.15) Write the equation for the reaction with water of
a) the phenolate ion, $C_6H_5O^-$
b) the acetate ion, CH_3COO^-
c) methylamine, CH_3NH_2
d) aniline, $C_6H_5NH_2$

13.16) Calculate the pK_b values for the following bases.
a) salicylate ion, $HOC_6H_4COO^-$ (see Table 13–4)
b) urea, H_2NCNH_2, if the K_a for $H_2NCNH_3^+$ is 0.10
            $\overset{\|}{O}$ $\overset{\|}{O}$
c) the hypochlorite ion, if the pK_a for its conjugate acid is 7.5
d) the sulfate ion (see Table 13–4)

13.17) Write the chemical equation for the following neutralization reactions, showing the products in ionic form in aqueous solution. Use Tables 13–4 and 13–5 if necessary.
a) citric acid, $H_3C_6H_5O_6$, and carbonate ion (one step only)
b) nitrous acid HNO_2 and methylamine CH_3NH_2
c) nitric acid, HNO_3, and lactate ion, $CH_3CHOHCOO^-$

13.18*) An unaware consumer confuses washing soda with baking soda and takes a glassful of Na_2CO_3 solution to help a hangover instead of the intended $NaHCO_3$. What are the likely results? Why?

13.4 AMINES

LEARNING GOAL 13J: Distinguish between primary, secondary, and tertiary amines.

13K: Write a balanced equation for the formation of an amide.

Amines are derivatives of ammonia, NH_3, in which one or more of the hydrogen atoms have been replaced by an organic group, such as a hydrocarbon chain. Like alcohols, amines are classified as

Primary: $R—\overset{..}{N}—H$ as in $CH_3—\overset{..}{N}—H$ or $C_6H_5—\overset{..}{N}—H$

methylamine   aniline

Secondary: $R—\overset{..}{N}—R'$ as in $CH_3CH_2—\overset{..}{N}—CH_3$

methylethylamine

Tertiary: $R—\overset{..}{N}—R''$ as in $CH_3—\overset{..}{N}—CH_3$

trimethylamine

In a primary amine, one hydrogen from ammonia has been replaced by an organic group. The two examples given above are both found in Table 13–5. Methylamine and aniline, along with the other amines, are organic bases.

In a secondary amine, two ammonia hydrogens have been replaced by organic groups, leaving only one hydrogen on the nitrogen. In a tertiary amine, all three ammonia hydrogens have been replaced.

As shown in the examples, all types of amines leave the nitrogen with an unshared electron pair. This electron pair can readily accept a proton, H^+, to form a positive ion similar to the ammonium ion, NH_4^+. All of the amines will thus neutralize acids to form salts:

$$CH_3NH_{2(aq)} + HCl_{(aq)} \longrightarrow CH_3NH_3^+ + Cl^-$$

methylamine   methylammonium chloride

While the basic properties of amines make them of interest in this chapter on acids and bases, this group of compounds is of critical importance to life processes as well. All proteins, as well as almost all of the molecules that regulate and control life processes, such as vitamins and hormones, contain nitrogen.

Properties and names of amines

Each primary or secondary amine has hydrogen attached to the fairly electronegative nitrogen atom and can thus form the type of strong intermolecular attractions we described in Section 11.4 as hydrogen-bonding. This gives such compounds relatively high melting and boiling points. Amines are fairly soluble in water, also because of hydrogen-bonding.

Tertiary amines can also react with alkyl halides to form quaternary ammonium salts *in which the nitrogen atom is surrounded by* four *alkyl groups. The common formula would be R_4NX. These are sometimes used as disinfectants.*

Purine

Pyrimidine

Purine and pyrimidine are organic amines that contain organic ring structures (discussed in Chapter 15). The flavor of meat is due primarily to derivatives of these two substances.

Amines of low molecular weight may smell like ammonia. Some of higher formula weight will remind you of decaying fish because the odor of fish is caused by amines. Now you will understand why lemon juice is often spread on fish in cooked dishes; the citric acid neutralizes the (basic) amines and removes some of the odor.

While there is a IUPAC system for naming amines, it is little used. Instead, common names are made by naming the groups attached to the nitrogen atom. The usual prefixes are used if two or three groups are identical, as in *trimethylamine,* shown earlier as an example of a tertiary amine.

Amide formation

Carboxylic acids neutralize amines to give salts. For example, acetic acid reacts with aniline:

$$CH_3COOH + H-N-C_6H_5 \longrightarrow CH_3C\underset{O}{\overset{O}{<}} \quad ^+H-N-C_6H_5$$

acetic acid   aniline   anilinium acetate

On heating the product, *water is lost* and a bond is formed between a carbon atom of the acetate and the nitrogen atom to form an **amide:**

$$CH_3C\underset{O}{\overset{O}{<}} {}^- + {}^+H-N-C_6H_5 \longrightarrow CH_3C-N-C_6H_5 + H_2O$$

acetanilide

The process is very similar to the formation of an ester (Chapter 9). The product in this particular case, *acetanilide,* was used for many years as an analgesic (pain-relieving) drug and as an antipyretic (fever-reducing) drug.

Since acetanilide is somewhat toxic, other safer drugs were sought. One result was *acetaminophen,* sold under such brands as Tempra, Tylenol, and at least 20 other* trade names:

$$CH_3COOH + H_2NC_6H_4OH \longrightarrow CH_3\overset{O}{\overset{\|}{C}}-\overset{H}{\overset{|}{N}}-C_6H_4OH + H_2O$$

acetaminophen

Another pain reliever, similar in structure to acetanilide and acetaminophen, is phenacetin, once commonly combined with aspirin and caffeine in APC (aspirin, phenacetin, caffeine) tablets such as Empirin and Anacin.

$$HN-\overset{O}{\overset{\|}{C}}CH_3$$

$$OC_2H_5$$

phenacetin

---

* Chemists often know a drug by its *generic,* or scientific, name. If the drug has been available long enough, its patent will have expired and it can often be purchased either by its generic name or by various trade names. Pentobarbital, a sedative and anesthetic, is also known by the trade names Nembutal, Embutal, Pentyl, Pentone, Sopental, Carbrital, Continal, Euthatal, Mebumal, Sagatal, Sotyl, Barpental, "844," and possibly others. The generic form of such a drug is often much less expensive than a "name" brand. If the patent is still held by a pharmaceutical company, then only the trade-name version made by that company will be available. An excellent reference to the generic and trade names of drugs, as well as an outstanding source of other information about compounds of medical interest, is the *Merck Index,* published by Merck & Co.

Most amides of pharmaceutical interest contain complicated ring structures; they will be discussed in Chapter 15. It is of interest to consider the diversity of such compounds: barbiturates, LSD, tetracycline antibiotics, thalidomide, and one form of niacin all contain amide linkages.

Under certain conditions, the amide linkage may be repeated over and over again in the same molecule to give polyamide (nylon) plastics (Chapter 16) and proteins (Chapter 19).

Amino acids

Proteins are the building materials of life, and the fundamental unit that makes up a protein by amide linkages is the **amino acid.** The simplest such compound is glycine:

$$H_2N—CH_2—COOH$$

which has an amino ($—NH_2$) group at one end and a carboxylic acid group ($—COOH$) at the other. There are over 20 such compounds, discussed more fully in Chapter 19.

Amino acids react with each other because the acid side of one molecule can react with the amine side of another to make an amide. Water is, of course, lost in the process. The two ends of the molecule that results again contain an amine and an acid group, so the formation of amide or *peptide* linkages can continue, resulting in long chains.

Amides can be *hydrolyzed* in the presence of added acid or base, resulting in the addition of water and the breaking up of the amide into the carboxylic acid and ammonium salt (in acid) or the acid anion and the amine (in base). In a way, this is the reverse of amide formation. Hydrolysis of proteins breaks them down into their component amino acids. This can be done so carefully that the exact sequence of amino acids can be determined.

Mild pain-killing drugs

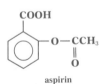

aspirin

The acetyl group on ASA seems to reduce its acidity and give it a more tolerable taste. Over 40 million pounds of ASA are manufactured each year in the United States. Total sales of analgesics in the United States are over a quarter of a *billion* dollars.

We have briefly discussed several amides that have proven effective in reducing pain and fever. Many of us have our favorite remedies for the treatment of headaches and colds. The most popular is undoubtedly aspirin (acetylsalicylic acid or ASA), which is an ester of acetic acid with salicylic acid.

Aspirin works by reducing inflammation and swelling of tissues. Since much pain is due to the pressure of swollen tissue on peripheral nerve endings, such pain is often relieved. The acetyl ($CH_3CO—$) group appears to make aspirin a better pain-killer than salicylic acid.

Aspirin is also taken in large dosages (12 to 16 tablets each day, or about 5 grams) by arthritics, who benefit not only from pain relief but also from the anti-swelling effect of aspirin on joint tissue. Since aspirin also tends to prevent blood platelets from forming clots, it may be useful in preventing strokes resulting from blood clots in the brain.

Many drugs have been tested, during the past 80 years, for their ability (in competition with aspirin) to reduce pain and fever. Phenacetin is an aniline derivative that was used for about 75 years but has recently been phased out of many products because of possible damage to kidneys and blood. It has often been replaced by acetaminophen. However, neither of these amides is of value to arthritics since neither reduces swelling or inflammation of tissues.

The main danger with pain-killers (as with antacids, Section 13.1) is overdose. We are all familiar with stories of children being rushed to the hospital from overdoses of aspirin. Acetaminophen is often claimed to be safer than aspirin, yet it is possible for a relatively low dose (12 tablets, or 6 grams) of acetaminophen to cause such damage to liver cells that death results in one to two weeks. Particular care must therefore be taken to avoid any kind of overdose with products containing this "aspirin substitute."

People who take large doses of aspirin sometimes experience stomach upset. One product, Bufferin, was developed in the late 1940's to combine an antacid with aspirin, and thus reduce the stomach problem. This antacid additive also speeded up the absorption of the aspirin.

On the other hand, most "combination of ingredients" drugs are not really intended to remedy one particular condition, and many provide unneeded medication. For example, some antacids also contain aspirin (Alka-Seltzer) or acetaminophen. The 1973 report of a panel of the U.S. Food and Drug Administration concluded that such combinations are "irrational for antacid use alone."

Many analgesic pills combine several other compounds with aspirin. At one time, a combination of aspirin, phenacetin, and caffeine (known as A.P.C.) was very widely sold. When phenacetin was shown to cause kidney damage, it was dropped from the formulation. Anacin, for example, now contains aspirin and caffeine. However, the amount of caffeine in one tablet, 32.5 mg, is about the same as that in ¼ cup of brewed coffee. According to *AMA Drug Evaluations,* the caffeine is of no value in an analgesic drug. Excedrin adds two more compounds: acetaminophen and salicylamide, the latter considered in the AMA report to be too weak and unreliable to be useful. An FDA advisory panel on internal analgesics has stated that, in general, the fewer ingredients in an over-the-counter product, the safer and more rational the therapy.*

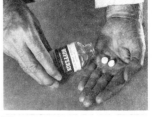

The antacid in Bufferin is similar to that in Rolaids (Table 13–3). It permits faster absorption of the ASA in the intestinal tract.

Antihistamines

Another popular family of drugs is the antihistamines. From their name, you might gather that amines are involved. In fact, histamine may be formed by removing the carboxyl group from an amino acid, histidine, leaving the amine end. It may therefore be considered a substituted ethylamine.

When histamine is formed in the body, as a result of tissue damage or a foreign substance, it sets off a chain of events that we call *inflammation.* One effect is to dilate (enlarge) the small blood vessels, allowing more blood to get through; the effect in the brain may be to bring on a headache, and in the lungs this dilation can cause asthma. Histamine also can cause swelling, itching, and increased formation of gastric fluids. While these reactions are all intended as a defense against "invasion" of the body by microbes and other foreign matter, the same response can apparently be triggered in an allergic person by very small amounts of protein in food, dust, pollen, or animal hairs.

The chemistry of a drug molecule is often directly related to the action of a natural substance in the body. A portion of the chemical structure of an antihistamine, the ethylamine section, is similar to that in histamine. This portion of the drug molecule competes with histamine for the "receptor site" that will trigger the problems associated with inflammation.

In addition to the direct effects of antihistamines, which are useful to many allergic people, the side effects may be useful. Some sleeping pills, such as Nytol, contain an antihistamine that causes drowsiness as a side effect.

Each of the antihistamine molecules is somewhat too large to dissolve easily in water (and in body fluids), even with the aid of hydrogen-bonding between the amine group and H_2O. These compounds are therefore sold not as the pure amine but as its ammonium salt. Benadryl is sold as the chloride (after reaction with HCl) or the ascorbate (after reaction with ascorbic acid). Pyribenzamine is prepared as the chloride or citrate, and Chlor-trimeton as the maleate.

Similarly, other drugs that must dissolve in body fluids and are composed of amines will be made up as ammonium salts. Otrivin nosedrops are sold as an am-

histamine

ethylamine

Benadryl
(diphenhydramine)

Pyribenzamine
(tripelennamine)

Chlor-trimeton
(chlorpheniramine)

---

* See *The Medicine Show,* 5th edition, Chapter 1 on analgesics and Chapter 2 on cold remedies, published by Consumers Union, Mount Vernon, NY, 1980.

monium chloride salt, as is Neo-Synephrine. Skin ointments are also sold as salts. The local anesthetic procaine (Novocain) is sold as either the chloride or the borate. It is not sufficient to be sure that a drug works. It is equally important to be sure that it dissolves in body fluids and reaches the point of action!

SELF-CHECK

13.19) The following structural formulas may seem complex, but they can be looked at in terms of the functional groups they contain. Does each compound contain a primary, secondary, or tertiary amine? (Note: The symbol

simply stands for a benzene ring (Chapter 15) containing six carbon atoms and generally five hydrogen atoms. No nitrogen atoms are involved.)

a) proline, an amino acid

e) Penicillin G

b) monosodium glutamate, a food additive

$$H_2N-CHCO_2H$$
$$\ \ \ \ \ \ \ \ \ \ \ \ \ \ \ \ CH_2CH_2CO_2Na$$

f) disulfiram, used to treat alcoholism

c) barbital, a barbiturate

g) mescaline, a hallucinogen

d) L-*dopa,* used in treating Parkinson's disease

h) procaine, a local anesthetic

13.20) Write an equation for the formation of an amide from propanoic acid and methylamine.

13.21*) How do antihistamines work?

13.5 BUFFER SOLUTIONS

> *LEARNING GOAL 13L: Explain how a given amphoteric species can act either as an acid or as a base.*
>
> *13M: Given a buffer solution, write balanced equations for the reaction of the buffer with added acid and with added base.*
>
> *13N: Describe, in general terms, how to make a buffer solution for a given pH.*

Human blood must be kept in a very narrow pH range or else the body will not function properly because enzymes will not have the correct environment for action. Normal blood has a pH of 7.4, which means a H^+ concentration of 0.000 000 04 M. That is very close to neutral, just slightly on the basic side.

If there were no system to control the pH of the blood, the blood would quickly become acidic and the pH would go down. For example, the breaking down of proteins and nucleic acids releases phosphoric acid, H_3PO_4, and sulfuric acid, H_2SO_4, into body fluids. Many organic acids are produced in the metabolic cycles we will discuss in Chapters 22 to 27. As we know from Section 13.2, acids like lactic acid, even though they dissociate only slightly, will liberate $H^+_{(aq)}$ and acidify the blood. Also, the carbon dioxide produced by the cells must be carried through the blood to the lungs. Dissolved CO_2 reacts somewhat in aqueous solution to form $H^+_{(aq)}$ and $HCO^-_{3(aq)}$. Such excess of H^+ ions must be neutralized or the blood would be acidic.

The average American diet liberates 0.040 to 0.080 moles of $H^+_{(aq)}$ each day. To cope with this acid, the body has a *buffer* mechanism that acts to keep the pH constant.

The transport of O_2 by hemoglobin and the dissolving of CO_2 in the blood stream are also essential body processes that are dependent on the proper blood pH.

Various natural sources of water are slightly acidic as a result of dissolved CO_2. When acidic waters pass through limestone (chalk, $CaCO_3$) they dissolve the stone to create caverns.

Amphoteric molecules and ions

An acid can donate a proton; a base can accept a proton. Some of the species we have discussed so far in this chapter can either give away or receive protons, and thus can act as either acids or bases. We call these **amphoteric** substances.

One example is the bicarbonate ion, HCO_3^-. If you use baking soda, $NaHCO_3$, to make a cake rise, it reacts with acid and releases carbon dioxide gas:

$$HCO^-_{3(aq)} + H^+_{(aq)} \longrightarrow H_2O_{(\ell)} + CO_{2(g)}$$

However, if you add sodium bicarbonate to an even stronger basic solution, such as that of lye, NaOH, the bicarbonate ion will act as an acid:

$$HCO^-_{3(aq)} + OH^-_{(aq)} \longrightarrow H_2O_{(\ell)} + CO^{2-}_{3(aq)}$$

A solution of sodium bicarbonate powder dissolved in water will be basic, since the pK_b of the HCO_3^- ion is 7.6. It will also tend to *resist* change in pH, by reacting with any added acid to form CO_2 or with any added strong base to form CO_3^{2-}. We can thus say that it **buffers** any change in pH by such reactions.

Aluminum hydroxide, $Al(OH)_3$, found in many antacids, is also a buffer, since it can react with either acid or base. The hydrogen sulfate ion provides a buffer on the acid side of the pH range. Two anions of phosphoric acid found in the body, $H_2PO_4^-$ and HPO_4^{2-}, are similarly amphoteric.

Amphoteric properties of amino acids

We have already described an amino acid as a substance that has a basic amine group, $-NH_2$, at one end of the molecule and a carboxylic acid group, $-COOH$, at the other end. This makes an amino acid both acidic and basic, and thus amphoteric.

To understand amino acids better, however, we must realize that in the solid state (as in the proteins of skin, hair, and other tissues) and in aqueous solution, we obtain not an uncharged molecule but a molecule with equal and opposite charges on the two ends. We can see this better if we imagine two glycine, H_2NCH_2COOH, molecules reacting with each other, first at one end:

$$\underset{\text{acid}}{H_2NCH_2COOH} + \underset{\text{base}}{H_2NCH_2COOH} \longrightarrow H_2NCH_2COO^- + \underset{\text{salt}}{{}^+H_3NCH_2COOH}$$

and then at the other end:

$$\underset{\text{acid}}{{}^+H_3NCH_2COOH} + \underset{\text{base}}{H_2NCH_2COO^-} \longrightarrow {}^+H_3NCH_2COO^- + \underset{\text{salt}}{{}^+H_3NCH_2COO^-}$$

We end up with two identical molecules, each of which has a cation end ($^+H_3N-$) and an anion end ($-COO^-$). The composition of glycine has not changed; it still consists of the same atoms. It is in a different form called the **zwitterion,** or *inner ion*. This form, like the original molecule, is amphoteric.

In a solution of pH = 6.0, slightly on the acidic side of neutral, all of the glycine molecules will be in the zwitterion form. This point is called the isoelectric ("equally charged") pH for glycine and is typical of most amino acids. If the pH is decreased by addition of acid, the anion side of glycine will react with the added acid:

$$^+H_3NCH_2COO^- + H^+ \longrightarrow {}^+H_3NCH_2COOH$$

bringing the pH back toward 6.0 and creating positively charged cations of glycine. If, on the other hand, a strong base is added to increase the pH, the cation side of the zwitterion reacts:

$$OH^- + {}^+H_3NCH_2COO^- \longrightarrow H_2O + H_2NCH_2COO^-$$

again shifting the pH back toward 6.0 and in the process creating glycine negatively charged anions.

For any amino acid, if it is in a solution with pH near its isoelectric point, it will exist in the ^+H_3N-----COO^-, or dipolar, form. If the solution is more basic, we will find the anion, the H_2N-----COO^- form. If the solution is more acidic, we will find the cation, the ^+H_3N-----$COOH$ form. This isoelectric point, sometimes called pI, ranges from 5.1 to 6.3 for the simpler amino acids.

Some amino acids have extra carboxyl groups on side chains. One example is glutamic acid (from which the food additive monosodium glutamate is derived). Such an amino acid has a pI shifted toward a lower value (2.7 to 3.2). Some amino acids have extra amino groups on side chains, shifting the pI to the basic side (7.6 to 10.8). You will see all of the amino acid structures in Chapter 19.

Proteins consist of chains of amino acid units from which water has been lost through formation of amide or peptide bonds. However, the *ends* of protein chains, and of some side chains, still behave in the fashion of the amino acid units that make them up. Thus, proteins help to buffer body fluids in the way described for glycine.

The pH of hair and skin

The outer layer of skin, hair, and nails forms protein structures made up mostly of *keratin,* dead cell material composed of the 20 different amino acids. Part of the toughness of such material is due to *ionic bonding* between —NH_3^+ and —COO^- ions on neighboring chains. This attraction is strongest at pH = 4.1 because glutamic acid groups are involved.

Anything that increases the pH of hair or skin above 4.1 will make it less tough by weakening the ionic bonds (since there will be fewer —NH_3^+ cations). Since water dilutes the solution involved, bringing the pH close to 7.0, wet hair can be stretched to 1.5 times its dry length and "moisturized" skin is soft and flexible.

Very strong acid, and relatively strong base, may permanently damage hair and skin and remove much of the ionic bonding. Chemicals used as depilatories (hair-removers) contain bases such as calcium sulfide, CaS, and calcium hydroxide, $Ca(OH)_2$. They work, but remember that the outer layer of skin can be damaged in exactly the same way as the hair being removed! Very curly hair is sometimes straightened using preparations that contain a strong base. Such preparations must be used with considerable care and expertise to avoid damaging both the hair and skin.

Many shampoo manufacturers proclaim the virtues of their "nonalkaline, pH-balanced" products. Consumers Union has tested a wide variety of shampoos and found that ". . . most of the tested shampoos have pH values between 5 and 8. Consumer Union's chemists consider the difference between a pH of 5 and a pH of 8 too small to affect the hair or scalp one way or another."* Even a pH of 4, as in the shampoo Earth Born,** is quickly diluted by the water you are using to wash your hair! Some people even find Ivory soap (pH = 9) to be safe and effective in soft water for cleaning hair and scalp.

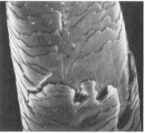

A highly enlarged view through an electron microscope of a human hair. Note the layers of keratinized cells. An excellent review of skin care preparations is in Jones et al, *Chemistry, Man and Society,* 3d edition, Saunders College Publishing, 1980, Chapter 16.

Buffer pairs

There are many situations in which we wish to maintain the pH of a solution within a certain range. In such cases, we can prepare a buffered solution of known pH by using a pair of substances, a weak acid and its conjugate base. If these two substances are in *equal* concentrations in an aqueous solution, the pH of that solution will be equal to the pK_a of the weak acid.

Using Table 13–4, we can see that, for example, at 25°C, equal amounts of HCOOH and $HCOO^-$ will give a solution with pH = 3.7 = pK_a of HCOOH, equal amounts of $H_2PO_4^-$ and HPO_4^{2-} will give a solution with pH = 7.2 = pK_a of $H_2PO_4^-$, and equal amounts of NH_4^+ and NH_3 will give a solution with pH = 9.3 = pK_a of NH_4^+. That immediately gives us three possible buffer solutions, one in the acidic region, one for a neutral solution (with pH very close to that of body fluids), and one in the basic region.

In each case, the acid that is present guards against a major increase in pH when a strong base is added. The conjugate base present in the buffer guards against a drop in pH when a strong acid is added.

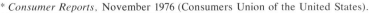

* *Consumer Reports,* November 1976 (Consumers Union of the United States).
** *Protect Yourself,* August 1978 (Office de la protection du consommateur, Government of Quebec, Canada).

Any combination of a weak acid and its conjugate base may be used to create a buffer solution.

EXAMPLE 13k: What will be the pH of each of the following buffer solutions at 25°C before addition of any other acid or base? Use Table 13–4.
i)   0.10 M H$_2$CO$_3$ with 0.10 M NaHCO$_3$
ii)   0.10 M Na$_2$CO$_3$ with 0.10 M NaHCO$_3$
iii)   0.10 M HF with 0.10 M NaF
iv)   0.10 M acetic acid with 0.10 M sodium acetate

– –

ANSWER: Since all have equal concentrations of acid and conjugate base, the pH of the solution is equal to the pK_a of the acid.

i)   The pK_a of H$_2$CO$_3$ = 6.4, thus the pH of this buffer is 6.4 .

ii)   The pK_a of HCO$_3^-$ = 10.2, so the pH of the buffer is 10.2 .
(Note that HCO$_3^-$ is the base in the H$_2$CO$_3$/NaHCO$_3$ buffer pair, but the acid in the Na$_2$CO$_3$/NaHCO$_3$ buffer.

iii)   The pK_a of HF = 3.2, so the pH of the buffer is 3.2 .

iv)   The pK_a of CH$_3$COOH is 4.7, so the pH of this buffer is 4.7 .

The pH of a buffer can be changed by varying the ratio of the acid concentration and the base concentration.

If the acid and base concentrations are equal, pH = pK_a of the acid.
If the acid concentration is ten times the base concentration, pH = (pK_a − 1.0).
If the acid concentration is one tenth the base concentration, pH = (pK_a + 1.0).

By varying the ratio of HF/NaF concentrations between 10/1 and 1/10, we can create buffer solutions in a range from pH = 2.2 to pH = 4.2. If you are asked to create a buffer solution, the ratio of acid and conjugate base concentrations should fall into this range between 10/1 and 1/10.

EXAMPLE 13l: Describe what kinds of solutions from Table 13–4 you might use to make buffers with pH of
i) 4.2   ii) 4.7   iii) 8.3

– –

ANSWER:
i)   A pH of 4.2 is exactly what we would get if we mixed equal concentrations of benzoic acid and sodium benzoate. A second choice would be to mix ten parts of F$^-$ base (as KF, say) with one part of hydrofluoric acid, HF, since in that case pH = pK_a + 1.0 = 3.2 + 1.0 = 4.2.
ii)   For a pH of 4.7, we could use equal concentrations of acetic acid and acetate ion or we could use one part of formic acid to ten parts of formate ion, since formic acid has a pK_a = 3.7.
iii)   For a pH of 8.3, the only candidate in Table 13–4 that could qualify using the rules we have learned is a ratio of ten parts NH$_4^+$ ion to one part NH$_3$, which would give a pH = pK_a − 1.0 = 9.3 − 1.0 = 8.3.

In reality, there are many other ways we could make these solutions. If you use the Henderson-Hasselbach equation on p. 388

$$pH = pK_a + \log_{10} \frac{[\text{weak acid}]}{[\text{conjugate base}]}$$

and use acid/base ratios in the range $\frac{1}{10} \leftarrow 1 \rightarrow \frac{10}{1}$, then buffer solutions for pH = 4.2 could also be made from nitrous acid/nitrite, formic acid/formate, lactic acid/lactate, ascorbic acid/ascorbate, and acetic acid/acetate. Other buffer pairs could likewise be used for the solutions mentioned in parts ii and iii.

The buffers in human blood

In order to create the most favorable environment for the transport of oxygen to the cells and for the action of enzymes in the red blood cells and elsewhere in the blood stream, the blood is buffered at pH = 7.4. There are only two buffer pairs we could choose from Table 13–4 to make buffers for pH = 7.4, H_2CO_3/HCO_3^- and $H_2PO_4^-/HPO_4^{2-}$. In fact, the carbonic acid/bicarbonate pair, usually referred to simply as the **bicarbonate buffer,** is the major non-protein buffer in blood plasma. The dihydrogen phosphate / monohydrogen phosphate pair is of some importance in blood plasma and of greater importance inside body cells.

The large protein molecule of hemoglobin, which carries O_2 to the cells, is responsible for about 70% of the buffering action in blood.

Carbon dioxide is a waste product of metabolism, since the production of energy in the body is one version of combustion, and a whole chain of very complex reactions can be summed up as

$$C_6H_{12}O_{6(aq)} + 6\ O_{2(g)} \longrightarrow 6\ CO_{2(g)} + 6\ H_2O_{(\ell)}$$

The excess CO_2 is carried by the blood plasma to the lungs and exhaled as described in Section 10.5.

Normally, CO_2 dissolved in a water solution is acidic, reacting somewhat as follows:

$$CO_{2(g)} + H_2O_{(\ell)} \rightleftharpoons HCO_{3(aq)}^- + H_{(aq)}^+$$

The body helps maintain the pH of plasma and many other body fluids by converting CO_2 to HCO_3^- until the ratio is 1:20, at which point the pH will be 7.4. While it would be difficult to keep a laboratory buffer system at a 1:20 ratio because of changing concentrations, the CO_2 in the blood stream is constantly being replenished at the cells and removed at the lungs, permitting the body to adjust the ratio. If the blood becomes too acidic (too much CO_2) and goes to pH = 7.2, the breathing rate increases and more CO_2 is exhaled. If the blood becomes too basic, more CO_2 is retained in the body. Not breathing for a minute will reduce the pH of blood plasma from 7.4 to 7.1. You are then required to breathe more often and more deeply to reduce the CO_2 concentration and bring the pH back to 7.4.

If the blood becomes too acidic, the body is in a state of acidosis; if the blood pH goes too high, the result is alkalosis. The causes and remedies for these conditions are discussed further in Section 24.1.

The processing of sugar in the body to produce energy and carbon dioxide also results in the production of acids. These can normally be handled by the body's buffer system in the same manner as CO_2. However, if the metabolic process goes haywire, as in diabetes mellitus, the body may shift from using sugars (which it cannot handle) to more processing of fats. The metabolism of fats causes extra formation of acids. The body's buffer system cannot handle these acids, so the pH falls. If the patient is left untreated, a coma and eventually death can result.

While the two inorganic buffer systems are important in the body fluids outside cells, the amphoteric protein molecules described earlier are most important *inside* cells.

In summary, the blood and extracellular fluids are kept very close to pH = 7.4 by a combination of hemoglobin and bicarbonate and hydrogen phosphate ion buffers. Inside tissue cells, the phosphate and protein buffers perform the same role for the fluids. The acids produced by the body are eventually excreted through the lungs and kidneys.

SELF-CHECK

13.22)   List three weak acids that are amphoteric.

13.23)   Threonine is an amino acid with the formula

$$\begin{array}{c} CH_3 \\ | \\ H-C-OH \\ | \\ H_2N-C-COOH \\ | \\ H \end{array}$$

a)   Draw a structural formula for the zwitterion of threonine.

b)   Write a chemical equation for the reaction of threonine with $H^+_{(aq)}$.

c)   Write a chemical equation for the reaction of threonine with $OH^-_{(aq)}$.

13.24)   If equal numbers of moles of ascorbic acid and sodium ascorbate (see Table 13–4) are dissolved in water, we have a buffer solution with pH = 4.1.

a)   Write a balanced equation for the reaction of this buffer with added $H^+_{(aq)}$.

b)   Write a balanced equation for the reaction of this buffer with added $OH^-_{(aq)}$.

13.25)   Using Table 13–4, explain how one could choose a buffer solution for pH = 12.0.

13.26*)   When a buffer solution reacts with added acid, the number of moles of weak acid in the buffer is increased and the number of moles of conjugate base in the buffer is decreased. Explain, using the bicarbonate buffer in blood plasma as an example.

13.27*)   When a buffer solution, such as the bicarbonate system, reacts with added acid, the pH does not remain constant, but decreases. It does not decrease as much as if the buffer were not present. Explain.

13.28*)   Clairol *Short & Sassy* shampoo was found by a Canadian testing laboratory to have a pH of 7.1. The same company's *Herbal Essence* had a pH = 6.7, while its *Natural pH* shampoo had pH = 4.8. On what basis should you choose between these shampoos?

13.29*)   Should a person with sensitive skin consider using a depilatory cream to remove unwanted hair? Explain.

13.30*)   Which buffer systems are most significant in the human body in

a)   blood plasma and red blood cells?

b)   the fluid inside tissue cells?

CHAPTER THIRTEEN IN REVIEW ■ Acids and Bases

13.1 STRONG ACIDS AND BASES   Page 374

13A: Write the chemical equations for dissociation (in aqueous solution) of three common strong acids and one strong base.

13B: Write a balanced equation for the neutralization of a strong acid by a strong base.

13C: Given the pH of a solution, describe it as acidic, basic, or neutral; given pH values for two solutions, state which is more acidic.

13.2 WEAK ACIDS
Page 384

13D: Given the formula of a weak acid, write the equilibrium equation for its partial dissociation.

13E: Given pK_a values for two different weak acids, decide which of them will form a more acidic aqueous solution if both are at the same concentration.

13F: Given the formula of a weak acid, identify its conjugate base.

13.3 WEAK BASES
Page 390

13G: Given the formula of a basic molecule or anion, write the equilibrium equation for its reaction with water.

13H: Given formulas of any acid and any base, write the neutralization equation.

13I: Given the pK_a of a weak acid, calculate the pK_b of its conjugate base.

13.4 AMINES
Page 394

13J: Distinguish between primary, secondary, and tertiary amines.

13K: Write a balanced equation for the formation of an amide.

13.5 BUFFER SOLUTIONS
Page 399

13L: Explain how a given amphoteric species can act either as an acid or as a base.

13M: Given a buffer solution, write balanced equations for the reaction of the buffer with added acid and with added base.

13N: Describe, in general terms, how to make a buffer solution for a given pH.

GLOSSARY FOR CHAPTER THIRTEEN

acid A proton (H^+) donor; a substance that produces an aqueous solution in which there are more H^+ ions than OH^- ions. (p. 374)

alkali A strong base. (p. 377)

amide A compound with the bonding

$$-\overset{|}{\underset{|}{C}}-\overset{O}{\overset{\|}{C}}-\overset{|}{\underset{|}{N}}-\overset{|}{\underset{|}{C}}-$$

formed by the loss of water in a reaction between a carboxylic acid and an amine. (p. 395)

amine An organic compound containing a nitrogen that has a pair of electrons free to accept a proton; a kind of organic base; an organic derivative of ammonia, NH_3; the amino group is $-NH_2$; amines may (like alcohols) be *primary, secondary,* or *tertiary.* (p. 394)

amino acid An organic compound containing both carboxylic acid ($-COOH$) and amino ($-NH_2$) groups; amino acids combine with each other through amide (peptide) linkages to form proteins. (p. 396)

amphoteric The ability to either lose a proton (act as an acid) or gain a proton (act as a base); examples include the bicarbonate ion, HCO_3^-, and any amino acid. (p. 399)

base A proton (H^+) acceptor; a substance that produces an aqueous solution in which there are more OH^- ions than H^+ ions. (p. 377)

bicarbonate buffer The combination of HCO_3^- ion, H_2CO_3, and dissolved CO_2 that keeps extracellular body fluids at a pH near 7.4. (p. 403)

buffer   A substance, or pair of substances, that can act to neutralize either added acid or added base and thus maintain a relatively constant pH; an amphoteric substance is a self-buffer. (p. 399)

concentrated   Describing an aqueous solution that has a relatively higher molarity of solute than a *dilute* solution; usually applied to *very* concentrated (12.0 M or higher) stock solutions of strong acids and strong bases. (p. 378)

conjugate acid-base pair   The pair of species related to each other by the gain or loss of one proton (H^+); the conjugate acid loses one proton to become its conjugate base. (p. 386)

dilute   Describing an aqueous solution that has a relatively lower molarity of solute than a *concentrated* solution; usually applied to a solution that is much safer to use than a concentrated solution; however, also applied to stock solutions of relatively high (6.0 M) concentration. (p. 378)

equilibrium constant   A number, expressed by the letter K, that expresses a relationship between the products and reactants of an equilibrium chemical equation; the constant K varies with temperature but does not depend on concentrations; one example is K_a, the acid constant; for a weak acid,

$$K_a = \frac{[H^+][A^-]}{[HA]}. \text{ (p. 388)}$$

K_w The equilibrium constant for water; at 25°C, $K_w = 1.0 \times 10^{-14} = [H^+][OH^-]$. (p. 379)

molarity   The concentration of a solute in moles/liter of solution; represented by the letter M; square brackets are often used to represent the molar concentration of an aqueous solute; [OH^-] represents M_{OH^-}, the molarity of the hydroxide ion in the solution. (p. 378)

neutralization   Reaction of an acid with a base to form an ionic salt. (p. 377)

pH   A measure of the acidity of a solution; low pH means a highly acidic solution; high pH indicates a basic solution; neutral is pH = 7.0;   pH = $-\log_{10}[H^+]$. (p. 379)

pK_a   A measure of the strength of an acid; a low pK_a indicates a relatively strong acid; a high value indicates a very weak acid; water has a p$K_a = 14.0$ at 25°C; p$K_a = -\log_{10} K_a$. (pp. 386, 388)

pK_b   A measure of the strength of a base; a low pK_b indicates relatively high base strength; may be calculated from pK_a of the conjugate acid at 25°C using the relationship p$K_b = 14.0 - pK_a$. (p. 391)

polyprotic   Having more than one ionizable hydrogen and thus able to form acid solutions in several stages, as H_3PO_4 and H_2SO_4; a substance with only one ionizable hydrogen is *monoprotic*. (p. 385)

strong acid   An acid that dissociates (ionizes) almost completely in aqueous solution to form $H_{(aq)}^+$ and a hydrated anion; includes only the acids HCl, HBr, HI, HNO_3, H_2SO_4, and $HClO_4$. (p. 375)

strong base   An ionic compound that contains OH^- ion and that ionizes in aqueous solution to produce hydrated hydroxide ions and metal cations; includes NaOH, KOH, $Mg(OH)_2$, and $Ca(OH)_2$. (p. 377)

weak acid   An acid that does not ionize completely in a relatively concentrated (0.1 M) solution; the opposite of a strong acid; an acid with a pK_a considerably greater than 1.0 (p. 385)

weak base   A substance that partially reacts with water to liberate OH^- ions and create a pH above 7.0; a substance whose conjugate acid has a pK_a higher than 7.0 and less than 14.0; the organic amines are weak bases. (p. 390)

zwitterion   The double ion or "dipolar" ion form $^+H_3N\text{-----}COO^-$, in which amino acids are found; the species as a whole is electrically neutral, but can form ionic bonds and react in an amphoteric manner. (p. 400)

QUESTIONS AND PROBLEMS FOR CHAPTER THIRTEEN ■ Acids and Bases

SECTION 13.1 STRONG ACIDS AND BASES

13.31) Write equations for the ionization of two different strong bases in aqueous solution.

13.32) Pick out each *strong* acid from the following list.
HF HNO$_3$ HCN CH$_3$COOH

13.33) Pick out each *strong* base from the following list.
C$_6$H$_5$NH$_2$ Ca(OH)$_2$
CH$_3$COO$^-$ KOH   H$_2$O

13.34) Is a weak base necessarily safer to use than a strong base? Explain your answer with reference to lye (NaOH) and aqueous ammonia (NH$_3$).

13.35) Write a balanced equation for the neutralization of nitric acid, HNO$_3$, by milk of magnesia, solid Mg(OH)$_2$.

13.36) A solution of borax used for washing clothes has a pH of 9.2; is it acidic or basic?

13.37) Carrot juice has a pH of 5.1, while asparagus juice has a pH of 5.6. Are they both acidic or both basic? Which juice is *more* so?

13.38*) Acidic drinks, such as colas, should not be stored in galvanized iron vats, which have a coating of zinc metal. Why?

13.39*) The laboratory stockroom shelf holds two bottles of aqueous nitric acid. One bottle is 6 M, the other is 16 M. Which should be labeled "concentrated"?

13.40*) What is the pH of a solution
a) that has [H$^+$] = 1 × 10^{-3} M?
b) that has [OH$^-$] = 1 × 10^{-5} M?

13.41*) An automobile battery contains sulfuric acid solution. If you try to "jump start" a dead battery with cables, the battery could explode. Could this be dangerous to your health? Why?

13.68) Write equations for the ionization of any two of the six *strong acids* in aqueous solution.

13.69) Pick out each *strong* acid from the following list.
HNO$_2$ CH$_3$CH$_2$COOH H$_2$SO$_4$ H$_2$CO$_3$

13.70) Pick out each *strong* base from the following list.
F$^-$ NaOH
CH$_3$NH$_2$ NH$_3$ Mg(OH)$_2$

13.71) Is a weak acid necessarily safer to use than a strong acid? Explain your answer with reference to HCl and CH$_3$COOH.

13.72) Write a balanced equation for the neutralization of stomach acid, HCl, with limewater, Ca(OH)$_2$, as is sometimes done in cases of gastric hyperacidity.

13.73) A solution of sodium silicate has a pH of 12.6; is it acidic or basic?

13.74) Gooseberry juice has a pH of 2.9, while blackberry juice has a pH of 3.4. Are they both acidic or both basic? Which juice is *less* so?

13.75*) Pewter is an alloy of lead. Acidic drinks, such as wine, should not be served from a pewter pitcher, or you may poison your guests! Why?

13.76*) The laboratory stockroom shelf holds two bottles of aqueous ammonia. One bottle is 15 M, the other is 6 M. Which bottle should be labeled "dilute"?

13.77*) What is the pH of a solution
a) that has [OH$^-$] = 1 × 10^{-10} M?
b) that has [H$^+$] = 1 × 10^{-8} M?

13.78*) Much sulfur dioxide (SO$_2$) gas from the burning of oil is converted to SO$_3$ in the atmosphere and mixes with water vapor in clouds. When the rain falls to earth, nylon stockings dissolve in this "acid rain." Write the equation for dissolving SO$_3$ in water, and explain.

13.42*) Explain exactly how Tums helps relieve heartburn. What danger is there in the long-term use of Tums in high dosages? Use Table 13-3.

SECTION 13.2 WEAK ACIDS

13.43) Write the equilibrium equation for the ionization of each aqueous *weak* acid in the following list.

HF   HCl HNO_2 CH_3COOH

13.44) Acetic acid has a pK_a of 4.7 at 25°C, while bromoacetic acid has a pK_a of 2.7. Which 0.1 M solution will be more acidic?

13.45) Write the formula of the conjugate base of
a) HF
b) HSO_4^-
c) C_6H_5COOH
d) HPO_4^{2-}

13.46*) Which of the following organic acids is polyprotic?
a) pyruvic acid, $CH_3COCOOH$
b) adipic acid, $HOOC(CH_2)_4COOH$
c) dibromoacetic acid, $Br_2HCCOOH$

13.47*) What species will be present in the greatest concentration if the following 0.10 M aqueous solutions are mixed? Use Table 13–4.
a) HF and Na_2CO_3
b) CH_3COOH and $KHSO_3$

13.48*) What will be the pH at 25°C of
a) 0.10 M formic acid (aq)
b) 0.010 M NH_4Br (aq)

13.49*) Which do you expect to have the higher pK_a, bromoacetic acid or tribromoacetic acid? Explain.

SECTION 13.3 WEAK BASES

13.50) Write the equilibrium equation for the reaction with water of
a) $CH_3CH_2NH_2$, ethylamine
b) HCOONa, sodium formate

13.51) Using Table 13–4, write the equation for neutralization of
a) ascorbic acid with Na_2CO_3
b) nitrous acid with $Mg(OH)_2$

13.79*) Explain exactly how Alka-Seltzer tablets help relieve heartburn. What danger is there in the long-term use of such products? Use Table 13–3.

13.80) Write the equilibrium equation for the ionization of each aqueous *weak* acid in the following list.

HNO_3 $NaHSO_4$
NH_4Cl $CH_3CH_2CH_2COOH$

13.81) Benzoic acid has a pK_a of 4.2 at 25°C, while o-hydroxybenzoic acid has a pK_a of 3.0 at the same temperature. Which 0.1 M solution will be less acidic?

13.82) Write the formula of the conjugate base of
a) NH_4^+
b) CH_3COOH
c) $H_2PO_4^-$
d) HNO_2

13.83*) Which of the following organic acids is polyprotic?
a) lactic acid, $CH_3CHOHCOOH$
b) valeric acid, $CH_3(CH_2)_3COOH$
c) malonic acid, $HOOCCH_2COOH$

13.84*) What species will be present in the greatest concentration if the following 0.10 M aqueous solutions are mixed? Use Table 13–4.
a) NH_4Cl and NaH_2PO_4
b) NH_3 and $NaHSO_4$

13.85*) What will be the pH at 25°C of
a) 0.010 M lactic acid (aq)
b) 0.10 M $NaHSO_4$ (aq)

13.86*) Which do you expect to have the higher pK_a, $CH_3CH_2CH_2COOH$ or $CH_3CH_2CHOHCOOH$? Explain.

13.87) Write the equilibrium equation for the reaction with water of
a) $CH_3CHOHCOOLi$, lithium lactate
b) $CH_3CH_2CH_2NH_2$, propylamine

13.88) Using Table 13–4, write the equation for neutralization of
a) ammonium bromide with NaOH
b) acetic acid with Na_3PO_4

13.52) Calculate the pK_b of the poisonous alkaloid strychnine, $C_{21}H_{22}N_2O_2$, if $pK_a = 8.26$ for the acid cation, $C_{21}H_{23}N_2O_2^+$. Is strychnine acidic or basic?

13.53) Amphetamines are dangerous. An overdose of "speed" may be treated by administering ascorbic acid (Table 13–4) to acidify the urine so that the neutralized drug is excreted. Write the equation for this neutralization of amphetamine,

$$C_6H_5CH_2\underset{\underset{CH_3}{|}}{C}HNH_2.$$

13.54*) Using Tables 13–4 and 13–5 as necessary, decide whether a 0.10 M solution of each of the following salts is acidic, neutral, or basic.
a) $NaNO_3$ d) CH_3NH_3Br
b) NH_4Cl e) $NaHCO_3$
c) KF

SECTION 13.4 AMINES

13.55) Give an example of a secondary amine. Write an equation for the reaction of that amine with acetic acid, CH_3COOH.

13.56) If the salt you formed in Problem 13.55 is heated, it may lose water and form an amide. Write an equation for this process, and show the full structural formula of the amide.

13.57*) What products will result from *basic* hydrolysis of the amide in Problem 13.56?

13.58*) Amphetamine, shown in Problem 13.53, is never dispensed medically as the pure amine. Benzedrine, for example, is in the form of the sulfate. Why?

13.59*) What is one advantage of aspirin over acetaminophen in reducing pain and fever?

13.60*) One brand of analgesic, Cope, combines caffeine, antacid, and an antihistamine with aspirin. Would Cope do a better job than plain aspirin? Explain.

13.89) Calculate the pK_b of the addictive painkiller *morphine*, $C_{17}H_{19}NO_3$, if $pK_a = 8.21$ for the acid cation, $C_{17}H_{20}NO_3^+$. Is morphine acidic or basic?

13.90) Bee and wasp stings hurt because of the injection of formic acid, HCOOH. The pain may be relieved by putting aqueous ammonia on the wound. Write the balanced equation for this neutralization.

13.91*) Using Tables 13–4 and 13–5 as necessary, decide whether a 0.10 M solution of each of the following salts is acidic, neutral, or basic.
a) $C_6H_5NH_3Cl$ d) $Mg(HSO_4)_2$
b) CaF_2 e) CH_3COOK
c) Na_3PO_4

13.92) Give an example of a primary amine. Write an equation for the reaction of that amine with formic acid, HCOOH.

13.93) If the salt you formed in Problem 13.92 is heated, it may lose water and form an amide. Write an equation for this process, and show the full structural formula of the amide.

13.94*) What products will result from *acid* hydrolysis of the amide in Problem 13.93?

13.95*) Before morphine (Problem 13.89) can be injected into a patient to relieve pain, it must be mixed with a dilute H_2SO_4 solution. Why?

13.96*) What is one advantage of aspirin over phenacetin in reducing pain and fever?

13.97*) One brand of analgesic, Excedrin PM, combines acetaminophen, salicylamide (similar to aspirin), and an antihistamine with aspirin. Would this do a better job on an "Excedrin headache" than plain aspirin? Explain.

13.61*) What precautions should be taken if you are taking an antihistamine for hay fever? Should you drive?

SECTION 13.5 BUFFER SOLUTIONS

13.62) Bacteria require an amino acid, *p*-aminobenzoic acid, $H_2NC_6H_4COOH$, for proper functioning. Some antibiotics work by blocking the function of this substance. Show how this molecule is amphoteric by writing chemical equations.

13.63*) One serious effect of the disease cholera is to destroy the bicarbonate buffer system in the blood. Would the body then suffer from excess acidity or from excess basicity?

13.64) Baking soda, $NaHCO_3$, may be combined with cream of tartar, $KHC_4H_4O_6$, in baking powders. Write the equation for combination of these two substances, after water is added, to produce the CO_2 gas that makes cakes rise.

13.65) Describe exactly how the $HPO_4^{2-}/H_2PO_4^-$ buffer system can stabilize the pH inside a cell.

13.66*) Plugged bathtub and bathroom sink drains are often a result of collected hair and soap. Products containing NaOH, like *Liquid Plumr* and *Drano*, can quickly break up this mass. Explain.

13.67*) Acid rain damages not only wildlife but also artwork. Marble statues and buildings are made of $CaCO_3$ (limestone). Write the equation for the reaction between nitric acid solution (one type of acid rain) and a marble sculpture. What will be the result?

13.98*) Most sleeping pills, such as barbiturates, are available only by prescription. Yet you can buy over-the-counter drugs like Nytol, Sominex, and Sleep-Eze that claim to help you sleep. Explain.

13.99) The buffering of the fluid inside body cells involves the salt K_2HPO_4, which is *amphoteric*. Write equations for the reaction of this substance, potassium monohydrogen phosphate, with strong acid and with strong base.

13.100*) Give two reasons the blood pH must be maintained near pH = 7.4 by buffer systems.

13.101) Bread can be made from "sour dough," which contains $NaHCO_3$ and the lactic acid, $CH_3CHOHCOOH$, from sour milk. How would these two substances combine (equation!) to provide the CO_2 gas that makes the bread rise?

13.102) Describe how a protein buffer can help stabilize the pH inside a living cell.

13.103*) Quicklime, CaO, is used in making cement and reacts with water to produce $Ca(OH)_2$. Should construction workers use gloves when working with cement? Explain.

13.104*) Aspirin can pass most easily through membranes in the form of acetylsalicylic acid. If converted to its carboxylate anion, it will be absorbed much more slowly and will be excreted in the urine. The treatment for a lethal overdose of aspirin is oral administration of sodium bicarbonate. Explain, with an equation.

Solution Calculations

14

We have discussed the properties of water solutions (in Chapter 12) and described what happens in acid and base solutions (in Chapter 13) so that you will understand the later discussions of biological reactions in the human body. To this point, we have avoided calculations of the exact masses or volumes of chemical substances in solution.

For some courses, solution calculations may be unimportant and this whole chapter may be skipped. Other classes may need to learn only how to do one or two types of calculations and then move on to Chapter 15. A few students require *all* of the skills discussed in this chapter. In order to give your instructor maximum flexibility in adapting this text to your needs, Chapter 14 is presented in such a fashion that you may learn needed skills directly and omit those that are not essential for your course.

You should realize that calculation skills are learned by *practice,* not by reading. Plan to use plenty of paper and a pencil as you proceed.

You may use the following list of sections as a checklist:

—— Section 14.1 How to prepare and use solutions of given concentration
—— Section 14.2 Dilution of already-prepared solutions and isotonic solutions
—— Section 14.3 Calculation of the pH of a buffer solution
—— Section 14.4 Writing a net ionic equation
—— Section 14.5 Using titration data

14.1 PREPARATION AND USE OF AQUEOUS SOLUTIONS

> LEARNING GOAL 14A: Describe how to prepare an aqueous solution of given
>   molarity from a pure solute and water.
>   14B: Describe how to prepare an aqueous solution of given
>   per cent concentration.
>   14C: Given the mass of solute dissolved in a known total
>   volume of solution, calculate the molarity or per cent concentration; given
>   the concentration and volume of a solution, calculate the mass of solute.

Much of the practical work in chemistry involves making up solutions. Druggists are often required to weigh out a small amount of a solid powder and dissolve it in pure water or in a water-alcohol mixture. The "kitchen chemist'' follows a similar procedure to prepare Kool-Aid or Jello. A laboratory technician must often prepare solutions of known concentration.

Molarity

The concentration can then be expressed, as in Section 13.1 as $[AgNO_3] = 0.150\ M$.

Suppose that, as an amateur photographer, you need to make up 500 mL of a solution that will have 0.150 moles of silver nitrate, $AgNO_3$, in each liter. Such solutions are also used in manufacturing mirrors, in silver plating, in inks, in dyeing hair, and for several medical purposes. For this job you need a bottle of $AgNO_3$ solid powder, a balance, pure water, and a 500-mL volumetric flask. You then proceed as shown in Figure 14-1.

Why is 12.8 grams the amount of silver nitrate powder used? One liter of this solution must contain 0.150 moles of silver nitrate. We are making only 500 mL = 0.500 L, so we need only half as many moles of $AgNO_3$, or 0.0750 moles. The solute, $AgNO_3$, has a mass of 170 grams per mole, so we need (0.0750 moles)(170 grams/mole) = 12.8 grams of silver nitrate.

This whole calculation can best be done by the conversion-factor method used throughout Chapter 5. Our two conversion factors are the molarity, $\dfrac{\text{moles}}{\text{liter}}$, and the weight of one mole, $\dfrac{\text{grams}}{\text{mole}}$:

$$0.500\ \text{L} \times \frac{0.150\ \text{moles AgNO}_3}{\text{L}} \times \frac{170\ \text{g AgNO}_3}{\text{mole AgNO}_3} = 12.8\ \text{grams AgNO}_3$$

This weighing procedure is only useful for solids that can be weighed accurately. Some solids, such as NaOH and $CaCl_2$, absorb water from the air while they are being weighed! Solutions of these solutes must be *standardized* after preparation if we are to know their real concentrations.

You will notice that, in Figure 14-1, the solution is shown darker when solid is first dissolved. It is indeed *more concentrated* than the final solution, since we are using 0.0750 moles of $AgNO_3$ in less than 0.500 L of solution. We then dilute the solution (containing dissolved silver nitrate) to a final volume of 0.500 L. The color in this diagram is meant only to show the relative concentrations; an actual silver nitrate solution is colorless and clear.

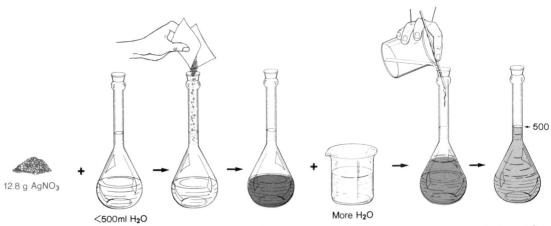

12.8 g $AgNO_3$ + <500ml H_2O More H_2O ← 500

FIGURE 14–1   Preparation of 500 mL of 0.150 *M* $AgNO_3$ aqueous solution. After 12.8 grams of silver nitrate powder have been carefully weighed out on a balance, the weighing paper is used to transfer the powder to the 500-mL volumetric flask. Water is added to wash the powder from the sides of the flask. After all solid is dissolved, more water is added until the bottom of the meniscus (Figure 11–3) is just at the mark on the neck of the flask.

If you are teaching someone how to prepare a solution of known concentration, starting from a solid and water, you should include the following steps.

1)   Calculate how many grams of solute are in one mole.
2)   Calculate how many moles of solute will be contained in the solution volume to be made, and then how many grams.
3)   Weigh out that many grams of solute on a precise balance.
4)   Carefully transfer the weighed powder to the proper volumetric flask.
5)   Add some water to wash down the flask and dissolve the solute.
6)   Finally, add water to fill the volumetric flask exactly to its mark.

After step 5 and after step 6, you must shake the flask to make sure that the solution is thoroughly mixed. **Volumetric flasks** come in convenient sizes, such as 10.00 mL, 25.00 mL, 50.00 mL, 100.00 mL, 250.00 mL, and, as shown in Figure 14–2, 1.00 L.

In the examples that follow, we will assume that you can calculate the mass of solute per mole (Section 5.3). We will find out how many grams of solute are needed, and what kind of flask.

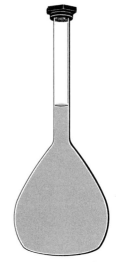

FIGURE 14–2 This volumetric flask is of the type used to prepare solutions. It holds exactly 1000 mL (1.000 liter) when filled to the mark on the neck.

EXAMPLE 14a: How can 250 mL of a 3.00 M NaCl solution be prepared from solid NaCl and water?

- -

ANSWER: The solution volume is 250 mL = 0.250 L.

$$0.250 \text{ L} \times \frac{3.00 \text{ moles NaCl}}{\text{L}} \times \frac{58.5 \text{ g NaCl}}{\text{mole NaCl}} = 43.9 \text{ grams NaCl}$$

Thus, our instructions would be, "Weigh out 43.9 grams of solid sodium chloride, carefully transfer to a 250-mL volumetric flask, add water to dissolve the solid, and then fill the flask to the mark."

SELF-CHECK

(*In this chapter, a self-check will generally be placed with each skill, rather than only at the end of a section.*)
14.1)   Determine the mass of solid solute and the size of volumetric flask needed to make each of the following solutions. If your course involves laboratory experiments, you should be ready to carry out each step to properly prepare a solution.
a)   Make 100 mL of 0.100 M KNO$_3$, sometimes used as a diuretic.
b)   Make 50.0 mL of 0.200 M HgCl$_2$, an antiseptic.
c)   Make 25.0 mL of a 2.32 M solution of lactic acid, CH$_3$CHOHCOOH.
d)   Make 500 mL of a saturated (0.021 M) solution of calcium sulfate, prepared from solid plaster of Paris, CaSO$_4 \cdot \frac{1}{2}$H$_2$O. The water of hydration (Section 11.6) must be included in the grams/mole calculation but has no other effect.

Chemists use molarity (moles/liter) as a concentration unit because it helps relate the amounts of substances that react with each other. The chemical equation tells us the *mole* ratio between two reactants. If we know the molarities of the two solutes in water solution, we can then perform calculations like those of Section 5.4.

The advantage of molarity as a concentration unit can be seen by comparing the ease with which we can answer the following two questions.

1) How many mL of 0.10 M HCl will react fully with 5.0 mL of 0.20 M KOH?

2) How many mL of 1.0% HCl will react fully with 5.0 mL of 2.0% KOH?

We can answer question 1 easily. The KOH solution is twice as concentrated as the HCl solution; it contains $(0.0050 \text{ L})(0.20 \text{ moles/L}) = 0.0010$ moles of KOH. We need the same number of moles of HCl: $(0.0010 \text{ moles HCl})(1 \text{ L HCl}/0.10 \text{ moles}) = 0.010 \text{ L} = 10 \text{ mL}$ of HCl. We need twice as much HCl solution as KOH solution. Since the number of moles of HCl reacting is equal to the number of moles of KOH reacting, we may write

> If the volumes are in liters, we are working in moles. However, we can also take the ratio of milliliters, and note that *millimoles* of HCl are equal to *millimoles* of KOH. In fact, any ratio of volumes will do, so long as both are measured in the same units.

$$V_{\text{HCl}} \times M_{\text{HCl}} = \text{moles}_{\text{HCl}} = \text{moles}_{\text{KOH}} = V_{\text{KOH}} \times M_{\text{KOH}}$$

$$\frac{V_{\text{HCl}}}{V_{\text{KOH}}} = \frac{M_{\text{KOH}}}{M_{\text{HCl}}}$$

What can we do with question 2? Not much! The answer is not 10.0 mL. The correct answer is 6.5 mL, but you can only obtain it after much calculation, using the weight of one mole of HCl and of one mole of KOH. If we want to relate two solutions that will react, we use molarity units.

Per cent w/v concentration

Almost all dilute clinical and drugstore solutions are prepared not by molarity but by **per cent concentration.** For example, the hospital NaCl solution used for injection into the veins is called a "0.9% saline" solution; the corresponding glucose solution is about 5%. The solution with which we began this section, silver nitrate, is used to treat urinary bladder irritation at 0.01% and for washing the eyes of newborn infants at 1%. As an antiseptic, $AgNO_3$ may be prepared in any concentration from 0.1% to 10%.

> When we calculate %, we usually use the same units for the parts measured and the total parts; for example, 5 grams of solute in 100 grams total is 5%. Since dilute solutions have densities very close to 1.0 g/mL, 100 mL of such a solution is just about 100 grams. For this reason, we will use the concentration unit % w/v only for dilute solutions, 5% w/v or less.

The concentrations of clinical solutions are stated in what, to a chemist, is an unusual kind of unit: **% w/v** (% weight/volume) such that

$$\text{Clinical \% concentration} = \frac{\text{mass of solute in grams}}{\text{volume of solution in mL}} \times 100$$

We can look upon % w/v as the number of grams of solute that will be found in 100 mL of solution.

The six-step procedure for preparing solutions of known molarity can be simplified for use in preparing % w/v solutions.

1) Calculate how many grams of solute will be contained in the solution volume.
2) Weigh out that many grams of solute on a precise balance.
3) Transfer to the proper volumetric flask, dissolve, fill.

> When weighing out small amounts of solute, *milligrams* are often used. Remember from Chapter 2 that 1 gram = 1000 milligrams.

EXAMPLE 14b: How would you prepare 10.00 mL of a 0.9% clinical saline (NaCl) solution?

- -

ANSWER:
$$10.00 \text{ mL} \times \frac{0.9 \text{ g NaCl}}{100 \text{ mL}} = 0.09 \text{ g NaCl} \approx \boxed{90 \text{ mg NaCl}}$$

Take 0.09 grams of solid NaCl (90 mg) and dissolve in a 10.00-mL volumetric flask. Fill to 10.00 mL with water.

14.2) Describe how you would prepare each of the following clinical solutions, all of which are used to treat cases of poisoning.
a) 50.00 mL of 3.0% sodium nitrite, $NaNO_2$ (for cyanide poisoning)
b) 250.0 mL of 1.0% boric acid, H_3BO_3 (a 5.0% solution of boric acid was once widely used as an eyewash but is now considered too toxic for general use)
c) 10.0 mL of 4.0% tannic acid, $C_{76}H_{52}O_{46}$
d) 5.00 mL of 0.10% epinephrine (adrenaline) hydrochloride, $C_9H_{13}NO_3 \cdot HCl$.

Converting from % w/v to molarity

If you need to know the molar concentration of a clinical solution for use in calculating the amount of products or reactants of a chemical reaction, you can easily find the number of moles per liter of solution. First multiply the number of grams per 100 mL (% w/v) by 10 to obtain the number of grams per liter. Then divide by the formula weight in grams:

$$\text{Molarity} = \frac{(10)(\% \text{ w/v})}{\text{mass of one mole of solute}}$$

EXAMPLE 14c: What is the molarity of a 1% $AgNO_3$ solution?

- -

ANSWER: This solution contains 1 g in 100 mL, or 10 g in one liter. That gives us

$$10 \text{ g AgNO}_3 \times \frac{1 \text{ mole AgNO}_3}{170 \text{ g AgNO}_3} = 0.06 \text{ moles AgNO}_3 \text{ in one liter.}$$

The concentration is $\boxed{0.06 \text{ M}}$.

14.3) Calculate the molarity of each of the four solutions in Self-Check 14.2.

If we know the mass of pure solute that has been dissolved in a given volume of solution, it is not difficult to determine either the molarity or the % w/v. This can be done even when the solute is a pure liquid instead of a solid.

Some liquid solutes in water have concentration expressed as % v/v (per cent volume of solute per volume of solution).

EXAMPLE 14d: The first-aid kit for poisoning suggested in the *Merck Index* includes, in addition to the four reagents in Self-Check 14.2, a solution of acetic acid. If we know that 50.0 mL of such a solution contains 1.00 gram of CH_3COOH, what is its concentration in % w/v and in M?

Vinegar is about 5.0% w/v acetic acid.

- -

ANSWER: If 1.00 gram of CH_3COOH is in 50.0 mL, then 2.00 grams of acetic acid are in (2)(50.0) = 100.0 mL. Since % w/v is the same as grams per 100 mL, this reagent is 2.0% w/v.
One liter of this solution contains (20)(1.00 gram) = 20.0 grams of acetic acid. One mole of CH_3COOH has a mass of 60.0 grams. One liter then contains 20.0 g × $\frac{1 \text{ mole}}{60.0 \text{ g}}$ = 0.333 moles CH_3COOH. The solution is 0.333 M in acetic acid.

Some very dilute solutions of drugs are described not in M or in % w/v but in a ratio of solute to solvent. A good approximation is to interpret such a ratio as one gram of solute for so many total mL of solution.

EXAMPLE 14e: Nocardamin is an antibiotic substance isolated from old bee honeycombs, and a 1:1000 aqueous solution will kill bacteria. What is the per cent concentration?

- -

ANSWER: If we interpret the 1:1000 ratio as being approximately one gram of nocardamin per liter of solution, that is, 0.1 grams of solute per 100 mL of solution, the concentration is $\boxed{0.1\% \text{ w/v.}}$

SELF-CHECK

14.4)   A 250-mL sample of Ringer's intravenous solution contains 2.15 grams of NaCl, 0.075 grams of KCl, and 0.083 grams of $CaCl_2$.
a)   Calculate the % w/v concentration of KCl.
b)   Calculate the molarity of Ca^{2+} ion in this solution.
c)   Calculate the *total* molarity of Cl^- ion in this solution.
14.5)   A 1:2000 solution of mercury(II) chloride, $HgCl_2$, is used as a surgical handwash. How many grams of this ionic salt must be dissolved in 5.00 liters of solution to give this concentration? What is the molarity of the solution?

Information about solutions can be used to calculate how much solute is contained in a given amount of solution or, in other words, how much solute would be obtained if a given amount of solution were evaporated to dryness.

EXAMPLE 14f: For people between the ages of 20 and 39, the average blood plasma level of cholesterol is about 0.20% w/v and the plasma level of copper (in the form of Cu^{2+} ion) is about $1.8 \times 10^{-5}\, M$. Calculate the number of grams of (i) cholesterol and (ii) Cu^{2+} in the 3.0 liters of plasma contained in a typical adult body.

- -

ANSWER: i)   The concentration of 0.20% w/v is equivalent to 0.20 grams in 100 mL (0.100 L) of plasma:

$$\frac{0.20 \text{ g cholesterol}}{0.100 \text{ L blood plasma}} \times 3.0 \text{ L blood plasma} = \boxed{6.0 \text{ grams cholesterol}}$$

ii)   Each liter of plasma contains 1.8×10^{-5} moles of Cu^{2+}:

$$\frac{1.8 \times 10^{-5} \text{ moles } Cu^{2+}}{1 \text{ L blood plasma}} \times 3.0 \text{ L blood plasma} \times \frac{63.5 \text{ g } Cu^{2+}}{1 \text{ mole } Cu^{2+}} =$$

$$0.0034 \text{ grams } Cu^{2+} = \boxed{3.4 \times 10^{-3} \text{ grams } Cu^{2+}}$$

We can turn this type of problem around to calculate how much solution is needed to obtain a given amount of solute.

EXAMPLE 14g: How many mL of 0.070 M $CuSO_4$ solution would be needed to give the mass of Cu^{2+} calculated in the previous example?

- - - - - - - - - - - - - - - - - - -

- -

ANSWER: The 0.070 M $CuSO_4$ solution is also 0.070 M in Cu^{2+}:

$$3.4 \times 10^{-3} \text{ g } Cu^{2+} \times \frac{1 \text{ mole } Cu^{2+}}{63.5 \text{ g } Cu^{2+}} \times \frac{1 \text{ L } Cu^{2+} \text{ soln}}{0.070 \text{ moles } Cu^{2+}} \times \frac{1000 \text{ mL}}{1 \text{ L}} =$$

$\boxed{0.76 \text{ mL}}$ of this solution

SELF-CHECK

14.6) One source of magnesium metal is sea water, which is typically 0.0520 M in Mg^{2+}. How many liters of sea water must be processed to obtain enough Mg^{2+} for eventual conversion to 1.00 gram of magnesium metal?

14.7) The typical iron cation content of human blood plasma is 1.1 milligrams per liter (1000 mg = 1 gram). Calculate, assuming all of the iron is present as Fe^{3+},
a) the per cent composition of Fe^{3+} (based on this information)
b) the molarity of Fe^{3+}
c) the average number of grams of Fe^{3+} in the blood stream of a person with 3.0 liters of blood plasma

14.8) How many liters of each of the following solutions would you need to evaporate to dryness to obtain one pound (454 grams) of sodium chloride?
a) · clinical saline solution, 0.9% w/v NaCl
b) sea water, typically 0.457 M NaCl
c) blood plasma, typically 0.10 M NaCl
d) saturated brine, 365 grams of NaCl per liter of solution

Other concentration units

The two concentration units we are using in this textbook, molarity and % w/v, are the most common in chemical laboratories and in practical work. However, there are other units that are often useful in describing concentrations. If you should run across any of these, it should not be difficult to make the necessary conversions.

The unit "ppm" is also used in air pollution reports to indicate the number of molecules of a pollutant gas in each million air molecules.

1) Weight per cent (% w/w) is $\dfrac{\text{mass of solute}}{\text{total mass of solution}}$. For a *dilute* aqueous solution, % w/w = % w/v.

2) Volume per cent (% v/v) is $\dfrac{\text{volume of solute}}{\text{total volume of solution}}$. In common usage in describing solutions of one liquid in another; for example, the level of ethanol in beer or wine and the amount of butterfat in milk are usually stated in % v/v.

3) Parts per million (ppm) is $\dfrac{\text{mg of solute}}{\text{kg of solution}}$. Units of ppm are often used to express very low impurity levels. You can think of ppm as mg of solute per liter of solution, in which case concentration in ppm = 10 000 times the % w/v.

4) Mol*a*lity is $\dfrac{\text{moles of solute}}{\text{kg of solvent}}$. This unit is used by physical chemists to calculate colligative properties (Section 12.6), such as the freezing point and boiling point of relatively concentrated solutions, and is sometimes applied to solutions in solvents other than water. For very dilute aqueous solutions, the molality is equal to the molarity.

Note that for mol*a*lity, we are using not kilograms of total solution (solute + solvent) but *only* kilograms of solvent, usually water. The molality of an aqueous solution is generally higher than its molarity.

5) Grams per deciliter (g/dL) is $\dfrac{\text{grams of solute}}{100 \text{ mL of solution}}$. Since "deci-" means 1/10, a deciliter is 0.10 L = 100 mL, as described in Section 2.1 and Example 2e on p. 22. This unit is commonly used to describe the solubility of inorganic compounds in water and also in measuring the amounts of some substances (such as hemoglobin) in blood. The concentration in g/dL is equal to the concentration expressed as % w/v:

milligrams per deciliter (mg/dL) is $\dfrac{\text{mg of solute}}{100 \text{ mL of solution}}$

micrograms per deciliter (μg/dL) is $\dfrac{\mu\text{g of solute}}{100 \text{ mL of solution}}$

nanograms per deciliter (ng/dL) is $\dfrac{\text{ng of solute}}{100 \text{ mL of solution}}$

picograms per deciliter (pg/dL) is $\dfrac{\text{pg of solute}}{100 \text{ mL of solution}}$

These four units may be used to express clinical measurements of very dilute substances. Remember from Section 2.1 that

"milli-" means one thousandth: 1 mg = 0.001 g = 1000 μg
"micro-" means one millionth: 1 μg = 1 $\times$ 10^{-6} g = 1000 ng
"nano-" means one billionth: 1 ng = 1 $\times$ 10^{-9} g = 1000 pg
"pico-" means one trillionth: 1 pg = 1 $\times$ 10^{-12} g (very small!)

For example, the blood serum level of calcium (Ca^{2+}) is typically 8.5 to 10.5 mg/dL. The normal level of thyroxine, from the thyroid gland, is 5 to 14 μg/dL. The female level of the sex hormone testosterone is typically 25 to 90 ng/dL. As more and more substances are found in extremely low (trace) amounts in the blood stream, we can expect reports at the picogram level. Many hospitals still use mass per deciliter on blood test reports.

Alcohol in the blood stream

The properties of ethanol were described in Section 9.6, and the means by which the body can use alcohol for energy will be covered in Chapter 25 on carbohydrate metabolism. Because ethyl alcohol is so important a part of daily human life, its use and abuse are of general interest. We shall here concentrate on the effects of various alcohol concentrations in the blood stream.

Alcohol is absorbed from the digestive tract extremely quickly in comparison with other foods and beverages. A given amount of alcohol taken without food and on an empty stomach will produce a peak (highest) concentration in the blood about 30 minutes after drinking.

Only small quantities (2 to 3% of the amount taken in) of alcohol can be eliminated in the breath, sweat, and urine. Almost all of the alcohol that enters the body must be oxidized in the liver, first to acetaldehyde, then to acetic acid, and finally to CO_2 and water. An average person oxidizes (metabolizes) about 0.5 ounces (15 milliliters) of ethanol in an hour. At that rate, it will take about two hours to break down the alcohol in a rather strong mixed drink, containing two ounces of whiskey, rum, gin, or vodka each of which is roughly 50% alcohol. Nothing is known that will increase this rate of oxidation—not exercise, steam baths, or coffee. Coffee will not counter the effects of alcohol. When you give a drunken person black coffee, all you get is a wide-awake drunk!

The concentration of alcohol in the breath of a person who has been drinking, although relatively small, is high enough to be noticed and measured. The concentration in the breath is proportional to the blood stream concentration. This permits the use of the *breathalizer test* to indicate blood alcohol concentration. Most states regard a blood level of 0.15% w/v to be evidence of drunken driving; this corresponds to 0.150 grams (150 milligrams) of ethanol in each 100 mL of blood.

Figure 14-3 shows the approximate effects of various blood alcohol concentrations on human health and abilities. Some large-scale studies have shown that in $^2/_3$ of fatal single-car auto accidents, the dead driver had a blood alcohol level above 0.05% w/v.

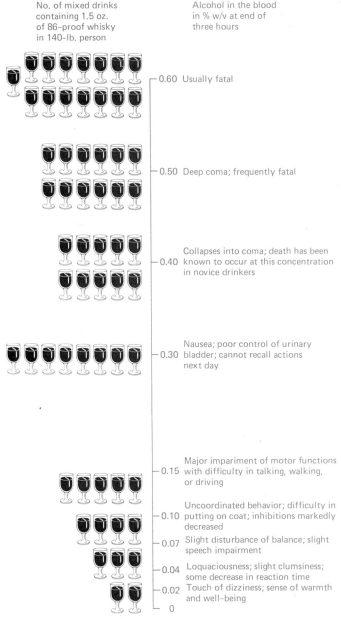

No. of mixed drinks containing 1.5 oz. of 86-proof whisky in 140-lb. person

Alcohol in the blood in % w/v at end of three hours

0.60 Usually fatal

0.50 Deep coma; frequently fatal

0.40 Collapses into coma; death has been known to occur at this concentration in novice drinkers

0.30 Nausea; poor control of urinary bladder; cannot recall actions next day

0.15 Major impairment of motor functions with difficulty in talking, walking, or driving

0.10 Uncoordinated behavior; difficulty in putting on coat; inhibitions markedly decreased

0.07 Slight disturbance of balance; slight speech impairment

0.04 Loquaciousness; slight clumsiness; some decrease in reaction time

0.02 Touch of dizziness; sense of warmth and well-being

0

FIGURE 14–3 The best measure of drunkenness is the concentration of ethanol in the blood. Although considerable variation exists in the rate of oxidation by the liver, the above calculations give some idea of the typical effects of drinking. Blood alcohol levels may also be expressed in milligrams per 100 mL. The occasionally fatal level of 0.40% w/v is the same as 400 mg of C_2H_5OH per 100 mL of blood.

14.2 DILUTION CALCULATIONS

LEARNING GOAL 14D: Describe how to prepare an aqueous solution of given molarity by dilution from a stock solution.

14E: Describe how to prepare a solution of a given osmotic pressure or one that is isotonic with another solution.

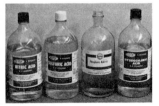

Four common laboratory stock acids.

In Section 14.1, we discussed the preparation of a solution from a solid and water. Similar methods may be used to prepare an aqueous solution of a liquid (such as ethanol or acetic acid) or a gas (such as ammonia).

It is very common, especially when using acids and bases, to use a commercially prepared stock solution as the starting material. In such cases, we are concerned with diluting concentrated solutions with water. It is expensive and complicated to dissolve ammonia gas in water every time we need a solution of aqueous ammonia. It is much simpler to use the 14.8 M solution available from supply houses (see Table 13–1).

Preparing solutions by dilution

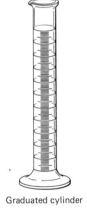

Graduated cylinder

The procedure in preparing a solution by dilution is to make sure that the proper *number of moles of solute* is placed in a volumetric flask. Once the number of moles is established, then we need only add water, as shown in Figure 14–4.

This correct number of moles is equal to the volume of the *final* solution times its molarity:

$$\text{moles solute} = (M_{\text{final}})(\text{liters}_{\text{final}})$$

To get the same number of moles, we must take an appropriate volume of the stock solution, which is more concentrated:

$$\text{moles solute} = (M_{\text{stock}})(\text{liters}_{\text{stock}})$$

Since the number of moles of solute is constant, we may write

$$(\text{molarity of final solution})(\text{liters}_{\text{final}}) = \text{moles of solute} =$$
$$(\text{molarity of stock solution})(\text{liters}_{\text{stock}})$$

large volume of solvent

8 particles

small volume of solvent

8 particles

Concentrated

Dilute

FIGURE 14–4   Dilution does not change the actual number of moles of solute present in a solution. By increasing the total volume of solution, we merely decrease the concentration in moles/liter.

Algebra can then be used to get the equation $M_1 V_1 = M_2 V_2$ or the more useful form

$$\frac{\text{volume of stock}}{\text{solution in liters}} = \frac{\text{volume of}}{\text{final solution}} \times \frac{M_{\text{final}}}{M_{\text{stock}}}$$

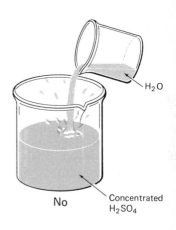

H₂O

No   Concentrated
H₂SO₄

EXAMPLE 14h: How could we prepare 250 mL of 0.50 M HNO₃ solution, starting with stock (concentrated) nitric acid at 16.0 M?

- -

ANSWER: There are two ways of doing the problem.
i) Find the number of moles of nitric acid needed:

$$0.250 \text{ L} \times \frac{0.50 \text{ moles HNO}_3}{\text{L}} = 0.125 \text{ moles HNO}_3 \text{ needed}$$

Then find the volume of stock solution that will give this amount:

$$0.125 \text{ moles HNO}_3 \times \frac{1 \text{ L stock}}{16.0 \text{ moles HNO}_3} = 0.0078 \text{ L} = \boxed{7.8 \text{ mL stock}}$$

or ii) Use the equation just given:

$$V_{\text{stock}} = (V_{\text{final}}) \left(\frac{M_{\text{final}}}{M_{\text{stock}}}\right) = (250 \text{ mL}) \left(\frac{0.50 \, M}{16.0 \, M}\right) = \boxed{7.8 \text{ mL}}$$

Either way, you need 7.8 mL of stock solution, generally measured in a 10-mL graduated cylinder. This is carefully poured into a 250-mL volumetric flask already containing some water (so that we will be following the rule "Always add acid to water, not water to acid, when working with concentrated acids"). The graduated cylinder is washed out with water, which is also added to the flask. After mixing, the flask is then filled to the 250-mL mark.

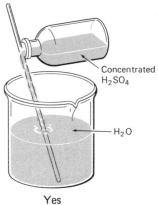

Concentrated
H₂SO₄

H₂O

Yes

The values in Example 14h can be easily checked. The volume of stock solution must be *much less* than the final volume! If you were to turn the equation in part ii upside down, so that you had by mistake

$$250 \text{ mL} \times \frac{16.0 \text{ M}}{0.50 \text{ M}} = 8000 \text{ mL}$$, you would know this to be an absurd answer! You cannot dilute 8000 mL of a concentrated solution to get 250 mL of a dilute solution.

In order to dilute concentrated acid safely, add the acid slowly to the water with constant stirring. Do NOT add water to the acid because the heat evolved may cause spattering.

14.9)   Calculate the number of mL of stock solution and the size of volumetric flask required to make each of the following.
a)   25.0 mL of 1.50 M H₂SO₄ from an 18.0 M stock solution
b)   500.0 mL of 0.17 M NH₃(aq) from a stock solution marked 14.8 M ammonium hydroxide
c)   100.0 mL of 1.0 M HCl (muriatic acid for cleaning brickwork) from the 11.6 M concentrated stock solution
d)   10.0 mL of 0.572 M HNO₃ from a 6.0 M "dilute" stock solution
e)   50.0 mL of 3.0 M acetic acid from 17.4 M glacial acetic acid solution

SELF-CHECK

It should be obvious that in medical and pharmacy work any gross error in calculating concentrations may result in serious harm or death to a patient. If you are entering a health field in which you may be called upon to prepare solutions, become especially proficient in this area!

Osmotic pressure and isotonic solutions

The osmotic pressure of urine is often measured to find the state of water balance in the body.

In Section 12.5, you learned about the very important role of osmosis in life processes. Inside the human body, osmotic pressure plays an essential part in establishing a *water balance*. If the concentration of dissolved solutes builds up in an area, water flows into that area by osmosis through cell membranes.

The most common application of osmotic pressure as it relates to the preparation of solutions is when we must insert an aqueous solution into the blood stream through a vein. The blood plasma must maintain its osmotic pressure or else the red blood cells traveling through it will gain or lose water. If the plasma solute concentration gets too low, body cells will swell with water (edema). If the plasma solute concentration, and osmotic pressure, become too high, the whole body will dehydrate its cells to dilute the plasma.

The average osmotic pressure of plasma at 37°C (body temperature) is 5453 torr, or 7.2 atm. Each particle dissolved in the plasma contributes to this osmotic pressure, by the (approximate) formula

$$\text{osmotic pressure (torr)} = 19\,300 \times \frac{\text{moles of particles in solution}}{\text{liters of plasma}}$$

The moles of particles may come from many different sources: dissolved salts (predominantly Na^+, Cl^-, HCO_3^-, and K^+), glucose, amino acids, proteins, urea, and other materials. Blood typically contains about 0.304 moles of such dissolved particles per liter of plasma.

The SI abbreviation for mole is *mol*. An *osmol* is then a mole of particles capable of exerting osmotic pressure.

Because it is awkward to refer continually to "osmotic pressure from total moles of particles," biochemists instead speak of **osmols** (Os) or, more often, of *milliosmols* (mOs) of pressure from dissolved solute. In these terms, blood plasma normally produces 304 mOs per liter, of which Na^+ ion contributes 144, Cl^- ion 107, and HCO_3^- ion 27 mOs. The relationship is

No other substance in blood plasma provides more than 6 mOs per liter.

$$\text{osmotic pressure (torr)} = 19.3 \times \text{number of milliosmols/L}$$

In the human body, the actual osmotic pressure, 5453 torr, is only about 93% of that calculated from this equation. We can verify this by calculating

$$5453 \text{ torr} \approx \left(\frac{93}{100}\right)(19.3)(304 \text{ mOs/L})$$

Remember, however, that not every intravenous solution is necessarily isotonic with plasma. If small amounts of drugs are to be injected, the effect of adding only a few milliliters of non-isotonic solution to the much larger volume of blood will not be drastic.

Osmotic pressure is a function of how many dissolved particles are in solution. It is not in any way a function of the nature of those particles. If we wish to add to the blood stream a solution that will be isotonic with the plasma and will cause no osmosis problems, we must make sure that our added solution gives 0.30 osmols/liter.

For a weak electrolyte, a substance that does not break up into ions, this would mean a concentration of 0.30 M. Each mole of such particles contributes 1 Os to the osmotic pressure.

EXAMPLE 14i: How would you prepare 100.0 mL of a glucose ($C_6H_{12}O_6$) solution that is isotonic with blood plasma? What is the % w/v of such a solution?

ANSWER: Glucose does not ionize, and therefore we are looking for a 0.30 M solution. We need (0.1000 L)(0.30 moles/L) = 0.030 moles of glucose. The mass of one mole is 180 grams. We must weigh out (0.030 moles) (180 g/mole) = 5.4 grams of glucose and dissolve in enough water to make 100.0 mL of solution in a volumetric flask.

The per cent concentration is 5.4 grams in 100 mL, or 5.4% w/v. This is, in fact, a solution used in hospitals for intravenous sugar feeding, administered to prevent shock.

The number of osmols in one liter is correctly known as the *osmolarity*. On some hospital forms, this colligative property is related to *osmolality*. Since we are dealing with dilute solutions, there is no significant difference between these terms. For reasons that are far too complex to worry about in this course, the osmotic pressure of a dilute solution is related to osmols per liter of solution, rather than osmols per kilogram of water.

SELF-CHECK

14.10) Ringer's intravenous solution is described in Self-Check 14.4 on p. 416. Determine the osmols/liter of that solution, assuming that all of the ionic salts are fully ionized. Is that solution isotonic with blood?

14.11*) Sea water contains the following ions in aqueous solution: Na^+, 0.457 M; Cl^-, 0.533 M; K^+, 0.010 M; Mg^{2+}, 0.052 M; SO_4^{2-}, 0.028 M; Ca^{2+}, 0.010 M. Calculate the osmotic pressure of sea water. Is it higher or lower than that of blood plasma? Do you lose water through your skin (shriveled skin on fingers) when you swim in the sea? What happens when a ship-wrecked sailor drinks sea water?

14.12) If the body fluids are too acidic (pH too low), a solution of sodium lactate, $CH_3CHOHCOO^-Na^+$, is administered intravenously. If the fluids are too basic (pH too high), a solution of NH_4Cl is administered. Each of these solutions should have the same molarity to be isotonic with plasma. What should that value be?

14.3 ACIDITY AND pH CALCULATIONS

LEARNING GOAL 14F: *Convert between [H⁺] and pH.*

14G: Calculate the pH of any buffer solution, given the pK$_a$ of the weak acid and the acid-base ratio.

pH and molarity of $H^+_{(aq)}$

The pH scale of acidity was described in Section 13.1. If the pH is a whole number, such as 6.0, the conversion between the $H^+_{(aq)}$ concentration and pH is quite easy:

$$\text{molarity of } H^+_{(aq)} = [H^+] = 10^{-pH}$$

For a pH of 6.0, $[H^+] = 1.0 \times 10^{-6}$.

The arithmetic involved in calculating pH values is not very difficult. You should realize, however, that pH values of real substances are generally not whole numbers like 6.0. They are more likely to be numbers like 8.13 or 6.48.

Acid-base indicators and test papers will give information on acidity to the nearest whole pH unit. We use a pH meter, a kind of voltmeter, to obtain more precise readings.

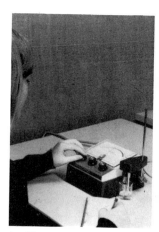

A pH meter is used to determine the pH of a solution.

If you have a calculator that converts between numbers, logarithms, and antilogarithms, the pH conversions are very easy. To find the pH, given the $[H^+]$, you calculate

$$pH = -\log_{10} [H^+]$$

EXAMPLE 14j: Using a calculator,
i)   find the pH if $[H^+] = 3.0 \times 10^{-4}$ for a sample of peach juice
ii)   Find $[H^+]$ if pH = 7.82 for a sample of drinking water

- -

ANSWER: i)   To find the pH, we must use the relationship $pH = -\log_{10}$ $[H^+]$. Punch the following on your calculator:

$\boxed{3}$ $\boxed{\cdot}$ $\boxed{0}$ $\boxed{EE}$ $\boxed{4}$ $\boxed{+/-}$ $\boxed{\log}$ $\boxed{+/-}$ and the answer, 3.5228788, should appear. Keep two decimal places: pH = $\boxed{3.52}$.

ii)   To find $[H^+]$, we use the relationship $[H^+] = 10^{-pH} =$ antilog $(-pH)$. Punch the following into the calculator:

$\boxed{7}$ $\boxed{\cdot}$ $\boxed{8}$ $\boxed{2}$ $\boxed{+/-}$ $\boxed{10^\times}$

or

$\boxed{\text{antilog}}$

and the value of $[H^+]$, $1.5135613 \times 10^{-8} M = \boxed{1.5 \times 10^{-8} M}$ should appear. It may help to consult the operating manual for your calculator. Remember that the key $\boxed{EE}$ (or $\boxed{EXP}$) means "times ten to the power. . . ."

In using your calculator to find $\log_{10}$, do not press the key marked "ln." That key will give you $\log_e$, the natural logarithm, which is not directly related to pH.

The calculator will always give you more digits than are needed or useful. In exact scientific work, the rules of significant digits (Appendix B) are used. In working with pH values, it is generally wise to keep two digits after the decimal point—for example, pH = 10.43 or pH = 5.77—using the rules for rounding off numbers.

If you do not have access to a calculator with logarithms, just use the following procedure to calculate pH. The concentration of H^+ has a *digit* part, which we shall call M, and a *power of ten* part, 10^{-N}.

$$[H^+] = 3 \cdot 0 \quad \times \quad 10^{-4}$$
$$\underset{\substack{\text{digit} \\ \text{part}}}{} \underset{\text{times}}{} \underset{\substack{\text{power of ten} \\ \text{part}}}{}$$

$$[H^+] = M \quad \times \quad 10^{-N}$$

You find the logarithm of the digit part by using Table 14–1. For example, to find the log of 3.0, you look down the left-hand column until you find 3, then

TABLE 14–1   TWO-PLACE LOGARITHMS

	0.0	0.1	0.2	0.3	0.4	0.5	0.6	0.7	0.8	0.9
1	0.00	0.04	0.08	0.11	0.15	0.18	0.20	0.23	0.26	0.28
2	0.30	0.32	0.34	0.36	0.38	0.40	0.41	0.43	0.45	0.46
3	0.48	0.49	0.51	0.52	0.53	0.54	0.56	0.57	0.58	0.59
4	0.60	0.61	0.62	0.63	0.64	0.65	0.66	0.67	0.68	0.69
5	0.70	0.71	0.72	0.72	0.73	0.74	0.75	0.76	0.76	0.77
6	0.78	0.79	0.79	0.80	0.81	0.81	0.82	0.83	0.83	0.84
7	0.85	0.85	0.86	0.86	0.87	0.88	0.88	0.89	0.89	0.90
8	0.90	0.91	0.91	0.92	0.92	0.93	0.93	0.94	0.94	0.95
9	0.95	0.96	0.96	0.97	0.97	0.98	0.98	0.99	0.99	1.00

Example of use: to find $\log_{10}$ of 4.7, read down to 4 and across to 0.7; this gives a logarithm of 0.67.

across the top until you reach 0.0. The logarithm of 3.0 is *0.48* from this table. You can then use the formula

$$pH = N - \log M$$

In this case, $[H^+] = 3.0 \times 10^{-4}$, $pH = 4 - 0.48 = 3.52$, which agrees with the answer in Example 14j, part i.

To find the value of $[H^+]$, given the pH, we must follow a different procedure. We must relate the pH value to the *next-higher* whole number. The next-higher whole number to 7.82 is 8, so $N = 8$. Subtract the pH value from that higher whole number:

$$
\begin{array}{ccc}
8 & - 7.82 = & 0.18 \\
\text{next-higher} & - \quad pH \quad = & \text{decimal} \\
\text{whole} & & \\
\text{number} & & \\
N & &
\end{array}
$$

Look up the decimal obtained by subtraction (here 0.18) in the *body* of Table 14–1. We can find the decimal 0.18 across from the number 1 and under the number 0.5. The *digit* part of our number (the antilog of 0.18) is 1.5, and corresponds to what we call M.

As before, $[H^+] = M \times 10^{-N}$. We have found in this particular case, Example 14j, part ii, that $M = 1.5$ and $N = 8$. Then $[H^+] = 1.5 \times 10^{-8}$ molar, which agrees with the answer given previously.

If we know the $[OH^-]$ value, we have to determine $[H^+]$ before we can calculate pH:

$$[H^+] = \frac{1.0 \times 10^{-14}}{[OH^-]} \text{ at } 25°C$$

It may be necessary to *interpolate* in the table if the value in a box does not correspond to the pH value. For example, suppose we wish to find $[H^+]$ if the $pH = 5.88$. This is $6 - 0.12$. When we look up "0.12" we find it is between log 1.3 and log 1.4, but closer to 1.3. The answer is then 1.3×10^{-6}.

Similar methods may be used to find pK_a or pK_b knowing K_a or K_b (or vice versa) for problems related to weak acids or weak bases (Sections 13.2 and 13.3).

SELF-CHECK

14.13)   Calculate the pH of each of the following solutions to two decimal places (for example, 7.82).
a)   saturated $Ca(OH)_2$ solution at 25°C, $[H^+] = 3.5 \times 10^{-13}$ *M*
b)   a sample of apple juice, $[H^+] = 7.4 \times 10^{-4}$ *M*
c)   a sample of maple syrup, $[H^+] = 1.5 \times 10^{-7}$ *M*
d)   0.010 *M* aqueous ammonia, $[OH^-] = 4.2 \times 10^{-4}$ *M* (Note: this is $[OH^-]$!)
14.14)   Calculate the value of $[H^+]$ to two significant digits (for example, 7.3×10^{-8} *M*) from the following pH values.
a)   0.010 *M* benzoic acid, $pH = 3.13$
b)   0.10 *M* sodium carbonate, $pH = 11.62$
c)   a sample of cherry soda, $pH = 2.87$
d)   a sample of human milk, $pH = 7.51$

Buffer solution calculations

The methods used in Section 13.5 for calculating the pH of buffer pairs are adequate for most general purposes. Having to look up or calculate logarithms is avoided by using the following formulas. Assuming HA is the weak acid and A^- its conjugate base,

if $\dfrac{[HA]}{[A^-]} = 1.00$, then $pH = pK_a$ of the weak acid HA if $\dfrac{[HA]}{[A^-]} = 10.0$, then pH = $pK_a - 1.0$

if $\dfrac{[HA]}{[A^-]} = 0.10$, then pH = $pK_a + 1.0$

In some cases, the use of logarithms cannot be so easily avoided. For example, in blood plasma the ratio of $CO_{2(aq)}$ and H_2CO_3 to HCO_3^- is about 1:20. In such a case, we must use the general Henderson-Hasselbalch equation in either of its two forms (p. 388):

$$pH = pK_a + \log \frac{[A^-]}{[HA]} \quad \text{or equivalently} \quad pH = pK_a - \log \frac{[HA]}{[A^-]}$$

buffer equation form I   buffer equation form II

To avoid arithmetic errors, it is safest to pick the **buffer equation** form that gives a positive logarithm, that is, the one where the *ratio is greater than one*. If there is more base than acid, use form I; if more acid than base, use form II. The answer can be checked if you remember that if there is more base than acid, the pH will be *higher* than the pK_a (higher pH means more basic). If there is more acid than base, the final pH will be lower than the pK_a (lower pH means more acidic).

If the ratio of acid to base or base to acid is between 1.0 and 9.9, we can use Table 14–1 to find the logarithm, and thus to calculate the pH.

EXAMPLE 14k: Find the pH of a buffer solution that contains 0.10 M acetic acid and 0.050 M sodium acetate. The pK_a = 4.7 for acetic acid.

- -

ANSWER: The acid-base ratio is 2:1. Use form II of the buffer equation: pH = pK_a − log [HA]/[A$^-$].
From Table 14–1, the logarithm of 2.0 is 0.30; then
pH = 4.7 − 0.30 = 4.4

SELF-CHECK

14.15)   Consulting Table 13–4 for pK_a values and Table 14–1 for logarithms, calculate the pH to one decimal place at 25°C of
a)   a buffer with a ratio of four HPO_4^{2-} ions to one $H_2PO_4^-$ ion
b)   a solution that is 0.010 M HCOOH and 0.030 M HCOONa
c)   a solution that is 0.30 M NaHCO$_3$ and 0.20 M Na$_2$CO$_3$
d)   a solution that is 0.020 M lactic acid and 0.010 M sodium lactate
e)   a bicarbonate buffer with a 1:20 acid-base ratio. (The logarithm of 20 is 1.30.)

14.4 NET IONIC EQUATIONS

LEARNING GOAL 14H: Given the reactants and products of a reaction in aqueous solution, write the net ionic equation.

Ionic equations were discussed earlier in Section 5.2. When ionic salts react in aqueous solution, it is much more accurate to show the ions present, such as $Na_{(aq)}^+$ or $SO_{4(aq)}^{2-}$, than to show something that does not exist, such as

$Na_2SO_{4(aq)}$. Molecular substances (which are covalently bonded) keep their identities when dissolved, so it is correct to write aqueous glucose, for example, as $C_6H_{12}O_{6(aq)}$.

In Section 12.3, we went a step further to describe a way in which we can distinguish experimentally between a strong electrolyte, which ionizes completely in aqueous solution, and a weak electrolyte, which ionizes only slightly, or a nonelectrolyte. We also wrote some very simple rules for predicting the solubility of ionic salts in water (Table 12–1 on p. 354).

Section 13.1 added another group of compounds to the list of strong electrolytes, the strong acids and bases. The weak acids and bases qualify as molecular compounds that ionize only slightly in water solution.

Strong electrolytes, written in ionic form when dissolved in aqueous solution, include soluble ionic salts, strong acids, and strong bases.

We write soluble ionic salts as ions: $Al_2(SO_4)_3$ when dissolved is written $Al^{3+}_{(aq)}$ and $SO^{2-}_{4(aq)}$; $CaCl_2$ when dissolved is written $Ca^{2+}_{(aq)}$ and $Cl^-_{(aq)}$.

Dissolved strong acids and strong bases ionize completely: $HNO_{3(aq)}$ is written $H^+_{(aq)}$ and $NO^-_{3(aq)}$; $Mg(OH)_{2(aq)}$ is written $Mg^{2+}_{(aq)}$ and $OH^-_{(aq)}$.

Pure solids, liquids, gases, and dissolved weak electrolytes or nonelectrolytes are not converted to ionic form.

If any of the following is a reactant or product in a reaction, we write it exactly as it appears in this list:

$Al_{(s)}$ $Mg(OH)_{2(s)}$ $C_6H_{12}O_{6(s)}$ $CH_3COOH_{(\ell)}$ $H_2O_{(\ell)}$ $Br_{2(\ell)}$
$CO_{2(g)}$ $NH_{3(g)}$ $H_{2(g)}$ $Cl_{2(g)}$ $CH_3COOH_{(aq)}$ $HF_{(aq)}$ $NH_{3(aq)}$ $O_{2(g)}$

As an example, the ionic salt aluminum fluoride is soluble in hot water. Suppose we take solid AlF_3 and place it in hot water. One way of expressing this process is

$$AlF_{3(s)} \longrightarrow AlF_{3(aq)}$$

However, this would not show that the final solution contains ions. The correct ionic equation is

$$AlF_{3(s)} \longrightarrow Al^{3+}_{(aq)} + 3\ F^-_{(aq)}$$

Do not write "F_3^{3-}" or "F_3^-"; the ions released should be those listed in Tables 4–1 and 4–2. The fluoride ion can only be written "F^-."

Chemists use different types of equations in different situations. If the emphasis is on what is actually present in an aqueous solution, we must write a **net ionic equation**. There is a three-step procedure for doing this:

1) Write and balance the conventional equation.
2) Replace all dissolved strong electrolytes in the conventional equation by the appropriate ions.
3) Eliminate any species that are in identical amounts on both sides of the equation.

While it is not strictly necessary to balance the conventional equation, it avoids some possible errors later. In any case, the final equation must balance charge and mass.

The state of each species—(s), (ℓ), (g), or (aq)—must be shown. Solid washing soda, $Na_2CO_{3(s)}$ is not the same chemical substance and is not written in the same way as dissolved sodium carbonate, $Na_2CO_{3(aq)}$ ($\rightarrow 2\ Na^+_{(aq)} + CO^{2-}_{3(aq)}$).

The word "net" in the term "net ionic equation" means that ions (and occasional molecules) that appear in equal amounts on both sides of the equation have been removed from the final equation. We shall call these nonparticipating ions and molecules **spectator ions.**

In the final equation, the number of atoms of each element must (as usual) balance on the two sides; also, the *charges* must add up to the same number on the two sides.

EXAMPLE 14l: (Cover the answer to each example as you do it on scratch paper. Don't simply read examples, *do* them!) Write the net ionic equation for the reaction between nitric acid solution and aqueous potassium hydroxide.

- -

ANSWER: Since HNO_3 is a strong acid and KOH is a strong base, both are strong electrolytes that are ionized in aqueous solution. This is a neutralization reaction, leading to water and KNO_3:

conventional equation: $HNO_{3(aq)} + KOH_{(aq)} \longrightarrow H_2O_{(\ell)} + KNO_{3(aq)}$

ionic equation: $H^+_{(aq)} + NO^-_{3(aq)} + K^+_{(aq)} + OH^-_{(aq)} \longrightarrow$
$$H_2O_{(\ell)} + K^+_{(aq)} + NO^-_{3(aq)}$$

The nitrate and potassium ions are present on both sides of the equation in the same numbers. They are thus spectator ions. To make the final ionic equation "net," we must remove them:

net ionic equation: $H^+_{(aq)} + OH^-_{(aq)} \longrightarrow H_2O_{(\ell)}$

This is the net ionic equation for any strong acid/strong base neutralization, as mentioned on p. 377.

EXAMPLE 14m: Potassium metal reacts violently with water to give hydrogen gas and a solution of potassium hydroxide (Figure 14–5). Write the net ionic equation.

- -

ANSWER: Remember that potassium metal is a solid and H_2 is a gas.

conventional equation: $2\ K_{(s)} + 2\ H_2O_{(\ell)} \longrightarrow 2\ KOH_{(aq)} + H_{2(g)}$

Potassium hydroxide is a strong base.

ionic equation: $2\ K_{(s)} + 2\ H_2O_{(\ell)} \longrightarrow 2\ K^+_{(aq)} + 2\ OH^-_{(aq)} + H_{2(g)}$

There are no spectator ions.

net ionic equation: Same as ionic equation. Note that the *charges* balance.

EXAMPLE 14n: Write the net ionic equation for the addition of vinegar, 5% $CH_3COOH_{(aq)}$, to lithium hydroxide, LiOH solution.

- -

ANSWER: Lithium hydroxide is a strong base, but acetic acid is a weak acid.

conventional equation: $CH_3COOH_{(aq)} + LiOH_{(aq)} \longrightarrow H_2O_{(\ell)} + CH_3COOLi_{(aq)}$

Lithium acetate is an ionic salt that dissociates completely.

ionic equation: $CH_3COOH_{(aq)} + Li^+_{(aq)} + OH^-_{(aq)} \longrightarrow$
$$H_2O_{(\ell)} + CH_3COO^-_{(aq)} + Li^+_{(aq)}$$

The Li^+ ions are spectators.

net ionic equation: $CH_3COOH_{(aq)} + OH^-_{(aq)} \longrightarrow H_2O_{(\ell)} + CH_3COO^-_{(aq)}$

Charges balance at -1 on each side.

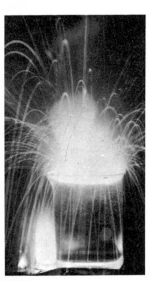

FIGURE 14–5 The reaction of potassium metal with water liberates enough heat to ignite the hydrogen gas produced by the reaction. (B.M. Shaub, Northampton, Mass.)

EXAMPLE 14o: Use aqueous hydrobromic acid (HBr) to neutralize ammonia solution.

- -

ANSWER: Hydrobromic acid is a strong acid, and ammonia is a weak base.

conventional equation: $HBr_{(aq)} + NH_{3(aq)} \longrightarrow NH_4Br_{(aq)}$

Ammonium bromide is an ionic salt that dissociates completely.

ionic equation: $H^+_{(aq)} + Br^-_{(aq)} + NH_{3(aq)} \longrightarrow NH^+_{4(aq)} + Br^-_{(aq)}$

The bromide ion is a spectator.

net ionic equation: $H^+_{(aq)} + NH_{3(aq)} \longrightarrow NH^+_{4(aq)}$

Charges balance at $+1$ on each side.

If we are dealing with a possible precipitation reaction, we must find out if any of the products are insoluble. Use Table 14–2 to make this decision.

EXAMPLE 14p: A solution of sodium carbonate is mixed with a solution of calcium chloride. Write the net ionic equation for any reaction.

- -

ANSWER: From Table 14–2, we see that calcium carbonate is insoluble in water. In fact, it makes chalk and limestone caverns.

conventional equation: $Na_2CO_{3(aq)} + CaCl_{2(aq)} \longrightarrow CaCO_{3(s)} + 2\ NaCl_{(aq)}$

The three dissolved ionic salts all ionize in solution. *Not* the solid!

ionic equation:

$2\ Na^+_{(aq)} + CO^{2-}_{3(aq)} + Ca^{2-}_{(aq)} + 2\ Cl^-_{(aq)} \longrightarrow CaCO_{3(s)} + 2\ Na^+_{(aq)} + 2\ Cl^-_{(aq)}$

The sodium and chloride ions are spectators.

net ionic equation: $Ca^{2+}_{(aq)} + CO^{2-}_{3(aq)} \longrightarrow CaCO_{3(s)}$

Charges balance, since each side is neutral.

EXAMPLE 14q: A solution of barium sulfide is mixed with a solution of aluminum nitrate. Write the net ionic equation for any reaction.

- -

ANSWER: The two salts that are mixed must be soluble in water, or they would not already be in solution. How about the possible products, Al_2S_3

TABLE 14–2   SOME GENERAL SOLUBILITY RULES

Generally Soluble in Water at 25°C	Generally Insoluble
All sodium (Na^+) and potassium (K^+) salts	—
All ammonium (NH_4^+) compounds	—
All nitrates (NO_3^-) and acetates (CH_3COO^-)	CH_3COOAg
Chlorides (Cl^-), bromides (Br^-), iodides (I^-)	Salts of Ag^+, Pb^{2+}
Sulfates (SO_4^{2-})	Salts of Ba^{2+}, Sr^{2+}, Ca^{2+}, Pb^{2+}, Ag^+
Na_2CO_3, K_2CO_3, $(NH_4)_2CO_3$	Other carbonates
Na_3PO_4, K_3PO_4, $(NH_4)_3PO_4$	Other phosphates
$NaOH$, KOH, $LiOH$, $RbOH$, $CsOH$	Other hydroxides
Na_2S, K_2S, CaS, BaS, SrS, Al_2S_3	Other sulfides

and $Ba(NO_3)_2$? According to Table 14–2, both are soluble. There is no reaction and no net ionic equation.

$$BaS_{(aq)} + Al(NO_3)_{3(aq)} \longrightarrow NO\ REACTION$$

Do not make the mistake of assuming that any two chemical solutions necessarily react with each other. Most don't!

SELF-CHECK

14.16) Write a balanced net ionic equation for the neutralization reactions that result from mixing the following solutions.
a) nitric acid with sodium hydroxide (lye)
b) calcium hydroxide (limewater) with hydrobromic acid (HBr) solution (HBr is a strong acid)
c) hydrochloric acid with methylamine, CH_3NH_2
d) lactic acid, $CH_3CHOHCOOH$, with ammonia
14.17) Write a balanced net ionic equation for any reaction that results from mixing the following solutions.
a) iron(III) nitrate, $Fe(NO_3)_3$, with sodium hydroxide
b) silver nitrate and hydroiodic acid, HI, solution (HI is a strong acid)
c) copper(II) chloride, $CuCl_2$, and potassium sulfide, K_2S
d) tin(II) nitrate, $Sn(NO_3)_2$, and potassium chloride, KCl
e) barium sulfide, BaS, and sulfuric acid

14.5 TITRATION CALCULATIONS

LEARNING GOAL 14I: Given the volumes of two solutions that exactly react with each other in a titration and given the concentration of one of the solutions, calculate the concentration of the other.

Titration is an *analytical* procedure that tells us *how much* of a substance is present. This technique may occasionally be used to determine the concentrations of substances in blood plasma, urine, drinking water, or an unknown drug. It provides excellent training for many types of laboratory work, since a student performing a titration must work carefully and precisely.

Titration is the very careful addition of one solution to another by means of a buret (Figure 14–6). A very careful worker can operate a 50-mL buret to complete a titration with as little as ¼ drop, or about 0.01 mL. An **indicator** is used to signal the **end point** of the titration. When an amount of the buret solution that has been added has *exactly* reacted with all of the substance in solution in the flask, we have the **equivalence point,** which should be as close as possible to the end point.

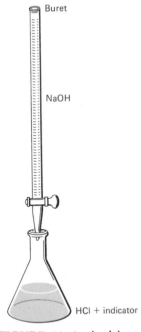
Buret

NaOH

HCl + indicator

FIGURE 14–6 A laboratory titration setup using NaOH solution in the buret to neutralize HCl solution in the flask. An indicator placed in the flask will change color when the acid is completely neutralized.

Strong acid/strong base titrations

A typical titration, shown in Figure 14–6, is that of a strong acid such as HCl with a strong base such as NaOH. When the end point of the titration is reached, the pH should be 7.0, since we have completed the reaction

$$HCl_{(aq)} + NaOH_{(aq)} \longrightarrow H_2O_{(\ell)} + NaCl_{(aq)}$$

TABLE 14–3   RANGE AND COLOR CHANGE OF SOME COMMON
ACID-BASE INDICATORS*

	pH Scale												
Indicators	1	2	3	4	5	6	7	8	9	10	11	12	13

Methyl orange	← red ⟶ 3.1–4.4 ⟵—————————— orange ————————⟶
Methyl red	⟵————— red ⟶ 4.4 ——— 6.2 ⟵———— yellow —————⟶
Bromthymol blue	⟵———— yellow ————⟶ 6.2 – 7.6 ⟵——— blue ——————⟶
Neutral red	⟵———— red ————————⟶ 6.8 — 8.0 ⟵——— yellow —————⟶
Phenolphthalein	⟵———— colorless ——————⟶ 8.0 ——— 10.0 ⟵—— red ——⟶ colorless beyond 13.0

* Adapted from Bates, R. *Determination of pH: Theory and Practice,* New York, John Wiley & Sons, 1964, pp. 138–139.

and should have salt water remaining in the flask. In net ionic form, the same reaction is

$$H^+_{(aq)} + OH^-_{(aq)} \longrightarrow H_2O_{(\ell)}$$

Ideally, we should have an indicator that changes color exactly at pH = 7.0, which is the equivalence point of this titration. Then the number of moles of H^+ in the flask at the start is exactly equal to the number of moles of OH^- added. One suitable indicator is *bromthymol blue,* an organic dye with a yellow acid form at a pH of 6.0 or less (acidic pH) and a blue basic form at a pH of 8.0 or more (basic pH). At the exact end point, the solution will look green with this indicator.

In fact, when we titrate a 1.0 *M* solution of a strong acid with a 1.0 *M* solution of a strong base, the pH is about 3.0 just a drop or so before the equivalence point and jumps to 11.0 with a very small amount of added base after equivalence. For this titration, then, we can use any indicator that changes color from its acid form to its base form between pH 3.0 and pH 11.0. Table 14–3 lists some common indicators with their color change from acid to base, along with the pH at which the change occurs. The most common indicator is phenolphthalein, which is colorless in a solution of pH 8.0 or less and bright pink at a pH of 10 or more. Its end point is at pH = 9.0.

Titration calculations

Since we know the balanced equation for reaction of a strong acid with a strong base, we have a conversion factor for moles of $OH^-_{(aq)}$ to moles of $H^+_{(aq)}$. This permits us to solve problems of the type discussed in Section 5.4.

EXAMPLE 14r: Into a flask we pipet 25.00 mL of stomach fluid containing HCl and add several drops of indicator. The indicator changes color after 11.37 mL of 0.1000 *M* NaOH have been added from a buret. What is the concentration of HCl in this sample of gastric fluid? Assume no other substances are present.

— —

ANSWER: The number of moles of NaOH used in the titration is

$$11.37 \text{ mL NaOH} \times \frac{1 \text{ L NaOH}}{1000 \text{ mL NaOH}} \times \frac{0.1000 \text{ moles NaOH}}{1 \text{ L NaOH}} =$$

$$0.001137 \text{ moles NaOH}$$

Because NaOH is a strong base, we have used 0.001137 moles of OH^-.

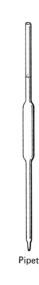
Pipet

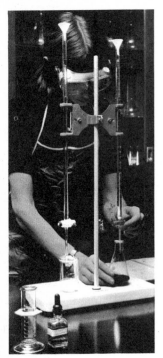

A student carrying out a titration. Note that she is (correctly) wearing safety glasses while dispensing NaOH solution.

Since the balanced equation is $H^+_{(aq)} + OH^-_{(aq)} \rightarrow H_2O_{(\ell)}$, we can calculate

$$0.001137 \text{ moles } OH^- \times \frac{1 \text{ mole } H^+}{1 \text{ mole } OH^-} = 0.001137 \text{ moles } H^+_{(aq)}$$

Because HCl is a strong acid, there were originally 0.001137 moles of HCl in the flask. Now find the molarity of the HCl. The 25.00-mL portion is 0.02500 L.

$$\frac{0.001137 \text{ moles } HCl}{0.02500 \text{ L } HCl} = \boxed{0.04548 \text{ } M \text{ } HCl_{(aq)}}$$

This whole calculation could be combined:

$$0.01137 \text{ L } OH^- \times \frac{0.1000 \text{ moles } OH^-}{1 \text{ L } OH^-} \times \frac{1 \text{ mole } HCl}{1 \text{ mole } OH^-} \times \frac{1}{0.02500 \text{ L } HCl} =$$

$$\boxed{0.04548 \text{ moles } HCl/L}$$

There are several things to note about this example.

1) The precision used in the titration is much greater (four digits) than what we usually use in calculations. Titrations are quite precise.
2) Water may be added to the flask containing HCl without affecting the titration. This is important because drops of NaOH solution stick to the buret tip and the sides of the flask. These drops must be washed down with distilled water to obtain a correct reading.

Other titrations

The same method may be used to titrate a weak acid using a strong base or a weak base using a strong acid, provided that an appropriate indicator is chosen.

EXAMPLE 14s: A student used 0.1013 M NaOH$_{(aq)}$ to titrate a sample of vinegar. The 5.00 mL of vinegar were put into a flask, and water with phenolphthalein indicator was added. It took 40.71 mL of base to reach an end point. Calculate the concentration of acetic acid, CH$_3$COOH, in the vinegar in i) molarity and ii) per cent (w/v) concentration.

ANSWER: Calculate the number of moles of NaOH (thus, of OH$^-$) used.

$$40.71 \text{ mL } OH^- \times \frac{1 \text{ L } OH^-}{1000 \text{ mL } OH^-} \times \frac{0.1013 \text{ moles } OH^-}{1 \text{ L } OH^-} =$$

$$0.004124 \text{ moles } OH^-$$

Now write the balanced net ionic equation to find the mole ratio.

conventional:
$$\text{NaOH}_{(aq)} + \text{CH}_3\text{COOH}_{(aq)} \longrightarrow \text{H}_2\text{O}_{(\ell)} + \text{CH}_3\text{COONa}$$

ionic:
$$\text{Na}^+_{(aq)} + \text{OH}^-_{(aq)} + \text{CH}_3\text{COOH}_{(aq)} \longrightarrow \text{H}_2\text{O}_{(\ell)} + \text{CH}_3\text{COO}^-_{(aq)} + \text{Na}^+_{(aq)}$$

net ionic:
$$\text{OH}^-_{(aq)} + \text{CH}_3\text{COOH}_{(aq)} \longrightarrow \text{H}_2\text{O}_{(\ell)} + \text{CH}_3\text{COO}^-_{(aq)}$$

The ratio is 1 mole of OH$^-$ to 1 mole of acetic acid. In that case, 0.004124 moles of OH$^-$ titrated 0.004124 moles of CH$_3$COOH.

i)   We had 5.00 mL = 0.00500 L of vinegar. Calculate the molarity.

Phenolphthalein is not only the most common laboratory indicator for acid-base titrations, but it is also the active ingredient (laxative) in the over-the-counter medication Ex-Lax. The titration of Example 14s is particularly common in college labs.

$$\frac{0.004124 \text{ moles CH}_3\text{COOH}}{0.00500 \text{ L solution}} = \boxed{0.825 \; M \text{ CH}_3\text{COOH}}$$

ii)   What is the mass of acetic acid? One mole weighs 60.0 grams. Then 0.004124 moles of CH_3COOH (in 5.00 mL) weighs (0.004124 moles)(60.0 grams/mole) = 0.247 grams in 5.00 mL. How many grams in 100 mL?

$$(0.247 \text{ grams}) \left(\frac{100 \text{ mL}}{5 \text{ mL}} \right) = 4.95 \text{ grams, so } \boxed{4.95\% \text{ w/v}} \; .$$

Similar techniques may be used for reactions other than acid-base neutralizations. For example, potassium permanganate solution, $KMnO_4$, may be used in the buret as an oxidizing agent. When the other reactant has been completely oxidized, the bright purple color of $KMnO_4$ gives a clear indication that the titration is complete.

EXAMPLE 14t: The concentration of oxalate ion, $^-OOCCOO^-$, in urine may be determined by titration with $KMnO_4$ solution. The net ionic equation in a strong acid solution is

$$5 \text{ H}_2\text{C}_2\text{O}_{4(aq)} + 2 \text{ MnO}_{4(aq)}^- + 6 \text{ H}_{(aq)}^+ \longrightarrow 10 \text{ CO}_{2(g)} + 8 \text{ H}_2\text{O}_{(\ell)} + 2 \text{ Mn}_{(aq)}^{2+}$$

The oxalate ions in 100 mL of urine required 1.79 mL of 0.003061 M permanganate solution. What is the concentration in moles/liter of oxalate in the sample?

The importance of the oxalate concentration in urine is related to the ability of the body to form urinary calculi (kidney stones) by precipitating calcium oxalate. If both the Ca^{2+} and $^-OOCCOO^-$ concentrations are high, stones may form.

- -

ANSWER: The conversion factor from the equation is 5 moles of $H_2C_2O_4$ for 2 moles of MnO_4^-. Be sure to use this in the setup.

$$0.00179 \text{ L MnO}_4^- \times \frac{0.003061 \text{ moles MnO}_4^-}{1 \text{ L MnO}_4^-} \times \frac{5 \text{ moles H}_2\text{C}_2\text{O}_4}{2 \text{ moles MnO}_4^-} =$$
$$1.37 \times 10^{-5} \text{ moles of H}_2\text{C}_2\text{O}_4,$$

which must have come from 1.37×10^{-5} moles of oxalate ion. Since this is the amount in 100 mL,

$$[\text{C}_2\text{O}_4{}^{2-}] = \frac{1.37 \times 10^{-5} \text{ moles}}{0.100 \text{ L}} = \boxed{1.37 \times 10^{-4} \; M} \; .$$

14.18)   Find the unknown concentration from the data given.

a)   A 25.00-mL sample of nitric acid is titrated with 37.51 mL of 0.2079 M NaOH solution. What is $[H^+]$ in the nitric acid?

b)   A 5.00-mL sample of lactic acid is titrated with 13.80 mL of 0.0890 M NaOH solution. What is the % w/v of the lactic acid, $CH_3CHOHCOOH$?

c)   A 100.0-mL sample of urine is analyzed with 5.69 mL of 0.00105 M $KMnO_4$ solution to determine dissolved oxalate, as in Example 14t. What is the molarity of the oxalate in the urine?

d)   A 10.00-mL sample of sulfuric acid, H_2SO_4, is completely neutralized by 41.07 mL of 0.1075 M NaOH solution. What is the molarity of the sulfuric acid?

SELF-CHECK

Normality

Chemists quite commonly use balanced equations, such as that in Example 14t, to do titration calculations. However, if such calculations must be done repeatedly,

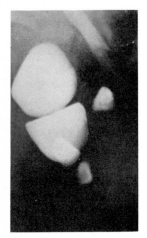

This X-ray photograph shows large kidney stones, possibly of calcium oxalate. Uric acid may also form hard deposits. (Indiana University Medical Center)

and if relatively untrained staff must perform the titrations, there is a chance of error. It is much too easy to forget the factor of "5 moles oxalic acid/2 moles MnO_4^-."It would be nice if nature could always provide us with one-to-one mole ratios, as in Examples 14r and 14s.

For this reason, some laboratories use concentrations of **normality** instead of molarity. The normality unit, with symbol N, is chosen so that equal volumes of solutions of equal normality will react exactly with each other. This allows use of the very simple equation

$$V_1 N_1 = V_2 N_2$$

where V_1 is the volume in mL of the solution in the buret and N_1 is its normality; V_2 is the number of mL of the solution being titrated and N_2 is its normality.

Let's rewrite the problem in Example 14t in terms of normality.

EXAMPLE 14u: An oxalate solution of volume 100 mL required 1.79 mL of 0.0153 N permanganate solution. What is the normality of the oxalate solution?

- -

ANSWER: Use the simple equation

$$V_1 N_1 = V_2 N_2$$
$$\text{for permanganate} \qquad \text{for oxalate}$$

$$(1.79 \text{ mL})(0.0153 \ N_1) = (100 \text{ mL})(N_2)$$

$$N_2 = N_1 \frac{V_1}{V_2} = 0.0153 \ N \times \frac{1.79 \text{ mL}}{100 \text{ mL}} = \boxed{2.74 \times 10^{-4} \ N}$$

While you learn much less chemistry from such a calculation (you do not even need to know the formula of either substance!), the calculation is quick and relatively error-free. In order to accomplish this, we have rewritten the concentration of MnO_4^-, formerly 0.003061 M (in Example 14t), as (5)(0.003061 M) = 0.0153 N.

The answer we obtained in Example 14u is not the molarity. It is the normality, which is *twice* the molarity obtained for oxalate in Example 14t. In this particular case, we are working with an oxidation-reduction reaction (Chapter 8). For all such *redox* reactions

$$\text{normality} = \text{molarity} \times \frac{\text{number of moles of } e^- \text{ gained or lost}}{\text{mole of solute}}$$

Permanganate gains five electrons per anion to go from MnO_4^- to Mn^{2+}. Its normality is thus five times its molarity. Oxalate loses two electrons per anion to go from $C_2O_{4(aq)}^{2-}$ to $CO_{2(g)}$. The oxalate normality is two times its normality.

Acid-base neutralization reactions follow a similar rule. For an acid-base reaction

$$\text{normality} = \text{molarity} \times \frac{\text{number of moles of } H^+ \text{ gained or lost}}{\text{mole of solute}}$$

For the following solutions, the molarity is equal to the normality: $HCl_{(aq)}$, $CH_3COOH_{(aq)}$, $CH_3CHOHCOOH_{(aq)}$, $NH_{3(aq)}$, $NaOH_{(aq)}$, and $HNO_{3(aq)}$. In each case, one formula unit gains or loses one proton, so one mole gains or loses one mole of protons.

For sulfuric acid, H_2SO_4, and oxalic acid, $HOOCCOOH$, in acid-base neutralization reactions (either can also participate in redox reactions) the normality is double the molarity. Each has two ionizable hydrogens. It is sometimes easy to tell the relationship between molarity and normality, but it is at times more difficult! It helps to have a balanced equation at hand, to be sure.

Equivalents and milliequivalents

The concept of **equivalents** comes from the ideas we have just discussed. If two substances, A and B, react with each other, then

One equivalent of A reacts with one equivalent of B.

Normality is the number of equivalents in one liter.

If we are working with relatively dilute solutions, as in the human body, an equivalent may be a rather large amount. Therefore, we refer to *milliequivalents*, such that 1000 meq = 1 eq, or 1000 milliequivalents make up one equivalent.

The **equivalent weight** of a substance is the mass in grams of one equivalent. It is related to the weight of one mole:

$$\text{equivalent weight} = \frac{\text{mass of one mole in grams}}{\text{number of equivalents in one mole}}$$

The equivalent weight is thus a number smaller than or equal to the mass of one mole.

For a substance in an oxidation-reduction reaction, the number of equivalents in one mole is equal to the number of electrons gained or lost by one formula unit.

For an acid or base in a neutralization reaction, the number of equivalents in one mole is equal to the number of $H^+_{(aq)}$ gained or lost per formula unit.

> Just as the mole is sometimes called a "gram molecular weight," the *equivalent* defined here is sometimes called a "gram equivalent." Similarly, the *equivalent weight* may be called the "gram equivalent weight."

EXAMPLE 14v: Determine the equivalent weight of
i) I_2 in a redox reaction where the product is I^-
ii) H_3PO_4 in a complete neutralization with strong base

- -

ANSWER: i) The I_2 molecule gains two electrons in going from I_2 to $2\,I^-$. The equivalent weight is one half the mass of one mole, or $(0.5)(254$ g/mole) = $\boxed{127 \text{ g/equivalent}}$.

Note that this is also the equivalent weight of the I^- anion!
ii) The H_3PO_4 molecule loses three $H^+_{(aq)}$ to go to PO_4^{3-}. The equivalent weight is one third the mass of one mole, or $(0.33)(98.0$ g/mole) = $\boxed{32.7 \text{ g/equivalent}}$.

Body fluid electrolytes

In order to keep track of the electrolytes in the various fluids of the body, biochemists have given a third definition to the word "equivalent." For electrolyte balance

An equivalent possesses one mole of + or − electrical charge.

Since a cation (Na^+, Ca^{2+}, etc.) is positively charged and an anion (Cl^-, HCO_3^-, $H_2PO_4^-$, HPO_4^{2-}, SO_4^{2-}) is negatively charged,

For electrical neutrality, the number of equivalents of cations must be equal to the number of equivalents of anions.

The equivalent weight as defined for a biological electrolyte is the mass of one mole divided by the amount of charge on one formula unit. For Na^+, the equivalent weight is the same as the mass of one mole, 23.0 grams. For Ca^{2+}, however, the equivalent weight is one half the mass of one mole, or $(0.5)(40.08) = 20.0$ grams.

Blood analyses frequently refer to the number of milliequivalents per liter of a particular cation or anion; for example, the normal Cl^- concentration in blood plasma is about 100 meq/L, or 0.100 M.

SELF-CHECK

14.19) Calculate the normality of each solution described.
a) 17.85 mL of this NaOH solution neutralize 34.03 mL of 0.100 N HCl
b) 3.98 mL of this NH_3 solution neutralize 17.86 mL of 0.0200 N H_2SO_4
c) 7.96 mL of this hydrogen peroxide solution are oxidized by 34.59 mL of 0.1010 N permanganate solution

14.20) Calculate the equivalent weight of
a) $Zn_{(s)}$ when used as a reducing agent
b) H_2NNH_2 when used as a base
c) C_6H_5COOH when used as an acid
d) HPO_4^{2-} when an electrolyte in body fluids

CHAPTER FOURTEEN IN REVIEW ■ Solution Calculations

GLOSSARY FOR CHAPTER FOURTEEN

buffer equation The equation for calculating the pH of a buffer solution, knowing the acid-base ratio and the pK_a of the weak acid; pH = pK_a + log $[A^-]/[HA]$;
the Henderson-Hasselbalch equation. (p. 426)

end point The titration stage at which an *indicator* changes color and the buret volume is recorded;

should be made as close as possible to the *equivalence point* by choice of a suitable indicator. (p. 430)

equivalence point The titration stage at which the number of moles of reagent added from the buret is exactly that needed to react fully with the number of moles of reagent in the flask. (p. 430)

equivalent An amount of one substance that reacts exactly with one equivalent of another substance; the number of moles of a substance that contains one mole of net electrical charge on its ions (clinical definition) or which gains or loses one mole of electrons (redox) or of protons (acid-base); the amount of substance in one liter of $1\,N$ solution. (p. 435)

equivalent weight The mass of one equivalent; the mass of one mole of a substance divided by a small whole number (1, 2, 3, etc.) that is the number of charges on an ion (clinical) or the number of electrons or $H^+_{(aq)}$ gained or lost by one formula unit. (p. 435)

indicator A substance dissolved in a solution being titrated, which changes color to signal the *end point* of the titration; usually an organic dye like phenolphthalein or bromthymol blue. (p. 430)

net ionic equation A chemical equation written to show the reactants and products in the forms (ionic or nonionic) present in the greatest amounts in an aqueous solution; an ionic equation with *spectator* ions removed. (p. 427)

normality A concentration unit of equivalents/liter; if two solutions have the same normality, equal volumes will react exactly; the normality of a solution is the molarity multiplied by a small whole number (see *equivalent weight*). (p. 434)

osmol (Os) A unit of numbers of particles related to osmotic pressure; one osmol is one mole of dissolved particles (of all kinds); often measured in milliosmols (mOs or mOsmol), where 1000 mOs = 1 Os; normal blood plasma averages 0.30 Os/L = 300 mOs/L. (p. 422)

per cent concentration (% w/v) A clinical concentration unit equal to the number of grams of solute in 100 mL of solution (g/dL); most commonly used for dilute solutions of solid solutes. (p. 414)

spectator A species in a balanced ionic equation that appears in equal amounts on both sides of the equation, and thus is neither a reactant nor a product; spectator ions are removed when writing *net ionic equations*. (p. 428)

titration The careful measurement of the number of milliliters of a solution of known concentration required to react exactly with a known volume of a solution of unknown concentration; uses a buret whose reading is taken at an *end point*, signalled usually by a color change; the reading desired is that of the *equivalence point*. (p. 430)

volumetric flask A piece of laboratory glassware used for the preparation of solutions of precise concentration; a flask on which a line has been marked to indicate precisely a total volume of 10.00 mL, 100.0 mL, etc. (p. 413)

QUESTIONS AND PROBLEMS FOR CHAPTER FOURTEEN

■ **Solution Calculations**

SECTION 14.1 PREPARATION AND USE OF AQUEOUS SOLUTIONS

14.21) Describe how you would prepare

a) 25.00 mL of 0.100 M $AgNO_3$

b) 5.00 mL of the common indi-

14.40) Describe how you would prepare

a) 250.0 mL of 0.0300 M NaCl

b) 10.00 mL of the common indicator solution *methyl orange*, 0.10% w/v $C_{14}H_{14}N_3NaO_3S$

c) 100.0 mL of 1.50 M sodium bicarbonate solution, $NaHCO_{3(aq)}$

d) 250.0 mL of a 5.0% w/v solution of *procaine (novocaine) hydrochloride*, $C_{13}H_{20}N_2O_2HCl$, used for spinal anesthesia

14.22) If you dissolve a pound (454 grams) of NaCl in 4.00 L of final solution, what will be the % w/v? the molarity?

14.23*) The noncaloric sweetener *saccharin* is 500 times as sweet as sugar. The sweet taste can be detected in a 1 : 100 000 aqueous solution. What is the % w/v of the solution? If saccharin is $C_7H_5NO_3S$, what is the molarity of this solution?

14.24) The following are typical blood plasma levels. If there are 3.0 liters of plasma, calculate the mass of each solute in the blood stream.

a) ammonia, $2.2 \times 10^{-5}\ M$

b) sulfate ion, 0.0010% w/v

c*) $H^+_{(aq)}$, 40 nM

d*) testosterone, 600 ng/dL (in males)

cator *alizarin yellow R*, 0.10% w/v $C_{13}H_8N_3NaO_5$

c) 25.00 mL of 0.870 M sodium carbonate solution, $Na_2CO_{3(aq)}$

d) 5.00 mL of a 0.40% w/v solution of *benoxinate hydrochloride*, $C_{17}H_{28}N_2O_3HCl$, used as an anesthetic for the eye

14.41) If you dissolve a single aspirin tablet (0.324 grams of $C_9H_8O_4$) in one glass (225 mL) of water, what will be the % w/v? the molarity?

14.42*) The noncaloric sweetner *sodium cyclamate* is about 30 times as sweet as sugar. The sweet taste can be detected in a 1 : 10 000 aqueous solution. What is the % w/v of this solution? If sodium cyclamate is $C_6H_{11}NHSO_3Na$, what is the molarity of this solution?

14.43) The following are typical blood plasma levels. If there are 3.0 liters of plasma, calculate the mass of each solute in the blood stream.

a) urea, H_2NCONH_2, $5 \times 10^{-3}\ M$

b) calcium ion, 0.0095% w/v

c*) glucose, $C_6H_{12}O_6$, 5.1 mM

d*) creatinine, 1.1 mg/dL

SECTION 14.2 DILUTION CALCULATIONS

14.25) Given a stock solution that is 11.6 M HCl, describe how to prepare

a) 50.00 mL of 1.50 M HCl

b) 250.0 mL of 0.735 M HCl

14.26*) What kind of measuring device do we use to obtain a precise *final solution* volume?

14.27) How many mL of water must you add to each of the following solutions to make a solution that is isotonic with blood plasma (0.30 Os/L)?

a) 50.0 mL of 6.00 M $NH_{3(aq)}$

b) 5.0 mL of 10.0% w/v $CaCl_2$

14.28*) Describe how you might prepare a CH_3COOH solution that has an osmotic pressure at 25°C of 1.00 atm.

14.44) Given a stock solution that is 14.8 M $NH_{3(aq)}$, describe how to prepare

a) 100.0 mL of 0.800 M NH_3

b) 10.0 mL of 3.50 M NH_3

14.45*) What kind of measuring device do we use to obtain a relatively precise volume of *stock solution* of concentrated acid or base?

14.46) How many mL of water must you add to each of the following solutions to make a solution that is isotonic with blood plasma (0.30 Os/L)?

a) 10.0 mL of 1.50 M $C_6H_{12}O_6$

b) 100.0 mL of 3.0% w/v NaCl

14.47*) Describe how you might prepare a sodium bicarbonate solution with an osmotic pressure at 25°C of 2000 mm Hg.

SECTION 14.3 ACIDITY AND pH CALCULATIONS

14.29) Calculate the pH of each of

14.48) Calculate the pH of each of

the following solutions to two decimal places.

a) 0.1 M lactic acid, $[H^+] = 4.0 \times 10^{-3}\ M$

b) saturated $Fe(OH)_2$ solution, $[H^+] = 3.2 \times 10^{-10}\ M$

c) a sample of beer, $[H^+] = 3.9 \times 10^{-5}\ M$

d) a sample of saliva, $[H^+] = 1.2 \times 10^{-7}\ M$

14.30) Calculate the $[H^+]$ of each of the following solutions.

a) carrot juice, pH = 5.11

b) sauerkraut, pH = 3.53

c) a 1% detergent solution of sodium tripolyphosphate, $Na_5P_3O_{10}$, pH = 9.74

d) saturated milk of magnesia, pH = 10.5

14.31) From Table 13–4, ascorbic acid (vitamin C) has a pK_a of 4.1; estimate the pH of each of the following buffer solutions.

a) 0.010 M ascorbic acid with 0.010 M sodium ascorbate

b) 0.010 M ascorbic acid with 0.0020 M sodium ascorbate

c) 0.010 M ascorbic acid with 0.030 M sodium ascorbate

14.32*) If 0.0050 moles of OH^- are added to one liter of solution (a) in Question 14.31, what will be the final pH? What would be the pH if the buffer were not present?

the following solutions to two decimal places.

a) 0.1 M acetic acid, $[H^+] = 1.34 \times 10^{-3}\ M$

b) saturated $CaCO_3$ solution, $[H^+] = 4.0 \times 10^{-10}\ M$

c) a sample of wine, $[H^+] = 1.9 \times 10^{-4}\ M$

d) a sample of urine, $[H^+] = 6.8 \times 10^{-9}\ M$

14.49) Calculate the $[H^+]$ of each of the following solutions.

a) hominy, pH = 7.47

b) cole slaw, pH = 5.37

c) a 10% solution of the oxidizing agent sodium dichromate, $Na_2Cr_2O_7$, pH = 3.56.

d) 2.5% pyribenzamine HCl, pH = 6.71

14.50) From Table 13–4, ammonium ion (NH_4^+) has a pK_a of 9.3; estimate the pH of each of the following buffer solutions.

a) 0.10 M NH_4Cl and 0.10 M NH_3

b) 0.10 M NH_4Cl and 0.050 M NH_3

c) 0.10 M NH_4Cl and 0.70 M NH_3

14.51*) If 0.020 moles of H^+ are added to one liter of solution (a) in Question 14.50, what will be the final pH? What would be the pH if the buffer were not present?

SECTION 14.4 NET IONIC EQUATIONS

14.33) Write net ionic equations for any reactions that occur on mixing the following solutions.

a) HI + NaOH

b) $Fe(NO_3)_3 + Na_3PO_4$

c) $NH_4Cl + CH_3COOH$

d) $NaHSO_4 + KOH$

e) $BaS + Na_2SO_4$

f) $LiOH + MgCl_2$

g) $Al(NO_3)_3 + Na_2S$

h) $NaHCO_3 + HCl$

i) $H_2NCH_2COOH + KOH$

14.52) Write net ionic equations for any reactions that occur on mixing the following solutions.

a) HCl + KOH

b) $Cu(NO_3)_2 + KBr$

c) $NH_3 + HNO_3$

d) $Na_2CO_3 + NH_3$

e) $AgNO_3 + CaCl_2$

f) $NH_4Cl + Pb(C_2H_3O_2)_2$

g) $H_3PO_4 + CuNO_3$

h) $NaHCO_3 + NaOH$

i) $H_2NCH_2COOH + HNO_3$

SECTION 14.5 TITRATION CALCULATIONS

14.34) Find the unknown concentration (molarity) from the information given.

a) a 10.00-mL sample of $HNO_{3(aq)}$

14.53) Find the unknown concentration (molarity) from the information given.

a) a 25.00-mL sample of $HCl_{(aq)}$

requires 15.67 mL of 0.100 M $NH_{3(aq)}$ to reach an end point

b) a 5.00-mL sample of $KOH_{(aq)}$ requires 7.89 mL of 0.500 M H_2SO_4 to reach a *final* end point

14.35*) From the list in Table 14.3, choose the indicator most likely to provide a good end point (near the equivalence point) for titration (a) in Question 14.34.

14.36*) Determine the *normality* of each of the following acid-base solutions.

a) 0.10 M HCl
b) 0.0050 M NH_3
c) 1.50 M H_3PO_4

14.37*) Calculate the unknown *normality* in the following solutions.

a) 15.78 mL of an acid solution neutralize 37.69 mL of 0.100 N base
b) 10.00 mL of a solution of a reducing agent react exactly with 17.79 mL of 0.0790 N permanganate solution

14.38*) Calculate the equivalent weight of

a) HOOCCOOH as an acid
b) Fe^{3+} ion in body fluids
c) F_2 as an oxidizing agent

14.39*) The following are typical blood plasma levels in meq/L (milliequivalents/liter). Convert each to moles/liter.

a) potassium ion, 4.2 meq/L
b) lactate ion, $CH_3CHOHCOO^-$, 1.3 meq/L
c) magnesium ion, 1.9 meq/L

requires 34.21 mL of 0.0500 M $NaOH_{(aq)}$ to reach an end point

b) a 10.00-mL sample of NaOH requires 26.79 mL of 0.1000 M H_3PO_4 to reach a *final* end point

14.54*) From the list in Table 14.3, choose the indicator most likely to provide a good endpoint (near the equivalence point) for titration (b) in Question 14.53.

14.55*) Determine the *normality* of each of the following acid-base solutions.

a) 0.10 M KOH
b) 0.0250 M H_2SO_4
c) 0.950 M HNO_3

14.56*) Calculate the unknown *normality* in the following solutions.

a) 25.96 mL of a base solution neutralize 19.78 mL of 0.0500 N acid
b) 33.69 mL of a permanganate solution react exactly with 25.00 mL of a 1.089 N solution of a reducing agent

14.57*) Calculate the equivalent weight of

a) Ca^{2+} ion in body fluids
b) H_2 as a reducing agent
c) NH_3 as a base

14.58*) The following are typical blood plasma levels in meq/L. Convert each to moles/liter.

a) pyruvate anion, CH_3COCOO^-, 0.05 meq/L
b) calcium ion, 5.0 meq/L
c) HPO_4^{2-} ion, 2.0 meq/L

Aromatic and Heterocyclic Ring Systems

In Section 7.3, we saw that carbon atoms can join together to form ring or cyclic compounds: the cycloalkanes. Except for the small, strained cycloalkanes, these cyclic compounds are similar to alkanes in properties and chemical reactivity. Cyclic compounds can also contain double bonds. For example, cyclohexene is a cyclic alkene of six carbon atoms:

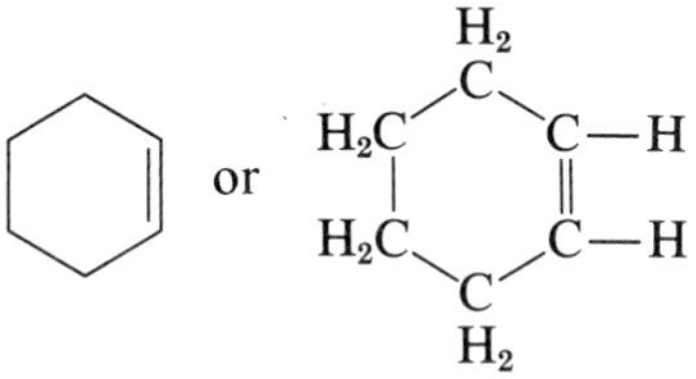

cyclohexene
C_6H_{10}

The physical and chemical properties of cycloalkenes are similar to those of the open-chain alkenes with the same number of carbon atoms. Many of the chemicals of importance to life, such as cholesterol (Figure 1–4), Vitamin A (the essential chemical of vision), and β-carotene (a vitamin found in carrots), contain a cyclohexene ring as part of their overall structures:

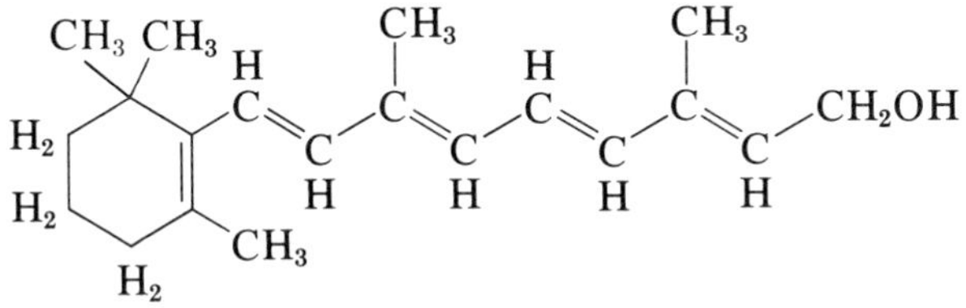

vitamin A (all-*trans*)

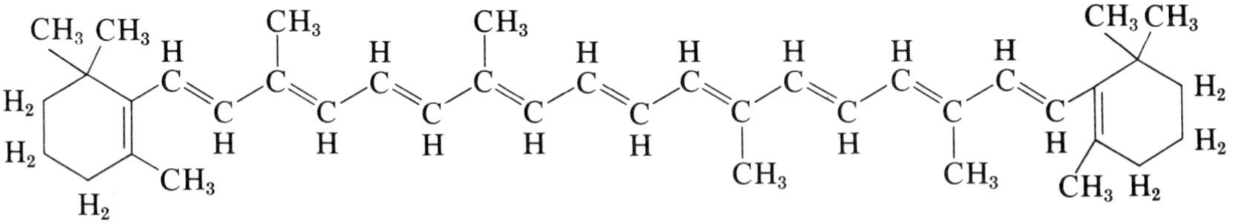

β-carotene (all-*trans*)

In earlier chapters, we distinguished between classes of hydrocarbons according to the type of bonding between the carbon atoms in the molecule. An alkane has only single bonds between carbon atoms, an alkene one double bond, and an alkyne one triple bond.

In this chapter, we will examine unsaturated cyclic compounds of a different type. Each will contain (in most cases) a six-membered carbon ring. However, the chemical and physical properties of this type of ring compound, called an *aromatic hydrocarbon,* are quite different from those of any type of hydrocarbon we have met so far.

15.1 BENZENE

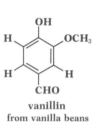

vanillin
from vanilla beans

Arene is another name for an aromatic hydrocarbon.

Benzene is not a pleasant-smelling substance. The original meaning of the term "aromatic" cannot be applied to benzene itself.

LEARNING GOAL 15A: Draw the structural formula of benzene, and explain how the pi electrons are delocalized.

Early in the 19th century, chemists isolated a particular type of hydrocarbon from substances such as oil of cloves and vanilla beans. These compounds were called "aromatic" because of their pleasant, persistent odors. Chemical examination of this class of compounds showed that they are not related to alkanes, alkenes, or alkynes. They form a new class of hydrocarbons—called **aromatic hydrocarbons** on the basis of their odor. This classification based on odor did not last very long. It was soon recognized that all the members of this class are related to a cyclic hydrocarbon called **benzene,** which has the molecular formula C_6H_6. Today, the term aromatic hydrocarbon means any substance that has certain chemical properties similar to benzene.

Benzene was first isolated in 1825 by Michael Faraday. When heated to high temperatures (1000°C) in the absence of air, soft coal breaks up to form coke and a black, viscous, gummy liquid (coal tar) that serves as a source of aromatic compounds. Today, many aromatic substances are obtained from petroleum.

Benzene was a puzzling and fascinating substance to these early chemists. The molecular formula (C_6H_6) requires that each carbon atom in the benzene molecule have only one hydrogen atom joined to it. This feature indicates benzene must contain multiple bonds.

However, chemists rapidly discovered that benzene did not easily add hydrogen the way ethene or ethyne did. It was *stable* under the normal conditions of catalytic hydrogenation and behaved pretty much like an alkane. Imagine how confused these chemists must have been when they found these properties for benzene!

Further chemical work finally gave some clues to the structure of benzene. When hydrogenation was carried out at high pressures in the presence of a catalyst, three moles of hydrogen added to one mole of benzene to give cyclohexane:

$$C_6H_6 + 3\ H_2 \xrightarrow[\text{high pressure}]{\text{Ni}}$$

cyclohexane, C_6H_{12}

This experiment showed that benzene contains a six-membered ring of carbon atoms. The addition of three molecules of hydrogen per mole of benzene showed that benzene contains unsaturation equivalent to three double bonds.

It was also found that benzene reacts with chlorine or bromine in the presence of an iron catalyst. However, addition does not occur. Instead, one of the hydrogen atoms of benzene is *substituted* by a halogen atom. The halogen *replaces* the hydrogen:

$$C_6H_6 + X_2 \xrightarrow{\text{Fe}} C_6H_5X + HX$$
$$(X = Cl, Br)$$

Only one organic compound with the molecular formula C_6H_5X has ever been isolated. No isomers are known. Thus, all six carbon-hydrogen bonds in benzene must be equivalent (have the same properties). If they were not equivalent, more than one isomer of C_6H_5X would be possible.

To account for these experimental observations, Friedrich Kekulé in 1865 proposed the following structure for benzene:

The **Kekulé structure** consisted of a hexagon with alternating single and double bonds between the carbon atoms. This structure nicely accounted for the addition of hydrogen to form cyclohexane. Also, substitution of any one of the six hydrogens by a bromine atom would give only *one* C_6H_5Br compound.

So finally, 40 years after its discovery, chemists knew the structure of benzene. Well, not exactly! The Kekulé structure doesn't explain why a halogen does not *add* to benzene, but instead undergoes a substitution reaction. More important, the Kekulé structure predicts two isomers for a 1,2-disubstituted benzene (I and II):

and

(I)   (II)

In isomer I, the two carbon atoms holding the chlorine atoms are joined with a double bond, whereas in isomer II they are joined with a single bond. However, only *one* dichlorobenzene with the chlorine atoms on adjacent carbons has ever been isolated. There are not two isomers. How can we account for this fact?

Kekulé modified his earlier theory to explain this situation. He proposed that the double bonds shift back and forth so rapidly that although I and II are isomers, the equilibrium is so rapid that they can never be separated.

Alkenes readily add Cl_2 or Br_2: $H_2C{=}CH_2 + Br_2 \rightarrow CH_2BrCH_2Br$

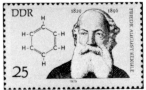

Friedrich Kekulé (1829–1896).

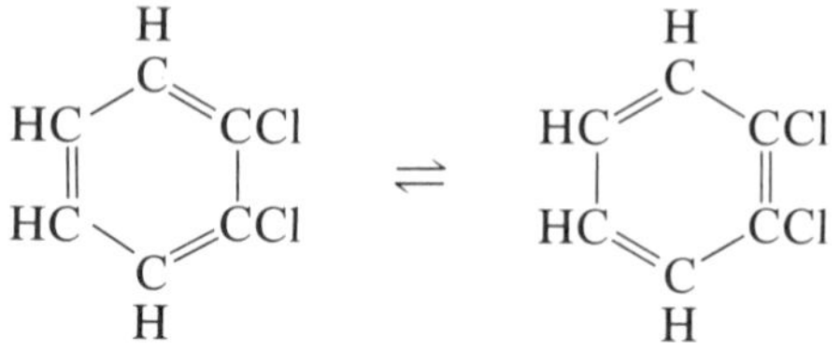

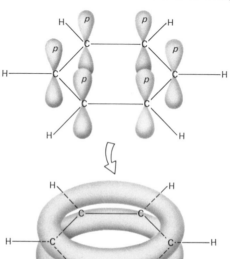

proposed very fast equilibrium

I   II

Benzene is stable to HBr, which normally reacts readily with alkenes (via addition) at room temperature (Chapter 7).

Although this modified theory persisted until the 1930's, it was not entirely adequate. It still did not account for the lack of reactivity of benzene or its preference for substitution reactions rather than addition reactions.

The modern concept of the structure of benzene has evolved from orbital theory. The measurement of bond lengths and bond angles of benzene by x-ray analysis has shown that benzene is shaped like a *planar* hexagon and that all the carbon-carbon bond lengths are *identical* and equal to 1.39 Å (Figure 15–1). This bond length is intermediate between that of a pure single carbon-carbon bond (1.54 Å) and that of a pure double carbon-carbon bond (1.33 Å). We know now that this is a result of *delocalized* electrons (Section 6.2).

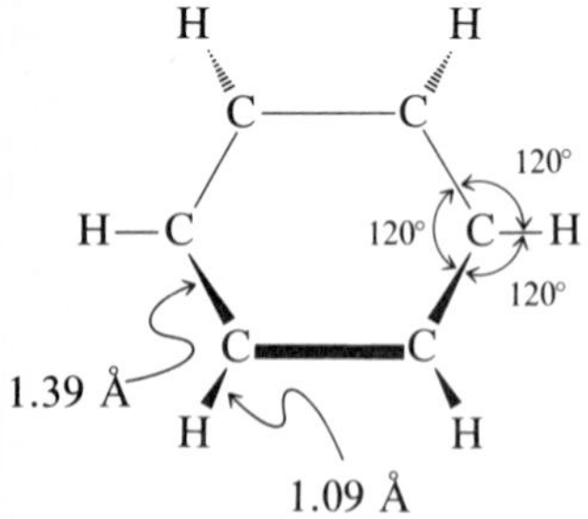

In Figure 15–2, the delocalized electron cloud of benzene is shown. The 30 valence electrons (4 for each carbon, 1 for each hydrogen) are distributed as follows: 24 are used for the 12 sigma bonds, leaving 6 electrons (30 minus 24) for the delocalized pi bond. These six delocalized electrons move freely around the planar hexagon ring.

The proposed ''equilibrium'' originally envisioned by Kekulé was thus almost correct. It is *not* an equilibrium, however. The two Kekulé structures (I and II) are *localized* electron structures. The true structure is not adequately represented by either Lewis diagram. The true delocalized structure is an average of these forms.

How can we conveniently represent the ''real'' benzene molecule in chemical reactions to indicate a compound with six equivalent carbon

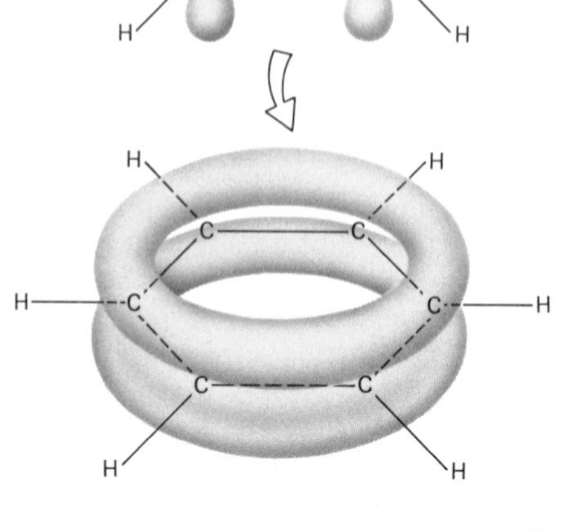

FIGURE 15–1   Benzene bond angles and lengths.

1.39 Å

1.09 Å

120°

Benzene is neither

nor

but an average of these two Lewis forms.

FIGURE 15–2   Delocalized π-electron cloud in benzene.

atoms, each bonded to a hydrogen atom and each participating in delocalized electron bonding? One possible way is to draw only one of the Kekulé structures and leave it to the reader to recognize that this is a localized form of the real structure. Another type of shorthand used by chemists to represent benzene is to draw a circle to represent the 6 delocalized pi electrons (Figure 15–3).

The delocalization of pi electrons in benzene helps to stabilize the molecule. Any reaction that will break up this delocalization will be resisted. Thus, if benzene underwent addition reactions, the delocalization over all six carbon atoms would be lost. However, when benzene undergoes substitution reactions, the delocalization and stability of the molecule are preserved. Except under extreme circumstances, benzene will undergo only substitution reactions, since this type of reaction costs the molecule least in terms of stability.

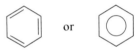

FIGURE 15–3 Alternate ways of drawing a benzene ring.

The delocalized structure of benzene has a lower energy and is more stable than either of the Kekulé structures.

15.2 SUBSTITUTED BENZENES

> *LEARNING GOAL 15B:* *Given the structural formula for a substituted benzene, write its name.*
>
> *15C:* *Use the* ortho, meta, para *system to name disubstituted benzenes.*
>
> *15D:* *Give three examples of aromatic substitution reactions.*

Names

For some simple aromatic compounds, the naming scheme has some order to it. A *prefix* for the substituent that has replaced hydrogen on the benzene ring is joined to the word "benzene."

> EXAMPLE 15a: What is the name of the compound
>
> [benzene ring with Br]
>
> -
>
> *SOLUTION:*   Bromine has replaced one hydrogen of the ring. The prefix "bromo-" is joined to the word "benzene." The name of this compound is bromobenzene .

The following examples also illustrate this naming system:

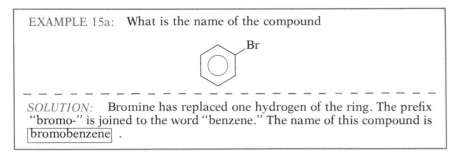

chlorobenzene   nitrobenzene   fluorobenzene   iodobenzene

Many of the monosubstituted (one-substituent) benzene compounds have common names that are always used. Some examples are

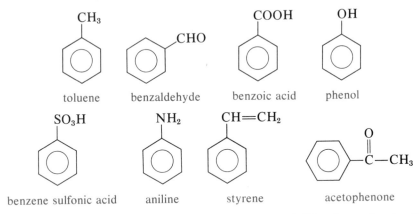

toluene benzaldehyde benzoic acid phenol

benzene sulfonic acid aniline styrene acetophenone

Note that it doesn't make any difference where the substituent is attached to the ring—all the positions are the same in benzene.

The removal of a hydrogen from benzene (C_6H_6) gives rise to the C_6H_5- group. This group is called the *phenyl group;* it is like an alkyl group (Section 7.1), which is derived by removal of a hydrogen from an alkane. The phenyl group is often used in naming aromatic compounds. For example:

The phenyl group can be written.

$$CH_3-\underset{\underset{H}{|}}{\overset{\overset{OH}{|}}{C}}-\bigcirc \text{ is 1-phenylethanol.}$$

The phenyl group is named as a substituent on the longest carbon chain of the alcohol and its location on the chain is given by the appropriate number. Similarly, $CH_3(CH_2)_5C_6H_5$ is 1-phenylhexane.

Disubstituted benzenes

The numbers used on the carbons of the ring in naming substituted benzenes are assigned to give the lowest possible numbers, as for substituted alkanes. The carbon atoms are numbered from the first substituent:

When two substituent groups are attached to a benzene ring, the positions on the ring are no longer all equivalent. The groups can be separated by zero, one, or two ring carbon atoms. The relative positions of the groups *must* be designated. Two methods are commonly used: either a numbering system or the prefixes *ortho*, *meta*, and *para*.

EXAMPLE 15b: Name the compound

Br
Br

- -

SOLUTION: Both the name of the substituents and their relative positions must be specified. The substituents are both bromine (bromo); their location is 1,2 relative to each other; the prefix "di-" is used to indicate two identical substituents. The name is $\boxed{\text{1,2-dibromobenzene}}$.

Often one of the groups alone on the ring would give the compound a common name. This common name may be used to designate the compound, with the second group named as a substituent.

EXAMPLE 15c: Write the common name of the compound

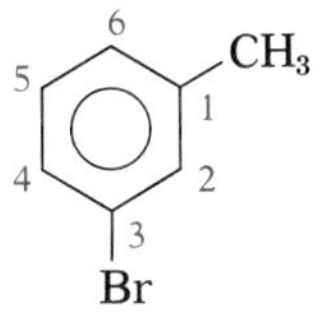

SOLUTION:

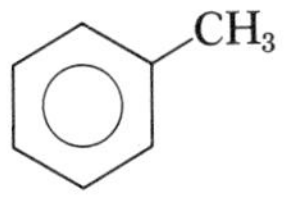

is toluene. This common name is used. The bromo group is located on carbon 3 relative to the methyl group. The name is 3-bromotoluene .

The prefixes **ortho, meta,** and **para** are also used to distinguish the 1,2, 1,3, and 1,4 relationships. These prefixes are usually abbreviated *o-*, *m-*, and *p-*, respectively. The use of these prefixes is illustrated below.

ortho: Two groups joined to adjacent (neighboring) ring carbon atoms are said to be *ortho* (*o-*) to one another.

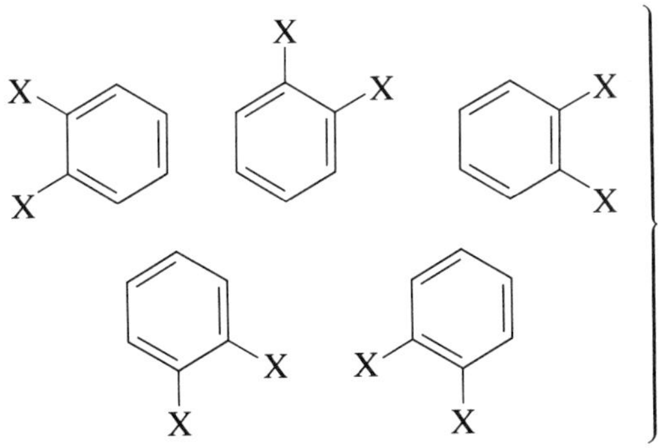

equivalent sets of *ortho* positions

meta: Two groups bonded to ring carbon atoms that are separated by one ring carbon are said to be *meta* (*m-*) to one another.

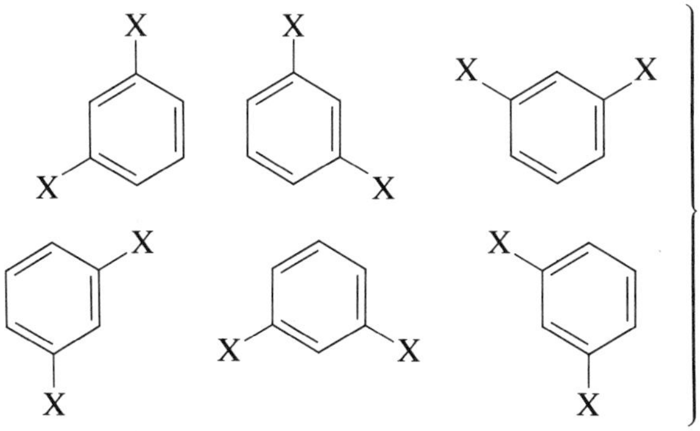

equivalent sets of *meta* positions

para: Two groups bonded to ring carbon atoms that are separated by two ring carbons are said to be *para* (*p-*) to one another. Two *para* groups are opposite each other on the ring.

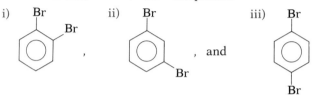

equivalent
sets of
para positions

EXAMPLE 15d: Name the compounds

i)

Br
Br

,

ii)

Br

Br

, and

iii)

Br

Br

by the *o-*, *m-*, *p-* system.

- -

SOLUTION: i)

Br
Br

The bromo groups are located *ortho* (1,2) to each other. The name is
o-dibromobenzene .

ii)

Br

Br

The bromo groups are located *meta* (1,3) to each other. The name is
m-dibromobenzene .

iii)

Br

Br

The bromo groups are located *para* (1,4) to each other. The name is
p-dibromobenzene .

EXAMPLE 15e: Name the compound

OH

Cl

by the *o-, m-, p-* system.

_ _

SOLUTION:

OH

is phenol. The chloro group is located *para* (1,4) relative to the hydroxy group. The name is $\boxed{p\text{-chlorophenol}}$.

If neither group on the ring is associated with a common name (if it were alone on the ring), then both groups are named and located in the name.

EXAMPLE 15f: Name the compound

Br

I

by the *o-, m-, p-* system.

_ _

SOLUTION: Neither the bromo- nor iodo- group on the ring has a common name associated with it. So both groups are named and their relative locations (1,3) indicated by the appropriate prefixes. The name is $\boxed{m\text{-bromoiodobenzene}}$.

When two methyl groups are attached to a benzene ring, three isomeric $C_6H_4(CH_3)_2$ compounds are possible. The common name for this benzene derivative is "xylene." The naming of the isomers is as shown:

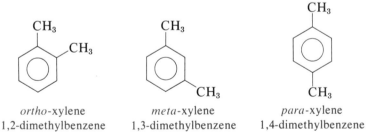

ortho-xylene	*meta*-xylene	*para*-xylene
1,2-dimethylbenzene	1,3-dimethylbenzene	1,4-dimethylbenzene

Polysubstituted benzenes

When three or more substituents are attached to a benzene ring, only the numbering system is used. Some examples are

1,3,5-trimethylbenzene   3-chloro-2-nitrotoluene

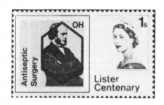

Joseph Lister (1827–1912) first proved the value of using phenol as an antiseptic.

2,4,6-trinitrotoluene
(TNT)

Important substituted benzenes

Benzene and some of its derivatives are important everyday chemicals. Benzene has been used as a building block for many other substituted aromatic compounds in the chemical industry.

Phenol has strong antiseptic properties. As a class of compounds, the phenols are active in killing germs. However, because of its extreme toxicity, phenol itself is now rarely used as an antiseptic. It is corrosive, causes blistering of the skin, and is a poison when taken internally. Dilute solutions of the cresols are used in hospitals as disinfectants. Other important commercial phenol derivatives are *hexylresorcinol,* used in mouthwashes, *pentachlorophenol (Pentachlor),* used as a wood preservative, and *pyrogallol,* used as a photographic developer:

o-cresol

m-cresol   *p*-cresol

Cresols (methyl phenols) are constituents of "creosote," a wood preservative. Lysol, a disinfectant solution, contains the phenol derivatives

OH   and

C₆H₅

Cl — OH

CH₂C₆H₅.

hexylresorcinol   pentachlorophenol   pyrogallol

Benzoic acid is used in the synthesis of organic compounds. Its sodium salt (sodium benzoate) is a common food preservative. *Para*-aminobenzoic acid is necessary in the diet of chickens, mice, and bacteria. As yet, it has not been proved essential to humans.

Salicylic acid (*o*-hydroxybenzoic acid), its salts, and its esters are used as fever-lowering agents and as painkillers in the treatment of rheumatism and arthritis. Salicylic acid itself is too irritating to be taken internally but its acetic acid ester, acetylsalicylic acid (*aspirin*) is widely used as a fever-lowering and analgesic agent.

Further discussion of these drugs can be found in Section 13.4.

Methyl salicylate is oil of wintergreen, a common ingredient of liniments.

salicylic acid   aspirin   sodium salicylate
(acetylsalicylic acid)

Diflunisal, an analgesic, is a substituted salicylic acid.

Recently, an aspirin substitute called *diflunisal* has appeared on the market. It is claimed to have none of the side effects of aspirin.

Aniline is made in large quantities in the chemical industry. Most of it is used in the manufacture of dyes, pharmaceuticals, and chemicals for the plastic industry. Substituted anilines, such as *phenacetin* and *acetaminophen,* have been used extensively as analgesic and antipyretic (fever-lowering) agents.

Reactions of aromatic hydrocarbons

As noted earlier, the most common reaction of aromatic hydrocarbons is a substitution reaction in which a ring hydrogen is replaced by another atom or group of atoms. In this section, we will examine the replacement of the ring hydrogen by an alkyl group, a halogen, a nitro group, and a sulfonic acid ($-SO_3H$) group.

Alkylation

The French chemist Charles Friedel and the American chemist James Craft discovered that when benzene reacts with an alkyl halide in the presence of an aluminum chloride catalyst, a ring hydrogen is substituted by an alkyl group in a process called **alkylation:**

| benzene | bromomethane | toluene |

| benzene | chloroethane | ethylbenzene |

This type of alkylation is called the *Friedel-Craft reaction* after its discoverers. It is a general reaction of benzene and its derivatives.

Halogenation

In **halogenation,** benzene reacts with chlorine or bromine in the presence of $FeCl_3$ or $FeBr_3$. A ring hydrogen is substituted by a chlorine or bromine atom:

Fluorine (F_2) is too reactive to use unless special precautions are taken. Iodine (I_2) is too inert.

| benzene | chlorobenzene |

| benzene | bromobenzene |

Reaction with Acids

Substitution of a ring hydrogen of benzene also occurs when a strong acid, such as nitric or sulfuric acid, is allowed to react with benzene:

benzene   nitric acid   nitrobenzene

Nitrobenzene has a harmful effect on the red blood cells and on the liver. Caution should thus be used in handling this material, and inhalation of its vapor should be avoided.

The introduction of a nitro (NO_2—) group is called a **nitration** reaction. The nitro group can be reduced with tin and hydrochloric acid to give the amino (NH_2—) group (Chapter 13). This two-step process is the most common way to introduce an amino group onto an aromatic ring:

nitrobenzene   aniline

The replacement of a ring hydrogen by a —SO_3H group is called **sulfonation.** Sulfur trioxide (SO_3) is used to speed up this reaction:

benzene   sulfuric acid   benzene sulfonic acid

TABLE 15–1   A FEW OF THE MORE EFFECTIVE SULFA DRUGS

Name	Structural Formula
Sulfanilamide	
Sulfapyridine	
Sulfadiazine	
Sulfathiazole	
Sulfaguanidine	
5-Sulfanilamido-3,4-dimethylisoxazole	
3-Sulfanilamido-6-methoxypyridazine	

Substituted sulfonic acid derivatives are among the oldest of the antibiotics. They are the *sulfa drugs*. Their antimicrobial action was first discovered in the early 1930's in Europe, when "prontosil," a dye, was found to be active against bacterial infections. It was quickly discovered that prontosil was broken down in the body to give a bacteria-killing compound called sulfanilamide:

$$H_2N \underset{\text{prontosil}}{\underbrace{\bigcirc \overset{\overset{\displaystyle NH_2}{|}}{\bigcirc} - N{=}N - \bigcirc - SO_2NH_2}} \xrightarrow[\text{body}]{\text{in}} H_2N \underset{\text{sulfanilamide}}{\underbrace{\bigcirc - SO_2NH_2}}$$

Sulfanilamide was effective against streptococcus infections, pneumonia, and gonorrhea. Unfortunately, sulfanilamide is only slightly soluble in water. When given orally, the drug is absorbed by the body and eventually carried to the kidneys for excretion. When the dosage is large, or under prolonged treatment, the kidneys may be damaged by deposited sulfanilamide. Chemists began a search for sulfanilamide derivatives that were less harmful. Over 5000 similar compounds were made and tested for biological activity and harmful side effects. Only a few of these compounds showed satisfactory properties and have been used with humans. Some of the more effective ones are listed in Table 15–1. Note that all are similar to sulfanilamide except for the type of group attached to the nitrogen atom. The sulfa drugs were early attempts by chemists to build compounds with specific application as drugs. Penicillin and other antibiotics have partially replaced the sulfa drugs as agents against infection in humans. However, sulfa drugs still find widespread use in medicine, particularly in diseases of the urinary tract and for treating infections in animals.

The chemist's shorthand

In Section 7.3 we started drawing diagrams of cyclic compounds, such as the cycloalkanes, without showing all the carbon atoms. For example, a simple hexagon

stands for the compound C_6H_{12}, with one carbon atom at each corner of the figure and two hydrogens bonded to it. Similar diagrams are drawn for the other cycloalkanes.

Since the beginning of this chapter we have been using a hexagon with a circle,

to represent a benzene ring. You see then that a simple geometric figure in organic chemistry is assumed to represent a carbon atom at each corner, with the appropriate number of hydrogen atoms. Sometimes such short-hand is extended so that a single line off the ring represents a methyl group. Some examples may make this type of shorthand clearer:

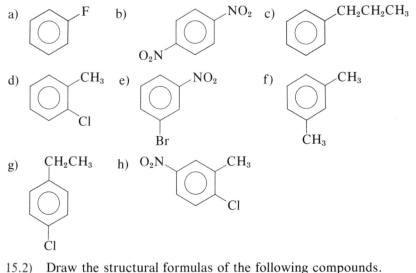

SELF-CHECK

15.1)   Name the following compounds.

a) F b) NO_2 O_2N c) $CH_2CH_2CH_3$

d) CH_3 Cl e) NO_2 Br f) CH_3 CH_3

g) CH_2CH_3 Cl h) O_2N CH_3 Cl

15.2)   Draw the structural formulas of the following compounds.
a)   iodobenzene
b)   o-nitrotoluene
c)   1,3,5-tribromobenzene
d)   p-xylene
e)   m-bromonitrobenzene
f)   p-chlorophenol
g)   o-fluorophenol
h)   p-nitrobenzene sulfonic acid

15.3) Draw the structural formula of the product expected from the reaction of benzene with bromoethane, using aluminum chloride as a catalyst.

15.3 FUSED-RING HYDROCARBONS

LEARNING GOAL 15E: Give three examples of fused-ring hydrocarbons.

So far, we have seen several examples of ring hydrocarbons, such as the cycloalkanes, cycloalkenes, and benzene. Many organic compounds have two or more rings in the molecule. These rings may be separated or they may be *fused* (joined) so that *each ring shares two carbons with another ring.*

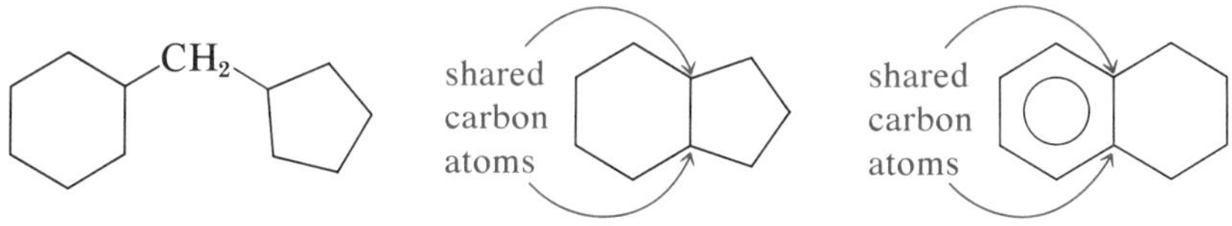

separated rings fused rings fused rings

The **fused rings** may be saturated, unsaturated, or aromatic. There are many kinds of compounds that contain two or more fused rings. In this section we will look at only a select few, but keep in mind that almost any combination is possible.

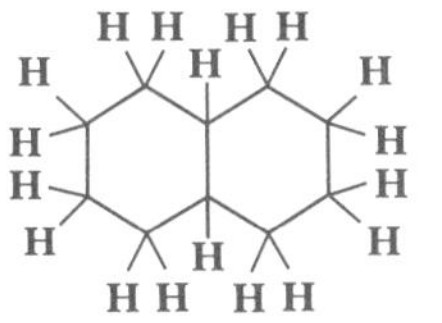

Steroids

The steroids are a group of compounds that contain four rings fused together. The typical **steroid nucleus** or ring system contains three six-membered rings and one five-membered ring (Figure 15–4). Steroids are molecules that play a variety of biological roles in humans. Depending upon the type and position of the functional groups placed on the steroid nucleus, they may be components of the bile, the brain, or the spinal tissue. Some of them are sex hormones, some vitamin D-related compounds, and some birth control agents. Figure 15–5 illustrates several common steroids. They are discussed in more detail in Chapter 18.

Fused-ring aromatic hydrocarbons

A number of fused-ring aromatic compounds are known. There has recently been an intensive research effort in this area, since some of these compounds may be the carcinogenic (cancer-causing) agents in cigarette smoke. The simplest fused-ring aromatic hydrocarbon is naphthalene, $C_{10}H_8$, commonly used in moth balls.

In terms of Kekulé-type diagrams, we can write three Lewis forms for naphthalene:

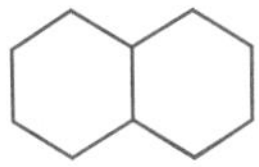

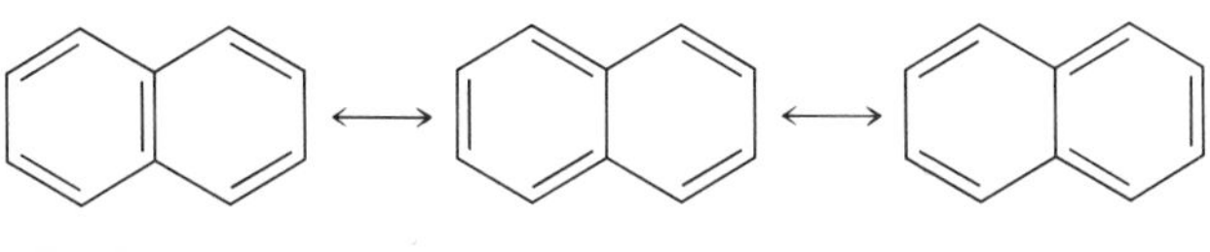

The fusion of two six-membered rings is called *decalin*.

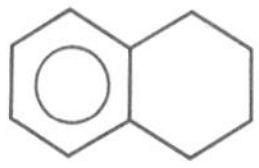

The fusion of a benzene ring and a cyclohexane ring is called *tetralin*.

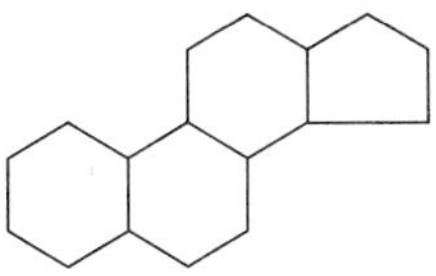

FIGURE 15–4 The steroid nucleus.

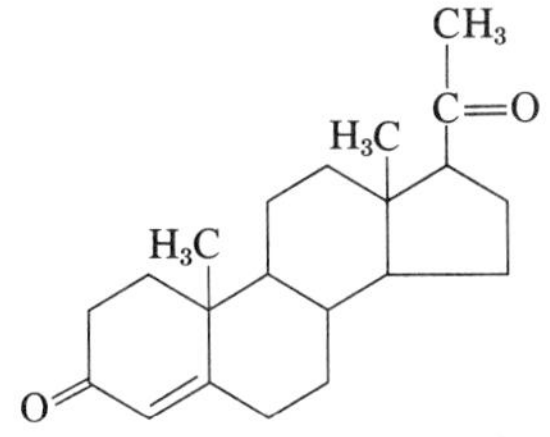

progesterone (pregnancy hormone)

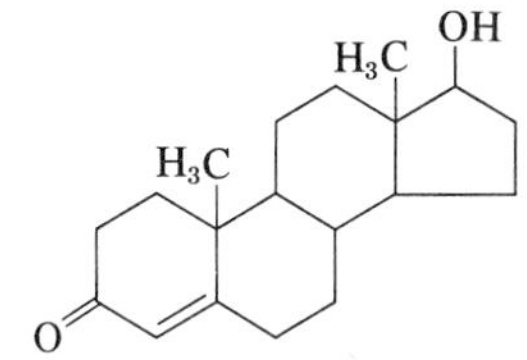

testosterone (male sex hormone)

FIGURE 15–5 Some steroid derivatives.

Benzene itself is suspected of being able to cause leukemia. The U.S. Occupational Safety and Health Administration (OSHA) has imposed a benzene workplace exposure limit of 10 parts of benzene per million parts of air (10 ppm).

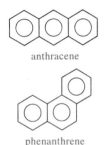

anthracene

phenanthrene

FIGURE 15–6 **Two possible ways to fuse three benzene rings.**

Naphthalene thus has a completely delocalized π-electron system.

When we join *three* benzene rings, there are two different ways to fuse the rings. Thus, anthracene and phenanthrene (Figure 15–6) are isomers. Anthracene is an important starting material in the manufacture of some dyes.

For many years it was known that coal tar workers had a high susceptibility to skin cancer. Recent investigation has shown that some aromatic fused-ring hydrocarbons can cause cancer when applied to the skin. Two of the compounds that have been demonstrated to cause cancer are 1,2-benzopyrene (BaP) and methylcholanthrene.

CH₃

1,2-benzopyrene   methylcholanthrene

1,2-benzopyrene is a component of cigarette smoke and is believed to be a major cause of lung cancer in smokers (Section 10.5).

SELF-CHECK

15.4) Which of the following are fused-ring hydrocarbons?

a)   b)   c)

15.4 HETEROCYCLIC RINGS

LEARNING GOAL 15F: Distinguish a heterocyclic compound from a carbocyclic compound.

15G: Give an example of a heterocyclic ring that contains an oxygen atom; a nitrogen atom; a sulfur atom.

15H: Give three examples of heterocyclic compounds each containing two hetero atoms per molecule.

Thus far in our discussion of cyclic compounds, we have restricted ourselves to those that have only carbon atoms in the ring. Such compounds are called *carbocyclic* compounds. Ring compounds having nitrogen, oxygen, sulfur, or other elements in the ring are called **heterocyclic** compounds (each noncarbon ring atom is called a **hetero atom**). In this section we introduce you to some of the heterocyclic ring systems that are important in biological compounds. These will then be familiar to you when you see them later as parts of more complex molecules.

Five-membered rings

Several important compounds include a heterocyclic ring made up of one oxygen and four carbon atoms. This ring system is known as *furan*. One of its important derivatives is the aldehyde *furfural*:

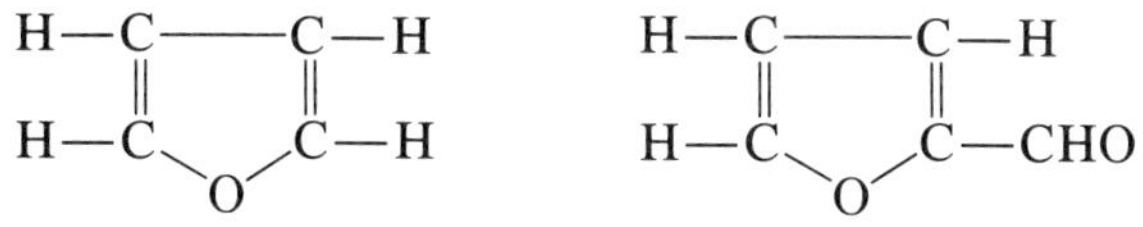

furan   furfural

For purposes of naming, the rings are numbered counterclockwise, generally starting from the hetero atom, as shown in Figure 15–7. When a heterocyclic ring contains only one hetero atom, Greek letters may also be used to designate ring positions. The carbon atom next to the heteroatom is the α (alpha) carbon; the next carbon is the β (beta) carbon.

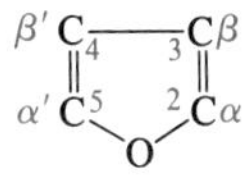

Furfural is produced commercially by the dehydration and ring closure of sugars found in corn cobs, oat hulls, and straw. This type of process shows how farm waste products can be used to produce commercial chemicals. Furfural is used in making plastics, as a solvent, and occasionally as an insecticide.

When passed over a hot catalyst, furfural can lose carbon monoxide to give furan. Catalytic hydrogenation of furan gives the saturated five-membered oxygen-containing heterocyclic ring called *tetrahydrofuran,* abbreviated THF. This compound is an important laboratory and industrial solvent:

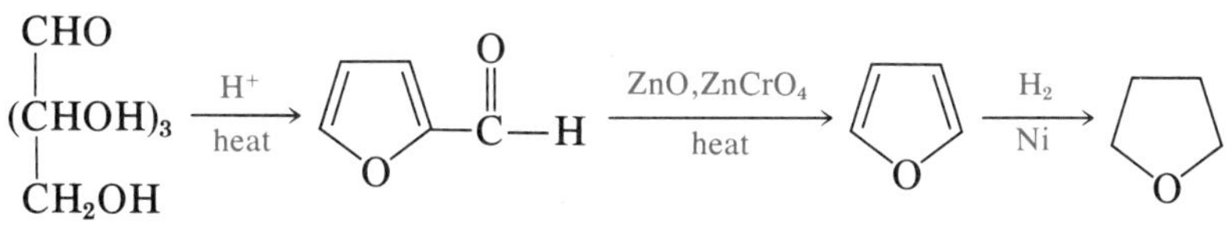

FIGURE 15–7 Numbering of a heterocyclic ring.

pentose sugar   furfural   furan   tetrahydrofuran (THF)

An important heterocyclic ring containing nitrogen is *pyrrole*. It can be readily obtained by the action of ammonia on a hydroxycarboxylic acid called *glycaric acid:*

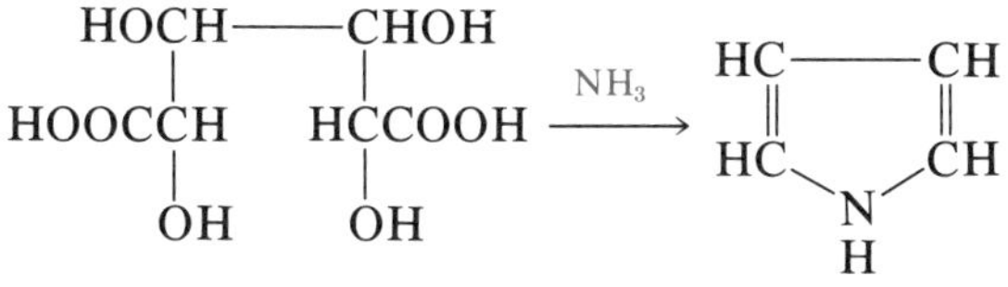

glycaric acid   pyrrole

Pyrrole is a liquid that gradually forms dark-colored resins on exposure to air. The pyrrole nucleus is a part of the ring systems called porphyrins, which are found in many biological molecules. One such system is that of protoporphyrin. The nitrogen atoms may share electrons with such metals as iron to form hemoglobin (Chapter 24) or magnesium to form chlorophyll (Chapter 25).

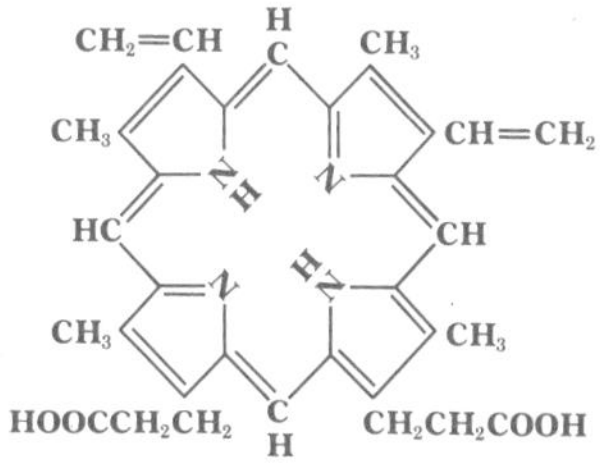

If pyrrole is fused to a benzene ring, another type of heterocyclic nucleus called *indole* is produced:

protoporphyrin

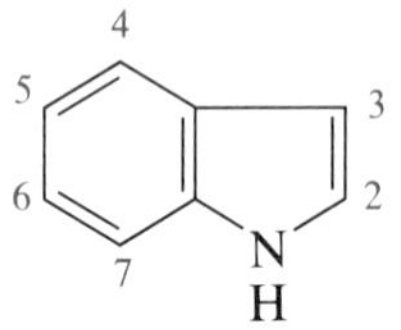

indole 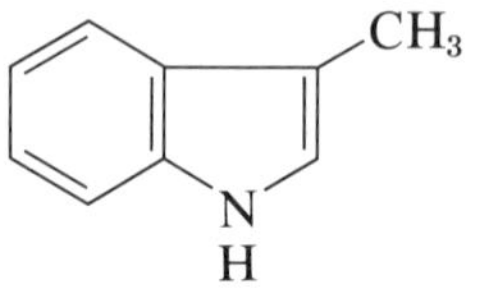   skatole 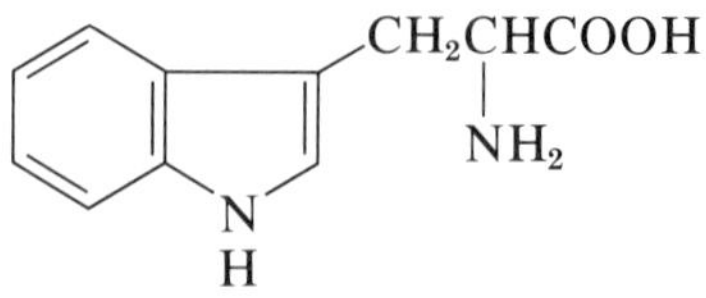   tryptophan

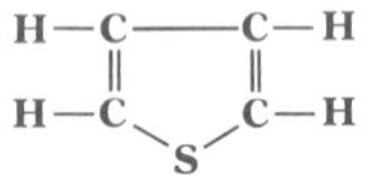

Indole and 3-methyl indole, called *skatole,* are formed during the decomposition of proteins in the large intestine. They are responsible for the characteristic odor of feces. One of the most important indole derivatives is the amino acid *tryptophan,* which is present in most proteins and is a necessary part of the diet of growing animals.

A five-membered heterocyclic ring that contains sulfur is *thiophene.* This compound occurs as an impurity in the benzene obtained from coal tar and is used as an industrial solvent and raw material.

thiophene

Five-membered rings with two hetero atoms

There are many examples of heterocyclic rings that contain two atoms of elements other than carbon. Oxazole, imidazole, pyrazole, and thiazole are similar to furan, pyrrole, and thiophene, except that each has a nitrogen atom in another position in the ring.

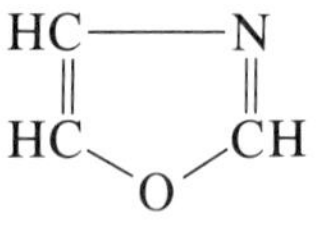

oxazole 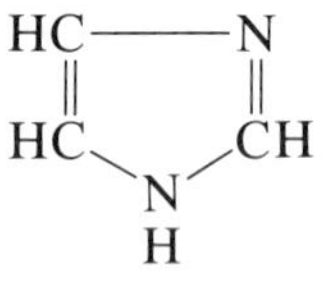   imidazole 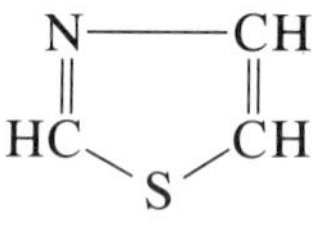   thiazole 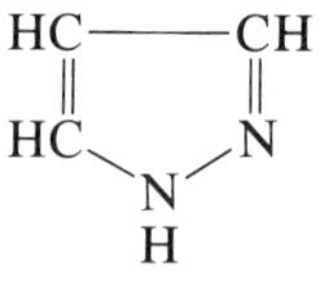   pyrazole

The imidazole ring is found in important substances such as the purines (Chapter 27) and the amino acid histidine (Chapter 19), which is essential to animal nutrition. The thiazole ring is present in the vitamin thiamine (Chapter 23) and in the penicillins, which are valuable antibiotic agents in medicine:

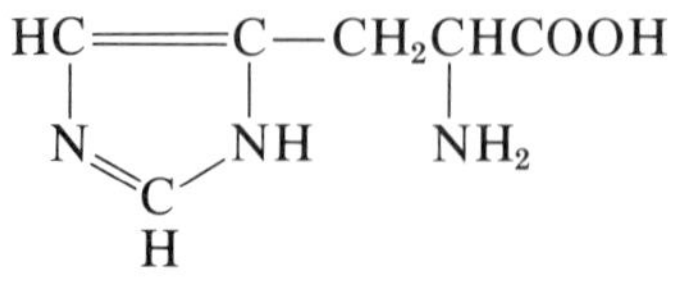

histidine 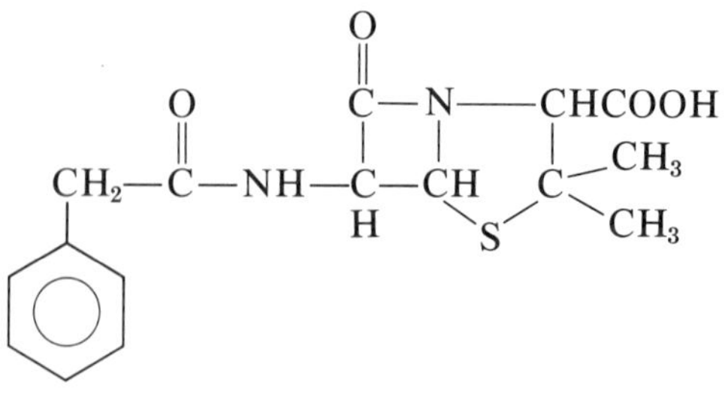   penicillin G

Six-membered rings

The most common six-membered rings containing one hetero atom are pyran and pyridine:

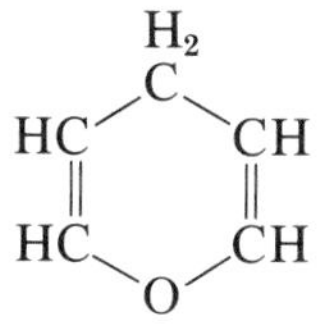

pyran 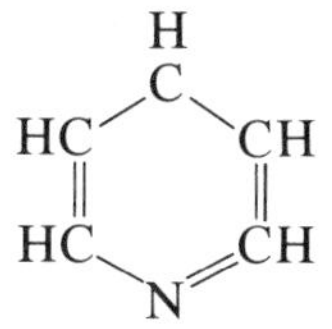   pyridine

The pyran ring is present in anthocyanidins, responsible for the color of flowers. The benzopyran ring is found in many plants and is part of the α-tocopherol (Vitamin E) molecule. (Chapter 23).

Pyridine is a liquid with a disagreeable odor. It is a good solvent for many organic and inorganic compounds and is used in large quantities in the manufacture of such pharmaceuticals as sulfa drugs and antihistamines. The methyl pyridines are *picolines;* they are easily oxidized to the corresponding carboxylic acids. The particular acid obtained from oxidation of 3-methyl pyridine is known as nicotinic acid:

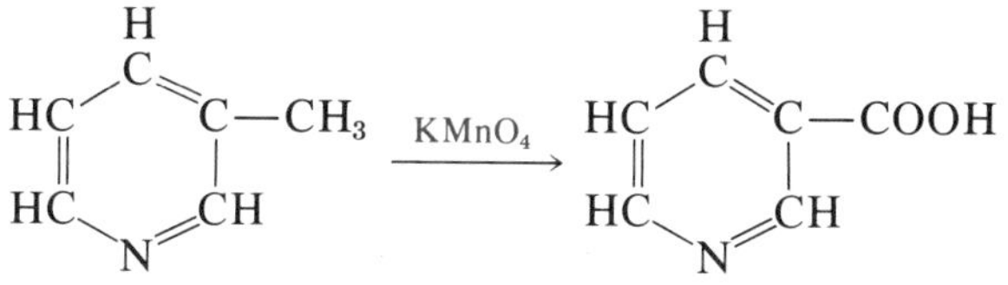

3-methyl pyridine   nicotinic acid
                                        (niacin)

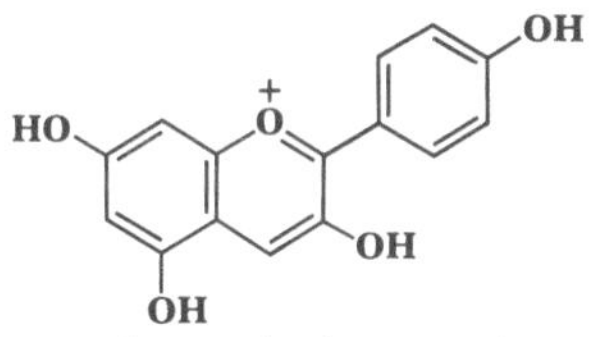

pelargonidin (geranium)

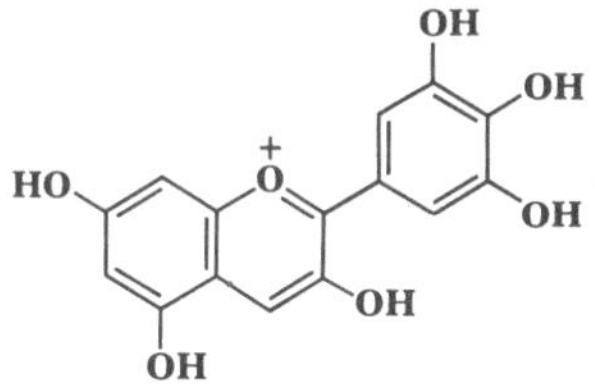

delphinidin (pansy, grape)
Two anthocyanidins.

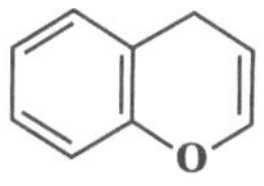

Nicotinic acid and some of its derivatives are parts of the Vitamin B complex (Chapter 23).

Six-membered rings with two hetero atoms

There are three aromatic six-membered rings containing two nitrogen atoms. *Pyridazine* contains the nitrogen atoms in the 1,2 position, *pyrimidine* in the 1,3 position, and *pyrazine* in the 1,4 position of the ring:

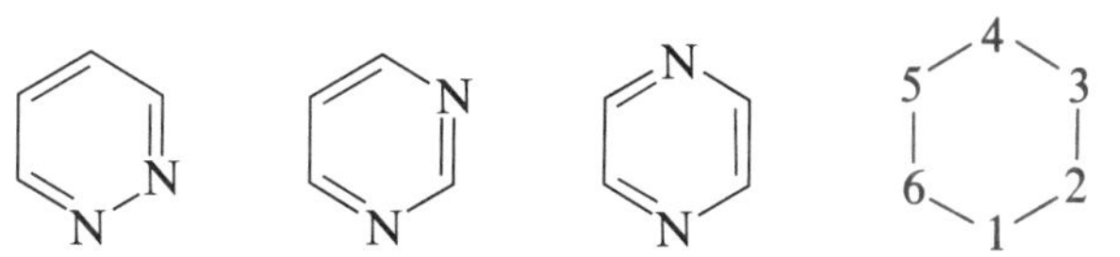

pyridazine   pyrimidine   pyrazine   ring positions

Pyrimidine is the most important of these heterocyclic rings. Its derivatives are found in nucleic acids, which are the carriers of the genetic codes in living systems. Nucleic acids will be discussed in detail in Chapter 20. Other common heterocyclic compounds found in nucleic acids are cytosine, thymine and uracil (pyrimidine derivatives) as well as adenine and guanine (purine derivatives) whose structures are illustrated in Figure 15–8.

The stimulants *theophylline* and *caffeine* are derivatives of purine. Theophylline is used to treat certain heart conditions and bronchial asthma. It is also in Dramamine, which is used for the prevention of motion sickness. Caffeine, a very active stimulant, is consumed in large quantities in coffee, tea, cocoa, and cola-based drinks.

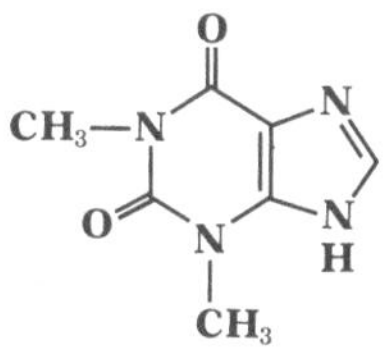

benzopyran

theophylline

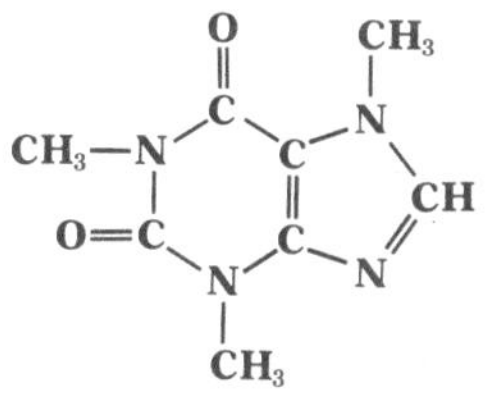

caffeine

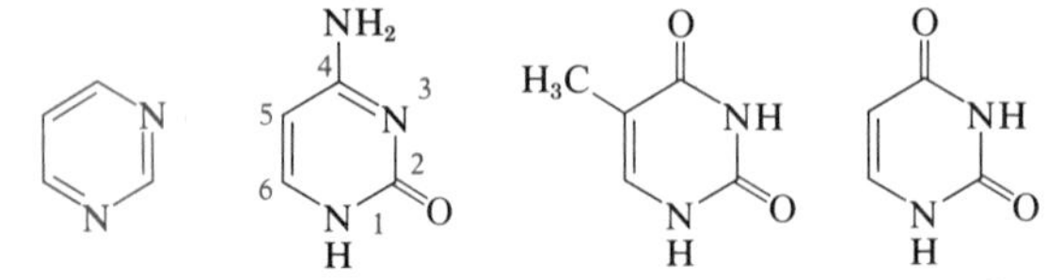

pyrimidine cytosine thymine uracil

substituted pyrimidines in DNA and RNA

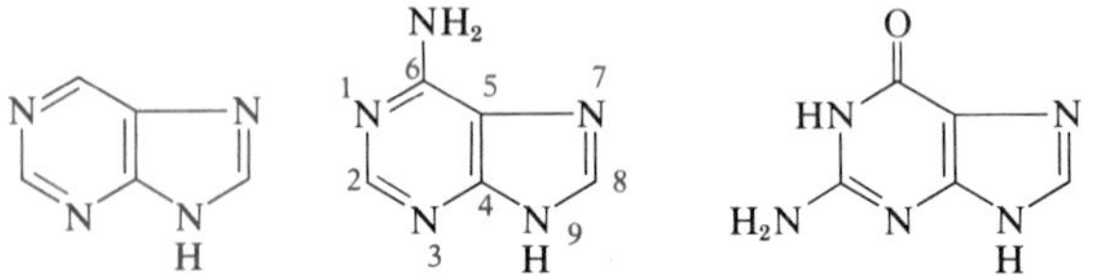

purine adenine guanine

substituted purines in DNA and RNA

FIGURE 15–8 Heterocyclic systems found in nucleic acids.

The *barbiturates* form an important group of pyrimidine derivatives. They are made by the following general type of reaction:

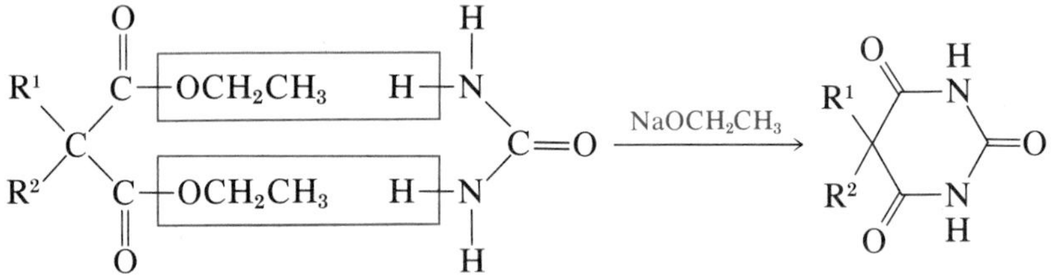

urea barbiturate

Barbiturates belong to a class of drugs that depress the central nervous system. When given in doses of 10 to 20 mg, they show beneficial sedative or hypnotic (sleep-inducing) effects. Unfortunately, they are habit-forming drugs, and habitual users develop a tolerance, thereby needing larger and

TABLE 15–2 COMMONLY USED BARBITURATES

R^1	R^2	Name	Trade Name
C_2H_5—	C_2H_5—	Barbital	Veronal
C_2H_5—	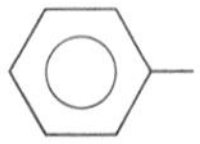	Phenobarbital	Luminal
C_2H_5—	$CH_3CH_2CH_2CH(CH_3)$—	Pentobarbital (Yellow Jackets)	Nembutal
C_2H_5—	$CH_3CH(CH_3)CH_2CH_2$—	Amobarbital	Amytal
$CH_2{=}CHCH_2$—	$CH_3CH_2CH_2CH(CH_3)$—	Secobarbital (Red Devils)	Seconal

larger doses. Excessive amounts of barbiturates (called "downers" in drug-culture terms) may cause deep sleep or coma and eventually death.

The different drugs differ only in the R^1 and R^2 groups in the barbiturate molecule. The nature of these groups changes the solubility of the barbiturate in body fats and plays an important role in the action of the drug. Some of the more commonly used barbiturates are shown in Table 15–2.

Fused aromatic heterocyclic rings

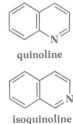

quinoline

isoquinoline

Quinoline and isoquinoline are fused heterocyclics that are similar in structure to naphthalene. Quinoline has a nitrogen at position 1. Isoquinoline is the 2-isomer.

Both quinoline and isoquinoline contain a pyridine ring fused to a benzene ring and are used as drugs to combat malaria, as well as in the manufacture of important dyes.

SELF-CHECK

15.5) Give a name to the compound

15.6) In oxazole, the oxygen and nitrogen hetero atoms have a 1,3 relationship in the ring. Isoxazole is an isomer of oxazole in which the oxygen and nitrogen hetero atoms have a 1,2 relationship in the ring. Draw the structural diagram of isoxazole.

CHAPTER FIFTEEN IN REVIEW ■ Aromatic and Heterocyclic Ring Systems

GLOSSARY FOR CHAPTER 15

alkylation Replacement of a hydrogen on an aromatic ring with an alkyl group. (p. 451)

aromatic hydrocarbon Any organic compound that contains the benzene ring system. (p. 442)

benzene The parent aromatic compound,

C_6H_6. (p. 442)

fused ring A molecule in which two (or more) rings share adjacent atoms. (p. 455)

halogenation Replacement of a hydrogen on an aromatic ring with a halogen (F, Cl, Br, I). (p. 451)

hetero atom In a ring, an atom other than carbon. (p. 456)

heterocyclic A compound in which at least one ring contains an atom other than carbon. (p. 456)

Kekulé structure A representation of the structure of benzene; consists of a hexagon with alternating single and double bonds:

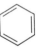

(p. 443)

meta A position on a benzene ring separated by one carbon from a reference position; symbol: *m*. (p. 447)

nitration Replacement of a hydrogen on an aromatic ring with the —NO₂ group. (p. 452)

ortho A position on a benzene ring next to a reference position; symbol: *o*. (p. 447)

para A position on a benzene ring opposite (separated by two carbons from) a reference position; symbol: *p*. (p. 447)

steroid nucleus A fused-ring system that contains three six-membered rings and one five-membered ring. (p. 455)

sulfonation Replacement of a hydrogen on an aromatic ring with the —SO₃H group. (p. 452)

QUESTIONS AND PROBLEMS FOR CHAPTER FIFTEEN ■
Aromatic and Heterocyclic Ring Systems

SECTION 15.1 BENZENE

15.7) How do aromatic hydrocarbons differ from alkenes?

15.8) Draw the two Kekulé structures of benzene.

15.30) Write the symbol most commonly used to represent the benzene ring. Describe what it means in terms of bonding between the carbon atoms.

15.31*) How many isomers are there of the compound

SECTION 15.2 SUBSTITUTED BENZENES

15.9*) When toluene is brominated, three isomeric monobromo products

15.32*) When chlorobenzene is nitrated, three isomeric mononitro

are obtained. One is

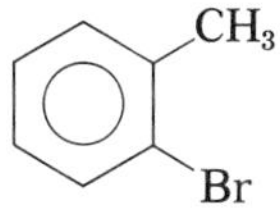

Draw the structural formulas of the other two isomers.

15.10) Name the three products in Question 15.9.

15.11) Name the compounds represented by these three structural formulas:

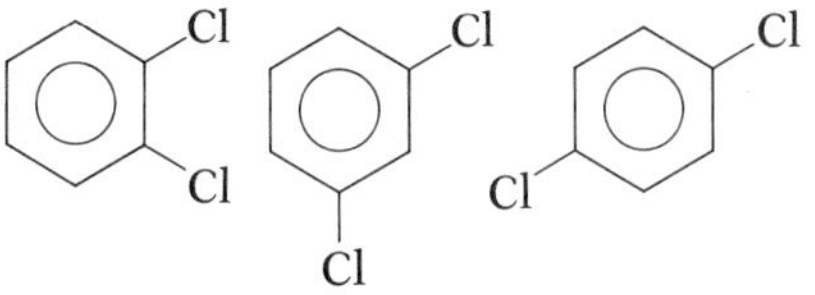

15.12) Draw the structural formula for *p*-nitrotoluene.

15.13) Name the compound represented by the structural formula

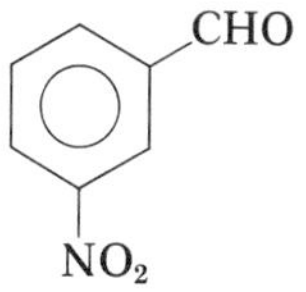

15.14*) Draw the structural formula for *m*-bromostyrene.

15.15*) Name the compound represented by the structural formula $C_6H_5CH_2CH_2CH_2CH_3$.

15.16*) Name the compound represented by the structural formula

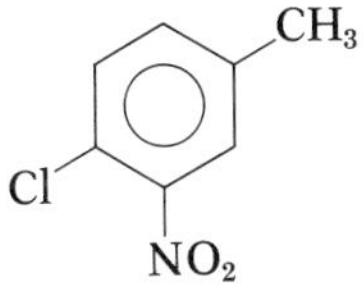

15.17*) Draw the structural formula of the product from the alkylation of benzene with ethyl iodide.

products are obtained. One is

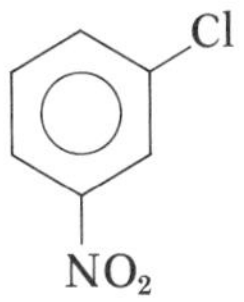

Draw the structural formulas of the other two isomers.

15.33) Name the three products in Question 15.32.

15.34) Name the compounds represented by these three structural formulas:

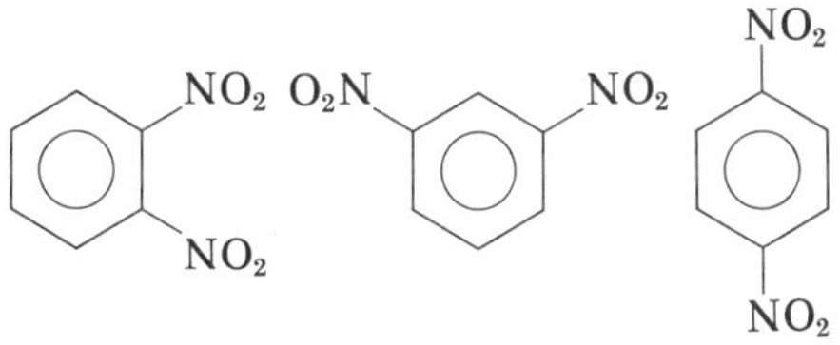

15.35) Draw the structural formula for *o*-bromophenol.

15.36) Name the compound represented by the structural formula

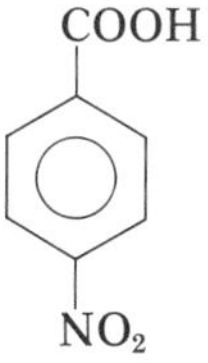

15.37*) Draw the structural formula for *p*-fluorobenzene sulfonic acid.

15.38*) Name the compound represented by the structural formula

$CH_3CH_2CHCH_2CH_2CH_3$

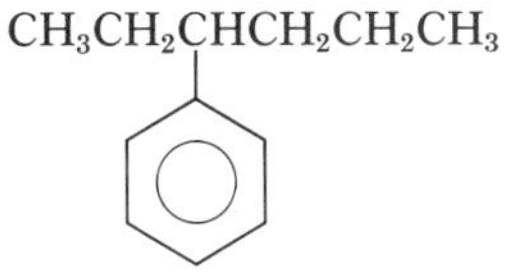

15.39*) Name the compound represented by the structural formula

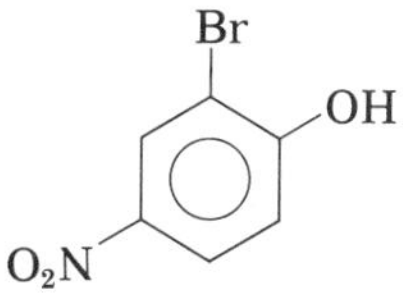

15.40*) Draw the structural formula of the product from the alkylation of benzene with 2-bromopropane.

15.18*) Nitration of toluene gives predominately the *ortho* and *para* isomers. Draw the structural formulas of these products.

15.19*) Sulfonation of 1,3,5-trimethylbenzene gives a monosulfonated product. Draw the structural formula of this product.

15.20*) Chlorination of nitrobenzene occurs predominately at the *meta* position. Draw the structural formula of the major product of chlorination of nitrobenzene.

15.41*) Nitration of 1,3,5-trimethylbenzene gives a mononitro product. Draw the structural formula of this product.

15.42*) Sulfonation of toluene occurs predominately at the *ortho* and *para* positions. Draw the structural formulas of the monosulfonated products of toluene.

15.43*) Bromination of benzene sulfonic acid occurs predominately at the *meta* position. Draw the structural formula of the major product of bromination of benzene sulfonic acid.

SECTION 15.3 FUSED-RING HYDROCARBONS

15.21) Draw the structural formula of a four-membered ring fused to a six-membered ring.

15.22*) Draw the five Kekulé structures for phenanthrene.

15.44) Draw the structural formula of a three-membered ring fused to a five-membered ring.

15.45*) Draw the four Kekulé structures for anthracene.

SECTION 15.4 HETEROCYCLIC RINGS

15.23*) Piperidine is a saturated six-membered heterocyclic ring containing a nitrogen atom. Draw its structural formula.

15.24*) Oxetane is a saturated four-membered ring containing an oxygen atom. Draw its structural formula.

15.25) Is the molecule

a heterocyclic or a carbocyclic compound?

15.26) The structural formula of camphor is

H$_3$C   CH$_3$

CH$_3$ O

Is camphor a heterocyclic or a carbocyclic compound?

15.27*) 1,4-dioxane is a saturated six-membered heterocyclic ring con-

15.46*) Azetidine is a saturated four-membered heterocyclic ring containing a nitrogen atom. Draw its structural formula.

15.47*) Oxirane (ethylene oxide) is a saturated three-membered ring containing an oxygen atom. Draw its structural formula.

15.48) Is the molecule

a heterocyclic or a carbocyclic compound?

15.49) Vitamin B$_1$, thiamine, has the structural formula

NH$_2$

N═C   C—CH$_2$—N$^+$═CCH$_3$ Cl$^-$

CH$_3$C═N   CH   HC   CCH$_2$CH$_2$OH.   S

Are the rings in thiamine heterocyclic or carbocyclic?

15.50*) 1,3-dithiane is a saturated six-membered heterocyclic ring containing two oxygen atoms. Draw its structural formula.

15.28*) Benzofuran, C_8H_6O, is a heterocyclic ring system made by fusing a benzene ring and a furan ring. Draw a possible structural formula for this compound.

15.29*) Draw the structural formula of an isomer of thiazole.

taining two sulfur atoms. Draw its structural formula.

15.51*) Benzothiophene, C_8H_6S, is a heterocyclic ring system made by fusing a benzene ring and a thiophene ring. Draw a possible structural formula for this compound.

15.52*) Draw the structural formula of an isomer of imidazole. What is its name?

Polymers

16

Thus far, all the organic molecules we have examined have been small ones containing only atoms of carbon, hydrogen, oxygen, and other nonmetal elements. Generally, their molecular weights range from 16 (CH_4) to several hundred atomic mass units.

Not all organic molecules, however, are quite so simple. Compounds such as starch and cellulose (Chapter 17) and nucleic acids (Chapter 20) are large, complex, naturally occurring substances. These compounds, called **polymers,** are very large molecules of high molecular weight with a common repeating structural unit that has been formed by the linking together of many small molecules called **monomers.** The process of joining many small molecules together is called **polymerization.**

Nature has been forming polymers for millions of years. Many of these natural polymers will be discussed in later chapters. They are essential to all forms of life. Cellulose is the main component of the cell membranes of plants. The human body contains proteins and nucleic acids (DNA and RNA) that are in our tissues, blood, and skin. Some natural polymers, such as wool, cotton, silk, paper, and rubber, have been used for thousands of years to improve our daily lives.

In this chapter, we will be mainly concerned not with natural polymers, but with *synthetic* organic polymers, which have been developed since about 1930 by the chemical industry. The polymer industry has become a multibillion dollar giant based on products such as polyethylene, polyvinyl chloride (PVC), Teflon, polystyrene, Dacron, nylon, Plexiglas, Orlon, and synthetic rubber. The synthetic polymers often provide superior and economical substitutes for such natural polymers as cotton and wool. They have become part of the daily existence of modern society. It would be difficult for most people to do without these substances. Applications include plastic cups, carpets, plastic food and garbage bags, clothing, phonograph records, nonstick pan coatings, electrical insulation, vinyl car tops, floor tiles, and recording tapes. Our lives would be dramatically changed without these polymer-based products. Our purpose in this chapter is to introduce you to some of the chemistry and technology of polymers. We hope you will obtain an appreciation of the contribution of chemistry to your standard of living and of the widespread role of polymers in your daily life.

> Polymer comes from the Greek *poly* and *meros*, meaning "many parts." It's not uncommon for polymers to have molecular weights of 100 000 to several million.

> A polymer is a molecule made up of a large number of smaller units (monomers) connected by covalent bonds. It is also known as a *macromolecule; macro-*, large, *micro-*, small.

> A larger proportion of industrial chemists work with polymers than with any other type of chemicals.

16.1 MONOMERS AND POLYMERS

LEARNING GOAL 16A: Describe how monomers join together to form homopolymers, block copolymers, and random copolymers.

The monomer units linked together in a polymerization reaction may or may not be identical. If only one monomer is used, the result from the polymerization process is called a **homopolymer.** All of the repeating structural units are identical:

All the monomer units [A] in a polymer are joined by covalent bonds.

$$A + A + A + A + A + ... \xrightarrow{\text{polymerization}} -A - A - A - A - A -$$

monomers of substance A   a homopolymer

If two different monomers are linked together, we obtain a **copolymer.** The two monomer substances, [A] and [B], may alternate in some systematic pattern with each other in the polymer. If large blocks of each monomer are back to back in the repeating unit, we obtain a **block copolymer:**

$$A \quad + \quad B \quad \longrightarrow$$

monomer   monomer

$$-A-A-A-A-A-A-B-B-B-B-B-A-A-A-A-A-A-B-B-B-B-B-$$

block copolymer

On the other hand, the monomers [A] and [B] may link together in a random manner with no definite pattern of monomer units. Polymers of this kind are called **random copolymers:**

A copolymer may have useful properties that are often superior to the properties of the homopolymer from [A] or [B].

$$A \quad + \quad B \quad \longrightarrow$$

monomer   monomer

$$-A-A-B-A-B-B-B-A-A-B-A-B-A-A-A-A-B-A-B-$$

random copolymer

Block copolymers and random copolymers have different physical properties. The properties of the copolymer will also be determined by the ratio of [A] to [B].

SELF-CHECK

16.1) Give an example of a copolymer prepared from monomer [A] and monomer [B] that is
a) a block copolymer with alternating groups of six [A] monomers and 3 [B] monomers
b) a random copolymer
c) a homopolymer

16.2 ADDITION POLYMERS

LEARNING GOAL 16B: Describe the three steps involved in any addition polymerization reaction.
16C: Give three examples of commercially important addition polymers.

There are two very important types of reactions used by the chemical industry to make polymers: addition reactions and condensation reactions. We will consider addition reactions first because they are more easily understood. In addition polymerization reactions, (a) the monomer units simply link together, (b) there are no reaction products other than the polymer itself, and (c) the addition polymer has the same weight per cent of each element as the monomer.

Most **addition polymers** are formed from monomer molecules containing carbon-carbon double bonds, the alkenes or alkene derivatives (Section 7.2). The most important such monomer is ethene (ethylene), which is sixth in importance among all commercial chemicals because of its use in the manufacture of *polyethylene*. All addition polymerization reactions include the following steps:

$$\text{Initiation} \longrightarrow \text{propagation} \longrightarrow \text{termination}$$

or the start, continuation, and ending of the polymer chain. We will look at each process in turn.

Initiation

Ethene left by itself will remain ethene, a stable molecule. We must start the polymerization process by *breaking the double bond* in the molecule. This can be accomplished in some cases by heat. For example, when ethene is heated under pressure in the presence of oxygen, polymers with formula weight of about 30 000 amu are formed. High-energy light (x-ray, ultraviolet) may also do the trick. However, the chemist prefers to have more control over the polymerization process.

The addition is therefore usually initiated by certain unstable chemicals, such as organic peroxides, that easily break apart into pieces with *unpaired electrons*. For example, benzoyl peroxide splits into two identical pieces, each of which is a *free radical:*

$\cdot CH_3$ is the methyl radical.

is the phenyl radical. Cl$\cdot$ would be a chlorine radical, a single gaseous chlorine atom.

benzoyl peroxide   (a free radical, R·)

Because a free radical contains an unpaired electron, it is extremely quick to react. It tries to find a "friend" for its unpaired electron and in the process creates *another* free radical. The polymerization process has begun. If the free radical R· hits ethene, we obtain

$$R\cdot + CH_2{=}CH_2 \longrightarrow R{-}CH_2{-}CH_2\cdot$$

reactive site

another free radical

On the other hand, if ethene is heated, it can create its own free radical through the breaking of the double bond:

reactive site

Each *reactive site* has an unpaired electron.

Propagation

The polymer grows as each free radical reacts with another ethene molecule, until a long hydrocarbon chain is formed:

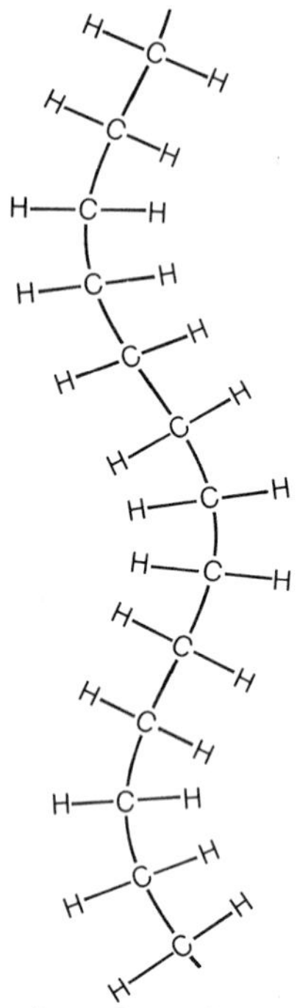

A portion of a polyethylene polymer. Ethylene is unsaturated; polyethylene is saturated.

$$R—CH_2—CH_2· + CH_2{=}CH_2 \longrightarrow R—CH_2—CH_2—CH_2—CH_2·$$

This addition is followed by

$$R—CH_2—CH_2—CH_2—CH_2· + \overset{·}{C}H_2{=}CH_2 \longrightarrow$$
$$R—CH_2—CH_2—CH_2—CH_2—CH_2—CH_2·$$

This process continues by adding one monomer unit ($H_2C{=}CH_2$) at each step until there are thousands of carbon atoms in the chain. Note that the carbons are connected to each other by *single* covalent bonds. We are actually creating a "polyalkane," a continuous-chain saturated hydrocarbon with thousands of —CH_2— units.

Termination

In theory, the polymer chain could grow indefinitely. In reality, this does not happen. Some time after the chain has begun to form, the chain growth is interrupted and the polymerization reaction stops or is *terminated*. An impurity may react with the active site or two growing chains may meet:

$$R—CH_2—(CH_2)_n—CH_2· + ·CH_2—(CH_2)_m—CH_2—R \longrightarrow$$

growing chain   growing chain

$$R—CH_2—(CH_2)_p—CH_2—R$$

terminated polymer

The letters n, m, and p represent numbers in the thousands. We end up with a polyethylene polymer. This process is called *coupling*, akin to joining (coupling) two railroad cars together.

The initiator free radicals R· or specific reagents, called *chain transfer agents*, may also terminate the chain.

Types of addition polymers

Initiation, propagation, and termination are present in all addition polymerization reactions. In many cases, the reactions may be more complex than those just outlined. Physical properties can be varied by chain *branching*. The continuous-chain or "linear" polyethylene molecules produce a tough plastic that is useful in making toys, bottles, and other items. Branched-chain polyethylene is less dense and more flexible; it is often used for squeeze bottles.

There are many ethene derivatives, created by replacing one or more of the four hydrogen atoms in $H_2C{=}CH_2$ with other groups. Table 16–1 shows some of the more common polymers produced by this group of monomers through addition polymerization.

Remember that the addition polymer chains we have been discussing consist of singly bonded carbon atoms. The geometry around each carbon atom is tetrahedral, so the chain actually follows a zigzag path, as shown in Figure 16–1. Addition polymers formed from ethene derivatives, such as styrene, can link together in any of three possible ways. The monomer $H_2C{=}CHR$ can form a head-to-head and tail-to-tail polymer:

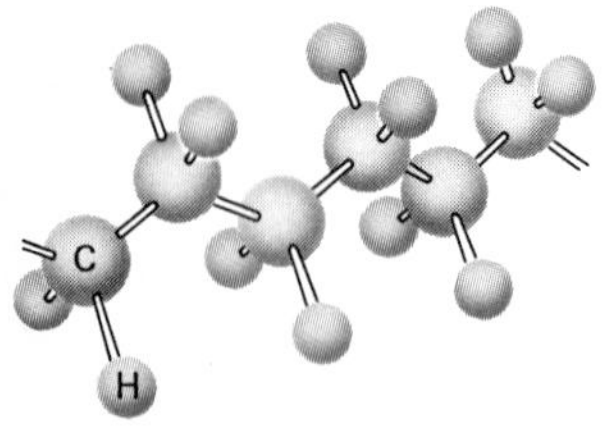

head-to-head   tail-to-tail

FIGURE 16–1 In polyethylene the carbon chain is zigzag. This gives a flexible, elastic polymer.

$$CH_2{=}CH + CH{=}CH_2 + CH_2{=}CH \longrightarrow —CH_2CHCHCH_2CH_2CH—$$
$$\quad\ | \qquad\qquad | \qquad\qquad\quad | \qquad\qquad\qquad\quad |\ \ | \qquad\qquad |$$
$$\quad\ R \qquad\qquad R \qquad\qquad\quad R \qquad\qquad\qquad\ R\ \ R \qquad\qquad R$$

TABLE 16–1 SOME COMMON ADDITION POLYMERS

Monomer	Monomer Formula	Polymer Unit	Trade Name	Common Uses
Ethylene	$H_2C{=}CH_2$	(–CH₂–CH₂–)ₙ chain of carbons each bearing H, H	Polyethylene	Molded toys and utensils, plastic bags and films
Propylene	$H_2C{=}CHCH_3$	chain of carbons bearing H and CH_3	Polypropylene, Herculon	Molded containers, indoor-outdoor carpeting, auto interior parts
Vinyl chloride	$H_2C{=}CHCl$	chain of carbons bearing H and Cl	PVC, polyvinyl chloride	Vinyl floor tiles, phonograph records, plastic garden hoses, car tops
Vinylidene chloride	$H_2C{=}CCl_2$	chain of carbons bearing Cl and Cl	Saran	Plastic food wrap
Acrylonitrile	$H_2C{=}CHC{\equiv}N$	chain of carbons bearing H and CN	Acrilan, Orlon, Dynel	Rugs and fabrics
Tetrafluoroethylene	$F_2C{=}CF_2$	chain of carbons bearing F, F	Teflon	Artificial body parts, non-stick coatings
Methylmethacrylate	$H_2C{=}\underset{\underset{\displaystyle CH_3}{\textstyle\vert}}{C}{-}\overset{\displaystyle O}{\overset{\|}{C}}{-}OCH_3$	chain of carbons bearing CH_3 and CO_2CH_3	Plexiglas, Lucite, Perspex	Car and airplane windows, latex paints, plastic combs and brushes
Styrene	$H_2C{=}CH{-}\text{C}_6\text{H}_5$	chain of carbons bearing H and phenyl group	Styrofoam, polystyrene	Food and drink coolers, building insulation, toys
Chloroprene	$H_2C{=}\underset{\underset{\displaystyle Cl}{\textstyle\vert}}{C}{-}CH{=}CH_2$	chain of carbons bearing H, Cl, –CH=	Neoprene	Synthetic rubber products, automobile tires

or a head-to-tail polymer as illustrated in Table 16–1 (most common):

tail head head tail

$$\underset{\displaystyle R}{CH_2{=}CH} + \underset{\displaystyle R}{CH_2{=}CH} + \underset{\displaystyle R}{CH_2{=}CH} \longrightarrow -CH_2\underset{\displaystyle R}{CH}CH_2\underset{\displaystyle R}{CH}CH_2\underset{\displaystyle R}{CH}-$$

or a random addition polymer with no regular pattern:

$$\underset{\displaystyle R}{CH_2{=}CH} + \underset{\displaystyle R}{CH}{=}CH_2 + \underset{\displaystyle R}{CH}{=}CH_2 + \underset{\displaystyle R}{CH_2{=}CH} \longrightarrow -CH_2\underset{\displaystyle R}{CH}\underset{\displaystyle R}{CH}CH_2\underset{\displaystyle R}{CH}CH_2CH_2\underset{\displaystyle R}{CH}-$$

Shorthand for writing polymer formulas

The polymerization reactions we have looked at are a bit unwieldly to write out. Chemists have a shorthand way of writing the structural formula for a polymer molecule and the equation for a polymerization reaction. The monomer is shown on the left-hand (reactants) side of the equation. On the right-hand (products) side, the repeating polymer unit is enclosed in brackets, and lines pass *through* the brackets to show that the chain continues in both directions. The subscript n shows how many times the repeating unit appears in the full polymer; generally the value of n is in the thousands.

$$\underset{\text{monomer}}{n\ H_2C{=}CHR} \longrightarrow \underset{\text{polymer}}{\left[CH_2-\underset{\displaystyle R}{CH} \right]_n}$$

Note that the monomer contains a double bond and the polymer does not. The electrons of the monomer pi bond have moved and are used to link one monomer unit to another by sigma bonds (Section 6.2) as indicated by the extended lines in the abbreviated polymer formula. The backbone of the polymer consists of the carbon atoms that originally formed the double bonds. Nothing is added; nothing is lost. The monomers are simply added together, in accord with our description of an *addition* polymer.

Giulio Natta of Italy and Karl Ziegler of Germany have devised catalysts for many addition polymerizations. They received the Nobel Prize in 1963 for this important work. One original catalyst was a mixture of aluminum triethyl and titanium tetrachloride.

Polypropylene is an addition polymer obtained by polymerization in the presence of a catalyst. This highly ordered polymer has a high melting point for a plastic (165 to 170°C), is very strong, and is easily converted to molded objects and fibers:

$$\underset{\substack{\text{propylene}\\ \text{(propene)}}}{n\ CH_3CH{=}CH_2} \xrightarrow{\text{catalyst}} \underset{\text{polypropylene}}{\left[\overset{\displaystyle CH_3}{CH}-CH_2 \right]_n}$$

Another important addition polymer is polytetrafluoroethylene (Teflon). This polymer is stable over a wide temperature range, is chemically unreactive, and slides very easily:

$$\underset{\text{tetrafluoroethylene}}{n\ CF_2{=}CF_2} \xrightarrow{\text{catalyst}} \underset{\text{Teflon}}{\left[CF_2-CF_2 \right]_n}$$

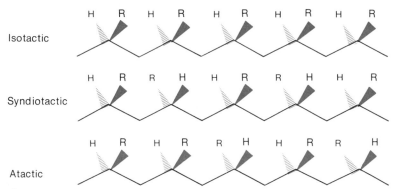

Isotactic

Syndiotactic

Atactic

FIGURE 16–2 Three possible structures for addition polymers of the head-to-tail type. The solid black line represents a carbon chain. The solid color wedge extends *toward* you, while the broken wedge is going away from you into the book. Depending on reaction conditions, the polymer obtained may have any of the three orientations shown.

Three-dimensional structure of addition polymers

When a substituted ethylene derivative ($H_2C\!\!=\!\!CHR$) is polymerized, the monomer units usually link in a head-to-tail fashion. There are three different ways that the R group ($-CH_3$, $-Cl$, $-CN$, $-COOCH_3$) can be joined to the chain in relation to the backbone of the polymer (Figure 16–2). In the first structure, called *isotactic,* all the R groups are in identical positions along the polymer chain. When the R groups extend in alternate directions away from the chain, a *syndiotactic* arrangement results. When there is a random arrangement of the R groups along the backbone of the polymer chain, an *atactic* arrangement results. Most free-radical-initiated polymerizations give atactic polymers. If a catalyst is used, the polymerizations can be controlled to give either isotactic or syndiotactic polymers. For polypropylene, all three types have been synthesized (Figure 16–3).

Atactic is from the Greek, *ataktos,* without order.

FIGURE 16–3 (*a*) Isotactic polypropylene. The bulky methyl groups are close to each other in this arrangement. (*b*) To eliminate crowding of the methyl groups on one side of the polymer chain, the chain flexes to produce a helical arrangement.

Interfering methyl groups

(a)

(b)

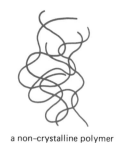

a non–crystalline polymer

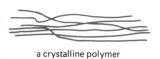

a crystalline polymer

The chemical composition of a polymer chain is called its **primary structure.** All three types of polypropylene have the same primary structure. How the chain is oriented in relation to itself and other chains is called the **secondary structure** of the polymer. The polymer chains can be a tangled mass of chains like a bowl of spaghetti. Such polymers usually are soft and rubbery. They are of limited practical use. Atactic polypropylene is of this type. The atactic polypropylene chains cannot approach each other closely because of the randomness of the methyl groups. There is little order to the polymer chain, and the polymer is considered "noncrystalline." On the other hand, the polymer may have continuous chains held together by hydrogen-bonding or other dipole-dipole attractions. Such polymers have much more order and are called "crystalline." Syndiotactic and isotactic polypropylene are more "crystalline" than atactic polypropylene. The chains can get close to each other. The polymer melts at 170°C and can be easily formed into fibers. As you can see, the secondary structure of a polymer is of great importance in determining its properties.

SELF-CHECK

16.2)   Vinyl chloride ($H_2C{=}CHCl$) forms the addition polymer polyvinyl chloride. Outline the three steps in the free-radical polymerization of vinyl chloride to form PVC.

16.3*)   The presence of too much peroxide initiator can cause an addition polymerization reaction to stop prematurely. Explain.

16.4)   Give three examples of alkene derivatives that form addition polymers useful in everyday life.

16.3 CONDENSATION POLYMERS

LEARNING GOAL 16D: Give two examples of condensation polymers.

To form a **condensation polymer,** two monomers are joined (condensed) together and a small molecule, such as water or alcohol, is split out (eliminated). Usually two different monomers are condensed; thus condensation polymers are really copolymers.

To give a high-molecular-weight molecule, the condensation reaction must occur over and over again. Thus *each monomer* used in a condensation polymerization requires *two functional groups* that can enter into the reaction that builds the polymer chain. Condensation polymerizations do not require the presence of carbon-carbon double bonds.

Polyesters

Most of the chemical reactions used in forming condensation polymers are simple reactions that form functional groups, such as esterification (Section 9.5):

$$R{-}O{-}\boxed{H + H{-}O}{-}\overset{\displaystyle O}{\overset{\displaystyle \|}{C}}{-}R' \longrightarrow R{-}O{-}\overset{\displaystyle O}{\overset{\displaystyle \|}{C}}{-}R' + H_2O$$

elimination of water

alcohol   acid   ester   water

In the formation of the ester, two organic functional groups are condensed into one and a molecule of water is eliminated. This is exactly what happens when a **polyester** is formed. The only difference is that the product of the first condensation is capable of additional condensations. It still contains the necessary functional groups for further reaction.

> The repeating unit in a polyester contains the ester functional group.

Dacron is a polyester formed from an aromatic dicarboxylic acid and a diol. One monomer has two —COOH groups, the other has two —OH groups:

terephthalic acid   ethylene glycol   ester   water

In the initial condensation reaction, an ester is formed and a molecule of water is split out. The product of this initial reaction still has a reactive group at each end of the molecule. At one end there is a carboxyl group (—COOH), which can react with a diol molecule. At the other end is a hydroxyl group (—OH), which can react with another dicarboxylic acid molecule. Thus, further reaction is possible. This process continues until we obtain a large polymer molecule containing many ester groups:

Dacron

Mylar film is used in recording and computer tapes.

Dacron fiber, also called Terylene or Teron, can be ironed into permanent creases. It finds widespread commercial use in combination with other fibers in wash-and-wear fabrics. When made into a thin film, called Mylar, it is used to make magnetic recording tapes.

> Most wash-and-wear clothing is made from a blend of Dacron and cotton.

Polyamides

When a carboxylic acid and an amine are condensed, a molecule of water is split out and a new functional group, an *amide*, is formed (Section 13.4):

carboxylic acid   amine   amide   water

If a dicarboxylic acid is condensed with a diamine, a **polyamide** can be formed. *Nylons* are the best known polyamides, initially developed during World War II as substitutes for silk. Different types of nylons are distinguished by the use of numbers, which refer to *the number of carbon atoms* in the monomer(s) used. For *Nylon 66*, hexamethylenediamine is condensed

> The repeating unit in a polyamide contains the
>
> (amide) functional group.
>
> Nylon 66 is the nylon used in women's hosiery.

with adipic acid. The initial condensation product is an amide, which still contains reactive amine and acid groups:

$$HO-\overset{\overset{O}{\|}}{C}-(CH_2)_4-\overset{\overset{O}{\|}}{C}-OH \quad + H_2N-(CH_2)_6-NH_2 \longrightarrow \quad HO-\overset{\overset{O}{\|}}{C}(CH_2)_4\overset{\overset{O}{\|}}{C}-\overset{\overset{H}{|}}{N}(CH_2)_6\overset{\overset{H}{|}}{N}-H$$

reactive ends

adipic acid   hexamethylenediamine   amide

Further reaction of this initial product with more diamine and diacid molecules gives the polyamide:

$$-\overset{\overset{O}{\|}}{C}-(CH_2)_4\left[\overset{\overset{O}{\|}}{C}-\overset{\overset{}{\underset{\overset{|}{H}}{N}}}\right](CH_2)_6\left[\overset{}{\underset{\overset{|}{H}}{N}}-\overset{\overset{O}{\|}}{C}\right](CH_2)_4\left[\overset{\overset{O}{\|}}{C}-\overset{}{\underset{\overset{|}{H}}{N}}\right](CH_2)_6-$$

Nylon 66

(amide groups boxed for emphasis)

Nylon was the first commercial fiber to be a huge economic success. This spurred the chemical industry to spend more money on polymer research. Since the discovery of nylon in 1935, the polymer industry has grown faster than any other segment of the chemical industry. Nylon fibers are widely used in carpets and, more recently, in water desalination units (Section 12.4).

Nylon 6 is prepared from caprolactam, which comes from aminocaproic acid. The monomer contains an amine group on one end of the molecule and an acid group on the other end. Each time two molecules condense, the resulting condensation product again contains an amino group and an acid group:

$$H_2N-(CH_2)_5-\overset{\overset{O}{\|}}{C}-OH \xrightarrow{-H_2O} (CH_2)_5\begin{array}{c}N-H\\ |\\ C=O\end{array} \xrightarrow{\text{polymerization}} -\overset{\overset{H}{|}}{N}-(CH_2)_5-\overset{\overset{O}{\|}}{C}-\overset{\overset{H}{|}}{N}-(CH_2)_5-\overset{\overset{O}{\|}}{C}-$$

aminocaproic acid   caprolactam   portion of nylon 6
                      (an intermediate)

Hydrogen-bonding is also of great importance in proteins, which are also polyamides (Chapter 19).

The condensation reaction can repeat many, many times.

Because of their ability to form hydrogen-bonds between the polymer chains (Figure 16–4), nylons show unusually high strength and make excellent fibers.

The carbohydrates starch and cellulose (Section 17.5) are condensation polymers formed by loss of water between sugar molecules. Their molecular weights range from 50 000 to 100 million amu. Similarly, proteins (Section 19.2) are the result of condensation polymerization of amino acids. Loss of water gives the peptide (amide) group, the repeating functional group in proteins:

$$2 \text{ R}-\overset{}{\underset{\overset{|}{NH_2}}{CH}}-\overset{\overset{O}{\|}}{C}-OH \longrightarrow \text{R}-\overset{}{\underset{\overset{|}{NH_2}}{CH}}-\overset{\overset{O}{\|}}{C}-\overset{\overset{H}{|}}{N}-\overset{}{\underset{\overset{|}{R}}{CH}}-\overset{\overset{O}{\|}}{C}-OH \longrightarrow \begin{array}{l}\text{protein}\\ \text{polymer}\end{array}$$

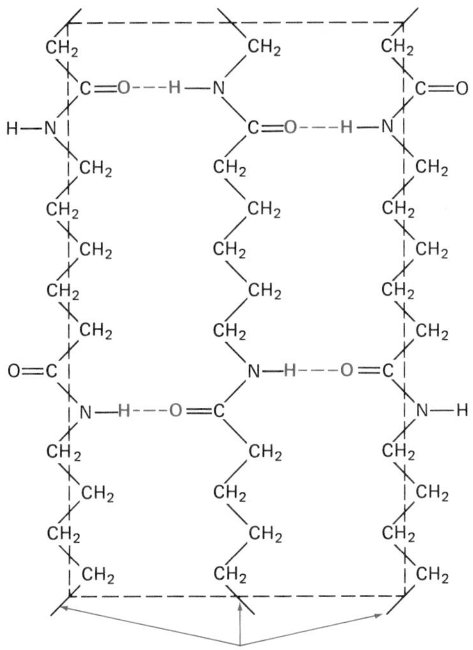

FIGURE 16–4   Structure and hydrogen-bonding in Nylon 6.

Animal and vegetable fats (Section 18.1) are triesters formed by condensation between fatty acids and a triol, glycerine.

SELF-CHECK

16.5)   What general principle governs whether two monomers can produce a condensation polymer?

16.4 CROSS-LINKED POLYMERS

LEARNING GOAL 16E: Give an example of a cross-linked polymer.

In simple polyesters and polyamides, the polymer chains are long continuous molecules without linkages (other than hydrogen-bonds) connecting the individual strands of the polymers. In some condensation polymers, however, covalent bond formation may occur *between* the polymer chains. These connections between the chains are called "cross-links" and the result is a **cross-linked polymer**. Cross-linking is shown in Figure 16–5.

An example of such cross-linking occurs when phthalic acid (a diacid) is copolymerized with glycerol (a triol). The third hydroxyl group is available to form a connection (cross-link) between the individual strands of the polymer chains:

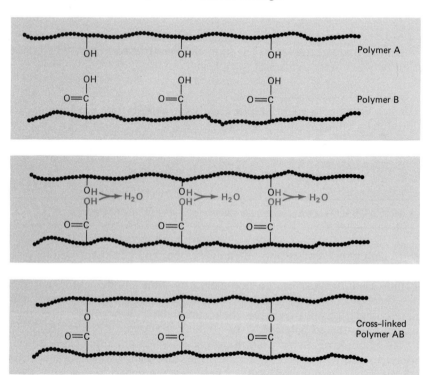

Glyptal, a cross-linked polymer

Polyester polymers with cross-links are called *alkyd resins*. Usually, cross-linked polymers are rigid, insoluble materials that do not soften when heated. They are hard and tough. When heated to melting, polymers of this type undergo a permanent change and set to a solid that cannot be remelted. They are called **thermosetting polymers.** On the other hand, polymers such as polyethylene and nylon can be softened on heating, molded into almost any shape, drawn out into fibers, and made into films. Polymers of this type, such as polystyrene, are called **thermoplastic polymers.** They can be remelted and reformed many times without change.

FIGURE 16–5   Cross-linking of two polymer chains.

The resin Bakelite is a cross-linked copolymer of phenol and formaldehyde. In the initial stage of polymerization, phenol condenses with formaldehyde to give a "phenol alcohol." Further condensation of the phenol alcohol with more phenol and formaldehyde gives the cross-linked polymer:

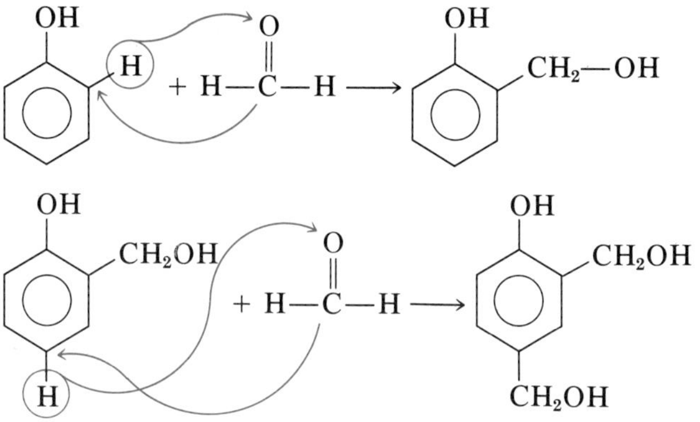

"phenol alcohol"

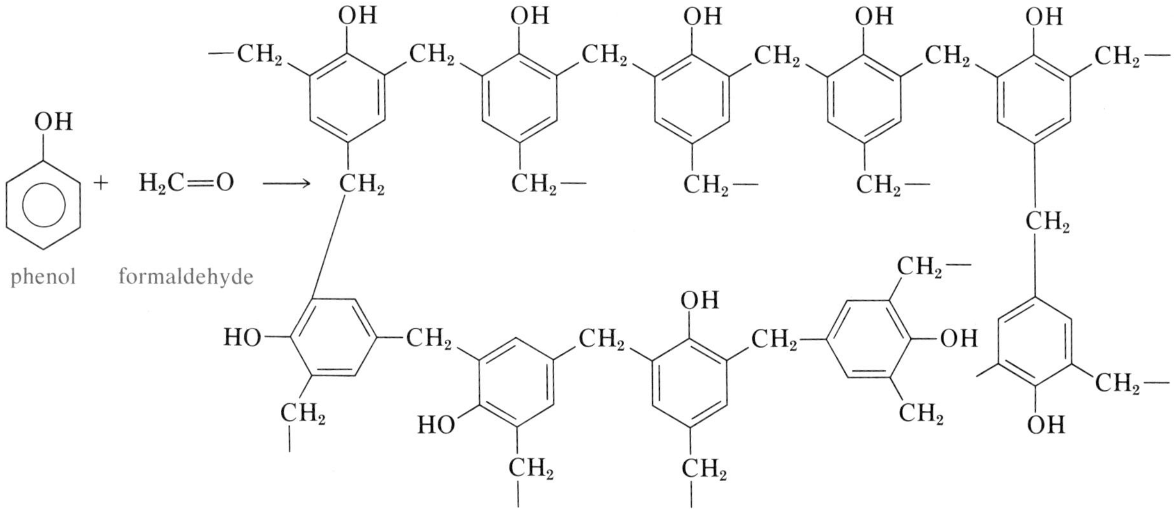

phenol   formaldehyde

Bakelite

Table 16–2 gives some examples of cross-linked polymers.

SELF-CHECK

16.6*) The first step in the preparation of a urea-formaldehyde polymer (Table 16–2) is the formation of an "amino alcohol." Suggest a structural formula for this "amino alcohol" intermediate.

16.5 ELASTOMERS

LEARNING GOAL 16F: Give an example of a synthetic elastomer.

Natural rubber is an *elastic* polymer. It stretches when a pull (tension) is applied and contracts when the tension is removed. Polymers that exhibit such elasticity are called **elastomers.** Natural rubber is made from the

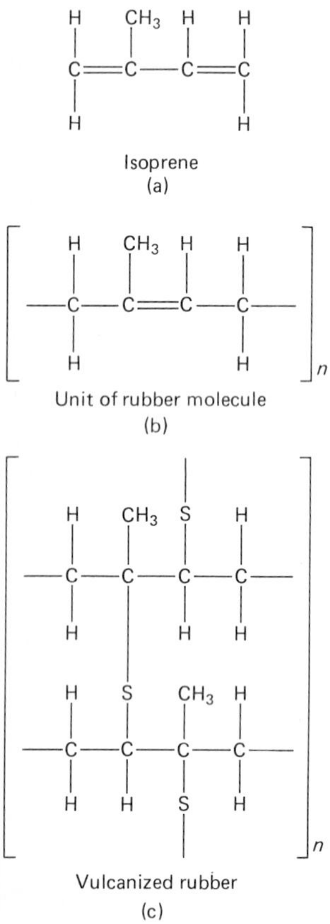

Isoprene
(a)

Unit of rubber molecule
(b)

Vulcanized rubber
(c)

FIGURE 16–6 The structural unit of natural rubber is isoprene (a). When thousands of these units are linked together, they form natural rubber (b). Vulcanization results in a cross-linked structure (c).

TABLE 16–2 SOME TYPICAL CROSS-LINKED POLYMERS

Monomers	Polymer Name	Uses
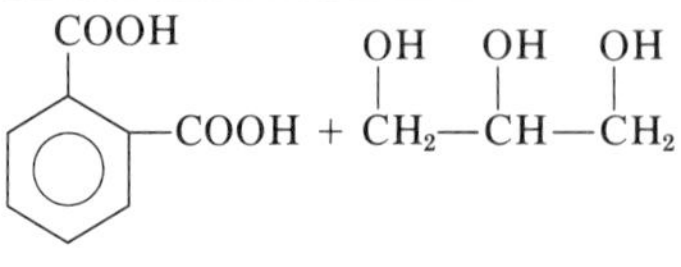 phthalic acid + glycerol	Glyptal	Molded plastic articles, alkyd paints
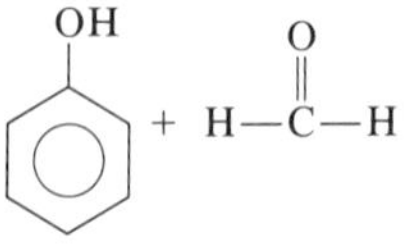 phenol + formaldehyde	Phenol-formaldehyde resin, Formica, Bakelite	Table tops, wall panels, handles, dials
urea + formaldehyde	Urea-formaldehyde resin	Translucent light panels, adhesives, enamels
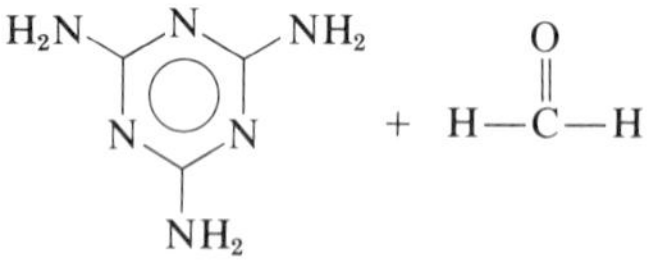 melamine + formaldehyde	Melamine-formaldehyde resin, Melmac	Dishes, buttons

monomer *isoprene* (Figure 16–6). It is found in the *latex* (an emulsion of sap particles in water) of the rubber trees of Southeast Asia.

Natural rubber is an addition polymer. It differs from those of Section 16.2 in one important respect. When isoprene polymerizes, its double bonds open up to form a long-chain addition polymer:

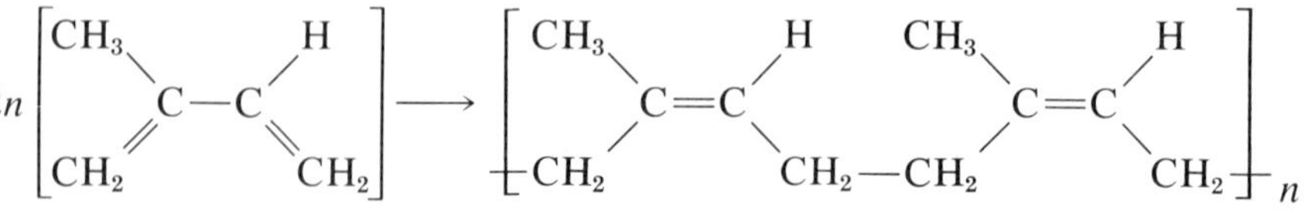

isoprene → natural rubber (poly-*cis*-isoprene)

However, there are double bonds left in the natural rubber. Polymerization reduces the number of double bonds but does not remove them all.

In the late 1930's, Charles Goodyear discovered that if he took the gummy, sticky mass of natural rubber obtained from latex and heated it with sulfur, he got a flexible, elastic, water-repellent material. This discovery was the start of the rubber industry. The process of heating with sulfur cross-links the polymer strands of rubber and removes some of the unsaturation (Figure 16–6). Cross-linking of rubber with sulfur is called *vulcanization*. The sulfur cross-links line up the long-chain molecules, so that when the rubber is stretched, it tends to spring or pull back the strands to their original position when the tension is removed (Figure 16–7). Rubber bands provide a common example of this type of elasticity.

One type of synthetic rubber is made by copolymerization of butadiene (H_2C=CH—CH=CH_2) with styrene. Typically, the monomers are mixed in a ratio of one mole of styrene to three moles of butadiene:

In natural rubber, the monomer units are arranged head-to-tail and all the —CH$_2$—groups are in the cis arrangement in relation to the double bond.

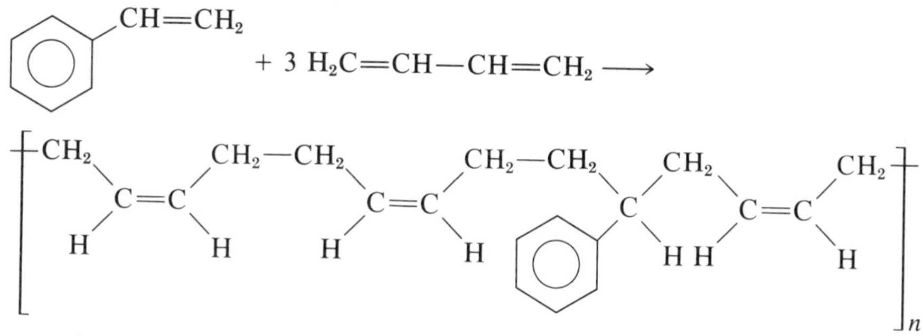

$$CH = CH_2$$
$$+ 3 H_2C = CH - CH = CH_2 \longrightarrow$$

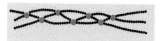

Polymer chains

Sulfur cross-link

a. Before stretching

b. Stretched

FIGURE 16-7   Stretched vulcanized rubber retains its elasticity.

butadiene unit   butadiene unit   styrene unit   butadiene unit

This copolymer is known as SBR (styrene-butadiene rubber) and accounts for over 50% of the total production of synthetic rubber. It is mainly used in making automobile tires.

Another synthetic elastomer, called Neoprene, was developed in the DuPont laboratories in the early 1930's. It is made by polymerizing chloroprene ($H_2C = CH - CCl = CH_2$):

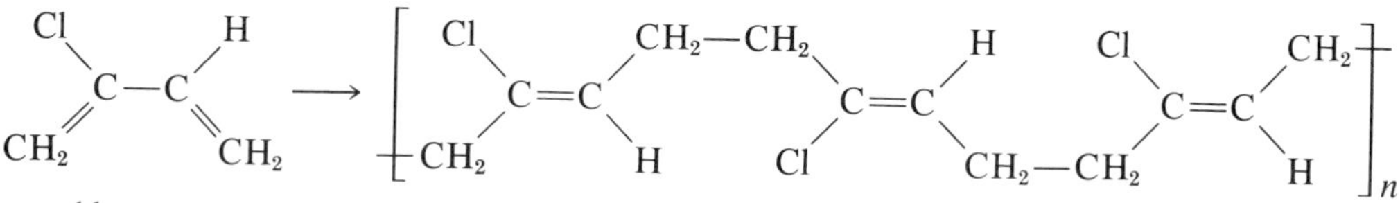

chloroprene   Neoprene

Neoprene is more resistant than natural rubber to attack by solvents, so it is used in such applications as gaskets and gasoline fuel lines.

From our discussions of addition and condensation polymers and elastomers, you can see that both the primary and secondary structure of the polymer play important roles in the properties of the plastic or synthetic fiber. Thus, a synthetic polymer chemist, by varying these factors, can potentially make a polymer with almost any desired properties. In a short 50 years, polymer chemistry has come a long way. The future will undoubtedly give us many new and exciting giant molecules of benefit to society.

Chloroprene (2-chloro-1,3-butadiene) is similar to isoprene, differing only in the chlorine at the 2 position.

Neoprene is more expensive than natural rubber and so is not used in automobile tires.

16.7*) Butadiene ($H_2C = CH - CH = CH_2$) can be polymerized to form a homopolymer that has properties similar to those of natural rubber. Sketch a portion of the butadiene polymer (include three monomer units).

SELF-CHECK

16.6 PLASTICIZERS

LEARNING GOAL 16G: Describe the use of a plasticizer.

Many addition polymers are hard and brittle and may be too stiff for certain applications. Chemists have found that these polymers can be made softer and more flexible by the addition of chemicals called **plasticizers**. Depending on the type of plastic, plasticizers may make up 30 to 50 per cent of the weight of the plastic. They are used in a variety of products ranging from

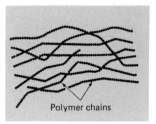

Di-(2-ethylhexyl)phthalate (DOP), a typical plasticizer.

blood-storage bags to construction products. Over one billion pounds of these chemicals are used annually in the United States.

The attractive forces between polymer strands give rigidity to the polymer. Plasticizers fit into these spaces between polymer strands. They reduce some of the attractive forces and increase the flexibility of the macromolecule (Figure 16–8).

The most common type of plasticizer is an ester of a diacid, such as phthalic acid. Plasticizers are usually lost from the polymer by evaporation. Thus, many plastics become brittle and crack with age.

Recent studies have shown that these substances find their way into our environment. Probably of all the chemicals developed by scientists, none is more widely dispersed in the environment than plasticizers. They have been found in the water we drink, the food we eat, and the air we breathe.

The use of plasticizers must be carefully controlled when polymer materials are used in medical applications. Plastic tubing is used in medicine for adding solutions to the blood by intravenous infusions. Liquids passing through such tubing can become contaminated with the plasticizers. In one case, kidney patients connected by plastic tubing to a dialysis machine became nauseated while patients connected to similar machines without plastic tubing were unaffected. The problem was finally traced to the plasticizers in the tubing, which were being washed out and were finding their way into the patient's blood stream. Similarly, it was found that human blood stored for three weeks in polyvinyl chloride plastic bags was contaminated with 5 to 7 milligrams of DOP plasticizer. Patients given transfusions of blood from these plastic bags showed significant amounts of DOP in the spleen, liver, lung, and abdominal fat. No DOP was found in the blood of patients who had not received the transfusions.

It should be emphasized that, as yet, plasticizers have not been proven to be the cause of any disease. However, the widespread use of these substances in large amounts does give some concern that risks do exist, and their effects might not appear until many years later after millions of people have been exposed to them. Much additional work needs to be done to determine the effects of plasticizers and to see if these substances aggravate illnesses in the body.

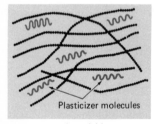

Polymer chains

Rigid

Plasticizer molecules

Less rigid

FIGURE 16–8 How a plasticizer works.

SELF-CHECK

16.8) The plastic material used in covering outdoor lawn furniture becomes brittle after a few years and begins to crack. Explain.

CHAPTER SIXTEEN IN REVIEW ■ Polymers

16.3 CONDENSATION POLYMERS   Page 474

    16D: Give two examples of condensation polymers.

16.4 CROSS-LINKED POLYMERS   Page 477

    16E: Give an example of a cross-linked polymer.

16.5 ELASTOMERS   Page 479

    16F: Give an example of a synthetic elastomer.

16.6 PLASTICIZERS   Page 481

    16G: Describe the use of a plasticizer.

GLOSSARY FOR CHAPTER 16

addition polymer A large molecule (polymer) formed by the continuing addition of an unsaturated compound to the growing end of the chain. (p. 469)

block copolymer A copolymer in which the monomer units alternate in some definite (systematic) pattern. (p. 468)

condensation polymer A copolymer in which the repeating unit is made by the removal of a small molecule (usually H_2O) by reaction of functional groups from two monomers. (p. 474)

copolymer A polymer prepared from two or more different monomers. (p. 468)

cross-linked polymer A polymer in which there are connections between the individual strands of a network. (p. 477)

elastomer A polymer that shows flexibility and elasticity, such as rubber. (p. 479)

homopolymer A polymer prepared from only one monomer; it contains a single repeating unit in the polymer chain. (p. 468)

monomer A small molecule used as a reactant to make polymers. (p. 467)

plasticizer An additive that makes a polymer soft and flexible. (p. 481)

polyamide A condensation polymer that contains an amide group in the repeating unit, as a result of the elimination of water. (p. 475)

polyester A condensation polymer that contains an ester group in the repeating unit as a result of the elimination of water. (p. 475)

polymer A large molecule made up of small, generally repeating units; a *macromolecule* with weight in the thousands of amu. (p. 467)

polymerization A chemical reaction used to make polymers from monomers. (p. 467)

primary structure The chemical composition of a polymer chain. (p. 474)

random copolymer A copolymer in which the monomer units are not joined in a definite pattern. (p. 468)

secondary structure The orientation of a polymer chain with respect to itself and to other chains. (p. 474)

thermoplastic polymer A polymer that can be softened by heating and then molded, drawn, or made into films; it can be remelted without any permanent change. (p. 478)

thermosetting polymer A polymer that undergoes a permanent change when heated to its melting point; it cannot be remelted. (p. 478)

QUESTIONS AND PROBLEMS FOR CHAPTER SIXTEEN ▪ Polymers

SECTION 16.1 MONOMERS AND POLYMERS

16.9) Draw a block copolymer that has alternating units of three parts [A] and two parts [B].

16.26) Draw a unit of a homopolymer of ethylene.

SECTION 16.2 ADDITION POLYMERS

16.10*) Saran Wrap is a head-to-tail homopolymer of $H_2C{=}CCl_2$. Draw a portion of its polymer chain.

16.11*) $F_2C{=}CFCl$ forms a head-to-tail polymer called Kel-F. Draw a portion of the Kel-F polymer chain.

16.12) Identify the monomer from which the following polymer can be made.

$$\left[\begin{array}{cccccccc} H & H & H & H & H & H & H & H \\ | & | & | & | & | & | & | & | \\ C & C & C & C & C & C & C & C \\ | & | & | & | & | & | & | & | \\ H & CN & H & CN & H & CN & H & CN \end{array}\right]_n$$

16.13*) $H_2C{=}CH{-}\overset{\displaystyle O}{\overset{\|}{C}}{-}OCH_3$ forms an addition polymer similar to Plexiglas. Sketch a portion of this head-to-tail polymer.

16.14) Outline the three steps in the peroxide initiated polymerization of propylene to form polypropylene.

16.15*) Show the isotactic structure of a portion of the polymer formed through the head-to-tail polymerization of $H_2C{=}CHCN$.

16.27*) Polystyrene (styrofoam) is a head-to-tail homopolymer of

$$\langle\!\bigcirc\!\rangle{-}CH{=}CH_2 .$$

Draw a portion of its polymer chain.

16.28*) $H_2C{=}CF_2$ forms a head-to-tail polymer. Draw a portion of the polymer chain of this addition polymer.

16.29) Identify the monomer from which the following polymer can be made.

$$\left[\begin{array}{ccccccc} H & H & H & H & H & H & H \\ | & | & | & | & | & | & | \\ C & C & C & C & C & C & C \\ | & | & | & | & | & | & | \\ Cl & H & Cl & H & Cl & H & Cl \end{array}\right]_n$$

16.30*) $CH_2{=}CHCl$ forms the addition polymer PVC. Sketch a portion of this head-to-tail polymer.

16.31) Outline the three steps in the peroxide initiated polymerization of styrene to form polystyrene.

16.32*) Show the syndiotactic structure of a portion of the polymer formed through the head-to-tail polymerization of $H_2C{=}CHCH_3$.

SECTION 16.3 CONDENSATION POLYMERS

16.16) Draw the structure of the monomer used to make the polymer

$$\left[\begin{array}{c} \overset{\displaystyle O}{\overset{\|}{C}}{-}(CH_2)_6{-}\overset{\displaystyle O}{\overset{\|}{C}}{-}\overset{\displaystyle H}{\overset{|}{N}}{-}(CH_2)_6{-}\overset{\displaystyle H}{\overset{|}{N}} \end{array}\right]_n$$

16.17*) Write an equation showing the formation of a condensation polymer by the reaction of

$$HOOC(CH_2)_3COOH$$

with

$$H_2NCH_2CH_2NH_2 .$$

16.18*) What functional group is present in the repeating unit of a polyamide?

16.33) Draw the structure of the monomer used to make the polymer

$$\left[\begin{array}{c} \overset{\displaystyle O}{\overset{\|}{C}}{-}\overset{\displaystyle H}{\overset{|}{N}}{-}(CH_2)_4{-}\overset{\displaystyle O}{\overset{\|}{C}}{-}\overset{\displaystyle H}{\overset{|}{N}}{-}(CH_2)_4 \end{array}\right]_n$$

16.34*) Write an equation showing the formation of a condensation polymer by the reaction of

$$HOOC(CH_2)_4COOH$$

with

$$HOCH_2CH_2OH .$$

16.35*) What functional group is present in the repeating unit of a polyester?

16.19) Consider each of the following pairs of compounds. Which pairs can react to form polyesters?

a) CH_3COOH and CH_3CH_2OH

b) $HOOCCH_2COOH$

and

$HOCH_2CH_2OH$

c) $HOOCCOOH$ and $HOCH_2CH_2OH$

16.20*) Lexan is a polyester. The monomers can be considered to be

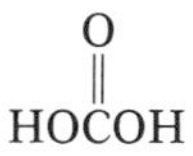

$$\overset{\displaystyle O}{\underset{\displaystyle \|}{HOCOH}}$$

(carbonic acid) and

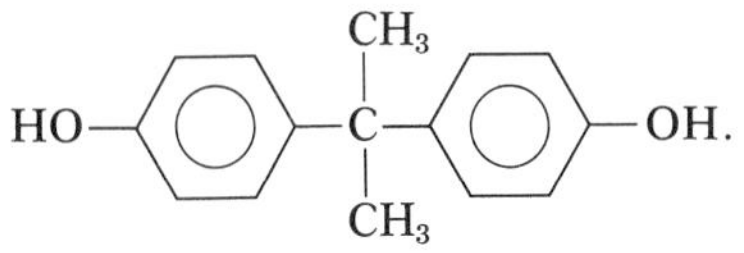

Draw a portion of the chain of this condensation polymer, called a *polycarbonate*.

16.21*) What are the starting materials for the preparation of Nylon 4?

SECTION 16.4 CROSS-LINKED POLYMERS

16.22) Give an example of a polymer that might be the result of the reaction between a trifunctional acid and a difunctional alcohol.

16.23) Describe the difference between a thermosetting polymer and a thermoplastic polymer.

SECTION 16.5 ELASTOMERS

16.24*) Natural rubber is poly-*cis*-isoprene. The poly-*trans*-isoprene occurs in the leaves and bark of the sapotacca tree and is known as *gutta-percha* rubber. It is used for golf ball covers. Sketch a portion of the polymer chain of gutta-percha rubber.

SECTION 16.6 PLASTICIZERS

16.25) Explain how a plasticizer can make a polymer more flexible.

16.36) Consider each of the following pairs of compounds. Which pairs can react to form polyamides?

a) $HOOCCOOH$ and H_2NCH_3

b) $HOOCCOOH$

and

$H_2NCH_2CH_2NH_2$

c) CH_3COOH and H_2NCH_3

16.37*) Kodel is a polyester made from the diacid

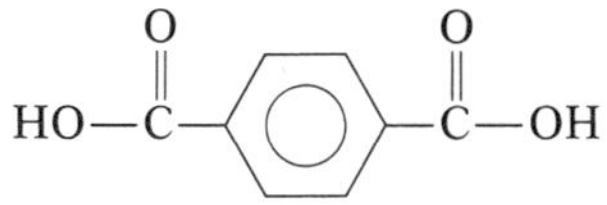

and the diol

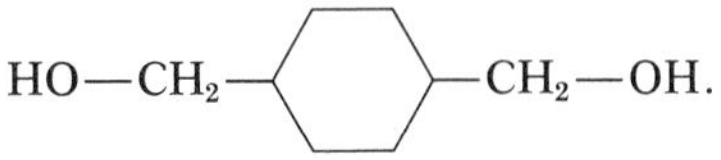

Draw a portion of the chain of this condensation polymer.

16.38*) Suggest a starting material for the preparation of Nylon 45.

16.39) Give an example of a polymer that might be the result of the reaction between a difunctional acid and a trifunctional alcohol.

16.40) If you accidentally placed an object made of a thermosetting polymer in an oven and it began to melt, would you be able to remold its shape?

16.41*) When polybutadiene is heated with sulfur, *vulcanization* of the polymer occurs. Explain. Sketch a portion of the vulcanized polymer chain.

16.42) Explain why it's not wise to use ordinary plastic tubing to connect a patient to a dialysis machine.

Carbohydrates   17

In the previous 16 chapters, we discussed some very general aspects of chemistry, using both inorganic and organic compounds and reactions as examples. In the introduction to this text, we compared the learning of chemistry to the learning of a language. Chapters 1 through 16 have provided you with the chemical alphabet (the element symbols), with an extensive chemical vocabulary of both technical terms and compound formulas, and with the basic principles of chemical reactivity.

Throughout those chapters, you saw applications to the everyday world and to the human body. It is now time to become more specific about the compounds and reactions that affect the living cell.

Let us consider briefly how the topics you learned in Chapters 1 through 16 apply to the biochemistry of the body.

Chapter 1 discussed the elements believed to play a role in life processes (Table 1-1) and gave brief examples of the nutrients in food (Figure 1–5). We will now describe the nutrients in more detail: *carbohydrates* in this chapter, *lipids* in Chapter 18, *proteins* in Chapter 19, *vitamins* in Chapter 23, and the *minerals* and *water* that go into body fluids in Chapter 24.

Chapter 2 was about measurement of mass, length, volume, and atoms. Biochemistry involves many such measurements.

Chapter 3 discussed electron configurations and how they relate to the families of elements in the periodic table. The roles of many elements in the human body were discussed briefly. In Chapters 17 through 28, you will see how certain elements perform particular functions in the body and how these functions are directly related to the electronic configurations of the elements.

Chapter 4 provided an introduction to simple chemical formulas. From such simple compounds are built the very complex and high-molecular-weight biochemicals of the cell. Many of the ions of Tables 4–1 and 4–2 play roles in the body. The continuous-chain carbon skeleton of hydrocarbons will be found in the carbohydrates and lipids of Chapters 17 and 18.

Chapter 5 presented some simple chemical reactions, such as acid-base neutralization and combustion. These will help you understand the considerably more complex reactions that generate energy for the body (Chapter 22) and break down food nutrients to create materials needed by the body (Chapters 25, 26, and 27).

Chapters 6 through 9 showed you how organic compounds are bonded and how they react. The oxidation-reduction reactions of Chapter 8 are of particular importance as they relate to biochemical energy (Chapter 22). The alcohols and carboxylic acids of Chapter 9 lead directly to the carbohydrates and lipids of Chapters 17 and 18.

Chapters 10 through 12 discussed the states of matter when pure and when mixed with other substances. Each chapter contained much material of importance to the body, as well as sections (10.5. The Breath of Life; 11.2. Blood Pressure; 12.5. Osmosis and Living Cells) with physiological information.

Chapters 13 and 14 presented the acid-base properties of solutions, which are directly related to the peptide linkages that convert amino acids to proteins (Chapter 19). The discussion of buffer solutions is of immense importance to our consideration of body fluids in Chapter 24.

Chapter 15 introduced some very important cyclic systems that are included in many of the more complex biochemical molecules to be discussed in the rest of this book.

Chapter 16 described how polymers are created from monomers. This should help you understand how the body synthesizes protein polypeptides, carbohydrate polysaccharides, and other natural polymers.

As you study more aspects of biochemistry, you will notice other relationships with the materials of Chapters 1 through 16.

The carbohydrates will be discussed first, since they possess the simplest chemical structures. As a class of compounds, they include sugars, starch, and cellulose. Such sugars as glucose, fructose, and sucrose are constituents of many fruits and vegetables.

While you are aware of the role of sugar and other carbohydrates in your food, you may not realize that *polymer* carbohydrates—cellulose and starch—account for more than half of the organic matter on the earth. Cellulose is the supporting structural material of all trees and other plants. Processed cellulose is used widely in textiles, the polymers *cellophane* and *celluloid,* and other industrial uses.

Another polymer or *polysaccharide,* starch, is a form in which living organisms store energy. *Glycogen* (Chapter 25) is built up in our muscles and liver to be called upon when the body needs calories for sudden activity.

The most important carbohydrate in the body is glucose, $C_6H_{12}O_6$, which circulates in the blood stream and is carried to tissues and cells. There, it provides energy for cell processes (Chapter 22) and for raw materials for building new carbohydrates, lipids, and proteins.

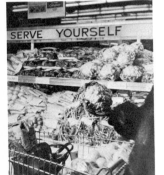

Cellophane, a polymer made from the carbohydrate cellulose, is a widely used packaging material for food products. (DuPont)

17.1 TYPES OF CARBOHYDRATES

> *LEARNING GOAL 17A:* Draw a structural formula for a triose and a hexose.
> *17B:* Describe what is shown in a projection formula, a perspective formula, and a Haworth structure of an organic molecule.
> *17C:* Given a Haworth structure for the ring form of a hexose, state whether the compound is the alpha or the beta form.

Consider the formula of the most common carbohydrate, glucose: $C_6H_{12}O_6$. Since there is twice as much hydrogen as oxygen, early chemists considered glucose to be a *hydrate* of carbon, $(C \cdot H_2O)_6$, containing water and carbon. This led to the name *carbohydrate.*

If you look at the structural formula for glucose (Figure 17–1), how-ever, you see that there is no water present; the repeating unit is actually

$$H—\overset{|}{\underset{|}{C}}—OH$$

Another carbohydrate present in nucleic acids, deoxyribose, has the molec-ular formula $C_5H_{10}O_4$ and is clearly not hydrated carbon. Carbohydrates are now defined as compounds that contain in each molecule a *carbonyl group* ($—\overset{|}{C}=O$) plus *several hydroxyl groups* ($—OH$). Glucose is a polyhydroxyal-dehyde, since the carbonyl carbon is at the end of the molecule. Other simple sugars are polyhydroxyketones. Some derivatives of these com-pounds are also classified as carbohydrates.

Aldoses and ketoses

A sugar containing an aldehyde group, $—CHO$, is called an **aldose.** Glu-cose is an aldose. A very common sugar in fruits and in honey is *fructose*, which like glucose has the molecular formula $C_6H_{12}O_6$. However, fructose is a **ketose** since its carbonyl group involves the second carbon rather than the first. Fructose and glucose are thus structural *isomers* (Section 7.2).

Monosaccharides

The simplest sugars are formed when continuous-chain polyhydroxy al-cohols are oxidized to create one carbonyl group on each molecule. Glycerol will be discussed as one of the two components of fats (Section 18.1). Oxida-tion of the end carbon of glycerol gives the aldose *glyceraldehyde*. Oxidation of the center carbon of glycerol gives a ketose, *dihydroxyacetone*.

$$\begin{array}{c} CHO \\ | \\ H—C—OH \\ | \\ HO—C—H \\ | \\ H—C—OH \\ | \\ H—C—OH \\ | \\ CH_2OH \end{array}$$

FIGURE 17–1 Glucose, $C_6H_{12}O_6$, is the most impor-tant simple sugar. Since it contains a $—CHO$ group, glucose is an *aldose*. The placement of the $—OH$ groups to the left or right of the central carbon spine is not random. It is specific and provides information about the three-dimensional struc-ture of the molecule.

$$\begin{array}{c} CH_2OH \\ | \\ C=O \\ | \\ HO—C—H \\ | \\ H—C—OH \\ | \\ H—C—OH \\ | \\ CH_2OH \end{array}$$

fructose

glyceraldehyde (aldose)

glycerol
(polyhydric alcohol)

dihydroxyacetone (ketose)

These two simple sugars containing three carbons are called *trioses* (tri = three). A sugar with five carbon atoms (such as ribose) is a *pentose* (penta =

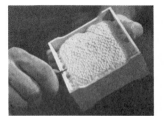

The fructose in honey ac-counts for its sweetness. Like glucose, fructose is $C_6H_{12}O_6$, but with a *keto* group. High-fructose corn syrup is increasing in use as a "natural" sweetener. (Photo from *American Bee Journal*)

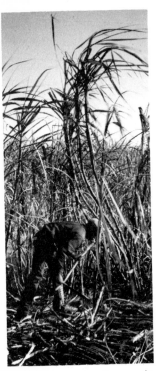

five). Glucose, fructose, and other six-carbon simple sugars are **hexoses** (*hexa* = six).

Each of these simple sugars with one carbonyl group is a **monosaccharide** (*mono* = one). The ending "-ose" is characteristic of sugars.

Polysaccharides

Table sugar, *sucrose*, $C_{12}H_{22}O_{11}$, is not a monosaccharide. If you analyze its formula, you will find that sucrose contains two hexose units minus one water. Sucrose is, in fact, a **disaccharide** (*di* = two), formed by reacting glucose with fructose and splitting out a molecule of water:

$$\underset{\text{glucose}}{C_6H_{12}O_6} + \underset{\text{fructose}}{C_6H_{12}O_6} \longrightarrow \underset{\text{sucrose}}{C_{12}H_{22}O_{11}} + H_2O$$

When sucrose is hydrolyzed in the body, we obtain the reverse of the above reaction, the formation of glucose and fructose.

A combination of from two to five simple sugars (monosaccharides) linked together is known by the general name *oligosaccharide*. When the pattern is repeated again and again, we obtain a polymer of monosaccharide monomer units. This polymer (starch and glycogen are two examples) is a **polysaccharide.**

Projection and perspective formulas

To this point in the course we have used molecular formulas (such as $C_6H_{12}O_6$ for glucose), condensed structural formulas (such as

$$CH_2OHCHOHCHOHCHOHCHOHCHO$$

for glucose), Lewis electron-dot diagrams, and written-out structural formulas (as in Figure 17–1). You learned earlier that these ways of writing the atoms in a molecule do not necessarily show anything about the real geometry. Certainly the glucose molecule is *not* in a straight line; all of the carbon atoms are at tetrahedral angles to each other as in an alkane.

In our discussion of carbohydrates, the real geometry of a molecule is of great significance because two different molecules can have identical structural formulas. *Galactose* is a hexose with the same molecular and condensed structural formula as glucose; it is found in milk sugar and in brain and nerve tissue. Chemists write structural formulas for D-glucose and D-galactose as follows:

Remember, however, that the central spine of carbon atoms does not go straight up and down, but follows a zigzag path. If you accept that, then for the monosaccharide hexoses with formula $C_6H_{12}O_6$, there are four —OH groups (on carbons 2, 3, 4, and 5) that may be on either the left or the right of the spine. Two possibilities for each of four —OH groups gives sixteen isomers, since $2 \times 2 \times 2 \times 2 = 16$. Because of three-dimensional geometry (Section 17.2), no two of the sixteen are exactly the same.

```
          H                        H
          |                        |
          C=O                      C=O
          |                        |
     H —  C — OH             H —  C — OH
          |                        |
    HO —  C — H             HO —  C — H
          |                        |
     H —  C — OH            HO —  C — H
          |                        |
     H —  C — OH             H —  C — OH
          |                        |
         CH₂OH                    CH₂OH
       D-glucose                D-galactose
```

What is the difference between these two molecules? Because the actual geometry is tetrahedral *at each carbon*, there are various ways the —OH groups can be placed with respect to each other. There are actually 16 possible compounds that are isomeric with glucose except for the relative positions in space of the bonds. These are the *stereoisomers* of glucose.

Chemists can show these differences by assigning a specific meaning to the placement of the —OH group to the *right* or *left* of its carbon in the structural formula. When used in this way, the diagram is called a *Fischer projection formula*. Figure 17–1 is a Fischer projection formula. Horizontal lines are used to indicate bonds to atoms that project (to some extent) *toward* the reader, above the plane of the paper. Vertical lines indicate bonds to atoms that project *away from* the reader, behind the plane of the paper. While it is difficult to actually visualize the geometry from these formulas, they do provide an easy way of differentiating between stereoisomers.

A more direct way to indicate the relative directions of bonds is to write a *perspective* formula. Essentially similar to the Fischer projection formula, the perspective formula tries to give a feel for what is coming up out of the paper by using heavy wedges for the bonds and for what is down behind the paper by using dotted lines for the bonds. To take a very simple example, the actual geometry of D-lactic acid, $CH_3CHOHCOOH$, can be visualized as shown:

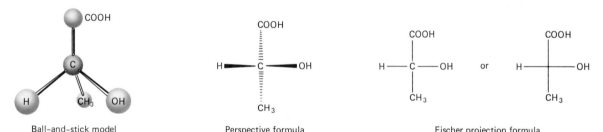

| Ball-and-stick model | Perspective formula | Fischer projection formula |

Both the projection and perspective formulas of sugars are written with the aldehyde or ketone group at the top. We will return to these formulas when we discuss *optical isomers* in the next section.

Haworth ring structures

To this point, we have considered a simple sugar as a continuous chain molecule with a carbonyl group. In reality, glucose and other monosaccharides exist mostly in a form obtained through reaction between the carbonyl group and the hydroxyl group on the fifth carbon of the *same* molecule. This ring or *hemiacetal* form will be seen frequently in the chapters to come.

The ring formed by glucose (Figure 17–2) can be considered a derivative of the heterocyclic *pyran* ring (p. 459). The ring form of glucose is known as **glucopyranose.**

In a structure first suggested by Sir Walter Haworth, the heavy lines in Figure 17–2 indicate that the five carbons and one oxygen of glucopyranose *all lie in the same plane*. If you think of this plane as being perpendicular to the page (sticking out toward you and going back into your desk), the thickly drawn bonds of the ring are closest to you and those drawn with thin lines are behind the paper.

Stereoisomers differ from each other only in their three-dimensional geometry, just as left-hand and right-hand gloves differ only in direction in space. The symbol "D" used for D-glucose and D-fructose will be explained in Section 17.2.

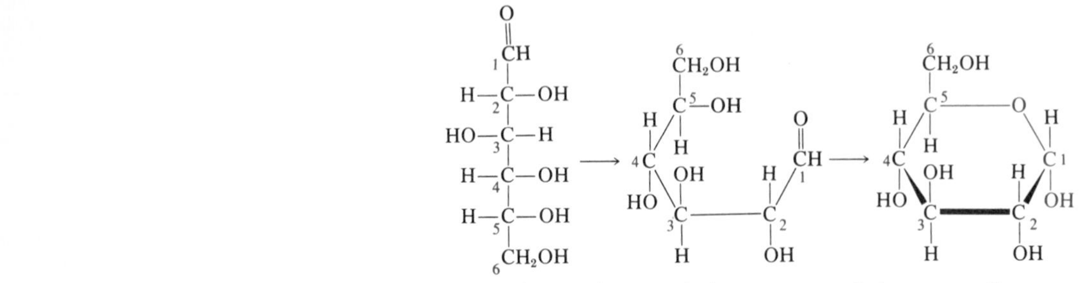

FIGURE 17-2 The continuous-chain structure of glucose easily reacts to form a ring called the *glucopyranose* structure. The form shown is alpha-D-glucopyranose. If the —OH on carbon 1 were above the plane of the ring, it would be beta-D-glucopyranose. Over 99% of the glucose in the body is in the ring forms.

Groups (—H, —OH) written to the *right* of a carbon in the projection or perspective formula are shown *below* the ring of the pyranose or furanose structure. Those written to the *left* of the carbon chain in a formula are shown *above* the ring in a Haworth structure, as in Figure 17-2.

Ring sugar structures are described as *alpha* or *beta* based on the positions of the groups bonded to the carbon that originally formed the carbonyl group, shown as carbon 1 for glucose in Figure 17-2. If the Haworth diagram shows the —OH on carbon 1 *below* the ring, it is an alpha (α) isomer. If the hydroxyl group is shown *above* the ring, it is a beta (β) isomer.

Fructose also forms ring structures similar to *furan* (p. 457). They are therefore *furanose* rings:

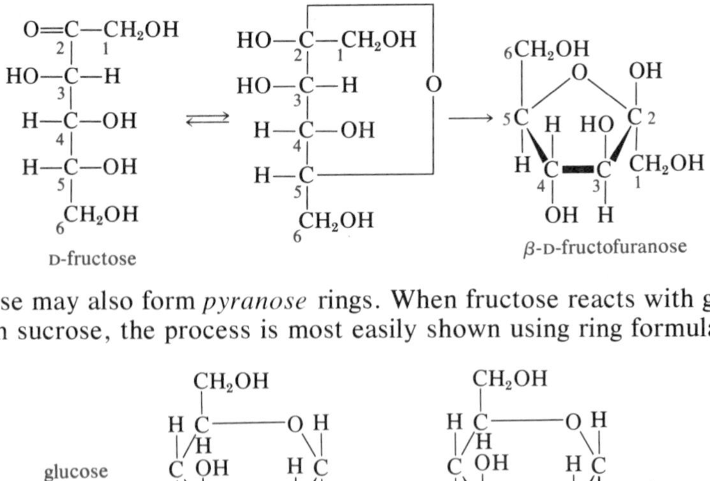

D-fructose

β-D-fructofuranose

Fructose may also form *pyranose* rings. When fructose reacts with glucose to form sucrose, the process is most easily shown using ring formulas:

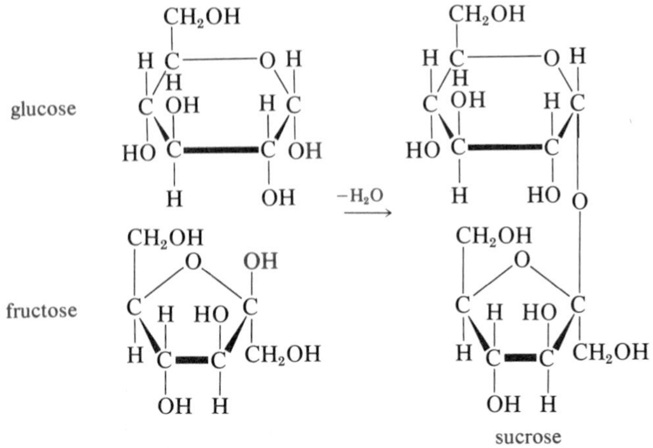

glucose

fructose

$-H_2O$

sucrose

Unfortunately, the Haworth ring structures may be somewhat mislead-ing, since they suggest that the five- and six-membered furanose and pyranose rings are planar. This is not the case. As is also true for cyclo-hexane (Section 7.3), the hexagon is not really planar but instead forms a "chair" that looks like this:

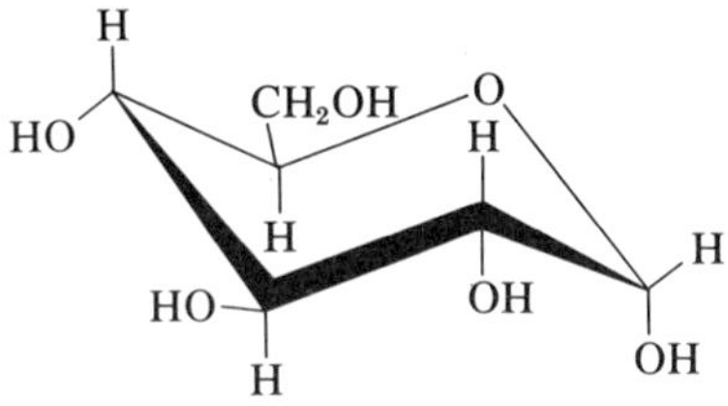

α-D-glucopyranose

However, the Haworth diagrams are convenient to use, and you will see them often in this text and elsewhere.

17.1) Draw a structural formula for a triose. Then, assuming that what you have drawn is a correct projection formula, draw a perspec-tive formula for the same molecule.

17.2) Given the following Haworth structure for a simple sugar:
a) is it a hexose or a pentose?
b) is it an alpha or beta form?

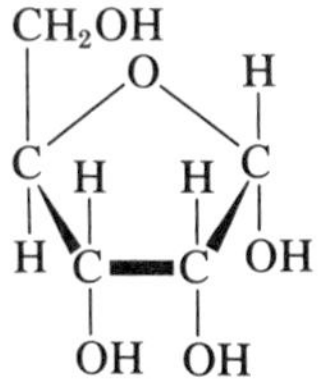

c) is it a monosaccharide or an oligosaccharide?
d*) write the correct projection formula for this molecule in its open-chain form.
e*) from the projection formula, is it an aldose or a ketose?

17.2 OPTICAL ACTIVITY

LEARNING GOAL 17D: Draw a pair of optical isomers and explain in what ways they differ; given the structural formula of a compound, state whether optical isomers can be expected.
     17E: Describe how the D, L, and racemic forms of a com-pound may be distinguished from each other experimentally.
     17F: Explain why optical isomerism is important in the biochemistry of the human body.

In Section 17.1 we mentioned that there are 16 different compounds with the same structural formula as glucose. However, there are only *eight* different sets of physical properties. For example, D-glucose melts at 150°C and D-galactose melts at 170°C, while another isomer, D-mannose, melts at

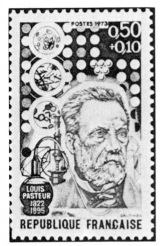

Louis Pasteur (1822–1895) was the first person to recognize the existence of optical isomers. He is perhaps best known for his development of vaccines against anthrax and rabies.

132°C and a fourth, D-altrose, melts at 104°C. By all criteria of organic chemistry, these are distinctly different chemical compounds.

However, one of the 16 isomers, called *L-glucose*, has exactly the same physical properties as D-glucose. The compound L-mannose has exactly the same melting point as D-mannose. The D and L forms of a compound differ from each other in a way that does not affect their physical properties.

In the 1850's, the famous French scientist Louis Pasteur examined some crystals of tartaric acid. He found that he could separate them into two piles, one of crystals that seemed to have faces shifted to the right and the other of crystals with faces apparently shifted to the left. They were alike in all other respects.

Suppose you were sorting through a pile of gloves, all the same size, color, and type. You would be able to divide them into two groups, one meant for right hands and the other meant for left hands. They would differ only in "handedness." Each glove would be the mirror image of the other because if you hold a right hand up to a mirror, you see a left hand. Mirrors change right to left but leave all other directions the same.

Lactic acid, $CH_3CHOHCOOH$, has two such *mirror-image* isomers (Figure 17–3):

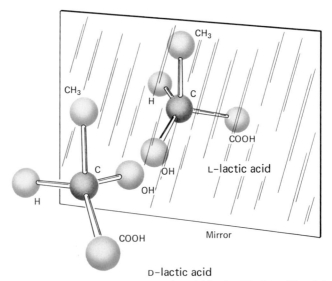

FIGURE 17–3   The D and L forms of lactic acid look alike but, like right-hand and left-hand gloves, cannot be exactly superimposed.

If we look at the image of D-lactic acid in a mirror, we see L-lactic acid. If we simply pluck the L-lactic acid molecule out of the mirror and set it alongside its isomer, we see that the four groups attached to the central carbon atom do not quite match. The two isomers cannot be lined up or *superimposed*, in the same way that a right-hand glove and a left-hand glove do not exactly match.

Mirror image (D, L) isomers are also known as *enantiomers*. Optical isomers that are not mirror images of each other, such as D-glucose and D-galactose, are known as *diastereomers* and have distinctly different physical properties.

Each of the simple sugars we have discussed in this chapter has optical isomers with D and L forms. The naming of D and L comes from glyceraldehyde (Figure 17–4). The D stands for "dextro" or right-handed and represents a compound with the same arrangement as D-glyceraldehyde around the next-to-bottom carbon atom. The L stands for "levo" or left-handed and comes from the configuration of L-glyceraldehyde. We will not ask you to determine if a given structure is D or L. However, the difference is very important in nature. Only the D forms of carbohydrates and only the L forms of amino acids are used by the body.

Chiral carbons

Most molecules we have studied do not have stereoisomers. The first requirement of a stereoisomer, which is satisfied by the sugars and amino acids we are considering, is that there be at least one carbon atom *with four different groups bonded to it*. Lactic acid, for example, has around the central carbon atom (1) —CH$_3$, (2) —H, (3) —OH, and (4) —COOH. The central carbon atom in lactic acid is thus **chiral** or **asymmetric.** The mirror image of one form of lactic acid will not be the same molecule.

A molecule with one chiral carbon atom will have D and L forms. Glucose has not one but four chiral carbon atoms (carbons 2, 3, 4, and 5), which increases the number of possible isomers, as we have seen. Tartaric acid, investigated by Pasteur, has two chiral carbons. You might thus expect it to have four different forms, but it does not. It has three forms, two of which are mirror images (D and L) and one that is the same as its mirror image and is called the *meso* form:

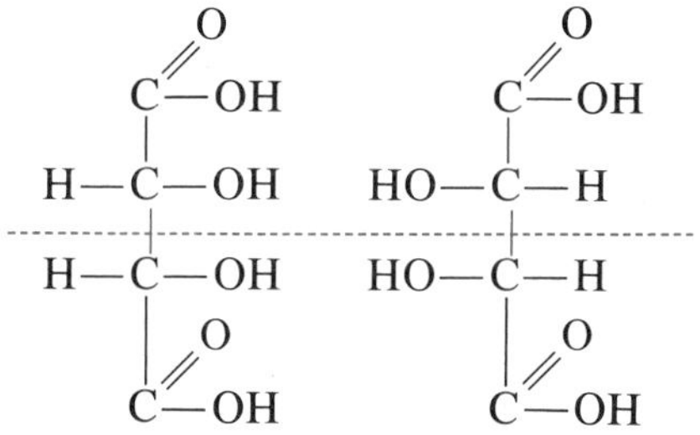

$$
\begin{array}{cc}
\overset{\displaystyle O}{\underset{|}{C}}\!\!-\!OH & \overset{\displaystyle O}{\underset{|}{C}}\!\!-\!OH \\
H\!-\!\underset{|}{C}\!-\!OH & HO\!-\!\underset{|}{C}\!-\!H \\
\text{-----------} & \text{-----------} \\
H\!-\!\underset{|}{C}\!-\!OH & HO\!-\!\underset{|}{C}\!-\!H \\
\underset{O}{C}\!\!-\!OH & \underset{O}{C}\!\!-\!OH
\end{array}
$$

meso-tartaric acid

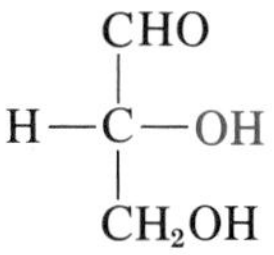

The polarimeter

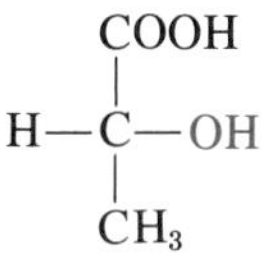

The only way to distinguish a solution of D-glucose from a solution of L-glucose is to take advantage of some property for which a right-handed molecule will differ from a left-handed molecule. If we were testing right-hand and left-hand gloves, we might see which one fit properly on each hand. For molecules, the method is to use a property of light.

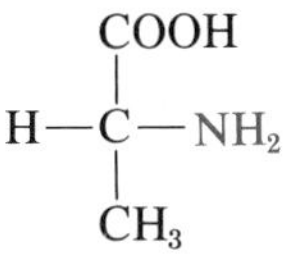

A "normal" light beam is transmitted in a straight line and has waves that vary to the left, to the right, and up and down with respect to that straight line. Certain crystals (as well as the polarizing plastic sheets invented by Edwin Land in 1928 and called *Polaroid*) can cut out all but one direction of wave motion, as shown in Figure 17–5.

As plane-polarized light passes through a sample tube and the electrons in a substance absorb and scatter some of the light, the wave properties of the polarized light will be changed. In water or a solution of a material that is not optically active, the only result will be to "depolarize" some of the light. However, in a solution of an optically active substance, the result will be to turn (rotate) the plane of polarization of the light (Figure 17–6). This capability is called **optical activity.**

If a second polarizing sheet is used to observe the light, it is turned until the light is at its brightest. Built into an instrument called a **polarimeter,** this

CHO
H—C—OH
CH$_2$OH

D-glyceraldehyde

COOH
H—C—OH
CH$_3$

D-lactic acid

COOH
H—C—NH$_2$
CH$_3$

D-alanine

—C—
H—C—OH
CH$_2$OH

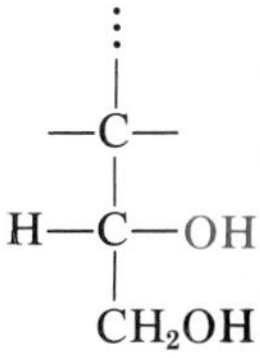

a D-sugar

FIGURE 17–4 In all D isomers, the configuration around the *second* carbon from the bottom is like that of D-glyceraldehyde. Each functional group attached to that carbon of a D compound is shown to the *right* in the Fischer projection. Note that D-glucose (Figure 17–1) and D-galactose are written similarly around carbon 5.

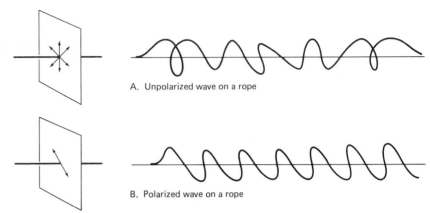

A. Unpolarized wave on a rope

B. Polarized wave on a rope

FIGURE 17–5 A rope analogy for polarized light. In (A), the rope goes in all directions, like an unpolarized beam. In (B), all parts of the rope line up in a single plane, like a polarized light beam.

Unfortunately, the direction of rotation *cannot* be predicted from the D or L geometry. A complete description of a hexose would thus include α or β, D or L, and (+) or (−), as in β-D-(+)-glucopyranose.

second filter can be turned in such a way that the direction and amount of rotation can be measured. For example, one typical glucose solution will rotate the plane of polarized light to the right by 52.5°. This is reported as a rotation of + 52.5°, and the direction of rotation is *plus,* symbolized by "(+)." If the rotation is to the left, the direction is indicated by a minus sign "(−)."

A substance that rotates the plane of polarized light to the right (+) is said to be *dextrorotatory.* One that rotates to the left (−) is *levorotatory.* If there are two optical isomers of a substance, D and L isomers, one will rotate polarized light to the right (not necessarily the D form) and one an equal

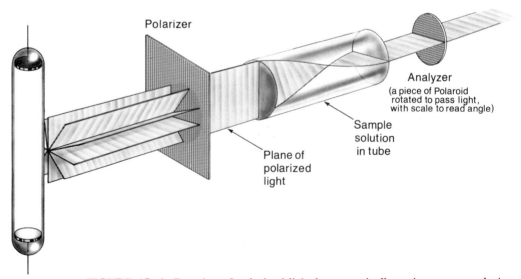

FIGURE 17–6 Rotation of polarized light by an optically active compound. As a beam of polarized light passes through the sample solution, the plane of polarization is rotated continuously. The direction of rotation (right or left) depends on the molecular structure of the compound. The amount of rotation that is observed will depend on the length of the sample.

amount to the left. This provides a way of distinguishing between the two mirror-image isomers of a compound.

Pasteur found that the solutions he made from the two different crystals of tartaric acid showed equal but opposite optical rotation. One was (+), the other (−). When he mixed equal amounts of the two forms and made a solution of the mixture, it was optically inactive.

When compounds containing asymmetric carbon atoms are synthesized in the laboratory, these compounds are often optically inactive. As Pasteur observed with tartaric acid, solutions of these compounds contain 50% D and 50% L and their optical activity is exactly balanced to zero. Such a mixture of optically active forms is known as a **racemic mixture.**

Biological activity of optical isomers

Optical isomers often differ in how they work in the body. As an example, the lactic acid formed during strenuous muscular exercise is D-lactic acid. The yeast used in fermenting sugar solutions to produce alcohol contains L-lactic acid, which can be isolated from the fermentation products. When milk sours, the lactic acid that is formed is a racemic mixture of equal amounts of the D and L forms. In his studies on tartaric acid, Pasteur discovered that he could separate the D and L forms in one particular racemic mixture by treating it with a mold from penicillin that selectively acted on the D form, leaving only the L form intact.

Another common example involves the hormone *epinephrine* (adrenalin). This hormone, which stimulates the heart, blood flow, and blood pressure and is involved in the burning of carbohydrates, is only active when in the L form.

The property of taste is also affected by optical forms. The amino acid asparagine is used by psychologists in checking taste sensation. It tastes sweet to most people when the L form is applied to the tongue. The D form gives no taste sensation. The flavor-enhancing agent monosodium glutamate only works when the L form is used.

For the remainder of this text, we will emphasize the forms used by the body, the D forms of carbohydrates and the L forms of amino acids. We will generally drop the D or L when writing such names in later chapters. Most enzymes will act only on one of the two optical isomers of a compound.

adrenalin
(epinephrine)

The C* indicates a *chiral* carbon atom.

$$H_2NCCH_2C^*COOH$$

asparagine

monosodium glutamate

SELF-CHECK

17.3) Draw a pair of optical isomers of an amino acid. Explain in exactly what way they are different. What properties would differ? Would both isomers be used by the body in building proteins?

17.4) One of the optical isomers of benzedrine ("speed," a potent and medically useful but dangerous drug) has the following perspective formula:

Draw the perspective formula of the other optical isomer.

17.5)   Which of the following molecules will have optical isomers?

$$CH_3-\overset{\overset{\displaystyle H}{|}}{\underset{\underset{\displaystyle Br}{|}}{C}}-H \qquad CH_3-\overset{\overset{\displaystyle Cl}{|}}{\underset{\underset{\displaystyle Br}{|}}{C}}-H \qquad CH_3-\overset{\overset{\displaystyle Cl}{|}}{\underset{\underset{\displaystyle Cl}{|}}{C}}-CH_3$$

(a)   (b)   (c)

$$\bigcirc-\overset{\overset{\displaystyle H}{|}}{\underset{\underset{\displaystyle NH_2}{|}}{C}}-\bigcirc \qquad \bigcirc-\overset{\overset{\displaystyle NH_2}{|}}{\underset{\underset{\displaystyle H}{|}}{C}}-CH_3$$

(d)   (e)

17.6)   Solution I contains L-mannose. Solution II contains a racemic mixture of D- and L-mannose. How could you tell these two solutions apart?

17.7)   Will a solution of L-glucose provide the body with some calories of energy? Can the L-glucose be used as a raw material for the building of body carbohydrates, fats, and proteins? Explain.

17.3 REACTIONS OF CARBOHYDRATES

> *LEARNING GOAL 17G: Explain why glucose is called a reducing sugar.*
> *17H: Describe the formation of a phosphorylated sugar.*

Carbohydrates undergo many of the reactions that you have already studied in earlier chapters. Dehydration, acetal formation, oxidation, and ester formation are some of the reactions we will consider in this chapter.

Reducing sugars

In Section 8.2 we discussed the various oxidation levels of organic compounds from alcohols through aldehydes and ketones to carboxylic acids and CO_2. Even a mild oxidizing agent will react with an aldehyde to produce a carboxylic acid.

In the Tollens (silver mirror) test, the Ag^+ ion reacts to give silver metal, which precipitates on the surface of the test tube:

$$Ag^+ + -CHO \longrightarrow \underset{\text{mirror}}{Ag_{(s)}} + -COO^-$$

The three test reagents for reducing sugars keep the metal cation (Ag^+ or Cu^{2+}) locked up or *complexed* until reduction takes place, Tollen's with ammonia, Benedict's with citrate ion and Fehling's with tartrate ion. Benedict's solution, which stores well, is the basis for *Clinitest* tablets, and will be discussed later in this chapter as a way of distinguishing between various carbohydrates.

Benedict's Test and Fehling's Test similarly use a mild oxidizing agent, here the copper(II) cation, to give a visible result:

$$\underset{\substack{\text{(blue} \\ \text{solution)}}}{Cu^{2+}} + -CHO \longrightarrow \underset{\text{red solid}}{Cu_2O_{(s)}} + -COO^-$$

Any carbohydrate that can react with Ag^+ to give a silver mirror or with

Cu^{2+} to give red copper(I) oxide is defined as a **reducing sugar.** Such tests, especially the Benedict's test, are often used to detect diabetes by checking for presence of glucose in the urine. It is thus important to know which substances can, in fact, give positive test results.

Since the open-chain form of glucose is an *aldose,* with a —CHO group, it is clearly a reducing sugar. Although monosaccharides in solution exist almost entirely in ring forms, there is an equilibrium with the open-chain isomer. As some of the open-chain molecules react, others are formed from the hemiacetal rings, which can thus be considered to contain *potential* aldehyde or ketone groups. Although ordinary ketones (such as acetone) will not reduce Cu^{2+} cation, a molecule with a —OH group on the carbon next to (*alpha* to) the carbonyl carbon will, indeed, become oxidized. The ketoses are thus also reducing sugars.

Since reducing sugars other than glucose (and reducing agents that are not sugars) would be measured in a total determination of reducing sugars in the blood, the enzyme *glucose oxidase* is now commonly used for testing because it affects only glucose.

$$
\begin{array}{c}
H \\
| \\
C{=}O \\
| \\
H{-}C{-}OH \\
| \\
HO{-}C{-}H \quad + \; H_2O \; + \; O_2 \xrightarrow[\text{oxidase}]{\text{glucose}} \\
| \\
H{-}C{-}OH \\
| \\
H{-}C{-}OH \\
| \\
CH_2OH \\
\text{glucose}
\end{array}
\qquad
\begin{array}{c}
COOH \\
| \\
H{-}C{-}OH \\
| \\
HO{-}C{-}H \\
| \quad + \; H_2O_2 \\
H{-}C{-}OH \\
| \\
H{-}C{-}OH \\
| \\
CH_2OH \\
\text{gluconic acid}
\end{array}
$$

The amount of hydrogen peroxide formed from the glucose is determined in a reaction that forms a colored compound. The intensity of the final color is proportional to the amount of glucose present. This reaction is the basis of the dip-sticks or test strips used by patients with diabetes or by laboratories to check the amount of glucose in urine.

If only the primary alcohol group of glucose is oxidized by chemical agents or enzymes, glucuronic acid is produced. Glucuronic acid is a very important physiological compound, since it combines with drugs and poisons in the body to convert them to soluble glucuronide complexes that are readily excreted in the urine.

Oxidation of glucose with concentrated nitric acid, a strong oxidizing agent, converts both the aldehyde and the primary alcohol group to carboxyl groups, producing the dicarboxylic acid, saccharic acid.

$$
\begin{array}{c}
H \\
| \\
C{=}O \\
| \\
H{-}C{-}OH \\
| \\
HO{-}C{-}H \\
| \\
H{-}C{-}OH \\
| \\
H{-}C{-}OH \\
| \\
COOH \\
\text{glucuronic acid}
\end{array}
$$

$$
\begin{array}{c}
COOH \\
| \\
H{-}C{-}OH \\
| \\
HO{-}C{-}H \\
| \\
H{-}C{-}OH \\
| \\
H{-}C{-}OH \\
| \\
COOH \\
\text{saccharic acid}
\end{array}
$$

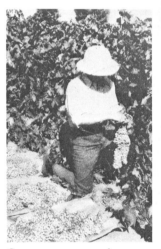

Grapes are a good source of glucose, formerly called "grape sugar." Fermentation of grape juice yields wine. (Photo from *Economic Botany,* A.J. Winkler, Agricultural Experimental Station, Davis, Calif.)

Fermentation

The enzyme mixture called zymase (present in common bread yeast) will act on some of the hexose sugars to produce alcohol and carbon dioxide.

$$
C_6H_{12}O_6 \xrightarrow{\text{zymase}} 2\,C_2H_5OH + 2\,CO_2
$$

Dry table wines result from fermentation alone. Appetizer wines (such as sherry or vermouth) and dessert wines (like port) may have up to 20% alcohol by volume since they are *fortified* through the addition of distilled alcohol or brandy.

The common hexoses (with the exception of galactose) ferment readily, but the pentoses are not fermented by yeast. Disaccharides, such as sucrose, must first be broken down into monosaccharides by other enzymes in yeast before they can be fermented. Malt syrup obtained from grains such as barley contains the disaccharide maltose. Fermentation of malt syrup produces beer and ale (4 per cent alcohol), while fermentation of fruit such as grapes is used to make wine (8 to 15 per cent alcohol). By distilling the products of these fermentations, the alcohol content can be increased, as in whiskey (40 to 50 per cent) and brandy (30 to 40 per cent). Wines may be "sparkling" as a result of natural CO_2 or may have CO_2 added under pressure. Reagent-grade ethyl alcohol (95%) can be made by distilling the products of the fermentation of sugars, syrups, grains, fruits, and other plants.

There are many other types of fermentation of sugars besides the common alcoholic fermentation. When milk sours, its lactose is converted to lactic acid by a fermentation process. Citric acid, acetic acid, butyric acid, and oxalic acid may all be produced by similar reactions.

Glycoside and ester formation

When monosaccharides are treated with an alcohol in a strong acid solution, they form *glycosides*. The hemiacetal structure reacts with the hydroxyl group of an alcohol to form a glycoside or acetal:

glucose
(hemiacetal)

α-methyl glucoside (acetal)

β-methyl glucoside (acetal)

You have already encountered some important esters formed by the reaction of organic acids and alcohols (Section 9.5). Monosaccharides also form esters with phosphoric acid. A molecule of water is split out between hydrogen of phosphoric acid and the hydroxyl group of a monosaccharide, such as glucose, to form an ester:

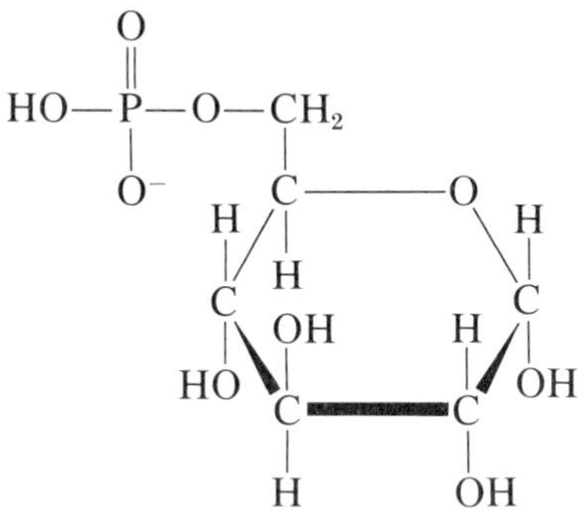

α-D-glucose-6-phosphate

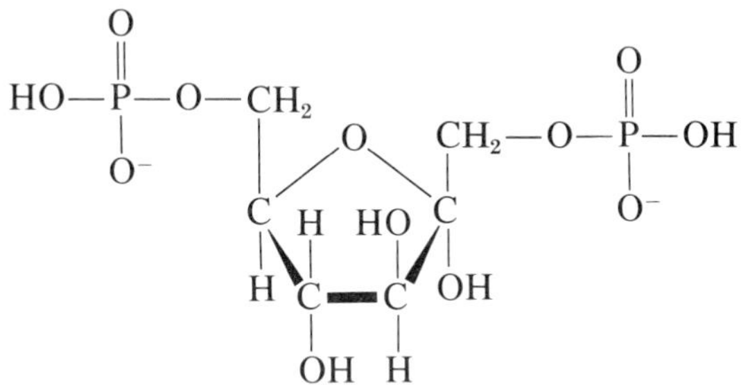

α-D-fructose-1,6-diphosphate

Later in the text, you will find that several of these phosphorylated sugars are produced in the metabolism of carbohydrates (Chapters 22 and 25). For example, glucose is phosphorylated before it can be used by cells and tissues.

17.8)   Why are monosaccharides good reducing agents?
17.9*) How is glucose oxidase used to measure glucose in blood and urine?
17.10*)   Draw the structure for β-D-ribose-5-phosphate.

17.4 DISACCHARIDES

LEARNING GOAL 17I: Describe the acetal or glycoside linkage between two monosaccharides.
                17J: Use the structure for sucrose to explain why it does not reduce Benedict's solution.

A disaccharide is composed of two monosaccharides whose linking together, between the hemiacetal form of one and a hydroxy group of the other, involves the splitting out of a molecule of water.

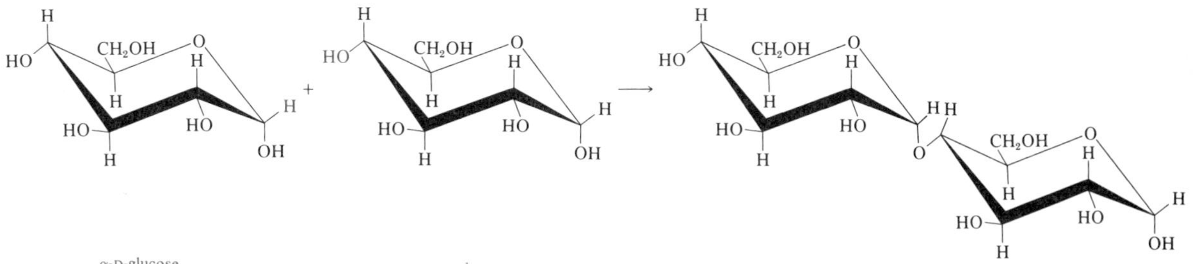

α-D-glucose   α-D-glucose   maltose

The **acetal linkage** is always made from the aldehyde group (on carbon 1) of one of the sugars to a hydroxyl or ketone group of the second. In the structure of the individual disaccharides, such as sucrose, lactose, and maltose,

Leslie Hough in London, England, has prepared a tetrachlorinated sucrose derivative that is 500 to 600 times sweeter than sucrose. Since its caloric value would be approximately the same, gram for gram, as that of sucrose, the same amount of sweetening could be obtained for essentially *zero* calories intake. This compound has no bitter aftertaste, a problem with saccharin, and no licorice-like taste typical of some sweeteners derived from amino acids.

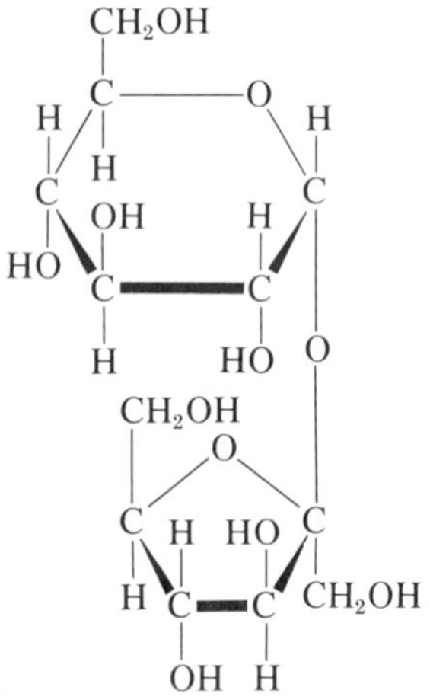

FIGURE 17–7 Sucrose, also known as α-D-glucopyranosyl-β-D-fructofuranose. The complete name for a disaccharide starts with the name of the first sugar and includes the particular isomers involved in the linkage.

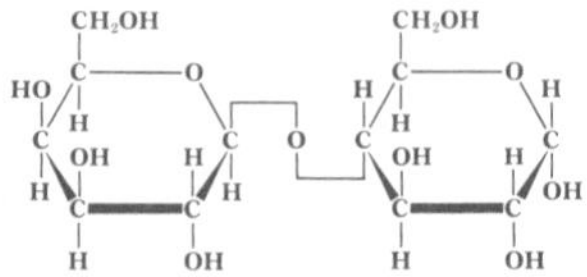

β-D-Galactopyranosyl-α-D-glucopyranose (lactose)

we must know the exact location of the acetal linkage and the isomeric forms involved. In order to reduce Benedict's solution, a disaccharide must have a ring structure containing an aldehyde or ketone group that is not involved in the acetal linkage between the two sugars.

Sucrose

Our distant ancestors used honey for sweetening purposes for thousands of years. It was not until the 17th century that plantations of sugar cane furnished material for the production of large quantities of sucrose (Figure 17–7), which is commonly sold as granulated sugar and is used for sweetening purposes in the home, in soft drinks, and in the food industry. It is found in many plants, such as sugar beets, sorghum cane, sugar cane, and the sap of the sugar maple. Commercially, sucrose is prepared from sugar cane and sugar beets, but purified granulated sugar from any source is the same as pure sucrose prepared in the laboratory.

Sucrose is produced when a molecule of glucose is joined to a molecule of fructose in an acetal linkage that involves the reducing groups (aldehyde and ketone groups) of both sugars. The structure is written in a way that emphasizes the linkage between the hemiacetal —OH on carbon 1 of glucose and the hemiacetal —OH on carbon 2 of fructose.

Sucrose is the only common mono- or disaccharide that will not reduce Benedict's solution. There is no aldehyde or ketone group available—all are tied up in the acetal linkage. When sucrose is hydrolyzed, either by the enzyme sucrase or by an acid, a molecule of glucose and a molecule of fructose are formed.

The fermentation of sucrose by yeast is possible, since yeast contains the enzymes sucrase and zymase. First the sucrase hydrolyzes the sugar, and then the zymase ferments the monosaccharides to form alcohol and carbon dioxide. The enzyme sucrase is sometimes called *invertase*, because during hydrolysis the (+) specific rotation of sucrose, is "inverted" to equal the (−) specific rotation of an equal mixture of glucose and fructose. This mixture is also called *invert sugar* and is used by candy manufacturers because it is sweeter than sucrose. Bees also supply their own invertase, and the sweet taste of honey is due to the presence of invert sugar.

Lactose

The disaccharide in milk is lactose, or *milk sugar*. It is produced in the mammary glands of animals from the glucose in the blood. Commercially, it is obtained from milk whey and is used in infant formulas and special diets. When hydrolyzed by the enzyme lactase or by an acid, lactose forms a molecule of glucose and a molecule of galactose. The enzyme lactase is essential in the digestion of certain carbohydrates in the body. You can readily see how important this enzyme would be in infant nutrition. Some adults have lost the ability to make lactase and have great difficulty digesting milk and other dairy products. Lactose will reduce Benedict's solution, but it is not fermented by yeast. From its reducing properties, it is obvious that the linkage between its constituent sugars does not involve both hemiacetal aldehyde groups (carbon 1 of galactose is connected to carbon 4 of glucose).

Maltose

Maltose commonly occurs in germinating grains (cereal going to seed). It is often called *malt sugar* because it is obtained as a product of the hydrolysis of starch by enzymes present in malt. It is also formed in animals by the action of enzymes on food starch during digestion. Commercially, it is made by the partial hydrolysis of starch by acid in the manufacture of corn syrup. Maltose reduces Benedict's solution and is fermented by yeast.

The structure of maltose is shown on p. 501.

SELF-CHECK

17.11)   Describe the acetal linkage between the two glucose molecules in maltose.

17.12)   Explain why maltose and lactose will reduce Benedict's solution but sucrose will not.

17.5 POLYSACCHARIDES

LEARNING GOAL 17K: Describe the difference in structure between amylose and amylopectin.

17L: Distinguish between the structures of cellulose and glycogen.

A polysaccharide is a polymer carbohydrate made up of many monosaccharide units. Because of this, its molecular weight is very high. In general, polysaccharides do not have a sweet taste. Because of their large size, they generally do not dissolve in water, but form colloids instead. Although most polysaccharides have terminal glucose monomers that may act as reducing sugars, the contribution of this portion of the molecule is extremely small. Most polysaccharides, therefore, will not reduce Benedict's solution.

There are polysaccharides formed from only pentoses or hexoses, and there are also mixed polysaccharides. The most important are composed of the hexose glucose and are called *hexosans* or, more specifically, *glucosans*. As we have seen for disaccharides, whenever two molecules of a hexose combine, a molecule of water is split out. For this reason, we may represent a hexose polysaccharide by the formula $(C_6H_{10}O_5)_n$. You should recognize this as $C_6H_{12}O_6$ minus H_2O, where the n represents the number of hexose units in the individual polysaccharide. The number of glucose units in any one polysaccharide is only an estimate. Thus, the molecular weights of the polysaccharides described in this section are approximations.

Starch

From a nutritional standpoint, starch is the most important polysaccharide. It is a glucosan containing only glucose units and is the storage form of carbohydrates in plants. Two types of polysaccharides are present in starch. One is amylose, composed of a continuous chain of glucose monomers. The other is amylopectin, a branched-chain polymer of glucose. The repeating structure of glucose monomers with C-1-alpha linkages in amylose is shown in Figure 17–8.

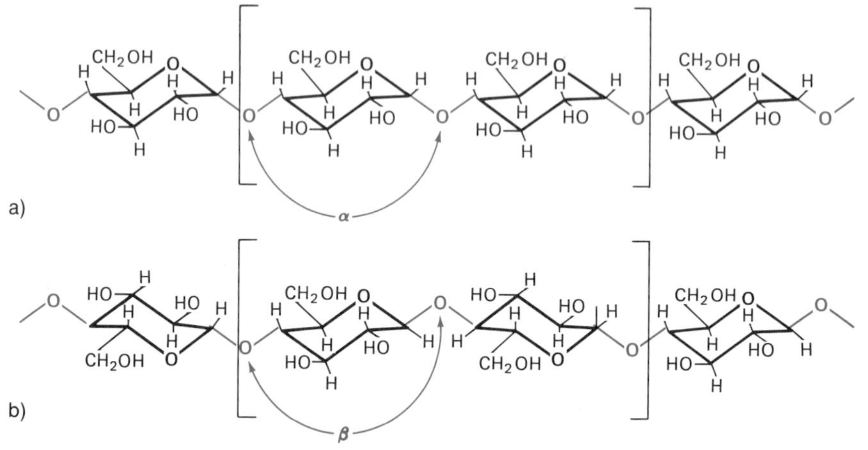

FIGURE 17–8 Two important polysaccharides. Amylose (a), present in starch, contains from 60 to 300 α-D-glucose units bonded by *alpha* linkages. Cellulose (b), the structural material of plants, contains about 2800 β-D-glucose monomer units bonded by *beta* linkages. (Notice that every other glucose unit is flipped over with beta linkages intact.)

Amylose chains may have 300 or more glucose units per molecule, whereas amylopectin chains have in excess of 1000 glucose units per molecule. The branching of the glucose chain in amylopectin occurs about every 24 to 30 glucose units. The molecular weights of various kinds of starch cover a range from 45 000 to over 10 million amu.

Starch will not reduce Benedict's solution and is not fermented by yeast. When hydrolyzed by enzymes or by an acid, it is split into a series of intermediate compounds containing smaller numbers of glucose units. Complete hydrolysis produces free glucose molecules. A characteristic of starch is its reaction with iodine to form a blue compound. This test is often used to follow the progress of the hydrolysis of starch, since the color changes from blue through red to colorless with decreasing molecular weight:

If an iodine solution is spilled on a starched uniform, it produces a blue spot.

starch ⟶ amylodextrin ⟶ erythrodextrin ⟶
blue   blue   red

achroodextrin ⟶ maltose ⟶ glucose
colorless   colorless   colorless

Dextrins

Dextrins are present in germinating grains, but are usually obtained by the partial hydrolysis of starch with enzymes or acid. The branched-chain hydrolysis products are erythrodextrins, which give a red color with iodine. The dextrins are soluble in water and have a slightly sweet taste. Large quantities are used in the manufacture of adhesives because they form sticky solutions when wet. An example of their use is the glue on the back of some postage stamps.

Glycogen

Glycogen is the storage form of carbohydrates in the body. It is found in liver and muscle tissue, is soluble in water, does not reduce Benedict's solution, and gives a reddish-purple color with iodine. The glycogen molecule is similar to the amylopectin molecule in that it has branched chains of glucose that occur about every six to ten glucose units. The branched-chain struc-

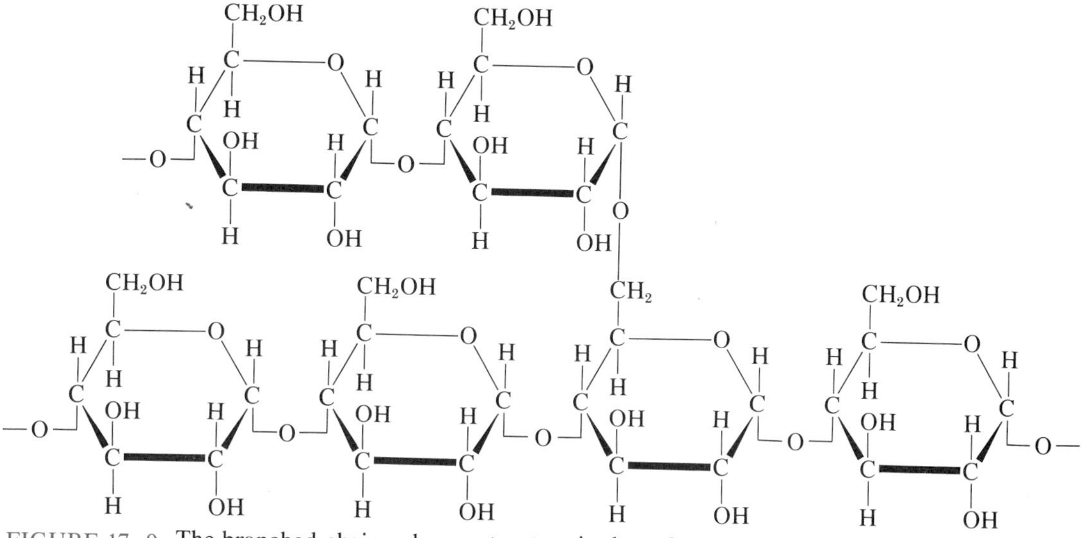

FIGURE 17–9 The branched-chain polymer structure in the polysaccharides amylopectin and glycogen.

ture common to both amylopectin and glycogen is illustrated in Figure 17–9. Glycogen is a large molecule whose molecular weight may exceed 5 million amu. When glucose is needed to maintain the normal sugar content of the blood, the glycogen stored in the liver is readily hydrolyzed to glucose. Another way to illustrate the glycogen molecule is shown in Figure 17–10, where each glucose unit is represented by a small circle.

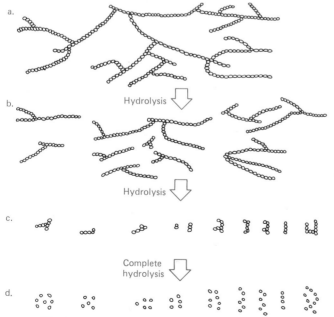

FIGURE 17–10 The hydrolysis of a branched-chain polysaccharide, such as glycogen. Each ring represents a glucose monomer unit. The polymer (a) breaks down into dextrins (b), which continue decomposing into oligosaccharides (c), which finally hydrolyze to yield D-glucose (d), which can be used by the body.

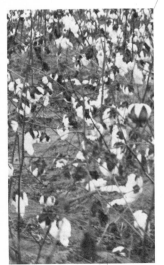

A field of cotton ready to be picked so that the cellulose it contains can be woven into clothing.

According to some recent research, cellulose from corn stalks and grass may be dissolved in a special solvent (cadmium oxide in 28% aqueous ethylenediamine). When enzymes from certain bacteria are added to the solution, 99% of the cellulose is hydrolysed to glucose. This process might become very important in finding ways to increase the world's food supply.

Cellulose

Cellulose is the polysaccharide that provides the supporting structure of trees and plants. It is composed of a straight-chain polymer of glucose units similar to that described earlier for amylose. The major difference concerns the linkage of the glucose units, which is C-1-alpha in amylose and C-1-beta in cellulose. A portion of a chain is shown in Figure 17–8.

Cellulose is insoluble in water, will not reduce Benedict's solution, and is not attacked by enzymes present in the human digestion tract. Ruminants, such as the cow, can use cellulose for food, since bacteria in the rumen (the first of four stomachs) have an enzyme called cellulase, which hydrolyzes cellulose to glucose. The molecular weight of cellulose in different species of trees and plants has been estimated to range from 50 000 to 2.5 million amu, which is equivalent to 300 to 15 000 glucose units.

Mixed polysaccharides

From our discussion of polysaccharides, it may appear that only those with glucose units joined by C-1-alpha linkages are of interest to the body. Mixed polysaccharides such as heparin, hyaluronic acid, and chondroitin sulfate are physiologically important molecules that also deserve a brief discussion.

Heparin prevents the clotting of blood by blocking the conversion of prothrombin to thrombin. Prothrombin is always present in the blood, but when it is changed to thrombin, the thrombin acts as a catalyst in converting plasma fibringen into the fibrin clot. The structure of heparin varies but we know it contains a repeating unit of glucuronic acid linked to glucosamine, with sulfate groups on some of the hydroxyl and amino groups.

Hyaluronic acid is a polysaccharide found in body tissues. It is sometimes called a mucopolysaccharide (from mucous tissue). It is an essential component of the intercellular "cement" of connective tissue. It has a high viscosity and a molecular weight in the millions. The molecule consists of repeating units of glucuronic acid and N-acetyl-glucosamine (glucosamine with an acetyl group on the —NH₂ group) joined in a C-1-beta linkage.

Chondroitin sulfates are polysaccharides found in the cartilage of mammals. Chondroitin sulfate is similar in structure to hyaluronic acid, except that galactosamine replaces the N-acetyl-glucosamine.

SELF-CHECK

17.13) Which two polysaccharides contain branched chains of glucose monomers?

17.14) Name one polysaccharide in which you find only the C-1-alpha linkage and one in which you find only the C-1-beta linkage.

CHAPTER SEVENTEEN IN REVIEW ■ Carbohydrates

17.1 TYPES OF CARBOHYDRATES   **Page 488**

17A: Draw a structural formula for a triose and a hexose.

17B: Describe what is shown in a projection formula, a perspective formula, and a Haworth structure of an organic molecule.

17C: Given a Haworth structure for the ring form of a hexose, state whether the compound is the alpha or the beta form.

GLOSSARY FOR CHAPTER SEVENTEEN

acetal linkage The bonding between the aldehyde group of one sugar and the hydroxy or ketone group of a second sugar, as in disaccharides or polysaccharides. (p. 501)

aldose A simple sugar (monosaccharide) containing an aldehyde (—CHO) group. (p. 489)

Benedict's Test A color test for a *reducing* sugar which uses a solution of complexed Cu^{2+} cation; a positive test gives a red precipitate of Cu_2O; sucrose is the only common mono- or disaccharide that will not give a positive test. (p. 498)

chiral or asymmetric carbon A carbon atom having four different atoms or groups of atoms attached to it, giving rise to the possibility of optical isomers. (p. 495)

disaccharide A carbohydrate, such as sucrose, lactose, or maltose, made up of two monosaccharides joined by an acetal linkage. (p. 490)

glucopyranose The ring (cyclic) structure of glucose. (p. 491)

hexose A monosaccharide containing six carbon atoms. (p. 490)

ketose A monosaccharide containing a ketone (—C=O) group. (p. 489)

monosaccharide A simple sugar with one carbonyl group and one carbon chain or ring; normally has up to six carbons, such as glucose. (p. 490)

optical activity The property of rotation of the plane of polarized light by an *optical isomer* of a compound containing a *chiral* carbon atom. (p. 495)

polarimeter An instrument used to measure the direction and degree of optical rotation. (p. 495)

polysaccharide A carbohydrate polymer made up of monosaccharide units joined by acetal linkages. (p. 490)

racemic mixture A mixture containing equal amounts of two optically active forms of a compound, resulting in overall optical inactivity. (p. 497)

reducing sugar A carbohydrate containing free carbonyl groups capable of reducing metal ions such as Cu^{2+} and Ag^+. (p. 499)

QUESTIONS AND PROBLEMS FOR CHAPTER SEVENTEEN ■ Carbohydrates

SECTION 17.1 TYPES OF CARBOHYDRATES

17.15) Are glyceraldehyde and di-hydroxyacetone aldoses or ketoses? trioses or hexoses?

17.16) Draw a ball-and-stick model of glyceraldehyde.

17.17) In the Haworth structure of glucose, how could you recognize the D form?

SECTION 17.2 OPTICAL ACTIVITY

17.18) Draw ball-and-stick models of the two optical isomers of glyc-eraldehyde. How do they differ?

17.19) How could you distinguish between L- and D-lactic acid using a polarimeter?

17.20*) A racemic mixture of as-paragine tastes sweet to most people. Explain why.

SECTION 17.3 REACTIONS OF CARBOHYDRATES

17.21) What form of glucose is responsible for its action as a re-ducing sugar?

17.22*) Draw the structure of β-ethyl glucoside. What type of compound is this?

SECTION 17.4 DISACCHARIDES

17.23) Describe the acetal linkage between two molecules of β-D-glucose to form a disaccharide.

17.24) How would you join two molecules of α-D-glucose so that the disaccharide will not reduce Bene-dict's solution?

SECTION 17.5 POLYSACCHARIDES

17.25) Describe the two types of polysaccharides in starch.

17.26) What is the essential dif-ference between the structure of starch and that of cellulose?

17.27) Give an example of a hexose that is a ketose and of one that is an aldose.

17.28) Draw the projection formula for the model in Question 17.16.

17.29) How does α-D-glucose differ from β-D-glucose?

17.30) Encircle the chiral carbons in the two structures in Question 17.18.

17.31) Would a racemic mixture of L- and D-lactic acid rotate the plane of polarized light? Explain.

17.32*) An industrial chemist of-fered a food processor a large quan-tity of D-monosodium glutamate at a very low price. Was it a bargain?

17.33) Would α-D-ribofuranose re-duce Benedict's solution? Explain.

17.34*) Draw the structure of α-D-glucose-1,6-diphosphate.

17.35) Draw an acetal linkage be-tween α-D-glucose and β-D-galac-tose.

17.36) Join α-D-glucose and β-D-fructose by an acetal linkage to pro-duce a disaccharide that will reduce Benedict's solution.

17.37) How do the α-1,6 linkages affect the shape of a polysaccharide molecule?

17.38) Starch can be hydrolyzed by enzymes. What products might re-sult from this treatment?

17.39*) With circles representing glucose units, draw a small portion of the glycogen molecule with α-1,6 linkages every six glucose units.

17.40*) Draw the Haworth structure of α-D-glucuronic acid-2-sulfate.

Lipids and Cell Membranes

In Figure 1–4 on p. 8 are shown four organic compounds found in the human body. Glucose, a carbohydrate, was discussed in Chapter 17. Alanine, an amino acid, is typical of the compounds that will be discussed in Chapter 19. The remaining two compounds , tristearin and cholesterol, are *lipids* or *fats*. Lipids are characterized by long chains of carbon atoms which make them relatively insoluble in water. Since much of the biochemistry of the human body takes place in water solution, much of lipid chemistry involves the way the body builds boundaries between lipid and aqueous regions.

Such boundaries are created by *membranes*, which enclose cells as well as the small organs (organelles) that function inside cells. If the membrane were soluble in water, the cell wall would disappear! Membranes are therefore composed of lipids, including particular molecules called *phospholipids.*

In order to absorb a lipid (as in digestion), the body must find a way to make one end of the lipid molecule soluble in water. This requires emulsifying agents (Section 12.1) such as bile salts (Section 18.4). The fats must be broken down, often to *fatty acids* (Section 9.5), the simplest lipids, which we will discuss in this chapter.

Among the more complex lipids that are important to the body, we will stress the role of the *steroids,* such as cholesterol, which are polycyclic compounds that act as hormones and fill other roles in human biochemistry.

Lipids are animal or plant substances that will dissolve in nonpolar solvents, such as acetone, diethyl ether, or benzene. Similar properties are shown by long-chain hydrocarbons.

18.1 MAJOR TYPES OF SIMPLE LIPIDS

LEARNING GOAL 18A: *Draw the structural formula for a given unsaturated fatty acid.*

18B: *Distinguish between a fat and a wax.*

Lipids are compounds that are familiar to us as vegetable oils in plants and seeds and as solid fats (lard, chicken fat) in animals and humans. Often to our dismay, we find that fatty foods contain more calories per gram than proteins or carbohydrates do and that poor dietary habits may lead to a bulging waistline. On the other hand, consumption of lipids in moderation is required for good nutrition. The detailed manner in which the body breaks down food lipids into raw materials and then converts some of these materials to energy and others to body lipids will be discussed in Chapter 26.

Lipids provide the most important means for long-term energy storage in the body. Fat deposits also help insulate the vital organs against shock and temperature change.

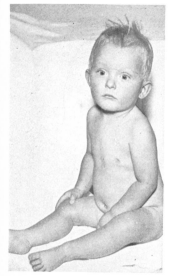

Linoleic acid is essential in the diet. The upper photo shows a six-month-old infant who had eczema that was very resistant to treatment. The lower photo shows the same child six months later, after a source of linoleic acid had been included in the diet. (Courtesy of A. E. Hansen)

TABLE 18–1   SOME NATURALLY OCCURRING FATTY ACIDS

Name	Formula	Number of Carbon Atoms	Position of Double Bonds	Common Source
Saturated				
Butyric	C_3H_7COOH	4		Butter fat
Caproic	$C_5H_{11}COOH$	6		Butter fat
Caprylic	$C_7H_{15}COOH$	8		Coconut oil
Capric	$C_9H_{19}COOH$	10		Palm kernel oil
Lauric	$C_{11}H_{23}COOH$	12		Coconut oil
Myristic	$C_{13}H_{27}COOH$	14		Nutmeg oil
Palmitic	$C_{15}H_{31}COOH$	16		Animal and vegetable fats
Stearic	$C_{17}H_{35}COOH$	18		Animal and vegetable fats
Arachidic	$C_{19}H_{39}COOH$	20		Peanut oil
Unsaturated				
Palmitoleic (1 =)*	$C_{15}H_{29}COOH$	16	Δ9†	Butter fat
Oleic (1 =)	$C_{17}H_{33}COOH$	18	Δ9	Olive oil
Linoleic (2 =)	$C_{17}H_{31}COOH$	18	Δ9, 12	Linseed oil
Linolenic (3 =)	$C_{17}H_{29}COOH$	18	Δ9, 12, 15	Linseed oil
Arachidonic (4 =)	$C_{19}H_{31}COOH$	20	Δ5, 8, 11, 14	Lecithin

* Number of double bonds.

† Δ9 indicates a double bond between carbons 9 and 10, Δ12 between carbons 12 and 13, and so forth.

Lipids generally contain five elements: carbon, hydrogen, oxygen, and (less frequently) nitrogen and phosphorus. There are several types of lipids containing a variety of functional groups.

We will begin our discussion with the simplest lipid units, the fatty acids and glycerol, and see how they are combined to make fats.

Fatty acids

You have already seen some of the shorter-chain members of the carboxylic acid family in Chapters 9 and 13. Fatty acids are like acetic acid, CH_3COOH, except that the carbon chain contains not 2 carbon atoms but 4, 6, 8, 10, or—more commonly—16, 18, or 20 carbon atoms. It helps to remember that almost all fatty acids have continuous (unbranched) chains and have an *even* number of carbon atoms in each molecule. They may be saturated or unsaturated, as shown in Table 18–1.

In the series of saturated fatty acids (no double bonds) shown in Table 18–1, those up to and including the ten-carbon *capric acid* are liquids at room temperature and have objectionable odors. *Butyric acid,* in fact, is present in body odor and in rancid butter. The melting point of the fatty acids increases with increasing length of the carbon chain (thus greater dispersion forces, Section 11.3).

The more important saturated fatty acids are *palmitic* (16-carbon) and *stearic* (18-carbon) acids, which are waxy solids at room temperature. These two compounds are found in most common animal fats and also in solid vegetable shortening.

Unsaturated fatty acids have lower melting points than saturated ones and are found in animal and plant oils such as liquid vegetable oil. *Oleic acid,* the most common unsaturated fatty acid, contains one double bond:

$$\underset{18}{CH_3}\underset{17}{CH_2}\underset{16}{CH_2}\underset{15}{CH_2}\underset{14}{CH_2}\underset{13}{CH_2}\underset{12}{CH_2}\underset{11}{CH_2}\underset{10}{CH}=\underset{9}{CH}\underset{8}{CH_2}\underset{7}{CH_2}\underset{6}{CH_2}\underset{5}{CH_2}\underset{4}{CH_2}\underset{3}{CH_2}\underset{2}{CH_2}\underset{1}{COOH}$$

oleic acid, $C_{17}H_{33}COOH$ ($\Delta 9$)

The symbol "$\Delta 9$" indicates that there is a double bond on carbon 9 in the molecule, counting the —COOH carbon as carbon 1.

Remember that the geometry around each carbon atom from carbons 2 to 8 and 11 to 18 is tetrahedral. The actual molecule has a zigzag shape, sometimes shown as

By drawing only lines, with each junction representing a —CH$_2$— unit, we are using the organic shorthand discussed on p. 454.

Unsaturated fatty acids show *cis-trans* isomerism (Section 7.2). The zigzag picture of oleic acid shows the bonds from carbon 8 to carbon 9 and from carbon 10 to carbon 11, both on the same (*cis*) side of the double bond. Only the *cis* configuration is found in nature, so all of the unsaturated fatty acids listed in Table 18–1 have the *cis* form.

Essential fatty acids

While most fatty acids required by the body can be synthesized from available raw materials (Chapter 26), *linoleic acid* must be included in the diet or poor growth and skin problems may result. There is insufficient evidence to call *linolenic acid* a dietary essential. Metabolically, the most important fatty acid seems to be *arachidonic acid*. These three vital lipids, the bottom three compounds in Table 18–1, are *poly*unsaturated. The double bonds are uniformly spaced at three-carbon intervals:

$$\underset{18}{CH_3}\underset{17}{CH_2}\underset{16}{CH_2}\underset{15}{CH_2}\underset{14}{CH_2}\underset{13}{CH}=\underset{12}{CH}\underset{11}{CH_2}\underset{10}{CH}=\underset{9}{CH}\underset{8}{CH_2}\underset{7}{CH_2}\underset{6}{CH_2}\underset{5}{CH_2}\underset{4}{CH_2}\underset{3}{CH_2}\underset{2}{CH_2}\underset{1}{C}\overset{O}{\underset{OH}{\diagup}}$$

linoleic acid ($C_{18}\Delta_{9,12}$)

$$\underset{18}{CH_3}\underset{17}{CH_2}\underset{16}{CH}=\underset{15}{CH}\underset{14}{CH_2}\underset{13}{CH}=\underset{12}{CH}\underset{11}{CH_2}\underset{10}{CH}=\underset{9}{CH}\underset{8}{CH_2}\underset{7}{CH_2}\underset{6}{CH_2}\underset{5}{CH_2}\underset{4}{CH_2}\underset{3}{CH_2}\underset{2}{CH_2}\underset{1}{C}\overset{O}{\underset{OH}{\diagup}}$$

linolenic acid ($C_{18}\Delta_{9,12,15}$)

$$\underset{20}{CH_3}\underset{19}{CH_2}\underset{18}{CH_2}\underset{17}{CH_2}\underset{16}{CH_2}\underset{15}{CH}=\underset{14}{CH}\underset{13}{CH_2}\underset{12}{CH}=\underset{11}{CH}\underset{10}{CH_2}\underset{9}{CH}=\underset{8}{CH}\underset{7}{CH_2}\underset{6}{CH}=\underset{5}{CH}\underset{4}{CH_2}\underset{3}{CH_2}\underset{2}{CH_2}\underset{1}{C}\overset{O}{\underset{OH}{\diagup}}$$

arachidonic acid ($C_{20}\Delta_{5,8,11,14}$)

The *prostaglandins* are fatty acids containing a ring. They were first described in the 1930's by Ulf von Euler, a Swedish chemist. They have been found in human semen and the prostate gland but apparently also have very important roles in the cell. They seem to have an effect on blood pressure and temperature, relaxation and contraction of smooth muscles, such as those of the uterus, and other body functions. Of the more than a dozen prostaglandins known, one example is

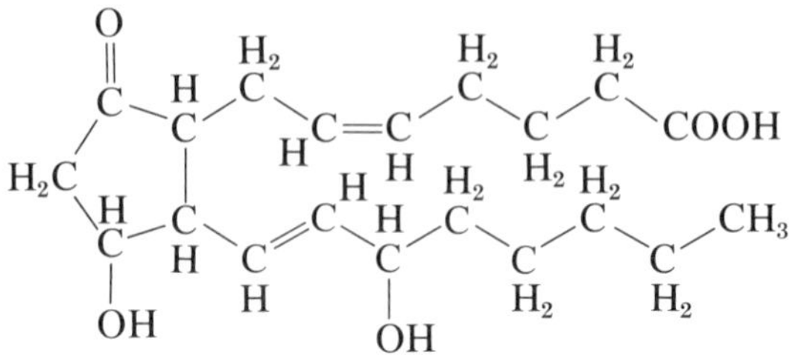

prostaglandin E$_2$

This compound contains exactly the same number of carbon atoms (20) as arachidonic acid and is presumed to be synthesized in the body from that acid. The relationship can be more clearly seen if we draw only the carbon skeleton of each molecule, curling the arachidonic acid chain around:

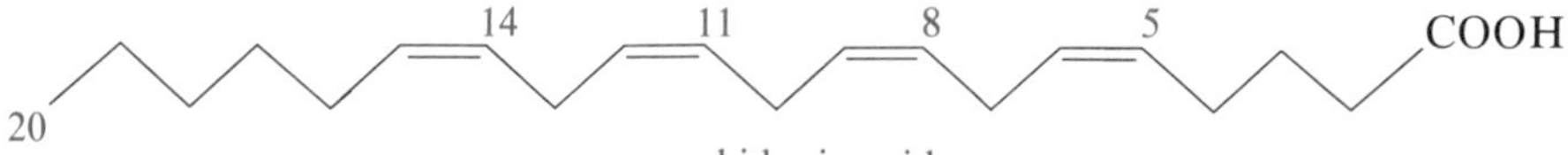

arachidonic acid

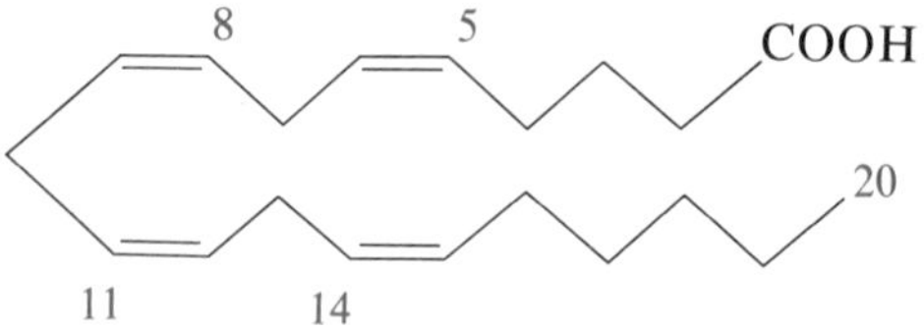

arachidonic acid

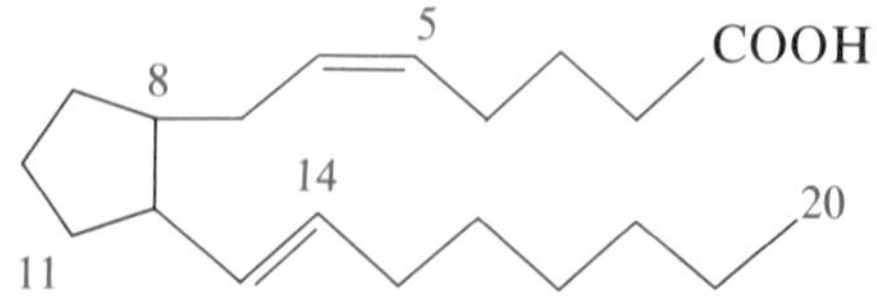

prostaglandin E$_2$

A major reason for the necessity of polyunsaturated fatty acids in the human diet may be the fact that arachidonic acid is formed in the body from linoleic acid.

Fats

Once commonly called *triglycerides*, fats are now officially known as *triacylglycerols*. Both terms should be learned. The term "acyl" refers to a carboxylic acid unit (RCOO—) in an ester.

A **fat** or **triacylglycerol** (sometimes called a **triglyceride**) is a triester combining three molecules of fatty acid(s) with one molecule of the triol *glycerol*. For example, *tristearin* (Figure 1–4) is formed from glycerol and stearic acid:

$$
\begin{array}{c}
\mathrm{H} \\
| \\
\mathrm{H{-}C{-}OH} \\
| \\
\mathrm{H{-}C{-}OH} \\
| \\
\mathrm{H{-}C{-}OH} \\
| \\
\mathrm{H}
\end{array}
\;+\;
\begin{array}{c}
\mathrm{O} \\
\| \\
\mathrm{HO{-}C{-}C_{17}H_{35}} \\
\mathrm{O} \\
\| \\
\mathrm{HO{-}C{-}C_{17}H_{35}} \\
\mathrm{O} \\
\| \\
\mathrm{HO{-}C{-}C_{17}H_{35}}
\end{array}
\;\longrightarrow\;
\begin{array}{c}
\mathrm{H} \qquad \mathrm{O} \\
| \qquad \| \\
\mathrm{H{-}C{-}O{-}C{-}C_{17}H_{35}} \\
| \qquad \mathrm{O} \\
| \qquad \| \\
\mathrm{H{-}C{-}O{-}C{-}C_{17}H_{35}} \;+\; 3\ \mathrm{H_2O} \\
| \qquad \mathrm{O} \\
| \qquad \| \\
\mathrm{H{-}C{-}O{-}C{-}C_{17}H_{35}} \\
| \\
\mathrm{H}
\end{array}
$$

| glycerol | 3 molecules of stearic acid | tristearin, a fat |

Tristearin is a *simple* triacylglycerol because the three fatty acid molecules are identical. Other examples of simple glycerides include *tripalmitin* (three palmitic acid + glycerol) and *triolein* (three oleic acid + glycerol).

In most naturally occurring fats, different fatty acid units are found in the same molecule. These are called *mixed* triacylglycerols and usually involve both saturated and unsaturated fatty acids.

The fats we have described are *neutral* lipids since their molecules are not charged. Fatty acids present in body fluids (pH = 7.4) are ionized to the carboxylate *anions*, which permits the —COO⁻ end to situate itself in the water solution and dissolve. In order to dissolve a fat in water, it is thus necessary to hydrolyze the ester linkages.

Beef fat, mutton fat, lard, and butter are common examples of mixed triacylglycerols in which saturated fatty acids predominate. These fats are solid at room temperature. Butter is easily distinguished from other animal fats by its relatively high content of short-chain fatty acid units.

Triacylglycerols that are found in plants usually exist as **oils,** which indicates a high degree of unsaturation. Table 18–2 shows the typical content of some common fats.

Coconut oil, like butter fat, contains a relatively high percentage of

TABLE 18–2 PROPORTIONS OF SATURATED AND UNSATURATED FATTY ACID UNITS IN COMMON DIETARY FATS

Fat	Per Cent of Total Fatty Acids by Weight		
	*Saturated**	*Monounsaturated*	*Polyunsaturated*
Coconut oil	93	6	1
Corn oil	14	29	57
Cottonseed oil	26	22	52
Lard	44	46	10
Olive oil	15	73	12
Palm oil	57	36	7
Peanut oil	21	49	30
Safflower oil	10	14	76
Soybean oil	14	24	62
Sunflower oil	11	19	70

Natural lipids may vary in fatty acid composition, depending on biological conditions. Just as the motor oil you put in your car in the summer is more viscous than that needed in the winter, linseed oils collected from plants in warm climates are more viscous (more highly saturated) than those collected in cold climates. Lard from corn-fed hogs is more highly saturated than that from peanut-fed animals.

* *Saturated* means no carbon-carbon double bonds; *monounsaturated* means one carbon-carbon double bond per fatty acid molecule; *polyunsaturated* means two or more carbon-carbon double bonds per fatty acid molecule. The chief unsaturated fatty acid is linoleic acid. Although derived from vegetable rather than animal fats, both coconut oil and peanut oil have been associated recently with hardening of the arteries when combined with a high cholesterol intake.

Vegetable oils are esters, but *mineral* oils are high-molecular-weight hydrocarbons, mainly alkanes, such as those in petroleum. The similarities between the two types of oils are great, since both contain long hydrocarbon chains. The longer-chain alkanes are solids at room temperature. They are called "paraffin" and resemble biological waxes, even to their possible use as candle wax.

short-chain fatty acids. This permits the oil to remain liquid at room temperature (but just barely!) despite its high saturated-acid content. We can thus see that longer carbon chains lead to higher melting points and to solids. The presence of polyunsaturated fatty acids, such as oleic and linoleic acids, leads to compounds with lower melting points, usually liquids at room temperature.

Waxes

A **wax** is a simple ester that combines a fatty acid with a very long carbon chain with an alcohol of very high molecular weight. The alcohol contains only one —OH group, rather than the three in glycerol. The fatty acid molecule and the alcohol molecule each contains from 24 to 36 carbon atoms.

Waxes are solids because of their long carbon chains. They may form protective, waterproof coatings on the skin and fur of animals and on the feathers of birds. Naturally occurring waxes that have commercial uses are *beeswax, lanolin* (from wool), *spermaceti* (from the sperm whale), and *carnauba wax* (from a wax palm tree). Lanolin is widely used as a base for medical ointments and creams. Spermaceti is used in cosmetics, some pharmaceutical products, and candles. Carnauba wax is widely used in floor, furniture, and automobile polishes.

SELF-CHECK

18.1)   Write the structural formula of any unsaturated fatty acid that contains one double bond and 16 carbon atoms. Your formula does not have to match a compound in Table 18–1.
18.2)   How does the chemical composition of a fat differ from that of a wax?

18.2 REACTIONS OF FATS

LEARNING GOAL 18C: Explain the possible relationship between hydrogenation of vegetable oils in our diet and human health.
          18D: Describe the difference between acid hydrolysis and saponification of a fat.

A fat can undergo any of the reactions normally associated with its functional groups (for example, the double bonds in an unsaturated fat can be hydrogenated as in Section 7.2). A fat can be hydrolyzed to its fatty acid and glycerol components. The glycerol can then be dehydrated and oxidized to form an unsaturated aldehyde called *acrolein*, $CH_2\!\!=\!\!CHCHO$. Acrolein vapors have a very sharp odor and can make your eyes tear. The formation of acrolein can thus be used as a test for fats.

Hydrogenation

We have just seen that the main difference between oils and fats lies in the number of unsaturated fatty acid units in one molecule. Vegetable oils may thus be converted to solid shortening by *hydrogenation*, the addition of hydrogen to the double bond, which results in solid margarine, Crisco, Spry, and other products.

Certain natural oils, such as coconut oils, and hydrogenated vegetable oils, such as solid margarine, are **saturated fats.** Such fats are thought to increase the risk of circulatory disease in some individuals by the formation of plaques (plugs) in arteries. The formation of these plaques is related to the level of cholesterol in the blood.

Since degree of hydrogenation can be controlled, the food industry now produces soft margarines and cooking oils that are high in *polyunsaturated* fatty acid units. This may help reduce the present very high level of heart disease in developed countries.

As a side effect, hydrogenation of vegetable oils tends to convert some of the naturally *cis* double bonds to *trans* positions. While the body can use *trans* fatty acids, there may be a relationship between these compounds and atherosclerosis. Food companies are thus seeking ways to harden vegetable oils without creating *trans* fatty acids.

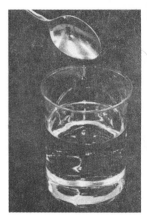

Rancidity

You may have noticed that some fats develop an unpleasant odor and taste when allowed to stand in contact with air at room temperature. This **rancidity** (spoiling) may be *hydrolytic* (due to hydrolysis) or *oxidative* (due to oxidation).

Hydrolytic changes are the result of food enzymes or bacteria hydrolyzing the fat to glycerol and free fatty acids. If these acids are of the short-chain variety, such as butyric acid, there will be an obnoxious odor and taste, as in rancid butter.

The most common type of rancidity is oxidative, with the formation of peroxides and eventually of aldehydes, ketones, and carboxylic acids by oxidation of the double bonds. Heat, light, moisture, and exposure to air all speed up the oxidation process. It is important to prevent rancidity of the lard and vegetable shortenings used in making crackers, pretzels, pastries, and similar food products. Modern packaging often has antioxidants such as BHT or propyl gallate added to the waxed paper liner or in some cases to the food. The formation of peroxides involves *free radicals* (Section 16.2). These antioxidants react with free radicals and stop the oxidation process. Certain natural products, such as ascorbic acid (Vitamin C) and lecithin, may be used for the same purpose.

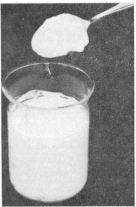

Fats can be obtained by hydrogenation of the double bonds in vegetable oils. The beaker in the top photo contains clear oil before hydrogenation. Below, the same oil is shown hardened by hydrogenation. (Courtesy Procter and Gamble)

Pure fats are colorless, odorless, and tasteless. Any tastes or odors you find in oils or waxes are due to dissolved impurities or oxidation products. Note that hydrocarbon (mineral) oils and waxes will generally be highly saturated and are thus less likely to be oxidized.

Saponification

In the laboratory, fats may be hydrolyzed to glycerol and free fatty acids (a) by acids, producing the carboxylic acids; (b) by superheated steam, with the same result; and (c) by bases, producing the salts of the carboxylate anions of the fatty acids. Acid hydrolysis with superheated steam is used to convert waste fats to a cheap source of glycerol for the manufacture of explosives (such as nitroglycerine) and pharmaceuticals.

Basic hydrolysis is usually carried out in an alcohol solution of NaOH or KOH and produces the sodium or potassium salt of the fatty acid, called a *soap:*

In the body, enzymes called *lipase* **(Chapter 26) act to speed up the hydrolysis of food lipids in the digestive system.**

OH

$(CH_3)_3C$ — ⬡ — $C(CH_3)_3$

CH$_3$

BHT

HO — ⬡ — OH

OH ... OH

$COCH_2CH_2CH_3$
‖
O

propyl gallate

$$\underset{\text{tristearin}}{\begin{array}{l} CH_2-O-\overset{\overset{\displaystyle O}{\|}}{C}-C_{17}H_{35} \\ CH-O-\overset{\overset{\displaystyle O}{\|}}{C}-C_{17}H_{35} \\ CH_2-O-\overset{\overset{\displaystyle O}{\|}}{C}-C_{17}H_{35} \end{array}} + 3\ NaOH \longrightarrow \underset{\text{glycerol}}{\begin{array}{l} CH_2OH \\ CHOH \\ CH_2OH \end{array}} + \underset{\substack{\text{sodium stearate} \\ \text{(soap)}}}{3\ C_{17}H_{35}\overset{\overset{\displaystyle O}{\|}}{C}-ONa}$$

This process, called *saponification,* was briefly discussed in Section 9.5. Sodium salts of fatty acids produce hard soaps, such as those used in the home. Potassium salts are found in soft soaps, such as the "tincture of green soap" used in hospitals.

Analysis of lipids

The *saponification number* is the number of milligrams of KOH required to saponify (turn to soap) 1.00 gram of a fat. The highest values (215 to 235 for butter) indicate shorter-chain fatty acids.

The actual compound used to add to the double bonds is IBr, iodine bromide.

The determination of the composition of a given fat or wax was a very difficult process for many years. Sometimes a factor called the *saponification number* is used to help roughly estimate the molecular weight of the lipid. This number is a relative measure of the amount of strong base required to saponify a known weight of fat.

The addition of I_2 to a double bond (Section 7.2) is used to find the degree of unsaturation of a fat. The *iodine number* is defined as the number of grams of iodine that would be absorbed by 100 grams of fat or oil. For linoleic acid, the iodine number is 181. A high iodine number indicates a high degree of unsaturation.

Although the iodine number is sometimes still used, thin layer and gas-liquid *chromatography* are currently the favored methods for finding out exactly what is present in a lipid.

Chromatography

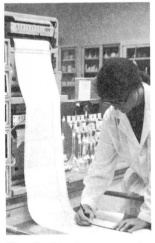

Gas liquid chromatography is a technique commonly used to detect trace amounts of substances. This particular apparatus is analyzing a lipid sample for traces of pesticides. (Photograph by Donald D. Dechert, Food and Drug Administration Laboratories, Los Angeles)

Most chromatography methods are based on the fact that different solutes tend to have different solubilities in a common solvent. The solvent is first mixed with several solutes. The solution then *moves* through a tube, up along a plate or piece of paper, or down through a column. The solute that is most soluble in the solvent will "stay with" the solvent, while those that are less soluble will "lag behind" the solvent front. The result is *fractionation,* or separation of the various solutes. The rate of passage through a chromatography column or plate may be a simple measure of molecular weight or it may be related to the intermolecular forces of the various solutes and the solvent(s). Such techniques are now used for analysis of all kinds of organic and biochemical substances and will be discussed again in Chapter 19 in relation to the separation of the amino acids of a protein.

Gas-liquid chromatography is a recently developed tool of the lipid chemist. Any substance that is volatile (evaporates easily), like simple alcohols and ketones, or can be made into a volatile derivative (for example, fatty acids converted to their methyl esters) can be separated and analyzed by this technique. The fatty acid derivatives dissolved in a nonpolar solvent are injected into a heated column that contains a nonvolatile liquid like ethylene glycol. Helium gas is passed through the column carrying the volatile derivatives to a detection device. Both chain length and degree of unsaturation of the methyl esters influence their rate of passage through the column. The detection device, often a hydrogen flame, is sensitive to ionization and structural differences and records these differences as peaks on a recorder chart (Figure 18–1). In a similar technique, the inert gas is replaced by a liquid in which the components to be analyzed are dissolved and the liquid is forced through the column

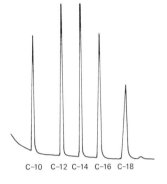

FIGURE 18–1   Fatty acids can be separated according to chain length by gas-liquid chromatography.

C–10   C–12   C–14   C–16   C–18

under a high pressure. This is known as *high-pressure liquid chromatography* (HPLC). Many compounds of physiological importance are now being analyzed by HPLC.

SELF-CHECK

18.3)   What is a possible health advantage to using cooking oils and soft margarine instead of solid fats?
18.4)   How do the products of the acid hydrolysis and base hydrolysis of a fat differ from each other?

18.3 PHOSPHOLIPIDS AND CELL MEMBRANES

LEARNING GOAL 18E: *Distinguish a phospholipid from a fat.*
                                18F: *Describe the most accepted model of a cell membrane.*

The **phospholipids** are found in brain and nerve tissue and are important compounds in cell membranes. They are made from glycerol and fatty acids (the two components of fats) plus phosphoric acid (H_3PO_4) and one of several nitrogen-containing compounds. Some may be considered derivatives of glycerol phosphate, an ester formed by an alcohol and phosphoric acid:

$$
\begin{array}{c}
H \\
| \\
H-C-OH \\
| \\
H-C-OH \\
| \\
H-C-OH \\
| \\
H
\end{array}
\;+\;
\begin{array}{c}
O \\
\| \\
HO-P-OH \\
| \\
OH
\end{array}
\longrightarrow
\begin{array}{c}
H \\
| \\
H-C-OH \\
| \\
H-C-OH \\
| \\
H-C-O-P-OH \\
| \;\;\;\;\; \| \\
H \;\;\;\; OH
\end{array}
\;+\; H_2O
$$

glycerol   phosphoric acid   glycerol phosphate

Similar linkages will be seen frequently in biochemistry, especially in the "high-energy" compounds like ATP and ADP, which provide energy for cell reactions (Section 22.1). *Phosphate group transfer* (the gain or loss of a $PO_4{}^{3-}$ with several hydrogens) is seen here in its simplest form.

If two fatty acids join with glycerol phosphate, the product is *phosphatidic acid,* shown here in the form of its 1- anion, the species commonly found in the body at pH = 7.4:

$$
\begin{array}{c}
\quad\quad\quad\quad\quad\quad\quad\quad\quad O \\
\quad\quad\quad\quad\quad\quad\quad\quad\quad \| \\
O \quad\quad\quad CH_2-O-C-R \\
\| \quad\quad\quad\quad | \\
R-C-O-CH \quad\quad\quad O \\
\quad\quad\quad\quad | \quad\quad\quad\quad \| \\
\quad\quad\quad\quad CH_2-O-P-OH \\
\quad\quad\quad\quad\quad\quad\quad\quad | \\
\quad\quad\quad\quad\quad\quad\quad\quad O^-
\end{array}
$$

L-α-phosphatidic acid

Several important phospholipids, called *phosphatides,* result when phosphatidic acid forms esters with choline or with ethanolamine and serine.

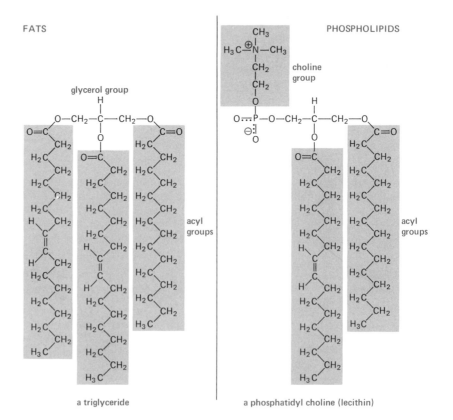

FATS   PHOSPHOLIPIDS

a triglyceride   a phosphatidyl choline (lecithin)

Choline has the formula $(CH_3)_3\overset{+}{N}CH_2CH_2OH$. It is a component of the compound *acetylcholine,* which is essential to the proper transmission of nerve impulses in the body.

FIGURE 18–2   The structure of a fat and a phospholipid. While both ends of the fat are water insoluble, the dipolar-ion end of the phospholipid is soluble in aqueous solutions. Note that there is a double nonpolar tail in lecithin; this will be important in our discussion of cell membranes. The three fatty acid units in the triacylglycerol (triglyceride) shown are from different compounds, as is usual in nature.

Lecithins

Choline is a quaternary ammonium compound (p. 394). When it reacts with phosphatidic acid, we obtain a lecithin, as shown in Figure 18-2.

The **lecithins** are used in the transport of fats from one tissue to another and in the structure and function of cell membranes. Notice that the fatty acid parts of the molecule are soluble only in nonpolar solvents, but the choline end is charged (a negative charge on the phosphate group and a positive charge on the nitrogen) and thus soluble in water. With a water-soluble "head" and two fat-soluble "tails," molecules like lecithin play vital roles in cell membranes.

Lecithin may be obtained commercially from soybeans and finds wide application as an emulsifying agent (like a detergent) because of its polar/nonpolar nature. It is useful in preparing such food products as chocolate candies.

If the fatty acid unit on the central carbon of lecithin is removed by hydrolysis, the resulting compound is *lysolecithin*. The venom of snakes such as the cobra contains an enzyme that speeds up exactly this conversion. The lysolecithin then causes disintegration of red blood cells and the loss of the ability to transmit oxygen from the lungs to the cells (Chapter 24). A few insects and spiders poison by the same mechanism.

Cephalins, sphingomyelins, and cerebrosides

The **cephalins** are esters of phosphatidic acid with serine or ethanolamine:

$$
\begin{array}{l}
\quad\quad\quad\quad\quad O \\
\quad\quad\quad\quad\quad \| \\
\quad\quad CH_2-O-C-R \\
O\quad\quad | \\
\| \quad\quad | \\
R-C-O-CH\quad\quad O \\
\quad\quad | \quad\quad \| \\
\quad\quad CH_2-O-P-OR^1 \\
\quad\quad\quad\quad\quad | \\
\quad\quad\quad\quad\quad O^-
\end{array}
$$

Basic cephalin structure

For phosphatidyl serine,

R^1 is $—CH_2CHNH_2$
$\quad\quad\quad\quad\quad |$
$\quad\quad\quad\quad COOH$

For phosphatidyl ethanolamine,

R^1 is $—CH_2CH_2NH_2$

The prefix *cephalo-* means "of the head," from the Greek *kephale*. A child suffering from *hydrocephalus* has excess pressure inside the skull caused by a buildup of fluid.

The name "cephalin" comes from the fact that these phospholipids are found in the head and in spinal tissue. They play a role in the blood-clotting process.

The **sphingomyelins** are also found in large amounts in brain and nerve tissue and are important compounds inside all cells. In both sphingomyelins and cerebrosides, the triol glycerol is replaced by a long-chain unsaturated amino alcohol *sphingosine:*

$$CH_3(CH_2)_{12}CH=CHCHCHCH_2OH$$
$$\quad\quad\quad\quad\quad\quad\quad | \quad |$$
$$\quad\quad\quad\quad\quad\quad HO\quad NH_2$$

sphingosine

The *plasmalogens* are also derivatives of phosphatidyl ethanolamine and are found in the cells of brain, nerve, heart, and liver tissue. Their exact function is not known.

Cerebrosides make up 7% of the solid matter in the brain and are named from the Latin *cerebrum*, meaning "the brain." Lipids such as the cerebrosides that combine fatty acid units *with carbohydrates* are called *glycolipids*.

Ceramide is formed when a fatty acid neutralizes the basic —NH₂ group on sphingosine to make an amide. Sphingomyelin is therefore ceramide joined to phosphate and to choline:

$$CH_3(CH_2)_{12}CH=CH—CH—CH—CH_2OH$$
$$\quad\quad\quad\quad\quad\quad\quad\quad | \quad\quad |$$
$$\quad\quad\quad\quad\quad\quad\quad OH \quad NH$$
$$\quad\quad\quad\quad\quad\quad\quad\quad\quad\quad\quad |$$
$$\quad\quad\quad\quad\quad\quad\quad\quad\quad\quad\quad R$$

ceramide

$$
Ceramide—O—P—O—CH_2CH_2N(CH_3)_3
$$

with phosphate group O=P, O⁻, and N⁺

sphingomyelin

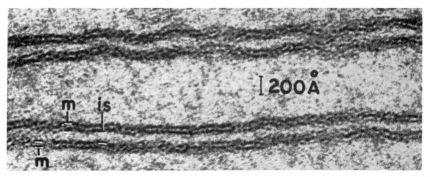

FIGURE 18–3 The cell membranes of intestinal cells are clearly shown in this electron micrograph in which all features are magnified 240 000 times. The membranes of animal, plant, and bacterial cells as well as the walls of many components inside the cell have a similar three-layer structure. The letter **m** indicates the membrane, while **is** shows the space between cells.

At least three diseases, all hereditary, involve the abnormal accumulation of certain types of lipids in the brain and other organs as a result of the absence of hydrolyzing enzymes. In Niemann-Pick disease, sphingomyelins build up in the brain, causing mental retardation and early death. In Gaucher's disease, the glycolipids contain glucose instead of galactose. In Tay-Sachs disease, glycolipids build up in the brain and eyes, usually causing death before two years of age. These diseases are called "inborn errors of metabolism" or "genetic diseases." Some of them will be discussed further in Chapter 28.

Cerebrosides differ from other phospholipids by not having phosphoric acid in their structures. They are formed by the reaction of a ceramide and a carbohydrate, such as glucose, galactose, or an amino derivative. A typical cerebroside is *kerasin:*

cerebroside

Cell membranes and the lipid bilayer

The membrane surrounding a cell determines the chemistry that will take place inside the cell in some very important ways. It permits water, nutrients, and other essential materials to enter the cell while keeping out unneeded or potentially harmful substances. It stops the loss of useful substances while encouraging the release from the cell of toxic or useless by-products of the biochemical reactions. It maintains the concentrations of all substances inside the cell at the proper levels. In addition, it may serve as a site for certain processes. Modern techniques using the electron microscope reveal the fine structure of cell membranes (Figure 18–3).

Human **cell membranes,** as well as the membranes of organelles inside the cell, typically consist of 50 to 75% proteins and glycoproteins (protein-carbohydrate combinations) and 25 to 50% lipids. Two types of lipids present in many animal cells are cholesterol and glycolipids, such as the cerebrosides. We will not be concerned here with the roles of these components.

The main lipids are the phospholipids we have just discussed: lecithins, cephalins, and sphingomyelins. What do these all have in common? **Every such molecule contains a dipolar end that is soluble in water plus one or two nonpolar hydrocarbon chains.** Look again at Figure 18–2 to see the "head plus two tails" molecular structure that we will need for our discussion of membranes.

Scientists are still not sure exactly how all of the compounds in the membrane are arranged in its three-dimensional structure. Our ideas about the molecular organization of membranes have evolved gradually as a result of research that was begun at the end of the 19th century and continues today.

When lecithin is added to water, it forms a **lipid bilayer** (Figure 18–4) that has many of the properties of actual cell membranes. The bilayer is made up of two layers of phospholipid molecules, with their water-soluble end facing the aqueous solutions outside and inside the cell and their non-polar tails hidden deep inside the membrane. It should be clear how such a membrane serves its main purpose of keeping what is *inside* the cell apart from what is *outside* the cell.

To the lipid bilayer model, we must add explanations for two facts:

1) Much of the membrane consists of protein, which is polar.
2) There has to be a way for the substances to pass through the membrane, into and out of the cell, in a highly controlled manner.

An early model for a cell membrane suggested that the core of lipid bi-

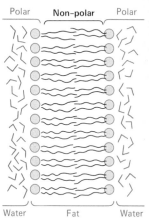

FIGURE 18–4 The lipid bilayer in a membrane. The polar ends of phospholipid molecules all face outward, providing a lipid wall to separate the contents of the cell from the external environment as well as a surface onto which proteins can be attracted.

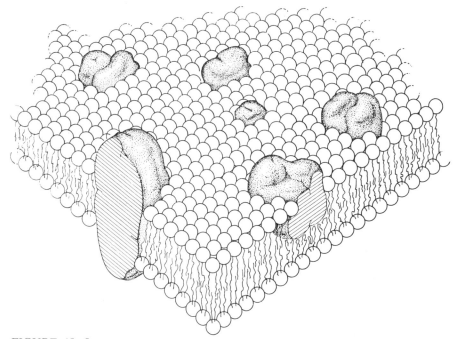

FIGURE 18–5 The fluid mosaic model of membrane structure. The large bodies are globular protein molecules, which are attached to (or through) a lipid bilayer. The pores (holes) in the membrane are not shown. (From Singer, S.J., and Nicolson, G.L., *Science,* 175: 723 [1972]. Copyright 1972 by The American Association for the Advancement of Science)

layers is coated with protein on both sides. The most modern version of this picture, the *fluid mosaic* model of S.J. Singer, was developed in 1971 and is shown in Figure 18–5. Singer's model presumes that the main wall or barrier is provided by a lipid bilayer and that proteins are attached at various places and play various roles. Some of the proteins go all the way through the bilayer and probably play a role as carriers of certain substances through the membrane. Others probably act as *enzymes,* serving as convenient "service stations" to make difficult chemical reactions proceed more easily.

The fluid mosaic model allows for wide variations in the relative amounts of proteins and lipids. It is sometimes called the "potato" model, since the globular proteins look a bit like different sizes of potatos embedded in a layer of marbles.

Passive diffusion across a membrane

The inside and outside of a membrane are exposed to aqueous solutions with different concentrations of various solutes. For example, the Na^+ ions in blood plasma are at a concentration averaging about 0.14 moles/liter. Inside a cell, the Na^+ concentration is only about 0.010 moles/liter. We call such a difference a *concentration gradient* from the region of high concentration to the region of low concentration.

The cell membrane contains small holes, or *pores,* which permit small molecules such as H_2O, O_2, CO_2, or H_2NCONH_2 (urea) as well as small ions such as Na^+ to travel across the membrane like small fish passing through a net. This process of *passive diffusion* (Figure 18–6) always occurs from a region of high concentration to a region of low concentration.

Transport across a membrane

We have just finished saying two things that seem to flatly contradict each other. The Na^+ concentration is about 0.14 M outside the cell and about 0.010 M inside the cell, yet Na^+ ions can pass freely from the outside of the cell membrane to the inside. Shouldn't the two concentrations very quickly reach identical values?

Indeed, if passive diffusion were the only factor, the two concentrations would very soon be the same. Since there is a significant biological reason for the Na^+ concentration gradient, the body must find a way to *pump* sodium cations out of the cell as fast as they stream in. Pumps require energy. Thus, metabolic reactions must provide enough energy, through coupling with the ATP/ADP mechanisms described in Chapter 22, to carry Na^+ out of the cell. One possible way this could be accomplished is shown in Figure 18–7. The same type of process keeps the K^+ concentration high in-

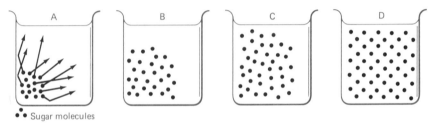

• • Sugar molecules

FIGURE 18–6 Passive diffusion. When a small lump of sugar is dropped into a glass of water, its molecules (colored circles) dissolve (A). Over a period of time, passive diffusion from regions of high sugar concentration to regions of low sugar concentration (B, C) will lead to an even distribution of sugar molecules throughout the water in the glass (D). At that point, the concentration gradient has disappeared.

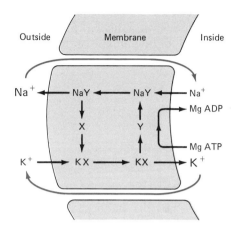

FIGURE 18–7 Active transport of Na$^+$ and K$^+$ cations across a membrane. The Na$^+$ ions flow easily through cell pores (colored arrow) from the high concentration outside the cell to the low concentration inside. The carrier Y is shown picking up the Na$^+$ and taking it back outside. The K$^+$ ions similarly diffuse through the pores to the outside of the cell and must be brought back in by the carrier X. The arrow with the MgATP shows one possible source of energy for this cell pump.

side the cell and low outside the cell (shown by large and small letters in Figure 18–7). In fact, to preserve electrical neutrality, it may often be essential for the pump, which we call *active transport,* to carry equal numbers of cations in both directions.

There are many biologically important molecules that are a bit too large to fit through the pores of the membrane. How do they get into and out of the cell? There must be a means of *facilitated diffusion,* which generally involves the proteins that pass all the way through the membrane (Figure 18–5).

For example, glucose is too large to fit through the membrane pores. To get into the cell, the glucose must first bind to a specific carrier protein on the outer surface of the cell membrane. The carrier protein might then move from one side of the membrane to the other; or it might rotate within the membrane, carrying the glucose with it (Figure 18–8); or it might even change shape in such a way as to move the section that carries the glucose to the inside of the membrane. We obviously have much to find out about the structure and function of cell membranes, but it will be a fascinating search.

There is a direct relationship between a Na$^+$ active transport system in the intestinal mucous membranes and the transport of glucose into the cells. A single carrier molecule combines with both a glucose molecule and a Na$^+$ cation and carries *both* into the cell. This more complex mechanism, called *symport,* is needed because there is more glucose inside the cell than outside it, which would make facilitated diffusion impossible.

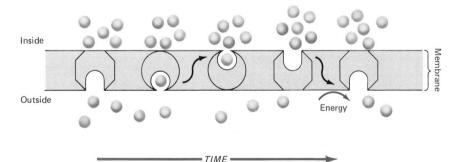

FIGURE 18–8 Protein carrier transport across a cell membrane. Only one possible manner of carrying molecules across the membrane is shown here. The carrier receives a nutrient molecule, turns, releases it on the opposite side, then returns empty for another, much like a revolving door. This specific picture shows molecules being transported *against* a concentration gradient. This requires energy from a coupled reaction (colored arrow).

SELF-CHECK

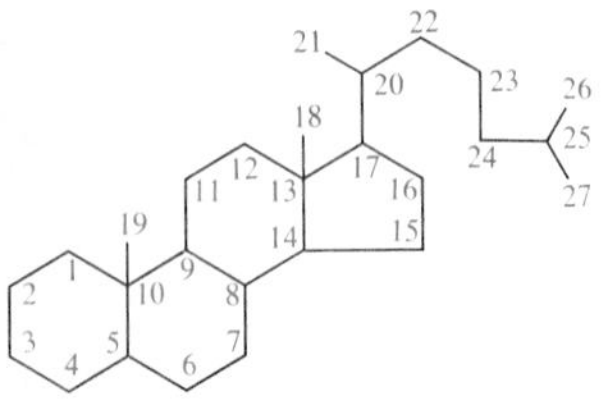

FIGURE 18–9 Steroid ring numbering system.

18.5) In what ways does a cerebroside differ from a fat?

18.6) Why must the fluid mosaic model of membrane structure accommodate the fact that some types of membranes contain a much greater proportion of proteins than others?

18.4 STEROIDS

LEARNING GOAL 18G: Recognize the steroid ring system in a given hormone.

cholesterol

The **steroids** (sterols) are special lipids in the cells and tissues that are derivatives of high-molecular-weight polycyclic alcohols. The parent cyclic hydrocarbon for all the steroids is the *sterol nucleus* or *steroid ring system* (Section 15.3). The numbering system for the carbon atoms is shown in Figure 18–9.

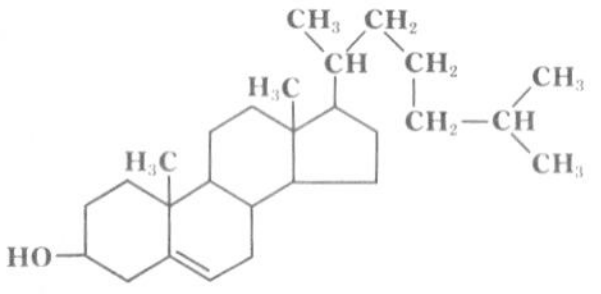

The most common steroid is **cholesterol,** which is found in brain and nerve tissue, cell membranes, and gallstones. Important points you should notice in cholesterol are the steroid ring system, the hydroxyl group at carbon 3, the unsaturation between carbons 5 and 6, the methyl groups on carbons 18 and 19, and the hydrocarbon chain starting with carbon 20. Many of the features of the cholesterol structure are also found in physiologically important derivatives of cholesterol. During the metabolism of cholesterol by the liver, the molecule is converted to bile acids—for example, *cholic acid,* which has —OH groups on the ring system at carbons 7 and 12. After carbons 25, 26, and 27 have been split off, carbon 24 is oxidized to a carboxyl group. When cholic acid combines with the amino acid glycine in a peptide linkage, a *bile salt* is formed.

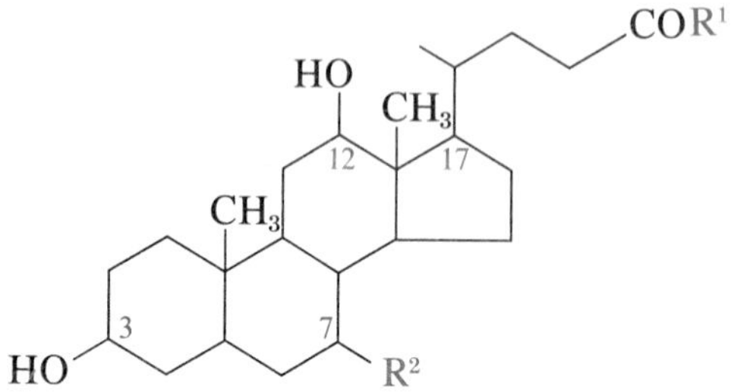

Basic structure of bile salts

cholic acid: R^1 is —OH and R^2 is —OH
deoxycholic acid: R^1 is —OH and R^2 is —H
glycocholic acid: R^1 is —NHCH$_2$COOH (glycine)
taurocholic acid: R^1 is —NHCH$_2$CH$_2$SO$_3$H (taurine)

Bile salts are detergent-like compounds that aid in the emulsification and absorption of lipids in the intestine (Chapter 26).

Steroid hormones

Hormones, such as the protein insulin, are chemical messengers that are formed in specialized glands in the body, the **endocrine glands,** and carried to other parts of the body to exert regulatory (stop and go) effects on physiological processes. The location of these endocrine glands is shown in Figure 18–10.

Adrenal hormones

The cortex (outer layer) of the adrenal gland produces a group of hormones with important physiological functions. If the adrenal cortex does not function normally, as in Addison's disease, electrolyte and water balance are abnormal. Also, the metabolism of both carbohydrates and proteins is hindered, and the individual is more sensitive to cold and stress. Typical steroid hormones of the adrenal gland are shown in Figure 18–11.

Corticosterone was the name given to the first adrenal cortical hormone identified by scientists. It is the parent compound for many members of this family of hormones. The biochemist is always interested in the relationship between the structure of a compound and its physiological activity. Corticosterone, cortisol (hydrocortisone), and aldosterone are the major hormones in the blood, with cortisol exerting the greatest effect on carbohydrate and protein metabolism and aldosterone the greatest effect on the body fluid electrolytes.

In the 1940's, *cortisone* was first tried clinically in the treatment of rheumatoid arthritis. It created excitement at the time, but it has since been replaced by steroid derivatives that have fewer negative side effects and increased therapeutic potency. *Prednisolone*, a steroid closely related to cortisol, has some of these properties. The 9-fluoro-16-methyl derivative of prednisolone is 100 to 250 times as potent as cortisone in the treatment of rheumatoid arthritis.

Female sex hormones

The female sex hormones (**estrogens**) are steroids formed in the ovaries, which are endocrine glands on either side of the pelvic cavity. The follicles and corpus luteum (yellow bodies) in the cortex of the ovary form hormones that regulate the *menstrual cycle* and function during pregnancy (Figure 18–12). Follicular hormones are also responsible for the development of the secondary sexual characteristics of females, which appear at puberty. The liquid within the follicle contains at least two hormones, estrone and estradiol (Figure 18–11). *Estrone* was the first hormone to be isolated from the follicular liquid, but *estradiol* is more potent than estrone and may be the principal hormone of the follicle. These two steroids are excreted in the urine in increased amounts during pregnancy.

The hormone produced by the corpus luteum is known as *progesterone* (upper left in Figure 18–11). The main function of progesterone is the preparation of the lining of the uterus for implantation of the fertilized ovum. If pregnancy occurs, this hormone is responsible for keeping the embryo in the uterus and for developing the mammary glands in the breasts prior to milk production. In the normal menstrual cycle, the injection of extra progesterone inhibits ovulation. In the 1950's, several laboratories attempted to make steroid pills with the properties of progesterone. *Norethindrone* and *norethynodrel*, used as the progesterone-like component of several *oral contraceptives*, resulted from these efforts. These compounds effectively stop ovulation in women. It was also discovered that when these drugs were made, they were contaminated with a small amount of estrogen. This extra estrogen apparently improved the effect of the progesterone.

A third synthetic steroid used in birth control pills is *mestranol*. Oral contraceptives ("the pill") now generally contain either norethindrone or

11-dehydro-17-hydroxycorticosterone
(compound E, cortisone)

prednisolone

9-fluoro-16-methyl prednisolone

norethindrone

norethynodrel

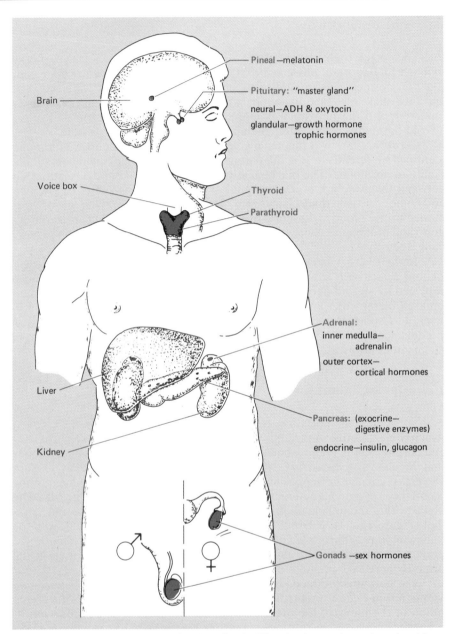

FIGURE 18–10 The human endocrine glands. The glands are shown in color. Note that the pancreas produces both digestive enzymes and hormones. Only the hormones from the gonads and the adrenal cortex are steroids. Most other hormones are proteins.

mestranol

norethynodrel and mestranol. A typical dose in early pills was 10 mg of norethynodrel and 0.15 mg mestranol. However, doctors doing studies of the long-range effects of oral contraceptives have been somewhat concerned about such side effects as nausea, dizziness, headaches, and thrombosis, the formation of clots in blood vessels. The dosage has recently been reduced,

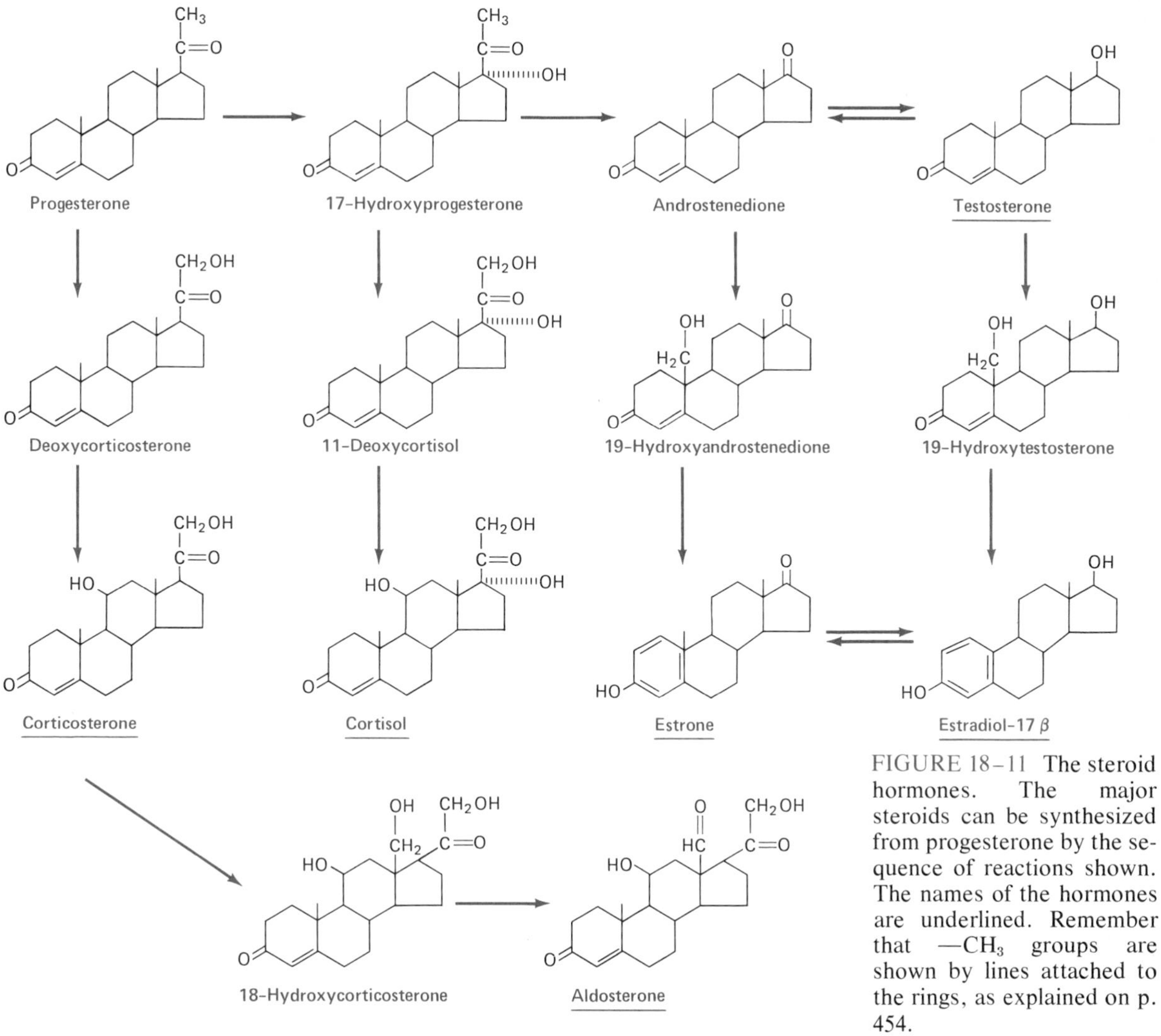

FIGURE 18–11 The steroid hormones. The major steroids can be synthesized from progesterone by the sequence of reactions shown. The names of the hormones are underlined. Remember that —CH₃ groups are shown by lines attached to the rings, as explained on p. 454.

toward a combination of 1 mg norethynodrel and 0.05 mg mestranol, as an example, to try to reduce the side effects.

Male sex hormones

The sex hormones of adult males are produced by the testes, two oval-shaped endocrine glands located in the scrotum. Spermatozoa (sperm cells), which are capable of fertilizing a mature ovum, are made in the testes. Between the cells that manufacture spermatozoa are the interstitial cells, which produce a hormone known as *testosterone* (Figure 18–11, upper right). The male sex hormones, also called **androgens,** have structures similar to the estrogens, the female sex hormones. In fact, estrogens and an-

OVARY

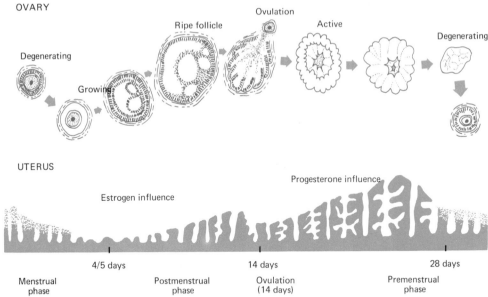

UTERUS

4/5 days		14 days	28 days
Menstrual phase	Postmenstrual phase	Ovulation (14 days)	Premenstrual phase

FIGURE 18–12 The sequence of events in the human menstrual cycle. Studies of oral contraceptives have concluded that their main effect is to inhibit the maturing of the follicle and thus prevent ovulation, the release of an egg.

drogens are found in both males and females, although the quantity of male hormones in a female or female hormones in a male is very low.

An important function of the androgens is the development of masculine sexual characteristics (deepening of the voice, growth of a beard, and distribution of body hair) at puberty. Androgens also control the function of the reproductive glands, such as the seminal vesicles, the prostate gland, and the testes.

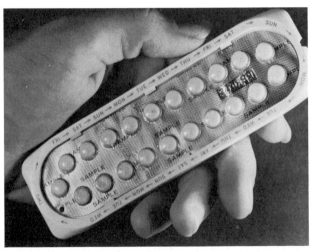

Contraceptive pills, designed to produce a regular 28-day menstrual cycle.

18.7)   What are the main characteristics of the cholesterol structure?

18.8*)   How is the structure of estrone similar to that of testosterone? How does it differ? (Use structural formulas in Figure 18–11.)

CHAPTER EIGHTEEN IN REVIEW ■ Lipids and Cell Membranes

18.1 MAJOR TYPES OF SIMPLE LIPIDS   Page 509

    18A: Draw the structural formula for a given unsaturated fatty acid.

    18B: Distinguish between a fat and a wax.

18.2 REACTIONS OF FATS   Page 514

    18C: Explain the possible relationship between hydrogenation of vegetable oils in our diet and human health.

    18D: Describe the difference between acid hydrolysis and saponification of a fat.

18.3 PHOSPHOLIPIDS AND CELL MEMBRANES   Page 517

    18E: Distinguish a phospholipid from a fat.

    18F: Describe the most accepted model of a cell membrane.

18.4 STEROIDS   Page 524

    18G: Recognize the steroid ring system in a given hormone.

GLOSSARY FOR CHAPTER EIGHTEEN

androgen   A male steroid hormone, formed in the testes; controls sexual development. (p. 527)

cell membrane   The wall or "skin" that surrounds a cell; contains a lipid bilayer of phospholipid molecules with embedded protein molecules. (p. 520)

cephalin   A phospholipid; an ester of phosphatidic acid with serine or ethanolamine. (p. 519)

cerebroside   A lipid found in brain and nerve tissue that contains a carbohydrate (such as galactose) joined to sphingosine and a fatty acid; one type of glycolipid. (p. 520)

cholesterol   The most common steroid; found in blood, some cell membranes, brain and nerve tissue, some gallstones, and fatty deposits in arteries; may be considered the "parent compound" of steroid hormones. (p. 524)

endocrine gland   Any of several glands in the body that produce hormones that control growth, development, and metabolic processes. (p. 524)

estrogen   A female steroid hormone, formed in the ovaries; controls sexual development and the menstrual cycle. (p. 525)

fat   A lipid that is a triester of glycerol with fatty acids; a triacylglycerol; a triglyceride. (p. 512)

lecithin   A phospholipid that is important in the formation of the lipid bilayer of cell membranes because of its having a polar head and nonpolar tails in each molecule. (p. 519)

lipid bilayer   A part of the cell membrane consisting of two layers of phospholipid molecules with their water-soluble ends facing toward the aqueous solutions inside and outside the cell and their water-insoluble ends buried inside the cell membrane. (p. 521)

oil   A fat that is liquid at room temperature; usually contains a high proportion of unsaturated fatty acid units; a hydrocarbon mixture (mineral oil, petroleum) with similar physical properties. (p. 513)

phospholipid A lipid found in all cells and especially in brain and nerve cells and in cell membranes; includes cephalins, lecithins, and sphingomyelins. (p. 517)

rancidity Decomposition of a fat, accompanied by unpleasant odors and taste, when left in contact with air. (p. 515)

saturated fat A fat that contains a very high proportion of fatty acid units that have only single bonds; a fully hydrogenated fat. (p. 515)

sphingomyelin A phospholipid found in brain and nerve tissue. (p. 519)

steroid A lipid based on the steroid ring system; one of several hormones produced by the gonads or by the adrenal glands; one of several drugs or other compounds chemically similar to *cholesterol*. (p. 524)

triacylglycerol A fat. (p. 512)

triglyceride A fat; former name for a *triacylglycerol*. (p. 512)

wax A lipid that is solid at room temperature; an ester of a long-chain fatty acid with a high-molecular-weight alcohol; a long-chain hydrocarbon with similar properties. (p. 514)

QUESTIONS AND PROBLEMS FOR CHAPTER EIGHTEEN ■

Lipids and Cell Membranes

SECTION 18.1 MAJOR TYPES OF SIMPLE LIPIDS

18.9) Draw the structure of linoleic acid ($C_{17}H_{31}COOH$) with double bonds at ($\Delta 9$, 12).

18.10) How could you distinguish between a fat and a wax by looking at the alcohol part of each molecule?

18.17) Use the structure of oleic acid, $C_{17}H_{33}COOH$ ($\Delta 9$), to show what is meant by a *cis* fatty acid.

18.18) How could you distinguish between a fat and a wax by looking at the fatty acid part of each molecule?

SECTION 18.2 REACTIONS OF FATS

18.11) What important steroid is often associated with consumption of saturated fats in the diet?

18.12) What is the major purpose of *saponification* of a fat? Why do we *not* obtain pure organic products from this reaction?

18.19) What specific health hazard might possibly be avoided by making sure that one's diet contains mostly polyunsaturated fats?

18.20) If you wish to find out what specific fatty acids are present in a fat, do you wish to saponify or to hydrolyze the fat? Why?

SECTION 18.3 PHOSPHOLIPIDS AND CELL MEMBRANES

18.13) What physical property clearly distinguishes a fat from a phospholipid?

18.14) Describe some functions of the proteins in cell membranes.

18.21) How does the molecular structure of a lecithin differ from that of a fat?

18.22) Describe the function of the lipid bilayer in cell membranes.

SECTION 18.4 STEROIDS (*Use Figure 18–11 as needed for these questions.*)

18.15) Is the bile salt *cholic acid* (p. 524) a steroid?

18.16*) What three functional groups are attached to the steroid ring system of cholesterol?

18.23) Is the birth control drug *mestranol* (p. 526) a steroid?

18.24*) What is the major difference between the molecular structure of aldosterone and that of corticosterone?

Amino Acids and Proteins 19

There are over 2000 different kinds of proteins making up the structure of the cell and its components. Some serve as enzymes, which are protein molecules that control the speed of chemical reactions that occur in the cell (Section 21.5). There are structural and supportive proteins, as in muscle, tendons, skin, and hair. There are proteins that function in transportation systems, such as hemoglobin for carrying oxygen (Section 10.5) and cytochromes for carrying electrons in energy production (Chapter 22). Other important proteins are the antibodies or gamma globulins that protect against bacterial invasion. Proteins are such essential biological molecules that their name, chosen by Mulder in 1839, means "of prime importance."

Protein molecules are large polymers composed of monomers called amino acids joined together in amide (peptide) linkages. Proteins could therefore be classified as *polyamides* or *polypeptides*. Five of the elements discussed in Chapter 1 (carbon, hydrogen, oxygen, nitrogen, and sulfur) are found in all naturally occurring proteins. Other elements, such as phosphorus, iron, iodine, and magnesium, are essential constituents of certain special proteins. Most cell and tissue proteins have molecular weights in the range from 10 000 to 500 000 amu. Some very large protein complexes have molecular weights as high as 50 000 000 amu (Figure 19–1).

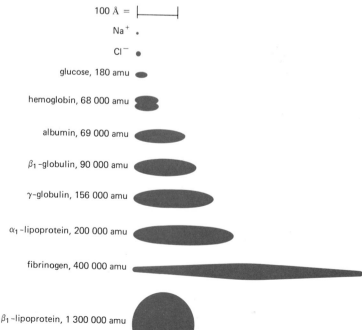

FIGURE 19–1 The relative sizes of some protein molecules. A length of 100 Å is given at the top for reference, along with the sizes of the Na^+ and Cl^- ions. (After Oncley, J.L., *Conference on the Preservation of the Cellular and Protein Components of Blood*, published by the American Red Cross, Washington, D.C.)

531

An idea of the numbers of atoms involved may be gained from an approximate formula for oxyhemoglobin, the oxygen-carrying protein in the red blood cells: $C_{2932}H_{4724}N_{828}S_8Fe_4O_{840}$. The molecular weight of oxyhemoglobin is about 68 000 amu.

19.1 AMINO ACIDS

> *LEARNING GOAL 19A: Draw the structural formulas for acidic, basic, aromatic, and sulfur-containing amino acids.*
>
> *19B: Describe how the isoelectric point of a protein is related to the amphoteric properties of amino acids.*
>
> *19C: Describe the use of chromatography to measure the relative amount of each amino acid in a protein.*

Protein molecules are more complicated than the polymers we studied in Chapter 16. The monomers that are formed by the complete hydrolysis of a protein are *amino acids* (Section 13.4). Common reagents used for the hydrolysis of proteins are aqueous acids (HCl and H_2SO_4), bases (NaOH), and enzymes (proteases).

Before considering the properties and complex structure of proteins, we will first look at the individual amino acids. In simple terms, an amino acid is a carboxylic acid that contains an amino group ($-NH_2$). If a hydrogen is replaced by an amino group on the carbon atom that is next to ("alpha" to) the carboxyl group in acetic acid, CH_3COOH, the simplest amino acid, *glycine*, is formed:

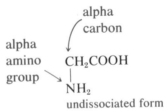

undissociated form

The amino acids are often divided according to their organic chemistry classification (aliphatic, aromatic, or heterocyclic). They are further separated into *nonpolar* and *polar* amino acids to help explain their influence on the properties and shapes of protein molecules (Table 19–1).

The abbreviation for each amino acid used in sequence and structure models is based on its common name.

Amphoteric properties

Amino acids and proteins may behave either as weak acids or as weak bases, since each contains at least one carboxyl group and one amino group. Proteins are thus *amphoteric* (Section 13.5). An example would be alanine, in which both the acidic and basic groups are normally ionized in solution to form a dipolar ion or zwitterion (German for "between ion," p. 400). The alanine molecule is electrically neutral since it contains an equal number of positive and negative ions. The zwitterion form of alanine is therefore *iso-electric*, that is, it has an equal number of positive and negative charges. The pH at which the molecule exists almost entirely as the zwitterion is called the **isoelectric point** (Table 19.2).

In a solution more acidic than the isoelectric point the amino acid (or protein) will be a positively charged cation. In a solution more basic than the isoelectric point the amino acid (or protein) will be a negatively charged anion:

$$CH_3—CH—COO^- \xleftarrow{OH^-} CH_3—CH—COO^- \xrightarrow{H^+} CH_3—CH—COOH$$

NH_2	NH_3^+	NH_3^+
anion	zwitterion	cation
in	at	in
base	isoelectric point	acid

At the neutral pH of body fluids, the acidic amino acids are present as anions and the basic amino acids as cations.

TABLE 19–1   THE STRUCTURES OF 20 COMMON AMINO ACIDS

Nonpolar (Hydrophobic) Amino Acids

Aliphatic

Glycine (Gly)

$$H—CHCOOH$$
$$\underset{NH_2}{|}$$

Alanine (Ala)

$$CH_3—CHCOOH$$
$$\underset{NH_2}{|}$$

Valine (Val)

$$CH_3CH—CHCOOH$$
$$\underset{CH_3}{|} \quad \underset{NH_2}{|}$$

Leucine (Leu)

$$CH_3CHCH_2—CHCOOH$$
$$\underset{CH_3}{|} \qquad \underset{NH_2}{|}$$

Isoleucine (Ile)

$$CH_3CH_2CH—CHCOOH$$
$$\underset{CH_3}{|} \quad \underset{NH_2}{|}$$

Aromatic

Phenylalanine (Phe)

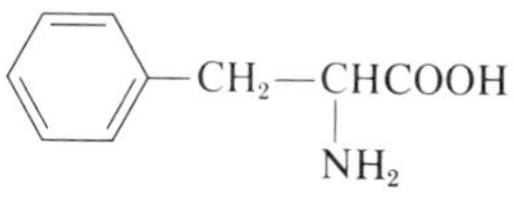

$$—CH_2—CHCOOH$$
$$\underset{NH_2}{|}$$

Heterocyclic

Tryptophan (Trp)

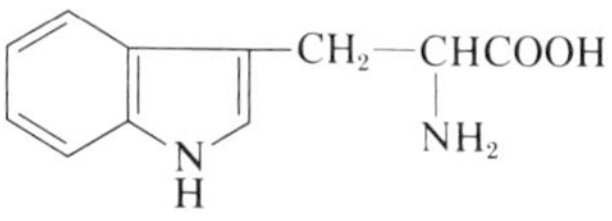

$$—CH_2—CHCOOH$$
$$\underset{NH_2}{|}$$

Proline (Pro)

$$H_2C \underset{H_2C}{\overset{\overset{H_2}{C}}{}} \underset{N}{\overset{H}{\underset{H}{}}} \overset{H}{C}—COOH$$

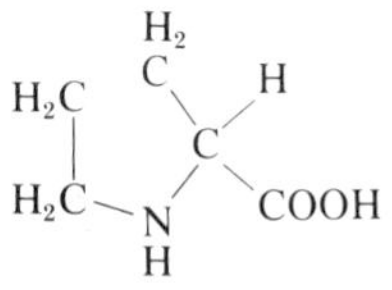

Sulfur-containing

Methionine (Met)

$$CH_3—S—CH_2CH_2—CHCOOH$$
$$\underset{NH_2}{|}$$

The term *hydrophobic* means "hating water." You know that nonpolar groups, such as long hydrocarbon chains, do not dissolve in water. *Hydrophilic* means "loving water." Polar molecules and zwitterions are soluble in water. The *aliphatic* hydrocarbons are those studied in Chapter 7, and the *aromatic* compounds are those of Section 15.2.

(Table continued on following page.)

TABLE 19–1 **THE STRUCTURES OF 20 COMMON AMINO ACIDS** (*Continued*)

Polar Amino Acids (Hydrophilic)

Acidic

Aspartic acid (Asp)

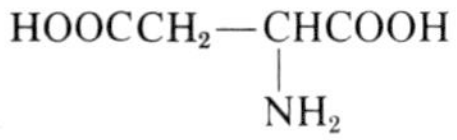

$$HOOCCH_2—CHCOOH$$
$$\underset{NH_2}{|}$$

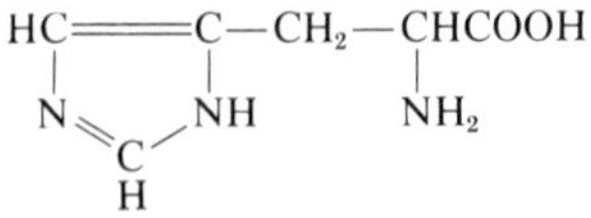

Acidic Amides

Asparagine (Asn)

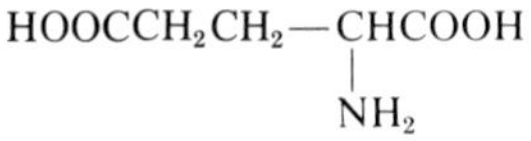

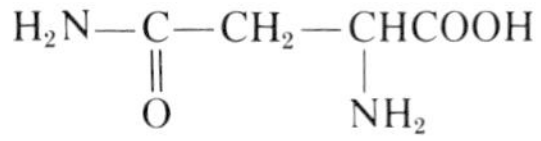

$$H_2N—\underset{\underset{O}{\|}}{C}—CH_2—\underset{\underset{NH_2}{|}}{C}HCOOH$$

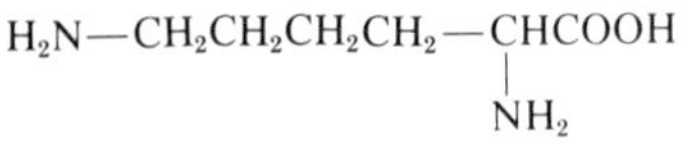

Glutamic acid (Glu)

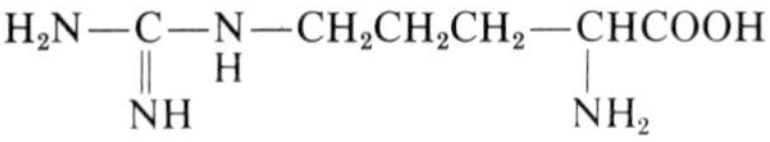

$$HOOCCH_2CH_2—CHCOOH$$
$$\underset{NH_2}{|}$$

Glutamine (Gln)

$$H_2N—\underset{\underset{O}{\|}}{C}—CH_2—CH_2—\underset{\underset{NH_2}{|}}{C}HCOOH$$

Basic

Lysine (Lys)

$$H_2N—CH_2CH_2CH_2CH_2—CHCOOH$$
$$\underset{NH_2}{|}$$

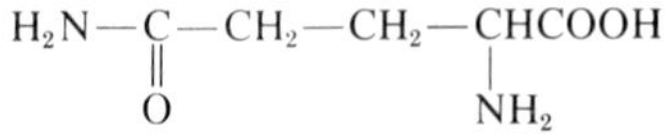

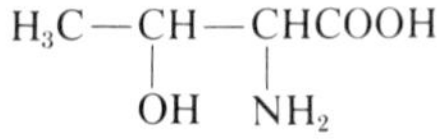

Hydroxy-containing

Serine (Ser)

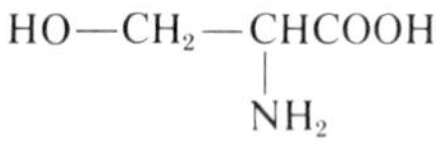

$$HO—CH_2—CHCOOH$$
$$\underset{NH_2}{|}$$

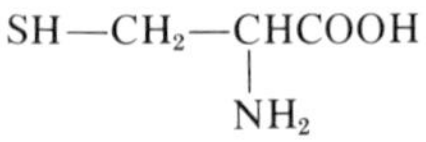

TABLE 19–2 **ISOELECTRIC POINTS OF AMINO ACIDS**

Arginine (Arg)

$$H_2N—\underset{\underset{NH}{\|}}{C}—\underset{H}{N}—CH_2CH_2CH_2—\underset{\underset{NH_2}{|}}{C}HCOOH$$

Threonine (Thr)

$$H_3C—\underset{\underset{OH}{|}}{C}H—\underset{\underset{NH_2}{|}}{C}HCOOH$$

Histidine (His)

Tyrosine (Tyr)

All aliphatic
  pI = 6.0

Hydroxy-containing
  pI = 5.6 to 5.7

Phenylalanine	5.5
Tryptophan	5.9
Proline	6.3
Methionine	5.7
Asparagine	5.4
Glutamine	5.7
Cysteine	5.1
ACIDS	
Aspartic acid	2.98
Glutamic acid	3.2
BASES	
Lysine	9.7
Arginine	10.8
Histidine	7.6

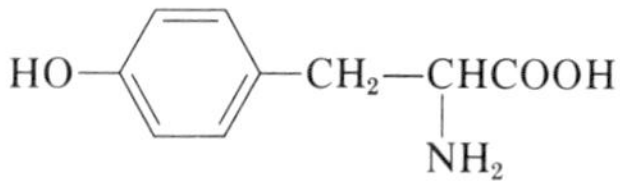

Sulfur-containing

Cysteine (Cys)

$$SH—CH_2—CHCOOH$$
$$\underset{NH_2}{|}$$

The amphoteric properties of proteins are used in a process called *electrophoresis.* An electric field is applied to a protein mixture. The cations move toward the negative electrode, the anions toward the positive electrode. Zwitterions do not move at all.

The process is similar to electrodialysis (Section 12.4).

The amphoteric properties of proteins are responsible for their action as buffers in blood and other body fluids.

Reactions of amino acids

Many of the common reactions of organic chemistry occur with amino acids. Certain amino acids, whether in a solution of hydrolyzed protein (the **hydrolysate** solution) or combined in proteins, take part in specific reactions that involve color changes, which aid in the detection and measurement of the amino acids. The *Millons test* for tyrosine gives a red color, and tryptophan produces a violet color in the *Hopkins-Cole test.* In the *Sakaguchi reaction,* arginine forms a red color. Cysteine yields a red color with sodium nitroprusside. A more general color test for amino acids is the **ninhydrin reaction,** in which all the amino acids in a protein hydrolysate form a bluish-purple colored compound. The intensity of the color may be used to determine the amount of amino acids.

Chromatography of amino acids

Before 1950, biochemists were convinced that it was not possible to determine the exact way in which the different amino acids make up a single protein. Protein hydrolysis and specific color reactions of amino acids were not sufficient to determine the sequence of amino acids in even a small protein molecule.

Several types of **chromatography** have been developed for the analysis of mixtures of molecules such as amino acids. *Paper chromatography* and *thin layer chromatography* are relatively simple methods that produce excellent separation, detection, and measurement of the individual amino acids. A small drop of a protein hydrolysate is placed on a strip of filter paper or a glass plate coated with a layer of cellulose powder or silica gel. The paper or plate is dipped into a mixture of solvents (such as butanol + acetic acid + water), which moves upward, carrying each amino acid to a spot that can be identified using a known sample of pure amino acids for comparison (Figure 19-2).

Chromatography has been improved by the use of long glass tubes or columns of cellulose powder or ion exchange resins. A mixture of amino acids (hydrolysate) in a small volume of buffer solution is placed on top of

Chromatography is now commonly used for many laboratory purposes. You may have seen it used for the detection of drugs and poisons in body fluids and tissues on the TV program "Quincy."

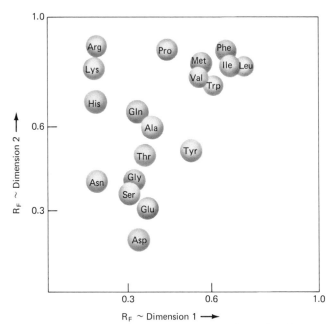

FIGURE 19-2 Separating amino acids through two-dimensional paper chromatography. Two different solvents are used. The value of R_F indicates how well an amino acid has been able to "keep up with" the movement of solvent. (White *et al., Principles of Biochemistry,* 4th edition, New York, McGraw-Hill, 1968, p. 114)

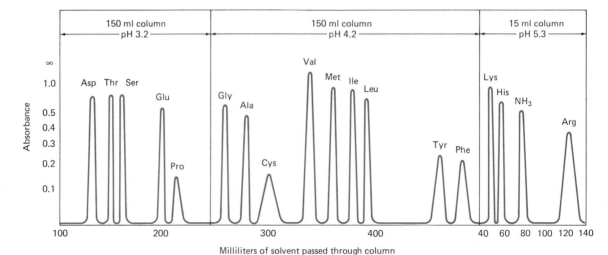

FIGURE 19–3 A mixture of amino acids can be separated by chromatographic fractionating. (Moore *et al., Anal. Chem.* 30: 1186, 1958)

the column, and the amino acids are washed down through the column by the addition of more buffer solution. The speed with which each acid passes down the column depends on its reaction either to the cellulose or to the positively or negatively charged groups on the ion exchange column. By the proper choice of ion exchange resins, buffers, column length, and flow rate, it is possible to separate a mixture of amino acids. First the acidic amino acids like aspartic and glutamic acids move through the column, followed by more neutral amino acids like alanine and leucine and finally by the basic amino acids like lysine and arginine, as shown in Figure 19–3. As each amino acid comes off the bottom of the column, it can be collected in a tube and transferred to an automatic analyzing instrument that determines the amount of the amino acid. With column chromatography, it is possible to obtain an amino acid analysis of a protein hydrolysate in a few hours.

SELF-CHECK

19.1) Give an example of an aliphatic, an aromatic, a heterocyclic, an acidic, and a basic amino acid.
19.2) Draw the structure for glycine as a zwitterion and use it to explain the *isoelectric point.*
19.3) Describe how paper chromatography can show which amino acids are in a given protein.

19.2 POLYPEPTIDES

LEARNING GOAL 19D: Draw a peptide linkage between any two given amino acids.

19E: Describe the importance and composition of the backbone structure of polypeptide chains.

19F: Describe the important contribution made by Sanger to our knowledge of protein structure.

19G: Explain the importance of the disulfide group in proteins.

Proteins are polymers of amino acids joined together by **peptide linkages** between the carboxyl group of one amino acid and the amino group of another amino acid, with the splitting out of a molecule of water. This type of linkage may be illustrated by the union of a molecule of alanine and a molecule of glycine:

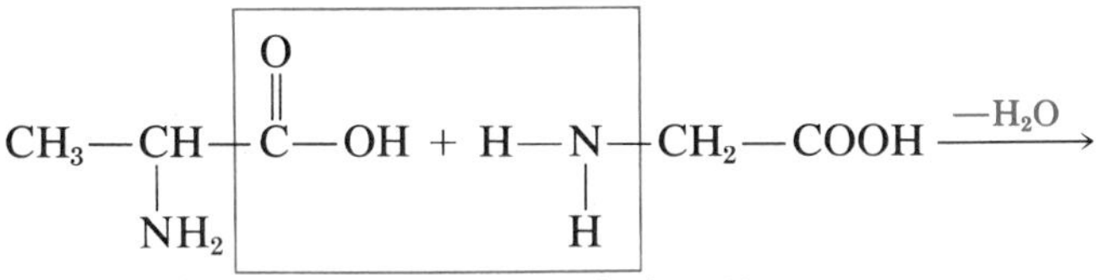

$$CH_3—CH—\boxed{\overset{\overset{\displaystyle O}{\|}}{C}—OH + H—N}—CH_2—COOH \xrightarrow{-H_2O}$$

$$\underset{\displaystyle NH_2}{|} \qquad\qquad \underset{\displaystyle H}{|}$$

alanine (Ala) glycine (Gly)

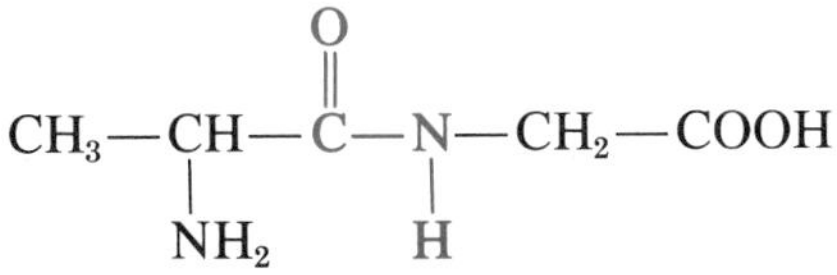

$$CH_3—\underset{\underset{\displaystyle NH_2}{|}}{CH}—\overset{\overset{\displaystyle O}{\|}}{C}—\underset{\underset{\displaystyle H}{|}}{N}—CH_2—COOH$$

alanylglycine (Ala·Gly)

The compound alanylglycine, which results from this linkage, is called a *dipeptide*. A combination of three amino acid monomer units results in a *tripeptide;* thus, we could join tyrosine to alanylglycine by a peptide linkage:

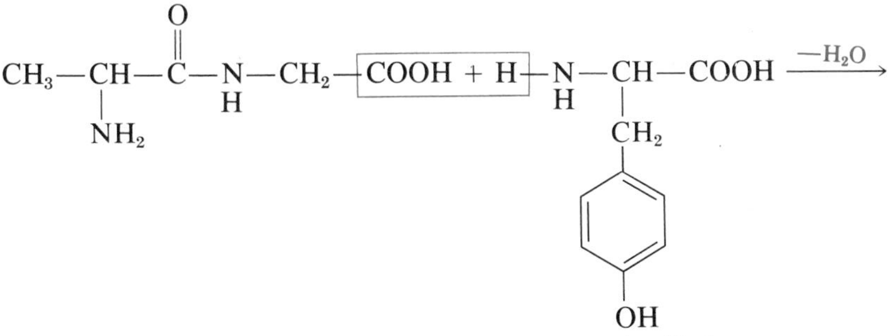

Some dipeptide esters, such as Asp-Phe-OCH$_3$, are very sweet and might be used as low-calorie sweetening agents. A di-, tri-, or polypeptide is often abbreviated by using the amino acid abbreviations, here "Asp" for aspartic acid, "Phe" for phenylalanine.

$$CH_3—\underset{\underset{\displaystyle NH_2}{|}}{CH}—\overset{\overset{\displaystyle O}{\|}}{C}—\underset{\underset{\displaystyle H}{|}}{N}—CH_2—\boxed{COOH + H}—\underset{\underset{\displaystyle H}{|}}{N}—\underset{\underset{\displaystyle CH_2}{|}}{CH}—COOH \xrightarrow{-H_2O}$$

alanylglycine (Ala·Gly) tyrosine (Tyr)

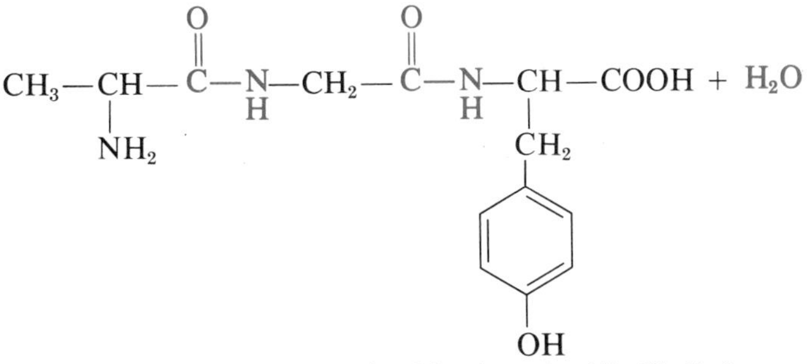

with CH$_2$ attached to a benzene ring bearing OH

$$CH_3—\underset{\underset{\displaystyle NH_2}{|}}{CH}—\overset{\overset{\displaystyle O}{\|}}{C}—\underset{\underset{\displaystyle H}{|}}{N}—CH_2—\overset{\overset{\displaystyle O}{\|}}{C}—\underset{\underset{\displaystyle H}{|}}{N}—\underset{\underset{\displaystyle CH_2}{|}}{CH}—COOH + H_2O$$

benzene ring bearing OH

alanylglycyltyrosine (Ala·Gly·Tyr)

A peptide is named starting with the amino acid with the free amino (NH$_2$—) group (alanine in the tripeptide shown). A combination of several amino acids with peptide linkages is called a **polypeptide.** Each amino acid loses water when it joins other amino acids in a polypeptide chain. The monomer unit is called an *amino acid* **residue.** In the primary structure of a protein, the backbone of the polypeptide chain consists of the alpha carbon, the carboxyl carbon, and the amino nitrogen.

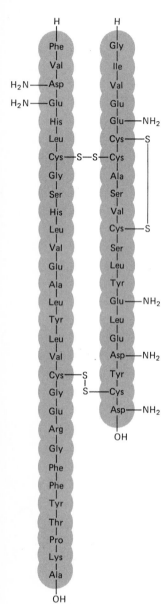

FIGURE 19–4 The amino acid sequence in beef insulin, containing 51 amino acid residues in two chains cross-linked by disulfide bonding.

Relaxin is an animal hormone that widens the birth canal to permit delivery of the young. It has three disulfide linkages identical to those in insulin. This suggests that a common gene may be responsible for these two hormones.

Examine the above structure closely and you find that 1 through 4 represent *side chains* from alanine, tyrosine, serine, and cysteine, respectively. Such a tetrapeptide segment would be named *alanyltyrosylserylcysteine* and abbreviated Ala-Tyr-Ser-Cys.

An important color reaction of proteins and polypeptides is the **biuret test,** which produces a violet color with proteins and peptides containing two or more peptide linkages. The intensity of the color may be used to measure the protein concentration in a solution.

Amino acid sequences

As chromatography has developed in recent years, biochemists have found that small sections of the polypeptide chain form definite spots on chromatograms. Fredrick Sanger in 1950 was the first biochemist to successfully tackle the problem of the **amino acid sequence** of a protein. He studied the small protein molecule *insulin,* a hormone that controls the use of glucose by the body. Methods available at the time established a molecular weight of about 6000 amu, so Sanger could calculate the approximate number of amino acid residues in the molecule. He found that insulin readily splits into two polypeptide chains and that he could identify both end amino acids on each chain. He solved the larger problem of the sequence in each chain by chopping the chain into small fragments by enzyme hydrolysis, separating the fragments by chromatography, and identifying the order of the two, three, or four amino acids in each fragment using specific color tests. As he identified and determined the sequence of more and more fragments from each polypeptide chain, he put them together like pieces of a jigsaw puzzle to establish the exact sequence of all the amino acid residues in the two chains.

Figure 19–4 illustrates the amino acid sequence in beef insulin, showing the two polypeptide chains established by Sanger held together by two linkages between cysteine molecules in each chain. This **disulfide linkage** is often seen in the structure of protein molecules, either as a bridge between two cysteine residues in a polypeptide chain or holding together two or more polypeptide chains (Figure 19–5).

Sanger's results stimulated other biochemists to study the amino acid sequences of other peptides and proteins. Vincent du Vigneaud soon established the sequence in two small peptide hormones, oxytocin and vasopressin. Oxytocin causes contraction of smooth muscles and is used in pregnancy to initiate labor. Vasopressin constricts blood vessels, raising blood pressure and affecting water and electrolyte balance (Chapter 24). Each peptide contains eight amino acid residues, with an internal disulfide bridge across four of the amino acid units:

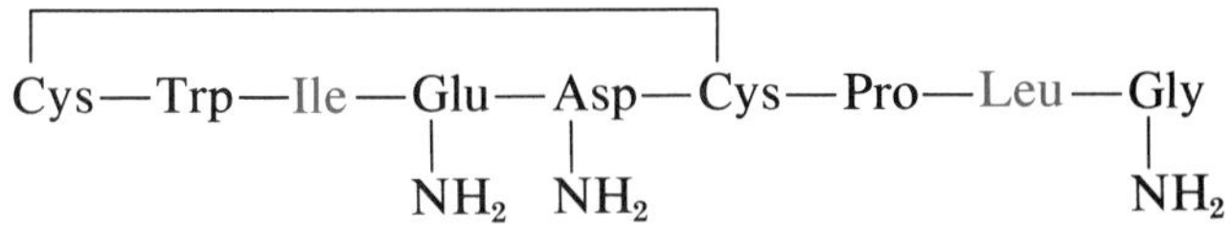

Cys—Trp—Ile—Glu—Asp—Cys—Pro—Leu—Gly
         | | |
        NH$_2$ NH$_2$ NH$_2$

oxytocin

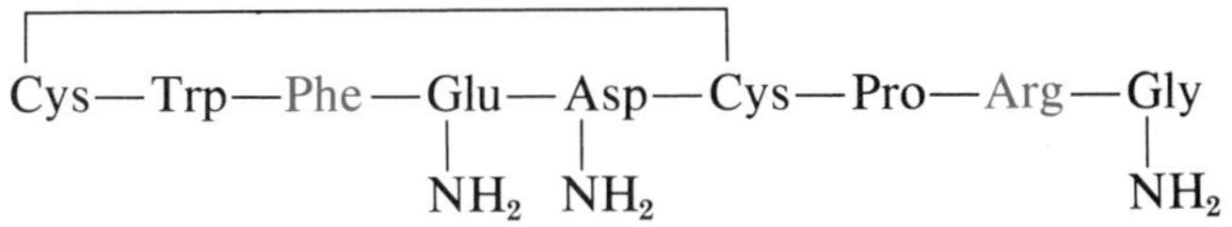

Cys—Trp—Phe—Glu—Asp—Cys—Pro—Arg—Gly
         | | |
        NH$_2$ NH$_2$ NH$_2$

vasopressin

Comparison of these two molecules indicates that having two *different* amino acids in such small polypeptides results in very different physiological activity.

The amino acid sequence has been determined for the adrenocorticotropic hormone, ACTH (Chapter 25), containing 39 amino acid residues, and the enzyme ribonuclease, with 124 residues. The α and β polypeptide chains of hemoglobin (Chapter 24), containing 141 and 146 amino acid residues, respectively, and the tobacco mosaic virus protein with 158 monomer units have also been characterized. It should be emphasized that these sequence studies are very time consuming and become more difficult as the protein molecule increases in size. In recent years, an automated solid-phase synthesis technique has been developed by Robert Merrifield to assist in determining the sequences of peptides and proteins.

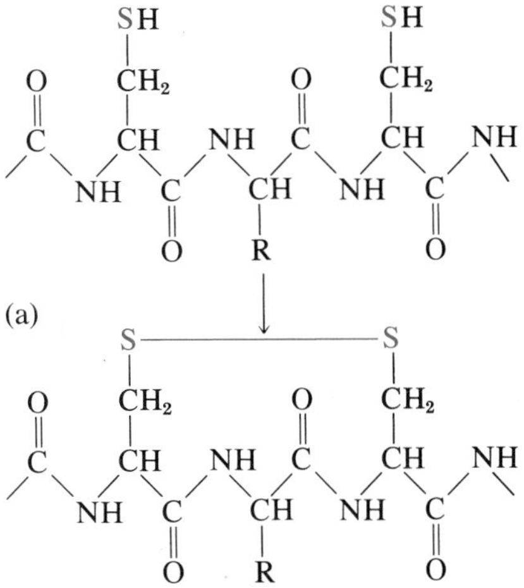

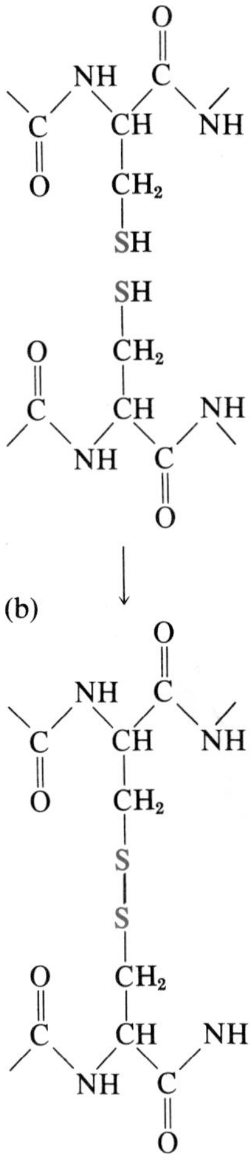

FIGURE 19–5 Formation of disulfide linkages in peptide chains: (a) within one chain (remember that the chain curls around to bring the two sulfur atoms close together); (b) between two chains.

SELF-CHECK

19.4) Draw the structure for the tripeptide glycylglycylalanine.
19.5) Draw the structure of the backbone of any polypeptide chain and circle the peptide linkages.
19.6) Why is the amino acid sequence of a protein important?
19.7*) Two of the three disulfide linkages in insulin are different from the third. Explain.

19.3 THE STRUCTURE OF PROTEINS

LEARNING GOAL 19H: Describe the difference between the primary and secondary structures of proteins.

19I: Describe the hydrogen-bonding in the α-helix and the pleated sheet structure.

19J: Explain the reason for the particular locations of polar and nonpolar amino acid residues in globular proteins.

All the properties of a specific protein depend on the structure of the molecule as it exists in its natural surroundings, that is, in body tissues or fluids. Proteins range in complexity from a small simple polypeptide, such as vasopressin, to a globular protein such as myoglobin, whose molecule includes three-dimensional features such as helix formation, cross-linkages, and the folding of peptide chains.

Primary structure

If only peptide (amide) bonds were involved in protein structure, the molecules would consist of long polypeptide chains coiled in random shapes. This is the *primary structure* of proteins described in Section 19.2. Most proteins, however, are either fibrous or globular (lumpy) and consist of polypeptide chains joined together or held in definite folded shapes by *hydrogen-bonding* (Section 11.4).

Secondary structure

The influence of hydrogen-bonding on the protein molecule is responsible for the *secondary structure* of the protein. Although hydrogen-bonding may form between several groups on the peptide side chains, the most common attraction occurs between the carbonyl and amide groups of the peptide backbone, as shown by the dotted lines in Figure 19–6:

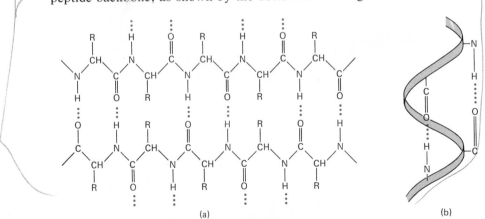

(a)   (b)

FIGURE 19–6   Hydrogen-bonding between adjacent chains in proteins: (a) two horizontal backbone structures with hydrogen-bonding at every possible location (this two-dimensional diagram might not represent the true shape of a protein); (b) a twisted backbone structure (often more realistic) with connecting hydrogen-bonds.

After studying the polypeptide structure of the fibrous protein *keratin* (in hair and wool), Linus Pauling concluded that the chains are regularly coiled to form a structure called the **α-helix.** This structure consists of a stretched-out chain of amino acid residues wound into a spiral which is held together by hydrogen-bonding between the carbonyl group of one amino acid and the amino group of an amino acid farther along the chain. Each amino acid residue is separated from the next residue by an equal space, and the helix makes a complete turn for each 3.6 residues. This relationship is illustrated in Figure 19–7. The keratins of hair and wool consist of bundles or cables of three or seven such α-helical coils twisted around each other.

In other proteins, such as fibroin (the fibrous protein of silk), the polypeptide chains are in an extended zigzag pattern similar to that of the peptide backbone. These chains are arranged alongside each other to form a **pleated sheet** structure, in which the adjacent polypeptide chains run in opposite directions. In addition, the chains are arranged so that the maximum hydrogen-bonding occurs between neighboring oxygen and nitrogen pairs of the backbone. In Figure 19–8, a side view of the pleated sheet is shown along with a top view that illustrates the extensive hydrogen-bonding in four such chains.

Tertiary structure

The polypeptide chains of *globular* proteins are more extensively coiled and folded than those of fibrous proteins. This results from several types of attractions that hold the structure in a more complex and rigid shape. These attractions are responsible for the *tertiary structure* of proteins, and they exert stronger forces than hydrogen-bonding in holding together polypeptide chains or folds of individual chains.

A strong covalent bond may be formed between two cysteine residues, resulting in the disulfide bond we have already described. **Salt linkages** of ionic bonds may be formed between the basic amino acid residues of lysine and arginine and the dicarboxylic amino acids, such as aspartic and glu-

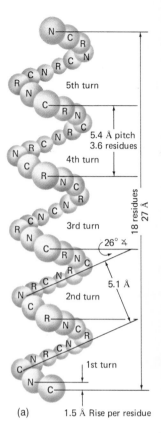

(a)

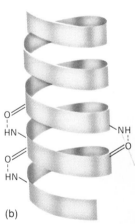

(b)

FIGURE 19–7 The alpha helix of a polypeptide: (a) a carefully measured chain (Pauling, L., and Corey, P., *Proc. Intern. Wool Textile Conf. N*, 249, 1955); (b) a drawing of the alpha helix as a spiral or "screw-shaped" structure, held in place by hydrogen-bonding.

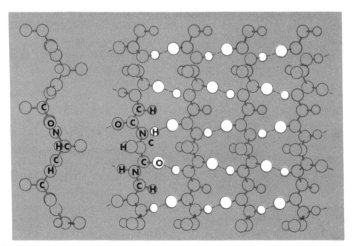

FIGURE 19–8 The pleated sheet structure of a polypeptide. Written in perspective, this drawing shows that the sheet is not flat. Atoms shown in white are involved in hydrogen-bonding.

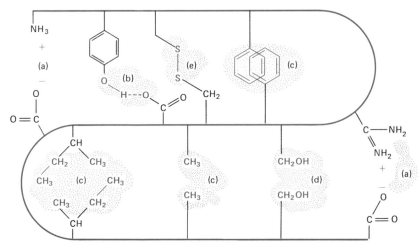

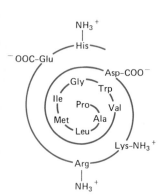

FIGURE 19–10   The hydrophobic effect. In globular proteins, the nonpolar side chains tend to be directed toward the inside of the structure, leaving the polar side chains on the surface, where they can attract water molecules. The overall effect is similar to that described for the lipid bilayer in Section 18.3.

FIGURE 19–9   The attractions that determine protein structure: (a) the ionic bonds of salt linkages; (b) hydrogen-bonding; (c) dispersion forces (hydrophobic attractions) between nonpolar side groups; (d) dipole-dipole attractions between polar side groups; (e) sulfur-sulfur covalent bonds in disulfide linkages. The various attractions are obviously not of equal strength. The strongest are the disulfide bonds (50 to 100 kcal/mole), then the salt linkages (5 to 10 kcal/mole), followed by hydrogen-bonding (2 to 5 kcal/mole). (After Anfinsen, C.B., *The Molecular Basis of Evolution*, New York, Wiley, 1959, p. 102)

tamic. There are also many examples of *hydrophobic attractions* that result from the closeness of nonpolar groups to each other, as shown in Figure 19–9. These attractions are dispersion forces (Section 11.3).

The tertiary structure of proteins is also strongly influenced by the location of polar and nonpolar amino acids (Table 19–1). Protein molecules with mixed polar and nonpolar regions will tend to fold in such a way as to place the polar side chains (hydrophilic) on the surface, where they can interact with water molecules. This tendency to bury the nonpolar side chains inside a globular protein molecule is illustrated in Figure 19–10.

Sanger's important contribution, the identification of the sequence of amino acids in the insulin molecule, was matched by the development of the first three-dimensional picture of the protein molecule *myoglobin* by Kendrew and his co-workers. Myoglobin has a molecular weight of 17 000 amu and consists of a single polypeptide chain with 153 amino acid residues. It functions as a carrier of oxygen within muscle fibers (Figure 19–11).

Quaternary structure

Another level of protein structure is the *quaternary structure,* in which the protein contains several polypeptide chains or subunits. The hemoglobin molecule is a good example of subunit structure in proteins. Hemoglobin has a molecular weight of 68 000 amu in a neutral solution. If the solution is made acidic, the molecular weight changes to 34 000 amu. This dissociation of subunits is due to the four polypeptide chains that exist in hemoglobin as two pairs. Each peptide chain is approximately the same size and shape as the single chain in myoglobin, and each chain is wrapped around a central molecular unit called "heme." Hemoglobin functions as a carrier of oxygen in the blood (Chapter 24).

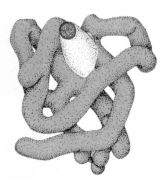

FIGURE 19–11   The globular structure of myoglobin. The dark disk at the top is the molecular subunit *heme,* which contains an iron cation and can bond with O_2. (After Kendrew, J.C., *Science*, 139:1261, 1963)

19.8) How would you describe the primary structure of a protein molecule?

19.9) Why is it more difficult to show all the hydrogen-bonds in an α-helix structure than in a pleated sheet structure?

19.10) In a globular protein, where would you expect to find a salt linkage? hydrophobic attractions? disulfide bonds?

19.4 DENATURATION AND PRECIPITATION

> LEARNING GOAL 19K: *Distinguish between denaturation and precipitation.*
> 19L: *Explain how the charges on a protein molecule are affected by addition of an acidic solution or of a heavy metal salt.*

One of the most important characteristics of a protein is the ease with which it is denatured or precipitated by any of several reagents. **Denaturation** of a protein molecule causes changes in the structure, which include the breaking of hydrogen-bonds and disulfide bonds and the unravelling of peptide chains in globular proteins. These structural changes result in loss of biological activity and solubility changes. New amino acid side chains are exposed at the surface of the protein molecule. Relatively mild changes, such as exposure to strong light, heating, shaking, or exposure to reagents such as detergents or organic solvents, may denature proteins in solution.

Precipitation of proteins usually requires more drastic conditions or stronger reagents and results in an insoluble solid. Some of the normal functions in the body are essentially precipitation reactions, for example, the clotting of blood. Since animal tissues are chiefly protein, reagents that precipitate protein will have a harmful effect if introduced into the body. Bacteria, which are mainly protein, are effectively destroyed when treated with suitable precipitants. Many of the common poisons and disinfectants act in this way.

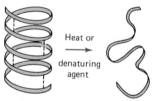

Denaturation of a protein. Heat and other agents break hydrogen-bonds and other attractions and allow the polypeptide chains to uncoil.

Heat coagulation

When most protein solutions are heated, the protein is first denatured and then becomes insoluble and precipitates, forming coagulated protein. Many protein foods coagulate when they are cooked. Tissue and bacterial proteins are readily coagulated by heat. Abnormal skin growths such as warts can be removed by heat coagulation with an electric needle. Routine examination of urine specimens for protein (present in kidney disease and infections) is done by heating the urine in a test tube to coagulate any protein that might be present.

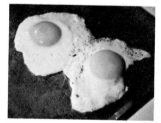

The heat coagulation of egg protein.

Alcohol

A 70 per cent by volume solution of ethyl alcohol is commonly used to sterilize the skin since it effectively penetrates bacteria and completely precipitates their protein. The alcohol breaks the hydrogen-bonds and removes the water needed to keep the protein in solution. A 95 per cent solution of alcohol is *less* effective because it coagulates the outer surfaces of the bacterial cells too rapidly and does not destroy all of their functional proteins.

Extreme cold will also result in coagulation and in the rupturing of cell walls through the freezing of cell contents. Liquid nitrogen at a temperature of 77 K (−196°C) is often used to treat warts and to destroy unwanted tissue.

Salts of heavy metals

Salts of heavy metals, such as mercury(II) chloride and silver nitrate, precipitate proteins. Since proteins behave as zwitterions, they ionize to negatively charged ions in neutral or alkaline solution and as positively charged ions in acidic solution. The reaction with silver or mercury ions produces an insoluble ionic salt:

$$R—CH—COO^-_{(aq)} + Ag^+_{(aq)} \longrightarrow R—CH—COOAg_{(s)}$$

NH₂		NH₂

$$\begin{array}{ccc} \text{NH}_2 & & \text{NH}_2 \\ \text{protein} & \text{silver} & \text{silver proteinate} \\ \text{anion} & \text{cation} & \text{solid} \end{array}$$

Such a silver-protein salt (Argyrol) is used to treat throat infections. Silver nitrate is used to remove warts from the skin, cauterize wounds, and prevent gonorrheal infection in the eyes of newborn babies. Both mercury(II) chloride and silver nitrate are used on skin for their disinfecting action but are very harmful when taken internally.

A protein suspension, such as egg white or milk, is given as an antidote in cases of poisoning with heavy metal cations such as silver. The protein combines with the metal ion to form a metal salt. The precipitate that is formed must then be removed from the body with an emetic (a substance that causes vomiting) before the protein is digested and the heavy metal cation is again free to act on tissue protein.

Acids

Tannic acid, $C_{76}H_{52}O_{46}$, is used for tanning leather by precipitating proteins. It is occasionally applied by prize-fighters to their skin to "toughen it." Tungstic acid, H_2WO_4, may be used to precipitate proteins in body fluids prior to clinical analysis.

Proteins can be precipitated with concentrated solutions of hydrochloric, sulfuric, and nitric acid, as well as some organic acids. Proteins of the skin are sometimes accidentally precipitated by nitric acid in the laboratory, producing an unsightly yellow area. Corns and warts on the skin are removed by proper treatment with salicylic acid (Compound W) or trichloroacetic acid.

SELF-CHECK

19.11) One student spilled vinegar on her hand, another spilled nitric acid. What probably happened to the protein of the skin in each case?
19.12) If a fellow laboratory worker accidentally swallowed a mercury salt solution, how might you treat the emergency?

CHAPTER NINETEEN IN REVIEW ■ Amino Acids and Proteins

19E: Describe the importance and composition of the backbone structure of polypeptide chains.

19F: Describe the important contribution made by Sanger to our knowledge of protein structure.

19G: Explain the importance of the disulfide group in proteins.

19.3 THE STRUCTURE OF PROTEINS   Page 540

19H: Describe the difference between the primary and secondary structures of proteins.

19I: Describe the hydrogen-bonding in the α-helix and the pleated sheet structure.

19J: Explain the reason for the particular locations of polar and nonpolar amino acid residues in globular proteins.

19.4 DENATURATION AND PRECIPITATION   Page 543

19K: Distinguish between denaturation and precipitation.

19L: Explain how the charges on a protein molecule are affected by addition of an acidic solution or of a heavy metal salt.

GLOSSARY FOR CHAPTER NINETEEN

alpha helix The shape of a polypeptide coiled into a spiral held together by hydrogen-bonding. (p. 541)

amino acid sequence The order of amino acid residues in a polypeptide chain. (p. 538)

biuret test A common color test for determining the amount of protein in a solution. (p. 538)

chromatography A process for the separation and determination of chemical compounds, as of amino acids in a protein hydrolysate. (p. 535)

denaturation A minor change in the structure of a protein that produces loss of biological activity and solubility changes. (p. 543)

disulfide linkage A covalent bond between the sulfur atoms of two cysteine units in a protein. (p. 538)

hydrolysate A solution that results when a protein is hydrolyzed to its component amino acids. (p. 534)

isoelectric point The pH at which an amino acid or protein will exist almost entirely as the zwitterion. (p. 533)

ninhydrin reaction A common color test for determining relative amounts of amino acids. (p. 535)

peptide linkage Amide bonding between the carboxyl group of one amino acid and the amino group of another; found in the polypeptide chains that make up proteins. (p. 537)

pleated sheet A polypeptide structure in which the chains are held together by hydrogen-bonding. (p. 541)

polypeptide A chain of several amino acid residues joined by peptide linkages. (p. 537)

residue An amino acid unit or monomer in a polypeptide chain. (p. 537)

salt linkage An ionic bond between a negatively charged group of an amino acid residue and a positively charged group. (p. 541)

QUESTIONS AND PROBLEMS FOR CHAPTER NINETEEN

■ **Amino Acids and Proteins**

SECTION 19.1 AMINO ACIDS

19.13) What products are formed by complete hydrolysis of proteins?

19.14) Write the formula and name of a basic amino acid.

19.26) Hydrolysis of a protein is the *reverse* of what process?

19.27) Write the formula and name of an aromatic amino acid.

19.15) What is meant by the isoelectric point of an amino acid?

19.16) How could you be sure that a spot resulting from paper chromatography was caused by tyrosine?

SECTION 19.2 POLYPEPTIDES

19.17) How many peptide linkages are there in a tripeptide?

19.18) How many alpha carbons, carboxyl carbons, and amino nitrogens are there in the backbone structure of a tetrapeptide?

19.19*) Would a fragment of a polypeptide chain that contained four amino acids give a positive biuret test? Explain.

19.20*) Which amino acid is capable of bonding *to itself* with a disulfide bond?

19.28) If you add NaOH to a solution of alanine at its isoelectric point, how will the charge be affected?

19.29) A peak obtained from column chromatography was labeled arginine. Explain.

19.30) Draw a peptide linkage between tyrosine and tryptophan.

19.31*) If two alanine molecules were added one at a time to a backbone consisting of four glycine residues, how would you name the new polypeptide?

19.32*) Would a tripeptide give a positive biuret test? Explain.

19.33*) If you broke a disulfide bond, would new amino acids be formed? Explain.

SECTION 19.3 THE STRUCTURE OF PROTEINS

19.21) Draw the primary structure of a protein.

19.22) Where might you find polar and nonpolar amino acids in a globular protein?

19.23*) Covalent bonds and ionic bonds are found *between* polypeptide chains. How could these be formed?

19.34) What would you add to the structure in Question 19.21 to represent the secondary structure of a protein?

19.35) How does the pleated sheet structure differ from the primary structure of a protein?

19.36) What kind of forces holds nonpolar side chains together?

SECTION 19.4 DENATURATION AND PRECIPITATION

19.24) A medical student was asked to draw a specimen of blood from a vein on a patient's arm. A nurse said to swab the arm with an alcohol solution. Why?

19.25*) Describe two procedures you could use to detect the presence of protein in a solution.

19.37) A bottle of insulin solution for injection was accidently placed on a mechanical shaker and shaken for 30 minutes. What might happen to the insulin?

19.38*) Mercury(II) chloride solutions were once used as antiseptics in hospitals. Why were they used?

19.39*) To what color tests would a tetrapeptide made up of Ala-Tyr-Cys-Trp give positive results?

19.40*) Imagine a polypeptide chain in an α-helix structure. Is it possible for this chain to bind to other α-helix structures in a protein molecule? Explain.

19.41*) How would you bring about the denaturation of the insulin molecule? Would your product have biological activity? Explain.

The Living Cell and Protein Synthesis

20

The goal of biochemistry is to understand the chemical reactions that occur in the living cell and their relation to cellular function and structure. The molecular components of the cell are formed from low-molecular-weight compounds, such as simple sugars, amino acids, and fatty acids. The large organic molecules that serve as structural building blocks for the cell include proteins, carbohydrates, lipids, and nucleic acids.

Whether we consider a single-cell organism like an amoeba or a complex living being like a person, life began from a single cell. The cell is the basic structure in which life processes are carried out. In this chapter, we will consider the various parts of a cell and the kinds of chemical substances that relate to each part. In later chapters, we will return to discuss the roles of certain cell structures in metabolism.

The human body contains about 75 trillion cells, which come in hundreds of basic types and are composed of many different kinds of inorganic and organic molecules. You will recognize the following from Chapter 1 as being, along with trace minerals and the vitamins to be discussed in Chapter 23, the components of a balanced diet.

Carbohydrates are taken in as food, broken down to monosaccharides (particularly glucose), and then used for energy and body-building. The energy-producing reactions will be discussed in Chapter 22, while those involving the synthesis, storage, and oxidation of body carbohydrates will be discussed in Chapter 25.

Lipids are consumed as fats in food, hydrolyzed to fatty acids, and used for energy and body processes. The metabolism of lipids will be discussed in Chapter 26.

Proteins (Chapter 19) are also food nutrients. While they may be used for energy, they mainly serve as raw materials for the amino acids needed for growth and maintenance of body tissues and for the synthesis of enzymes and hormones.

Inorganic cations and anions, such as Na^+, K^+, Ca^{2+}, Mg^{2+}, Cl^-, and HCO_3^-, fill vital roles in the body fluids. This topic will be discussed in Chapter 24.

Water is the most important substance in the body, permitting all cell reactions to take place in the aqueous solutions of the body fluids.

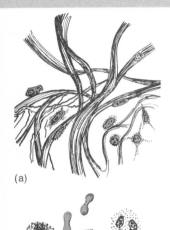

(a)

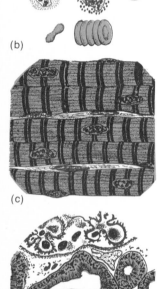

(b)

(c)

(d)

FIGURE 20–1   Some examples of human body cells: (a) connective tissue; (b) red and white blood cells; (c) muscle cells; (d) kidney tissue, showing tubules lined with *epithelial* cells.

20.1 THE LIVING CELL

> LEARNING GOAL 20A: *Draw a typical human cell, labeling at least four major organelles; show where nucleic acids and proteins are synthesized in the cell.*
>
> 20B: *Describe the primary function of the mitochondria in a cell.*

A living cell (Figure 20–1) is not simply a collection of molecules and ions in a bag. It has a shape, fixed by an outside cell wall or membrane, and several types of smaller internal bodies called **organelles.** Each organelle is enclosed in its own membrane and floats in the aqueous solution (*cytoplasm* or *intracellular fluid*) that fills the cell.

To help us understand the living cell, we might begin by putting each organelle into a diagram of the total cell (Figure 20–2). Carbohydrates are found in the *cytoplasm* and the *mitochondria*. The various *membranes* and

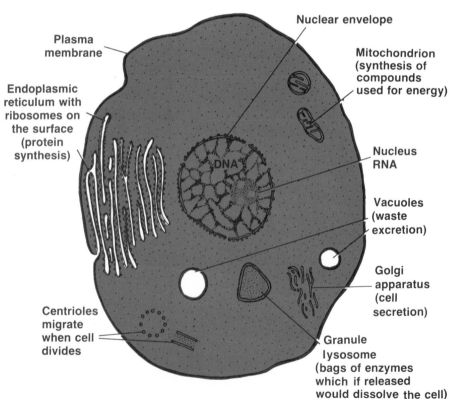

FIGURE 20–2   A typical human tissue cell showing the various organelles and membranes. Although the various organelles are shown separated from each other for clarity, most actually interact in the cell and function together.

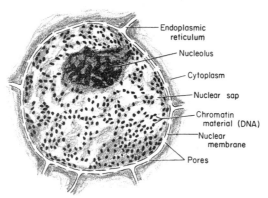

FIGURE 20–3 The parts of a nucleus, the control center of the cell.

Labels: Endoplasmic reticulum, Nucleolus, Cytoplasm, Nuclear sap, Chromatin material (DNA), Nuclear membrane, Pores

endoplasmic reticulum are made of lipids, especially phospholipids; lipids are also found in the cytoplasm and the mitochondria. Proteins are found everywhere in the cell. The transmission of hereditary information from the nucleic acids in the nucleus is carried out through protein synthesis. The enzymes that regulate the rate of cell reactions are all proteins. Protein synthesis is thus the most important function of a living cell.

One definition of biochemistry is "The chemistry of the living cell in health and disease." We must therefore attempt to relate the structure, function, and chemical reactions of a living cell to the larger organism.

The nucleus

The importance of the **nucleus** (Figure 20–3) to cell function and reproduction has been known for many years. In a sense, life starts with DNA and RNA, the nucleic acids of the nucleus. The genetic information stored in the chromosomes of the nucleus directs the synthesis of cell and tissue proteins needed for normal growth and functioning of the body.

Ribosomes

The **ribosomes** are ball-like structures on which proteins are synthesized. They are composed of roughly half nucleic acid and half protein. Ribosomes floating free in the cytoplasm make proteins that are used in the cell. The majority of the ribosomes, however, are attached to a network of flattened tubelike structures (Figure 20–4) called the "rough" **endoplasmic reticulum.** These ribosomes make proteins that are packaged by the Golgi

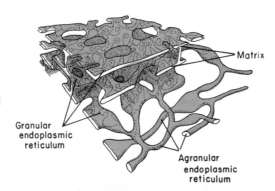

FIGURE 20–4 The endoplasmic reticulum, a chemical factory inside the cell.

Labels: Matrix, Granular endoplasmic reticulum, Agranular endoplasmic reticulum

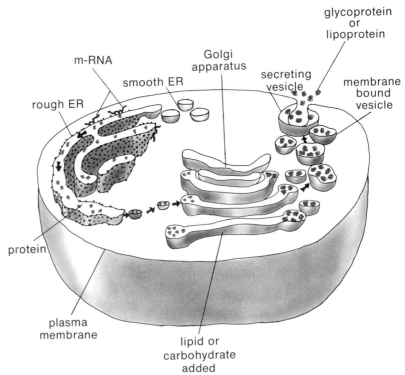

FIGURE 20-5   The roles of the endoplasmic reticulum and the Golgi bodies in synthesizing and packaging protein for shipment out of the cell. The function of m-RNA will be described in Section 20.5.

apparatus and shipped out of the cell for use in tissues and fluids throughout the body. The "smooth" endoplasmic reticulum (without ribosomes on the surface) makes lipids, phospholipids, and carbohydrates. These compounds may either be used to construct the cell membranes or be combined in the Golgi bodies to make *glycoproteins* (carbohydrate + protein) or *lipoproteins* (lipids + protein).

Golgi apparatus

As shown in Figure 20-5, the polypeptides synthesized in the ribosomes on the "rough" endoplasmic reticulum pass into small tubes (tubules) in another organelle, the **Golgi apparatus.** There we find a series of flattened tubes similar to those of the endoplasmic reticulum. In a factory, this would be called a "shipping room." The proteins, glycoproteins, and lipoproteins are packaged in small containers called *vesicles*, which eventually pass through the cell wall and release their contents to the fluid outside the cell. The enzymes for the digestive system and the hormone insulin are prepared in this manner.

Lysosomes

Some of the proteins manufactured inside the cell are kept for further use by the same cell. An example is the group of enzymes enclosed in **lyso-**

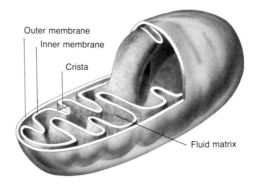

FIGURE 20–6 A mitochondrion, with part cut away to show the internal membranes.

somes. These organelles, shown in Figure 20–2, provide a system that allows the cell to digest (hydrolyze) and remove unwanted substances and structures. These might include worn-out cell parts as well as unneeded tissue, such as that of the uterus after pregnancy. If a cell is damaged, its complete hydrolysis by lysosomes allows a new cell to take its place. Foreign substances, such as bacteria, are also destroyed in this manner, especially by the white blood cells.

Mitochondria

Many of the processes in the body require an on-the-spot source of energy. This energy is needed to break the chemical bonds in the reactants, as described in Section 21.4. More than 95% of the energy for the cell—and for the body—comes from the **mitochondria** (Figure 20–6).

These organelles are large, football-shaped structures that float in the cytoplasm. The energy-providing series of reactions begins in the cytoplasm with *glycolysis* (Section 22.2), which converts glucose to pyruvate, and continues in the mitochondria with the *Krebs cycle* (Section 22.3) and the *electron transport system* (Section 22.4), which together convert pyruvate to carbon dioxide and water, with the release of energy.

Mitochondria have both outer and inner membranes. The inner layer is folded into many projections called *cristae* or "crests," which provide a large surface area on which reactions can take place.

The mitochondria are self-sufficient and contain enough DNA, RNA, ribosomes, and enzymes for the manufacture of the many proteins needed to maintain the functions of this organelle.

Cytoplasm

The *intra*cellular fluid or **cytoplasm** is a protein-rich aqueous solution in which nutrients are dissolved and the cell organelles are suspended. The synthesis of many essential molecules, such as fatty acids and amino acids, occurs in the cytoplasm, along with the energy-producing process of *glycolysis*. The detailed composition of the cytoplasm will be briefly described in Section 24.4. It is kept buffered at normal body pH (about 7.4) by protein and phosphate buffers, as noted in Section 13.5.

It is important to remember that the cytoplasm inside the cell is separated from the *interstitial* fluid (lymph, tissue fluids) by the cell membrane. Each cell organelle is also surrounded by a similar kind of membrane, composed of phospholipid bilayers and proteins that effectively keep certain

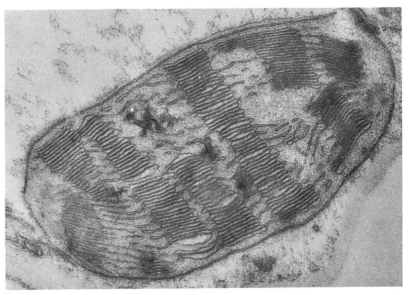

Photograph of a chloroplast taken by an electron microscope (enlarged about 20 000 times).

molecules and ions out of and others inside the organelle while allowing nutrients and products to pass through.

Chloroplasts

Green plants have additional organelles called *chloroplasts,* which are not found in animal cells. A series of flattened membrane structures called *grana* contain the green substance chlorophyll, which plays a major role in photosynthesis (Section 25.5).

Chloroplasts are often compared with mitochondria because, in addition to having a somewhat similar appearance, chloroplasts also contain the DNA and RNA needed to synthesize protein. The major difference between these two kinds of organelles is that mitochondria *oxidize* complex molecules to release CO_2, H_2O, and energy, while chloroplasts use the sun's energy along with CO_2 and H_2O to manufacture complex molecules.

SELF-CHECK

20.1)   Make a list of the organelles contained in a typical human tissue cell. Which organelles are involved in the synthesis of proteins for ''export'' to other tissues?

20.2)   Explain why mitochondria are sometimes called ''the power-houses of the cell.''

20.2 NUCLEIC ACIDS

LEARNING GOAL 20C: Describe the difference in composition between DNA and RNA.

20D: Compare the chemical structure of ATP with that of a nucleotide.

In our discussion of the cell and its contents, we briefly mentioned the DNA and RNA in the nucleus, mitochondria, and chloroplasts. These **nucleic acid** molecules are responsible for genetic characteristics and the flow of information from the nucleus to all parts of the cell.

Of prime importance is the role of nucleic acids in the synthesis of *all* the proteins used by the body. **DNA,** **d**eoxyribonucleic acid, is contained in the chromosomes of the nucleus. It sends a message by way of *messenger* **RNA**, a type of **r**ibonucleic acid, to the ribosomes. The message says that a specific protein (for example, the hormone *insulin*) must be synthesized. The flow of information is

DNA $\longrightarrow$ messenger RNA $\longrightarrow$ ribosomes $\longrightarrow$ protein for export

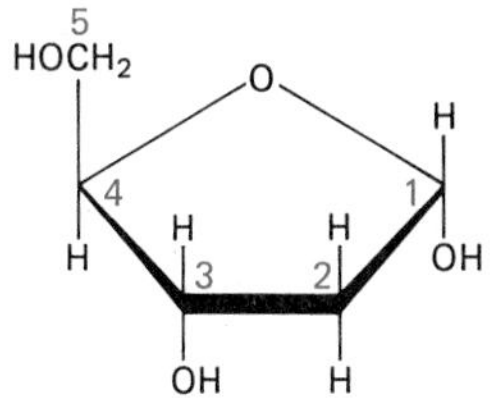

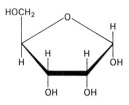

α-2-deoxy-
D-ribose

α-D-ribose

FIGURE 20–7   The two pentoses in nucleic acids. The only difference between them is the presence on carbon 2 of a hydrogen atom or a hydroxyl group. The term *deoxy* means "removal of oxygen." These sugars are always shown in the furanose (ring) form.

The nucleic acid pentoses

The hydrolysis of a large biochemical molecule gives the small monomer units that make up its structure. The hydrolysis of a nucleic acid produces phosphoric acid (H_3PO_4), nitrogen-containing bases, and five-carbon monosaccharides (sugars) called pentoses.

The two important types of nucleic acid, DNA and RNA, differ in the sugars they give on hydrolysis. DNA gives *deoxyribose* and RNA gives *ribose* (Figure 20–7). You may recall the D-ribose structure from Self-Check 17.2 (p. 493). The ribose unit should be learned well since it is a part not only of RNA but also of the energy-containing molecule ATP and other extremely important compounds in the cell.

Pyrimidine and purine bases

Pyrimidine and purine rings were discussed in Section 15.4. Both contain nitrogen as part of the heterocyclic ring and are thus basic amine-like compounds. The five important bases produced in the hydrolysis of nucleic acids are shown in Figure 20–8.

The DNA structure involves two pairs of purine and pyrimidine bases, the purines adenine and guanine and the pyrimidines cytosine and thymine (Section 20.3). RNA is built with the same purine bases, but its pyrimidines are cytosine and uracil (Section 20.4).

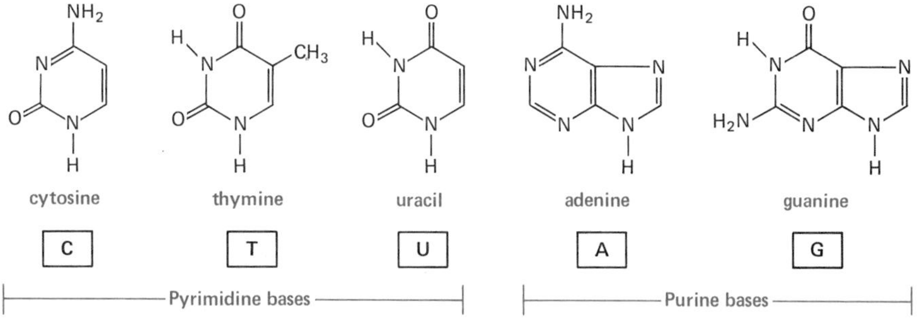

| cytosine | thymine | uracil | adenine | guanine |
| C | T | U | A | G |

—————— Pyrimidine bases ——————   —————— Purine bases ——————

FIGURE 20–8   The bases in DNA and RNA. The boxed initial letter of each base is commonly used as its symbol. The bases A, T, G, and C are found in DNA; A, U, G, and C are found in RNA.

Nucleotides

Nucleic acids are natural polymers created by condensation polymerization, the splitting out of water between monomer units. The formation of a repeating pattern is shown in Figure 20–9.

When a pyrimidine or purine base combines with ribose or deoxyribose (as at the upper right of Figure 20–9), the result is a **nucleoside** molecule. When phosphoric acid then combines with a hydroxyl group of the sugar in an ester linkage, the complete molecule is a **nucleotide.** The combination in Figure 20–9, adenine + ribose, leads to the nucleoside *adenosine*. This name will become familiar when we discuss ATP, adenosine **tri**phosphate, and ADP, adenosine **di**phosphate, in Chapter 22. The complete molecule shown in Figure 20–9 is often called AMP, adenosine **mono**phosphate.

AMP has an extremely important property: additional phosphate units can combine with it. Adding one more phosphate gives ADP, and adding a third phosphate gives ATP (Figure 20–10). AMP, ADP, and ATP are found in every cell. ADP and ATP are the source of unique bonds, shown by the wavy lines (∿) between phosphorus and oxygen in Figure 20–10, which

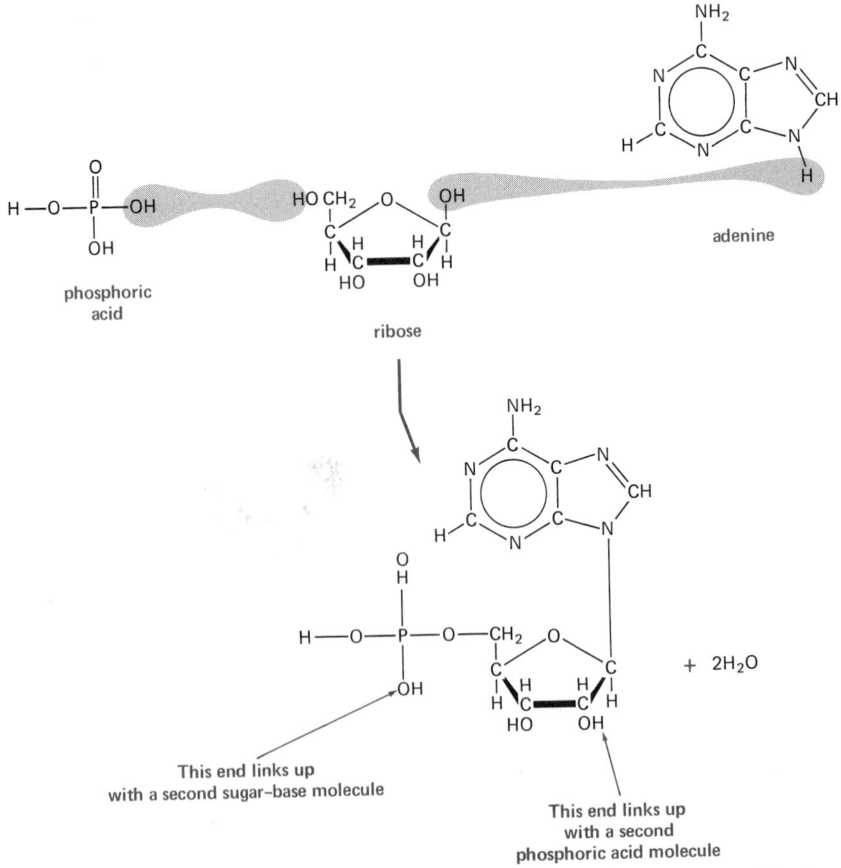

AMP, also called adenylic acid, is important in muscle tissue. A derivative of ATP called *cyclic* AMP has the phosphate linked to *two* carbons of the ribose ring and is important in carbohydrate metabolism

FIGURE 20–9 The repeating structure in DNA and RNA is a nucleotide, formed by condensing a base, a sugar, and phosphoric acid. The adenine + ribose combination gives a nucleoside called adenosine. The further reaction with phosphoric acid gives AMP, adenosine **mono**phosphate, which can then join with other nucleotides to form DNA and RNA polymers.

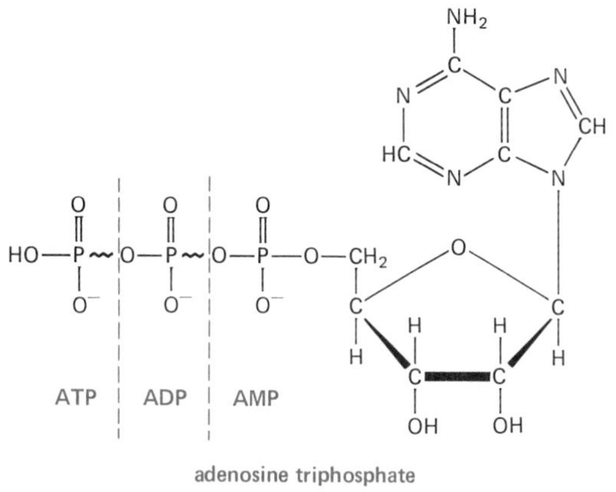

FIGURE 20–10   The structure of ATP. Remove one phosphate unit and you obtain ADP. Remove another and you arrive at AMP, a nucleotide. The wavy lines indicate bonds between phosphorus and oxygen that can be used in energy transfer to fuel metabolic reactions.

adenosine triphosphate

when broken provide energy for many metabolic reactions, as described in Chapter 22.

A number of different nucleotides are possible. The base may be any of the five we have discussed (as well as a few others); the sugar may be ribose or deoxyribose; and the phosphoric acid may condense with the hydroxyl group at carbon 2, 3, or 5 of ribose (or carbon 2 or 3 of deoxyribose). We will soon see that these diverse combinations give rise to the genetic information that regulates life.

Nucleotides also combine with some vitamins to form *coenzymes*, which will be discussed in Section 23.3.

SELF-CHECK

20.3)   What compounds are formed by the complete hydrolysis of DNA? How would the result differ for RNA?
20.4)   Starting with adenosine, what reactions must occur to arrive at ATP?

20.3 THE STRUCTURE OF DNA

LEARNING GOAL 20E: Describe the backbone structure of a polynucleotide chain.

20F: Explain how hydrogen-bonding between complementary bases is essential to the double helix structure of DNA.

The nucleic acids DNA and RNA are polymers of nucleotides or *polynucleotides*. The monomer units are joined when the phosphate group of one monomer forms an ester linkage with the sugar of the next nucleotide, as shown in Figure 20–11 (see page 556).

The purine and pyrimidine bases project out from the backbone. Note that in Figure 20–11 the symbol that represents the base adenine (A) has a V-shaped opening, and the symbol for the base thymine (T) has a V-shaped projection that exactly matches that opening. These two bases fit together very well and form strong hydrogen-bonding attractions. Similarly, you can see that the symbol for cytosine (C) fits into the symbol for guanine (G). We therefore say that thymine is *complementary* to adenine and cytosine is complementary to guanine. One side is always a purine base, the other side a pyrimidine base. The hydrogen-bonding attractions between two backbone chains are shown in Figure 20–12.

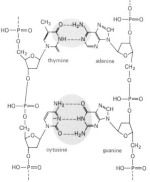

FIGURE 20–12
Hydrogen-bonding between parallel strands of DNA stabilizes the overall structure. Thymine always pairs with adenine, cytosine always with guanine.

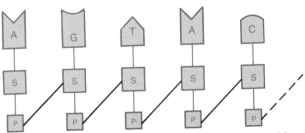

FIGURE 20–11 The polymer structure of a strand of DNA. Nucleotide monomers are joined together by phosphate groups (P) linked to the deoxyribose sugars (S). The purine bases adenine (A) and guanine (G) are larger than and *complementary to* the pyrimidine bases thymine (T) and cytosine (C). This allows two such strands to lie parallel, attached to each other by hydrogen-bonding.

Between 1950 and 1953, many scientists tried to determine the exact structure of the DNA molecule. It was found that there were equal numbers of purine and pyrimidine bases.

Hydrogen-bonding between complementary base pairs is essential to the DNA structure.

DNA molecules have molecular weights ranging from one million to one billion amu. Experimental work by Franklin and Wilkins indicated that DNA might consist of two or more polynucleotide chains arranged in a helix or spiral structure. In 1953, Watson and Crick constructed a molecular model

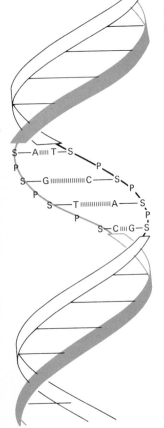

FIGURE 20–13 The double helix structure of DNA proposed by Watson and Crick. As usual, S = sugar, P = phosphate. Compare this spiral structure with that shown in Figure 19–7 for certain proteins.

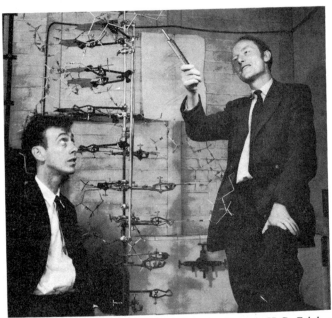

The double helix structure of DNA is pointed out by Francis H.C. Crick, with James D. Watson looking on. These two scientists built scale models of DNA based on the x-ray data on distances between atoms and bond angles obtained by Maurice H.F. Wilkins. They have compared this task to the working of a three-dimensional jigsaw puzzle. For this work, Watson, Crick, and Wilkins received the 1962 Nobel Prize in chemistry.

for DNA that included all of the facts known to that time. They twisted the two chains into a *double helix* (Figure 20–13).

It turns out that this double-stranded model fulfills all of the requirements. At each monomer unit, there must be hydrogen-bonding between a purine base and a pyrimidine base. A pair of purines (A + G) would be too large and bulky; a pair of pyrimidines (T + C) would be too small and would have weak attractions. The fit has to be perfect.

The nucleus of each cell contains hereditary information in the form of DNA. Since each such DNA molecule has a weight of roughly *one billion* amu, there are many, many possible sequences of bases that could be found along the backbone. We now know that these sequences provide the *genetic code* that tells the rest of the cell what proteins need to be synthesized.

The cell biologist is aware of the existence of chromosomes in the nucleus of each tissue cell. Each chromosome contains *genes* that make us what we are. Each gene has the recipe for a specific protein molecule. The chemist therefore describes a biological gene as a *portion* of the DNA double helix chain. The total DNA in a single human cell is estimated to contain an average of 5.5 billion base pairs and to have a stretched-out length of about two meters. Inside the cell, it must be coiled very tightly!

The process by which DNA is reproduced during cell division (*replication*) will be discussed in Section 28.1.

Some bacteria, single-celled organisms, have only one chromosome with one molecule of DNA. This single spiral then contains all of the genetic information for that organism.

20.5) What base pairs are found in the DNA polynucleotide chain?
20.6) What holds the double helix structure of DNA together?

SELF-CHECK

20.4 THE STRUCTURE AND ROLE OF RNA

LEARNING GOAL 20G: Describe the process of transcription.
20H: List the three different kinds of RNA and briefly describe the role of each.

RNA differs from the DNA double helix in three respects: the sugar unit is ribose instead of deoxyribose (Figure 20–7), the thymine on DNA is replaced by uracil (Figure 20–8) on RNA, and RNA consists not of a double helix but of a single strand or chain of nucleic acid monomers, forming a polymer considerably shorter than DNA. RNA molecules have molecular weights from 25 000 to about one million amu.

There are three types of RNA that participate in the process of protein synthesis in the cell. All are produced using information from the DNA in the cell nucleus by a process called **transcription.**

Messenger RNA (m-RNA) carries the genetic code, which specifies the sequence of amino acids in a protein. It goes from the nucleus into the cytoplasm and threads its way through ribosomes.

Transfer RNA (t-RNA) is a small molecule that serves as a "shuttle" to bring amino acids to the m-RNA in a process called *translation.*

Ribosomal RNA (r-RNA) provides the site for protein synthesis by combining with protein to make a ribosome surface that can accept the m-RNA molecule.

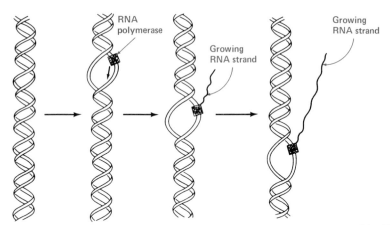

FIGURE 20–14   Transcription involves the unraveling of a DNA strand by RNA polymerase and the formation of a single strand of RNA.

Transcription from DNA to RNA

The DNA molecule is a tightly held double helix. How does it transmit information? An enzyme (a large protein that helps make and break bonds) called *RNA polymerase* is involved.

By random collisions between RNA polymerase and the DNA double helix, the RNA polymerase eventually runs into certain sequences of bases on the DNA strands and latches onto them. These sequences of DNA bases are recognized by the enzyme as "start" positions for transcription. The enzyme then begins to *unravel* part of the DNA double helix, as shown in Figure 20–14.

The RNA polymerase moves down the DNA, unraveling the strands as it goes. Nucleoside triphosphates like ATP are available in the solution and pair up with the newly revealed DNA bases. In this way, a sequence involving adenine, uracil, guanine, and cytosine is built up in a pattern complementary to that in DNA (Figure 20–15). The RNA sequence is, in fact, identical to that in one of the DNA strands except that thymine has been replaced by uracil. In that way, the genetic message has been recorded or transcribed into the RNA chain, just as a phonograph record may be used to transcribe a musical performance already on a master disk.

The unwound DNA strand serves as a *template* or stencil for synthesis of the RNA strand. As the enzyme moves down the strand, the DNA rewinds back into its original double helix. Finally, the enzyme reaches a base sequence that signals the end of transcription. At that point, the enzyme and the newly formed RNA molecule separate completely from the DNA. The net result is an RNA strand with a base sequence complementary to that of the DNA strand that served as a template. The three types of RNA are prepared from different sections of the DNA strand.

The genetic code

The DNA provides the exact sequence of bases in messenger RNA. However, there are only four bases. This cannot provide full information to set the sequence of the amino acid residues in a polypeptide, since there are 20 amino acids.

DNA with **DNA**   **DNA** with m-RNA   m-RNA with **t-RNA**

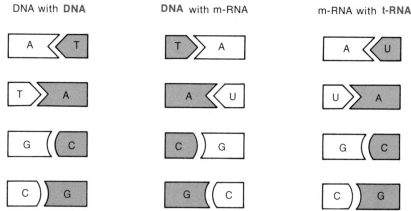

FIGURE 20–15 Base-pairing in three different situations related to protein synthesis: (left) the DNA double helix is held together by hydrogen-bonding between complementary bases on the two strands; (center) *transcription* occurs when complementary bases are formed on a messenger RNA strand; (right) *translation* of the genetic code occurs when the correct type of transfer RNA is fitted to the m-RNA. Note that the t-RNA sequence (shown in color) carries the same information as the original DNA strand (shown in color, with *T* replaced by *U*).

Instead, the information regarding the particular amino acid is contained in a "triplet" of three adjacent bases, as listed in Table 20–1. This triplet, called a **codon,** determines which amino acid will be inserted in a protein. There are 64 (4 × 4 × 4) possible three-base sequences (codons), and each one has a specific function, shown in Table 20–1. For example, there is only one codon for the amino acid tryptophan. When the m-RNA strand has the sequence uracil-guanine-guanine, we will end up with tryptophan in the polypeptide chain.

After transcription, the messenger RNA strand passes out of the cell nu-

A *codon* carries a code for a particular amino acid unit in a polypeptide. Unfortunately, and contrary to what may be implied in Figure 20–16, there is *no spacing* between codons. If a DNA strand is damaged by the addition or removal of a nucleotide, the entire m-RNA base sequence could be affected, and the new protein might be different from the original. This may be one of the causes of genetic defects. The codons listed in Table 20–1 are thought to be universal, that is, valid for all types of organisms.

TABLE 20–1 CODONS FOR SPECIFIC AMINO ACIDS

Amino Acids	Codons for m-RNA
Alanine	GCA, GCC, GCG, GCU
Arginine	AGA, AGG, CGA, CGG, CGC, CGU
Asparagine	AAC, AAU
Aspartic acid	GAC, GAU
Cysteine	UGC, UGU
Glutamic acid	GAA, GAG
Glutamine	CAG, CAA
Glycine	GGA, GGC, GGG, GGU
Histidine	CAC, CAU
Isoleucine	AUA, AUC, AUU
Leucine	CUA, CUC, CUG, CUU, UUA, UUG
Lysine	AAA, AAG
Methionine	AUG—Chain initiation
Phenylalanine	UUU, UUC
Proline	CCA, CCC, CCG, CCU
Serine	AGC, AGU, UCA, UCG, UCC, UCU
Threonine	ACA, ACG, ACC, ACU
Tryptophan	UGG
Tyrosine	UAC, UAU
Valine	GUA, GUG, GUC, GUU
Chain termination	UAA, UAG, UGA

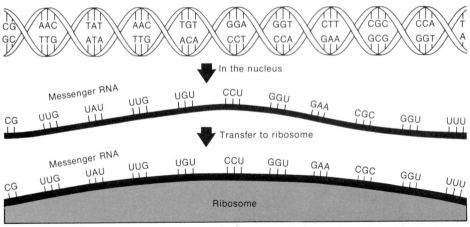

FIGURE 20–16 Transcription carries a genetic message from the DNA in the nucleus to the m-RNA on a ribosome. Each triplet of bases is a *codon* and matches one particular amino acid. There is no spacing between codons in a real molecule. The m-RNA section shows codes for (from left to right) leucine-tyrosine-leucine-cysteine-proline-glycine-glutamic acid-arginine-glycine, as listed in Table 20–1.

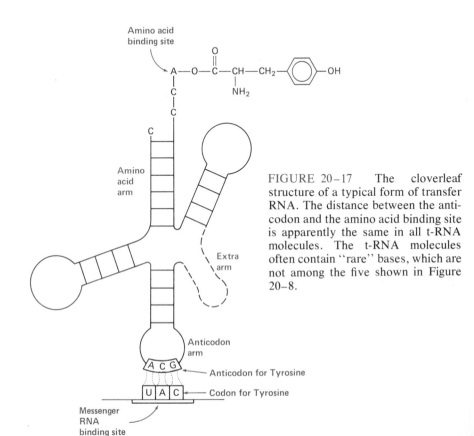

FIGURE 20–17 The cloverleaf structure of a typical form of transfer RNA. The distance between the anticodon and the amino acid binding site is apparently the same in all t-RNA molecules. The t-RNA molecules often contain "rare" bases, which are not among the five shown in Figure 20–8.

cleus and into the cytoplasm, where it latches onto a ribosome. It then serves as a template for protein synthesis, as shown in Figure 20–16.

Transfer RNA

Transfer RNA plays the role of carrier of individual amino acids onto the messenger RNA template (Figure 20–16). Each t-RNA molecule is small, with molecular weight from 25 000 to 40 000 amu. In contrast to m-RNA, which consists of a single long strand, the t-RNA molecule folds up into a cloverleaf shape as a result of hydrogen-bonding between different parts of the same strand, as shown in Figure 20–17.

At one end of the t-RNA chain is a grouping of nucleotides, C—C—A in the case shown in Figure 20–17, which serves to bind an amino acid carried by ribosomal RNA. At the opposite end of the cloverleaf is a triplet of bases that are complementary to the corresponding bases in the codon of m-RNA. The t-RNA triplet is called the **anticodon.** There is one t-RNA molecule for each anticodon. This assures that the t-RNA will line up properly to assemble the polypeptide strand of the protein.

SELF-CHECK

20.7)   Name three different compounds that are essential to the process of transcription in a cell.
20.8)   How does m-RNA differ from t-RNA?

20.5 PROTEIN SYNTHESIS

LEARNING GOAL 20I: Describe the process of translation in protein synthesis.

We have already described how the genetic code is *transcribed* from the DNA double helix in the chromosomes of a cell onto messenger RNA, and how the m-RNA forms a template on a ribosome. We will now concern ourselves with the formation of a polypeptide chain that follows the same genetic code.

Transfer RNA serves as an ideal "errand runner" to fetch the proper amino acid and bring it into position. In this process, ATP first reacts with the amino acid to form an "activated" ATP-amino acid complex. This

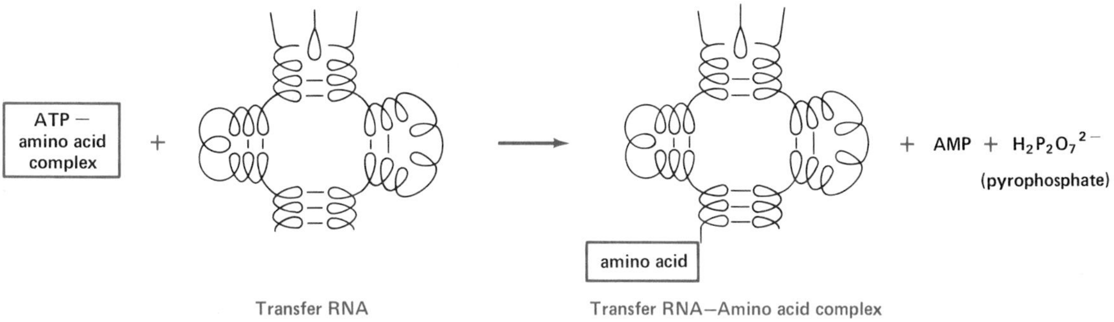

FIGURE 20–18   An amino acid is bonded to a t-RNA molecule with the help of energy-rich ATP.

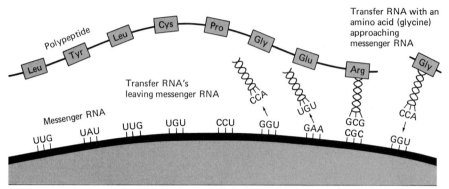

FIGURE 20–19 Translation of the genetic code involves the transport by t-RNA molecules of amino acids to their proper positions above the m-RNA template. The template arrived on the ribosome earlier, as shown in Figure 20–16.

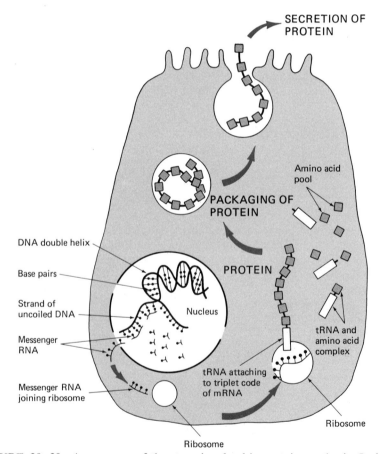

FIGURE 20–20 A summary of the steps involved in protein synthesis. Inside the nucleus (lower left), a strand of uncoiled DNA serves as a template for the lining up of nucleotides to make a strand of messenger RNA. The messenger RNA goes to the ribosomes. The transfer RNA forms a complex with amino acids from the amino acid pool (floating amino acids in the cytoplasm) and links up with the m-RNA to form the protein. The protein is then packaged in the Golgi apparatus and secreted from the cell.

species then reacts with the t-RNA carrier, as shown in Figure 20–18. The products of that reaction are AMP and a form of phosphoric acid. This reaction could not occur in the absence of the energy-carrier ATP. It is thus *coupled* with a phosphate transfer reaction in order to make it go, as described more fully in Section 22.1.

The base sequence of the anticodon on the t-RNA is the same as the sequence on the original DNA strand except that thymine is replaced by uracil. The process by which the amino acid residues are set up in the proper order is called **translation.** This process is shown in Figure 20–19, which shows a polypeptide chain being continued. A new t-RNA for glycine is arriving with its load, while two earlier t-RNA molecules are no longer needed and can go off to pick up new loads.

Each step is controlled by specific enzymes, using ATP or similar triphosphate molecules as energy sources. It almost seems as though the t-RNA molecules "know where they are going." This is, of course, not true. There are so many millions of molecular collisions each second that some of those collisions must be the correct ones to carry out the chemical reaction.

Eventually, we reach the m-RNA codon for chain termination (UAA, UAG, or UGA) and the polypeptide chain is a complete protein molecule. It can then leave the ribosome to perform its function, as shown in Figure 20–20.

SELF-CHECK

20.9)   Describe how, in the process of translation, amino acids are brought together to form a polypeptide chain.
20.10*)   Under some conditions, amino acids will react to form polypeptides. Why do we need such a complicated system involving m-RNA and t-RNA? Why not simply have enzymes to facilitate the formation of peptide bonds?
20.11*)   From Table 20–1, choose the two codons for phenylalanine. Describe the anticodons on the t-RNA molecules that could be used to add phenylalanine to a growing polypeptide chain.

CHAPTER TWENTY IN REVIEW ■ The Living Cell and Protein Synthesis

20.1 THE LIVING CELL

Page 548

20A: *Draw a typical human cell, labeling at least four major organelles; show where nucleic acids and proteins are synthesized in the cell.*
20B: *Describe the primary function of the mitochondria in a cell.*

20.2 NUCLEIC ACIDS

Page 552

20C: *Describe the difference in composition between DNA and RNA.*
20D: *Compare the chemical structure of ATP with that of a nucleotide.*

20.3 THE STRUCTURE OF DNA

Page 555

20E: *Describe the backbone structure of a polynucleotide chain.*
20F: *Explain how hydrogen-bonding between complementary bases is essential to the double helix structure of DNA.*

GLOSSARY FOR CHAPTER TWENTY

anticodon A group of three adjacent bases on transfer RNA complementary to a codon on messenger RNA. (p. 561)

codon A group of three adjacent bases on messenger RNA that specifies a particular amino acid unit in sequence in a polypeptide chain to be formed by *translation*. (p. 559)

cytoplasm The viscous aqueous solution inside the cell that contains the organelles; the intracellular fluid. (p. 551)

DNA Deoxyribonucleic acid, a polymer of nucleotide monomers arranged in a double helix; provides genetic information; found in the cell nucleus. (p. 553)

endoplasmic reticulum A network of tubelike structures in the cytoplasm; contains ribosomes used in protein synthesis. (p. 549)

Golgi apparatus Organelles in the cell that receive proteins from the ribosomes, sometimes add carbohydrate or lipid to them, and prepare them for shipment out of the cell. (p. 550)

lysosomes Organelles containing enzymes capable of hydrolyzing waste and foreign matter in the cell. (p. 550)

messenger RNA (m-RNA) Nucleic acid molecules with single strands formed by *transcription* from DNA in the nucleus; used on the ribosomes to synthesize polypeptide chains; contains codons. (p. 557)

mitochondria Organelles that contain all the necessary compounds for 95% of the energy provided to the cell as ATP; the site of several important metabolic cycles. (p. 551)

nucleic acid A polymer of nucleotide units; a polynucleotide, such as DNA or RNA. (p. 553)

nucleoside A molecule formed by combining a purine or pyrimidine base with a pentose. (p. 554)

nucleotide The monomer that forms a nucleic acid; a nucleoside combined with phosphoric acid in an ester linkage. (p. 554)

nucleus, cell A spherical organelle that contains DNA and is the site of transcription. (p. 549)

organelle A small organ inside a cell that performs specialized functions; examples include the nucleus, mitochondria, ribosomes, lysosomes, endoplasmic reticulum, and Golgi apparatus. (p. 548)

ribosomes Small round organelles, mainly on the rough endoplasmic reticulum, that serve as sites for the synthesis of proteins through *translation*; contain ribosomal RNA (r-RNA). (p. 549)

RNA Ribonucleic acid, polynucleotide molecules involved in the synthesis of proteins. (p. 553)

transcription The construction of a strand of messenger RNA containing the proper genetic code (codons) from the complementary bases on a strand of DNA in the nucleus. (p. 557)

transfer RNA (t-RNA) A small RNA molecule that carries a specific amino acid to a ribosome for protein synthesis. (p. 557)

translation Transport by t-RNA of amino acids to m-RNA on the ribosomes to synthesize a protein containing a definite sequence of amino acid units. (p. 563)

QUESTIONS AND PROBLEMS FOR CHAPTER 20 ■ The Living Cell and Protein Synthesis

SECTION 20.1 THE LIVING CELL

20.12) Draw a picture that shows the difference between the Golgi apparatus and the nucleus of a cell.

20.13) Compare the functions of mitochondria and ribosomes.

SECTION 20.2 NUCLEIC ACIDS

20.14) How does the full name of RNA relate to the five-carbon sugar in its molecule?

20.15) What purine and five-carbon sugar are present in ATP?

SECTION 20.3 THE STRUCTURE OF DNA

20.16) What are the roles of the five-carbon sugar and phosphoric acid in the polynucleotide chain of DNA?

20.17) Equal numbers of purine and pyrimidine bases are essential to the double helix structure of DNA. Explain.

SECTION 20.4 THE STRUCTURE AND ROLE OF RNA

20.18) Name the molecules produced by the process of transcription.

20.19) Which kind of RNA consists of relatively short chains? What is its role?

20.20*) Which amino acid in Table 20–1 has a single codon? What is the codon?

SECTION 20.5 PROTEIN SYNTHESIS

20.21) How does t-RNA connect to m-RNA in the translation process?

20.22*) What is the special role of the codon AUG? (See Table 20–1.)

20.23) Use a drawing to show how lysosomes differ from free ribosomes.

20.24) Compare the functions of lysosomes and mitochondria.

20.25) Do RNA and DNA differ in their purine or pyrimidine bases? Explain.

20.26) How does ATP differ from AMP?

20.27) Why doesn't adenine pair with guanine in the polynucleotide chain of DNA?

20.28) How many hydrogen-bonds connect each pair of bases in DNA? Explain.

20.29) What energy-rich molecule is essential for the production of RNA from DNA in transcription?

20.30) Which kind of RNA moves out of the nucleus and onto ribosomes? Why?

20.31*) Why are there more codons than amino acids?

20.32) How are amino acids attached to t-RNA in the translation process?

20.33*) What happens to a t-RNA molecule after its amino acid is attached to the growing polypeptide chain?

Energy and Reaction Rates

21

The cell and its component parts and membranes contain carbohydrates, lipids, proteins, and nucleic acids. We have just considered the chemical properties of these substances. To maintain life, the cell must also have a source of energy. The chemical reactions that will liberate energy from food are thus vital.

In Chapter 1, we briefly discussed how fats and carbohydrates can be used in the human body to provide energy. Section 3.3 discussed the ionization energy of individual atoms, a concept that was seen again in Section 6.1, where we introduced the energy units of *kilocalories*.

In addition to the Law of Conservation of Mass (Sections 2.4 and 5.1), there is a Law of Conservation of Energy:

In normal chemical and physical processes, energy is neither created nor destroyed. It can only be converted from one energy form to another.

In this chapter, we will discuss how *heat energy* (enthalpy) can be gained and lost in several kinds of processes. We will see how energy is gained from food and how it is used in body activity. Finally, we will look at some factors that affect the rate of a chemical reaction and will briefly discuss the role of enzymes, the biological catalysts, in regulating body processes. Along the way, we will introduce in as simple a manner as possible the idea of *free energy*, which is commonly used in biochemistry. It is a measure of the "driving force" that makes a chemical reaction happen.

The SI energy unit is the joule (J). One kilocalorie is exactly 4184 joules.

21.1 HEAT TRANSFER

> *LEARNING GOAL 21A: Given the mass of a pure substance, the specific heat, and a temperature change, calculate the heat flow, ΔH.*
>
> *21B: Given the mass of a pure substance changing between the liquid and gas states (or between solid and liquid) and given the heat of vaporization (or fusion), calculate the heat flow, ΔH.*

In Section 10.2, we defined temperature as the *average energy of motion* of the particles in a sample. We also showed how temperature determines the direction of heat flow:

Heat flows from a hotter (higher-temperature) body to a colder (lower-temperature) body.

567

Heat is simply the total energy of motion of particles. However, it is not possible to measure the amount of heat actually contained in a sample. Instead, we often measure the heat flow, the gain or loss of heat (kinetic energy) required to raise or lower the temperature of a substance.

Heat energy corrected for pressure and volume effects is called **enthalpy,** with the symbol H. While we cannot measure directly the amount of enthalpy, we will often refer to the **enthalpy change,** ΔH, of a reaction or process. In this text, we express ΔH in units of kilocalories.

Specific heat

At this point, we will discuss the amount of heat that is needed to raise the temperature of a sample or the amount of heat that must be removed to lower the temperature. The easiest substance to deal with is liquid water.

The kilocalorie is defined as follows:

One kilocalorie is the amount of heat needed to raise the temperature of one kilogram of pure liquid water by exactly one Celsius degree.

Specific heat is a measure of how many kilocalories of heat energy are required for the heating process. For water, we can say that the specific heat is 1.00 kilocalorie for each kilogram* for each Celsius degree of temperature rise, or SH = 1.00 kcal/kg-K, where K stands for a change in temperature in either Celsius or Kelvin degrees (p. 272).

In general, the specific heat is the heat flow in kilocalories required to increase or decrease the temperature of a substance by one degree. Table 21–1 gives the specific heat values of some common substances. There is some variation in specific heat with temperature. For liquid water, the specific heat varies from 0.998 kcal/kg-K at 35°C to 1.007 kcal/kg-K at 100°C.

If you know something about specific heats, you can better understand some everyday events. For example, when the temperature drops at sundown, which cools off more quickly, the land or a body of water? The land does: water maintains its temperature because it has a *high* specific heat. For the same reason, it takes a long time for the oceans to warm up in the spring. The seas, lakes, and rivers help keep the temperature of the environment relatively constant between day and night and between winter and summer.

Would you prefer a frying pan made of aluminum or of cast iron if you wish to cook a hamburger quickly? Both are metals and thus have low specific heats. However, iron will heat up almost twice as fast as aluminum. Iron has a specific heat of 0.106 kcal/kg-K, while that of aluminum is 0.21 kcal/kg-K.

If you leave a silver spoon in a cup of hot coffee, the temperature of the spoon quickly rises (SH = 0.057 kcal/kg-K), while a stainless steel spoon (SH = 0.106) takes longer to heat up. You are more likely to burn your mouth using a silver spoon than using one made of stainless steel!

The chemist's kilocalorie is the same as the "Calorie" (with a capital C) used when discussing food and dieting. Some texts give ΔH values in joules, where one joule is 0.000239 kcal. Other units you may run across include Btu (British thermal units), ergs, and eV (electron volts). Any of these may be converted to kilocalories.

Remember from Chapter 10 that one degree interval in Celsius (from 25° to 26°, for example) is the same as one degree interval in Kelvin (from 298 K to 299 K). The symbol K is used to indicate the number of degrees of temperature *difference* on either scale.

TABLE 21–1   SELECTED SPECIFIC HEATS IN kcal/kg-K
(at 25°C unless noted)

Aluminum	0.21
Copper	0.092
Gold	0.031
Iron	0.106
Silver	0.057
Liquid water	1.00
Ice (0°C)	0.49
Steam (100°C)	0.48
Ethanol	0.59
Acetone	0.51
Liquid mercury	0.0332
Oxygen gas	0.219

---

* Specific heat is usually defined as the heat flow to change one *gram* of a substance by one degree and is then measured in calories (with a small c) per gram-degree. Rather than create confusion over which kind of "calorie" is meant, we will use a slightly different interpretation of specific heat, which uses numbers identical to those found in common tables. This permits us to use only one unit, the kilocalorie, for all heat calculations.

Changes of state and heat flow

In Section 11.5 we discussed the difference between endothermic and exothermic processes, using changes of state as an example. Let's review these terms.

Endothermic means "taking in heat." Processes that absorb heat from the surroundings include increasing a temperature, melting, evaporating, and boiling.

Exothermic means "giving off heat." Processes that emit heat to the surroundings when they occur include decreasing a temperature, freezing, condensing a vapor, and burning a fuel.

The equilibrium between the solid and liquid forms of water at its freezing point can be shown using a double arrow:

$$H_2O_{(s)} \rightleftharpoons H_2O_{(\ell)}$$

The liquid state has a greater total energy of motion than the solid state. We will realize this if we remember that the liquid molecules are moving about, while the ice molecules are fixed in position. We can show this by adding heat as a reactant to the same equation:

$$heat + H_2O_{(s)} \rightleftharpoons H_2O_{(\ell)}$$

Heat must be added to ice to convert it to liquid water. When liquid water freezes, heat is given off. The process from left to right is *endothermic* (ice absorbs heat on melting), while the process from right to left is *exothermic* (liquid releases heat on freezing). This is shown graphically on a "heating curve" such as Figure 11–13 (p. 324).

The heat required to melt a solid (such as ice at 0°C) is the **heat of fusion** at that temperature. We usually describe a heat of fusion in terms of heat flow or change of enthalpy, ΔH_{fus}.

The word *fusion* comes from Latin and means "melting." A *fuse* protects the wiring in a house by melting (and breaking the circuit) if the current gets too great.

The meaning of ΔH

The Greek capital letter *delta* (Δ) is used by scientists most commonly to mean "the change in," and it is calculated as *final minus initial* or *products minus reactants*. For example, suppose the temperature of a patient in a hospital suddenly increases from 37.0°C to 40.0°C. We can show this change in temperature as

$$\text{temperature rise} = \Delta T = T_{final} - T_{initial} = 40.0°C - 37.0°C = +3.0 \text{ K}$$

Since the final temperature is higher than the beginning temperature, this is a positive temperature change. If, instead, there were a drop in temperature, ΔT would be negative.

Change in enthalpy (heat) is defined in the same way:

$$\Delta H = H_{final} - H_{initial} \qquad \text{or} \qquad \Delta H = H_{products} - H_{reactants}$$

For example, if 1.00 kg of water were heated from 25°C to 26°C, the water would have *absorbed* 1.00 kcal of heat. The products (water at 26°C) would have more H, more heat, than the reactants (water at 25°C). In that case,

$$\Delta H = H_{water\ at\ 26°C} - H_{water\ at\ 25°C} = +1.00 \text{ kcal}$$

We see that when heat is absorbed (an endothermic process), the sign of ΔH is positive (+).

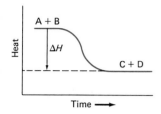

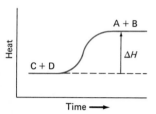

FIGURE 21–1 The top diagram shows an *exothermic* process. The reactants (A + B) contain more enthalpy (*H*) than the products (C + D). The bottom diagram shows the reverse reaction, a typical *endothermic* reaction, in which the reactants (C + D) have less energy than the products (A + B) and thus require heat input.

Suppose we are going from liquid water at 100°C to gaseous water (steam) at 100°C, again using 1.00 kg of water:

$$\Delta H = H_{\text{steam at 100°C}} - H_{\text{liquid at 100°C}} = +540 \text{ kcal}$$

Again the sign of ΔH is positive, since boiling is an endothermic process. But suppose 1.00 kg of steam condensed to liquid water:

$$\Delta H = H_{\text{liquid at 100°C}} - H_{\text{steam at 100°C}} = -540 \text{ kcal}$$

This is an exothermic process, and ΔH is negative. The products have less heat than the reactants, so heat has been given off.

The heat (enthalpy) required to change one kilogram of liquid to gas is the **heat of vaporization, ΔH_v.** For water, it has a value of 540 kcal/kg at 100°C. The heat of vaporization is a very direct measure of the strength of intermolecular forces in a liquid, as described in Section 11.5.

The relationship between the terms *exothermic* and *endothermic* and the sign of ΔH for a process is summarized in Figure 21–1.

Calculations using ΔH

You should be able to calculate the heat flow, ΔH, under constant pressure (as in an open pot) for the heating or cooling of any substance for which you know the specific heat (Table 21–1). The heat flow will increase with increasing mass of the sample. It will also increase with a greater temperature change. It takes more heat to change a substance with high specific heat than to change one with low specific heat. This leads us to the equation

$$\text{heat flow} = \Delta H = H_{\text{final}} - H_{\text{initial}} = (\text{mass})(\text{specific heat})(\Delta T)$$

Remember that ΔT is the final temperature minus the initial temperature. As a check, the sign of ΔH must be the same as the sign of ΔT.

EXAMPLE 21a: How many kilocalories of heat energy are required to heat 2000 g of liquid water from room temperature (25°C) to its boiling point (100°C)?

- -

ANSWER: The specific heat of liquid water is 1.00 kcal/kg-K.

$$\Delta T = T_{\text{final}} - T_{\text{initial}} = 100°C - 25°C = +75 \text{ K}$$

A mass of 2000 g is 2.00 kg, so

$$\Delta H = (2.00 \text{ kg } H_2O_{(\ell)})(1.00 \text{ kcal/kg-K})(+75 \text{ K}) = \boxed{+150 \text{ kcal}}$$

Check that the sign of ΔH (+) is the same as that of ΔT (+).

EXAMPLE 21b: An iron sword weighing 5.00 kg (about 10 pounds) has been forged in a fire and is now cooling from 350°C to 25°C. Calculate the heat flow from the sword.

- -

ANSWER: The specific heat for iron (from Table 21–1) is 0.106 kcal/kg-K.

$$\Delta T = T_{\text{final}} - T_{\text{initial}} = 25°C - 350°C = -325 \text{ K (a negative value!)}$$

The sword weighs 5.00 kg.

$$\Delta H = (5.00 \text{ kg Fe})(0.106 \text{ kcal/kg-K})(-325 \text{ K}) = \boxed{-172 \text{ kcal}}$$

Check again: ΔT is negative, and ΔH is negative.

Remember that mass and specific heat must both be positive numbers.

TABLE 21-2 MELTING AND BOILING DATA FOR SOME
PURE SUBSTANCES

Substance	Melting point (MP), °C	Boiling point (BP), °C	Heat of fusion, kcal/kg at MP	Heat of vaporization, kcal/kg at BP
H_2O	0	100	80	540
Na	98	892	27	1020
NaCl	801	1413	124	—
Cu	1083	2595	49	1150
C_2H_5OH	−114	79	25	204
Hg	−39	357	3	71
CCl_4	−24	77	4	46

To calculate heat flows for changes of phase, we must be sure we know which change is involved so that we may look up the appropriate heat of fusion or heat of vaporization. While a change of phase is taking place (as shown in Figure 11–13), there is no temperature change. That simplifies the calculation. Heat of fusion and vaporization values for some common substances are given in Table 21–2. Remember that the heat of an exothermic change is negative but has the *same value* as the heat of the reverse process, which is an endothermic change. If it takes 80 kcal to melt 1 kg of ice at 0°C, then the freezing of 1 kg of water at 0°C gives off the same 80 kcal.

Heats of fusion and vaporization are sometimes called *latent heats*. "Latent" means "hidden." The heat of fusion is "hidden" in the liquid, waiting to be produced when the solid is formed.

EXAMPLE 21c: A soft drink contains 100 g of ice at 0°C. The ice gradually melts. How much heat has it absorbed while melting?

- -

ANSWER: The heat of fusion of water at 0°C is 80 kcal/kg. We have 100 g of ice, which is 0.100 kg.

$$\Delta H = 0.100 \text{ kg ice} \times \frac{80 \text{ kcal}}{\text{kg ice}} = \boxed{+8.0 \text{ kcal}}$$

The heat of fusion is used as a simple conversion factor.

EXAMPLE 21d: Liquid sodium is used in many nuclear reactors as a coolant to keep the uranium fuel elements from melting. Since sodium melts at 98°C and boils at 892°C (at 1 atm pressure), the whole reactor core must be kept at several hundred degrees. What is ΔH if we convert 1.00 tonne (1000 kg) of sodium from liquid to solid at 98°C?

- -

ANSWER: From Table 21–2, the heat of fusion of Na is 27 kcal/kg at 98°C. We have 1.00×10^3 kg of Na metal. Using the heat of fusion as a conversion factor,

$$\Delta H = (1.00 \times 10^3 \text{ kg Na})(- 27 \text{ kcal/kg Na}) = \boxed{-2.7 \times 10^4 \text{ kcal}}$$

The value is negative since freezing is an exothermic process.

We can use the same methods to tackle a more complicated problem.

EXAMPLE 21e: What is the value of ΔH when 25.0 g of ethanol vapor at 79°C are condensed and cooled to 25°C?

- -

ANSWER: The heat of vaporization of ethanol at 79°C can be read from Table 21–2. It is 204 kcal/kg. As a first step, see what the value of ΔH is for the condensation step:

$$\Delta H = (0.0250 \text{ kg ethanol})(-204 \text{ kcal/kg ethanol}) = -5.10 \text{ kcal}$$

Now see how much heat is given off in cooling. The specific heat of liquid ethanol (Table 21–1) is 0.59 kcal/kg-K, and $\Delta T = 25°C - 79°C = -54$ K.

$$\Delta H = (0.0250 \text{ kg ethanol})(0.59 \text{ kcal/kg-K})(-54 \text{ K}) = -0.80 \text{ kcal}$$

Add up the values of ΔH: $-5.10 \text{ kcal} + (-0.80 \text{ kcal}) = \boxed{-5.90 \text{ kcal}}$

Heats of reaction

Every chemical equation has a heat flow attached, of the type shown in Figure 21–1. Only rarely does the total enthalpy of the products equal that of the reactants.

One obvious heat flow comes from the combustion reaction of a hydrocarbon fuel, such as methane in natural gas:

$$CH_{4(g)} + 2 O_{2(g)} \longrightarrow CO_{2(g)} + 2 H_2O_{(g)} + \text{heat}$$

The amount of heat released to heat your home or cook your food, 213 kcal for each mole of methane, may be shown as a product of the reaction. To do so converts an ordinary chemical equation to a **thermochemical equation:**

$$CH_{4(g)} + 2 O_{2(g)} \longrightarrow CO_{2(g)} + 2 H_2O_{(g)} + 213 \text{ kcal}$$

Or, we can write the equation and put next to it the value of ΔH. Since this is an exothermic reaction, $\Delta H = -213$ kcal/mole CH_4.

The **heat of reaction** is the energy released as bonds are made in the products minus the energy required to break the bonds in the reactants. If a gas must be expanded or compressed, the work involved also enters into calculation of ΔH.

It is important to remember that the heat of reaction for a process such as the burning of methane is calculated for the number of moles of reactant shown in the equation. Table 21–3 gives you heats of reaction for a number of organic combustion processes. These may be used as conversion factors in calculations.

TABLE 21–3 VALUES OF ΔH FOR SOME COMBUSTION REACTIONS IN kcal/mole AT °25C

Hydrogen gas	−68
Carbon (coal)	−94
Methane	−213
Ethane	−373
Propane	−531
Ethene	−337
Ethyne	−311
Acetic acid (ℓ)	−209
Ethanol (ℓ)	−327
Acetone (ℓ)	−428
Benzene (ℓ)	−781
Lactose (s)	−1350
Sucrose (s)	−1348
Arachidic acid (s)	−3026
Palmitic acid (s)	−2385
Glycine (s)	−233
Tyrosine (s)	−1070

EXAMPLE 21f: Calculate the heat of reaction if 1.00 liter (789 g) of liquid ethanol burns completely to CO_2 and H_2O at 25°C.

ANSWER: From Table 21–3, the heat of combustion of ethanol is −327 kcal/mole. One mole of C_2H_5OH weighs 46.0 g. Using the conversion-factor method

$$789 \text{ g } C_2H_5OH \times \frac{1 \text{ mole } C_2H_5OH}{46.0 \text{ g } C_2H_5OH} \times \frac{-327 \text{ kcal}}{\text{mole } C_2H_5OH} = \boxed{-5.61 \times 10^3 \text{ kcal}}$$

Such a heat output makes alcohol lamps very useful for home chemistry kits and field laboratories. It also provides the heat for flaming desserts, such as crêpes suzette.

Figure 21–2 is much like Figure 21–1, except that we have shown more details of the enthalpies of reactants and products. This type of **enthalpy-**

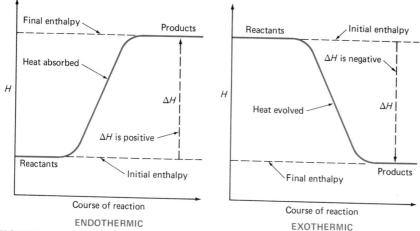

FIGURE 21–2 Diagrams plotting enthalpy against the course of an endothermic reaction (left) and an exothermic reaction (right).

reaction graph, plotting enthalpy (H) against the course of the reaction, will be discussed again in Section 21.4.

Coupled reaction energies

One important chemical principle can be stated:

The heat of a reaction depends only on the products and the reactants, not on the manner in which the reaction was carried out.

This principle allows us to add together the heats of known reactions to obtain a previously unknown reaction heat. For example, from Table 21–3, we can write

$$H_{2(g)} + {}^1/_2 O_{2(g)} \longrightarrow H_2O_{(\ell)} \qquad \Delta H = -68.3 \text{ kcal/mole } H_2O$$

Using Table 21–2, and noting that $\Delta H_v = 540 \text{ kcal/kg} \times 0.018 \text{ kg/mole} = 9.72 \text{ kcal/mole}$, we can write the process for vaporization of water:

$$H_2O_{(\ell)} \longrightarrow H_2O_{(g)} \qquad \Delta H = +9.72 \text{ kcal/mole } H_2O$$

Suppose we want to know the heat of reaction for the burning of hydrogen to give steam. We can simply add together these two equations:

Combustion equation:
$$H_{2(g)} + {}^1/_2 O_{2(g)} \longrightarrow H_2O_{(\ell)} \quad \Delta H = -68.3 \text{ kcal/mole } H_2O$$

+

Vaporization equation:
$$H_2O_{(\ell)} \longrightarrow H_2O_{(g)} \quad \Delta H = +9.72 \text{ kcal/mole } H_2O$$

New equation:
$$H_{2(g)} + {}^1/_2 O_{2(g)} + H_2O_{(\ell)} \longrightarrow H_2O_{(\ell)} + H_2O_{(g)}$$

or

$$H_{2(g)} + {}^1/_2 O_{2(g)} \longrightarrow H_2O_{(g)} \quad \Delta H = -58.6 \text{ kcal/mole } H_2O$$

To obtain the heat of the coupled reaction, we add together the two values of ΔH. This principle is widely applied in biochemistry to see how the energy-carrying molecule ATP helps make biological reactions go.

Predicting the effect of temperature

Most of the processes we have discussed in this chapter are reversible, that is, they can go from right to left or from left to right. For example, the melting of ice is represented by, from left to right,

$$\text{heat} + H_2O_{(s)} \rightleftharpoons H_2O_{(\ell)}$$

and the freezing of water is shown by the same reaction going from right to left.

If we add heat to a combination of ice and water, we will melt some ice. The effect of the extra heat is to shift the equilibrium toward the direction of more water. If we put the ice and liquid water into a freezer, we are removing heat. The result will be to shift the equilibrium in the direction that will produce more ice. In both cases, the equilibrium has shifted to produce more reactants or more products in such a way as to partially counteract any change. If we add heat, the reaction uses some of it up. If we remove heat, the reaction shifts to provide some more heat. This effect is known as **Le Chatelier's Principle.**

The same principle tells us that if we add more reactant to a system in equilibrium, there will be a shift to form more product. If we add more ice to an ice-water mixture, some of the newly added ice will melt and more liquid water will be formed, until the system returns to a new position of equilibrium. If we add product to the system, there will be a shift in the reverse direction to make more reactant. Adding liquid water to ice and water in equilibrium will result in the formation of more ice.

The effect of Le Chatelier's Principle in the body is often to regulate how much product is formed in biochemical reactions. Where one of the products is *heat*, we can predict the effect of a temperature increase, which effectively provides more heat to the system.

For the reaction

$$A + B \rightleftharpoons C + D + \text{heat}$$

an increase in temperature will shift the equilibrium toward A and B; a decrease in temperature will shift the reaction toward C and D. An increase in temperature thus favors an endothermic process and hinders an exothermic process.

SELF-CHECK

21.1) Use Tables 21–1, 21–2, and 21–3 to determine ΔH for the following processes.
a)   heat 0.250 kg of aluminum metal from 25°C to 100°C
b)   cool 50.0 g of O_2 gas from 30°C to 0°C
c)   melt 1.00 pound (0.454 kg) of NaCl at 801°C
d)   condense 0.500 g of mercury vapor into liquid mercury at 357°C
*e)   burn 1.00 g of CH_4 to CO_2 and liquid water
*f)   burn 30.0 g of palmitic acid to CO_2 and liquid water

21.2*)   Write out the thermochemical equations for the combustion of ethanol and of acetic acid (use Table 21–3). Then add these equations and their associated ΔH values in such a way that you determine the heat of reaction for converting ethanol to acetic acid by air oxidation (the process that turns good wine into vinegar).

21.3*) Dissolving sucrose in water is an endothermic process:

$$C_{12}H_{22}O_{11(s)} + heat \rightleftharpoons C_{12}H_{22}O_{11(aq)}$$

Will table sugar dissolve more easily in hot coffee or in iced coffee? Why?

21.2 FOOD ENERGY

LEARNING GOAL 21C: Given the amount of carbohydrate, protein, and fat in a particular food item, use the approximate fuel energy values of 4, 4, and 9 kcal/g, respectively, to calculate the total fuel value of the food.

21D: Explain why and how the body gets rid of the excess heat created by the metabolism of nutrients.

When we move from measured heats of reaction in a chemical laboratory to a discussion of energy needs in the human body, we can continue to use many of the techniques of the previous section. In Table 21–3 you see the heat of combustion of several substances that go into foods. The table includes lactose and sucrose, representing carbohydrates (sugars); tyrosine and glycine, two amino acids that link together to make proteins; and arachidic and palmitic acids, two fatty acids that make up food oils and fats.

The value for each heat of combustion given in Table 21–3 was measured by direct burning, not by the complex mechanism used by the body. However, we know (from p. 573) that the way the reaction is carried out does not affect the value of ΔH. Thus, if the products are carbon dioxide and water, the heat released in the body should be the same, mole for mole, as that given in Table 21.3.*

However, knowing a heat of combustion *per mole* is of little use in calculating food energy because we measure the *weight* of foods. Table 21–4 shows the heats of combustion of the carbohydrates, amino acids, and fatty acids of Table 21–3 divided by the weight in grams of one mole to give kcal *per gram*. Ethyl alcohol has been added to the table because it is clearly a source of body energy when it is consumed. Average values for carbohydrates, proteins, and fats in the diet are also given.

Depending on composition, there is some variation in the energy values of carbohydrates, proteins, and fats. However, in all cases, the carbohydrates already contain as much oxygen as needed to combine completely with the hydrogen they contain to form water, as in sucrose, $C_{12}H_{22}O_{11}$. It is effectively only the carbon contained in the carbohydrate (in this case, 42% of the weight) that actually burns, and this fact leads to a low heat of combustion. Fats, on the other hand, contain long hydrocarbon chains, so their heats of combustion are closer to those of long-chain alkanes and alkenes.

However, the energy value of food to the human body does not reach the levels of Table 21–4 because not all of each type of food is actually digested. Accounting for this loss, the average physiological food values are

TABLE 21–4 VALUES OF ΔH FOR THE COMBUSTION OF SOME NUTRIENTS IN kcal/g AT 25°C

Lactose	−3.94
Sucrose	−3.94
Carbohydrates	−4.1 *avg.*
Tyrosine	−5.91
Phenylalanine	−6.73
Proteins	−5.65 *avg.*
Arachidic acid	−9.68
Palmitic acid	−9.30
Fats	−9.45 *avg.*
Ethyl alcohol	−7.11

* In the body, nitrogen from amino acids is converted to ammonia, NH_3, rather than to nitrogen gas, N_2. This will make a small difference (1.3 kcal/g) in the average ΔH value for amino acids.

considered to be

Carbohydrate: 4.0 kcal/g **Protein:** 4.0 kcal/g **Fat:** 9.0 kcal/g
Ethyl Alcohol: 7.0 kcal/g

These fortunately give nice round numbers that can be easily remembered. They are sufficiently accurate to determine the **food energy value** in kcal ("Calories") for practical estimates, as in the following example.

EXAMPLE 21g: A 250-mL portion of milk contains 12.3 g of carbohydrate, 8.7 g of protein, and 9.2 g of fat. Calculate its approximate fuel value.

ANSWER: Remembering the values of 4, 4 and 9 kcal/g for the three types,

for carbohydrate: 12.3 g × 4.0 kcal/g = 49 kcal
for protein: 8.7 g × 4.0 kcal/g = 35 kcal
for fat: 9.2 g × 9.0 kcal/g = 83 kcal

Total fuel value: 167 kcal   = 167 "Calories"

A person on a low-calorie diet to lose weight will start using some of the fat in the body's fat deposits as fuel. Let us see what the theoretical value would be if one pound of body fat is lost as energy. We must use 9.45 as the fuel value of fat, since none is lost in digestion; it's already in the body!

EXAMPLE 21h: Calculate the fuel value of 454 g of pure fat already stored in the body.

ANSWER: 454 g fat × 9.45 kcal/g fat = 4290 kcal
By this calculation, you would need to reduce your diet (or do extra exercise) by 4290 Calories to lose a pound of weight. Actually, since there is water stored with the fat and other factors are involved, the correct figure is close to 3500 Calories.

Use of energy by the body

Except for the amino acids and small amounts of carbohydrate and fat used for raw materials in the manufacture of proteins and other cell materials, the three chief energy nutrients of the body are oxidized in the cells, using oxygen supplied by the blood. During this process, bond energy holding the large molecules together is converted to work (in the muscles) and heat.

The body is like a "heat engine" (such as the gasoline engine that drives an automobile or the jet engine that propels an airplane) in several respects. Energy for work is obtained by *oxidation* of fuel. Heat is a by-product of the reactions by which energy is released, since no engine is capable of converting all available energy to work. We measure the amount of energy that actually does get converted to work in terms of the *efficiency* of the heat engine. In these terms, the efficiency of the body is about 20%, roughly the same as that of the automobile gasoline engine and half that of a diesel engine. Thus, four fifths of the kilocalories produced by the body in the process of oxidizing food are emitted as heat; only one fifth fuels the work of the muscles. Now you will understand why strenuous physical activity

TABLE 21-5 ENERGY COST OF SOME ACTIVITIES IN RELATION TO BASAL METABOLISM RATE = 1.00

Sleeping	0.9	Weeding, raking	3.1
Reading	1.2	Washing a car	3.5
Sitting and writing	1.4	Making beds, vacuuming	3.7
Using desk calculator	1.7	Playing with children	4.0
Light domestic work	1.9	Painting a house	4.5
Sitting and eating	2.1	Dancing a waltz	5.0
General laboratory work	2.1	Climbing stairs	6.0
Playing piano	2.3	Playing tennis	6.5
Walking 2.0 mph (on level ground)	2.7	Sawing wood	7.0
Washing dishes	2.7	Digging ditches	7.5
Dressing, bathing	2.9	Cross-country skiing	8.0

Note: most values are very approximate.

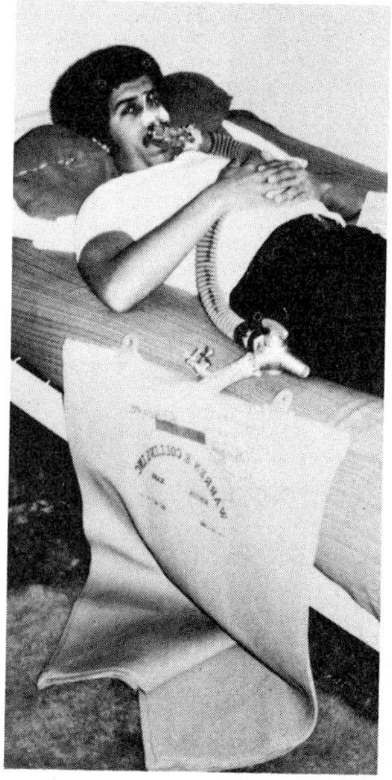

FIGURE 21-3 Basal metabolism can be measured by measuring the O_2 and CO_2 content of exhaled air.

leaves you sweating! You warm up the body with four times as much energy as you use in your work.

Energy needs vary widely among individuals. A range for adults of 1800 to 3600 kcal/day is typical. It is difficult to measure the number of calories actually consumed, so an indirect measurement of energy use is made.

Basal metabolism

The word *metabolism* is a general term used to cover all of the chemical changes that occur in the tissues of the body. Under *energy metabolism* we include the chemical changes by which fat, carbohydrate, and protein are oxidized to release energy as well as the changes by which these substances are converted to compounds in which unneeded energy is stored, as in the fatty "adipose" deposits of the body. A limited amount of carbohydrate is stored in the liver and muscles as animal starch or glycogen to provide a short-term supply of energy when needed.*

The **basal metabolism rate** represents the amount of energy required to maintain life at rest. The internal work of the body involves nervous system and brain activity (about 20% of the basal metabolism energy occurs in the brain), the work of the liver and kidneys, and the work of the heart, lungs, diaphragm, stomach, intestines, and glands. There is even some muscle activity when sleeping, and this is included. Figure 21-3 shows how basal metabolism is measured.

An average adult metabolizes about one kcal/hour for each kilogram of body weight, or perhaps 1800 kcal/day. Because the amount of oxygen needed to oxidize energy sources (and produce heat) is known, we can relate the energy rate to the volume of oxygen consumed.

When we are not resting, we naturally consume more energy in muscle activity, which is added to the basal metabolism rate to give the total energy cost. Table 21-5 gives the ratio of the energy cost of certain activities to the metabolic rate while sleeping.

The measurement of metabolic rate while exercising is shown in Figure 21-4. There is wide variation among individuals, so the values in Table 21-5

Intake by the body of 1.0 liter of oxygen is equivalent to 4.8 kcal of energy use. An average resting adult consumes about 200 mL of O_2 per hour for each kilogram of body weight. You might compare this human value with the very low 55 mL/kg for a frog and the very high 4500 mL/kg for a bird like a parakeet.

---

* Muscles and internal organs are rich in protein, which may be drawn upon for energy after the glycogen (stored carbohydrate) is exhausted or after about 16 to 20 hours without food. A healthy adult can live without food (but given water) for several weeks because of the varied ways the body stores energy.

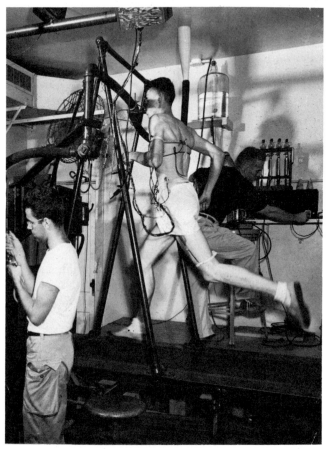

FIGURE 21–4   A treadmill measures the metabolic rate while exercising. The subject is running while breathing into equipment that tests the gases being exchanged in his lungs. His heart rate and skin temperature are also being monitored. (Courtesy S. Robinson, Indiana University, Bloomington)

should be considered only as rough guides. The daily level for a typical student has been calculated at about 1.4 to 1.9 times the resting rate, or for 70 kg of body weight, roughly 2500 to 3300 kcal/day.

Heat regulation

Cold-blooded animals, such as reptiles and insects, assume the temperature of their surroundings. Humans are warm-blooded, and our bodies only function properly within a fairly short range of temperatures, as shown in Figure 21–5. No particular temperature is "normal" for everyone; the familiar 98.6°F (37.0°C) is an average for oral thermometer readings. We mentioned earlier that roughly four fifths of the energy cost of daily life goes into producing heat, and only one fifth into doing work. Since the specific heat of the body averages 0.83 kcal/kg-K and the total energy cost of a typical 70-kg student is 2500 to 3300 kcal/day, there is enough energy given off as heat to raise the body temperature by 43 to 57 degrees each day. Clearly, we must have a way of getting rid of a lot of extra heat.

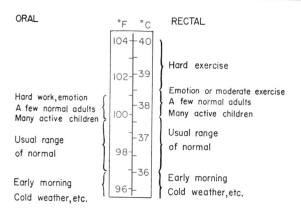

FIGURE 21–5 Ranges of body temperature under different "normal" conditions. "Normal" does not always turn out to be 37.0°C (98.6°F).

The balance between heat production and heat loss is shown in Figure 21–6. About 80% of the excess heat is lost through the skin, which results in sweating and flushing on a hot day. If additional muscle work is needed to cope with a cold environment, the body may shiver.

Since sweating loses heat through the evaporation of water from the surface of the skin, you can calculate how much water must be lost in sweat to get rid of a given number of kilocalories as heat of vaporization.

Flushing of the skin means that more blood is being sent into skin capillaries, where it can be cooled by exposure to the air temperature. In extremely cold situations, the reverse happens. Blood is held back from the skin and frostbite may result as skin cells freeze.

EXAMPLE 21i: How much water must a 70-kg person lose as sweat in order to lower the body temperature by one degree? The ΔH_v for water is 540 kcal/kg.

- -

ANSWER: The amount of heat to be lost is

$$70 \text{ kg body} \times \frac{0.83 \text{ kcal}}{\text{kg body-K}} \times 1.0 \text{ degree} = 58 \text{ kcal}$$

Then the amount of water converted from liquid to steam must be

$$58 \text{ kcal} \times \frac{1 \text{ kg water}}{540 \text{ kcal}} = \boxed{0.11 \text{ kg}} \quad \text{(about one half cup)}$$

Of course, we saw earlier that the extra heat generated inside the body each day would be enough to raise the body temperature by 43 to 57 degrees. If all of that heat had to be lost by sweating, you would need to lose 43 to 57 times 0.11 kg, or 4.7 to 6.3 kg of water, which is 5 to 7 quarts!

Luckily, not all of that heat loss must be accomplished by evaporating sweat, which only takes care of 25% of the heat loss for a nude person in a 25°C room. Radiation of heat from the skin (60%) and conduction of heat away from the skin to warm the air around the body (15%) also help. Thin people radiate about 50% more heat relative to body weight than fat people and thus tend to be more affected by cold temperatures in winter and more comfortable in summer.

The body cannot afford to have biochemical processes take place too quickly or too slowly. A high temperature speeds up a reaction, while a low temperature slows it down. Furthermore, the body enzymes only function well within a very strict temperature range. The body thus has a mechanism

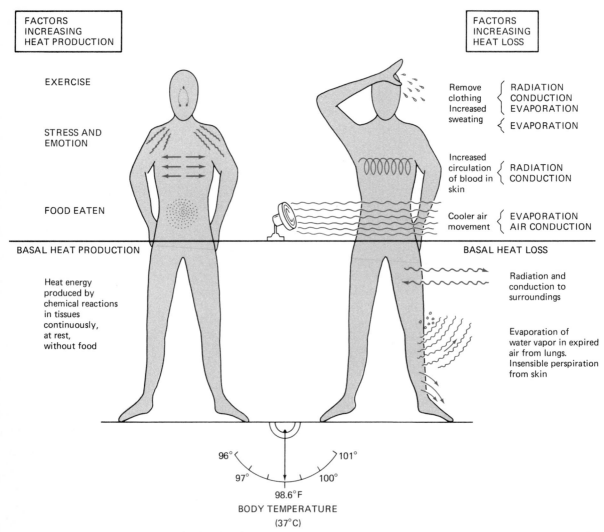

FIGURE 21–6 Heat balance in the human body. Some factors (left) increase the production of heat in the body, others (right) increase the rate at which heat can be lost from the body.

(the hypothalamus section of the brain, as well as some spinal cord reflexes) to keep body temperature in the proper range.

SELF-CHECK

21.4) One slice of whole-wheat bread contains about 2.5 g of protein, 0.8 g of fat, and 12 g of carbohydrate. Using the approximate fuel energy values for the different kinds of food, calculate the fuel value of a slice of this bread.

21.5) Why do people generally take off most of their clothes when they are hot? Wouldn't running around on a sunny beach in a skimpy bathing suit tend to heat up the body rather than cool it down?

21.3 WHAT MAKES REACTIONS GO?

LEARNING GOAL 21E: Give an example of an endothermic process that occurs in nature because of an increase in entropy.
                   21F: Explain the meaning of a negative, zero, or positive free energy change (ΔG) for a particular process.

We previously described the tendency of some chemical systems to give off energy and go to a *lower energy state.* An atom that contains an electron in a higher (excited) energy state will give off energy in the form of light as the electron falls to a lower energy state (Section 2.4). All else being equal, reactants with higher enthalpy (*H*) lose heat to go to products of lower enthalpy. Exothermic reactions are preferred in nature. In everyday language, "what goes up must come down."

We use the term **spontaneous** to mean "happens by itself with no outside forcing." For example, the reaction

$$2\ H_{2(g)} + O_{2(g)} \longrightarrow 2\ H_2O_{(g)}$$

is spontaneous once it has started. In fact, if you touch a match to a hydrogen balloon, you will obtain either a fire or an explosion. *Spontaneous* combustion does not even need a match; it happens by itself. Laughter of a studio audience at a TV show is spontaneous if the people find the show funny; it is forced if it only happens when a sign is displayed. Since an endothermic reaction requires an outside source of heat and an exothermic reaction gives off heat, we might conclude that *only* exothermic processes are spontaneous and happen by themselves. However, that is not true.

The need for a spark or flame to begin a combustion reaction or explosion does not mean that the reaction is nonspontaneous. The starting or *ignition* step simply provides a high temperature and a source of high-energy molecules that can overcome E_a.

Entropy

There is another major consideration in deciding whether or not something will happen by itself. All else being equal, molecular systems go to a lower energy state. However, if energy changes are neglected, then any change is likely to be in the direction of greater disorder, confusion, mixing, randomness. We call this the direction of greater **entropy.** The symbol for entropy is *S.*

Suppose a person wearing perfume enters a small room. The vapors of the perfume will soon mix with the air in the room. The mixing of two gases occurs spontaneously. However, if the gases are ideal, there is no energy change. The "driving force" that makes it easy to mix the gases (and almost impossible to separate them) is the *entropy* of mixing. The entropy of a mixture is greater than that of the pure substances taken separately.

Some salt crystals dissolve in water while giving off heat; they have negative heats of solution. Others take in heat while dissolving; they have positive ΔH of solution and dissolving them is endothermic. The process of dissolving sodium nitrate has a ΔH of + 4.90 kcal/mole, yet this salt dissolves very easily. Only the high entropy of mixing can allow this.

Some phase changes—gas to liquid (condensation), liquid to solid (freezing)—are exothermic and easily understood. How about the spontaneous melting of ice at temperatures above 0°C? Heat is being absorbed. Why? The liquid has a higher entropy than the solid, and *at certain temperatures*

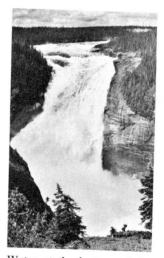

Water at the bottom of the waterfall has less potential energy (because of the force of gravity) than that at the top. Water thus flows *spontaneously* downhill, as in Churchill Falls, Labrador, Newfoundland, Canada, and provides much hydroelectric power.

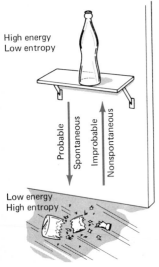

High energy
Low entropy

Probable | Spontaneous | Improbable | Nonspontaneous

Low energy
High entropy

The bottle on the shelf has a higher potential energy than the one on the floor. Since it is in one piece, the unbroken bottle also has a lower entropy. It is probable, and spontaneous, for the bottle to fall (go to lower energy). It is also probable and spontaneous for it to break and go to a state of higher entropy.

As reactants in the battery are converted to products, the reverse reaction (products → reactants) becomes more important. Eventually, equilibrium is reached. At that point, the cell voltage is zero and $\Delta G = 0$. The reaction is then being "driven" neither to the left nor to the right.

the entropy factor is more important. At temperatures lower than 0°C, liquid water spontaneously turns into ice. There clearly is competition between energy changes, ΔH, and entropy changes, ΔS. At 0°C, there is an equilibrium between freezing and melting, so the two factors must be in balance.

Free energy

At constant temperature and pressure, as is the case inside the body, we can express the competition between the tendency to lower enthalpy (ΔH negative) and higher disorder or entropy (ΔS positive) by writing the Gibbs equation:

$$\Delta G = \Delta H - T\,\Delta S \qquad \text{(T is the Kelvin temperature)}$$

The letter G represents the **free energy.** It measures the probability that a reaction will go spontaneously. If we consider a general type of process:

$$A \longrightarrow B \qquad (\Delta G = G_B - G_A = ?)$$

we note that, if the reactants have more free energy than the products, then

ΔG is negative, and the reaction $A \longrightarrow B$ is spontaneous.

If the products have more free energy than the reactants, then

ΔG is positive, and the reaction $A \longrightarrow B$ is *not* probable unless forced.

In fact, the reverse reaction $B \rightarrow A$, with a negative ΔG, is spontaneous. Finally, if $\Delta G = 0$, then both directions are equally likely. Therefore,

if ΔG is zero, then there is equilibrium: $\quad A \rightleftharpoons B$

You should note that the determining factor in deciding which direction is favored is the *temperature*, which weights (multiplies the effects) of ΔS. Table 21–6 lists the four possibilities for the signs of ΔH, ΔS, and ΔG.

Think of the work done by a storage battery running a watch, calculator, or electronic game. If the battery has a charge, then it can do work. No voltage across the battery terminals means no functioning of the battery-powered device. The voltage of a battery can be directly related to the free energy of the reactants inside it in relation to the free energy of the products:

$$\Delta G \propto \text{battery voltage}$$

The free energy difference ($G_{\text{products}} - G_{\text{reactants}}$), the driving force for a reaction to occur, is proportional to the voltage that can do work.

Although there are rarely any batteries inside the human body, we can still define ΔG as the energy "free" to do work in the body. If ΔG is negative, we have a process "itching to happen." All it needs is a way to happen

TABLE 21–6 HOW TO PREDICT THE SPONTANEITY OF PROCESSES GIVEN THE SIGNS OF ΔH AND ΔS

If process is	and the sign of ΔH is	ΔS is	then the sign of ΔG is	and the process is
Exothermic	−	+	always −	always spontaneous
Exothermic	−	−	either + or −	spontaneous at low temperatures
Endothermic	+	+	either + or −	spontaneous at high temperatures
Endothermic	+	−	always +	never spontaneous

and it will go. It is a spontaneous process. If ΔG is positive, then we must find a way to *drive* the reaction. To a biochemist, ΔG (rather than ΔH) represents the amount of energy that can do work under the conditions present in the living cell.

21.6)   Choose from the following list an endothermic process that happens in nature only because of an increase in entropy.
a)   a natural gas explosion at 25°C
b)   boiling liquid water to steam at 100°C
c)   freezing liquid water to ice at 0°C
21.7)   For the conversion of graphite to the diamonds used for jewelry and for industrial drills, ΔG is positive. What does this mean?

21.4 RATES OF REACTION

LEARNING GOAL 21G: Explain why some molecular collisions result in chemical reaction and others do not.
21H: On an enthalpy-reaction graph for a given reaction, interpret the reaction as exothermic or endothermic, identify the activated complex, and calculate the activation energy.
21I: Explain why an increase in temperature always causes an increase in reaction rate.

The word *rate* refers to the number of events in a given period of time. The speed of a car is a rate; if you are traveling 60 miles/hour (or 100 km/hour), you are relating a distance traveled (in miles or km) to the amount of time it takes. Your rate of progress in this course might be one chapter per week, or faster or slower. A **reaction rate** is therefore the number of changes from reactant to product in a given time. It can be measured in molecules/second, moles/minute, or any other ratio of amount to time.

A spontaneous chemical reaction may progress so quickly (at a *high* rate) that all of the reactants are converted to products in a fraction of a second. One example of such a quick reaction is an explosion. On the other hand, a reaction may be spontaneous but take years or centuries (a *low* rate) at room temperature. The conversion of a sparkling diamond to the graphite that we find in pencils is spontaneous. However, the rate is so low that diamond rings may be passed down from generation to generation without visible change.

Collision theory

Chemical reactions occur through collisions between molecules. The energy of the collision may be sufficient to break bonds in the reactants. However, even then not every collision between reactants will result in products being formed.

Figure 21–7 shows the gas reaction $A_2 + B_2 \rightarrow 2\ AB$. Only if the colliding molecules have the proper position *and* adequate collision energy can reaction occur. The position is important, not only because a glancing blow does not provide enough energy to break reactant bonds but also because an intermediate structure, a *transition state*, must be formed. This transition

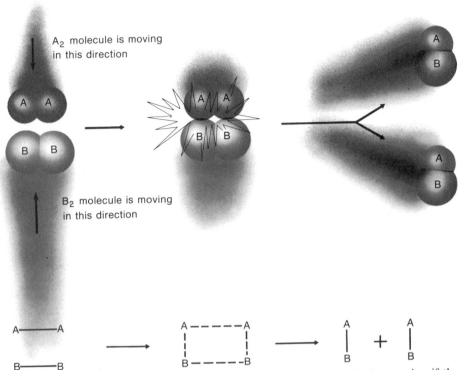

FIGURE 21-7 A collision between A_2 and B_2 molecules results in reaction if the molecules possess adequate energy *and* strike each other at the right angle. If the orientations (positions) are wrong, no reaction will occur.

state is often called an **activated complex** because it has higher energy than either reactants or products, as shown in Figure 21-8.

Reactants in an exothermic reaction do not simply evolve heat while going to the products. Instead, they require an initial amount of heat, a "push," to reach the activated complex, in this case the species A_2B_2. The activated complex may then break apart into the products *or*, if the energies are not right, separate as the reactants again.

The **activation energy,** E_a, can be obtained by collision with a molecule that is moving very fast. This is the reason so many chemical reactions need a spark or flame for *ignition*. Once ignited, a combustion reaction (exothermic) will generally produce enough heat to produce more high-speed molecules and keep the process going until all the fuel (reactants) is used up. The uphill effort of the sledder in Figure 21-9 provides a good analogy.

So far, we have been discussing exothermic reactions. Once we have *added* energy to the internal heat (enthalpy) of the reactants and have formed the activated complex, we can drop to an even lower energy state in the products and end up with a *net loss* of energy. The reverse reaction, reading from right (2 AB) to left ($A_2 + B_2$) in Figure 21-9, is therefore endothermic. The activation energy needed for that process is quite large, being equal to the activation energy for the forward reaction plus the ΔH of the reaction.

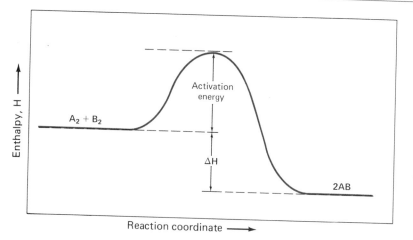

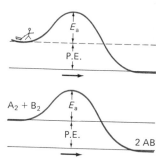

FIGURE 21–9   The activation energy (E_a) of getting to the top of the hill must be overcome before the sledder can slide all the way to the bottom and lose potential energy (PE). Similarly, reactants must first gain activation energy before a reaction, even an exothermic one, can proceed. Once the reaction is started, heat released can activate other reactant molecules.

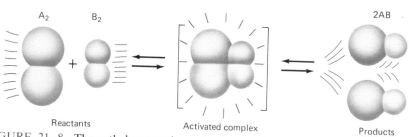

FIGURE 21–8   The enthalpy-reaction path diagram for a reaction shows the importance of the activated complex, which can be reached from the reactants ($A_2 + B_2$) *or* from the products (2 AB). Compare this figure with Figure 21–2, which does not show the intermediate energy.

The rate of a reaction depends on the number of molecular collisions that can overcome the activation energy barrier and reach the activated complex per unit of time. Figure 21–10 shows the fraction of molecules with sufficient energy to overcome the activation energy barrier at two different temperatures.

Temperature and reaction rate

As you can see from Figure 21–10, an increase in temperature results in having more molecules with adequate energies to react and overcome the activation energy barrier. The increase is not simply proportional to the temperature; it goes up very quickly. An increase from room temperature (27°C or 300 K) to body temperature (37°C or 310 K) is only a 3% overall temperature increase. Yet, for a typical biochemical reaction, the number of molecules with adequate kinetic energy to reach the activated complex will be roughly *doubled* (a 100% increase!) by this temperature increase, and thus the reaction rate will be doubled.

For this reason, doctors who wish to lower the rates of biochemical processes during a risky surgical operation think immediately of lowering the body temperature.

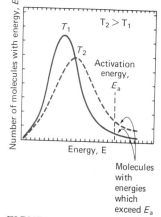

FIGURE 21–10   A small increase in temperature from T_1 to T_2 produces a large increase in the number of molecules with energies greater than the activation energy. The reaction thus has a much higher rate at the higher temperature.

Equilibrium and reaction rate

We have to this point discussed several types of equilibrium situations. Now we can define equilibrium in terms of reaction rates:

A system is in equilibrium if the rate of the forward reaction is the same as the rate of the reverse reaction.

In each unit of time, the number of reactant molecules being converted to products is the same as the number of product molecules becoming reactants. This fact emphasizes that equilibrium is not a situation in which "nothing is changing." In fact, the changes are simply equal and opposite.

SELF-CHECK

21.8) Two high-speed reactant molecules collided and yet no activated complex resulted. What could have happened?
21.9) How does the activation energy for an endothermic process compare with the activation energy for the reverse process? Explain, using an enthalpy-reaction graph.
21.10) Why does a decrease in temperature result in lower reaction rates?

21.5 INTRODUCTION TO ENZYMES

LEARNING GOAL 21J: Describe the effect of a catalyst in increasing reaction rate by comparing a catalyzed and uncatalyzed reaction on the same enthalpy-reaction graph.
21K: Describe the overall function of an enzyme.

A **catalyst** has a very simple role. It provides a way of obtaining an activated complex that is of *lower energy* than an activated complex obtained without the catalyst. It thus lowers the activation energy of the reaction (in both directions) and makes it easier for molecules to collide with sufficient energy to react (Figure 21–11).

If you have been accustomed to driving from one city to another using two-lane roads, most likely your rate of travel has been relatively low. If a superhighway is suddenly open to you, you can take it and go faster because obstacles that used to slow you down (traffic lights, slow-moving trucks, hills) have been removed. The catalyst similarly provides an alternative "route" (Figure 21–12).

The amount of catalyst present at the end of the reaction is exactly the same as the amount present before the reaction started, and it appears in exactly the same form. It probably becomes an important part of the activated complex and then is released unchanged when the products are formed.

There are many different kinds of catalysts. Acids often serve as catalysts in organic reactions. Certain metals, such as platinum, seem to be able to provide surfaces on which the reactants can "stick" and collide more successfully than they would be able to without the catalyst. For these metal catalysts, the surface area available to reactant molecules becomes very important.

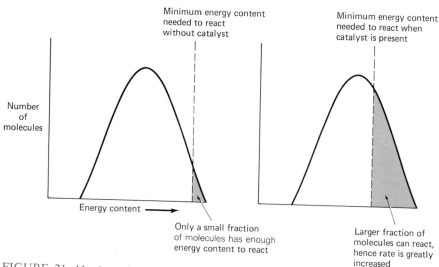

FIGURE 21–11 A catalyst lowers the activation energy for a reaction. The fraction of molecules with adequate energy to reach E_a is thus higher and the rate is greatly increased.

Since the presence of a catalyst does not affect the energies of the reactants or products, it cannot turn a nonspontaneous reaction into a spontaneous one. It does not at all change the position of equilibrium, but increases both the forward and reverse reaction rates and thus may allow a chemical system to reach equilibrium more quickly. In catalytic converters, for example, hydrocarbons and CO gas in automobile exhaust are converted to

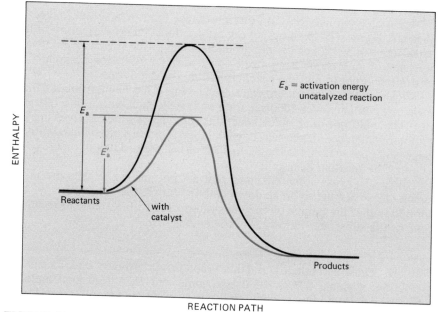

FIGURE 21–12 A catalyst lowers the activation energy of a reaction and thus increases the rate.

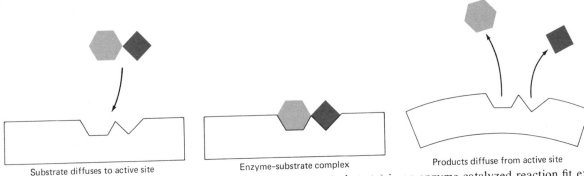

Substrate diffuses to active site   Enzyme–substrate complex   Products diffuse from active site

FIGURE 21–13 The reactants (substrate) in an enzyme-catalyzed reaction fit exactly into the enzyme protein molecule. The arrangement makes the breaking of substrate bonds easier. The products then leave the enzyme.

CO_2; this reaction would take place in the atmosphere, but at a much lower rate.

Enzymes

Enzymes are proteins that act as catalysts for the metabolic processes inside the living cell. For example, amylase, an enzyme found in saliva, speeds up the conversion of the polysaccharide starch to disaccharide sugar. In the laboratory (without a catalyst), this conversion takes several weeks; in the body, the conversion takes only a few *minutes* because of the amylase. Since each enzyme, like any other catalyst, can be used over and over again, only a trace of enzyme is needed to convert a large amount of reactant to product.

Each enzyme acts only on one particular kind of reactant, called the **substrate.** Figure 21–13 shows a very crude "lock-and-key" picture of how a substrate can be broken up into products by an active site on an enzyme. If the shape of an enzyme is changed—by too much heat, for example—the substrate will not fit and the reaction will not be catalyzed.

Close to 2000 different enzymes are known. It has been estimated that a single cell contains over 1000 separate enzymes, each with a different purpose. The multitude of chemical reactions catalyzed by the enzymes in a cell are not completely independent of each other. They are often linked into sequences of consecutive reactions. In such cases, the product of one reaction becomes the reactant of another.

Table 21–7 lists some enzymes that act not inside the cells but in the human digestive tract to break down carbohydrates, fats, and proteins. You will notice that the names of enzymes often start with a stem based on the name of the substrate, followed by the ending *-ase*.

TABLE 21–7 SOME
DIGESTIVE ENZYMES
AND THEIR SUBSTRATES

Enzyme	Substrate
Amylase	Amylose sugars
Pepsin	Proteins
Lipase	Lipids
Trypsin	Proteins
Sucrase	Sucrose
Lactase	Lactose
Maltase	Maltose
Dipeptidase	Dipeptides

Chapter 23 will discuss enzymes in much more detail. The digestive process will be reviewed in Section 25.1.

SELF-CHECK

21.11) Draw an enthalpy-reaction graph for an ordinary endothermic reaction. Assume ΔH is +5.0 kcal/mole and E_a = 15.0 kcal/mole. Now use a dotted line to show the type of curve that would result if a catalyst were present. What is the effect of the catalyst on E_a?

21.12) Why are enzymes needed in the digestive tract?

CHAPTER TWENTY-ONE IN REVIEW ■ Energy and Reaction Rates

GLOSSARY FOR CHAPTER TWENTY-ONE

activated complex A transition state; in a chemical reaction a species that is intermediate between reactants and products and has a higher energy than either. (p. 584)

activation energy The collision energy between reactants that will permit the formation of an activated complex; an important factor in determining the rate of reaction. (p. 584)

basal metabolism rate The amount of energy (measured as intake of O_2 gas) required to sustain life in a resting body. (p. 577)

catalyst A substance that speeds up a reaction by providing a reaction path with a lower activation energy; increases the reaction rate without itself being consumed in the reaction. (p. 586)

enthalpy (H) Heat content. (p. 568)

enthalpy change (ΔH) Heat flow at constant pressure; enthalpy of products minus enthalpy of reactants; ΔH is negative for an exothermic process, positive for an endothermic one. (p. 568)

enthalpy-reaction graph A diagram that shows the enthalpies of the reactants, activated complex, and products of a reaction so that the changes in enthalpy along the reaction path may be seen. (p. 572)

entropy A measure of molecular disorder or randomness (symbol S); the most important factor at high temperatures in determining the direction in which a reaction will be spontaneous. (p. 581)

enzyme A protein molecule that acts as a catalyst for a biochemical reaction. (p. 588)

food energy value Fuel value of a nutrient; the number of kilocalories per gram given off by a particular food when metabolized in the body. (p. 576)

free energy (G) A property of a chemical system that takes into account both enthalpy and entropy; reflects the ability of a system to do useful work; if ΔG for a change is negative, the change is spontaneous; if ΔG is zero, the system is at equilibrium. (p. 582)

heat of fusion (ΔH_{fus}) The value of ΔH for the change from solid to liquid (melting) for a pure substance, may be expressed in kilocalories per kilogram. (p. 569)

heat of reaction The ΔH value for a chemical reaction. (p. 572)

heat of vaporization (ΔH_v) The value of ΔH for the change from liquid to gas (vaporization) for a pure substance, may be expressed in kilocalories per kg. (p. 570)

Le Chatelier's Principle An important chemical law; states that if an equilibrium situation is disturbed, the reaction will shift to partially counteract the original change and thus bring the system to a new position of equilibrium. (p. 574)

reaction rate The amount of reactants being converted to products in a given time; usually approximated by dividing the number of moles of reactants that disappear in a given time by the time. (p. 583)

specific heat The heat flow in kilocalories required to increase the temperature of one kilogram of a substance by one Celsius degree. (p. 568)

spontaneous A term applied to a process that will happen by itself, with no outside "forcing"; the value of ΔG for a spontaneous process is negative. (p. 581)

substrate The reactants in a biochemical reaction being catalyzed by an enzyme; must "fit" the enzyme to be catalyzed. (p. 588)

thermochemical equation A chemical equation in which the heat of reaction is shown, either by being added as a reactant or product, or by having a value of ΔH shown; in either case, the heat flow shown is for the number of moles indicated by the coefficients of the equation. (p. 572)

QUESTIONS AND PROBLEMS FOR CHAPTER TWENTY-ONE ■

Energy and Reaction Rates

SECTION 21.1 HEAT TRANSFER

Use Table 21–1 to answer the following questions.

21.13) How many kilocalories are needed to heat 255 g of acetone from 20°C to 45°C?

21.14) What temperature will be reached by the pressing surface of a 500 g electric iron, initially at 23°C, if the Fe surface absorbs 2.81 kcal?

21.42) How many kilocalories are given off when a 2.25-kg bar of pure gold cools from 100°C to 25°C?

21.43) A piece of copper absorbs 58.6 kcal while being heated from −10.0°C to +13.7°C. What is the mass of the piece of copper?

Use Table 21–2 to answer the following questions.

21.15) How many kilocalories are needed to melt 1.00 tonne (1000 kg) of copper wire at 1083°C?

21.16) How many kilocalories will be given off as 2.00 kg of liquid water freeze to ice at 0°C?

21.17*) The naphthalene ($C_{10}H_8$) commonly used in mothballs melts at 80°C. If 7.20 kcal melt 200 g of naphthalene, what is the heat of fusion?

21.18*) Air temperatures below −2°C will damage grape vines. Grape growers spray a mist of liquid water on the vines when frost threatens the crop. How might this prevent damage?

21.19*) A dentist's high-speed drill produces a lot of heat through friction. Will the patient feel that heat earlier if the dentist is drilling tooth enamel or a silver filling? Why?

21.20*) Assuming specific heat is constant, what is ΔH when 150 g of liquid copper at 1550°C are cooled to 25°C (and form a solid)?

21.44) How many kilocalories are needed to evaporate 175 g of liquid mercury at 357°C?

21.45) How many kilocalories will be given off (to give you a bad scald) if 50.0 g of steam condense on your hand to liquid water at 100°C?

21.46*) Solid benzene is removed from a freezer and begins to melt at 5°C. If 0.750 kg of C_6H_6 requires 24.5 kcal for melting, calculate ΔH_{fus} for benzene.

21.47*) Hospitals often use alcohol rubs to cool the skin of feverish patients. How does putting alcohol on the skin help cool the body?

21.48*) In hot, humid weather, people enjoy iced drinks. An aluminum cup filled with iced tea quickly develops a layer of liquid water (condensation) on the outside of the cup, while a cup made of glass or china tends not to. Why?

21.49*) Assuming specific heat is constant, what is ΔH when 555 g of mercury cool from a liquid at 27°C to a solid at 77 K?

Use Table 21–3 to answer the following questions.

21.21*) Write the thermochemical equation for the combustion of propane, showing heat as a product.

21.22*) Calculate ΔH for the complete combustion of 3.45 kg of propane.

21.23*) As you will see in Chapter 22, the value of ΔH is −9.0 kcal/mole for the conversion of ATP to ADP in the body. When doing work, a muscle uses about 5×10^{-7} moles of ATP per kilogram of muscle per minute. What is the heat output for 25.0 kg of muscle working an 8-hour day?

SECTION 21.2 FOOD ENERGY

21.24) One medium-sized apple with its skin contains 20 g of carbo-

21.50*) Write the thermochemical equation for the combustion of acetone, showing heat as a product.

21.51*) Calculate ΔH for the complete combustion of 785 g of acetone.

21.52*) One gram of a new sweetening agent, aldoxime ($C_9H_{14}O_2N$), provides as much sweetening as 450 g of sucrose. The heat of combustion of aldoxime is 1360 kcal/mole. Calculate ΔH in kcal if 1.00 g of aldoxime is consumed, and compare this with the caloric value of 450 g of sucrose. $C_{12}H_{22}O_{11}$.

21.53) A typical portion of scrambled eggs contains 30 g of carbohyhydrate, 0.3 g of protein, and 0.8 g of fat. Calculate its fuel value in kcal.

21.25) Cranberry sauce derives its fuel value almost entirely from carbohydrate. If one serving provides 50 kcal, how many grams of carbohydrate are in the portion?

21.26*) Explain why carbohydrates have less fuel value per gram than fats.

21.27) Explain how sweating cools the body.

21.28) Why does an athlete sweat more than a spectator?

21.29*) What effect does exercise have on a weight-reduction program?

21.30*) What is the meaning of the "basal metabolism rate"?

drate, 12 g of protein, and 14 g of fat. Calculate its fuel value in kcal.

21.54) Whipped cream derives its fuel value almost entirely from fats. If one dollop on a piece of pumpkin pie provides 210 kcal, how many grams of fat are in the portion of cream?

21.55*) Which would you expect to have the greater fuel value per gram, ethanol, C_2H_5OH, or ethylene glycol, $C_2H_4(OH)_2$? Why?

21.56) Will taking a both in cool water help the body get rid of excess heat? How?

21.57) How does breathing help the body get rid of excess heat?

21.58*) What effect does the drinking of alcoholic beverages have on a weight-reduction program?

21.59*) The volume of oxygen used by the body in a given time can be used as a measure of metabolism rate. Why?

SECTION 21.3 WHAT MAKES REACTIONS GO?

21.31*) The vaporization of carbon tetrachloride is endothermic but has a positive ΔS. Using Table 21–2, decide at what temperatures this process is spontaneous, nonspontaneous, and at equilibrium (at one atmosphere pressure).

21.32) Which of the following processes are spontaneous? nonspontaneous? at equilibrium?
a) the expansion of gas into a vacuum
b) climbing Mount Washington
c) freezing water at 0°C and 1 atm

21.33) What would be the sign of ΔG for each of the three processes in Question 21.32?

21.34) Predict the sign of ΔS for each of the following processes.
a) synthesis of a protein from amino acids
b) scrambling an egg
c) the process that occurs when a soft-drink bottle is opened

21.35*) Equations may be added

21.60*) The melting of NaCl is endothermic but has a positive ΔS. Using Table 21–2, decide at what temperatures this process is spontaneous, nonspontaneous, and at equilibrium.

21.61) Which of the following processes are spontaneous? nonspontaneous? at equilibrium?
a) exploding of the gas-air mixture in an automobile engine
b) removing pollutants from water
c) dissolving sugar in a solution already saturated with sugar

21.62) What would be the sign of ΔG for each of the three processes in Question 21.61?

21.63*) Predict the sign of ΔS for each of the following processes.
a) polymerization of ethylene to form polyethylene film
b) formation of a gelatin dessert from the hot mixture of ingredients
c) osmosis

21.64*) In principle, glucose may

together to obtain not only enthalpy changes but also ΔG. An automobile manufacturer wishes to reduce $NO_{(g)}$ emissions from exhaust gases by reducing the NO to N_2 by

$$CH_{4(g)} + NO_{(g)} \longrightarrow CH_3OH_{(g)} + N_{(g)}$$
$$\Delta G = +61.6 \text{ kcal}$$
$$NO_{(g)} + N_{(g)} \longrightarrow N_{2(g)} + O_{(g)}$$
$$\Delta G = -74.18 \text{ kcal}$$

Would this work? Explain.

react with ADP directly by the reaction

$$C_6H_{12}O_{6(s)} + ADP_{(aq)} +$$
$$H_3PO_{4(aq)} + 6 O_{2(g)} \longrightarrow$$
$$6 CO_{(g)} + ATP_{(aq)} + 7 H_2O$$

Find the ΔG of this "coupled" reaction using the following data:

$$C_6H_{12}O_{6(s)} + 6 O_{2(g)} \longrightarrow$$
$$6 CO_{2(g)} + 6 H_2O$$
$$\Delta G = -686.4 \text{ kcal}$$

$$ATP + H_2O \longrightarrow ADP + H_3PO_4$$
$$\Delta G = -7.3 \text{ kcal}$$

SECTION 21.4 RATES OF REACTION

21.36) Even though a collision between reactants may involve energy that is high enough to break bonds, products may not form. Why?

21.37) Sketch an enthalpy-reaction graph for an exothermic reaction, showing the activated complex position, the activation energy, and the value of ΔH.

21.38) Why does an increase in temperature result in a higher reaction rate?

21.65) A collision between reactants may form the activated complex, yet products may not result. Why?

21.66) Sketch an enthalpy-reaction graph for an endothermic reaction, showing the activated complex position, the activation energy, and the value of ΔH.

21.67) To perform some delicate heart operations, the patient's body is cooled to lower the blood temperature. The operation is then safer. Why?

SECTION 21.5 INTRODUCTION TO ENZYMES

21.39) Why does a catalyst increase the rate of a reaction? Refer to an enthalpy-reaction graph.

21.40) What purpose is served by an enzyme?

21.41*) What is a carbohydrase? (Consider its name.)

21.68) If a catalyst increases the rate of the forward reaction, what happens to the rate of the reverse reaction? Why?

21.69) Even if there is an inorganic catalyst that speeds up a particular reaction, the resultant rate is still much lower than if an enzyme is used. Explain.

21.70*) What is a protease? (Consider its name.)

Biochemical Energy

22

We are all very much aware of the energy crisis in the world today. Wasteful use of the world's supply of oil and natural gas must soon come to an end because a supply that took nature millions of years to produce takes us only a few decades to consume. In Chapter 3 we briefly discussed some aspects of nuclear power, which holds great promise for providing energy for our future (especially in the form of nuclear *fusion*) but also holds great dangers. Renewable, nonpolluting sources of energy, such as solar energy, wind, and tidal power, are also being studied. To do work, each of these sources of power must be converted to mechanical or electrical energy.

Consider the conversion of the chemical energy stored in oil, coal, or natural gas to work to turn the wheels of a car or heat a home in winter. The fuel must be burned (*oxidized*) to liberate some of the energy stored in the chemical bonds. The molecules produced, such as CO_2 and H_2O, are simpler than those of the fuel and contain a higher proportion of oxygen. Heat is given off, since any combustion reaction is *exothermic*. Some of that heat can be used to do work. Unavoidably, some is also wasted, since no machine works at 100% efficiency.

The body converts chemical energy to work in a process that, in its broad outlines, is similar to the burning of a fuel. The basic ideas were discussed in Section 21.2, where we noted that carbohydrates, proteins, and fats can all provide energy to the body. We also mentioned that the body uses only about 20% of the liberated chemical energy *to do work*, the rest being given off as heat; these figures are about the same as for an automobile engine. The *metabolism rate* (Table 21–5) when an activity is being performed shows you how much oxidation of food sources must be taking place in the body.

However, the detailed manner in which the body uses chemical energy to do work, especially in the cells, differs from the way an automobile engine works. Generally speaking, our bodies require heat from an outside source for comfort in winter, and at other times produce large amounts of heat, which must be lost. The living cell, however, must operate at a constant temperature, a constant liquid pressure, and a constant pH. For this reason, a very complex series of chemical reactions has evolved to generate and store usable energy. The cell must be able to manufacture (synthesize) and break down (degrade) carbohydrates, lipids, proteins, and nucleic acids. Energy must be made available when and where it is needed. Surplus energy must be stored or removed, and energy shortages must be remedied. The cell cannot survive a "power blackout."

The energy cycle in a cell can be seen as a combination of three processes:

1) Carbohydrates and other energy sources become available through

digestion and enter the cell. These foods originally gained their energy (directly or indirectly) from the sun through plant *photosynthesis*. Thus, CO_2, H_2O, and other simple compounds from the air and soil went into making the complex materials we eat.

2) *Cell respiration* transforms the chemical energy of the nutrients (by oxidizing carbohydrates, fats, and, possibly, proteins) into energy that can do work in the cell:

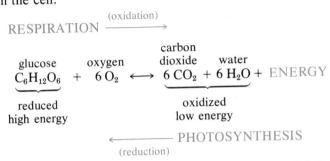

3) The cell can then do work involved in transporting materials into and out of the cell, including the *active transport* of ions described in Section 18.3, the mechanical work of muscle contraction, the electrical work of transmitting nerve impulses, and the chemical work of forming the bonds of the molecules that must be synthesized in the cell.

A significant portion of the energy produced in the cell is stored in extremely important *high-energy* compounds, such as adenosine triphosphate (ATP). These compounds provide immediate energy to drive essential reactions in the cycles that transform carbohydrates, lipids, and proteins into useful products. ATP also provides the immediate energy needed for muscle contraction. We now turn our attention to the way these high-energy compounds operate.

22.1 HIGH-ENERGY COMPOUNDS

LEARNING GOAL 22A: Describe and recognize the functional group that permits a high-energy molecule like ATP to store and release energy.

22B: Write a chemical equation for the release of free energy from a given high-energy molecule or the storage of free energy in a given low-energy molecule.

22C: Describe the role of the ATP/ADP system in coupling to a second reaction to either absorb (and store) energy or to deliver energy for work in the cell.

22D: Given the ΔG value for a nonspontaneous process, calculate whether coupling with the ATP/ADP system will be able to drive the desired reaction. If so, write the coupled equation.

22E: Describe the process of phosphate group transfer.

One of the major differences in composition between the fluid inside the cell and that outside the cell is the presence of large amounts of HPO_4^{2-} ion inside the cell. There must be something special about phosphates!

High-energy phosphate bonds

We have already discussed the phosphate ion, PO_4^{3-} (Chapter 4), and phosphoric acid, H_3PO_4 (Chapter 13). Section 13.5 pointed out that the phosphate buffer $HPO_4^{2-}/H_2PO_4^-$ plays a role in buffering the intracellular fluid. However, that is not its most important characteristic. Unlike the other common inorganic acids, phosphoric acid can form condensation polymers by the splitting out of water to produce acids such as $H_4P_2O_7$ or $H_5P_3O_{10}$. In fact, the sodium tripolyphosphate used in industrial detergents comes from such a polymer:

sodium tripolyphosphate

The "extra" phosphorus-oxygen bonds in such molecules, shown in color for $Na_5P_3O_{10}$, are sometimes called *anhydride* linkages. Any of these *meta*phosphoric acids may form salts and esters. The esters that these acids form with important biological alcohols are the high-energy storage molecules we will discuss in this section.

You should be aware that, since several hydrogens are attached to oxygen in each of these acids, any or all of the hydrogens may be lost (neutralized), depending on the pH of the solution. In some cases you may see these molecules in their acid forms (all —H present) and in other cases they may appear as anions. Do not concern yourself with this difference, which is more apparent than real. At the close-to-neutral pH levels of the body, some of the hydrogens will be attached to each phosphate group and others will be ionized, with the number ionized varying from molecule to molecule.

An *anhydride* is a molecule that has lost water. For example, the anhydride of sulfuric acid, H_2SO_4, is SO_3 gas, since $SO_3 + H_2O \rightarrow H_2SO_4$.

Hydrolysis of high-energy phosphate bonds

The two "extra" bonds in sodium tripolyphosphate are formed by the condensation of three PO_4^{3-} groups, with the splitting out of two water molecules. In fact, this is how *all* large natural molecules are formed. Proteins are made by peptide linkages, carbohydrates by hexose chains, and fats by esterification; all of these involve the splitting out of water. The breaking down of biological macromolecules into smaller units (amino acids, glucose, fatty acids) involves the addition of water (hydrolysis) to the chain. The digestive enzymes speed up this process.

The biological molecules that have phosphate groups on them are similarly formed by condensation and can be broken apart by hydrolysis. For example, the simplest organophosphate is acetyl phosphate:

acetyl phosphate hydrolyzes to acetic acid and phosphoric acid

When a bond is broken, energy is absorbed by the acetyl phosphate molecule. However, a greater amount of energy is given off when, in hydrolysis, new bonds are formed. Thus, there is a net release of energy; the reaction is exothermic.

However, the body cannot simply use the heat given off in a reaction (ΔH) to do work. Automobile engines can use heat to increase the pressure and temperature of gases in the cylinders, but the body cannot do the same. It must exist at a *constant* temperature. For a cell process, ΔH is not a very good measure of how much work can be done by the hydrolysis of a molecule.

Free energy of hydrolysis

In Section 21.3 we discussed the free energy (ΔG) of a reaction as a way of taking into account not only heat given off but also the entropy or "randomness" of the molecules. The breaking down of a complex molecule into two smaller ones is generally spontaneous because there is an increase in entropy, S, regardless of the exact value of ΔH. Since $\Delta G = \Delta H - T\,\Delta S$ (p. 582), ΔG becomes more negative (and the reaction happens to a greater extent) if there is a greater increase in entropy (randomness). As noted at the end of Section 21.3, the value of $-\Delta G$ represents the amount of energy that *can do work* under the constant-temperature conditions of a living cell. A compound that can store large amounts of usable energy should therefore have a *highly negative* ΔG of hydrolysis, which we will denote ΔG_h. One such compound is ATP.

> For an increase in entropy (disorder), ΔS is positive and therefore $-T\,\Delta S$ is negative, making the reaction more spontaneous.

ATP, ADP, and AMP

The most important energy-controlling compound in the body is **ATP, a**denosine **tri**phosphate (Figure 20–10). Adenosine can combine with one H_3PO_4 molecule in an ester linkage, in which case we obtain the nucleotide AMP, **a**denosine **mono**phosphate, found throughout the body and especially in muscle tissue.

If AMP again reacts with phosphoric acid, we obtain **ADP, a**denosine **di**phosphate. Reaction with a third phosphate produces ATP. ADP and ATP* are found in all cells and will be leading "actors" in the upcoming chapters. The overall structures of AMP, ADP, and ATP are shown in Figure 22–1.

ATP, ADP, and AMP can be hydrolyzed according to the following reactions. Values for ΔG_h are given so that you may see the relative amounts of usable energy contained in the phosphate bonds at 25°C.

$$\text{ATP} + H_2O \longrightarrow \text{ADP} + H_3PO_4 \qquad \Delta G_h = -7.3 \text{ kcal/mole}$$

---

* Why does *adenine* play this extremely important role, and not one of the other bases shown in Figure 20–8? One possibility is that adenine was relatively easy to synthesize in the natural conditions on earth hundreds of millions of years ago, when the first life forms were produced. We believe that HCN, hydrogen cyanide, molecules existed at that time. Since these can form polymers of the form —HCN—HCN—HCN— because of hydrogen-bonding, five such units could then relatively easily be converted to adenine, $C_5N_5H_5$. (See Arms, K., and Camp, P.S., *Biology,* 2nd edition, Philadelphia, Saunders College Publishing, 1982.)

The ATP molecule is now rather expensive for biochemists to study in the laboratory, costing about $2500 per mole. Dr. George Whitesides has devised a new way to synthesize ATP from acetone and phosphoric acid, which could reduce the cost to roughly $5 per mole.

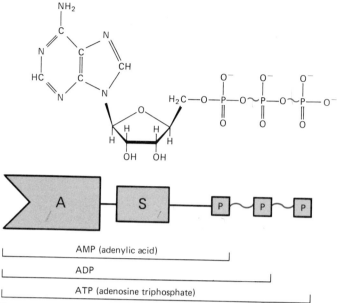

FIGURE 22–1 The structures of five molecules of importance to life can be seen within the overall formula of ATP. The base at the upper left is adenine, found also in DNA and RNA. Condensation with ribose (a sugar, S) gives adenosine, discussed on p. 554 as a *nucleoside*. Reaction with a single phosphoric acid molecule gives the *nucleotide* AMP. The energy-storage system ADP/ATP is built by addition of more phosphate units (P), with high-energy bonds (shown by colored wavy lines) between phosphorus and oxygen.

$$\text{ADP} + \text{H}_2\text{O} \longrightarrow \text{AMP} + \text{H}_3\text{PO}_4 \qquad \Delta G_h = -7.3 \text{ kcal/mole}$$
$$\text{AMP} + \text{H}_2\text{O} \longrightarrow \text{adenosine} + \text{H}_3\text{PO}_4 \qquad \Delta G_h = -2.2 \text{ kcal/mole}$$

A **high-energy compound** has a ΔG_h more negative than -5 kcal/mole. Such compounds are useful as sources of immediate energy, and also for energy storage. Using this definition, ATP and ADP are both high-energy compounds and AMP is a low-energy compound. (Creatine phosphate is another high-energy compound. It provides the driving force for muscle movement.)

The pathways we will see in Section 22.2 and in Chapter 25 involve such organophosphate compounds. Table 22–1 lists some of these compounds in order of decreasing importance as energy-storage units. Those high in the table tend to lose their phosphate groups; those toward the bottom tend to keep them. The compounds in Table 22–1 are shown in their partially ionized forms for consistency with other literature sources you may consult. The actual ionization state will vary with the pH and with the characteristics of the individual molecule.

These equations and their associated ΔG_h values have been simplified to represent "laboratory" standard conditions. The situation in living cells is somewhat different; for example, ΔG_h for ATP may be nearer -12 kcal/mole in a cellular reaction. (See Lehninger, A.L., *Bioenergetics*, 2nd edition, Menlo Park, Calif., W.A. Benjamin, 1971, Chapter 3.)

Phosphate group transfer

Since it indicates the relative ability of an organophosphate compound to lose its phosphate group, Table 22–1 may be used to predict phosphate group *transfer* from one molecule to another. The high-energy compounds at the top of the table can transfer their phosphate groups to the hydrolyzed forms of the low-energy compounds. For example, creatine phosphate can react with adenosine to give creatine plus AMP.

TABLE 22–1   SOME BIOLOGICALLY IMPORTANT
ORGANOPHOSPHATE COMPOUNDS

High-energy		ΔG_h (kcal/mole)
Phosphoenolpyruvate (glycolysis)		−14.8
1,3-Diphosphoglycerate (glycolysis)		−11.8
Creatine phosphate (in muscles)		−10.3
ATP		−7.3
ADP		−7.3

Low-energy		
Glucose-1-phosphate (glycogen production)		−5.0
Fructose-6-phosphate (glycolysis)		−3.8
Glucose-6-phosphate (glycolysis)		−3.3
3-Phosphoglycerate (glycolysis)		−2.4
AMP		−2.2

It is important to note that ADP occupies a *middle* position in the table with respect to its ability to transfer phosphate groups. The ATP/ADP system thus acts as a kind of bridge or link between high-energy and low-energy compounds. As an example, both phosphoenolpyruvate and 1,3-diphosphoglycerate are formed during the breakdown of glucose in the cell. Since their ΔG_h values are more negative than that of ATP, either can transfer a phosphate group to ADP (to give ATP). The ATP thus formed has a more negative ΔG_h than fructose, glucose, or glycerol, which may be present in the cell, and can react to form one of the bottom three (low-energy) organophosphate compounds in Table 22–1.

Coupled reactions

A reaction that proceeds spontaneously has a negative ΔG. We call such a reaction *exogonic* (similar to the term *exo*thermic for a negative ΔH). A reaction that must be "driven" needs a supply of free energy; its ΔG is positive. Such a reaction is *endo*gonic. It will not go by itself.

In many biological systems, a nonspontaneous reaction with a positive ΔG may be combined with a second (spontaneous) reaction with a negative ΔG, so that the exogonic reaction may provide the energy to drive the endogonic step. The two values of ΔG must add up to a negative total for the combined (*coupled*) reaction to go. The stored energy in ATP is often used to drive biological reactions with positive ΔG values.

For example, about 5.5 kcal/mole of free energy are needed to drive the formation of sucrose from glucose and fructose. Coupling with the ATP/ADP system and formation of an intermediate, glucose-1-phosphate, can be written

$$\text{glucose} + \text{ATP} \longrightarrow \text{glucose-1-phosphate} + \text{ADP}$$
$$\text{glucose-1-phosphate} + \text{fructose} \longrightarrow \text{sucrose} + \text{phosphoric acid}$$

The two reactions to be coupled are

$$\text{ATP} \longrightarrow \text{ADP} + \text{phosphoric acid} \qquad \Delta G_h = -7.3 \text{ kcal/mole}$$
$$\text{glucose} + \text{fructose} \longrightarrow \text{sucrose} \qquad \Delta G_h = +5.5 \text{ kcal/mole}$$

The coupled (net) reaction is

$$\text{ATP} + \text{glucose} + \text{fructose} \longrightarrow \text{ADP} + \text{sucrose} + \text{H}_3\text{PO}_4$$
$$\Delta G = -1.8 \text{ kcal/mole}$$

As with determining ΔH values (p. 573), the exact path of a coupled reaction does not affect the value of ΔG. However, the *speed* of a reaction is not given by ΔG. A spontaneous reaction may proceed very slowly. The presence of enzymes in the cell permits the coupled reaction to occur at a useful rate, as shown in Figure 22–2. The reaction pathway must therefore follow whatever route can use the enzymes present.

More generally, the ATP/ADP system first couples with an energy-producing system (such as oxidation of energy-producing nutrients) to *store* energy and then couples with a system that does work, which *needs* energy. It is the middle agent or "broker" in many processes, as shown in Figure 22–3. Here, and in the rest of this chapter, **P** will be used to represent any of the various forms of phosphoric acid (H_3PO_4, $H_2PO_4^-$, HPO_4^{2-}, or PO_4^{3-}).

Our society is becoming very much aware of the need to conserve and recycle raw materials. Many millions of years ago, living organisms discovered the same principle. A coupled reaction uses the "raw materials" of

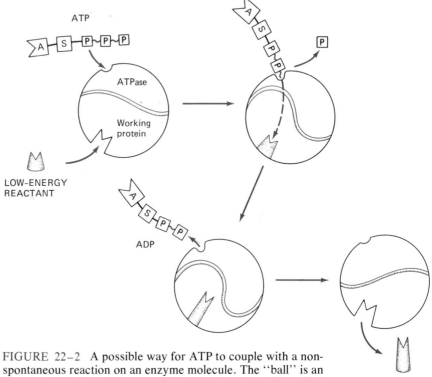

FIGURE 22–2 A possible way for ATP to couple with a non-spontaneous reaction on an enzyme molecule. The "ball" is an enzyme molecule with one part that receives the ATP (called *ATPase*) and another that catalyzes the transformation of a low-energy reactant to a high-energy product. While the ATP loses a phosphate group to become ADP, the enzyme *changes shape,* transfers the energy to the active site where the high-energy product will be formed, and completes the reaction. Some evidence for this idea comes from the observation that ATPases seem to be included in enzyme proteins.

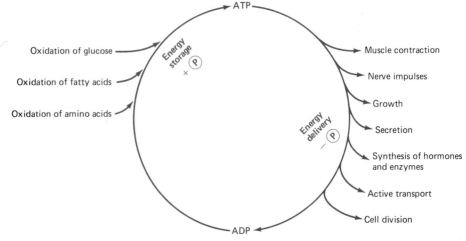

FIGURE 22–3 The cycle of energy in living cells. Energy-producing reactions change ADP to ATP. Coupling with other biological reactions permits them to work while converting ATP to ADP.

phosphate and adenosine over and over again by continually recycling ADP to ATP and ATP to ADP. There is no great need for constant addition or synthesis of adenine or phosphate, nor is there any "pollution" from surplus ADP or phosphate. It is difficult to imagine any modern-day machine that could perform in such harmony with its environment.

SELF-CHECK

22.1*) An electrical power plant normally uses heat to convert water to steam and then uses the steam to do work. Why can't the cell similarly use heat produced from oxidation in the cell to do work?

22.2) Write a chemical equation that illustrates the storage of energy in an AMP molecule.

22.3) If a cell reaction has a free energy change of $\Delta G = +2.0$ kcal/mole, will the reaction occur spontaneously? If not, will coupling with the ATP/ADP system possibly make the reaction work? Explain, using chemical equations.

22.4) Will creatine be able to remove a phosphate group from ADP? Explain, using Table 22–1.

22.5*) One feature of ATP is its ability to lose *two* phosphate groups, liberating a total of 14.6 kcal/mole. What other compound in Table 22–1 can similarly lose two phosphate groups? Would it liberate more or less free energy than ATP?

22.2 ENERGY PRODUCTION WITHOUT OXYGEN: GLYCOLYSIS

LEARNING GOAL 22F: Describe the initial reactants, the products, and the overall function of glycolysis in the cell.

22G: Account for the energy production that results from glycolysis.

22H: Describe the similarities in structure of NAD+, FAD, and ATP.

22I: Name the three major pathways that produce energy in the cell.

Scientists know of many species of bacteria that can survive and produce energy with no oxygen present. We call these *anaerobic* organisms, from *an-*, "not," plus *aero-*, "air," plus *bios*, "life"; these are life forms that do not need air. It is possible that such organisms were the remote ancestors of animals, such as humans, whose cells can often function either in the presence of oxygen or in its absence. Parts of a cell may produce energy using anaerobic reactions while other parts are using reactions that are *aerobic* and require oxygen.

Possible fuels for energy production include glucose, amino acids, and fatty acids. In general, our cells rely mostly on glucose as a source of energy. In this chapter, we will concentrate on the *anaerobic* process that uses glucose, **glycolysis,** and on the *aerobic* energy-producing processes that follow it.

The word *glycolysis* is from the Greek *glykys*, "sweet," plus *lysis*, "loosening" or "breaking apart." The process results in the overall conversion of glucose (a hexose, $C_6H_{12}O_6$) to two pyruvate anions, CH_3COCOO^-. This process is not, however, a simple change from a six-carbon molecule to two three-carbon molecules with the liberation of heat. In light of the discussions in Section 22.1, you would expect some coupled reactions using ATP. We also need some reactions that *produce* ATP to insure its recycling within the cell. All of these reactions (there are ten of them in glycolysis) use different enzymes to speed them up. With the exception of the first reactant (glucose) and the final product (pyruvate, CH_3COCOO^-), all of the (intermediate) compounds contain phosphate groups like those in Table 22–1. The series of reactions is often named the *Embden-Meyerhof pathway,* after two biochemists who first demonstrated the use of this process in the cell.

NAD^+ and FAD

Before discussing the ten steps of glycolysis, we should discuss the roles of two coenzymes that play a major part in the process. Recall from p. 588 that an enzyme is an important biological catalyst. Many enzymes contain *cofactors,* additional chemical groups required for their activity. The cofactor may be a metal, such as Mg, Zn, Mn, Fe, or Cu, in the cation form or it may be an organic molecular group bound to the enzyme protein. In such a case, the cofactor is called a **coenzyme.**

Many vitamins form coenzymes, as you will see in Chapter 23. However, in this chapter we will be concerned only with two interesting and important molecules that come from B-complex vitamins: NAD^+, **n**icotinamide **a**denine **d**inucleotide, (from the vitamin niacin or nicotinamide) and FAD, **f**lavin **a**denine **d**inucleotide, (from the vitamin riboflavin), which are shown in Figure 22–4.

On the left in both parts of Figure 22–4 is ADP. The coenzyme NAD^+ is formed when ADP bonds to ribose and then to the vitamin nicotinamide; FAD is the vitamin riboflavin connected by an ester linkage to ADP.

Both NAD^+ and FAD serve as parts of the enzyme structure that *oxidize* the substrate. Each removes two electrons and gains energy. For example, NAD^+ is often involved in the oxidation of an aldehyde group to a carboxyl:

$$NAD^+ + R—CHO \rightleftharpoons NADH + RCOO^-$$

or of a hydroxyl (alcohol) to a carbonyl:

$$NAD^+ + R_2CHOH \rightleftharpoons NADH + R_2C{=}O$$

as well as in many more complicated oxidation processes. The active part of the molecule is transformed to make NADH:

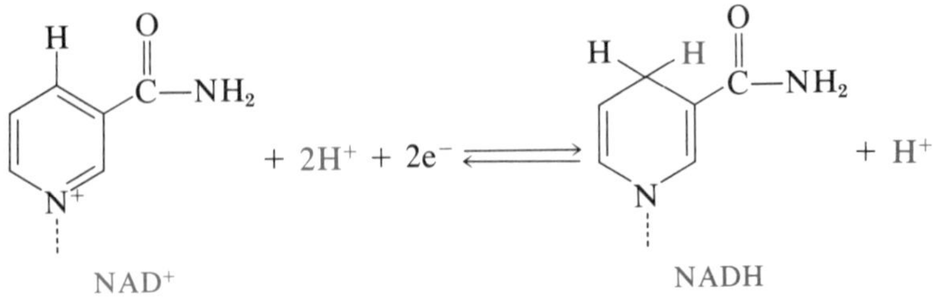

FAD similarly oxidizes the substrate, but retains *two* hydrogens instead of one. That makes it ideal for forming a double bond:

$$FAD + R\!-\!CH_2CH_2\!-\!R' \rightleftharpoons FADH_2 + R\!-\!CH\!=\!CH\!-\!R'$$
$$FAD + R\!-\!CH_2OH \rightleftharpoons FADH_2 + R\!-\!CH\!=\!O$$

It accomplishes this by conversion to $FADH_2$:

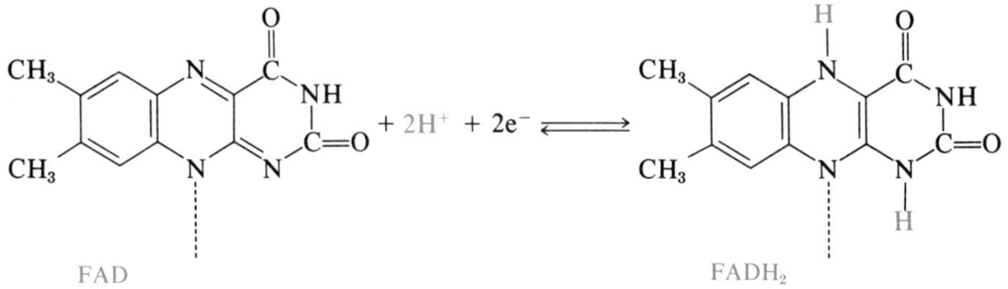

FAD   FADH$_2$

The reduced forms, NADH and $FADH_2$, are constantly being oxidized back to NAD^+ and FAD, giving up energy in the process. Most important, each can react with an oxygen molecule to give up large amounts of energy. At the pH of cell contents:

$$NADH + H^+ + \tfrac{1}{2}\,O_2 \longrightarrow NAD^+ + H_2O \qquad \Delta G = -52.7 \text{ kcal/mole}$$
$$FADH_2 + \tfrac{1}{2}\,O_2 \longrightarrow FAD + H_2O \qquad \Delta G = -36.2 \text{ kcal/mole}$$

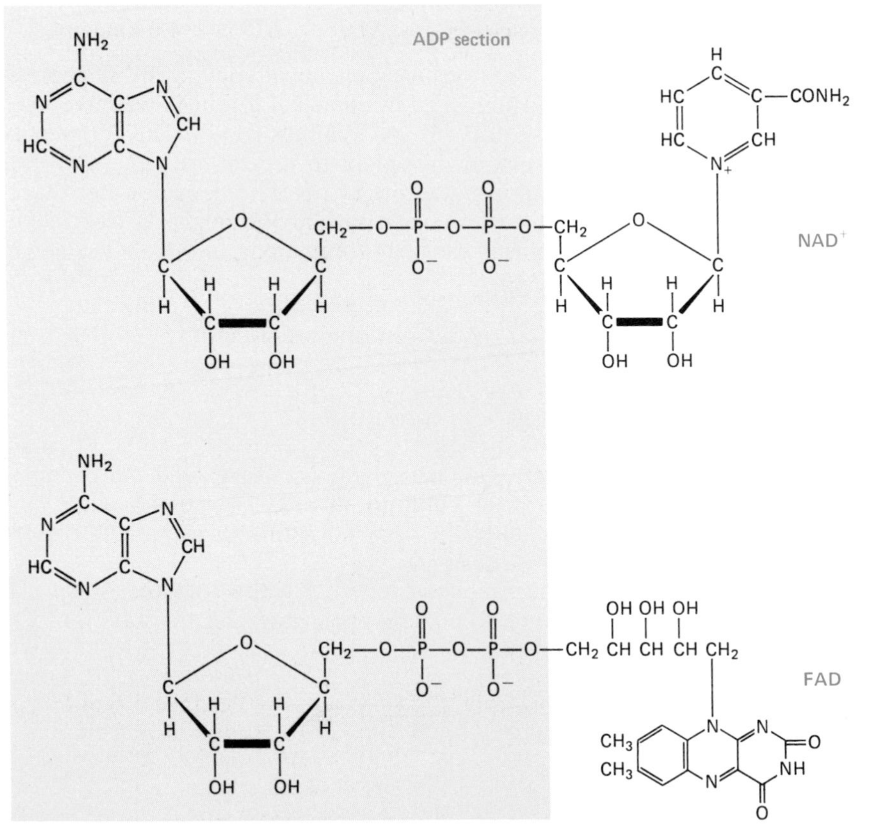

FIGURE 22–4 The structures of the coenzymes NAD^+ and FAD link molecular sections derived from vitamins (niacin for NAD^+, riboflavin for FAD) to the ADP molecular unit (shown in color).

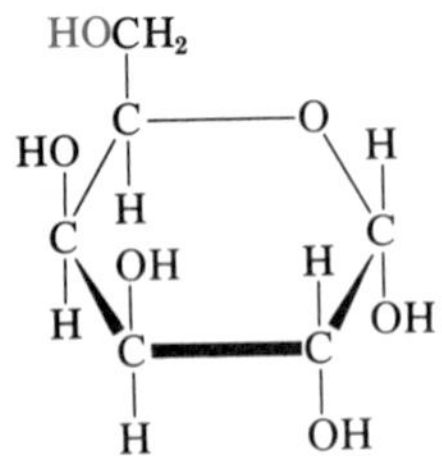

glucose

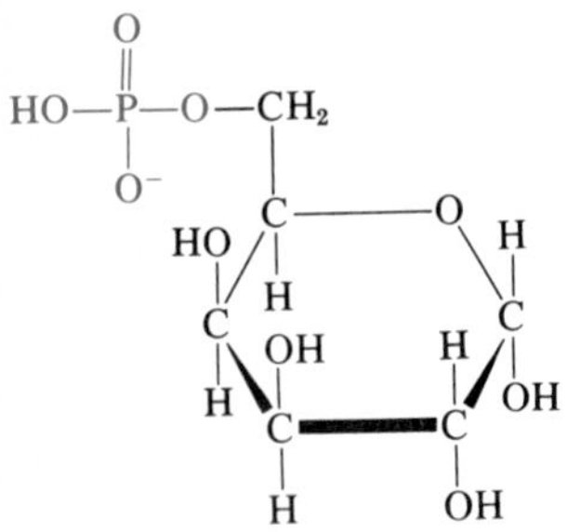

glucose-6-PO$_4$

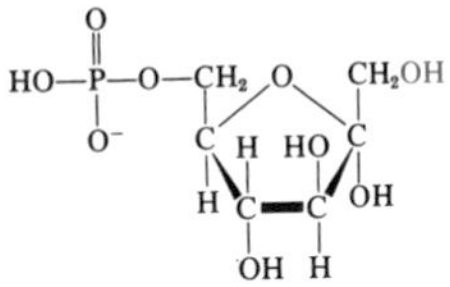

The free energy change for the hydrolysis of glucose-6-PO$_4$ is -3.3 kcal/mole at 25°C (Table 22–1). The value for the *formation* of glucose-6-PO$_4$, the reverse reaction, is therefore $+3.3$ kcal/mole.

fructose-6-PO$_4$

fructose-1,6-diPO$_4$

We therefore think of NADH and FADH$_2$ as *carriers* of usable energy from the place where a substance is being oxidized to where O$_2$ is being reduced. Each also serves as a reducing agent for other important metabolic steps.

This continual interchange of energy and hydrogens using NAD$^+$/NADH and FAD/FADH$_2$ as energy porters or "shuttles," is very important in the pathways which follow.

Glycolysis priming reactions

The first reaction in the Embden-Meyerhof pathway converts glucose to glucose-6-phosphate in a coupled reaction that also converts ATP to ADP. This is a "bare-bones" phosphate group transfer that can be written

$$\text{glucose} + \text{P} \longrightarrow \text{glucose-6-PO}_4 \qquad \Delta G = +3.3 \text{ kcal/mole}$$
$$\text{ATP} \longrightarrow \text{ADP} + \text{P} \qquad \Delta G = -7.3 \text{ kcal/mole}$$

Remember that we are using P to represent any of the several inorganic phosphate species we might encounter. The values of ΔG are taken from Table 22–1.

If we add the coupled reaction equations together, we obtain

$$\text{glucose} + \text{ATP} \longrightarrow \text{glucose-6-PO}_4 + \text{ADP} \qquad \Delta G = -4.0 \text{ kcal/mole}$$

To this point, we have used ordinary chemical equations, but there is not much point to that because instead of chemical formulas we have been reduced to the use of names (glucose) and symbols (ATP). The complexity of the molecules makes it very inconvenient to use the true chemical formulas. We have also saved time and effort by not writing each water that is added in hydrolysis or split out in condensation. We might as well move, then, to the use of biochemical shorthand equations in which the above chemical equation is expressed

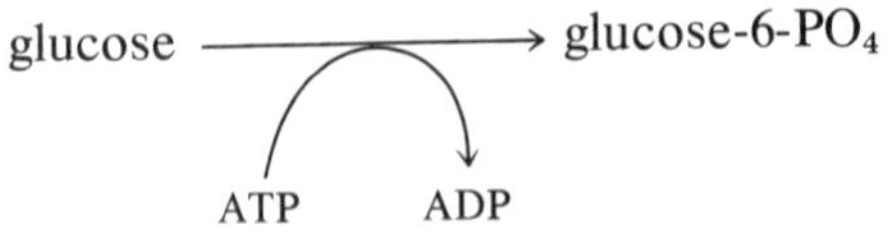

glucose $\longrightarrow$ glucose-6-PO$_4$

ATP ADP

This shorthand is read exactly the same way we would read the chemical equation: "Glucose reacts with ATP to give glucose-6-phosphate and ADP." The use of arrows makes the coupled nature of the reaction more apparent.

The next reaction in the Embden-Meyerhof pathway is the isomerization of glucose-6-phosphate to fructose-6-phosphate and the addition of a second phosphate:

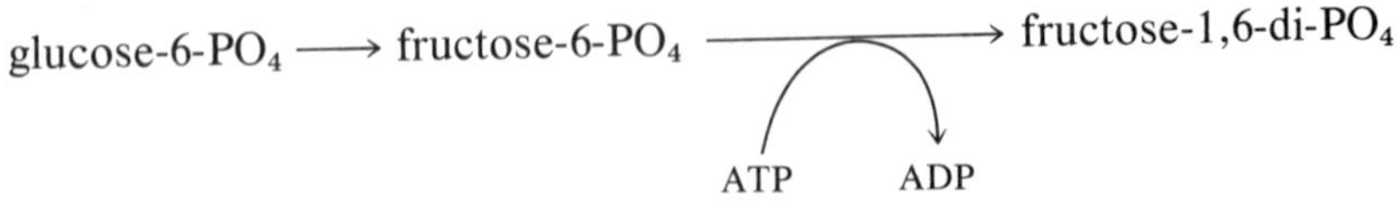

glucose-6-PO$_4$ $\longrightarrow$ fructose-6-PO$_4$ $\longrightarrow$ fructose-1,6-di-PO$_4$

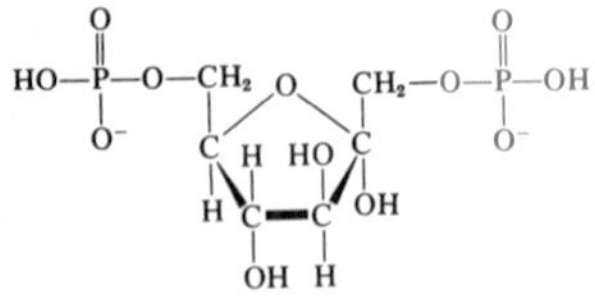

ATP ADP

The reactants now have enough energy to carry them the rest of the way without further ATP-to-ADP conversion. That is why these reactions are called *priming* reactions.

The glycolysis pathway

The manner in which one glucose molecule is converted to two molecules of pyruvate in the Embden-Meyerhof pathway is shown in Figure 22–5. The priming reactions are shown along the left. The splitting of the six-carbon sugar into two three-carbon molecules appears at the top, along with the oxidation of the aldehyde to the anionic form of a carboxylic acid. The phosphate groups are then moved off the three-carbon molecules until pyruvate is formed.

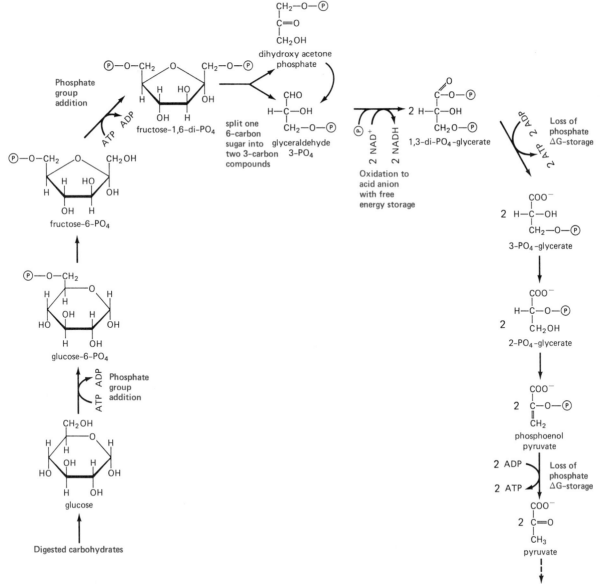

FIGURE 22–5 The Embden-Meyerhof glycolysis pathway.

Energy from glycolysis

The priming steps require two ATP molecules. However, along the right-hand side of Figure 22–5 we see that *four* ATP's are produced, for a *net gain* of two ATP units of stored energy.

When we discuss the electron transport system in Section 22.4, you will observe that each NADH molecule that enters that system can produce three ATP molecules. Since two NADH molecules are formed in glycolysis for each glucose processed, there is a *potential* of six additional ATP units of free energy, for a grand total of eight.*

Energy loss occurs, however, if there is a lack of oxygen in the cells. The glycolysis process is anaerobic; no oxygen is needed. However, the pyruvate formed generally moves along into an oxygen-rich environment to enter subsequent pathways. If the oxygen level is low, as during periods of severe muscle exertion, the pyruvate formed in glycolysis reacts with NADH to produce lactate:

$$
\begin{array}{ccc}
\text{COO}^- & & \text{COO}^- \\
| & & | \\
\text{C}=\text{O} & \longrightarrow & \text{H}-\text{C}-\text{OH} \\
| & \text{NADH} \quad \text{NAD}^+ & | \\
\text{CH}_3 & & \text{CH}_3 \\
\text{pyruvate} & & \text{lactate}
\end{array}
$$

This lactate may produce muscle fatigue and perhaps cramps. Each NADH converted to NAD^+ in this process represents a loss of three ATP energy units. Luckily, the cell has a way of converting lactate back to pyruvate and regaining the lost energy.

Stages of cell respiration

We have now briefly mentioned the three pathways that normally produce energy for the cell. These phases of **cell respiration** are summarized in Table 22–2.

As we will see in the next section, the pyruvate molecules from phase I (glycolysis) feed into the Krebs cycle, producing more ATP energy plus molecules of the reduced (energy-carrying) coenzymes NADH and $FADH_2$. These "carrier molecules" flow into the electron transport system, producing molecules of ATP and reducing O_2 to form water. Because oxygen must be present to relieve the NADH and $FADH_2$ of hydrogen, the Krebs cycle and the electron transport system are *aerobic* processes. There are obviously many intermediate chemical compounds involved, but all of them are recycled as the cell breaks down glucose to produce energy, carbon

---

* The glycolysis reaction produces two NADH molecules in the cytoplasm of the cell. In order for these energy carriers to enter the electron transport system to give up their energy, the hydrogens they carry must pass into the mitochondria. Since NADH cannot cross the membrane, special "shuttle" systems transfer the hydrogens to either NAD^+ or FAD inside the mitochondria. If NAD^+, as in liver and heart tissue, then no energy is lost. If FAD receives the hydrogens, as in nerve and muscle tissue, there is a reduction of two ATP energy units per glucose molecule, lowering the overall stored energy from glycolysis to six ATP units. Much more energy comes from the processes described in the following sections. See also the detailed discussion in the chapter on "Respiration" in Arms, K. and Camp, P.S., *Biology,* 2nd edition, Philadelphia, Saunders College Publishing, 1982.

TABLE 22-2 SUMMARY OF THE THREE STAGES
OF CELL RESPIRATION

Phase	Reactions	Energy yield
Glycolysis (cytoplasm)	No oxygen present Glucose split in two Atoms rearranged	2 ATP

Krebs cycle
(mitochondrial matrix)
	Water added to three-carbon
	    molecules
	H carried off by NADH and
	    FADH$_2$
	CO$_2$ produced
		2 ATP

Electron transport chain
(mitochondrial cristae)
	H atoms from NADH split into
	    H$^+$ and e$^-$
	Electrons pass down cyto-
	    chrome chain
	H$^+$ and e$^-$ combine with oxygen
	    to form H$_2$O
		Approx. 34 ATP

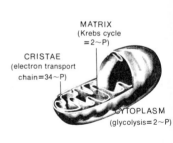

MATRIX
(Krebs cycle
=2~P)

CRISTAE
(electron transport
chain=34~P)

CYTOPLASM
(glycolysis=2~P)

dioxide, and water. Some differences between the anaerobic and aerobic processes in the cell are listed in Table 22–3.

There are many checks and balances in these systems, as in all biochemical processes. The amount of stored energy (as ATP) present in the cell regulates the amount of glucose processed in glycolysis, as will be seen in Chapter 25. Thus, the cell receives "feedback" on how much energy it is producing and how much is being used to do work.

SELF-CHECK

22.6) How do two pyruvate molecules result from one glucose entering the glycolysis pathway?
22.7) If 1.00 g of glucose, C$_6$H$_{12}$O$_6$, enters the glycolysis pathway, how many ATP molecules will be *directly* produced? how many NADH energy carriers? Remember that one mole contains 6.02×10^{23} molecules.
22.8) Describe the change in the NAD$^+$ ion when it is reduced to NADH.
22.9) Briefly describe the role of a coenzyme.
22.10) List the three stages of energy production in a cell, and state whether each occurs in the cytoplasm or the mitochondria.

TABLE 22-3 SOME DIFFERENCES BETWEEN AEROBIC
AND ANAEROBIC RESPIRATION

Aerobic respiration (oxidative phosphorylation)	Anaerobic respiration (fermentation)
Uses molecular O$_2$	Does not use O$_2$ as an electron acceptor
Degrades glucose to CO$_2$ and H$_2$O	Degrades glucose to trioses and other complex organic compounds
Exergonic	Exergonic
Recovers almost 50% of chemical energy	Recovers less chemical energy
Enzymes localized in mitochondria	Enzymes localized in the cytoplasm
Yields 36 ATP units per glucose molecule	Yields 2 ATP units per glucose molecule

22.3 ENERGY PRODUCTION FROM THE KREBS CYCLE

> *LEARNING GOAL 22J: Describe the role of acetyl coenzyme A in the Krebs cycle.*
>
> *22K: Describe how ATP molecules are produced in the Krebs cycle and how the hydrogen-carrier molecules NADH and FADH₂ are passed on to the electron transport chain.*

The second process is called the **Krebs cycle,** after Hans Krebs, the biochemist who first worked out the details in 1937. The series of reactions starts with the end product of glycolysis, pyruvate. Unlike glycolysis, which we represent with a U-shaped pathway, the Krebs reactions form a complete cycle.

Acetyl coenzyme A

As one pyruvate molecule moves into and around the Krebs cycle, one ATP, three NADH's, and one $FADH_2$ are produced. However, pyruvate cannot go directly into the cycle. The two pyruvate molecules resulting from the one glucose molecule entering glycolysis are converted (as usual, with the help of enzymes) to acetate for the trip around the Krebs cycle. However, the cycle does not accept the acetate ion directly. It must first be converted to an *activated* molecule known as **acetyl coenzyme A** (Figure 22–6), which contains a phosphate group on a ribose carbon and a long chain that contains a vitamin, *pantothenic acid*. We can abbreviate this rather complex chain (which for *coenzyme A* ends with an —SH group) HSCoA. Acetate ion can then react with coenzyme A:

$$CH_3COO^- + HSCoA \longrightarrow CH_3COSCoA$$
acetate ion   coenzyme A   acetyl coenzyme A

Acetyl coenzyme A

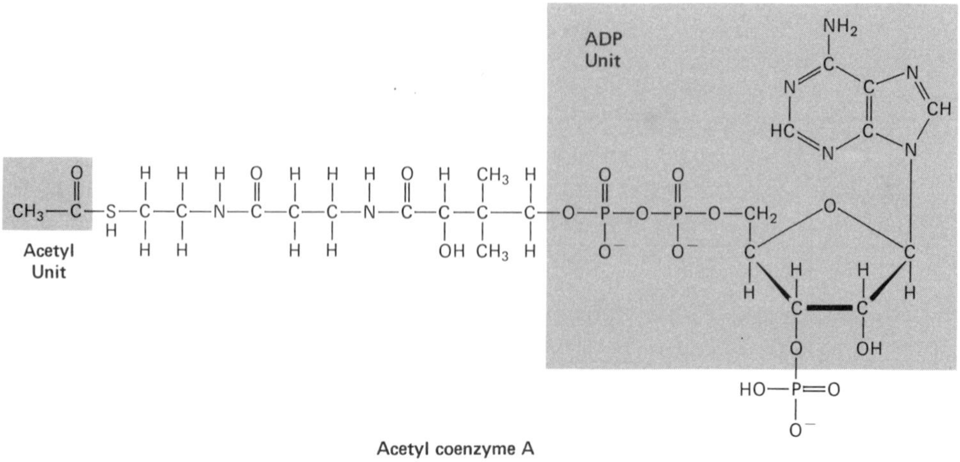

FIGURE 22–6 Acetyl coenzyme A includes a portion of the molecule common to ADP, NAD⁺, and FAD.

The acetyl coenzyme A formed in this reaction can transport acetyl groups anywhere in the body.

The conversion of pyruvate to acetyl coenzyme A is more complex than the simple reaction between the coenzyme and an acetate ion. It involves oxidation by NAD^+ (and thus storage of energy in NADH) and the release of carbon dioxide:

$$\underset{\text{pyruvate}}{\overset{\displaystyle COO^-}{\underset{\displaystyle CH_3}{\overset{\displaystyle |}{\underset{\displaystyle |}{C=O}}}}} \; + \; NAD^+ \; + \; \underset{\text{coenzyme A}}{HSCoA} \; \longrightarrow \; NADH \; + \; CO_2 \; + \; \underset{\text{acetyl coenzyme A}}{CH_3\overset{\displaystyle O}{\overset{\displaystyle \|}{C}}-S-CoA}$$

This step alone will send one NADH per pyruvate (and thus two NADH per glucose) into the electron transport chain for conversion to ATP. The yield will be six ATP per original glucose.

The Krebs Cycle

Now that we have made the link between the product of glycolysis (pyruvate) and the substance that can enter the Krebs cycle (acetyl coenzyme A), the cycle is primed. We can now refer to Figure 22–7 and follow the reactions of the cycle as energy is given off in the form of ATP and carrier molecules (NADH and $FADH_2$). You will notice oxaloacetate ion entering the cycle from reaction 9. Its four carbons combine with the two carbons of the acetyl group to give a six-carbon tricarboxylic acid anion, citrate, in reaction 2.*

In reactions 3 and 4 of the cycle, the six-carbon citrate ion is changed in several steps to the five-carbon ketoglutarate ion. In these reactions, the NAD^+ has effectively oxidized one of the carbon atoms of citrate to CO_2 and carried off the energy as NADH. This section of the Krebs cycle will therefore result in one NADH per pyruvate (two NADH per glucose) and thus six ATP energy units. In reactions 5 and 6 of the cycle, still another carbon is oxidized by NAD^+ and lost as CO_2, so we end up with a four-carbon acid anion, succinate. This is an extremely complex reaction involving oxidation by NAD^+ and a phosphate group transfer, which ends up producing one molecule of ATP directly. Coenzyme A is also involved in this process, forming succinyl coenzyme A. The energy gain will be one direct ATP plus three from NADH once it proceeds through the electron transport chain, for a total of four ATP per pyruvate, or eight ATP for each glucose.

Reactions 7 and 8 of the cycle involve a coenzyme that we saw in Figure 22–4, FAD. Each $FADH_2$ molecule will, like NADH, proceed to the electron transport chain, where it produces two ATP units per pyruvate, or four per glucose.

Reaction 9 of the Krebs cycle completes the recycling process because it produces the oxaloacetate we used in the beginning. Since one NADH is given off in this step, we will end up with three more ATP units, or six additional ATP units for each glucose processed at the beginning of the glycolysis pathway.

Any lactate ion present in the mitochondria can be oxidized to pyruvate (again giving off NADH), which can react in the normal manner.

Because citrate, the anion of citric acid, is the first product inside the cycle, the Krebs cycle is often called the *citric acid cycle*. To describe the group of compounds that includes citric and isocitric acids, it may also be called the *tricarboxylic acid cycle*.

---

* Remember that at the pH of the body (roughly 7.4) most organic acids exist mainly as anions. In some texts, you may see these reactions written in terms of acid molecules (pyruvic acid, oxaloacetic acid, citric acid).

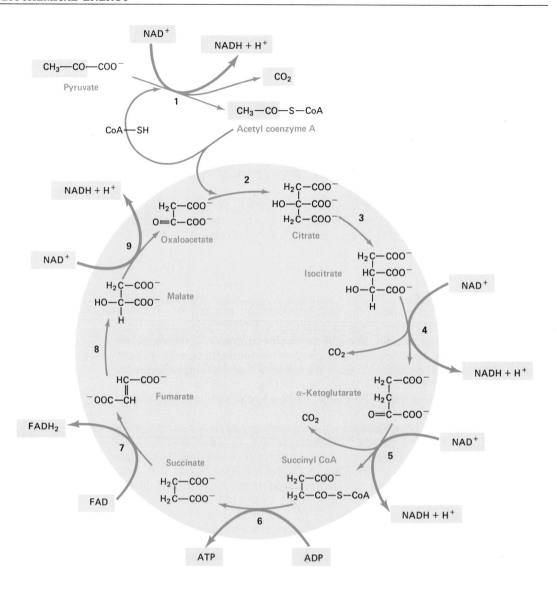

STEPS IN THE CITRIC ACID CYCLE

1. Pyruvate is oxidized to acetate, which is given extra energy by combining it with coenzyme A. Energy is saved as NADH.
2. Acetyl coenzyme A is combined with oxaloacetate from the cycle to make citrate and release coenzyme A for recycling.
3. Citrate is rearranged into isocitrate in preparation for subsequent reactions.

4. Isocitrate is oxidized to α-ketoglutarate, with the release of CO_2 and the saving of energy in the form of NADH.
5. α-Ketoglutarate is oxidized to succinate with release of CO_2; some of the energy is saved as NADH and some is stored temporarily by combining succinate with coenzyme A.
6. Succinyl coenzyme A loses its

coenzyme, and the energy released is ultimately stored as ATP.
7. Succinate is oxidized to fumarate, with the storage of energy in $FADH_2$.
8. Fumarate is rearranged to malate.
9. Malate is oxidized to oxaloacetate with the saving of energy as NADH. Oxaloacetate then is ready to participate in another turn of the cycle.

FIGURE 22–7 The Krebs or citric acid cycle. Adapted from Dickerson, R.E., and Geis, I., *Chemistry, Matter and the Universe*, Menlo Park, W.A. Benjamin, Inc., 1976, p. 565.

TABLE 22–4   ENERGY GAIN FROM THE KREBS CYCLE

Part of cycle	Energy storage products	Eventual free-energy gain in ATP units	
		For one Krebs cycle	*For one original glucose*
Priming (pyruvate to $CH_3COSCoA$)	NADH	3	6
Reaction 2	None	—	—
Reactions 3 and 4	NADH	3	6
Reactions 5 and 6	NADH + ATP	4	8
Reactions 7 and 8	$FADH_2$	2	4
Reaction 9	NADH	3	6
Total	4 NADH, 1 $FADH_2$, 1 ATP	15	30

The energy gain in the Krebs cycle is summarized in Table 22–4. Notice that the energy carriers NADH and $FADH_2$ carry off hydrogen atoms from the other reactants, thus oxidizing them. These hydrogen atoms are given up in the electron transport chain to reduce oxygen and form water; the NADH and $FADH_2$ return to their NAD^+ and FAD forms.

From Table 22–4, it is apparent that the Krebs cycle produces much more energy per molecule of glucose than glycolysis does. Furthermore, the conversion of NADH and $FADH_2$ to ATP units is quite efficient and reliable because all of the reactants are contained within a mitochondrion instead of being dispersed in the cytoplasm as is the case for glycolysis.

As a *very* rough calculation: if we assume that each mole of ATP can store (at 37°C, the temperature of the body) about 8 kcal of free energy, we will obtain about 48 kcal from glycolysis and 240 kcal from the Krebs cycle (after processing all carrier molecules through the electron transport chain), for a total of about 288 kcal for each mole of glucose entering glycolysis. Since there are 686 kcal of free energy available, that gives an overall efficiency of around 40%, making the cell an efficient machine for doing work. The remaining 60% of the glucose free energy is lost as heat, as described in Section 21.2, and provides most of the basal metabolism rate.

SELF-CHECK

22.11)   Describe the priming or preparatory reaction in the Krebs cycle.
22.12)   Most of the ATP molecules produced as a result of the Krebs cycle do not appear directly, but only after some coenzymes have undergone additional reactions. Explain.
22.13)   Why are two CO_2 molecules lost from the Krebs cycle? Where were those two carbon atoms originally?
22.14)   Would you consider oxaloacetate an important compound in the citric acid cycle? Explain.

22.4   ENERGY PRODUCTION FROM THE ELECTRON TRANSPORT SYSTEM

LEARNING GOAL 22L: *Explain how hydrogen atoms flow into the electron transport system.*

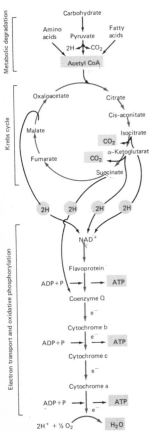

FIGURE 22-8 A general diagram of aerobic respiration, showing the hydrogens carried from the Krebs cycle into the electron transport chain and indicating the coupling reactions that produce new ATP molecules through oxidative phosphorylation.

22M: *Describe the role of the central iron cation in cytochrome c.*

22N: *Describe the role of coenzyme Q.*

The energy flow inside the cell begins with glycolysis or the Embden-Meyerhof pathway, goes through the Krebs cycle, and ends when the **electron transport process** is completed. Electron transport involves oxidation-reduction processes (Chapter 8). Much oxidation has taken place by the time the energy-transfer molecules, NADH and $FADH_2$, reach the electron transport system. One function of the system is then to oxidize these molecules *back* to NAD^+ and FAD, using the electrons gained and the hydrogen atoms released to combine with oxygen and form water. Figure 22-8 emphasizes the transfer of hydrogen atoms by NADH and $FADH_2$. These hydrogen atoms removed during glycolysis and the Krebs cycle pass into a series of colored proteins located on the folds of the *cristae*, the membranes of the mitochondria.

The first protein is *flavoprotein,* which is yellow and contains the vitamin riboflavin. It removes the hydrogen atoms from NADH and $FADH_2$, oxidizing these two carriers back to NAD^+ and FAD. In addition, it splits each hydrogen atom up into a hydrated H^+ ion and a high-energy electron.

The electrons then pass in sequence along the remaining four proteins, the **cytochromes,** which are red. The oxidized form of a cytochrome contains iron in its 3+ state, and the reduced form contains the Fe^{2+} cation, as shown in Figure 22-9.

At three steps in the electron transport chain, sufficient energy is available for the synthesis of ATP in a process called **oxidative phosphorylation.** Finally the electrons combine with oxygen molecules to produce the O^{2-} anions needed to combine with H^+ cations to form water.

Coenzyme Q

The flow of electrons along the transport chain involves a special transfer molecule, coenzyme Q, between the flavoprotein and the first cytochrome. Coenzyme Q has an oxidized *quinone* form and a reduced *hydroquinone* form:

$$H_3CO \quad \overset{O}{\underset{O}{\overset{\|}{C}}} \quad CH_3 \longrightarrow H_3CO \quad \overset{OH}{\underset{OH}{C}} \quad CH_3$$

coenzyme Q (quinone form)   coenzyme Q (hydroquinone form)

The multistep process in the electron transport chain is necessary because the energy stored in the carrier is greater than what can be received by ATP in one step. The sequence of operations is shown in Figure 22-8.

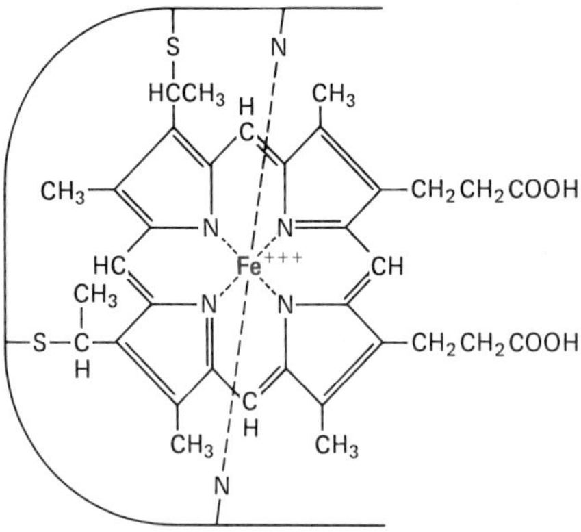

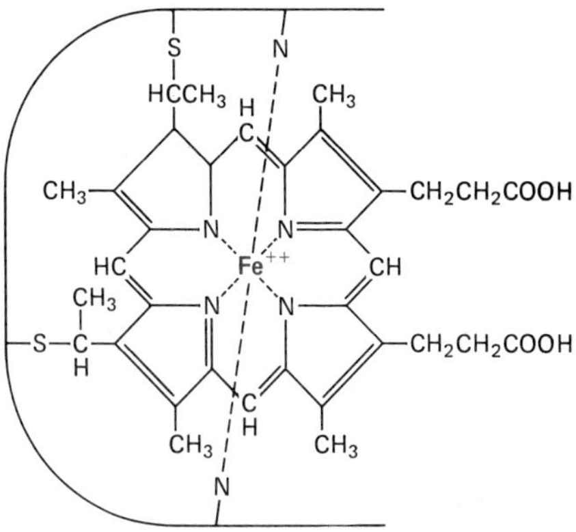

FIGURE 22–9 The oxidized (Fe^{3+}) and reduced (Fe^{2+}) forms of cytochrome c in the electron transport chain. The structure shown, called *heme,* is also found in the hemoglobin molecule (Section 24.2).

Summary of energy-producing reactions

The overall equation for the oxidation of glucose, given all the intermediate stages and enzyme-catalyzed reactions, becomes

$$C_6H_{12}O_6 + 6\ H_2O + 6\ O_2 \longrightarrow 6\ CO_2 + 12\ H_2O + energy$$

The oxygen for the CO_2 does not come from O_2 in the air, as is the case if one burns sugar, but from the oxygen in water. This turns out to be exactly the reverse of the reaction used by plants in photosynthesis.

Other energy-producing substances

In Chapter 1 we mentioned that the body can use many different kinds of foods for energy sources, including proteins, fats, and various kinds of carbohydrates. Our emphasis on the oxidation of glucose is not meant to imply that the body always uses glucose for energy. Other hexoses may enter the glycolysis pathway at various points, helped out by specific enzymes. Fats are broken down into acetate units and enter the Krebs cycle in the same manner as pyruvate. Amino acids from proteins are generally broken down (if needed as energy sources) into molecules that are intermediates in glycolysis or the Krebs cycle. Thus, all types of foods may be used for energy by the same path of cell respiration, as shown at the top of Figure 22–8.

There are many alternative pathways for specific situations, which are of interest to the biochemist but will not be treated here. Chapters 25 through 27 will return to these and other pathways with less emphasis on their value as a source of energy for the body and more emphasis on their role as a source of raw materials for the cell.

SELF-CHECK

22.15) How are hydrogen atoms obtained from NADH?
22.16) Describe that part of the structure of the cytochrome c molecule that permits it to transport electrons.

22.17)   Iron can relatively easily change from its 3+ "ferric" state to its 2+ "ferrous" state. How does this affect the body?

22.18)   Coenzyme Q, like all other coenzymes discussed in this chapter, has a very specific role in energy production. What is this role?

22.19*)   Why are only *two* molecules of ATP produced when $FADH_2$ is oxidized? (See Figure 22–8.)

22.20*)   What is the most important factor that permits the Krebs cycle and electron transport process to conserve energy far more efficiently than glycolysis?

CHAPTER TWENTY-TWO IN REVIEW ■ Biochemical Energy

GLOSSARY FOR CHAPTER TWENTY-TWO

acetyl coenzyme A An intermediate formed by coenzyme A and the pyruvate produced during glycolysis; this intermediate is necessary if pyruvate is to enter the Krebs cycle; involved also in fatty acid oxidation and synthesis. (p. 610)

ADP Adenosine diphosphate, a high-energy molecule that is converted to ATP by oxidative phosphorylation. (p. 598)

ATP Adenosine triphosphate, a high-energy molecule that supplies the energy for biological reactions; formed from ADP. (p. 598)

coenzyme A substance that attaches to an enzyme protein and is essential for its work; usually an organic molecule related to a vitamin; examples are NAD^+, FAD, coenzyme A, and coenzyme Q. (p. 604)

cytochrome A protein molecule containing an iron cation; the cation permits the cytochrome to gain and lose electrons in the electron transport chain. (p. 614)

electron transport process A series of reactions that takes electrons from an energy carrier (NADH, $FADH_2$) and carries them to oxygen (to make water) with the formation of ATP. (p. 614)

glycolysis The anaerobic process by which glucose is converted to pyruvate and CO_2, with the production of small amounts of energy in the form of ATP; occurs in the cytoplasm; the Embden-Meyerhof pathway. (p. 603)

high-energy compound A compound containing one or more removable phosphate groups, which on hydrolysis will yield a large amount of free energy. (p. 599)

Krebs cycle The most important process of *cell respiration*, by which energy is provided in the form of ATP molecules for use in the cell; the citric acid cycle; the tricarboxylic acid cycle. (p. 610)

oxidative phosphorylation The formation of ATP by means of the electron transport system. (p. 614)

respiration, cell The combined action of glycolysis, the Krebs Cycle, and the electron transport chain to produce energy for the cell while combining nutrient carbon atoms with O_2 molecules to produce CO_2. (p. 607)

QUESTIONS AND PROBLEMS FOR CHAPTER TWENTY-TWO ■

SECTION 22.1 HIGH-ENERGY COMPOUNDS

Biochemical Energy

22.21) Draw a structure that illustrates an anhydride linkage, splitting out water between two phosphoric acid molecules.

22.22) How does a high-energy compound differ from a low-energy compound?

22.23) Give an example of a coupled reaction.

22.24) If the $\Delta G = +8.9$ kcal/mole for a cell reaction, would coupling with the ATP/ADP system make the reaction go? Explain.

22.38) How many high-energy phosphorus-oxygen bonds are present in ATP? in AMP?

22.39) Write a chemical equation that illustrates the release of free energy from ADP.

22.40) The formation of glucose-6-PO_4 from glucose and phosphate has a free energy change of $\Delta G = +3.3$ kcal/mole. Would coupling with the ATP/ADP system make the reaction go? Explain.

22.41) Why are ATP and ADP ideally suited for coupled reactions in a cell?

22.25) What is the function of the ADP/ATP system in a cell?

22.42) Why is the direction of phosphate group transfer important in a coupled reaction? (Use Table 22–1.)

SECTION 22.2 ENERGY PRODUCTION WITHOUT OXYGEN: GLYCOLYSIS

22.26) What are the two priming reactions in glycolysis?

22.43) How many molecules of ATP are used in the glycolysis priming reactions? Explain why they are needed.

22.27*) How many molecules of ATP are produced as 1,3-di-PO_4 glycerate is converted to pyruvate?

22.44*) If we start with glyceraldehyde-3-PO_4 instead of 1,3-di-PO_4 glycerate, six additional molecules of ATP are produced. Explain.

22.28) How is NAD^+ related to ADP?

22.45*) Describe the change in FAD as it is reduced to $FADH_2$.

22.29*) Why is glycolysis important in cell respiration?

22.46*) How does NAD^+ relate glycolysis to the last stage of cell respiration?

SECTION 22.3 ENERGY PRODUCTION FROM THE KREBS CYCLE

(Use Figure 22–7 as needed.)

22.30) Why is the formation of acetyl coenzyme A called the priming reaction in the Krebs cycle?

22.47) How is the structure of coenzyme A related to ADP? Explain.

22.31) In what part of the Krebs cycle are ATP molecules directly produced? Explain.

22.48) Reactions 5 and 6 of the Krebs cycle produce more energy than any other part. Explain.

22.32) What compound is formed when the first molecule of CO_2 is lost in reaction 4 of the Krebs cycle?

22.49) What is formed when the second molecule of CO_2 is lost in reaction 5 of the Krebs cycle?

22.33) What chemical reaction connects glycolysis and the Krebs cycle?

22.50) Compare the ATP production in glycolysis and in the Krebs cycle.

SECTION 22.4 ENERGY PRODUCTION FROM THE ELECTRON TRANSPORT SYSTEM (Use Figure 22–8 as needed.)

22.34) What happens to the hydrogen atoms removed during glycolysis and the Krebs cycle?

22.51) Which coenzymes bring hydrogen atoms to the electron transport system?

22.35) How many ATP molecules are produced as electrons flow from cytochrome b to c to a and form water?

22.52) What part of the cytochrome molecule is involved in the oxidation-reduction reactions in the electron transport system?

22.36) How does the reduction of coenzyme Q differ from that of the cytochromes?

22.53) Coenzyme Q is sometimes called the "transfer molecule" in the electron transport system. Explain.

22.37) Each molecule of NADH produces more energy than a molecule of $FADH_2$ in the electron transport system. Explain.

22.54) How many NADH molecules feed into the electron transport system for each turn of the Krebs cycle?

22.55*) In the Embden-Meyerhof pathway, explain the need for the ATP/ADP system in order to convert fructose-6-PO_4 to fructose-1,6-di-PO_4.

Enzymes and Vitamins

23

Enzymes are so important in biological processes that we could not avoid discussing them in each chapter pertaining to human physiology. This would be a good occasion for you to review the structure of proteins (Section 19.3), since enzyme activity depends very much on three-dimensional structure. We mentioned in Section 17.2 that, in many cases, an enzyme will only act on one optical isomer, generally the D form of a carbohydrate or the L form of an amino acid. This emphasizes the importance of geometry in enzyme action. The membranes that form the wall of a cell (Section 18.3) and, more significant, the membranes that surround the internal parts of a cell (Section 20.1) provide solid support for enzymes so that they can assume the proper geometry.

In Chapter 21 we discussed the relationship between heat energy (ΔH) and reaction rate. In Section 21.4 you learned to draw an enthalpy-reaction graph for an exothermic or endothermic reaction and to recognize the *activation energy*. Section 21.5 gave you an introduction to the role and function of an enzyme, a catalyst that lowers the activation energy of a reaction so it may occur at a faster rate. In this chapter, we will pursue in more detail the manner in which an enzyme does its job. We will also look at the effects of pH, temperature, and the concentrations of various substances on the rate of a biological reaction.

Chapter 22 gave you a brief introduction to the role of a coenzyme. Four of the important molecules involved in energy transfer are coenzymes: NAD^+, FAD, coenzyme A, and coenzyme Q. Several of these are derived from vitamins. The link between vitamins and the coenzymes they form will be discussed later in this chapter.

Since enzymes are necessary for *all* body reactions to work at speeds that are useful, they are obviously involved in all the reactions discussed in Chapter 22 (glycolysis, the Krebs cycle, and the electron transport chain) as well as in all processes to be discussed in Chapters 25 to 27 on metabolism.

23.1 ENZYMES IN THE BODY

LEARNING GOAL 23A: *Explain why a specific enzyme is needed for every kind of physiological reaction.*

23B: *Describe the geometry changes that occur as a substrate molecule is converted to a product.*

23C: *Describe the use of the Michaelis constant, K_m.*

619

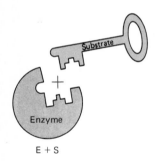

E + S

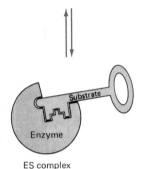

ES complex

The lock-and-key model of the fit between an enzyme and a substrate.

Living cells can function as effective chemical "machines" because they contain enzymes. As discussed in Section 21.5, enzymes are biological catalysts whose role is to greatly increase the rate of cellular reactions.

Many of the cellular reactions that can be carried out in the laboratory can be speeded up by inorganic catalysts, such as platinum. Enzymes are far more effective than inorganic catalysts because

1) each enzyme is *specific* to a particular reaction and is thus designed to most efficiently convert reactants (substrate) to products.
2) each enzyme functions particularly well in the temperature range (around 37°C) and low H^+ concentration (neutral pH) found in the living cell.

In Figure 21–13 you saw one way of illustrating the "lock-and-key" relationship between an enzyme and its substrate. The **active site** of the enzyme exactly fits the three-dimensional geometric structure of the substrate, including its right-handed or left-handed (D or L) isomeric form.

Structure of an enzyme

All known enzymes are protein molecules and include the same amino acids found in all proteins. Their characteristic shapes and properties are determined by the sequence of amino acids in the polypeptide chain as fixed by the genetic code (Section 20.5). Their reactive groups (active sites) are thus found in definite positions. The relationships in three-dimensional space between the active sites control their catalytic effect in a manner not seen in an inorganic catalyst. The proper amino acid sequence is thus essential to enzyme action. Any treatment that denatures the protein (Section 19.4) destroys the enzyme.

Naming of enzymes

In the early days of biochemistry, enzymes were named from the substance in which they were discovered (such as the amylase *ptyalin,* found in saliva, from the Greek *ptyalon,* "spittle") or from the method by which they were separated. As the number of known enzymes grew, the names were given in a more orderly fashion by adding the ending -*ase* to the root of the name of the substrate (sucrase = "sucr-" + "-ase" catalyzes the hydrolysis of sucrose; urease = "ure-" + "-ase" catalyzes the splitting of urea) or to the general type of reaction (a lipase = "lip-" + "-ase" catalyzes the hydrolysis of a lipid), as shown in Table 21.7 (p. 588).

As the list of enzymes increased to over 1000, an international commission suggested retaining earlier names, but in addition devised a complex code number that would identify each known enzyme plus any discovered in the future. It also divided all of the enzymes into six main classes according to the kind of reaction catalyzed:

Oxidoreductases are sometimes called oxidases.

1) *Oxidoreductases* are involved in oxidation-reduction (electron transfer or H atom transfer) reactions, such as those of Chapter 22 that produce and oxidize NADH. *Alcohol dehydrogenase* speeds up the conversion of ethanol to acetaldehyde (Chapter 8, p. 233), which causes the uncomfortable effects of a "hangover."
2) *Transferases* are needed to transfer a chemical group from one substrate to another. For example, a *kinase* is needed for each phosphate group

transfer discussed in Section 22.1. *Transaminases* (Chapter 27) are involved in transferring amino groups from one amino acid to produce another needed by the body.

3) *Hydrolases* speed up the very important hydrolysis reactions that happen in digestion and in various stages of metabolism. The types of hydrolases are obvious from their names: *lipase, carbohydrase, protease.*

4) *Isomerases* help change one isomer of a substance to another, such as in the second reaction of glycolysis (Figure 22–5), which changes glucose-6-phosphate to fructose-6-phosphate.

5) *Lyases* catalyze the addition of a group (such as water) to a double bond.

6) *Ligases* are involved in the formation of new bonds to a carbon atom.

Action of an enzyme

Recall from Chapter 21 that *activation energy* must be given to reactants before they can go "over the hill" to products. This is true not only for endothermic reactions, those that absorb energy, but also for highly exothermic reactions, which give off heat. (This is fortunate because otherwise paper would burn *without* our touching a match to it!)

The activation energy of a reaction (unlike the heat of reaction, ΔH) depends very much on the *way* the reaction is carried out. The role of a catalyst is to lower the activation energy. The rate of a reaction depends on the number of molecular collisions with sufficient energy to get over the activation "barrier." The lower the barrier, the easier it is to jump over it.

Figure 23–1 shows the enthalpy-reaction graph for the decomposition of hydrogen peroxide to water and oxygen:

$$H_2O_{2(\ell)} \longrightarrow H_2O_{(\ell)} + \tfrac{1}{2}O_{2(g)}$$

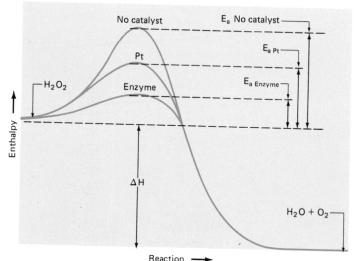

FIGURE 23–1   The activation energy of the decomposition of hydrogen peroxide is highest with no catalyst. A platinum catalyst lowers E_a somewhat and thus speeds up the reaction. With an enzyme, the reaction path is even more favorable and only a small amount of activation energy is needed, so the rate is very high.

The activation energy, E_a, without a catalyst is 18.0 kcal/mole. This is high enough to keep drugstore H_2O_2, bottled as a 3% solution, from exploding. On platinum metal, the value of E_a drops to 12.0 kcal/mole. The rate of the reaction will increase greatly if platinum is present, and in fact will go about 17 000 times as fast at 37°C. The enzyme *catalase* reduces the activation energy to only 3.0 kcal/mole, a value so low that the rate increases again by a factor of two million. The difference between this reaction happening in a drugstore bottle and in the body is (in molecules reacting per second) about 30 billion (3×10^{10}) under identical conditions. Although most biological reactions are somewhat more complicated than the decomposition of H_2O_2, the principle is the same. An enzyme lowers the activation energy of a reaction to the point where the reaction can be carried out efficiently under the conditions of the living cell.

Geometric factors

For many chemical reactions, the activation energy is needed to stretch or twist certain bonds so they will break and allow new bonds to form. One of the ways an enzyme works is to position the substrate in three-dimensional space in such a way that the bond is stretched or distorted. Thus, a pathway is created that does not require extra heat energy. This is one reason the lock-and-key relationship between the active site on the enzyme and the substrate geometry is essential to the enzyme action, as shown in Figure 23–2.

However, this exact fit between enzyme and substrate, which we call a *complementary* relationship, also makes the enzyme very *specific* in its action. It only recognizes one particular type of substrate. The protein structure of the enzyme is folded in such a way as to "fit" in only one manner.

Our senses of smell and taste rely on a similar "fit" of molecules inside the sensing membranes of the nose and tongue. Molecules with similar shape or charge may then smell or taste the same.

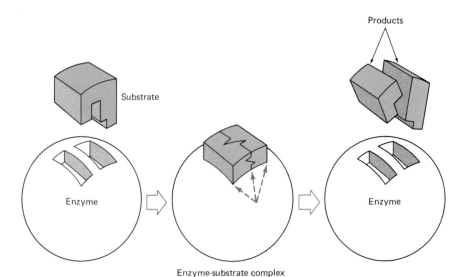

FIGURE 23–2 The exact fit or *complementarity* of geometric shape between the substrate and the active site on an enzyme is essential to enzyme action. Forces within the enzyme molecule, shown by the thin, dashed-line arrows, put a strain on the chemical bonds in the substrate, causing them to break. Other bonds are then formed. The energy source for this process is ATP, as shown in Figure 22–2.

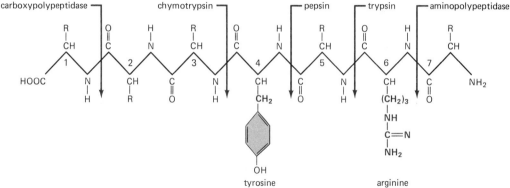

FIGURE 23–3 An enzyme is specific to a particular kind of reaction. The numbers on the polypeptide chain of this protein indicate amino acid residues, only two of which are shown in full. The enzyme *carboxypolypeptidase* hydrolyzes the residue at the —COOH end only; at the —NH₂ end of the chain, *aminopolypeptidase* does its work. *Pepsin* is specific to the amino side of a tyrosine or phenylalanine residue inside the chain; *chymotrypsin* works only on the carboxyl side of such residues, and *trypsin* hydrolyzes only the carboxyl side of arginine or lysine. The selectivity of enzymes helps researchers determine the sequence of amino acid residues in a protein.

Some enzymes are so specific that they fit only one or two very closely related molecules. Others may speed up the reactions of a whole class of substrates that all have a particular functional group, such as a peptide linkage or a double bond (Figure 23–3).

When the reactive groups (the active site) on the enzyme attract the substrate and (temporarily) bond with it, the shape of the enzyme molecule changes, as does the shape of the substrate. The bonds of the substrate are strained into a position that allows them to break more easily; thus, the new shape is more reactive. We call this special shape of the enzyme-substrate combination the **active intermediate complex;** "active" because it can lead to reaction, "intermediate" because it is a short-lived chemical substance, and "complex" because it is a combination molecule of enzyme + substrate.

The active intermediate may shift back to the original enzyme-substrate complex (and generally release the substrate, in which case no reaction occurs) or it may be converted to products of the reaction plus the original enzyme molecule:

$$\text{E} \; + \; \text{S} \; \rightleftharpoons \; \text{E·S} \; \rightleftharpoons \; \text{E·S†} \; \rightleftharpoons \; \text{E} \; + \; \text{P}$$

enzyme   substrate   E S   active   enzyme   products
complex   intermediate
complex

The three processes shown are all *reversible*. There is always an equilibrium between the left and right sides. On the other hand, the products of the reaction may be quickly removed to enter another process, in which case the enzyme released at the right can quickly take in another substrate molecule. In one minute, a single enzyme molecule may carry out as many as several million such cycles.

Once the ES complex is formed, the actual job of breaking and forming bonds can be helped by such "standard" catalysts as acid or strong base.

As an example of a catalytic process, let us consider the splitting up of a protein by hydrolysis. In Figure 23–4, we have an aspartic acid (Asp) residue with a partial negative charge, a histidine (His) residue with a partial

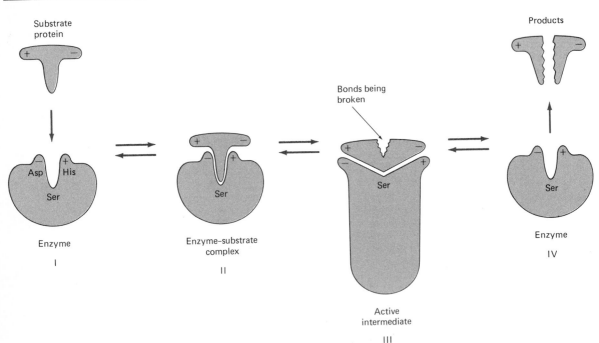

FIGURE 23–4 The action of a hydrolase in breaking apart a protein. The charges on the polypeptide chain being opposite those on the enzyme, the substrate is drawn into the active site. Some enzymes use arginine instead of histidine as a positively charged site. The active intermediate uses a changed enzyme shape to stretch bonds and a conventional catalyst (here serine) to help break them. The forces that break the bonds are all short-distance effects, so the fit must be exact. If the protein substrate is too large or too small, it will not fit into the enzyme and no reaction will occur.

positive charge, and a serine (Ser) group at the active site. A protein substrate with a positively charged residue fits with aspartic acid, and one with a negatively charged residue fits with histidine. These residues will be attracted by the charges on the enzyme and drawn into the active site. The serine group then acts as a conventional catalyst to form the products. An uncharged protein, or one with the wrong distribution of charges, will most likely bounce off the enzyme without forming a complex.

It is apparent why an enzyme works more efficiently than an inorganic catalyst. The active groups of the enzyme can be "stuck" right next to the reactive part of the substrate to be of maximum help in breaking bonds.

Effect of substrate concentration

The rate of an ordinary inorganic chemical reaction depends on the concentration of reactants. Since a chemical reaction happens because of collisions between reactant molecules, if one of the reactants isn't there at all, the rate must be zero!

The exact relationship of reaction rate to concentration depends on the way the reaction happens, that is, on its *mechanism* or pathway. Some mechanisms give a rate that is proportional to the concentration of each reactant. In some cases, where several steps happen in a row, the rate may depend largely on the concentration of one reactant and only slightly on the concentration of the other(s). It is of interest to the biochemist to be able to relate the rate of a biological process to the amount of raw material (substrate) present.

Consider the very simple reaction shown in Figure 23–4. Suppose we keep the amount of enzyme constant and vary the concentration of substrate, in this case a protein that is to be hydrolyzed and split. At very low substrate concentration, the number of substrate molecules that collide with the enzyme and are processed must also be very low. The rate (v) is very low. As the amount of substrate increases, the rate increases proportionately. However, as shown in Figure 23–5, as the substrate concentration increases even more, the effect of extra substrate on the rate becomes reduced and eventually a maximum rate, v_{max}, is reached.

For each constant amount of enzyme present in a cell (or in a test tube), the rate cannot increase beyond the point where the enzyme molecules are saturated with substrate. This happens if a new molecule of substrate combines with the active site of the enzyme as soon as the "old" products are released. Any extra substrate present cannot find enzyme molecules to react with.

The biochemists J. Michaelis and M. Menten first proposed the concept of an enzyme-substrate complex in 1913 and studied the rates of simple enzyme-catalyzed reactions. They found that a particular substrate concentration, K_m in Figure 23–5, which corresponds to *one half* the maximum rate ($v_{max}/2$), is characteristic of each enzyme. This concentration is called the **Michaelis constant.**

The details of the graph in Figure 23–5 are not important in this course. It is of interest, however, that the value of K_m obtained from this graph can tell us something about the functioning of an enzyme. At a substrate concentration equal to K_m, the enzyme molecules in a cell are *half* saturated with substrate. Many enzymes have K_m values very similar to the real-life concentrations of their substrates, assuring that they will be effective catalysts. At a substrate concentration of 100 times the K_m value, the enzyme will have the maximum rate of activity (v_{max}). There is leeway, so that if the cell needs more products, increasing the concentration of substrate will to some extent make up the need.

The value of K_m also indicates how tightly the enzyme holds its substrate. A high value of K_m indicates that the enzyme can gain and lose a substrate molecule easily, while a low value of K_m indicates that the substrate tends to stick in the active site.

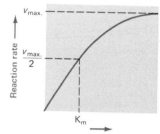

FIGURE 23–5   The Michaelis constant, shown on a graph of reaction rate vs. substrate concentration.

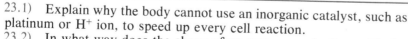

SELF-CHECK

23.1)   Explain why the body cannot use an inorganic catalyst, such as platinum or H^+ ion, to speed up every cell reaction.

23.2)   In what way does the shape of an enzyme make it specific for only one type of substrate?

23.3)   Would an enzyme that can process millions of substrate molecules each minute have a *high* or *low* value of K_m? Explain.

23.2 FACTORS AFFECTING ENZYME ACTIVITY

LEARNING GOAL 23D: Describe the effect on the rate of an enzyme-catalyzed reaction of enzyme concentration, pH, temperature, and concentration of end products.

> *23E: Describe a situation in which an enzyme inhibitor is helpful to the body and one in which it is harmful.*

Variation in enzyme activity is important in two ways. First of all, the body must have a way of regulating its production of biochemicals. Otherwise, it might have a surplus of "raw materials" for one key reaction and too little substrate for another. This is particularly important when we consider a series of *consecutive* reactions that must follow each other in turn. The regulation and control of metabolic processes is thus as important for life as the existence of those processes.

In the healthy body, enzyme activity is turned "up" and "down" as needed. There are ways in which enzyme activity can be increased or decreased by external agents. A second important aspect we will consider in this section is unhealthy or *pathological* changes in enzyme activity caused by disease and some poisons.

Concentration of enzyme

It is obvious that the amount of enzyme present can have an effect on the rate of an enzyme-catalyzed reaction. If there is no enzyme present, the reaction will happen very slowly indeed!

Figure 23–6 shows that at a substrate concentration of 100 K_m, the rate of a reaction is proportional to the concentration of enzyme. Such a situation is commonly used as a test in clinical laboratories to measure the amount of a certain enzyme present in the body. For such a test to be valid, however, both the pH and temperature of the solution must be strictly controlled.

Effect of pH

As shown in Figure 23–4, the partial charges on portions of the enzyme protein molecule are important in binding the substrate to the active site. As

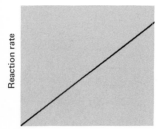

FIGURE 23–6 If an excess of substrate is present, then reaction rate depends on the amount of enzyme.

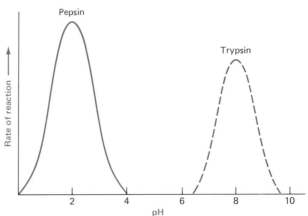

FIGURE 23–7 Enzyme activity depends on pH. The optimum pH for pepsin activity under laboratory conditions is about 2; in the body, pepsin operates best in an acidic environment, such as in the stomach, and stops working entirely in the basic solutions of the small intestines. Trypsin, on the other hand, works best in a basic (high pH) solution.

you know from Section 19.1, amino acids (and amino acid residues in proteins) have both acidic and basic character, and their particular charges depend on pH. In Figure 23–7 you can see that the maximum rate of an enzyme-controlled reaction occurs in a very narrow pH range. The middle of this range is called the **optimum pH** and generally corresponds to the normal acidity (generally pH = 7.4) of the body fluid in which a particular enzyme operates. There is a considerable decrease in reaction rate if the solution becomes too acidic (lower pH) or too basic (higher pH). As shown in Figure 23–7, the activity of pepsin, a protein-splitting hydrolase found in stomach fluids, is greatest at pH = 1.5 to 2.0. Trypsin works well in the intestines, since its optimum pH is 8.2.

Effect of temperature

An increased temperature leads to more molecules having enough energy to get over the activation energy barrier. This is true regardless of the pathway used in the reaction. We thus expect that, *so long as the enzyme is effective*, the rate of an enzyme-controlled reaction will increase with increasing temperature. It may be doubled for each ten-Celsius-degree rise (depending on the value of the activation energy) until the temperature rise itself changes enzyme performance.

There are many biological applications of this very strong effect of temperature. For example, when the body temperature is lowered, all reactions happen at a lower rate. The cells thus have less need for oxygen than they do at 37°C, normal body temperature. A person who is drowning in very cold water thus can survive longer than someone who sinks in warm water. There are cases of people who have been revived after being underwater for almost a half hour because the water was very cold. A similar technique is often used in dangerous surgical operations to reduce the risk of brain damage caused by lack of oxygen. The patient is immersed in cold water or ice to lower the body temperature during the operation.

On the other hand, a *fever* speeds up all body reactions. It also helps

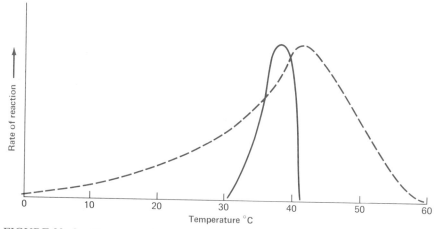

FIGURE 23–8   Enzyme activity depends on temperature. Two enzymes with somewhat different temperature dependence are shown, but each has maximum activity near the temperatures of the human body (36 to 38°C). Neither will function at freezing temperatures or under very hot conditions.

destroy bacteria by speeding up their reactions. A fever of 43°C (110°F) is generally fatal because the speeded-up reactions go out of control.

Enzymes are proteins, and proteins are affected by extreme cold (especially freezing) and heat. We should thus not be surprised to find enzymes functioning only within a narrow temperature range, about 10°C to 50°C, often with an **optimum temperature** of about 37°C, normal body temperature (Figure 23–8).

Effect of product concentration

The concentration of the end products of an enzyme-catalyzed reaction often affects the rate of reaction. Notice that all of the reactions in Figure 23–4 are reversible. As the concentration of end products builds up, the rate at which products go to active intermediate complex will also go up, leading to some formation again of the original reactants.

A catalyst works *both ways*. If it lowers the activation energy of the forward reaction, it also lowers the activation energy of the reverse reaction (Figure 23–1, read from right to left) by the same amount. It thus necessarily speeds up both the forward and reverse reactions. This causes no difficulty if the products are rapidly removed from the system.

Reduction of the overall rate of the (forward) reaction because products are undergoing the reverse process is sometimes called *inhibition* of enzyme activity, although what is actually happening is that the enzyme is working perfectly well, but in the wrong direction! This condition is also called *negative feedback,* especially in a situation in which there is a series of reactions and the products can enter the first step to inhibit further processing of substrate.

If the reactions shown in Figure 23–4 happen in a test tube, an equilibrium will eventually be set up. A biochemist may use this fact to measure the concentration of enzyme present. For example, the enzyme *lipase* catalyzes the hydrolysis of fat molecules to fatty acids and glycerol. The concentration of fatty acids formed from a given amount of fat is proportional to the concentration of lipase present in the solution at equilibrium.

Effect of chemical inhibitors

The effectiveness of an enzyme may be lowered (inhibited) by a variety of chemical substances that may enter the cell. Anything that will precipitate protein, such as a strong acid or base, will naturally destroy the enzyme.

Certain metal cations that occupy important spots on the active sites of some enzymes, such as Mg^{2+} or Cu^{2+}, may be bound up by negative ions such as F^- or CN^-. You may have heard that a cyanide salt is very poisonous. The CN^- ion is found in the seeds of cherries, plums, peaches, apples, and apricots. These fruit seeds contain amygdalin, a substance that hydrolyzes to HCN. There are a few recorded cases of poisoning from eating large numbers of apple seeds!

Cyanide can kill within a few minutes, and the lethal dose of CN^- ions is only a few milligrams. This ion can bind (tie up) Fe ions wherever they are in the body. The main poisoning effect of cyanide is to react with the iron atom in cytochrome *c* (Figure 22–9), an important link in the electron transport system. The Fe cations that are locked up in cyanide complexes cannot provide electrons for the reduction of O_2 and production of ATP. Cell respiration thus stops, causing death in minutes.

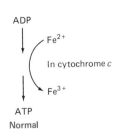

ADP

Fe^{2+}

In cytochrome *c*

Fe^{3+}

ATP
Normal

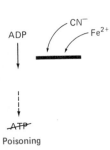

ADP

CN$^-$ Fe^{2+}

ATP
Poisoning

The effect of cyanide poisoning is to block the enzymes of the electron transport chain.

What is the connection between cytochrome c (Section 22.4) and enzymes? In fact, cytochrome c is actually an enzyme, since it shifts back and forth between its oxidized and reduced forms, speeding up electron transport in the process. It is sometimes called a cytochrome oxidase for that reason. Cyanide poisoning is thus one example of active site inhibition.

Certain functional groups of an enzyme protein that are required for activity, such as —SH (sulfhydryl) groups, may be removed or locked up by certain poisons such as *p*-chloromercuribenzoate, a mercury organic compound. Lead ions, Pb^{2+}, reacting with the —SH groups of enzymes, are the cause of lead poisoning. The arsenate ion, AsO_3^{3-}, also ties up the —SH groups, which explains why arsenic compounds are used to poison insects, and occasionally people.

Each of the above inhibitors combines with some group at the active site of an enzyme. No amount of additional substrate can make up for the destroyed enzyme. These compounds are called **noncompetitive inhibitors,** since the amount by which the reaction rate is reduced is *not* related to the amount of substrate present.

Some compounds may actually compete with substrate molecules in getting to the active site of the enzyme and forming the enzyme-substrate complex. They imitate the substrate and are called **competitive inhibitors.**

In Section 9.3 (p. 251), we discussed the causes of a "hangover." One treatment for alcoholism is to create an artificial hangover through the use of disulfiram, a sulfur-containing substance that competes with acetaldehyde for an oxidase that is necessary for the metabolism of acetaldehyde in the Krebs cycle. The result is a buildup of acetaldehyde (Figure 23–9) and a person too sick to want a drink.

Competitive inhibition can also be illustrated by the action of an antibiotic drug, sulfanilamide. This time, inhibition is used to help the body rather

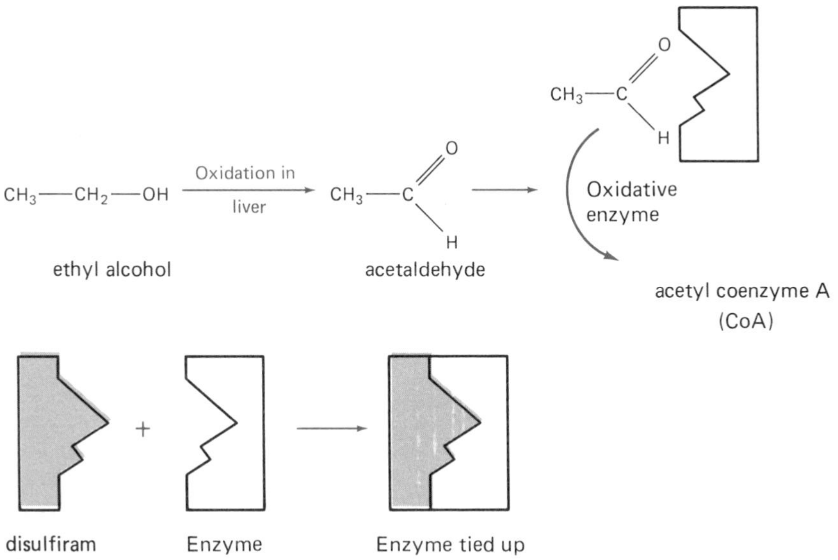

Melittin, a basic polypeptide with **26** amino acid residues, is the main toxin in honeybee venom. This substance, like similar ones in cobra venom and poisonous mushrooms, activates enzymes that then destroy the lipid bilayer of cell membranes.

FIGURE 23–9 Disulfiram can create an artificial hangover by blocking conversion of acetaldehyde to acetyl coenzyme A for processing in the Krebs cycle. Alcohol in the bloodstream then oxidizes to acetaldehyde, which builds up and causes discomfort. This effect can help a "problem drinker" abstain from alcohol, through competitive inhibition of an enzyme.

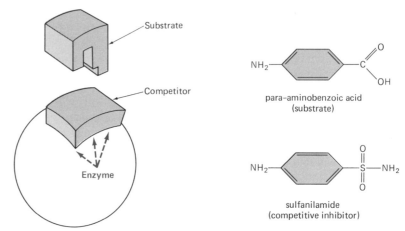

FIGURE 23–10 Competitive inhibition of bacterial enzymes by a sulfa drug. The competitor not only replaces the normal substrate (*p*-aminobenzoic acid) but also sticks in position, since it cannot itself be changed by the enzyme.

than to poison it. The substrate *p*-aminobenzoic acid, shown in Figure 23–10, is essential to the life support system in bacteria. The sulfanilamide molecule, as you can see, very much resembles that substrate and so can occupy the active site on the bacterial enzyme. This prevents the *p*-aminobenzoic acid from reacting with the enzyme, and the bacteria die.

Naturally, the binding of the competitor to the enzyme is reversible as is any reaction that follows the pattern shown in Figure 23–4. Thus, an excess of substrate, in this case extra *p*-aminobenzoic acid, will eventually displace the inhibitor.

Various other antibiotics may also inhibit enzyme action in bacteria. For example, penicillin seems to affect the construction of cell membranes in bacteria, thus destroying their enzyme activity.

All substances that inhibit enzyme action are called *antienzymes*. A parasite that must live in the intestine of an animal, such as the tapeworm, must release antienzymes that inhibit the action of proteases. Otherwise, the parasite (being made of protein) would be digested like anything else in the intestine. Substances that inhibit the action of both pepsin and trypsin have indeed been isolated from the tapeworm.

TABLE 23–1   SERUM ENZYMES USEFUL IN MEDICAL DIAGNOSIS

Symbol in Figure 24–1	Name of Enzyme	Increase Above Normal Levels May Indicate Presence of
Amylase	Amylase	Acute infection of the pancreas
Acid phosphatase	Acid phosphatase	Cancer of the prostate gland in men
Alk. phosphatase	Alkaline phosphatase	Rickets or liver disease
SGPT (ALT)	Alanine transaminase	Viral hepatitis (liver disease) or myocardial infarction
SGOT (AST)	Aspartate transaminase	Myocardial infarction
CPK (CK)	Creatine phosphokinase	Myocardial infarction
LDH	Lactate dehydrogenase	Myocardial infarction or muscle disease

(breakdown of heart muscle, thus, "heart attack")

Serum enzymes in medical diagnosis

In addition to the enzymes found in a cell under normal conditions, there are other enzymes that are released into the blood plasma by the breakdown of body tissues. Table 23–1 indicates what a marked increase in the concentration of each enzyme might indicate.

Of course, as with all clinical tests, high enzyme levels must be interpreted with caution. For example, the CPK level may be high in anyone who has just exercised or who has tensed muscles. The fact that one form of cancer can be detected by a blood test for acid phosphatase is an encouraging sign that *screening,* examination of a large number of individuals by a simple test, may be possible for other forms of this dread disease.

Low levels of the enzyme monoamine oxidase have been linked to chronic schizophrenia, the most common form of mental disorder. The disease itself may thus be due to an enzyme deficiency in the brain cells.

Other uses of enzymes

Have you ever used an ''enzyme presoak'' in a washing machine? In the late 1960's, there was a fad to use protease enzymes for laundry because they could remove food stains. The dangers of such enzymes (including skin rashes and environmental pollution effects) outweigh any possible value, and so they have disappeared from most laundry products.

If you have used papaya juice to tenderize beef steak, you've made use of enzyme action. Meat tenderizers contain *papain,* which can soften tough meat by breaking apart protein linkages. Another enzyme, pectate lyase, quickly degrades vegetable matter in household garbage. Perhaps liquified garbage will someday be used as fertilizer or as animal feed supplement.

Urokinase (prepared from urine) is used to dissolve blood clots in patients with pulmonary embolisms (blood clots blocking the action of the lungs).

However, the most important, and most controversial, use of enzymes is probably their potential in genetic engineering, the redesign of the hereditary material of the genes. *Recombinant DNA* research, now in its most primitive stages, involves certain bacterial enzymes that can make and break bonds inside the DNA molecule as discussed in Section 28.4.

Sperm from bulls is treated with an enzyme, beta-glucuronidase, before being used to artificially inseminate cows. Treated sperm fertilize eggs almost immediately, compared with an 8 to 10 hour waiting period without enzyme treatment.

SELF-CHECK

23.4) Glycine oxidase has an optimum pH of 8.8. Does it work best in an acidic or basic medium? Would it work in the stomach? in the small intestine?

23.5) The rate of a typical body reaction will increase somewhat if the temperature rises slightly but then drops if the temperature rises to, say, 50°C. Explain.

23.6) Describe the difference between a competitive and a noncompetitive inhibitor.

23.7*) What effect does lead (Pb^{2+}) cation have on body cells?

23.8*) What effect does sulfanilamide have on bacteria?

23.3 COENZYMES AND VITAMINS

LEARNING GOAL 23F: *Distinguish between a proenzyme and a coenzyme.*
        23G: *Describe the usual role of a water-soluble vitamin in the body.*
        23H: *List three water-soluble vitamins, and describe the function of each in the reactions of the cell.*

In Section 22.2, we briefly discussed some enzyme *cofactors.* Also in

Chapter 22, you saw how four important coenzymes—NAD$^+$, FAD, coenzyme A, and coenzyme Q—play roles in energy production in the cell. Two of these coenzymes come from B-complex vitamins. We shall see that other vitamins play similar roles as cofactors in enzyme action.

Proenzymes

Enzymes are rather complex protein molecules since they must have, in addition to the normal polypeptide strands of any protein, the catalytic groups that make up the active site. Therefore, it is somewhat complicated for the cell to synthesize enzymes, especially if cofactors must be added to the protein molecule.

A **proenzyme** is a large protein molecule that can react to form an enzyme but is folded over to ''hide'' the active site. In some cases, we would not wish to convert too much of the proenzyme to enzyme, for fear of digesting the membranes of the cell itself! Thus, the stomach wall secretes the protein *pepsinogen*. The ending ''-ogen'' means that it can be made into pepsin. As needed, the stomach acid converts pepsinogen to pepsin. Too much pepsin might result in a peptic ulcer. Similarly, the pancreas secretes trypsinogen, an inactive form. The enzymes in the small intestine then convert trypsinogen to trypsin, a protease. Proenzymes are sometimes called precursors, ''molecules that come before.''

Cofactors

Some enzymes consist not only of protein but also of metal cations (Mg^{2+}, Zn^{2+}, Mn^{2+}, Fe^{2+}, Fe^{3+}, Cu^{2+}). For example, the enzyme that converts ethanol to the ''hangover poison'' acetaldehyde (Figure 23–9) is alcohol dehydrogenase. Alcohol dehydrogenase consists of a protein part, called the *apoenzyme* (with no enzyme activity), plus a zinc (Zn^{2+}) cation as a *cofactor*. Only the combination of the two is effective as an enzyme. In general, a cofactor converts an enzyme protein molecule into its catalytically active form.

A *coenzyme* is an organic molecule that is necessary as part of the enzyme for catalysis to occur. You have already seen very large coenzymes like NAD$^+$, FAD, and coenzyme A in Chapter 22. In comparison, coenzyme Q (p. 614) is a relatively small organic molecule. Some enzymes require both a metal cation cofactor and an organic (but non-protein) coenzyme. A coenzyme actively participates in the enzyme reaction by accepting or donating a specific ion (like H$^+$) that is to be added to or removed from the substrate.

Vitamins

Many coenzymes are synthesized from **vitamins,** especially the water-soluble family of B vitamins. As mentioned in Chapter 1, vitamins are essential in our diet to prevent such deficiency diseases as beriberi, scurvy, and rickets. We will concentrate here on water-soluble vitamins and will discuss

TABLE 23–2   VITAMINS B AND C AS COENZYMES

Vitamin	Coenzyme Formed	Role in Enzyme Function
Thiamine	Thiamine pyrophosphate	Decarboxylation of keto acids (pyruvate)
Riboflavin	Flavin mononucleotide Flavin adenine dinucleotide (FAD)	Oxidation-reduction (Krebs cycle)
Niacin	Nicotinamide adenine dinucleotide (NAD$^+$)	Oxidation-reduction (glycolysis, Krebs cycle)
Pyridoxine	Pyridoxal phosphate Pyridoxamine phosphate	Amino group transfer
Pantothenic acid	Coenzyme A	Acetyl group transfer (Krebs cycle)
Folic acid	Tetrahydrofolic acid	One-carbon transfer
Vitamin B$_{12}$	Deoxyadenosyl cobalamin	Alkyl group transfer
Vitamin C (ascorbic acid)	(a cofactor)	Oxidation-reduction and hydroxylation reactions

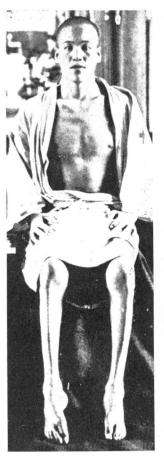

fat-soluble vitamins in Section 23.4. Table 23–2 lists the water-soluble vitamins and some coenzymes that result from them.

Thiamine

Thiamine, vitamin B$_1$, combines with two phosphate units to form the coenzyme *thiamine pyrophosphate* (*TPP*):

thiamine pyrophosphate (cocarboxylase) (TPP)

Beriberi, a result of a thiamine deficiency, can cause paralysis of the legs because of muscle atrophy. (Courtesy Herzog and *Philippine Journal of Sciences*)

The TPP coenzyme plays a part in the Krebs cycle, helping convert pyruvate to acetyl coenzyme A in the priming step. It also converts pyruvate to acetaldehyde. If, because of a thiamine deficiency, this reaction does not happen at a normal rate, pyruvate accumulates in the blood and tissues and produces the pain (*neuritis*) that is a symptom of *beriberi*. Thiamine occurs in cereal grains and as the coenzyme TPP in eggs, meat, and yeast.

Riboflavin

We have already discussed the role of FAD in the Krebs cycle. Riboflavin consists of a pentose alcohol, *ribitol,* linked to a yellow pigment called flavin. It forms FAD and a second coenzyme, FMN:

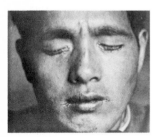

Inflammation of the eyes and cracks at the corners of the mouth are symptoms of riboflavin deficiency. (Bicknell, F., and Prescott, F., *The Vitamins in Medicine,* London, Heinemann Medical Books Ltd.)

flavin mononucleotide (FMN)

The flavoprotein shown in Figure 22–8 (the electron transport chain) involves FMN as a coenzyme. Riboflavin is found in foods as the complete coenzymes FAD and FMN. Foods such as yeast, liver, eggs, and leafy vegetables are rich in riboflavin. Cereals that are milled lose both thiamine and riboflavin, so the only way to obtain these vitamins in bread made from milled flour is to use *enriched* flour, which has these vitamins added to it.

Niacin

Niacin is a general name for either of two pyridine derivatives, nicotinic acid or nicotinamide:

pyridine   nicotinic acid   nicotinamide

Like riboflavin, niacin forms two different coenzymes. We have already seen NAD^+ in Chapter 22. The second is **NADP,** essentially NAD^+ with an extra phosphate group on the ribose ring:

nicotinamide-adenine
dinucleotide phosphate (NADP)

Niacin is found in liver and lean meat. Deficiency of niacin results in *pellagra,* with such symptoms as skin problems, sore tongue, loss of appetite, diarrhea, and nervous disorders. Pellagra was once very common in the southern United States, at a time when corn, molasses, and fatty meat made up much of the diet; all three foods are very low in niacin. One way of relieving this deficiency was to fortify flour with nicotinic acid, but people confused that vitamin with *nicotine,* the very different compound found in tobacco, and refused to eat the "tobacco bread." Once the name of the vitamin was changed to niacin, all objections disappeared.

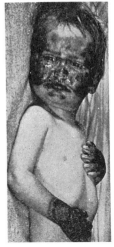

Pellagra in a child, showing the typical red rash on face and hands. (Courtesy John A. McIntosh)

Pyridoxine

Vitamin B_6 is a general name for three closely related compounds, whose phosphate derivatives are coenzymes involved in protein metabolism (Chapter 27). Deficiency leads to skin problems, irritability, and infections.

pyridoxal phosphate

pyridoxamine phosphate

Pantothenic acid

Pantothenic acid, an amide, is the vitamin that is part of the structure of coenzyme A (Figure 22–6):

$$HO-CH_2-\underset{\underset{CH_3}{|}}{\overset{\overset{CH_3}{|}}{C}}-\underset{\underset{}{\overset{OH}{|}}}{CH}-\overset{\overset{O}{\|}}{C}-\underset{\overset{H}{|}}{N}-CH_2-CH_2-COOH$$

pantothenic acid

In recent research on the effect of deficiency of this vitamin in humans, symptoms such as emotional problems, intestinal discomfort, and a burning sensation in the hands and feet have been noticed. Pantothenic acid is so widespread in nature that it was named from the Greek *pantos,* "everywhere." It functions mainly as acetyl coenzyme A, both in the Krebs cycle and in the synthesis of fats and steroids, as well as in the metabolic reactions of Chapters 25 to 27.

There is no truth to the advertising claim that pantothenic acid will restore the original color to gray hair.

Folic acid

Folic acid is a complex molecule consisting of three major parts:

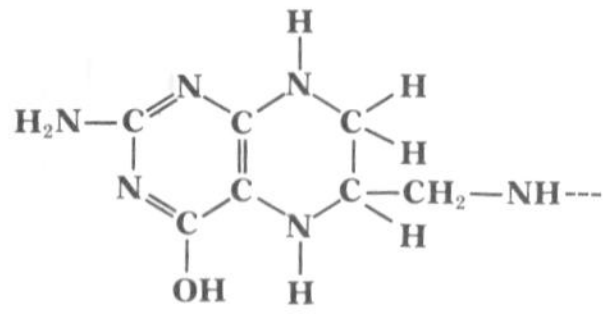

tetrahydrofolate

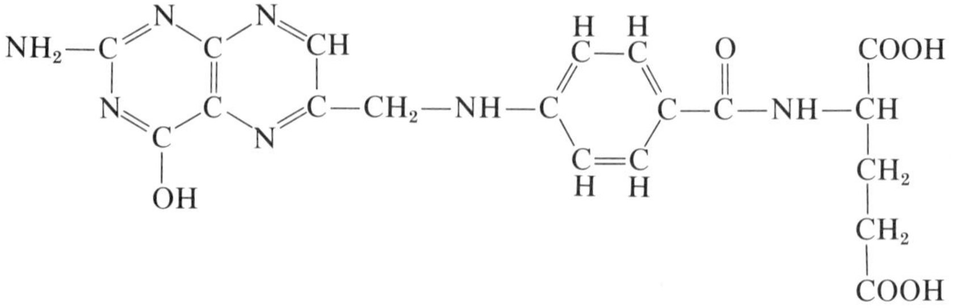

folic acid

The left-hand ring system is a yellow pigment called pteridine; it is bonded to *p*-aminobenzoic acid (Figure 23–10), which is connected by an amide linkage to glutamic acid. To function as a coenzyme, folic acid must be reduced to tetrahydrofolate.

Notice that this is the first coenzyme in our discussion that is *not* a high-energy molecule, that is, it does not have the phosphate groups described in Section 22.1.

Folic acid is found in many plants (*folic* from "*fol*iage") and animal tissues. A deficiency in this vitamin is apparently linked with red blood cell

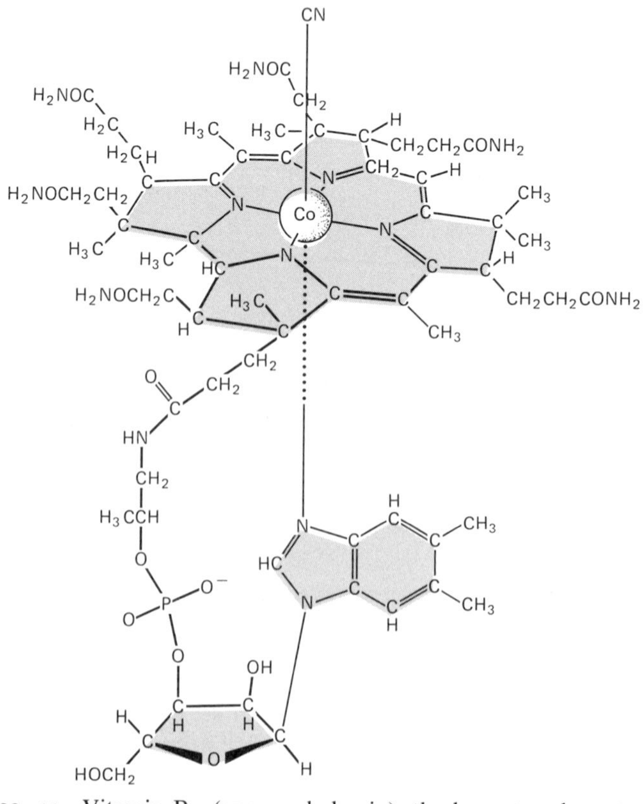

FIGURE 23–11 Vitamin B_{12} (cyanocobalamin), the largest and most complicated vitamin molecule known. It was first isolated in 1948 and finally synthesized in 1973 by a team led by Robert Woodward (Nobel Prize 1965) and Albert Eschenmoser and involving 99 scientists from 19 countries. The —CN group, normally poisonous, is held *very* tightly when it is bonded to a metal ion, such as the central cobalt cation in vitamin B_{12}.

disorders. The main function of the coenzyme is as a carrier of one-carbon ($HCOO^-$) units in the synthesis of amino acids. When acting as vitamins, folic acid and tetrahydrofolic acid are called *folacin*.

Vitamin B$_{12}$

The very complex structure of vitamin B$_{12}$, cyanocobalamin, is related both to the ADP structure and to the heme ring system with the central iron atom in cytochrome c. As can be seen in Figure 23–11, there is a cyanide (—CN) group sitting right on top of the cobalt cation. In the coenzyme form, the —CN group is replaced by the adenosine nucleoside that we saw for ADP (as well as NAD$^+$, FAD, and coenzyme A).

Vitamin B$_{12}$, like folic acid, is useful in the treatment of certain kinds of *anemia*. Pernicious anemia responds particularly well to treatment with vitamin B$_{12}$, which increases the amount of hemoglobin and the red blood cell count.

The best source of vitamin B$_{12}$ is beef liver. Liver extracts also contain a similar cobalt complex in which the —CN group is replaced by an —OH group on the cobalt atom. Coenzyme B$_{12}$ is a high-energy compound that is involved in the synthesis of nucleosides and in the conversion of dicarboxylic acids to their isomers.

Vitamin B$_{12}$

coenzyme B$_{12}$

Vitamin C

Vitamin C, ascorbic acid, is a hexose derivative that can be easily oxidized to dehydroascorbic acid:

ʟ-ascorbic acid   dehydroascorbic acid

Both compounds are biologically active. Ascorbic acid, like almost all of the vitamins we have discussed, functions as a cofactor in oxidation-reduction systems in the cell. The richest sources of this vitamin are citrus fruits, tomatoes, and green leafy vegetables. Most animals can synthesize their own vitamin C, but humans, monkeys, and guinea pigs cannot and must have it in their diet.

As early as 1720, scurvy was recognized as a disease of sailors and travelers. All British ships were required to carry limes on board, which led to the sailors' being called "limeys." Serious cases of scurvy are not common today, although mild cases with such symptoms as sore gums, mouth sores, fatigue, low resistance to infections, and joint pain are known.

A large proportion of the ascorbic acid in foods is destroyed in cooking. On the other hand, extra ascorbic acid is added to some foods to act as an

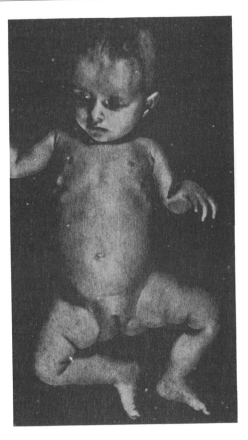

A serious case of infant scurvy. This photo shows a characteristic position with the legs flexed at hips and knees and the thighs turned back.

antioxidant, a substance that prevents the food from oxidizing and losing its normal flavor or color. The sodium and calcium salts of ascorbic acid can also be used for this purpose.

The biochemistry of vitamin C deficiency and use in the body is not well understood. Two-time Nobel Prize winner Linus Pauling has suggested that the common cold, and possibly other diseases, can be prevented or treated by large doses of ascorbic acid. Clinical trials, while not generally supporting his contention, have suggested that *some individuals* may benefit from such use of vitamin C.

SELF-CHECK

23.9) What is the difference between a proenzyme and a coenzyme?
23.10) Why are all coenzymes water soluble?
23.11*) What vitamins are associated with NAD^+, FAD, and coenzyme A?
23.12) What vitamins may be used to treat certain cases of anemia?
23.13) Why is vitamin C sometimes added to processed foods?

23.4 FAT-SOLUBLE VITAMINS

LEARNING GOAL 23I: Describe the main functions in the body of vitamin A, vitamin D, and vitamin K.

23J: Describe the similarities in structure of the four lipid-soluble vitamins.

Although scurvy and beriberi had already been recognized as vitamin-deficiency diseases for many years, it was nearly 1920 before experiments on the growth of young rats demonstrated the existence of fat-soluble vitamins. These vitamins, which include vitamins A, D, E, and K, are not coenzymes. They are fat soluble, so can only be found in body lipids like those of cell membranes. They therefore cannot combine with the enzymes that are dissolved in the cell fluid (cytoplasm).

Vitamin A

Carotene is a substance found in some yellow and orange fruits and vegetables. If a carotene molecule is split in the middle and oxidized, two vitamin A molecules may result:

β-carotene (all-*trans*)

vitamin A (all-*trans*)

Since vitamin A is soluble in lipids, you might expect its role to be very different from that of vitamins B or C. One of its most important functions is as part of the visual pigment (called *rhodopsin*) in the retina of the eye. Rhodopsin is made up of *retinal* (vitamin A aldehyde) and *opsin* (a protein). The eye is thus one of the first organs to show symptoms of vitamin A deficiency, first through night-blindness and eventually through major eye infections.

In night-blindness, the light receptors of the rod cells in the retina fail to respond normally. The nerve impulses in the retina are triggered by a shift in a double bond in the retinal of the visual pigment from a *cis* to a *trans* position (p. 204). The relation between rhodopsin, retinal, and vitamin A in the visual cycle is shown in Figure 23–12. To regenerate the rhodopsin pigment, vitamin A is used up. The blood must then supply additional vitamin A.

Another principal function of vitamin A is to maintain the health of mucous membranes and other *epithelial* tissues (such as the skin) and the ducts from external glands. The ear, nose, and throat mucous membranes are the first to suffer from a deficiency in vitamin A, which tends to result in infections. The vitamin is also essential for the production of tooth enamel and the maintenance of healthy gums and sex glands.

The active form of vitamin A in the sex glands, as in the eye, is an

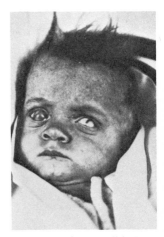

The eyes of this child show the effects of a vitamin A deficiency in a condition known as *xerophthalmia*.

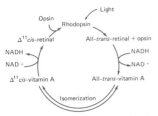

FIGURE 23–12 Vitamin A is involved in the nerve signals that accompany detection of light. When there is vitamin A deficiency, one of the first symptoms is night-blindness.

aldehyde form, produced from an alcohol by oxidation. The enzyme that catalyzes this oxidation is the same enzyme that converts ethyl alcohol to acetaldehyde (p. 629). Consumption of alcoholic beverages thus creates competition for the active sites on this enzyme between ethanol and vitamin A; a result can be reduced sperm production and sterility in male alcoholics. Female alcoholics will presumably be subject to some of the same problems found in cows fed a diet low in vitamin A: abnormal growth of the embryo, premature births, and miscarriages.

Uninformed people learning about these deficiency symptoms might be tempted to dose themselves with high levels of vitamin A, even to ward off winter colds and infections. Unfortunately, vitamin A is one of the few nutrients that is poisonous in large amounts. Even eating the liver of some wild animals, such as the polar bear, which builds up large concentrations of vitamin A, may cause poisoning over a long period.

There are many good sources of vitamin A, including fish liver oils. The body can store some vitamin A in the liver. Infants obtain a starting amount of the vitamin in the first milk (colostrum) from the mother's breast, which is 10 to 100 times richer in vitamin A than the later milk.

Vitamin D

Although there are several forms of vitamin D, the two most useful to humans are designated D_2 and D_3:

vitamin D_2 (calciferol)

vitamin D_3

Both forms may be obtained from other steroids by exposure to ultraviolet light. In fact, vitamin D_3 is the product of absorption of ultraviolet light by 7-dehydrocholesterol, which illustrates how humans may manufacture some of the vitamin D they need by exposing the skin to sunlight.

The main function of vitamin D is to help the assimilation of calcium and phosphorus in the normal formation of bones and teeth (Figure 23–13). Deficiency of this vitamin thus results in poor bone and tooth formation, a condition called *rickets*. Serious cases of rickets in childhood may result in bowed legs, abnormal rib formation, and other symptoms (Figure 23–14). Rickets does not occur in adults, although women may suffer from osteomalacia (softening of the bones) after several pregnancies.

Fish liver oils are potent sources of vitamin D for children who cannot be exposed to enough sunlight to manufacture the vitamin themselves. Milk is often fortified with vitamin D by the addition of small amounts of calciferol.*

---

* Recent studies suggest that "vitamin D" is actually a hormone, as implied in Figure 23–13, rather than a vitamin. It is activated in the liver before it can function in calcium and phosphorus metabolism in the bone and tissues. It is also related to the hormone *insulin;* a deficiency of vitamin D decreases the amount of insulin secreted by the pancreas.

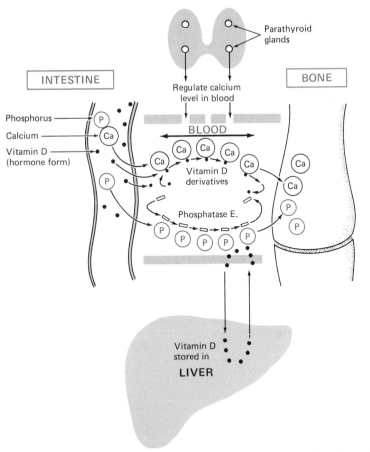

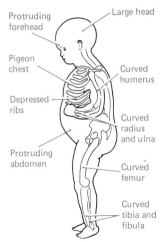

FIGURE 23–14 A diagram showing the deformities that are symptoms of a severe case of rickets. (From Harris, L.J., *Vitamins in Theory and Practice*, 4th edition, London, Cambridge University Press, 1955)

FIGURE 23–13 Vitamin D functions in the body by increasing the absorption of calcium and phosphorus from the intestine and promoting their deposition in bone. Reserves of this vitamin are stored in the liver.

Vitamin E

A group of compounds called *tocopherols* all have vitamin E activity. The most potent member of the group is alpha tocopherol:

$$H_3C-C \quad \begin{matrix} CH_3 \\ | \\ C \end{matrix} \quad \begin{matrix} O \\ \end{matrix} \quad C-(CH_2)_3-CH-(CH_2)_3-CH-(CH_2)_3-CH-CH_3$$

α-tocopherol

There is very little evidence that a lack of vitamin E has any great effect on humans. It seems to be needed for normal creatine excretion and for prevention of some blood disorders, including anemia. There is no evidence

Vitamin E reduces a form of heart damage associated with one kind of cancer treatment. *Adriamycin* is an antibiotic used to treat several types of cancer. Large amounts of vitamin E can reduce the harmful effects of the drug without reducing its anticancer effect.

that it has any effect on human sexual potency. However, many animals develop very serious symptoms when deprived of this substance.

The richest source of vitamin E is wheat germ oil. Other vegetable oils, meat, and green leafy vegetables often have considerable amounts.

The role of vitamin E in the body seems to be related almost entirely to its ability to be oxidized and thus to protect other substances from oxidation. For example, it seems to protect vitamin A and carotene from oxidation in the digestive system and thus helps the body avoid a deficiency of vitamin A. It may possibly also protect the polyunsaturated fats we consume and thus play some part in preventing heart disease. In smoggy cities, it may also prevent lung tissue from damage by oxidizing agents.

Vitamin K

A diet lacking in vitamin K will cause an increase in blood clotting time.

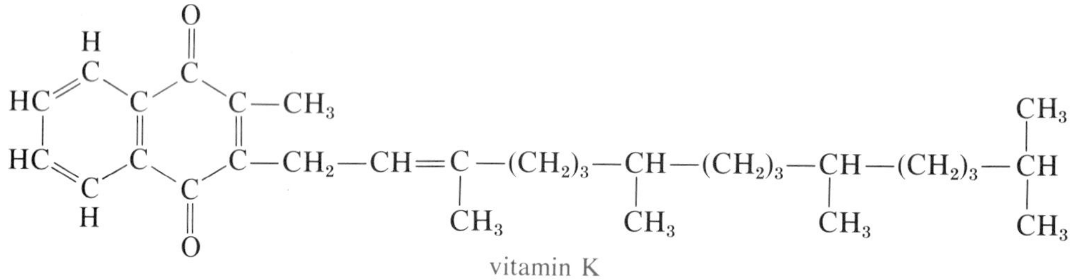

vitamin K

The vitamin is essential for the synthesis of prothrombin by the liver. The prothrombin is then involved in the clotting process. Green leafy vegetables are rich in vitamin K. Deficiencies are quite rare.

SELF-CHECK

23.14) What molecular features in vitamins A, D, E, and K make these vitamins soluble in lipids but not in water?
23.15*) Why would rickets be more of a problem in an urban ghetto in a northern climate than on a country farm located in a southern climate?
23.16) What is the main function of vitamin A in the eye?
23.17*) Will taking vitamin E increase your sexual drive?

CHAPTER TWENTY-THREE IN REVIEW ■ Enzymes and Vitamins

23.1 ENZYMES IN THE BODY **Page 619**

23A: Explain why a specific enzyme is needed for every kind of physiological reaction.

23B: Describe the geometry changes that occur as a substrate molecule is converted to a product.

23C: Describe the use of the Michaelis constant, K_m.

23.2 FACTORS AFFECTING ENZYME ACTIVITY **Page 625**

23D: Describe the effect on the rate of an enzyme-catalyzed reac-

tion of enzyme concentration, pH, temperature, and concentration of end products.

23E: Describe a situation in which an enzyme inhibitor is helpful to the body and one in which it is harmful.

23.3 COENZYMES AND VITAMINS   Page 631

23F: Distinguish between a proenzyme and a coenzyme.

23G: Describe the usual role of a water-soluble vitamin in the body.

23H: List three water-soluble vitamins, and describe the function of each in the reactions of the cell.

23.4 FAT-SOLUBLE VITAMINS   Page 638

23I: Describe the main functions in the body of vitamin A, vitamin D, and vitamin K.

23J: Describe the similarities in structure of the four lipid-soluble vitamins.

GLOSSARY FOR CHAPTER TWENTY-THREE

active intermediate complex The special shape assumed by the enzyme-substrate complex to serve as an intermediate in enzyme reactions. (p. 623)

active site The portion of an enzyme molecule to which the substrate binds. (p. 620)

inhibitor, competitive A compound that directly competes with a substrate for the active site on an enzyme surface. (p. 629)

inhibitor, noncompetitive A compound that bonds at the active site of an enzyme and cannot be displaced by additional substrate. (p. 629)

Michaelis constant The substrate concentration that will yield half the maximum rate in an enzyme reaction; designated K_m. (p. 625)

NADP Nicotinamide adenine dinucleotide phosphate, an important coenzyme in carbohydrate and lipid metabolism. (p. 634)

optimum pH The pH at which the maximum rate of an enzyme reaction occurs. (p. 627)

optimum temperature The temperature at which the maximum rate of an enzyme reaction occurs; about 37°C for most enzymes in the body. (p. 628)

proenzyme An inactive molecule synthesized by a cell; can be converted to an enzyme. (p. 632)

vitamin An organic compound essential in the diet in trace amounts to prevent deficiency diseases, such as beriberi and scurvy. (p. 632)

QUESTIONS AND PROBLEMS FOR CHAPTER TWENTY-THREE ■

Enzymes and Vitamins

SECTION 23.1 ENZYMES IN THE BODY

23.18) Describe the chemical nature of an enzyme.

23.19) Explain how an enzyme may be specific for only a single substrate.

23.20) What is meant by the active site on an enzyme?

23.33) How does an enzyme differ from an inorganic catalyst?

23.34) What happens to the shape of an enzyme and its substrate when the active intermediate complex is formed?

23.35) How do the charges on the amino acids at the active site of an enzyme help produce the changes in geometry that break bonds?

23.21) How is the Michaelis constant related to the substrate concentration in an enzyme reaction?

SECTION 23.2 FACTORS AFFECTING ENZYME ACTIVITY

23.22) Most enzymes that act inside the cell have an optimum pH of 7.2 to 7.6. Explain.

23.23) What would be the effect on reaction rate of a temperature drop from 37°C to 25°C? Refer to Figure 23–8.

23.24*) A drink containing cyanide rapidly causes death. Explain how.

23.25) Give an example of and explain the action of a competitive inhibitor.

SECTION 23.3 COENZYMES AND VITAMINS

23.26) Why are many digestive enzymes synthesized as proenzymes?

23.27) Name and describe two types of cofactors for enzyme action.

23.28) Why is niacin an important water-soluble vitamin?

23.29) Why is pantothenic acid an important water-soluble vitamin?

SECTION 23.4 FAT-SOLUBLE VITAMINS

23.30) Describe some of the important functions of vitamin A in the body.

23.31) What happens to children and adults whose diets lack vitamin D?

23.32) Why is vitamin K essential to body function?

23.36) What would be the effect on an enzyme reaction of a high value for K_m?

23.37) Explain why pepsin and trypsin should have different values for their optimum pH.

23.38) How would the rate of a biochemical reaction be affected by raising the body temperature from 37°C to 50°C, considering the information in Figure 23–8?

23.39*) Arsenic compounds are sometimes used to poison people. How do they work?

23.40) Why is a noncompetitive inhibitor usually more of a poison than a competitive inhibitor?

23.41*) Describe a way in which the body can convert proenzymes to enzymes.

23.42) What type of cofactor is represented by the water-soluble vitamins?

23.43) Enriched flour contains added niacin and riboflavin. What is the function of riboflavin?

23.44) Describe the function of ascorbic acid.

23.45) What might be the result if a person took large doses of vitamin A to prevent colds and sore throat?

23.46) What are the major functions of vitamin D in a growing child?

23.47) How are the structures of vitamins K, A, and E related?

23.48*) If hexokinase has a K_m of $1.5 \times 10^{-4}\,M$, what concentration of the substrate glucose would you use to measure the enzyme concentration in the reaction glucose $\rightarrow$ glucose-6-PO$_4$?

23.49*) How might the end products of an enzyme reaction affect the original reaction or another enzyme reaction in a series?

Fluids of the Human Body 24

Most of us are considered "solid citizens," yet our bodies are mainly water! Body fluids make up about 60% of the weight of an average woman and 70% of an average man. Water provides the basis for several kinds of body fluids that will be discussed in this chapter. These fluids have the properties of aqueous solutions (Section 12.3), since they contain dissolved molecules such as CO_2, glucose, and amino acids. They are also colloids (Section 12.1), since they contain large protein particles and fat globules, which are not fully dissolved. Suspended in various body fluids we also find cells and, inside cells, organelles (Section 20.1).

A 70-kilogram (154-pound) man contains about 50 liters, or 13 U.S. gallons, of body fluids. Of this, about 35 liters (70%) are inside the cells. Another 10 liters (20%) are **interstitial fluid,** which lies between the cells and includes lymph and body tissue fluids. Within the arteries, capillaries, and veins of the circulatory system, there are about 5 liters (10% of total body fluid) of blood, of which 2 liters represent cells and similar materials and 3 liters are *plasma*. The plasma and interstitial fluid are together considered **extracellular fluids,** along with all of the other fluids outside the cells, such as cerebrospinal fluid, intraocular fluid, digestive fluids, sweat, and tears.

When a person feels ill and visits a doctor or hospital for diagnosis, samples of blood and urine are often tested to see if their composition is normal or not. We will discuss both the normal composition of body fluids and some of the conditions that may lead to abnormal blood and urine test results.

Remember throughout this chapter that it is the role of all body fluids to promote the chemical reactions of metabolism by bringing reactants where the reaction will take place, by providing appropriate conditions (temperature, pH) for the enzymes to function, and by removing the waste products of the reaction.

The difference in the per cents for men and women is due to the greater proportion of body fat in adult women. Lipid-filled tissues contain relatively low levels of body fluids.

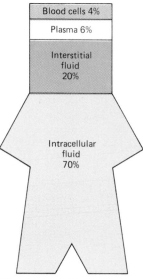

Distribution of body fluids in an average adult.

24.1 BLOOD

LEARNING GOAL 24A: *List five important functions of blood, and indicate which part of the blood performs each function.*

24B: *Describe how blood can be prevented from clotting.*

24C: *Describe how water and nutrients move between capillaries and the interstitial fluid.*

24D: *Describe the causes of metabolic acidosis and metabolic alkalosis.*

The **blood** is, as you know, the main transport system of the body. It makes up about 8% of lean body weight and is often an extremely important indicator of health or disease.

A living cell functions in a very complex manner. One of its most important roles is protein synthesis, which requires that the fluid inside the cell maintain an adequate supply of amino acids, enzymes, ATP, and other essentials. In order to supply necessary nutrients to the cell, the interstitial fluid must itself contain them in adequate concentrations. In higher animals, such as humans, a circulatory system is needed to carry nutrients and other substances (such as vitamins and hormones) to the tissues and to carry off wastes to the organs of excretion.

The *lymph,* a slow-moving fluid similar to blood plasma, is carried through the body in a system of tubes called "lymphatic vessels." It plays a small part in the body's overall transport system. The tissue fluid, resembling lymph but not contained in vessels, also plays a part. However, the most important transport system is necessarily the blood stream.

Functions of blood

If all of the trucks in the nation suddenly stopped moving, the cities would quickly become disaster areas. Truck transport brings food, clothing, and other needed items into the city and carries garbage away for disposal.

The blood performs similar vital functions for the tissues:

1) The blood carries amino acid, carbohydrate, and lipid molecules to the tissues for use in cell reactions.
2) It brings oxygen from the lungs to the cells so that oxidation processes (such as those of the electron transport chain) can occur.
3) It distributes substances that regulate and control metabolic reactions, such as hormones, vitamins, and some enzymes.
4) It keeps the body at constant temperature.
5) It provides the proper environment for metabolic reactions in the tissues by maintaining the proper pH and proper concentration of molecules and ions.
6) It carries waste products of metabolism to the organs of excretion, including the transport of CO_2 to the lungs.
7) It contains white blood cells and antibodies that protect the body against invasion by bacteria and viruses, as well as a clotting mechanism that protects against serious loss of blood.

In addition, the body forms the other extracellular fluids from blood plasma and keeps all of these fluids in equilibrium with each other.

The composition of blood

When blood is taken from your arm for tests, the test results are reported on a form such as the one shown in Figure 24–1. The form seems somewhat complex, since any of 32 different tests may be used in diagnosis. We will refer to this form in later chapters on metabolism to help you under-

DOCTOR: D. Smith

DIAGNOSIS: Diabetes

DATE: 3/8/82 TIME: 10:40 ROOM: 215

SERUM

ANALYSIS	RESULT		NORMAL
☐ SMA-7 (Na+, K+, Cl-, CO₂, Glu, Urea N, Creat)			
☐ ELECTROLYTES (Na+, K+, Cl-, CO₂)			
☐ SODIUM	130	m mol/L	135–148
☐ POTASSIUM	10	m mol/L	3.6–4.8
☐ CHLORIDE	87	m mol/L	96–105
☐ CO₂ Content	10	m mol/L	21–29
☐ GLUCOSE, AC	1200	mg/dL	65–105
☐ GLUCOSE, PC		mg/dL	
☐ GLUCOSE, Random or PCL		mg/dL	
☐ UREA N	30	mg/dL	10–20
☐ CREATININE	1.5	mg/dL	0.8–1.5
☐ ACETONE (Qual.)	Positive		
☐ OSMOLALITY	325	m mol/kg	280–295
☐ CALCIUM	6.0	m Eq/L	4.5–5.5
☐ PHOSPHORUS	4.0	m Eq/L	1.7–2.5
☐ URIC ACID	8.0	mg/dL	2.5–7.0
☐ CHOLESTEROL	225	mg/dL	150–275
☐ BILIRUBIN, TOTAL	1.0	mg/dL	0.2–1.0
☐ BILIRUBIN, DIRECT	0.4	mg/dL	0.1–0.4

☐ PROTEIN, TOTAL	8.0	g/dL	6.0–8.0
☐ AMYLASE	125	Som. u/dL	80–150
☐ ACID PHOSPHATASE	2.2	Gut. u/dL	0.5–3.0
☐ ALK. PHOSPHATASE	12	K-A u/dL	3–13
☐ SGPT (ALT) - Ala transferase	20	U/L	4–25
☐ SGOT (AST) - Asp transferase	17	U/L	5–19
☐ CPK (CK) - Creatine kinase	75	U/L	0–83
☐ LDH - Lactate dehydrogenase	150	U/L	52–142
☐ DIGOXIN (TOXIC> 2.2)		ng/mL	
☐ THYROXINE (T₄)		μg/dL	4.5–11.5
☐ LITHIUM (TOXIC> 1.8)		m mol/L	
☐ SALICYLATE (TOXIC> 14)		mg/dL	

☐ **GLUCOSE TOLERANCE TEST, 100 g p.o.**

	AC	½	1	1½	2	3 h
SERUM (mg/dL)						
URINE (Qual.)						

Signed: _[signature]_

BIOCHEMISTRY - BLOOD

FIGURE 24–1   A typical blood test form used in a hospital for a patient with diabetes.

TABLE 24–1   THE MAJOR COMPONENTS OF BLOOD

Component	Principal Functions
Cells and Cell Fragments	
Erythrocytes (red blood cells)	O_2 transport; buffering
Leucocytes (white blood cells)	Defense against infection
Thrombocytes (platelets)	Blood clotting
Plasma Components	
Water	Solvent
Inorganic ions (mainly Na^+, Cl^-)	Buffering and CO_2 transport (HCO_3^-); cell nutrients; maintaining overall osmotic pressure
Small organic molecules (glucose, amino acids, lipids)	Cell nutrients
Proteins: fibrinogen	Blood clotting
globulins	Immune reactions; carrying lipids
albumin	Water balance between capillaries and interstitial fluids; carrying fatty acids
Nitrogenous waste products	Waste disposal into urine

stand how each test relates to the normal and abnormal functioning of the body.*

The form in Figure 24–1 shows values for a typical patient with *diabetes*. The "normal" range of values for each test is printed on the form. For this particular patient, many of the tests have given "abnormal" results. However, you should be aware that no one is 100% "normal." The ranges shown are averages obtained from large numbers of people. You are quite unlikely to be "average" for every blood test, just as you are unlikely to be of average weight, height, intelligence, and driving ability *all at the same time*. The normal range is wide enough to accommodate most results. However, a single test value slightly above or below normal might not in itself indicate disease. It may tell the doctor that another test should be taken later. *Consistent* test results outside the normal range would generally be cause for concern.

Table 24–1 lists the main components of blood and some functions of each.

Formed "elements" in blood

As you can see from Figure 24–1, blood contains a large variety of substances. It is a suspension of about 40 to 45% cells or other *formed "elements"* and 55 to 60% plasma (fluid). The exact percentage of cells is called the *hematocrit value*.

When whole blood is separated in a centrifuge, we find three major layers (Figure 24–2). Roughly 1% of the volume is occupied by *leucocytes*, or white blood cells. White blood cells fight infection from bacteria, at a

---

* The red and white blood cell counts are reported separately in numbers of cells per cubic millimeter. You may wonder why so many different units are used in measuring blood components. The medical laboratory technologist uses units that correspond most conveniently to the apparatus readings on routine tests, which leads to a variety of sample sizes (1 liter, 100 mL = 1 dL, 1 mL) and a diverse assortment of units of "amount": millimoles (mmol), milligrams (mg), milliequivalents (mEq), micrograms (μg), nanograms (ng), and standard units (u or U). The metric prefixes are summarized in Table 2–1. For the purposes of this text, we will occasionally convert the analysis unit to a more convenient and familiar unit, such as moles/liter.

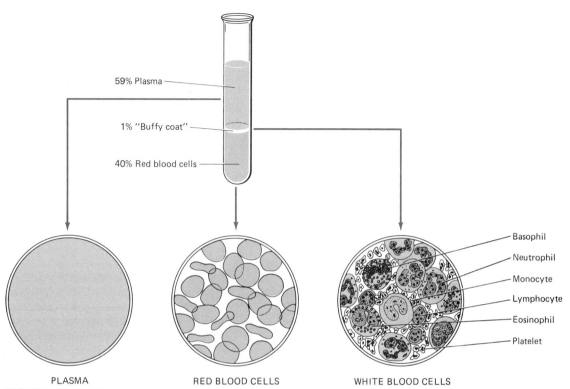

PLASMA   RED BLOOD CELLS   WHITE BLOOD CELLS

FIGURE 24–2   The major components of blood can be separated into red blood cells, a variety of white blood cells and platelets ("buffy coat"), and clear plasma. The percentage values given are normal averages.

normal level of 5000 to 10 000 cells in each cubic millimeter, or 5 to 10 billion cells in each liter of blood. An elevated white blood cell count, for example 20 000 cells per mm³, indicates that some tissue in the body is inflamed and possibly infected. The white blood cell count is commonly used to check for suspected appendicitis. If a large number of white blood cells engulf bacteria or dead tissue, they themselves die and form *pus*. In the form of cancer known as *leukemia*, white blood cells are produced in an uncontrolled manner and use up most of the nutrients needed for normal growth and development.

In leukemia cases, the white blood cell count may increase from a normal 5000 to as much as 500 000/mm³.

In the same layer with white blood cells we find the blood platelets, or *thrombocytes*, which are smaller than cells and function in the clotting of blood. There are normally 250 000 to 400 000 thrombocytes per cubic millimeter of blood.

The remaining 40 to 45% of the blood volume is taken up by the red blood cells, or *erythrocytes*, which are smaller than the white blood cells and do not contain cell nuclei. These extremely important cells (seen in Figure 24–2) contain hemoglobin, which carries O_2 to the cell and aids in the transport of CO_2 from the tissues to the lungs. The red blood cells also take care of 70% of the pH control (buffering) in the blood. The detailed ways in which hemoglobin accomplishes its tasks will be the subject of Section 24.2. A normal red blood cell count for a 70-kg man would be around 5 000 000 per mm³, or 5 trillion (5×10^{12}) per liter.

Plasma and serum

When blood is freshly drawn from a vein and allowed to stand, it clots and a pale yellow fluid separates from the clotted material. This fluid is called *serum* and is whole blood minus its formed elements and *fibrinogen,* a protein involved in the clotting process. If an anticoagulant is added to the whole blood to prevent clotting, the fibrinogen remains in solution and the fluid portion is then called **plasma.** The distinction between serum (no fibrinogen) and plasma (contains fibrinogen) is thus trivial for most purposes, and a reported "blood serum" level of some substance can be considered to be its concentration in blood plasma.

Blood plasma contains about 70 grams/liter of various types of **plasma proteins.** The most important of these are *fibrinogen,* the *globulins,* and *albumin,* formed mostly in the liver.

Fibrinogen and blood clotting

When tissue is damaged, blood platelets (thrombocytes) clump together and stick to the blood vessel wall at the site of the injury. They then disintegrate, releasing an enzyme, *thrombokinase,* in the presence of Ca^{2+} ion.

We mentioned on p. 642 that vitamin K is essential to blood clotting. It is apparently needed for the synthesis of a protein called *prothrombin,* which at the site of injury is converted by thrombokinase to its active enzyme form, *thrombin:*

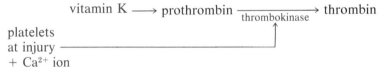

Thrombin then catalyzes the conversion of the soluble blood plasma protein fibrinogen to an insoluble substance *fibrin,* which actually forms the clot:

$$\text{fibrinogen} \xrightarrow[\text{thrombin}]{} \text{fibrin clot}$$

Because of a genetic defect, persons suffering from *hemophilia* are missing any one of several proteins that permit platelets to release thrombokinase. Instead of clotting within 5 minutes, as happens with normal blood, the blood of a hemophiliac may take as long as 50 minutes to clot. Blood loss from a nosebleed, tooth extraction, or minor injury can then be life-threatening. One of the most painful experiences for a hemophiliac is a bruise, since blood then collects under the skin and in joints, putting extreme pressure on nerves.

An anticoagulant is a substance that interferes with the clotting reaction. Blood-sucking leeches secrete a substance called *hirudin,* which prevents the conversion of fibrinogen to fibrin. Mosquitos also use anticoagulants to make our blood flow freely for their feast!

Any process that removes calcium ions will prevent clotting. Fortunately, in the living body, the calcium ion concentration never falls low enough to affect the clotting process. Long before it reaches such a level, the reactions that cause muscle movement will be affected.

On the other hand, when blood is removed for transfusion, it is impor-

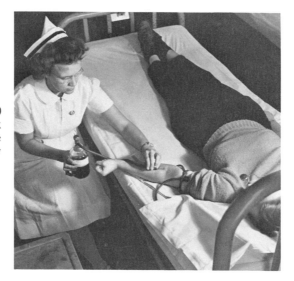

An occasional donation of 500 mL of blood to a blood bank has no serious effect on the body since the blood is rapidly replaced.

tant to prevent clotting. If citrate ion is added (the same ion we saw in the Krebs cycle), it will react with Ca^{2+} and prevent it from becoming involved in clotting. If oxalate is added, then insoluble calcium oxalate will be formed and again the action of Ca^{2+} will be blocked.

An abnormal clot that develops in a blood vessel is called a *thrombus*. Freely moving clots, called *emboli,* may become wedged in a narrow part of the circulatory system and cause damage to a section of tissue. If the tissue is heart, brain, or lungs, death may quickly result. Medical anticoagulants, such as *heparin* and *dicumarol,* interfere with the coagulation (clotting) process and find many uses in modern therapy.

Globulins and albumins

Fibrinogen makes up only 5% of the total protein in the blood. Globulins (40%) and albumins (55%) are more abundant. A technique called *electrophoresis* may be used to separate the various protein types (Figure 24–3). When this is done, the globulins can be separated into three subclasses, called "alpha," "beta," and "gamma."

FIGURE 24–3 Electrophoresis is used to separate plasma proteins by means of an electric field. The general method is similar to that of chromatography (Section 19.1).

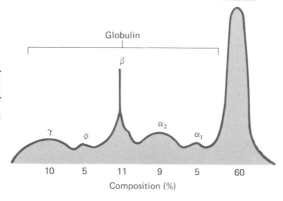

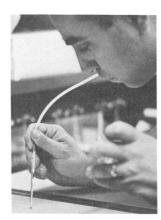

The α- and β-globulins help transport normally insoluble fats through the body. Cations such as Cu^{2+} and Fe^{2+} would normally form insoluble hydroxides at the slightly basic pH of the blood stream. These two globulins help keep the metal cations dissolved until they are needed. The γ-globulins contain antibodies that combat certain diseases caused by viruses, such as diphtheria, influenza, mumps, and measles.

Albumins also serve to help transport materials through the body. About 70% of the (unesterified) fatty acid molecules in the blood plasma are carried by albumins, which are also important for their ability to buffer the blood and to transport certain water-insoluble drugs in the blood stream.

The serum albumin level is often measured in medical diagnosis. Changes in the relative amounts of plasma proteins may be caused by diseases such as cirrhosis (of the liver) or nephrosis (of the kidneys). Figure 24–1 shows *total* protein analysis.

Albumins and oncotic pressure

The major function of albumins in the blood is to maintain osmotic pressure. In Section 12.5 we discussed how osmotic pressure controls the movement of water across semipermeable membranes, such as those of cells and organelles. If a person drinks too much water, the blood plasma becomes diluted and some excess water passes into the cells, which become swollen. Consuming excess NaCl raises the osmotic pressure of the blood plasma and causes water to move from the cells, thus dehydrating them. Under normal conditions, it is the plasma proteins, particularly the albumins, that provide the osmotic pressure to control this water "balance."

While the concentrations of the various solutes in the body fluids remain relatively constant, an incredible amount of water is constantly passing from the capillaries into the interstitial spaces, estimated at about 1500 liters each minute for our 70-kilogram man. The same amount of water must reenter the capillaries so that equilibrium is maintained.

The osmotic pressure due to dissolved inorganic salts in the blood plasma may be calculated by the methods in Section 14.2. It is quite high, averaging about 5450 torr (7.2 atm). However, the osmotic pressure of the interstitial fluid due to dissolved inorganic salts is *just as high*. There is *no* movement of water due to these substances.

On the other hand, the presence in the plasma of proteins that are not present in the interstitial fluid creates a "drawing power" of approximately 23 torr. This force, called the **oncotic pressure,** works to push water from the interstitial fluids into the capillaries.

Opposing the oncotic pressure is the fluid (blood) pressure, discussed in Section 11.2. At the end of the capillary nearest the heart, the arterial end, the blood pressure for a normal person averages about 32 torr higher than that in the interstitial space. Since the blood pressure is higher than the oncotic pressure by $32 - 23 = 9$ torr, the pressure difference forces water out of the capillary into the spaces between cells, as shown in Figure 24–4.

In the middle of the capillary, the blood pressure equals the oncotic pressure, so no water passes through the capillary wall. However, at the end of the capillary farthest from the heart, the venous end, the blood pressure difference has dropped to 14 torr but the oncotic pressure is still 23 torr. This draws water into the capillary by a difference of $(14 - 23) = -9$ torr. This mechanism or "colloidal osmotic machine" is responsible for the normal exchange of water between the blood stream and the tissue fluid.

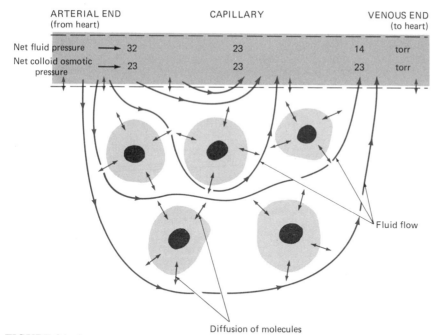

ARTERIAL END (from heart)	CAPILLARY	VENOUS END (to heart)	
Net fluid pressure → 32	23	14	torr
Net colloid osmotic pressure → 23	23	23	torr

Fluid flow

Diffusion of molecules

FIGURE 24-4 At the arterial end of a capillary, fluids flow from the blood stream into the interstitial spaces as a result of higher blood pressure. The nutrients then diffuse into cells. At the venous end of the capillary, the oncotic pressure is higher than the blood pressure and fluids flow from the interstitial fluid into the capillary.

So long as the concentration of plasma proteins remains normal, this system works properly. A decrease in plasma protein, such as occurs in serious protein malnutrition (kwashiorkor) or in kidney disease (proteinuria), provides a lower oncotic pressure. The result is *edema,* excess water entering the spaces between cells. Edema also occurs in cases of weak blood circulation or any other condition that increases blood pressure in a particular area of the body.*

A loss of body fluids may occur from diarrhea or from sweating. The concentration of plasma proteins then becomes higher than normal, increasing the oncotic pressure and causing cell dehydration, that is, loss of water from the cytoplasm.

Plasma electrolytes

An electrolyte is a dissolved substance present in the form of its ions. Figure 24-1 shows the levels of three electrolyte ions (Na^+, K^+, and Cl^-) in units of millimoles/liter and a fourth (Ca^{2+}) in units of milliequivalents/liter, where one mole is two equivalents. The total CO_2 content, measured in milli-

---

* Edema frequently results at the end of a long airplane journey. After sitting for a long time, passengers arrive with swollen feet because of excess venous blood pressure caused by gravity. Persons who are fasting may also suffer edema because of low levels of plasma proteins. Other causes of edema may be allergic reactions ("hives"); blockage of lymph channels, as in *filariasis* or certain types of cancer surgery; and even emotional upset, which can cause hoarseness as a result of edema of the larynx.

TABLE 24–2   ELECTROLYTE CONCENTRATIONS IN BLOOD PLASMA

Ion	Normal Concentration Range in Moles/Liter	Approx. Average Concentration in Moles/Liter	Average Concentration in mEq/Liter
Cations			
Na^+	0.135–0.148	0.144	144
K^+	0.0036–0.0048	0.0044	4.4
Ca^{2+}	0.0022–0.0028	0.0025	5.0
Mg^{2+}	0.0012–0.0018	0.0015	3.0
			(Total: 156 mEq/L)
Anions			
Cl^-	0.096–0.105	0.100	100
HCO_3^-	0.025–0.030	0.027	27
HPO_4^{2-}	0.0008–0.0011	0.001	2
$H_2PO_4^-$	0.0002–0.0004	0.0003	0.3
SO_4^{2-}	0.0004–0.0006	0.0005	1
Carboxylate anions			
$RCOO^-$	0.005–0.007	0.006	6
Protein anions	0.016–0.025	0.020	20
			(Total: 156 mEq/L)

Note: See p. 435 to review the calculation of mEq/liter.

moles/liter, includes bicarbonate ion, HCO_3^-. Together, these ions represent the greater part of inorganic dissolved solutes, as shown in Table 24–2.

Any major change in ion concentration upsets the water balance of the body, as described earlier. If the blood contains a higher-than-normal level of solutes, it stimulates thirst. The water we drink dilutes the body fluids, and concentration levels return to normal. The kidneys further regulate electrolyte levels by retaining ions for reabsorption into the blood stream or releasing them into the urine to maintain an **electrolyte balance.**

Table 24–3 shows how increased or decreased concentrations of certain plasma electrolytes might indicate abnormal conditions in the body.

TABLE 24–3   CONDITIONS RESULTING IN CHANGES IN ELECTROLYTE CONCENTRATION

Electrolyte	Increased Concentration May Accompany	Decreased Concentration May Accompany
Sodium, Na^+	Dehydration	Diarrhea, vomiting, metabolic acidosis
Potassium, K^+	Kidney failure, underactive adrenal glands	Metabolic alkalosis, vomiting
Chloride, Cl^-	Dehydration	Vomiting, metabolic alkalosis, kidney failure
Bicarbonate, HCO_3^-	Metabolic alkalosis	Metabolic acidosis, kidney failure, starvation
Calcium, Ca^{2+}	Overactive parathyroid	Tetany, rickets, underactive parathyroid
Magnesium, Mg^{2+}	Dehydration, kidney failure, diabetic coma	Diarrhea, chronic alcoholism, hyperthyroidism

Acid-base balance

Several of the ions in Table 24–2 were discussed in Section 13.5 as part of the **acid-base balance** system that keeps body fluids buffered at pH 7.4. These are the bicarbonate ion and the dihydrogen phosphate/monohydrogen phosphate pair. Since the proteins in all body fluids are amphoteric, having acidic (—COOH) and basic (—NH$_2$) ends, they play a major role in buffering, as described on p. 400. Hemoglobin is of particular importance in buffering the blood through its reactions in red blood cells.

Why are these buffers needed? The normal metabolic processes of the body result in the continuous production of acids. For example, the Krebs cycle results in the release of CO$_2$ into the cell fluids as part of the oxidation of energy nutrients. As discussed in Section 13.2, carbon dioxide is a weak acid, involved in the following equilibria:

$$CO_{2(aq)} + H_2O_{(\ell)} \rightleftharpoons H_2CO_{3(aq)} \rightleftharpoons H^+_{(aq)} + HCO^-_{3(aq)}$$

Between 10 and 20 moles of CO$_2$ are produced by the cells each day. If this CO$_2$ stayed dissolved in the roughly 50 liters of body fluids, the effect would be to change the pH from the normal slightly basic pH of 7.4 to an acidic solution of pH 3! This extra acid must be neutralized and removed. Other metabolic reactions, such as those described in Chapters 25 to 27, also release acids that must be carried to the kidneys and excreted without change in the blood pH.

The excess CO$_2$ is carried by red blood cells to the lungs for excretion. This process will be described in the next section.

Acidosis and alkalosis

On p. 403 we noted that if your body goes for one minute without breathing, the pH of the blood plasma can fall from its normal value of 7.4 to the more acidic pH of 7.1. This is due to the accumulation of CO$_2$, which is not being exhaled from the lungs. Such a situation is called respiratory *acidosis*, an over-acidic state of the blood plasma. If an athlete *hyperventilates* (breathes quickly and deeply), the pH of the blood will rise to perhaps 7.7 because of the quick removal of CO$_2$. This is called respiratory *alkalosis* because the blood is slightly more basic or alkaline than normal.

Hyperventilation can also be caused by excitement or panic.

Acidosis occurs more frequently in cases of diabetes mellitus, where extra acids are produced through lipid metabolism. If the body pH falls below about 6.9, the patient will go into a coma and will die unless treated quickly. The main effect of **metabolic acidosis** is thus depression of the central nervous system.

Severe fasting diets can result in metabolic acidosis, as can starvation.

Alkalosis occurs less often but can be caused by continued vomiting or by taking too much antacid (particularly sodium bicarbonate). The major effect of **metabolic alkalosis** is overexcitability of the nervous system. The muscles may go into a state of *tetany,* or uncontrolled spasms. A high degree of nervousness or even convulsions may also result. Death could come from tetany of the muscles of the lungs.

Figure 24–5 shows some of the possible causes of acidosis and alkalosis, along with the extreme pH changes that could result.

Acidosis is diagnosed by noting hyperventilation, as the patient attempts to get rid of CO$_2$ through the lungs, as well as a urine more acidic than usual. Alkalosis shows the opposite symptoms, hypoventilation (shallow breathing) and possibly basic urine.

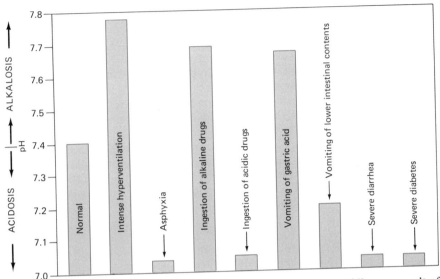

FIGURE 24–5   The pH of the extracellular fluids may become acidic as a result of breathing blockages, diabetes, diarrhea, or acidic drugs. It may become basic because of hyperventilation, antacid medications, or loss of stomach acid through vomiting. The bars indicate how a prolonged disorder may lead to a pH different from the normal blood pH of 7.4.

Treatment of acidosis resulting from diabetes is an immediate injection of insulin, a hormone that regulates carbohydrate metabolism. Most other cases of acidosis and alkalosis may be treated with intravenous solutions that are isotonic with blood plasma. Two such solutions were described in Self-Check 14.12 (p. 423).

SELF-CHECK

24.1)   Which part of the blood performs each of the following functions: (a) fighting infection? (b) carrying oxygen? (c) maintaining water balance?
24.2)   South American vampire bats feed on sleeping cattle. How do you suppose the bats keep the blood from clotting?
24.3)   How does a *decrease* in plasma protein concentration affect the movement of water between a capillary and the interstitial spaces?
24.4)   Describe one cause and one symptom of metabolic acidosis.

24.2 RESPIRATION AND HEMOGLOBIN

LEARNING GOAL 24E: Describe how O_2 is carried from the lungs to the cells and how CO_2 is transported from the cells to the lungs.
        24F: Describe how hemoglobin can deliver varying amounts of oxygen to the cells depending on the blood pH (Bohr effect).
        24G: Describe how hemoglobin can act as a buffer, and explain the chloride shift.
        24H: Describe the role of myoglobin in storing oxygen.

Section 10.5 briefly described the process of breathing, with special attention to the amount of O_2 and CO_2 present at each stage. The important compound *hemoglobin* contains Fe^{2+} cations that can accept oxygen molecules and carry them along in the blood stream. In this section, we will discuss the function of the hemoglobin molecule in detail.

Hemoglobin

We mentioned earlier the very important red blood cells, erythrocytes, which transport oxygen. Each red blood cell is saucer-shaped with a very thin center that allows gases to easily enter the cell. About one third of the total mass of a red blood cell is hemoglobin, about 3×10^8 molecules in each cell.

The most important structure in the hemoglobin molecule, *heme,* was shown in Figure 22–9 (p. 615). The electron transport chain uses one important property of the iron cation, its ability to gain and lose electrons, to provide energy to the body. To accomplish this, the iron cation must be held in position by the six nitrogen atoms surrounding it. Four of those nitrogens are arranged in a square around the iron as part of a *porphyrin* grouping (p. 457). This grouping is also found in vitamin B_{12} with cobalt as the central cation (Figure 23–11) and in the chlorophyll molecule (Section 25.5) with magnesium as the central cation. In cytochrome *c*, nitrogens from the surrounding protein are found above and below the central iron cation.

Figure 24–6 shows a heme grouping of the hemoglobin molecule. The drawing shows that the heme structure is *flat*. There is nothing above the central Fe^{2+} ion, which is thus able to form a bond in that direction. This bond may be formed with any substance that can *donate* an electron pair to the bond. Such substances, called *ligands* or *Lewis bases,* include $:NH_3$ (ammonia), $:OH_2$ (water), $C\equiv N:$ (cyanide, as in vitamin B_{12}), $C\equiv O:$ (carbon monoxide, which poisons by bonding with the Fe^{2+}), and, most important, $O=O:$ (the oxygen molecule in air).

Hemoglobin is a large molecule of about 68 000 amu. It consists of a protein section (globin) wrapped around and carrying *four* heme groups. The general structure is shown in Figure 24–7. An O_2 molecule may perch above and bond to the iron cation in the center of each heme "disk."

The three-dimensional structure of the whole hemoglobin molecule is quite complex. A molecular model is shown in Figure 24–8.

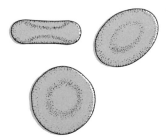

Red blood cells are flattened so that gases may easily be exchanged with the hemoglobin in the cell.

These are not Lewis electron-dot diagrams because they show *only*, for each ligand, the lone electron pair that bonds to the metal cation.

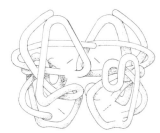

FIGURE 24–7   The broad outlines of the hemoglobin molecule, showing the tertiary structure of the globular protein surrounding the four heme groups. The exact folding pattern of the protein is *very* important to the manner in which hemoglobin carries oxygen and buffers the pH of blood.

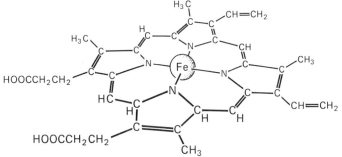

FIGURE 24–6   The heme grouping that carries oxygen in red blood cells consists of an iron(II) cation held in position by a porphyrin ring system. One hemoglobin molecule contains four heme groupings.

Blood circulation and gas transfer

Figure 24–9 shows a simplified picture of the human blood system. Oxygen enters the hemoglobin of the red blood cells when the blood passes through the lungs:

$$Hb + O_2 \longrightarrow HbO_2 \qquad \text{in the lungs}$$

We will let Hb be an abbreviation for a hemoglobin molecule with its four heme groups, in which case HbO_2 will be used to symbolize *oxyhemoglobin*,

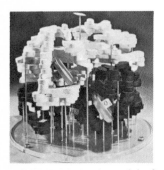

FIGURE 24–8   A model of the hemoglobin structure that resulted in the 1962 Nobel Prize in chemistry for Max F. Perutz. (From *Science*, 140:863, 1963)

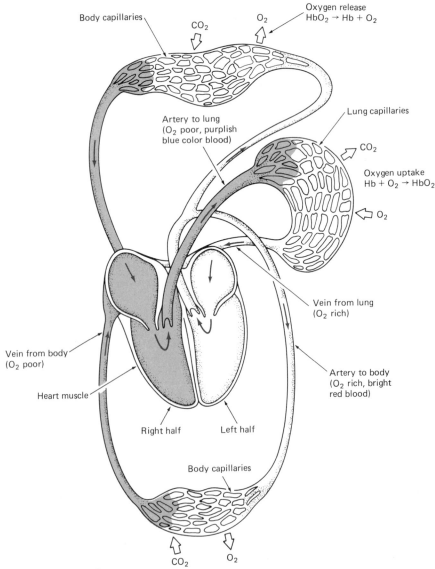

FIGURE 24–9   The human circulatory system. The white sections indicate the presence of oxygenated hemoglobin (HbO_2) in red blood cells, while the colored areas would be blue in the body and carry CO_2 back to the lungs for excretion.

a hemoglobin with one, two, three, or four oxygen molecules bonded to iron cations.

When the oxygenated blood reaches the capillaries, the interstitial fluid has relatively little oxygen. This causes O_2 to be released from the red blood cells and to diffuse from the capillary into the tissues where it is needed:

$$HbO_2 \longrightarrow Hb + O_2 \quad \text{in the tissues}$$

Why is hemoglobin necessary in blood? Couldn't the plasma itself carry enough oxygen to nourish the cells? No, because the solubility of oxygen in water, and thus in blood plasma, is very limited. One liter of plasma can carry only 0.0001 moles of O_2 at the temperature and pressures of the lungs. To satisfy the body's needs for oxygen, we would need over 300 liters of aqueous fluids, instead of the approximately 5 liters of blood! The blood can carry about 60 times as much oxygen as the same volume of simple plasma (because of the Fe^{2+} cations in heme), up to 0.008 moles of O_2 for each liter of blood.

Each minute, the heart pumps an average of five liters of blood. This delivers about 0.01 moles of O_2 to the tissues each minute for a resting person, and up to 20 times as much for a highly trained athlete, enough for the oxygen demands of the tissues.

Metabolic reactions within the cell, such as the Krebs cycle and electron transport, are continually using up O_2 to make water and producing CO_2 from nutrients. The CO_2 must be transported back to the lungs for excretion, as shown in Figure 24–9. As is the case with oxygen, the amount of CO_2 that can dissolve in plasma is relatively small, about 8% of what is actually present. Most of the CO_2 must be carried by other mechanisms, which are somewhat more complex than those for oxygen and which were briefly referred to on p. 403. We will cover these other mechanisms later on in this section.

Carbonated beverages contain CO_2 forced into water under pressure. Even so, the concentration of dissolved CO_2 in such drinks is less than that present in human veins.

Control of oxyhemoglobin saturation

Hemoglobin is called a respiratory *pigment* because it is colored; it contains "pigmentation" as a result of the electronic properties of the Fe^{2+} cation. Hemoglobin is purplish blue, the color of your veins. Oxyhemoglobin is bright red, the color of your arteries, as shown in Figure 24–9. When blood from a cut vein first reaches the air, it receives enough oxygen to turn red; otherwise we would all bleed "blue blood." People suffering from blood diseases or certain types of poisoning that prevent O_2 from reaching the hemoglobin often have blue lips and a bluish tinge to the skin and fingernails.

When hemoglobin is *completely* converted to oxyhemoglobin with *four* O_2 bonded to each hemoglobin molecule, the molecules are said to be *saturated* with oxygen.

There are several factors that affect the percentage saturation of hemoglobin, the most important of which is the amount of O_2 in the plasma, usually referred to as the "oxygen tension" or partial pressure, P_{O_2}. The very high concentration of oxygen in the lungs creates a situation of high saturation; in the tissues, there is less oxygen, so the O_2 molecules leave the hemoglobin and create a low-saturation condition.

However, this is a very rough description. As with all other mechanisms in the body, there is regulation and control of O_2 saturation so that the cells receive *exactly* as much O_2 as they need, no more and no less. For this

The word "saturated" can be understood in a sense similar to the use of the same term in Section 12.2. Hemoglobin is saturated when it cannot hold any more oxygen. Since adding oxygen to an organic compound is a type of *oxidation*, the reverse process (removal of oxygen) is reduction. Hb is thus also called *reduced* hemoglobin or *deoxy*hemoglobin, where "deoxy" means "without oxygen," as in *deoxy*ribose (Figure 20–7).

The partial pressure of a gas, as defined in Section 10.3, is the pressure that gas would exert if it were alone. The gas tension in a fluid is defined on p. 298 as the *dissolved* gas concentration that corresponds to fluid at equilibrium with the pure gas at the given partial pressure. In practice, the gas will diffuse from a region of higher "tension" or partial pressure to a region with lower values.

reason, the blood entering the lungs from veins, which we have considered "pure Hb," is actually 75% saturated!

The regulation of the O_2 saturation of hemoglobin is accomplished by the following factors:

1)   The concentration of O_2 (P_{O_2}) in tissues outside the blood stream;
2)   The concentration of CO_2 (P_{CO_2}) in tissues outside the blood stream;
3)   The pH of the tissues;
4)   The amount of DPG (2,3-diphosphoglycerate) in the tissues;
5)   The temperature of the tissues.

Each of these factors affects the plasma because there is relatively free flow of materials through the capillary walls. Thus, a low P_{O_2} in the tissues quickly creates a low P_{O_2} in the plasma, and a warm tissue quickly warms up the plasma. The primary effect on hemoglobin O_2 saturation levels, the amount of O_2 present, can be illustrated by a graph, as shown in Figure 24–10.

In the lungs, the O_2 level is high, so the hemoglobin becomes almost entirely saturated with O_2. As it passes through the capillaries, where the O_2 levels are lower, about 25% of the O_2 is lost, so the blood in veins is only 75% saturated in tissues with no working muscles.

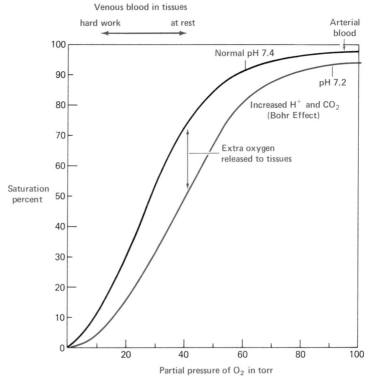

FIGURE 24–10 Hemoglobin saturation with oxygen at varying oxygen tension values. At the top of the graph, arrows show the saturation level in arterial blood and the range in venous blood between the resting and hard-working levels. The colored curve represents *decreased* oxygen saturation at lower pH and at higher CO_2 concentrations. The result is the release of extra oxygen to the tissues as a result of the *Bohr effect*.

Let us now consider muscles working very hard. During exercise, the mitochondria inside the cells demand more O_2 and produce more CO_2. The level of O_2 in extreme cases can drop to one fourth the level in a resting cell. The following effects all provide more oxygen to the cell:

1) Instead of leaving the capillaries that lead into the veins with 75% of the O_2 still in the hemoglobin, the saturation level drops. Thus, instead of receiving 25% of the oxygen being carried by the blood stream, the tissue receives more (Figure 24–10).

2) The high CO_2 level in the tissues makes the hemoglobin *less* able to retain its O_2 (that is, it shifts the curve in Figure 24–10 to the right and down a bit). This increases the amount of oxygen released to the tissues beyond the above effect.

3) In the process of generating energy in the muscles (and using up oxygen while producing CO_2), acids are produced by the cells. The pH of the tissue fluids becomes slightly more acidic than normal, say from pH 7.4 (normal) down to pH 7.2. This also shifts the curve in Figure 24–10 to provide a little extra oxygen to the tissues. The combined results of effects 2 and 3 are the *Bohr effect*. Recall that CO_2 dissolved in water is acidic, so the extra CO_2 *also* slightly lowers the pH, thus causing more release of oxygen to the cells.

4) A small ion, DPG, shown in Figure 24–11, fits inside the protein of deoxygenated hemoglobin and helps keep oxygen off. The three-dimensional structure of the protein is not fixed but can "flip" and turn to receive more O_2, especially once a single O_2 is present. This "flipping" is most effective if there is no DPG present. The more DPG there is, the less able is hemoglobin to efficiently keep its O_2. The DPG thus works cooperatively with the above three effects by keeping the hemoglobin from gaining back the oxygen that has left.

5) As muscles work, they heat up. Thus, the tissues that need more oxygen are warmer than tissues that need only normal amounts of oxygen. Any increase in temperature shifts the curve in Figure 24–10 to the right, just as a decrease in pH does. This effect again works to provide more O_2 to the cells.

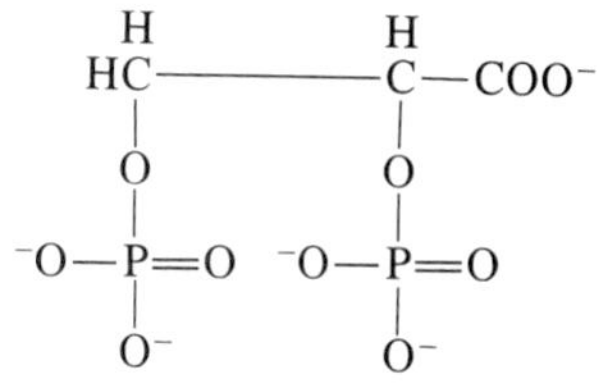

In this manner, an exercising muscle can pull just about all of the available O_2 from its blood supply.

Abnormal forms of hemoglobin

More than 50 000 black Americans suffer from a disease called *sickle cell anemia*. In a sickle cell, shown in Figure 24–12, a difference of one ("wrong") amino acid on a particular protein chain causes a change in the three-dimensional globin molecule structure. This change decreases the solubility of hemoglobin. Being less soluble, the hemoglobin molecules tend to clump together and form solid cystals, distorting the red blood cells into a "sickle" (curved) shape that can no longer carry adequate amounts of oxygen. In addition, the rigid sickle cells have great difficulty squeezing through small capillaries and often become blocked or tear the cell membrane. This hereditary disease causes many deaths and much pain, especially in tropical regions.

Sickle cell anemia is one example of a *genetic defect*, caused when the DNA in the genes, which carries the hereditary information for the manufacture of all proteins in the body, contains an error. The transmission of

2,3-diphosphoglycerate

FIGURE 24–11. 2,3-Diphosphoglycerate. This ion with five negative charges fits exactly between the heme units of hemoglobin, keeping it in a deoxygenated form. It thus regulates the three-dimensional structure of the globular protein.

A substance similar to DPG, that we have seen previously is 1,3-diphosphoglycerate, formed during glycolysis (Figure 22–5) and considered one of the important high-energy compounds (Table 22–1).

genetic information in the cell will be discussed in Chapter 28. You should realize that perhaps 5 out of every 1000 people carry a gene for an abnormal or *mutant* form of hemoglobin. We know of roughly 150 different mutant forms, each generally containing only one amino acid error. For example, in one form, the central iron atom in heme, which is normally present as an Fe^{2+} ion, can become an Fe^{3+} ion by oxidation. When the iron is in its 3+ state, the heme does not carry oxygen effectively.

The role of myoglobin

We have already discussed two very important compounds in the body that contain the heme unit with a central iron cation: cytochromes and hemoglobin. The muscles have a very important hemoglobin-like molecule known as **myoglobin.** In fact, myoglobin is essentially one fourth of a hemoglobin molecule, with one heme group and one polypeptide chain. It serves two functions, both related to those we have already seen for hemoglobin: (a) myoglobin can carry oxygen from an oxygen-rich area *inside* a cell to an oxygen-poor region, therefore helping to distribute oxygen evenly, and (b) myoglobin can store oxygen when the muscle is at rest, to be used when the muscle suddenly becomes active.

Effects of poisoning

Both hemoglobin and myoglobin have heme groups that bond with oxygen molecules. There are other molecules that can imitate oxygen and thus block the sites on the hemoglobin molecule that carry oxygen to the cells. The most important of these is carbon monoxide (CO), present in automobile exhaust and the fumes from gas space heaters. The CO molecule occupies a bonding site on the heme group more effectively than O_2 does and in essence reduces the useful amount of hemoglobin in the blood (Table 24–4). The cyanide ion (CN^-) can do the same thing, but, what is much more serious, it can block the similar coordinating position in cytochromes and other enzymes that speeds up oxygen-using processes inside the cell (p. 628).

Hemoglobin as a buffer

Each heme group (Figure 24–6) has two —COOH parts, which can serve as acids (proton donors). With four heme groups, a hemoglobin molecule can thus lose any or all of eight protons. In theory, then, there are many possible buffer systems. However, at the particular pH range of blood, not all of the eight possible forms will be important. We shall concern ourselves here with only four species, two for ordinary (reduced) hemoglobin,

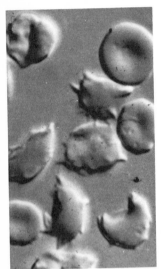
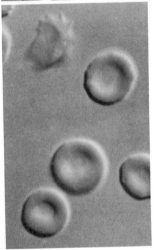

FIGURE 24–12 The effect of cyanate on sickle cells. Top: red blood cells in sickle cell anemia; bottom: after treatment with 0.03 *M* KNCO for 1 hour at 37°C (courtesy A. Cerami, Rockerfeller University, *Proc. Nat. Acad. Sci.* 68:1180, 1971). Recently, a laboratory-made tetrapeptide, Phe-Phe-Phe-Arg, has also been found to prevent formation of the hemoglobin clumps and crystals associated with this disease.

TABLE 24–4 CONCENTRATION OF CO IN ATMOSPHERE VERSUS PERCENTAGE OF HEMOGLOBIN (Hb) SATURATED*

CO concentration in air	0.01% (100 ppm)	0.02% (200 ppm)	0.10% (1 000 ppm)	1.0% (10 000 ppm)
Percentage of hemoglobin molecules saturated with CO†	17	20	60	90

* A few hours of breathing time is assumed.
† Normal human blood contains up to 5% of the hemoglobin as carboxyhemoglobin (HbCO).

one with an acidic hydrogen (HHb) and one without (Hb$^-$), and two for oxy-hemoglobin, again one with an acidic hydrogen (HHbO$_2$) and one without (HbO$_2^-$).

One buffer pair is therefore a combination of HHb and Hb$^-$. Excess acid can react with Hb$^-$ to give HHb:

$$Hb^- + H^+ \longrightarrow HHb$$

Excess base can react with the acid form of hemoglobin to give Hb$^-$:

$$HHb + OH^- \longrightarrow Hb^- + H_2O$$

Similar reactions can be written for the HHbO$_2$/HbO$_2^-$ buffer pair. To this point in our discussion, we have avoided any distinction between the acidic and basic forms of Hb or the acidic and basic forms of HbO$_2$. We must clearly distinguish between these forms, however, when we discuss how CO$_2$ is transported.

Carbon dioxide transport

When carbon dioxide is produced inside the cell, it dissolves in the cytoplasm (intracellular fluid), effectively forming a solution of CO$_2$ gas in water, which we usually write CO$_{2(aq)}$. The CO$_2$ molecule, surrounded by a number of water molecules, is *hydrated*.

One way to express this hydration is to pick *one* water molecule arbitrarily and join the CO$_2$ to it. Since the carbon is less electronegative than the oxygen, the CO$_2$ molecule has partial charges (Section 6.4). Water, as we know, is also a polar molecule with partial charges, so the CO$_2$ lines up:

Hydrated carbon dioxide   Carbonic acid

If one of the water oxygens forms a bond with the carbon and a hydrogen atom then moves to another oxygen, we obtain the carbonic acid molecule. Carbonic acid, in fact, has the same atoms as CO$_2$ + H$_2$O. The formation of such a molecule between water and CO$_2$ is speeded up by an enzyme, *carbonic anhydrase* (which also speeds up the breaking up of the pair).

Carbonic acid is a weak acid, dissociating slightly:

$$H_2CO_3 \rightleftharpoons H^+ + HCO_3^-$$

However, body fluids are all slightly basic, so the H$^+$ (hydrated proton) produced is quickly linked to some available base, such as a hemoglobin or other protein —COO⁻ or —NH₂ group. The result is that the dissolving of CO_2 in the red blood cells gives, in the end, some $CO_{2(aq)}$ and a good deal of bicarbonate ion (HCO_3^-).

The carbonic anhydrase is located only in the red blood cells, not in the plasma. Thus, the $CO_{2(aq)}$ passes into the plasma, enters the red blood cells, and is largely (67%) converted to bicarbonate ions, which then pass back into the plasma. Since the passing of HCO_3^- ions from the red blood cells into the plasma of capillaries creates a charge imbalance, chloride (Cl^-) ions must pass from the plasma into the red blood cells to maintain the total amount of negative charge in each cell. This is called the *chloride shift*.

Carbon dioxide can link up not only with an oxygen atom of water, but also with the nitrogen of an amino group (which, like oxygen, contains an unbonded pair of electrons). Since proteins contain many :NH₂— groups on side chains, *carbamino* compounds of the type O_2CNH_2— can be formed. Hemoglobin has a particularly strong tendency to form this kind of bond, which creates the species carbaminohemoglobin, $HbCO_2^-$. The transport of CO_2 from the cell into the blood stream is shown at the top of Figure 24–13. The movement of oxygen is also shown.

To complete the picture, oxyhemoglobin arrives in the tissues in its basic form, HbO_2^-, so that when it gives up oxygen it is in the basic form of hemoglobin, Hb^-. That base can then remove the proton from the carbonic acid provided by dissolved CO_2:

$$Hb^- + H_2CO_3 \longrightarrow HHb + HCO_3^-$$

This step provides a link between the CO_2 transfer process and that of oxygen.

Most comments related to what happens in the tissues apply in reverse to the process at the alveoli of the lungs. For example, there is a reverse chloride shift, this time from the red blood cells to the plasma to compensate for the movement of HCO_3^- ions into the red blood cells. The acidic form of oxyhemoglobin reacts with the bicarbonate in the red blood cell to produce the basic form and carbonic acid, which is transformed to the CO_2 that we exhale with every breath. The complete process is often called the **isohydric cycle** because it carries O_2 from the lungs to the tissues and CO_2 from the tissues to the lungs with no change in the overall pH of the blood.

The process shown in Figure 24–13 is complicated by the fact that other acids and bases present can neutralize HCO_3^- and H_2CO_3 or any of the hemoglobin forms. There may be numerous side reactions. Remember also that each hemoglobin (or oxyhemoglobin) molecule may actually have from one to four H's and we are intentionally simplifying the situation as much as possible.

The term *isohydric* comes from *iso* ("same") + *hydric* ("amount of hydrogen") and thus means "at constant pH."

Formation and destruction of red blood cells

Red blood cells are produced in the bone marrow, circulate for an average of four months, and are then destroyed and excreted. The heme portion of hemoglobin is made basically from two familiar compounds, acetic acid and glycine, mostly in the cell mitochondria.

As red blood cells get older, they become more fragile. A cell may rupture as it tries to squeeze through a very narrow capillary, especially in the spleen, an organ that stores and cleanses blood. Cells that break in the

FIGURE 24–13   Transport of gases and ions through capillary walls and red blood cell membranes in tissue (top) and the lungs (bottom). Chemical reactions are indicated by the thick black arrows and movement through fluids and across membranes by the thin arrows. The products of the reactions in the tissues ($HbCO_2^-$, HHb, HCO_3^-, and O_2) are the reactants in the alveoli of the lungs. The products of the lung reactions (HbO_2^-, Hb^-, and CO_2) are the reactants of the processes that take place in the tissues.

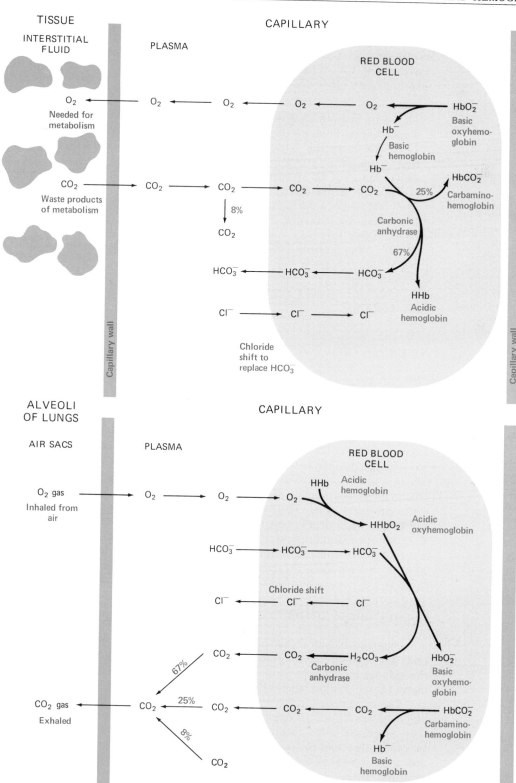

spleen are absorbed there by cells that also remove bacteria, parasites, and dirt from the blood. Similar cells are found in the liver. The Fe^{2+} from heme is released into the blood for possible use in new-cell production in the bone marrow. The rest of the heme is converted to a bile pigment, *bilirubin*, that combines with other substances.

SELF-CHECK

24.5) In Section 24.1 we discussed metabolic acidosis. What effect does acidosis have on the oxygen-carrying properties of hemoglobin?
24.6) Describe the major differences in the way O_2 and CO_2 are carried by the blood stream.
24.7) Why is CO_2 converted to bicarbonate ion in the red blood cells and not in the plasma?
24.8) How does the formation of basic oxyhemoglobin, HbO_2^-, in the lungs help the isohydric cycle?
24.9) What role does myoglobin play in the body?
24.10) Why is there a chloride shift if Cl^- plays no part in the chemistry of this chapter?

24.3 URINE

LEARNING GOAL 24I: Describe the role of the kidneys in regulating water balance to prevent edema.
24J: List three abnormal constituents of urine, and explain why each is significant.
24K: Describe the role of the kidneys in preventing metabolic acidosis.

The importance of the kidneys to the fluids of the body is shown by the fact that about one fourth as much blood passes through the kidneys each minute as passes through the heart! It is the job of the kidneys to remove the waste products of metabolism that are not excreted from the lungs or skin and to eliminate drugs, poisons, and excess water, acids, bases, and salts. The kidneys maintain fluid volume and normal osmotic pressures.

Just as we considered the diagnostic value of a blood test form (Figure 24-1) in Section 24.1, we can use a urinalysis form (Figure 24–14) as our guide to the normal and abnormal species found in the urine.

Formation of urine

TABLE 24–5 SOME SUBSTANCES NORMALLY FOUND IN URINE

IONS
Na$^+$ K$^+$ Ca^{2+}
Mg^{2+} NH$_4^+$ Cl$^-$
H$_2$PO$_4^-$ SO$_4^{2-}$

MOLECULES
Urea
Uric acid
Creatinine
Bile pigments

The liter of blood that passes through the kidneys every 50 or 60 seconds has been filtered to remove some of the waste products. It enters one of the kidneys through the kidney arteries and eventually finds its way through many of one million small filtering units called **nephrons** (Figure 24–15).

The most generally accepted theory for urine formation is as follows: As blood passes through a nephron, the plasma with its dissolved matter (other than proteins) filters through the capillary walls and enters excretory tubules. As this fluid passes down the tubules, a large proportion of the water and any substances useful to the body (such as glucose and amino acids) are returned to the blood stream. The waste products of metabolism, such as urea and uric acid, are only partially reabsorbed and continue down into collecting tubules for excretion. Thus, more material is filtered out at the start of the process than is actually lost from the blood stream at the end.

Some idea of the scale of this process may be gained from these daily values for a normal person: About 180 liters of water, 1000 g of NaCl, 170 g of glucose, and 360 g of $NaHCO_3$ are filtered through the kidneys. Slightly less water, 988 g of NaCl, 360 g of $NaHCO_3$, and 170 g of glucose are reabsorbed by the capillaries around the tubules. All of this is in order to excrete about 30 g of urea, 12 g of NaCl, and other waste products in 1.5 liters of urine. Table 24-5 lists some substances normally found in urine. The urea comes from the metabolism of proteins and the uric acid from purines.

Abnormal constituents of urine

Glucose

The concentration of glucose in the urine is normally so small that it will not give a positive test with Benedict's reagent (p. 498), Clinitest tablets, or a glucose test strip. Since routine examinations of urine always include a test for glucose, it may be useful to list the conditions that cause *glycosuria* (glucose in the urine). In addition to diabetes mellitus, the most common causes would be alimentary glycosuria (rapid excess ingestion of sugar, as by eating several candy bars in a short time) and emotional glycosuria (perhaps caused by fear of an extremely difficult examination for which you are not prepared). If a urine specimen is collected from a calm individual several hours after eating, alimentary and emotional glycosuria can be ruled out as reasons for a high glucose count. If large amounts of glucose are present in the urine at this time, diabetes mellitus is strongly suspected. Pregnant or nursing women sometimes excrete lactose in the urine, which gives a positive Benedict's test. Paper test strips that use *glucose oxidase* are specific for glucose

SPECIMEN/LAB. RPT. NO.

URINALYSIS

URGENCY	PATIENT STATUS
☑ ROUTINE	☑ BED ☐ AMB.
☐ TODAY ☑	☐ OUTPATIENT
☐ PRE-OP	☐ NP ☐ DOM.
☐ STAT	SPECIMEN SOURCE
	☐ ROUTINE
	☐ OTHER (Specify)

TEST(S)
SPECIMEN TAKEN

DATE 2/29/81	TIME 10 15 A.M. P.M.

RESULTS	REQUESTED	(X)
/////	ROUTINE	
Light	COLOR	
1.007	SPECIFIC GRAVITY	
	UROBILINOGEN	
negative	OCCULT BLOOD	
	BILE	
positive	KETONES	
positive	GLUCOSE	
negative	PROTEIN	
5.0	pH	
/////	MICROSCOPIC	
	WBC	
	RBC	
	EPITH. CELLS	
	WBC	C A S T S
	RBC	
	HYALINE	
	GRANULAR	
	BACTERIA	
	CRYSTALS	
	MUCUS	
	NITRITE	
	BENCE-JONES PROTEIN	
	HEMOSIDERIN	
	HCG	

URINALYSIS
Standard Form 550 (Rev. 4-77)
General Services Administration and Interagency
Committee on Medical Records FPMR 101-11.80F.8

FIGURE 24–14 Report form for urinalysis.

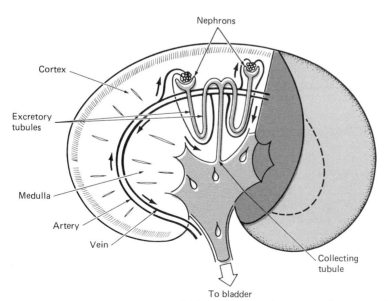

FIGURE 24–15 Diagram of a human kidney. Two nephrons are shown much enlarged. The direction of blood circulation is indicated by the arrows.

Labels: Nephrons, Cortex, Excretory tubules, Medulla, Artery, Vein, Collecting tubule, To bladder

and may be used to check for the excretion of glucose in these urine samples.

Protein

Normal urine does not contain protein because the nephrons do not permit these large molecules to filter into the urine. In cases of a kidney disease called *nephritis,* protein escapes from the blood into the urine and causes *proteinuria* (protein in the urine). Protein is sometimes found in the urine of a person who stands for several hours at a time (orthostatic proteinuria) or in the later stages of problem pregnancies. Paper test strips with the indicator *bromphenol blue* on their surface are used to test for the presence of protein in urine.

Acetone bodies

Acetone or *ketone bodies* (acetoacetic and β-hydroxybutyric acids and acetone) are formed in the liver and oxidized in the muscle tissue. In diabetes mellitus that is not properly controlled with insulin and in starvation or extreme dieting, these substances build up in the blood and are excreted by the kidneys.

Before excretion, the two acids must be neutralized by bases in the plasma. This may decrease the HCO_3^- level in the plasma and cause acidosis. To a limited extent, the tubular cells of the kidneys can use ammonia to excrete the acids as ammonium salts (NH_4^+ acetoacetate). Since a diabetic patient excretes acetone bodies in addition to glucose, a positive test for glucose and acetone bodies would tend to confirm the presence of the disease. A paper strip used to test for acetone bodies in the urine contains *sodium nitroprusside.*

Blood

The abnormal condition in which blood is present in the urine is called *hematuria* and can result from bleeding in the kidneys or in the urinary tract.

Any condition that causes hemolysis (swelling and bursting) of red blood cells, such as scurvy, extensive burns, or injection of hypotonic solutions, results in the excretion of hemoglobin and is known as *hemoglobinuria.* Fresh blood in the urine gives it a red color. Small amounts of blood or hemoglobin can be detected with a test strip similar to that used for glucose.

Bile or bilirubin

Bile or the pigment *bilirubin* may be found in the urine of patients with liver disease or with blockage of the bile duct (which goes from the liver to the small intestine). Normal urine does not contain either of these substances. There are special tablets (called *Ictotest,* from ''bile'' test) or test strips available to test urine for the presence of bile or bilirubin.

A urine specimen is often collected from a patient entering a hospital and is checked with a paper test strip containing spots of different reagents that will react with *all* the above abnormal constituents in one test. This simple procedure rapidly checks for indications of several disease processes.

Water balance and electrolytes

We have already discussed both the effect on oncotic pressure of high and low amounts of water in the body and the possible resultant edema or cell dehydration. The important hormone *vasopressin,* which triggers the sensation of thirst, also cuts down on urine production if the salt concentration (osmotic pressure) of the blood is high. This "fine control" of urine volume responds to changes in the osmotic pressure of blood plasma.

In a similar fashion, increase or decrease in urine production has a direct effect on electrolyte concentration. The excretion or retention of electrolytes will depend on the water balance.

Acid-base balance

In Chapter 12, p. 360, we considered some ion-exchange resins used to soften hard water. In a sophisticated laboratory demineralizer, even Na^+ ions can be removed by passing them through a column that exchanges them for hydrated H^+ ions. The kidneys can accomplish the same thing! The plasma contains HCO_3^- from the processes described in Section 24.2, plus large amounts of Na^+ ions. The urine in the tubules contains these ions, plus HPO_4^{2-} ion and many others. If the body loses too much bicarbonate ion, the system may become acidified. The kidney itself may add CO_2 (from its own metabolic reactions) to the blood or to the urine. If it adds the CO_2 to the urine, the urine becomes acidic (as it normally is) and there is no effect on the blood. However, if the CO_2 is changed (using carbonic anhydrase in the tubule cells) to H_2CO_3 and delivered to the blood, the blood is acidified and the acid-base balance is upset.

It is also possible for the kidney to return HCO_3^- to the blood by exchanging Na^+ ions for H^+ ions across the tubule walls. This process is called *acidifying the urine.* Instead of Na^+ ions going out in the urine and CO_2 in the blood (Figure 24–16), we end up with H^+ in the urine and Na^+ and HCO_3^- in the blood. This then provides another way for the body to control blood pH. At the same time, the sodium ion level can be controlled. The amount of sodium bicarbonate gained from the urine and reinserted into the blood may be as much as one pound per day.

On the other hand, the body may find itself short of base. The kidneys may respond as just described, or they may synthesize ammonia molecules. For example, in conditions of metabolic acidosis that might result from diabetes mellitus, acidic *acetone bodies* are produced. The bicarbonate ions in the blood stream neutralize these bodies, but once again the HCO_3^- can be replaced by carbon dioxide made in the kidneys.

However, that raises the problem of needing additional base. The kidney can synthesize the base NH_3 from glutamine or amino acids in the tubule cells, and the NH_3 can react with the acids to form NH_4^+ ions (Figure 24–16). The amount of NH_4^+ ion excreted by an average person on a normal diet is 0.030 to 0.070 moles/day. In conditions of severe metabolic acidosis, this may increase to over 0.200 moles/day.

Thus, you can see that the kidneys are definitely not simple organs of excretion. It has been said that what they retain is more important than what they eliminate from the body. When kidneys are severely injured, life is

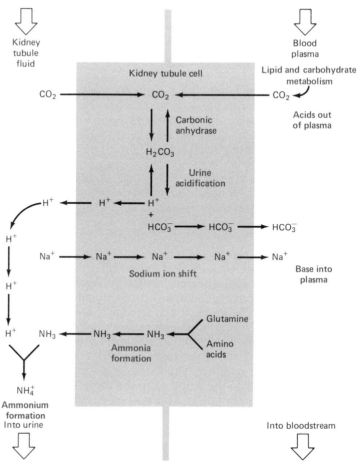

FIGURE 24–16 Kidney processes that help maintain acid-base balance in the body. Only the cations of the kidney tubule fluid are shown. Various anions are present, such as acetoacetate, hydrogen phosphate, and chloride. By the process of urine acidification, excess acids (in the form of CO_2) are removed from blood plasma and bases (HCO_3^-) are returned, while the hydrated H^+ ions proceed to the urine. The Na^+ ions must first pass from the tubule fluid into the cell to compensate for loss of positive ions (H^+) and then continue to accompany the HCO_3^- ions into the plasma to maintain electrical neutrality. The role of Na^+ in the kidneys is thus similar to the chloride shift shown in Figure 24–13.

threatened. Heavy-metal poisons, such as lead and mercury, may damage blood vessels and tubules. Some infections, metabolic diseases, and heart disease may also cause the tubules to stop functioning and allow too much of the filtered material to seep back into the blood.

In cases of nonfunctioning kidneys, the patient must use external hemodialysis to remove waste materials from the blood, as shown in Figure 12–23.

SELF-CHECK

24.11) List two ways in which the kidneys will respond to the imbalance created when a person drinks water containing dissolved NaCl.
24.12) If albumin protein is found in a patient's urine, what dysfunction might be present?

24.13)   How do the kidneys prevent all of the bicarbonate ion from being excreted from the body?

24.4 INSIDE THE CELL

LEARNING GOAL 24L: Describe the most important differences in composition between intracellular fluid and blood plasma.

We mentioned earlier that all body fluids are ultimately made from and related to blood plasma. Figure 24–17 shows the organs that transfer materials into and out of the body fluids, along with the ways in which the various fluids are related to each other. In this section, we will be concerned mainly with the activities shown in the bottom part of Figure 24–17, those inside the cell. First, however, let us summarize some of the very general details about body fluids that relate all the parts of Figure 24–17.

Water balance

If water balance is to be maintained in the body, fluid intake and excretion must be equal. The gain and loss of water for a normal adult of average

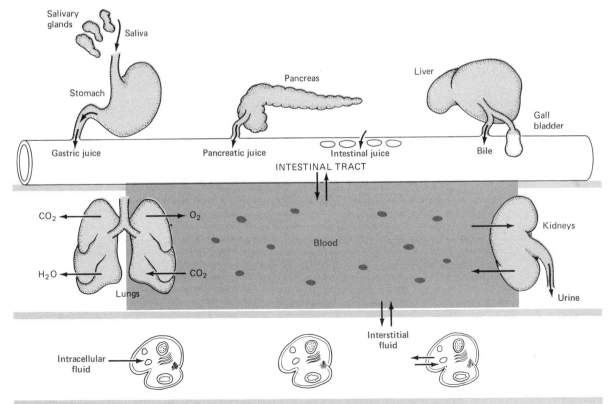

FIGURE 24–17   Some fluids and organs of importance to the metabolic processes in the human body. The fluids are named in color.

Average Intake in Liters/day	
In beverages	1.20
In food	1.50
From cell metabolism	0.30
Water gain	3.00

Average Output in Liters/day	
Evaporation from lungs	0.70
Evaporation from skin	0.30
Perspiration	0.30
In feces	0.20
In urine	1.50
Water loss	3.00

TABLE 24-7 DAILY FORMATION OF DIGESTIVE FLUIDS BY THE BODY

Fluid	Liters Formed Per Day
Saliva	1.50
Gastric fluid	2.50
Pancreatic and intestinal fluid	4.00
Liver bile	0.50
Total	8.50

(Compare with the total plasma volume of 3.50 liters!)

size is shown in Table 24–6, which shows that about three liters per day goes into and out of the body. There are about 50 liters of fluid in the body at any one time. Some of it is always in the process of being converted to digestive fluids (Table 24–7), which will be discussed in Section 25.1. These fluids are continually recycled.

As a general rule, if fluid intake is greater than fluid excretion for any significant length of time, edema (fluid retention in tissues) will result. This is often a problem for pregnant women and people with certain types of hormonal imbalances. Excessive loss of body fluid leads to dehydration of the body. Many people on "crash" diets are delighted to find an immediate drop in weight. This initial drop is due to loss of water from the body, not to any decrease in fat! By drinking less fluid than usual, the dieter has caused some

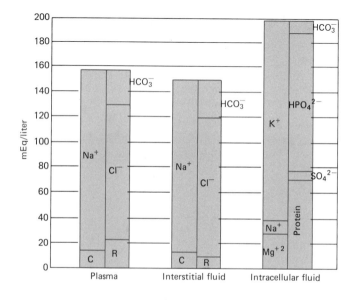

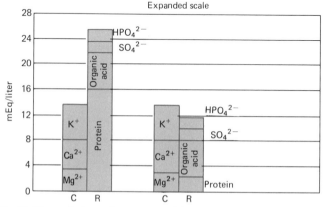

FIGURE 24–18 Normal electrolyte composition of some body fluids. The expanded scale shows the concentrations of the electrolytes in the bar regions marked "C" and "R." On a bar graph, you read a concentration by noting how far up the scale a particular bar extends. For example, in the interstitial fluid, the bar marked HCO_3^- extends from the 120-mEq/liter line up to the 150-mEq/liter position. We would therefore interpret the concentration of bicarbonate ion in normal interstitial fluid as being approximately $150 - 120 = 30$ mEq/liter.

dehydration. Since water alone represents more than half your weight, the results can seem significant.

Intracellular fluid

We discussed the intracellular fluid, the cytoplasm, briefly in Section 20.1. Because so many particles of widely varying sizes are dissolved, dispersed, or suspended in the cytoplasm, it behaves not like a simple solution but like a colloid. The portion immediately below the cell membrane is a semisolid *gel* (p. 344), while the rest of the cytoplasm is a *sol* and behaves like a liquid. If we look at the chemical composition of the sol section of the cytoplasm, we find it quite different from that shown in Table 24–2. Figure 24–18 compares plasma, interstitial fluid, and cytoplasm.

To summarize some of the major differences:

	In Extracellular Fluid (*Blood Plasma*)	In Intracellular Fluid (*Cytoplasm*)
Cations:	Almost entirely Na^+	Mostly K^+; relatively little Na^+; more Mg^{2+}
Anions:	Mostly Cl^-, some HCO_3^-	Essentially no Cl^-; considerable HPO_4^- and protein anions

In some cases, the reasons for these differences are obvious. The high HPO_4^- level inside a cell is related to the phosphate group transfer processes discussed in Section 22.1. The Mg^{2+} ion is an essential part of many enzymes inside the cell.

The differences between the Na^+ concentration (high outside the cell) and the K^+ concentration (high inside the cell) are created by the active transport system (Na^+/K^+ pump) described on p. 523. This difference creates an electrical ''potential'' across cell membranes that may be needed by all cells and is required for the normal functioning of muscle and nerve cells.

The functions of the intracellular fluid are similar to those of blood plasma and other body fluids. It must carry raw materials and waste products where they need to go, while providing an environment in which the chemical reactions can best be carried out.

24.14) One Group 1 cation and one Group 2 cation are present in much higher concentrations in the cytoplasm than in blood plasma. Name these two ions.

SELF-CHECK

CHAPTER TWENTY-FOUR IN REVIEW ■ Fluids of the Human Body

24.1 BLOOD   Page 645

24A: List five important functions of blood, and indicate which part of the blood performs each function.
24B: Describe how blood can be prevented from clotting.
24C: Describe how water and nutrients move between capillaries and the interstitial fluid.

24D: Describe the causes of metabolic acidosis and metabolic alkalosis.

24.2 RESPIRATION AND HEMOGLOBIN   Page 656

24E: Describe how O_2 is carried from the lungs to the cells and how CO_2 is transported from the cells to the lungs.

24F: Describe how hemoglobin can deliver varying amounts of oxygen to the cells depending on the blood pH (Bohr effect).

24G: Describe how hemoglobin can act as a buffer, and explain the chloride shift.

24H: Describe the role of myoglobin in storing oxygen.

24.3 URINE   Page 666

24I: Describe the role of the kidneys in regulating water balance to prevent edema.

24J: List three abnormal constituents of urine, and explain why each is significant.

24K: Describe the role of the kidneys in preventing metabolic acidosis.

24.4 INSIDE THE CELL   Page 671

24L: Describe the most important differences in composition between intracellular fluid and blood plasma.

GLOSSARY FOR CHAPTER TWENTY-FOUR

acid-base balance The maintenance of the normal pH of the blood by the combined action of the lungs, kidneys, and body fluid buffers. (p. 655)

blood A fluid, the primary transport system of the body, containing blood cells suspended in plasma. (p. 646)

electrolyte balance The normal concentrations of the positively charged cations and negatively charged anions in the plasma. (p. 654)

extracellular fluids Body fluids outside cells, such as blood, plasma, lymph, spinal fluid, digestive juices, bile, and urine. (p. 645)

hemoglobin The respiratory compound of red blood cells; a molecule containing four polypeptide chains and four heme units. (p. 657)

interstitial fluid The fluid, similar to blood plasma, that lies outside the cells; tissue fluid; has the same composition as lymph. (p. 645)

isohydric cycle The process of transporting O_2 and CO_2 between the lungs and tissues with little change in blood pH. (p. 664)

metabolic acidosis A condition caused by the increased production of acids; may occur in diabetes mellitus and starvation. (p. 655)

metabolic alkalosis An alkaline condition caused by persistent vomiting or excessive use of antacids. (p. 655)

myoglobin A heme-containing protein in muscle tissue; stores oxygen. (p. 662)

nephron The filtration unit of the kidney; important in urine formation. (p. 666)

oncotic pressure The extra osmotic pressure of the plasma proteins; pulls water into the capillaries from the spaces between cells. (p. 652)

plasma The fluid portion of the blood, containing proteins and the clotting factors but no cells. (p. 650)

plasma proteins A mixture of proteins, consisting of albumins, several globulins, and fibrinogen. (p. 650)

QUESTIONS AND PROBLEMS FOR CHAPTER TWENTY-FOUR ■

Fluids of the Human Body

SECTION 24.1 BLOOD

24.15) What two major types of cells are found in blood? What is the function of each?

24.16) Name two common causes of edema in the body.

24.17) What is the effect on blood clotting of Ca^{2+} deficiency in the blood stream?

24.18) What makes water and nutrients pass from the plasma into the interstitial fluid at the arterial end of a capillary?

24.19) What would happen to the acid-base balance of a sick child who vomited all meals?

SECTION 24.2 RESPIRATION AND HEMOGLOBIN

24.20) Describe in general fashion how O_2 is carried to the tissues.

24.21) How does acidosis affect the oxygen-carrying capacity of hemoglobin? Explain the effect on body cells.

24.22) Oxyhemoglobin is found in two forms, basic and acidic. Why?

24.23) In which direction does Cl^- move in the tissues? Explain.

24.24) Why do muscles need a way of storing oxygen?

24.25*) If the blood did not contain red blood cells, how would the O_2 and CO_2 transport be affected?

SECTION 24.3 URINE

24.26) What will the kidneys do if you drink a tremendous amount of fluid?

24.27) Plasma proteins are found in the urine of an alcoholic hospital patient. What might this mean?

24.28*) What general method is used to detect proteins in urine?

24.34) Some compounds, such as fats and fatty acids, are insoluble in blood plasma. How does the blood transport these compounds to tissues?

24.35) The "48-hour flu" accompanied by diarrhea may cause dehydration if you do not consume adequate amounts of liquids. Explain.

24.36) Under what circumstances might a doctor prescribe an anticoagulant?

24.37) What makes water and the waste products of metabolism pass from interstitial fluid into plasma at the venous end of a capillary?

24.38) An overweight student eats nothing for three days. What happens to the acid-base balance? Are fasting diets wise?

24.39) Describe in general fashion the most important mechanism for transporting CO_2 from the tissues to the lungs.

24.40) How does alkalosis affect the oxygen-carrying capacity of hemoglobin? Explain the effect on body cells.

24.41) Hemoglobin is found in its basic form in arterial blood. Why?

24.42) In which direction does Cl^- ion move in the lungs? Explain.

24.43) What method is used for storing oxygen in muscle tissue?

24.44*) What happens to the O_2-carrying capacity of the blood in victims of sickle cell anemia? Explain.

24.45) What will the kidneys do if you drink nothing for a day?

24.46) Glucose is found in the urine of a child who just played in a championship Little League game. What might this mean?

24.47*) What general method is used to detect glucose in urine?

24.29) How may the kidneys respond to an alkaline condition of the blood plasma caused by an overuse of antacids?

24.30*) In cases of severe shock, the kidneys may stop functioning for a full day. What will happen to the water balance in the body?

SECTION 24.4 INSIDE THE CELL

24.31) What are the major differences between the concentration of anions in blood plasma and in the cytoplasm?

24.32*) Give one reason why there might be higher concentrations of HCO_3^- in blood plasma than inside the cell.

24.33*) Digestive fluids (Table 24–7) are recycled each day. What would be the effect on water intake if we had to replace the amount used daily in manufacturing saliva, stomach fluids, bile, and intestinal fluids?

24.48) How may the kidneys respond to the production of ketone bodies in cases of diabetes mellitus?

24.49*) After a beer-drinking contest, the electrolyte content of a drinker's urine changes. Why? (Note: alcohol tends to stimulate urine production even further.)

24.50) What are the major differences between the amount of protein anions in blood plasma and in the cytoplasm? In which of these fluids might proteins play an important role in pH buffering?

24.51*) Give one reason why there might be higher concentrations of Ca^{2+} cation in blood plasma than inside the cell.

24.52*) After three sets of tennis in sunny hot weather, what might temporarily happen to a player's water balance? What might be the remedy? (Gatorade?)

Synthetic blood has, in fact, been used as a temporary measure to save the lives of people who refused transfusions of human blood for religious reasons. These fluorocarbons could also be of immense value in emergencies when a needed blood type for transfusion is not available, and possibly in cases of aplastic anemia. In a highly dramatic experiment, Dr. Leland Clark once prepared a fluorocarbon liquid with dissolved oxygen and immersed mice in it for one hour. The mice survived and remained healthy.

24.53*) Since they carry oxygen, certain fluorocarbons similar to freons (p. 110), but with long chains or large rings of —CF_2—linkages, have been tested for use as synthetic red blood cells. These compounds can absorb and release O_2 and CO_2 as much as 15 times as well as can blood plasma.

What functions are fulfilled by hemoglobin which would *not* be served by these synthetic fluids?

24.54*) How could a normal person develop a mild condition of metabolic acidosis?

24.55*) Why would a diabetic person tend to excrete more ammonia in the urine than a normal person?

24.56*) The average composition of sea water at 25°C is as follows:

Cations	Anions
Na^+ 0.457 M	Cl^- 0.533 M
Mg^{2+} 0.052 M	SO_4^{2-} 0.028 M
Ca^{2+} 0.010 M	HCO_3^- 0.002 M
K^+ 0.010 M	Br^- 0.001 M

plus many other substances at lower concentrations. Considering only the above major constituents of sea water and using information from this chapter:
a) Does sea water most resemble blood plasma or cytoplasm?
b) Are there any major constituents of body fluids that are absent from sea water? Are there any major ions in sea water that are not found in body fluids?
c) How would you respond to the suggestion, made by many biologists, that the similarity in composition between sea water and body fluids is evidence that all life on earth is descended from single-cell organisms that lived in the sea hundreds of millions of years ago? (There is no "right" or "wrong" answer to this question.)

Carbohydrate Metabolism 25

In this chapter, we begin a detailed discussion of the manner in which nutrients are converted to substances useful to the body. We usually call these processes and those of Chapter 22 the *metabolism* of carbohydrates, lipids, and proteins. One simple definition of metabolism might be **"all of the enzyme-controlled reactions occurring in the living cell."** This is a very general definition that includes thousands of different processes. The word *metabolism* thus really means "biochemical reaction."

In Section 25.1 we will subdivide cell reactions into meaningful types. The remainder of the chapter will consider the reactions that convert carbohydrates to glucose, glycogen, and energy.

While you are reading Chapters 25, 26, and 27, remember that one of the most important aspects of metabolic reactions is their *interrelationships*. The body is kept in balance by many systems of regulation and control, which we will refer to at various points.

25.1 PREVIEW OF METABOLISM

LEARNING GOAL 25A: *Describe the difference between anabolism and catabolism.*

25B: *Describe what happens to food components at each major stage of digestion.*

The biochemical reactions of the cell, **metabolism,** may be divided into **anabolism,** those reactions that build up (synthesize) more complex molecules from simple nutrients, and **catabolism,** the breaking down or degrading processes that convert large molecules to small molecules and energy. Anabolism is thus *con*struction of large molecules, and catabolism is their *de*struction. A metabolite is simply a product of any of these reactions.

Digestion

The chemical compounds needed by the cell are taken in by the body as large molecules of food. Figure 25–1 shows the regions of the human digestive tract, which can be summarized as follows:

1) The *mouth* receives and chews food.
2) The *esophagus* carries the food to the stomach.

677

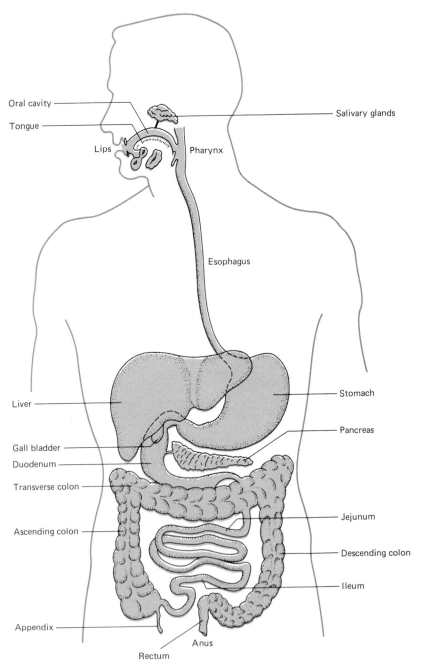

Oral cavity

Tongue

Lips

Pharynx

Salivary glands

Esophagus

Liver

Stomach

Pancreas

Gall bladder

Duodenum

Transverse colon

Jejunum

Ascending colon

Descending colon

Ileum

Appendix

Anus

Rectum

FIGURE 25–1   The human digestive system.

3)   The *stomach* liquifies the food and begins digestion.
4)   The *small intestine* does the major job of breaking down the food molecules into smaller units, which can then be absorbed into the blood stream.
5)   The *large intestine* removes water and forms the feces from waste food matter.

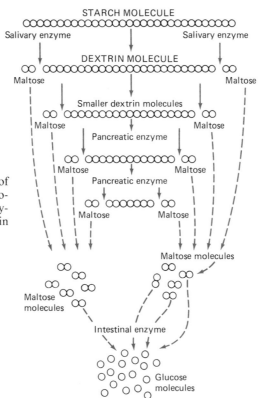

STARCH MOLECULE

Salivary enzyme   Salivary enzyme

DEXTRIN MOLECULE

Maltose   Maltose

Smaller dextrin molecules

Maltose   Maltose

Pancreatic enzyme

Maltose   Maltose

Pancreatic enzyme

Maltose   Maltose

Maltose molecules

Maltose
molecules

Intestinal enzyme

Glucose
molecules

FIGURE 25–2 The digestion of starch involves hydrolysis, producing smaller and smaller carbohydrate molecules. The end product in the intestine is glucose.

Recall that the bonds in protein are peptide bonds, created by the splitting out of water (Section 19.2). Starch, a typical carbohydrate, is a polysaccharide chain of glucose units, as described in Section 17.5, with water having been split out at each connection. A fat is an ester of a fatty acid and glycerol (Section 18.1), again water having been split out when the ester linkage was formed. Thus, all three kinds of food macromolecules—proteins, carbohydrates, and fats—are formed by the loss of water.

All of these condensation reactions can be reversed under the right conditions. To reverse them, that is, to break down the large molecules into small ones (amino acids, hexoses, and fatty acids), we must add water to each kind of linkage (peptide, acetal, or ester). The digestive enzymes (Table 21.7, p. 588) are thus *hydrolases* (hydrolytic enzymes) because they speed up the hydrolysis of food in the process of **digestion.** The end products of digestion then move across the intestinal lining into the blood stream, a process called **intestinal absorption.** Following this process, the blood stream carries the amino acids, hexoses, and lipids to the tissues.

As soon as food is received by the mouth, it comes into contact with *saliva,* which contains mucus to lubricate food and an enzyme, amylase, to hydrolyze starches. About 1.5 liters of saliva are secreted each day.

When food is swallowed, it passes through the esophagus into the stomach. The glands in the stomach wall secrete about 2.5 liters each day of a solution that is $0.160 M$ in hydrochloric acid. The pH of this solution is 0.8, and it is isotonic (Section 12.5) with other body fluids. Other secretions, food, and mucus then dilute this stomach acid to an average concentration of about $0.02 M$ (pH 1.6 to 1.8). This acidity is important because it destroys many harmful bacteria and thus protects the body. The first protease (peptide-linkage-splitting enzyme), *pepsin*, works in the stomach and functions best at acidic pH levels, as shown in Figure 23–7 (p. 626).

The mixing action of the stomach muscles produces a liquid called *chyme*, which passes very slowly into the small intestine. When this liquid hits the duodenum, the first part of the small intestine, it triggers the secretion of several hormones that stimulate the flow of *pancreatic juice, intestinal juice,* and *bile*. These three fluids are all basic. The intestinal enzymes all work best in a basic environment having an average pH of about 8.0.

The pancreatic and intestinal juices contain hydrolytic enzymes, such as amylopsin (which breaks starch down to maltose, as shown in Figure 25–2), as well as sucrase, lactase, and maltase, which break disaccharides down to hexoses. The hexose molecules can pass through the intestinal lining into the blood stream.

The function of **bile** is not to digest food, since it has no enzymes, but to emulsify fats with bile salts as described in Sections 12.1 and 18.4. It thus allows *lipase* to work directly on dietary fats. Table 25–1 summarizes the processes we have just discussed.

Intermediary metabolism

Figure 25–3 gives an overview of metabolism in the body, beginning with digestion. If you follow the middle of the diagram from polysaccharides down through pyruvate to oxaloacetate, you see the familiar processes of glycolysis (Section 22.2) and the Krebs cycle (Section 22.3). The lipids are converted in digestion to fatty acids and glycerol; the fatty acids then can enter the Krebs cycle as described in Chapter 26. Proteins are broken down to amino acids and similarly enter metabolic cycles described in Chapter 27. Both fatty acids and amino acids can, in fact, form acetyl coenzyme A and enter the Krebs cycle. These are the processes we call *catabolism*.

The arrows pointing the way back to lipids, polysaccharides, and proteins indicate the biosynthesis (*anabolism*) of large molecules in the body, which we will study in Chapters 25 to 27.

Recall that ATP and several coenzymes are extremely important for the Krebs cycle and the electron transport system (Sections 22.3 and 22.4).

TABLE 25–1 SUMMARY OF DIGESTION

Substrate	Enzyme	Final Products Formed
Starch	Salivary amylase (ptyalin)	Dextrins, maltose
Glycogen	Pancreatic amylase	Maltose
Disaccharides		Monosaccharides
Maltose	Maltase	Glucose
Sucrose	Sucrase (invertase)	Glucose and fructose
Lactose	Lactase	Glucose and galactose
Protein	Pepsins (gastric)	Polypeptides
Protein and polypeptides	Trypsin (pancreatic)	Small polypeptides
	Chymotrypsin (pancreatic)	Small polypeptides and
	Carboxypeptidase (pancreatic)	Amino acids
	Aminopeptidase (intestinal)	
Dipeptides	Intestinal dipeptidases	Amino acids
Fats emulsified with bile	Pancreatic lipase	Mono- and diglycerides, fatty acids
Monoglycerides	Intestinal lipase	Glycerol and fatty acids

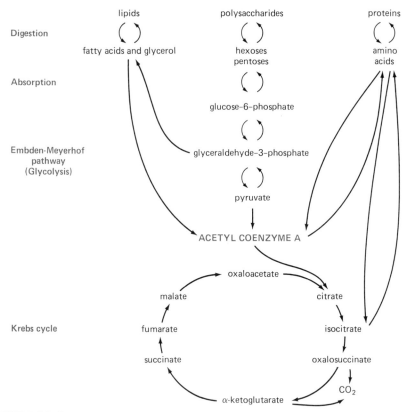

FIGURE 25–3   An overview of intermediary metabolism, stressing the interrelationships of the various processes.

Changes in ATP concentration in the cell can thus speed up or slow down the rate of metabolism simply by supplying more or fewer molecules to the coupled reactions of Figures 22–7 and 22–8. This role in regulating metabolic processes is shown in Figure 25–4.

We discussed briefly in Section 23.2 how enzymes may be inhibited by the products of a reaction. Sometimes the final product of a series of reactions may inhibit the enzyme catalyzing the first reaction in the series. This process is called *negative feedback,* and it cuts off further formation of product if there is a product surplus in the cell. There are several other sources of regulation and control; especially important are *hormones* (next section).

SELF-CHECK

25.1)   How does anabolism differ from catabolism?
25.2)   What is the role of the stomach in digestion?
25.3*)   What well-known coenzyme is common to the metabolism of lipids, carbohydrates, and proteins?

25.2   HORMONES AND THE BLOOD SUGAR LEVEL

LEARNING GOAL 25C: Outline the processes involved in returning the blood sugar level to normal after a meal.

> *25D: Explain how insulin lowers the blood sugar level.*
> *25E: Describe what happens to the hormone balance in a patient with diabetes mellitus.*

After the monosaccharide end products of carbohydrate digestion are absorbed into the blood stream, they are carried to the liver. The metabolism of carbohydrates is essentially the metabolism of glucose.

The concentration of glucose in the blood 6 to 12 hours after a meal is 70 to 90 mg/dL, which is considered the *normal fasting* **blood sugar level.** After a meal containing carbohydrates, the glucose content of the blood increases, causing a temporary condition of **hyperglycemia** (high amounts of glucose in the blood). In cases of severe exercise or prolonged starvation, the blood sugar value may fall below the normal fasting level, resulting in a mild **hypoglycemia** (lower-than-normal levels of glucose in the blood).

After an ordinary meal or several candy bars, the glucose in the blood reaches hyperglycemic levels (Figure 25–5). The glucose level is then brought back to normal by the following processes:

> One deciliter = $^1/_{10}$ liter = 100 milliliters. Although mg/dL may seem awkward, it is the standard unit for reporting glucose level in the blood. A normal concentration of 90 mg/dL corresponds to 0.90 g of glucose per liter, or 0.0050 moles/liter.

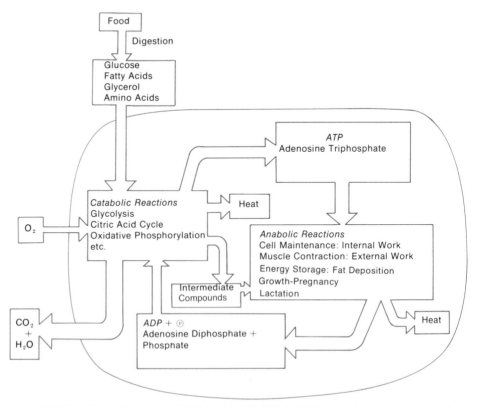

FIGURE 25–4   The role of ATP in the cell. While ATP provides energy by coupling with many cell reactions, the rate of production of ATP can be controlled in order to regulate the speed of metabolic processes. Catabolic reactions, those that release energy to form the high-energy bonds of ATP, were discussed in Chapter 22. The ATP then carries that energy to fuel the body's anabolic reactions. Heat is a necessary by-product of metabolism, since the body is not 100% efficient.

1) Storage as glycogen or fat.
2) Oxidation by tissues to produce energy.
3) Excretion by the kidneys (only occurs at very high glucose levels).

In an effort to bring the glucose concentration back to normal, the liver removes glucose from the blood stream and converts it to glycogen for storage. The muscles also take glucose from the blood and convert it to glycogen or oxidize it to produce energy. If the sugar intake is high, the glucose may be converted to fat and stored in the fat depots. These processes usually control hyperglycemia, but if the blood sugar level rises above about 160 mg/dL, the excess is excreted by the kidneys and *glucosuria* (glucose in the urine) occurs. The blood sugar level at which the kidney starts excreting glucose is known as the *renal threshold* and has a value of 150 to 170 mg/dL.

Hormones that control the blood sugar level

In addition to the above factors, there are specific reactions of the liver (and several hormones) to help control the blood sugar level. The liver is a marvelous organ, the site of many important metabolic reactions that can remove or add glucose to the blood to keep the level normal.

During periods of hyperglycemia, the liver stops pouring sugar into the blood stream and starts storing it as liver glycogen. Between meals the liver supplies glucose to the blood by breaking down its glycogen and by forming glucose from other food materials, such as amino acids or glycerol.

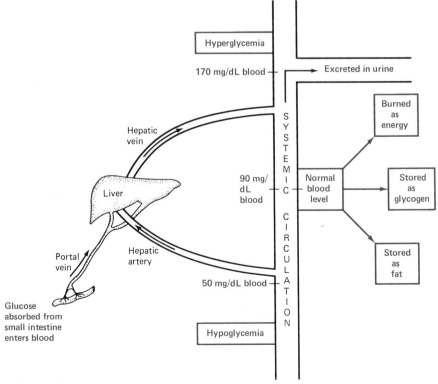

FIGURE 25–5 Factors affecting the glucose concentration in the blood plasma.

There are several hormones that assist the liver in this control process. In the regulation of body processes, a single hormone probably has control over several reactions. Essential cell processes generally depend on the balanced action of more than one hormone. A disturbance in this *hormone balance* can result in diseases such as diabetes.

Insulin

Diabetes mellitus, or sugar diabetes, which usually occurs when the body cannot produce sufficient amounts of insulin, has been recognized in humans for over 100 years. As early as 1889 it was demonstrated that removal of the pancreas of an animal would result in diabetes mellitus. In 1922 Fredrick Banting and Charles Best developed a method for obtaining active extracts from the pancreas. **Insulin** was isolated from these extracts and soon became available for the treatment of diabetes.

The insulin molecule consists of two polypeptide chains and has a molecular weight of 6000 amu (Figure 19–4). The molecule synthesized by the *islet cells* of the pancreas is a long single-chain polypeptide called *proinsulin*. Since insulin is a protein, it is not effective when taken by mouth, because the enzymes of the gastrointestinal tract would hydrolyze it to amino acids. Insulin given to a diabetic is thus usually injected under the skin.

There are two major types of diabetes. The more serious is the juvenile-onset type, where the pancreas does not produce sufficient insulin to control glucose. The more common type is the maturity-onset diabetes, which occurs in older people and in overweight individuals. The younger person with diabetes requires daily injections of insulin and often shows great variation in blood sugar levels during any 24-hour period. As the young diabetic grows older, the eyes, kidneys, and circulatory system all show abnormalities. Blindness may occur from diabetic retinopathy (a disease of the retina of the eye). Heart disease and strokes may occur because the arteries become clogged with cholesterol plaques (arteriosclerosis).

Many efforts are being made to help diabetics control this disease. Normal islet cells from a healthy pancreas may be injected into the blood stream of a diabetic and may attach themselves to tissues in the body and start producing insulin to help the abnormal pancreas. Small mechanical pumps containing insulin are being experimentally implanted (like pacemakers for the heart) so controlled bursts of insulin can be used to help control the blood sugar level. There are oral insulin substitutes that often help the maturity-onset diabetic who may need just a little additional insulin action to keep the blood sugar under control. Planned diets will also help diabetics, especially those that are grossly overweight.

Insulin lowers the blood sugar level by increasing the rate at which glucose is converted to liver and muscle glycogen, by regulating the oxidation of glucose in tissues, and by blocking the breakdown of liver glycogen to glucose. In muscle and adipose tissue (fat deposits), insulin increases the rate of transport of glucose across membranes into the cells. In liver tissue, insulin controls the phosphorylation of glucose to form glucose-6-phosphate, which is the first step in glycolysis and in the formation of glycogen.

Glucagon

The hormone *glucagon* is produced by the *alpha cells* of the pancreas. It is a polypeptide of known amino acid sequence with a molecular weight of

Proinsulin must be converted to insulin before it can act as a hormone, just as proenzymes must be converted to enzymes (p. 632)

At least 8.5 million Americans have diabetes. The average diabetic spends about $2500 per year for insulin. There is a real possibility, however, that this cost may soon be lowered by use of insulin manufactured by bacteria whose genetic material has been specifically altered to produce human insulin. Small amounts of active insulin have already been produced by this method, discussed in Chapter 28.

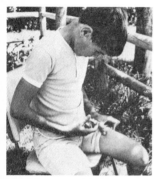

This diabetic boy has learned to give himself hypodermic injections of insulin. (Photo by Michal Heron)

about 3500 amu. Glucagon secretion causes a rise in the blood sugar level by increasing the activity of the enzyme *liver phosphorylase,* which functions in the conversion of liver glycogen to free glucose.

Epinephrine

A hormone produced by the central portion (medulla) of the adrenal glands (Figure 18–10), **epinephrine** counteracts the action of insulin in that it causes the breakdown of liver glycogen with the liberation of glucose. Secretion of epinephrine (adrenalin) occurs when a person feels such strong emotions as fear or anger. This mechanism is often used by the body as an emergency way to provide instant glucose for muscular work. Amazing feats of strength, like lifting a car off an accident victim, have been demonstrated by normal people in an emergency. The hyperglycemia that results from the secretion of epinephrine often exceeds the renal threshold, so glucose is excreted in the urine (glycosuria). Indeed, there have been college examinations so difficult that some students exhibited glycosuria!*

Adrenal Cortical Hormones

Hormones such as *cortisone* and *cortisol* are produced by the outer layer or cortex of the adrenal gland. These hormones stimulate the production of glucose in the liver by increasing the formation of glucose from amino acids. The cortical hormones therefore also counteract the effects of insulin.

Anterior pituitary hormones

Of the many hormones secreted by the anterior lobe of the pituitary gland, two—the growth hormone and ACTH—affect the blood sugar level. The action of the growth hormone is not completely understood. One of its effects is to stimulate the formation of glucagon by the pancreas. ACTH stimulates production of the adrenal hormones, such as epinephrine.

Figure 25–6 shows the very complicated interrelationships among the various hormones that affect blood sugar level. It also illustrates the fact that hormones can shift the body toward or away from the metabolism of glucose and stimulate or block the metabolism of lipids and amino acids.

The action of hormones in the body

You have now seen how hormones act to regulate one of the many types of metabolic processes. We first discussed hormones in Chapter 18, where the *steroids,* such as sex hormones and cortical hormones, were studied.

---

* Because so many different factors can influence the blood glucose level, people should be hesitant to suppose that something is seriously wrong if an abnormal blood sugar level is obtained during a single glucose tolerance test. Some physicians have been perhaps too quick to diagnose "hypoglycemia" in patients who were not really suffering from a disease but rather were in a "swing" of a hormonal cycle. Health food advocates have also tended to blame a variety of ills on "low blood sugar." The April 1979 issue of *Prevention* magazine claims that "an estimated 50 million Americans suffer from hypoglycemia." In fact, functional hypoglycemia is quite rare and can only be diagnosed if the blood sugar level falls below 45 mg/dL. See *Health Quackery,* Consumers Union of the United States, 1980, Chapter 4, "Low Blood Sugar: Fiction and Fact."

FIGURE 25–6 The hormonal regulation of blood sugar levels. When insulin is deficient, the blood glucose level increases, "spilling over" into the urine. Cortisone, glucagon, and thyroxin stimulate the breakdown of proteins and fat tissue to release fatty acids for oxidation as energy sources. The same hormones also stimulate conversion of the released amino acids to glucose in the liver. While insulin is clearly the key hormone in regulating blood sugar level, the overall process is controlled by a balance of several hormones.

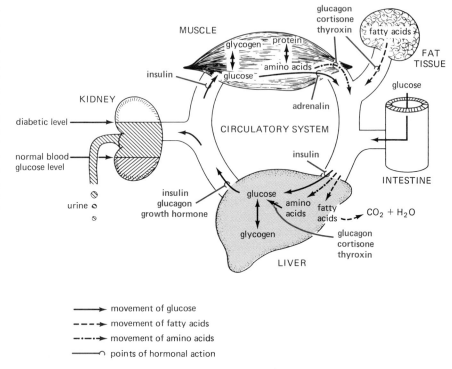

Figure 18–10 shows the locations of the hormone-producing or *endocrine* glands in the body. Table 25–2 lists the most important hormones and gives you some indication of their roles.

As we discussed the role of the nucleotide AMP (p. 598), we noted that another form of this compound exists. *Cyclic AMP* is called an intracellular hormonal *mediator* because it is formed from ATP inside a cell each time certain hormones exert their influence. This cyclic AMP remains in the cell and performs any of several functions, depending on the nature of the cell:

1) Cyclic AMP can activate enzymes from proenzymes.
2) It can make it easier for substances to pass through cell membranes.
3) It can cause smooth muscle to expand or contract.
4) It can activate protein synthesis.
5) It can cause the secretion of fluids by the cell.

In this manner, cyclic AMP can apparently "carry out the commands" issued by the original hormone.

A second important hormone action is to trigger the synthesis of certain specific proteins in "target" cells by stimulating the formation of the appropriate messenger RNA molecules. This process is called "activation of genes."

SELF-CHECK

25.4) Is hyperglycemia ever found in a normal person? Explain.

25.5) If there is too much insulin, what happens to the blood sugar level? What term is used to describe the result? Is this a *condition* or a *disease?*

25.6) What hormone is specifically lacking in cases of diabetes? Is there any other hormone in the body that can take over and do its work?

TABLE 25–2   SOME IMPORTANT HORMONES
AND THEIR PRINCIPAL EFFECTS

Hormone	Gland	Major Actions
Melatonin	Pineal	Inhibits ovaries; may regulate day-night cycle
ACTH	Anterior pituitary	Stimulates adrenal cortex to produce hormones (cortisol)
Prolactin		Stimulates breast development and milk production
Growth hormone		Stimulates growth of all body cells; increases protein synthesis, fat usage, and blood sugar level
Gonadotropic Thyrotropic		Stimulate thyroid and gonads to produce hormones
Oxytocin	Posterior pituitary	Stimulates uterus contraction
Vasopressin		Causes thirst in order to increase blood volume; acts to retain water in kidneys
Thyroxine	Thyroid	Stimulates cell respiration and protein synthesis
Calcitonin		Moves Ca^{2+} from blood stream and deposits it in bone
Parathormone	Parathyroid	Regulates phosphorus and Ca^{2+} metabolism
Aldosterone	Adrenal cortex	Stimulates recovery of Na^+ and Cl^- and excretion of K^+ from kidney
Cortisol		Increases blood sugar level and formation of glucose from amino acids and liver protein
Epinephrine (adrenalin)	Adrenal medulla	Produces "fight or flight" response; increases blood sugar level
Glucagon	Pancreas (alpha)	Stimulates conversion of liver glycogen to glucose; raises blood sugar level
Insulin	Pancreas (beta)	Stimulates use and storage of glucose; lowers blood sugar level
Estrogen Progesterone Testosterone	Ovaries or testes and adrenal cortex	Stimulate development and maintenance of sex characteristics and behavior
Gastrin Secretin Cholecystokinin	Digestive system Mucous membranes	Stimulate release of digestive fluids and enzymes

25.3 THE ROLE OF GLYCOGEN

> *LEARNING GOAL 25F: Explain why liver glycogen is important in controlling the blood sugar level.*
> *25G: Describe the importance of gluconeogenesis.*

Glycogen is a polysaccharide with a branched structure consisting of chains of glucose units. During the intestinal absorption of carbohydrates, any excess glucose is stored in the liver as glycogen. Normally the liver contains about 100 g of glycogen, but it may store as much as 400 g. The gly-

The reactions of glycogenesis.

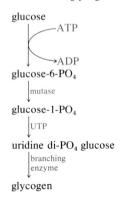

cogen in the liver is readily converted to glucose and serves as a reservoir from which glucose may be drawn if the blood sugar level falls below normal. The formation of glycogen from glucose is called **glycogenesis,** and the conversion of glycogen to glucose is known as **glycogenolysis.**

The muscles also store glucose as glycogen, but muscle glycogen is not so readily converted to glucose as is liver glycogen.

Glycogenesis

The process of glycogenesis is not just a simple conversion of glucose to glycogen. As we learned in Section 25.2, insulin is involved in the phosphorylation of glucose to glucose-6-PO_4. This starts the process. Then glucose-6-PO_4 is converted to the glucose-1-PO_4 isomer with the help of a *mutase* enzyme. The compound is then activated (by forming uridine diphosphate glucose) by reaction with UTP (like ATP but with uracil replacing adenine). In the presence of the proper enzymes, this activated molecule is converted to glycogen.

Glycogenolysis

The process of glycogenolysis liberates glucose into the blood stream to maintain the blood sugar level during fasting and to supply energy for muscular contraction.

First, in the liver, phosphorylase and a debranching enzyme convert glycogen to glucose-1-PO_4. Mutase then reverses glycogenesis to form glucose-6-PO_4. A specific enzyme in the liver called glucose-6-phosphatase acts on glucose-6-PO_4 to produce glucose. This enzyme is not present in muscle tissue, so muscle glycogen does not serve as a source of blood glucose. These reactions may be outlined as follows:

$$\text{glycogen} \xrightarrow[\text{debranching enzyme}]{\text{phosphorylase}} \text{glucose-1-}PO_4$$

$$\text{glucose-1-}PO_4 \xrightarrow{\text{mutase}} \text{glucose-6-}PO_4$$

$$\text{glucose-6-}PO_4 \xrightarrow[\textit{(liver only)}]{\text{glucose-6-phosphatase}} \text{glucose}$$

Gluconeogenesis

The glycogen stores of the liver are used up in less than a day if a person is not eating. Since muscle glycogen is not readily available to pour glucose into the blood stream, there must be other sources of glucose to maintain the blood sugar level.

Amino acids and acetyl groups may undergo the process of **gluconeogenesis** (making glucose). Liver cells are the main sites for gluconeogenesis because they contain enzymes that will convert phosphoenolpyruvate to glucose. Energy is required to reverse glycolysis from pyruvate back to phosphoenolpyruvate. With the help of ATP, pyruvate and CO_2 are converted to oxaloacetate. This is then changed to phosphoenolpyruvate and CO_2.

This reversal near the end of the glycolysis pathway makes possible the formation of glucose from any product of metabolism that can form pyruvate or oxaloacetate, as shown in Figure 25–7. The glucose that is formed by this

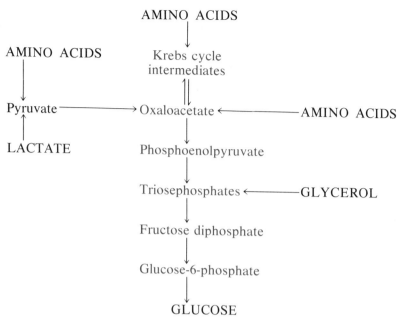

FIGURE 25–7   Major compounds in the process of gluconeogenesis. Any compound that can enter the Krebs cycle can serve as a starting compound for carbohydrate synthesis.

process may be either temporarily stored as glycogen in the liver or used directly to adjust the blood sugar level. Evidence that this process works is given by the number of people who have starved for two to four weeks without developing disastrous hypoglycemia. During such a fast, not only are the fat deposits reduced in size but body proteins, such as muscle tissue, are broken down to form amino acids, which may then be converted to glucose.

SELF-CHECK

25.7)   Why is liver glycogen more important than muscle glycogen in glycogenolysis?
25.8)   Compare the meaning of the terms *glycogenesis* and *gluconeogenesis*.

25.4 THE OXIDATION OF CARBOHYDRATES

LEARNING GOAL 25H: Compare the oxidation of glucose in resting and in working muscle tissue.
        25I: Outline the Cori cycle.
        25J: Explain why the metabolism of the brain and that of the heart are different from the metabolism in other tissues.

In Chapter 22 we learned how glucose was broken down in the Embden-Meyerhof pathway and how the resulting pyruvate fed into the Krebs cycle to ultimately form CO_2, H_2O, and energy as ATP. Glucose-6-PO_4 is a principal compound in the metabolism of glucose. It is formed by the phosphorylation of glucose under the control of insulin. Once it is formed, it may be converted to glycogen or back to free glucose in the liver, or it may take part in a metabolic process, as in the Embden-Meyerhof pathway.

Fatty acids can also be converted to acetyl coenzyme A and fed into the Krebs cycle. Resting muscles obtain most of their energy from fatty acids, but very active muscles also use glucose, converting it to pyruvate, which can either be fed into the Krebs cycle or converted to lactic acid.

In a 100-meter dash, for example, sprinters use the anaerobic glycolysis pathway to provide extra ATP energy to supplement that available from the oxidation of fatty acids. This high-power, short-term burst of energy may last for about 20 seconds. Some sprinters hold their breath to assure anaerobic conditions in the muscle. Unfortunately (for setting track records), lactic acid buildup soon causes fatigue, and a tremendous oxygen deficit occurs. Long-distance runners must start at (and maintain) a slower pace, since the energy required for the race must be generated through the Krebs cycle.

In the presence of oxygen, a working muscle regains its glycogen, loses lactic acid, and recovers its ability to contract. The high-energy compound creatine phosphate present in the muscle supplies more ATP for muscular contraction and is regenerated when the muscle is at rest. The ATP is the source of energy for muscular work and may be obtained from fatty acid or glucose oxidation, or directly from creatine phosphate.

The lactic acid that is formed in very active muscles returns to the liver, where it is converted to glucose by gluconeogenesis. This glucose may be returned to the circulatory system and to the working muscle, or it may first be changed to liver glycogen. This cycle that takes place between a working muscle and the liver is called the **Cori cycle,** after Carl and Gerty Cori, who first described its function. The Cori cycle, sometimes called the lactic acid cycle, is illustrated in Figure 25–8.

The metabolism in heart muscle is different from that we have just described. Since the heart is continuously active and always completely aerobic, lactic acid is not produced as the end product of glycolysis and the Krebs cycle is the main source of ATP. Heart muscle does not store gly-

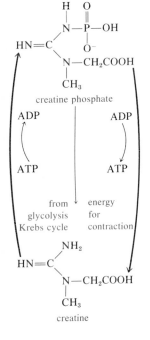

creatine phosphate

ADP   ADP

ATP   ATP

from   energy
glycolysis   for
Krebs cycle   contraction

creatine

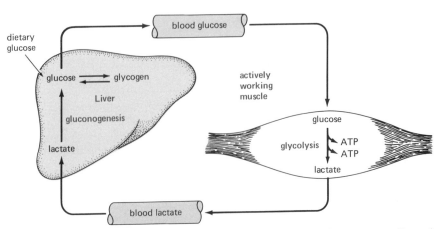

FIGURE 25–8 The Cori cycle. This diagram shows how reactions are coordinated between the liver and working muscles.

cogen; instead, it obtains its energy from blood glucose, fatty acids, and ketone bodies.

The metabolism of the brain is also very special, since it requires glucose as its major fuel. The fact that the brain contains very little glycogen makes it dependent on the glucose concentration in the blood. Symptoms of brain disturbance may be observed after short periods of severe hypoglycemia. The brain and the nervous system require a constant supply of ATP for the normal transmission of nerve impulses, and this ATP must be formed from blood glucose.

We have already considered the Embden-Meyerhof pathway of glycolysis (Section 22.2). Recall that it does not produce large amounts of energy. The *Krebs cycle*, starting with pyruvic acid or acetyl coenzyme A from any source, is an excellent source of energy. There are pathways involved in the oxidation of carbohydrates other than glycolysis and the Krebs cycle. One alternate is called the **pentose phosphate pathway** (Figure 25–9) because of the formation of phosphorylated pentose sugars. Another name for this pathway is the hexose monophosphate shunt, so called because glucose-6-PO_4 is ''shunted'' through a path other than the Embden-Meyerhof pathway. The key metabolic compound, glucose-6-PO_4, is oxidized in a series of reactions to 6-PO_4-gluconic acid. Then, through the loss of CO_2, a pentose phosphate is formed.

In another series of reactions, the pentose phosphate molecules are eventually converted to glyceraldehyde-3-PO_4 and fructose-6-PO_4. The primary purpose of this pathway in most cells is not to oxidize glucose but to generate reducing power in the cytoplasm in the form of the coenzyme NADPH (p. 634). This coenzyme is active in tissues that synthesize fatty acids and cholesterol, such as the liver, mammary glands, fat depots, and adrenal cortex. The pentoses that are formed, especially ribose, are used in the synthesis of nucleic acids, and the glyceraldehyde-3-PO_4 and fructose-6-PO_4 enter the Embden-Meyerhof pathway.

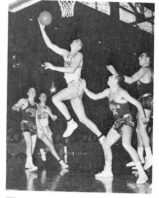

The major function of dietary carbohydrates is to supply energy for physical movement and exercise.

FIGURE 25–9   The pentose phosphate pathway.

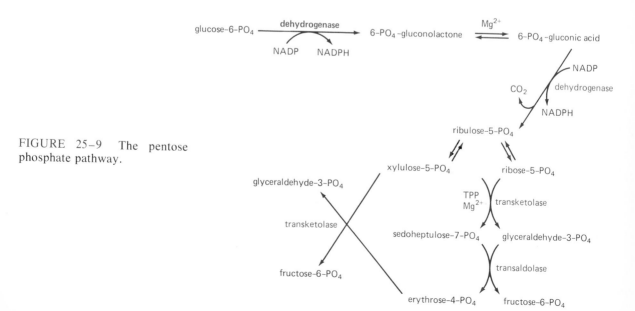

SELF-CHECK

25.9)   What is the main source of energy in resting muscles? in active muscles?

25.10)   What happens to the lactic acid that is formed in working muscles?

25.11)   Why is the glucose level in the blood important to the brain?

25.5 PHOTOSYNTHESIS

LEARNING GOAL 25K: Explain how photosynthesis is indirectly very important to human metabolism.

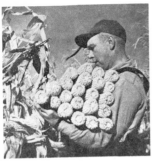

Photosynthesis produces carbohydrates, which we consume in edible grains such as corn. (J. C. Robinson Seed Company)

Solar energy is a very newsworthy subject when we discuss sources of energy to heat and cool our homes. Nature has for eons been using light energy from the sun to synthesize glucose from carbon dioxide and water. This process, **photosynthesis,** may be carried out in the cells of green plants or in one-cell organisms, such as the green and purple bacteria and the blue-green algae. Plants and algae use water as a hydrogen source to reduce carbon dioxide and produce glucose. A very simple equation for the process of photosynthesis is

$$6\ CO_{2(g)} + 6\ H_2O_{(\ell)} \xrightarrow{\text{sunlight}} C_6H_{12}O_{6(s)} + 6\ O_{2(g)}$$

This is exactly the *reverse* of the overall equation for animal respiration!

Although we may represent photosynthesis as a simple chemical reaction, it is actually very complex and involves reactions that require light as well as others that can occur in the absence of light. The first stage involves the absorption of light by *chlorophyll,* a molecule similar to the heme unit of hemoglobin or cytochrome *c.* (Chlorophyll is what makes green plants green.)

chlorophyll a

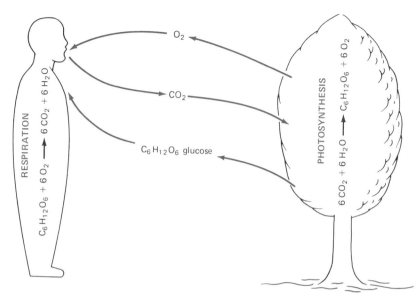

FIGURE 25–10 Respiration and photosynthesis are complementary processes. Oxygen is released by plants and used in respiration by animals; the carbon dioxide waste products of animal respiration are essential nutrients for plants. The carbohydrates that result from photosynthesis are, directly and indirectly, the main sources in our food supply of glucose for the energy-providing reactions of Chapter 22 and this chapter.

With the extra energy the chlorophyll gains from light, a molecule of water is split, oxygen is given off, and energy-rich molecules of ATP are produced, along with the important coenzyme, NADPH, which we saw earlier in Figure 25–9.

The energy trapped in ATP is then used to add carbon atoms, one at a time, to organic molecules already present in the plant cell. This process is called *carbon dioxide fixation,* since the carbon comes from CO_2.

Plants use H_2O and CO_2 to produce O_2 and glucose; animals use O_2 and glucose to produce H_2O, CO_2, and energy. This is a complete recycling process (called the carbon-oxygen cycle), part of which is shown in Figure 25–10. The complete cycle includes the combustion of fossil fuels to add CO_2 to the atmosphere. Human respiration, providing about 30 billion kg of CO_2 per year to the atmosphere, plays its part in providing nutrients for photosynthesis. More important to us, the plants provide the oxygen we breathe and the carbohydrates we consume as the major energy source for the body.

25.12) What products of photosynthesis are nutrients essential to humans?

SELF-CHECK

CHAPTER TWENTY-FIVE IN REVIEW ■ Carbohydrate Metabolism

GLOSSARY FOR CHAPTER TWENTY-FIVE

absorption, intestinal The process by which the end products of digestion are transported to the blood. (p. 679)

anabolism The process by which the body constructs large, complex molecules from simple nutrient molecules. (p. 677)

bile A fluid, formed by the liver and stored in the gallbladder, that emulsifies fats. (p. 680)

blood sugar level The concentration of glucose in the blood; related to carbohydrate metabolism. (p. 682)

catabolism The biodegradative (breaking down) processes in the cell that result in the release of chemical energy. (p. 677)

Cori cycle The conversion of muscle lactic acid to liver glycogen and glucose. (p. 690)

diabetes mellitus A disease characterized by poor carbohydrate oxidation and ordinarily caused by lack of insulin; symptoms include high blood sugar levels as well as glucose and ketone bodies in the urine. (p. 684)

digestion The action of hydrolytic enzymes in digestive fluids to convert large food molecules into smaller nutrient molecules used by the cell. (p. 679)

epinephrine A hormone produced by the adrenal glands that, among other functions, triggers glycogenolysis in the liver with the liberation of glucose into the blood; adrenalin; $C_9H_{13}NO_3$. (p. 685)

gluconeogenesis The formation of glucose in the liver from noncarbohydrate sources, such as amino acids and acetyl groups. (p. 688)

glycogen A polysaccharide used by the body for storage of energy through glucose units. (p. 687)

glycogenesis The synthesis of glycogen from glucose in the liver and in muscle tissues. (p. 688)

glycogenolysis The breakdown of glycogen in the liver to form glucose, which is liberated into the blood. (p. 688)

hyperglycemia A blood sugar level higher than the normal fasting level. (p. 682)

hypoglycemia A blood sugar level lower than the normal fasting level. (p. 682)

insulin A hormone produced by the beta cells of the pancreas; functions in the normal metabolism of glucose to maintain the proper blood sugar level. (p. 684)

metabolism The combination of all the processes of anabolism and catabolism in the cell; all cell reactions. (p. 677)

pentose phosphate pathway An alternate pathway for the oxidation of carbohydrates; products are pentose sugars and NADPH. (p. 691)

photosynthesis The formation of carbohydrates in the cells of green plants from carbon dioxide and water in the presence of sunlight and chlorophyll. (p. 692)

QUESTIONS AND PROBLEMS FOR CHAPTER TWENTY-FIVE ■

Carbohydrate Metabolism

SECTION 25.1 PREVIEW OF METABOLISM

25.13) Why is digestion important to anabolism?

25.14*) In Figure 25–3 glycolysis appears to be important in anabolism. Explain why.

25.24) Could catabolism proceed without the process of absorption? Explain.

25.25*) What coenzyme links glycolysis, the Krebs cycle, catabolism, and anabolism?

SECTION 25.2 HORMONES AND THE BLOOD SUGAR LEVEL

25.15) What normal processes reduce hyperglycemia after a meal?

25.16*) What is usually wrong with a person with diabetes?

25.17) Which hormone is involved in emotional hyperglycemia? What does it do?

25.26) How could a normal person produce a mild condition of hypoglycemia?

25.27*) How could one treat a condition of maturity-onset diabetes?

25.28) Could a normal person exhibit glycosuria? Explain.

SECTION 25.3 THE ROLE OF GLYCOGEN

25.18) Describe what happens to liver glycogen in a typical 24-hour period.

25.19) Why is glucose-6-PO_4 important in glycogenesis?

25.29) How does the liver try to maintain a balance between glycogenesis and glycogenolysis?

25.30*) What is the importance of liver glucose-6-phosphatase?

SECTION 25.4 THE OXIDATION OF CARBOHYDRATES

25.20) What limits a sprinter's effort to break track records?

25.21) What would happen to the brain if severe hypoglycemia lasted for more than an hour?

25.22*) What is one role of an alternate path like the pentose phosphate pathway?

25.31) What happens to muscle lactic acid in the Cori cycle?

25.32) Why must the heart obtain its energy in a manner different from other muscles?

25.33*) What important coenzyme is produced by the pentose phosphate pathway? What vitamin is needed to synthesize this coenzyme?

SECTION 25.5 PHOTOSYNTHESIS

25.23) Would our bodies be able to function properly if there were no plants on earth? Explain.

25.34) Future space colonies might maintain green plants in hydroponic gardens, where the plants would live not in soil, but in water enriched with mineral nutrients. What survival value to humans would these plants have?

25.35*) Could the concentration of ATP in a cell be used to control the rate of a metabolic process? Explain.

25.36*) What would you expect to find in the blood and urine of a severe diabetic?

25.37*) Why do marathon runners sometimes drink a very dilute glucose solution or eat orange sections during a run?

Lipid Metabolism

26

The major sources of energy-rich fuel in the body are carbohydrates and fats. The energy for many activities is derived from the metabolism of carbohydrates, as described in Chapters 22 and 25. Fats are also excellent sources of energy since they have a caloric value more than twice that of carbohydrate or protein (p. 575). In a normal diet, up to 40 per cent of the caloric requirement is provided by dietary fat. In fasting individuals or hibernating animals, the fat stores supply almost all the energy required by the body.

The metabolism of lipids also involves phospholipids, glycolipids, and sterols. These three types of lipids are not stored in the fat depots but are essential constituents of the tissues involved in fat transport and metabolic reactions in the cells. These lipids also function as components of cell membranes, nerve tissue, and the chloroplasts of green leaves. In this chapter, we will consider the anabolism and catabolism of fats and the role of such tissue lipids as cholesterol and the phospholipids.

26.1 BLOOD LIPIDS

> *LEARNING GOAL 26A: Describe the role of bile salts in fat digestion.*
> *26B: Describe the absorption of lipids in the intestine.*
> *26C: Name the three types of blood lipids.*

Before lipids can be used by the body, they must be present in the blood in a form that can be metabolized by the tissue cells. The whole process starts with the fat in our food. Unfortunately for some of us, the foods banned from weight-reducing diets are those we crave most. Rich desserts, ice cream, pastries, fast-food items, and fried foods are often loaded with fats that must be first digested, then absorbed into the blood, and finally disposed of by lipid metabolism.

Fats present a further problem because body fluids are aqueous solutions and fat is insoluble in water. Before dietary fat can be digested, it must be broken into very fine droplets to form an emulsion that can be attacked by the enzyme *pancreatic lipase*. *Bile salts,* formed by the liver and poured into the small intestine during digestion, are detergents. They not only form

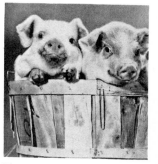

Pigs are superior to all other animals in their ability to store fat.

If the fats we ate contained only short-chain fatty acids (fewer than ten carbons), we could digest and absorb them without bile salts, since such fats are soluble enough to be carried in the body fluids. Artificial mixtures of fats made with short-chain fatty acids are fed to patients who lack bile salts because of gallbladder removal, or who have intestinal absorption difficulties.

emulsified fat droplets but also provide a charged surface that allows lipase (a protein) to combine with the fat to initiate hydrolysis.

A fat molecule, as you recall, is a triacylglycerol or triglyceride (p. 512) involving three fatty acids combined with glycerol. During digestion, the pancreatic lipase rapidly splits away the outer two fatty acids, leaving a monoglyceride with the fatty acid on the central glycerol carbon atom. This is a product of fat digestion that can be absorbed through the walls of the small intestine. Bile salts help keep these compounds in solution during absorption. In the cells of the intestinal walls, fatty acids are reattached to the monoglyceride, producing new fat molecules that can be used by the body. These new fats move out of the cells into the lymph and eventually into the blood.

In a way, blood lipids act in the same manner as blood sugar. Their concentration in the blood increases after a meal, and the level returns to normal through the processes of storage, oxidation, and excretion. The *normal fasting level* of blood lipids, shown in Table 26-1, is usually measured in the plasma.

The fats, phospholipids, and cholesterol in the plasma are combined with protein as *lipoprotein complexes* for transport in a more water-soluble form. A small amount of *free fatty acids* (*FFA*) is always present in the blood. These FFA molecules are bound to the albumin fraction of the plasma for transport and are thought to be the most active form of the lipids involved in metabolism. Their concentration is affected by the action of hormones that regulate the release of fat from fat storage depots.

TABLE 26-1 NORMAL FASTING LEVELS OF BLOOD LIPIDS

	mg/dL
Total lipids	510*
Fats	150
Phospholipids	200
Cholesterol	160

* Values are averages for a healthy young adult.

SELF-CHECK

26.1) Name the three types of blood lipids.
26.2) Describe the products of lipase action in fat digestion.
26.3) Why are lipid molecules modified for transportation in the blood?

26.2 SYNTHESIS OF FATTY ACIDS

LEARNING GOAL 26D: Describe how the cytoplasm and mitochondria cooperate in the synthesis of fatty acids.
26E: Describe the overall process of fatty acid synthesis from acetyl coenzyme A.

A typical diet of today is rich in fats and carbohydrates, so the body obtains dietary fatty acids and fat to store in the fat depots. The carbohydrates we eat are changed to glucose and proceed through the Embden-Meyerhof pathway to pyruvate. As you recall, the pyruvate can enter the mitochondria and yield energy by way of the Krebs cycle. When our carbohydrate intake exceeds our need for energy and even our need for liver glycogen, the excess pyruvate moves into the mitochondria and forms excess acetyl coenzyme A. Instead of going through the Krebs cycle, this acetyl CoA can migrate back to the cytoplasm of the cell and serve as the starting material for the synthesis of fatty acids:

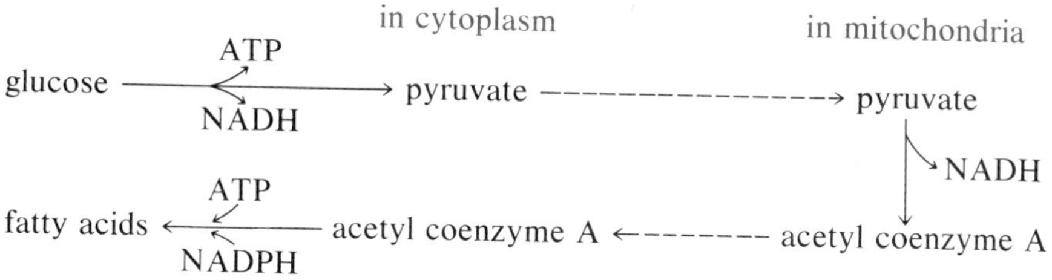

in cytoplasm   in mitochondria

glucose $\xrightarrow[\text{NADH}]{\text{ATP}}$ pyruvate $----------\rightarrow$ pyruvate

$\downarrow$ NADH

fatty acids $\xleftarrow[\text{NADPH}]{\text{ATP}}$ acetyl coenzyme A $\longleftarrow-----$ acetyl coenzyme A

The fatty acid molecules are constructed by condensing acetyl groups obtained from acetyl CoA:

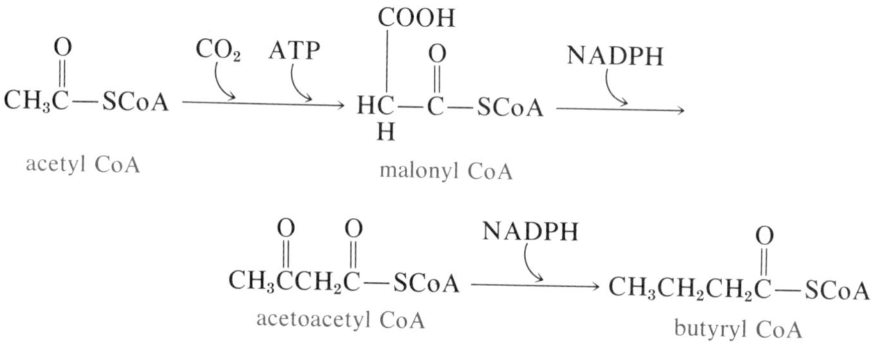

$$\underset{\text{acetyl CoA}}{CH_3\overset{O}{\overset{\|}{C}}-SCoA} \xrightarrow{\quad CO_2 \quad ATP \quad} \underset{\text{malonyl CoA}}{\overset{COOH}{\underset{H}{\overset{|}{HC}}}-\overset{O}{\overset{\|}{C}}-SCoA} \xrightarrow{\quad NADPH \quad}$$

$$\underset{\text{acetoacetyl CoA}}{CH_3\overset{O}{\overset{\|}{C}}CH_2\overset{O}{\overset{\|}{C}}-SCoA} \xrightarrow{\quad NADPH \quad} \underset{\text{butyryl CoA}}{CH_3CH_2CH_2\overset{O}{\overset{\|}{C}}-SCoA}$$

The conversion of acetyl groups to fatty acids is almost a reversal of the oxidation of fatty acids, but the processes are separated, with oxidation occurring in the mitochondria and synthesis in the cytoplasm. The fatty acid chains are built by transferring one acetyl group at a time from CoA. With the help of ATP and the proper cofactors, acetyl CoA is converted to acetoacetyl CoA, which is then changed to butyryl CoA. The four-carbon butyryl CoA then goes through the same series of reactions to form caproyl CoA, a six-carbon compound. This process continues, adding two carbons at a time until palmitic acid (16 carbons) and stearic acid (18 carbons) are formed.

26.4)   What two compounds initiate fatty acid synthesis from glucose in the cell?

26.5)   How do the cytoplasm and mitochondria serve different roles in the synthesis of fatty acids?

SELF-CHECK

26.3 SYNTHESIS OF FATS

LEARNING GOAL 26F: *Explain the advantages of fat as a stored fuel.*
          26G: *Describe the nature and distribution of adipose tissue.*
          26H: *Explain what is meant by activated forms of glycerol and fatty acids.*

Before discussing the mechanism of fat synthesis, we should consider the nature and advantage of stored fat in our bodies. As we saw in Chapter 25, glucose and glycogen are rapidly used by the body. However, fat is a fuel

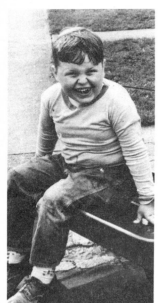

Obesity is a kind of "malnutrition of affluence." (Courtesy World Health Organization and P. Almasy)

that can be put into long-term storage. The average person contains enough liver glycogen to maintain activity for about one day, but stored fat can sustain life for over a month. If you eat a light meal in the evening and skip breakfast, you will be using about twice as many calories from (stored) fatty acid oxidation as from glucose oxidation to carry on your daily activities.

There are several advantages of fat as a stored form of energy. First, it yields more calories per gram than glucose or amino acids when oxidized for energy. Second, it is very compact when stored. The total mass of the body's fat depots is only about one fifth of the glycogen mass required to yield the same energy (in the form of ATP). That means that a normal individual with 8 kg of body fat would need 40 kg of glycogen to replace it for energy purposes. A third advantage of fat storage is the ability to withstand starvation. In such situations, obese individuals would still be living on the energy from their fat stores long after their weight-conscious friends had expired. Hibernating animals prepare for their long nap by building up their fat stores.

The fat stored in fat depots is called **adipose tissue.** The adipose region may contain over 90 per cent fat, but it is a definite tissue formed of specialized connective cells. It has a blood supply, a network of nerves, and an active metabolism that converts glucose to fat and releases fatty acids to provide energy for the body. The distribution of adipose tissue includes storage under the skin, around essential organs (kidneys, heart, lungs, and spleen), around deep blood vessels, and in the abdominal cavity.

Fats are synthesized in the tissues from *activated* forms of glycerol and fatty acids. The active form of glycerol is glycerol-3-PO_4, which is formed from *dihydroxyacetone phosphate,* an intermediate in the Embden-Meyerhof pathway:

$$\text{dihydroxyacetone-}PO_4 \xrightarrow[\substack{\\ \text{NADH} \quad \text{NAD}^+}]{\text{dehydrogenase}} \text{glycerol-3-}PO_4$$

The glycerol-3-PO_4 reacts with two activated fatty acid molecules (as fatty acid coenzyme A derivatives):

glycerol-3-PO_4 + 2 fatty acid CoA $\longrightarrow$ diglyceride phosphate + 2 CoASH

The diglyceride phosphate then loses its phosphate group and reacts with another molecule of activated fatty acid to complete the synthesis:

diglyceride + fatty acid CoA $\longrightarrow$ fat + CoASH

The above scheme points out the importance of coenzymes such as NAD^+ and CoA in biosynthesis and the interrelationships between glucose and lipid metabolism.

SELF-CHECK

26.6)   Fat depots are more dense than glycogen stores. How is this an advantage?

26.7)   What might be the disadvantage of having only one third the normal amount of fat storage depots?

26.8)   How is the activated form of glycerol related to glucose metabolism?

26.4 SYNTHESIS OF TISSUE LIPIDS

> *LEARNING GOAL 26I:* Explain why phospholipids are important in the body.
> *26J:* Name three compounds that are important in the synthesis of cholesterol.
> *26K:* Explain why the blood cholesterol level is important.

Phospholipids, glycolipids, and sterols are necessary in all of the cells and tissues of the body. We have already discussed cell membranes and the bilayers of phospholipids (Section 18.3). Cholesterol and protein-lipid (lipoprotein) combinations are also present in cell membranes.

The organ most concerned with lipid synthesis is the liver, which makes phospholipids and cholesterol. The liver can modify all blood fats by lengthening or shortening, and saturating or unsaturating, the fatty acid chains. Special fats and oils in the body, such as milk fat, various sterols, the natural oil of the scalp, and the wax of the ear, are examples of lipids synthesized from the fats of food.

Because of their structure and chemistry, *phospholipids* serve many important functions in the body. Their molecules are more strongly dissociated than any of the other lipids. They tend to be more soluble in water, to lower the surface tension of oil-water mixtures, and to be involved in the electron transport system in the tissues. They are found in large amounts in cell membranes, form lipoproteins for the transport of lipids in the blood, and are essential components of the blood clotting mechanism.

The biosynthesis of phospholipids and the biosynthesis of fats share some common reactions. For example, the first two reactions are the same in both schemes: dihydroxyacetone-PO_4 forming glycerol-3-PO_4 and two fatty acid CoA plus glycerol-3-PO_4 forming diglyceride phosphate. Diglyceride phosphate is activated for phospholipid synthesis by reacting with the high-energy compound cytidine triphosphate, CTP (similar to ATP). The activated molecule is then used as a starting material for the synthesis of lecithins and the cephalins (Section 18.3).

Our interest in the synthesis of sterols is mainly with cholesterol and its derivatives. The starting material for cholesterol synthesis is the familiar two-carbon compound acetyl CoA. Looking at the structure of cholesterol (p. 524) and that of acetyl CoA (p. 610) and realizing that cholesterol is built from the two-carbon acetyl groups, it is clear that the details of the reactions are rather complicated. They start with the formation of *mevalonic acid* (a six-carbon acid) from three molecules of acetyl CoA. The mevalonic acid is then phosphorylated and proceeds through a series of reactions to the formation of squalene, an open-chain hydrocarbon, which is converted to cholesterol by a ring-forming reaction.

Although the synthesis of cholesterol occurs in many tissues in the body, the liver is the main site. As mentioned in Chapter 18, cholesterol is a key compound in the synthesis of such essential steroids as bile acids, sex hormones, adrenal cortical hormones, and vitamin D. Cholesterol is not only converted to bile acids by the liver but is also excreted in the bile. Unfortunately, the cholesterol in the bile can form gallstones by coating insoluble particles in the gallbladder (the bile storage organ) and growing coat by coat until the stones will not flow out of the gallbladder into the small intestine. If the stones lodge in the bile duct, which connects the liver to the intestine, a

Phosphatidic acid, shown on p. 518, would be a natural starting material for the synthesis of lecithins and cephalins.

squalene

cholesterol

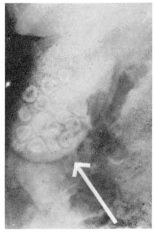

The arrow is pointing to gall-stones in a dye-filled gall-bladder and bile duct. (J. Edward Tether and J.E. Harrity)

TABLE 26–2
CHOLESTEROL
LEVELS IN THE
BLOOD

Age group, years	Cholesterol range, mg/dL
0–19	120–230
20–29	120–240
30–39	140–270
40–49	150–310
50–59	160–330

serious liver condition called "obstructive jaundice" occurs and surgery may be required to remove the stones.

The concentration of cholesterol in the blood depends on the dietary intake of steroids and fats and on the synthesis of cholesterol by the liver and body tissues. The normal level in the blood gradually increases with age and ranges from 150 to over 300 mg/dL. Our population enjoys a carbohydrate- and lipid-rich diet, and the different age groups show a range of blood cholesterol values (Table 26–2). If the cholesterol level in the blood is maintained at an abnormally high concentration, such as 300 mg/dL, cholesterol plaques may become deposited in the arterial walls, especially in the aorta and arteries of the heart (p. 315). This condition, known as **atherosclerosis,** is commonly seen in older persons and often results in arteriosclerosis (hardening of the arteries) and circulatory problems that end in heart disease or heart failure. The increasing incidence of heart disease in people of all ages has resulted in more and more research on the subject. Dietary fats, especially those with saturated fatty acids, and dietary cholesterol are high on the list of risk factors in coronary artery disease. As you have perhaps learned from TV or radio, other risk factors are hypertension (high blood pressure), smoking, obesity, high caffeine intake (from coffee, tea, or cola beverages), lack of exercise, and stressful occupations. From a dietary standpoint, the risks can be lowered by reducing the intake of fat and perhaps by substituting unsaturated vegetable fats for saturated animal fats. Hypertension can be controlled by drugs, and the other risk factors are largely controlled by individual effort. One very important fact to keep in mind when anyone discusses the possible lowering of blood cholesterol through a restricted diet is that the starting material in cholesterol synthesis, acetyl CoA, can readily be formed from carbohydrates, fatty acids, and amino acids.

In Section 26.1 we mentioned that cholesterol is combined with plasma protein to form *lipoprotein* for transport through the body. It turns out that of the various types of lipoproteins that contain cholesterol, those with low density (LDL, normally about 70% of the total) seem to be related to atherosclerosis. When we relate human health to a measurement of total blood cholesterol, we may actually be looking at the effect of the LDL level.

High density lipoproteins (HDL) that contain cholesterol seem, in contrast, to protect the body in some fashion from the effects of LDL cholesterol. People with plasma levels of HDL cholesterol above 45 mg/dL have been found to have a lower incidence of coronary heart disease and atherosclerosis. Normal males under 45 years of age tend to have a higher total plasma cholesterol level and lower HDL levels than females. There may thus be an effect of sex hormones. Sustained muscular activity may increase HDL levels; this may explain the apparent effect of some types of exercise in reducing the risk of heart attack.

The reasons for these relationships are not understood. We will require considerable further research into the relationship between cholesterol in the blood plasma and the development of circulatory diseases.

SELF-CHECK

26.9) List three functions of phospholipids in the body.
26.10) Where do the six carbons of mevalonic acid come from in cholesterol synthesis?
26.11) If your blood cholesterol level were 160 mg/dL, what would this imply?

26.12) What would you suggest to a person whose blood cholesterol level was over 300 mg/dL?

26.5 OXIDATION OF FATTY ACIDS

LEARNING GOAL 26L: *Describe Knoop's theory of the beta oxidation of fatty acids.*

26M: *Describe the chemical changes that occur on the alpha and beta carbon atoms in fatty acid oxidation.*

We have already mentioned that fat stores are a good source of energy for the body. It has been estimated that the oxidation of fatty acids provides about one half the energy normally required by the body's organs and tissues. Hibernating animals and migrating birds obtain practically all of their energy from fat stores. Fat molecules released from fat depots during fasting or from dietary fat after a meal must be hydrolyzed to glycerol and fatty acids to start the oxidation process. The glycerol is phosphorylated in the liver and then oxidized to dihydroxyacetone phosphate:

$$\text{glycerol} \xrightarrow[\text{ATP} \quad \text{ADP}]{\text{glycerokinase}} \text{glycerophosphate} \xrightarrow[\text{NAD}^+ \quad \text{NADH}]{\text{dehydrogenase}} \text{dihydroxyacetone phosphate}$$

Dihydroxyacetone phosphate is also formed in the Embden-Meyerhof pathway, which means that fat as well as glucose can produce energy through glycolysis.

The oxidation of fatty acids occurs in the mitochondria, which contain the necessary enzymes and coenzymes for the process. As is common in the cell, before the process can begin the fatty acid molecules must be activated and moved inside the mitochondria. It should be no surprise that both ATP and coenzyme A are involved in the activation of fatty acids. Early research on the oxidation scheme by Franz Knoop in 1904 established the fact that fatty acids were oxidized on the beta carbon atom (the second from the —COOH group) with the splitting off of two-carbon fragments. In his theory of **beta oxidation,** Knoop stated that acetic acid was split off in each stage of the process that reduced an 18-carbon fatty acid to a 2-carbon acid. The detailed reactions with their enzymes and coenzymes have been worked out, and Knoop's theory has been essentially confirmed. Instead of acetic acid, the key compound in the reactions is acetyl CoA. Five reactions are involved in the conversion of a long-chain fatty acid to a CoA derivative having two fewer carbons and a molecule of acetyl CoA (Figure 26-1). Although this series of reactions may appear complex, if you look carefully at the alpha and beta carbon atoms of the CoA derivative of the fatty acid (in Figure 26-1, we are using palmitic acid as our example), you can follow the changes. First the palmitic acid is activated through reactions involving ATP and CoASH, then it is oxidized to give a double bond between the alpha and beta carbons. Water is then added and the beta carbon is oxidized to a keto group. The oxidized derivative is split into a fatty acid molecule with two fewer carbons, and acetyl CoA is formed. As shown in the scheme, palmitic acid, a 16-carbon fatty acid, requires seven turns of the cycle to form eight acetyl CoA molecules.

During the oxidation of palmitic acid, seven $FADH_2$ and seven NADH molecules are formed. When these coenzymes enter the electron transport system, they form a total of $(7 \times 2) + (7 \times 3) = 35$ molecules of ATP. In the seven turns of the cycle, you can see that eight acetyl CoA molecules are formed. As it feeds into the Krebs cycle, each acetyl CoA yields 12 ATP's for a total of $8 \times 12 = 96$ molecules of ATP. The sum of $35 + 96 - 2$ ATP (for activation) is a gain of 129 molecules of ATP for the complete oxidation of palmitic acid. The energy yield from this process in the form of ATP is about 48%, a relatively high level of efficiency.

SELF-CHECK

26.13) What is the main difference between the modern fatty acid oxidation scheme and Knoop's theory of beta oxidation?

26.14) What happens to the acetyl CoA molecules that are formed in the oxidation of fatty acids?

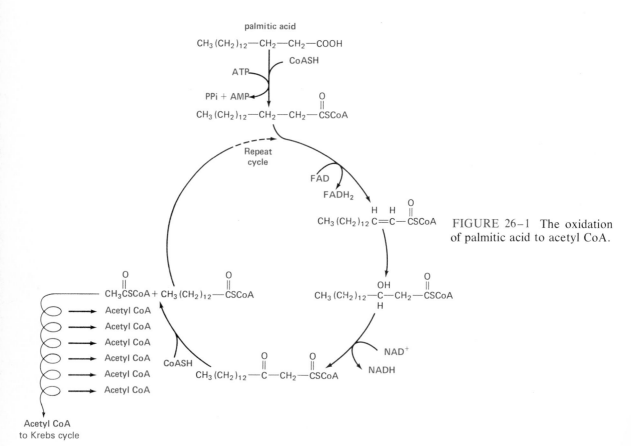

FIGURE 26–1 The oxidation of palmitic acid to acetyl CoA.

26.6 FORMATION OF KETONE BODIES

LEARNING GOAL 26N: Describe the formation of acetoacetic acid in the liver.

26O: Describe the effects of excess ketone bodies in the blood.

The ketone or acetone bodies formed during fat metabolism are *acetoacetic acid, β-hydroxybutyric acid,* and *acetone*. They are present in the blood of normal individuals, but only in small amounts, averaging about 0.5 mg/dL. Also, about 100 mg of ketone bodies are excreted per day in the urine. This low concentration in the blood and the small amount excreted in the urine cause no problems to the body. However, large amounts may be present in the blood and urine during prolonged starvation and in a person with diabetes mellitus. In general, any condition that results in a blocking or restriction of carbohydrate metabolism, thus an increase in fat metabolism to supply the energy requirements of the body, will produce extra ketone bodies.

The precursor of the **ketone bodies** is acetoacetic acid, which is formed in the liver from acetoacetyl CoA, a normal intermediate in the beta oxidation of fatty acids. Two molecules of acetyl CoA may, in fact, condense to form acetoacetyl CoA:

$$2 \underset{\text{acetyl CoA}}{CH_3\overset{O}{\overset{\|}{C}}CoA} \xrightarrow{\text{enzyme}} \underset{\text{acetoacetyl CoA}}{CH_3\overset{O}{\overset{\|}{C}}CH_2\overset{O}{\overset{\|}{C}}CoA} \xrightarrow{\text{deacylase}} \underset{\text{acetoacetic acid}}{CH_3\overset{O}{\overset{\|}{C}}CH_2COOH}$$

The other ketone bodies are formed from acetoacetic acid, acetone (by decarboxylation), and β-hydroxybutyric acid (by the action of a specific dehydrogenase enzyme):

$$CH_3\overset{O}{\overset{\|}{C}}CH_2COOH$$

$$\underset{\text{acetone}}{CH_3\overset{O}{\overset{\|}{C}}CH_3} \qquad \underset{\text{β-hydroxybutyric acid}}{CH_3\overset{H}{\underset{OH}{C}}-CH_2COOH}$$

After the ketone bodies are formed by the liver, they enter the blood stream and are carried to the muscle tissue, where they are converted back to acetyl coenzyme A and fed into the Krebs cycle. The muscles normally have a high capacity for using the ketone bodies, but the rate of formation by the liver

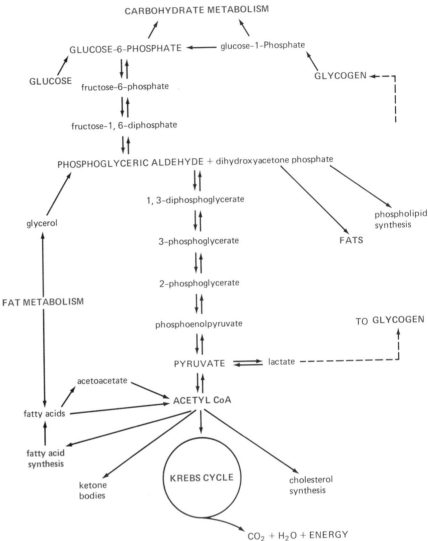

FIGURE 26–2   Relationships between lipid metabolism and the carbohydrate metabolism of Chapter 25.

may overcome the "using up" capacity of the muscles in cases of prolonged starvation, diabetes mellitus, abnormal increase in metabolism (as in hyperthyroidism, a disease of the thyroid gland), and even in a high-fat diet. If the liver overproduces ketone bodies, they build up in the blood and are excreted in large amounts in the urine (ketonuria).

If you look carefully at the structure of acetoacetic acid and β-hydroxybutyric acid, you will understand how increased concentrations in the blood will strain the capacity of the blood buffers. At the pH of the blood, 7.4, these acids are neutralized by the bicarbonate buffer and circulate as carboxylate anions. If the excess persists, they are excreted in the urine after partial neutralization by ammonia (p. 669). This results in a decreased concentration of sodium in the plasma, producing an electrolyte imbalance, acidosis, ketosis, and a loss of water from the body (dehydration) because the kidneys are using water to excrete the neutralized ketone bodies. All of these conditions can occur in a severe diabetic if carbohydrate metabolism is not properly controlled by diet and injections of insulin.

Some of the relationships between carbohydrate and lipid metabolism are shown in Figure 26–2.

SELF-CHECK

26.15) Are ketone bodies normally formed by the liver? Explain.
26.16) Describe two sources of acetoacetic acid in the liver.
26.17) In what forms are ketone bodies excreted in the urine of a severe diabetic?

CHAPTER TWENTY-SIX IN REVIEW ■ Lipid Metabolism

26.1 BLOOD LIPIDS   **Page 697**
  26A: *Describe the role of bile salts in fat digestion.*
  26B: *Describe the absorption of lipids in the intestine.*
  26C: *Name the three types of blood lipids.*
26.2 SYNTHESIS OF FATTY ACIDS   **Page 698**
  26D: *Describe how the cytoplasm and mitochondria cooperate in the synthesis of fatty acids.*
  26E: *Describe the overall process of fatty acid synthesis from acetyl coenzyme A.*
26.3 SYNTHESIS OF FATS   **Page 699**
  26F: *Explain the advantages of fat as a stored fuel.*
  26G: *Describe the nature and distribution of adipose tissue.*
  26H: *Explain what is meant by activated forms of glycerol and fatty acids.*
26.4 SYNTHESIS OF TISSUE LIPIDS   **Page 701**
  26I: *Explain why phospholipids are important in the body.*
  26J: *Name three compounds that are important in the synthesis of cholesterol.*
  26K: *Explain why the blood cholesterol level is important.*
26.5 OXIDATION OF FATTY ACIDS   **Page 703**
  26L: *Describe Knoop's theory of the beta oxidation of fatty acids.*
  26M: *Describe the chemical changes that occur on the alpha and beta carbon atoms in fatty acid oxidation.*
26.6 FORMATION OF KETONE BODIES   **Page 705**
  26N: *Describe the formation of acetoacetic acid in the liver.*
  26O: *Describe the effects of excess ketone bodies in the blood.*

GLOSSARY FOR CHAPTER TWENTY-SIX

adipose tissue A body tissue in which fat is stored, usually found under the skin and around essential organs; fat depots. (p. 700)

atherosclerosis The deposit of cholesterol plaques in arterial walls, especially in the aorta and arteries of the heart; can lead to serious heart disease. (p. 702)

beta oxidation In the Knoop theory, the oxidation of a fatty acid with the subsequent splitting off of a two-carbon fragment as acetyl CoA. (p. 703)

ketone bodies Molecules, including acetone, acetoacetic acid, and β-hydroxybutyric acid, normally produced in fatty acid oxidation; found in increased amounts in the blood and urine in cases of diabetes mellitus; may cause acidosis. (p. 705)

QUESTIONS AND PROBLEMS FOR CHAPTER TWENTY-SIX ■

Lipid Metabolism

SECTION 26.1 BLOOD LIPIDS

26.18) How is it possible for lipase, a water-soluble protein, to act on fat molecules during digestion?

26.19) Why are fats that contain short-chain fatty acids easier to digest than those containing long-chain fatty acids?

26.20) What happens to the blood lipids after a meal rich in fat?

SECTION 26.2 SYNTHESIS OF FATTY ACIDS

26.21) What role do the mitochondria play in fatty acid synthesis?

26.22) What compound is formed when an acetyl group is transferred to acetyl coenzyme A?

SECTION 26.3 SYNTHESIS OF FATS

26.23) How does adipose tissue compare with normal connective tissue?

26.24) What might happen if a hibernating animal had failed to build up its fat stores?

26.25) How is glycerol-3-PO_4 used in fat synthesis and what is its source?

SECTION 26.4 SYNTHESIS OF TISSUE LIPIDS

26.26) What is the relationship between fat and phospholipid synthesis?

26.27) What does the body use as starting material for cholesterol synthesis?

26.28*) List four factors possibly contributing to coronary heart disease.

26.35) What is the function of bile salts in absorption in the intestine?

26.36) Why don't food fats just pass directly into the blood?

26.37) How are different types of lipids transported in the blood?

26.38) How does the formation of pyruvate by glycolysis control fatty acid synthesis?

26.39) What role does malonyl CoA play in fatty acid synthesis?

26.40) Why does it take so long for an overweight person to lose weight on a low-calorie diet?

26.41) Prisoners of war in the Philippine Islands were secretly supplied with large jars of peanut butter. How did this help them survive?

26.42) What role does the fatty acid — coenzyme A complex play in fat synthesis?

26.43) How is diglyceride-PO_4 activated for phospholipid synthesis?

26.44) What happens to the mevalonic acid formed in cholesterol synthesis?

26.45) A 60-year-old man has been a vegetarian for many years. What kind of blood cholesterol value might he have?

SECTION 26.5 OXIDATION OF FATTY ACIDS

26.29) What happens to the glycerol from the hydrolysis of fat (before fatty acid oxidation)?

26.30) What is significant about the term "beta oxidation" in the Knoop theory?

26.31*) What coenzymes are involved in the process of fatty acid oxidation?

SECTION 26.6 FORMATION OF KETONE BODIES

26.32) How does acetone differ chemically from the other ketone bodies?

26.33) Acetoacetyl CoA is formed in two other processes involving fatty acids. Explain.

26.34) Describe two ways you could increase the production of ketone bodies in a normal person.

26.46) How are fatty acids activated for fatty acid oxidation?

26.47) Which two carbons on the fatty acid molecule are most involved in the oxidation process?

26.48) How many acetyl CoA molecules are formed in the complete oxidation of palmitic acid, $C_{15}H_{31}$ COOH? What happens to them?

26.49) Would you call β-hydroxybutyric acid a true ketone body? Explain.

26.50*) What processes are involved in the conversion of acetoacetic acid to acetone? to β-hydroxybutyric acid?

26.51) What changes are produced in the body by a prolonged increase in the number of ketone bodies in the blood?

Protein Metabolism 27

The chemistry of living organisms is very much the chemistry of the proteins of the cells. Proteins make up about half of the solid matter in the body and are deeply involved in the processes by which the body carries out anabolism, catabolism, tissue synthesis, transport of materials, and protection against invasion by bacteria and viruses. Recall that enzymes are proteins. Other proteins we have discussed include the *keratin* of skin, hair, and nails; *hemoglobin* in red blood cells; *albumin*, which transports fatty substances; and the *myoglobin* of muscle tissues, which contain about 20% (by weight) protein and 70% water.

Proteins are made by plant cells in a process that starts with photosynthesis (Section 25.5). Animals, including humans, can synthesize only a limited amount of protein by using purely inorganic sources of nitrogen, such as nitrate or ammonium salts. We are mainly dependent on plants or other animals for the raw materials—the amino acids—that we use to build the body proteins that are needed for growth, for maintenance of existing tissue, and for energy. When we use amino acids for energy, we excrete simple substances that are then used by growing plants as food (Figure 27–1). Animals provide fertilizer for plants and plants provide food for animals in a cycle of growth and decay that continually reprocesses the nitrogen in living matter.

A picture that shows the *complete* nitrogen cycle in nature becomes rather complex. Nitrogen compounds are added to the air by bacteria, volcanos, and pollution and to the ground by sewage and fertilizer runoff. Lightning plays a part in converting atmospheric N_2 to nitrogen oxides. However, the cycle shown in Figure 27–1 plays a substantial role in living systems and is of particular interest to the biochemist. No animals and only a few plants can use N_2 from the air to make amino acids.

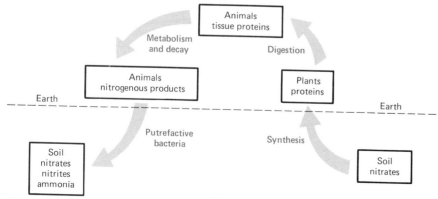

FIGURE 27–1   Nitrogen exchange between plants and animals.

27.1 THE AMINO ACID POOL

LEARNING GOAL 27A: *Describe the source and function of the body's amino acid pool.*

27B: *Describe the relationship between the amino acid pool and a protein already in place in body tissue.*

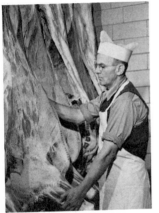

Beef is an excellent source of dietary proteins.

The body's proteins are made by the condensation polymerization of amino acid monomers, as described in Chapter 19. We get these amino acid molecules largely from food protein, which is hydrolyzed in the digestive system (Section 25.1). The enzyme *pepsin* starts the process in the stomach. Hydrolysis continues in the small intestine using the enzymes *trypsin*, *chymotrypsin*, and *polypeptidase* to break polypeptide chains down to dipeptides. While the dipeptides are being absorbed through the walls of the intestinal membranes, they are hydrolyzed to free amino acids by *dipeptidase* and then pass directly into the blood stream. This sequence is shown schematically in Figure 27–2.

These amino acid molecules from food, plus those from the breakdown of tissue proteins, make up a temporary collection of monomers called the **amino acid pool,** which the body uses to build new polypeptide chains. Protein metabolism is unlike that of carbohydrates and lipids in that there are no storage depots for raw materials. The pool of monomers in the blood stream is available to all tissues and serves as the source of raw materials for the synthesis of structural tissue proteins, blood proteins, hormones, enzymes, and other nitrogen-containing compounds, such as creatine and nucleic

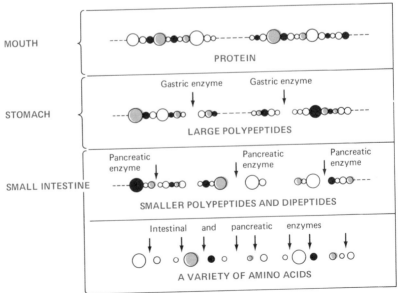

FIGURE 27–2 Hydrolysis of proteins during digestion provides amino acids for the pool used by the body to build new proteins.

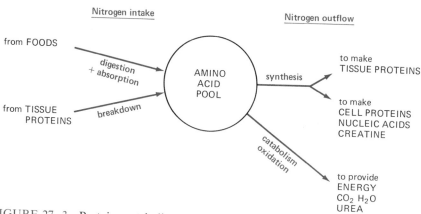

Nitrogen intake

Nitrogen outflow

from FOODS

digestion + absorption

AMINO ACID POOL

from TISSUE PROTEINS

breakdown

synthesis

to make TISSUE PROTEINS

to make CELL PROTEINS NUCLEIC ACIDS CREATINE

catabolism oxidation

to provide ENERGY CO_2 H_2O UREA

FIGURE 27–3   Protein metabolism and the role of the amino acid pool.

acids. The amino acids may also be oxidized directly for energy. An overview of protein metabolism is given in Figure 27–3.

In the early days of biochemistry (before the 1930's), it was believed that once a polypeptide chain was formed in the processes that synthesize tissue proteins, the amino acid units remain in place for life. If this were true, most of the amino acids we obtain from food would be used to produce energy. However, we now know that protein chains are not ''fixed'' for life but instead are in a state of dynamic equilibrium.

Isotope studies by Schoenheimer and his associates have found that when food amino acids were ''tagged'' with nitrogen-15, about 50% of the isotope found its way into the tissues of the test animal. Furthermore, most of the nitrogen was found in amino acid residues that were *different from* the amino acids in the food. This indicated that the amino acids of tissue proteins are constantly changing places with those in the amino acid pool. Furthermore, amino groups are being shifted from one carbon chain to another, a process we will discuss later in this chapter.

More recent studies have found that some tissue proteins change their amino acids more readily than others. Liver and blood plasma proteins change about half of their amino acid residues every 2 to 10 days, compared with about 180 days for muscle protein.

27.1)   Where does the body store the raw materials it needs to make proteins? Where do these raw materials come from?

27.2)   What would be the effect on your muscle tissue if your amino acid pool suddenly disappeared? Would this effect be noticeable right away, or only after some months? Would it be reversible, that is, would your muscles be able to regain what they had lost?

SELF-CHECK

27.2 FOOD AND PROTEIN SYNTHESIS

LEARNING GOAL 27C: Explain the nutritional importance of an essential amino acid.

27D: Describe the conditions under which the body falls into a negative nitrogen balance.

> *27E: Describe the difference between an active and an inactive protein.*

Some 20 different amino acids are known to be fairly common in the proteins that occur in nature. The number of different amino acids in the molecule of a specific protein may vary from 8 to 18. In order to synthesize that protein, the cell must find all of the necessary amino acid monomers in the body's amino acid pool. If the protein to be synthesized contains 15 different amino acids, but only 14 of them are available from the pool, that protein simply *cannot* be synthesized, no matter what else is present. The amino acid pool must therefore contain not only an adequate total amount of amino acids but also the necessary amount of *each type*.

Essential amino acids

More than half of the amino acids needed by the body can be synthesized inside the body from other materials at a rate that will satisfy the needs for normal growth in children and maintenance in adults. In studies between 1935 and 1955, W.C. Rose and his co-workers at the University of Illinois found that young rats must be fed ten different amino acids in adequate amounts to support normal growth. Those amino acids, the structures of which are shown in Table 19–1, are

arginine	histidine	isoleucine	leucine	lysine
methionine	phenylalanine	threonine	tryptophan	valine

Similar experiments by Rose on young men seemed to indicate that arginine and histidine can be made in adequate amounts by the human body.

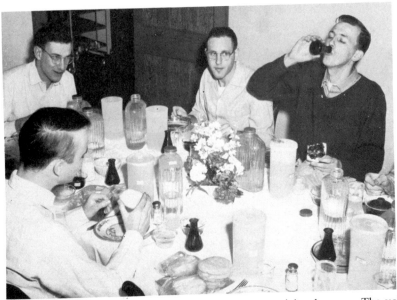

The classic study to find out which amino acids are essential to humans. The volunteer students are shown consuming their experimental diet. (Courtesy W. C. Rose, University of Illinois)

However, later studies* have shown that histidine is essential to human infants and perhaps, in the long run, to adults as well. While arginine can be made in the body, some question remains as to whether the rate of synthesis can always keep up with the need.

Those amino acids that *must* be consumed in food because the body cannot synthesize them are called **essential amino acids.** There are two additional amino acids, tyrosine and cysteine, that we might call "semiessential" because they must be synthesized from essential amino acids. Tyrosine can be made only from the essential amino acid phenylalanine and cysteine only from methionine. Thus, the amount of methionine that must be obtained from food is reduced if cysteine is present in the diet; the need for phenylalanine is lowered if tyrosine is available from food. Table 27-1 shows the minimum daily requirement of each essential amino acid as established in 1973 by the Food and Agriculture Organization (FAO) and the World Health Organization (WHO) of the United Nations. The table also shows the results of a 1970 study by the U.S. National Research Council (NRC) on how much of each amino acid is present in a typical U.S. diet. It seems clear that a typical American consumes more-than-adequate amounts of the essential amino acids.

The synthesis of protein in the body is constantly going on, especially in those tissues with a rapid turnover rate, such as the liver. The individual amino acids required for protein synthesis are sorted out by the cell and used to build polypeptide chains, as described in Section 20.5. If one essential amino acid is lacking in the diet, the use of all other amino acids will be lowered by a corresponding amount (Figure 27-4). If this condition persists for

Protein synthesis in the cell requires a great deal of energy, most of which is apparently used for "proofreading" and checking the exact sequence of amino acids. The transfer RNA molecules are very fussy about which amino acids they pick up to make a protein.

---

* This change in the nutritionist's list of essential amino acids illustrates the need for health-care personnel to keep abreast of current literature and research.

TABLE 27-1   MINIMUM DAILY REQUIREMENTS (FAO/WHO) OF ESSENTIAL AMINO ACIDS AND ESTIMATED AMOUNTS (NRC 1970) IN THE AVERAGE AMERICAN DIET

Essential amino acid	Minimum daily requirement (grams)			Amount in normal U.S. daily diet (grams)
	10-kg infant	*25-kg schoolchild*	*70-kg adult*	
Histidine	0.28	?	?	n.a.
Isoleucine	0.70	0.75	0.70	5.3
Leucine	1.61	1.1	1.0	8.2
Lysine	1.03	1.5	0.84	6.7
Methionine and cysteine	0.58	0.68	0.91	2.1
Phenylalanine and tyrosine	1.25	0.68	1.0	3.5
Threonine	0.87	0.88	0.49	4.7
Tryptophan	0.17	0.10	0.25	n.a.
Valine	0.93	0.83	0.70	4.1
				1.2
				5.7

Values adapted from Briggs, G.M., and Calloway, D.H., *Bogert's Nutrition and Physical Fitness,* 10th edition, Philadelphia, W.B. Saunders, 1979, p. 85. Chapter 5 in that text is highly recommended for additional details on the nutritional requirements for protein.

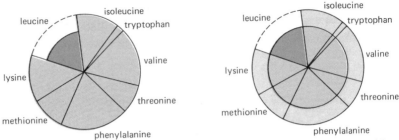

FIGURE 27-4 For optimal protein synthesis, all of the essential amino acids must be present in correct proportions, as shown on the left by the "slices" of the amino acid "pie." If one amino acid is partially absent (here, leucine), the use of the other amino acids will be reduced proportionately, as shown by the gray areas in the pie on the right.

a long time, there will be weight loss, a lowered blood plasma protein level, and edema in an adult. In a child, inadequate protein will, of course, result in very poor growth and will often lead to the protein-deficiency disease called "kwashiorkor" (Figure 27-5).

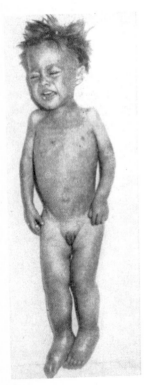

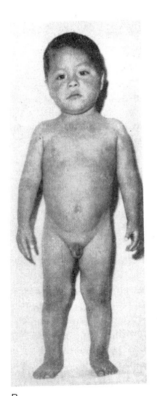

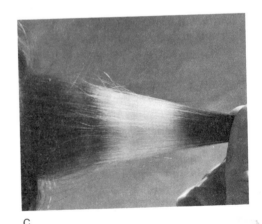

A　　　　　　　　　　　　　B　　　　　　　　　　　　　C

FIGURE 27-5 Protein-calorie malnutrition. (A) A child, 32 months old, on admission to hospital. (B) The same child 19 weeks later, after treatment with a high-protein vegetable diet. (C) The so-called "flag sign," when hair color is changing from orange back to black, often seen during recovery from kwashiorkor. (Courtesy Institute for Nutrition for Central America and Panama)

Nitrogen balance

A measurement of the body's **nitrogen balance** is one way of detecting a diet that is not providing adequate protein. An adult should normally be in *nitrogen equilibrium,* which means that the size of the amino acid pool remains constant over a period of time. A *positive* nitrogen balance means that the intake (in food) of amino acid nitrogen, symbolized by NI in Figure 27-6, is greater than the amount excreted by the body (its output or NO). We expect a positive nitrogen balance in a growing child, in an adult recovering from a prolonged illness, and in an athlete who is increasing muscle size through training.

A *negative* nitrogen balance is a sign of malnutrition. It means that more nitrogen is being excreted by the body than is being taken in. While body proteins are decomposing, new polypeptide chains are not being built at the same rate and so there will be loss of body tissue, as shown in Figure 27-6.

Complete and incomplete proteins

The United Nations has also determined the ideal amount of each essential amino acid that should be contained in food protein (this is called the *reference pattern*). This ideal amount can be compared with the amount provided by each common food source of protein, as shown in Table 27-2.

It is clear that animal proteins—eggs, dairy products, and meat—are generally quite satisfactory. These are called **complete proteins** because they contain adequate amounts of every essential amino acid. A child fed exclusively on any complete protein will suffer no deficiency, provided the total amount of protein is adequate for the body's needs. A vegetarian diet that includes adequate amounts of milk or eggs will not cause any protein-deficiency problems.

In contrast, the proteins in vegetables, legumes (beans), and grains are generally unbalanced in amino acid content and are called *incomplete pro-*

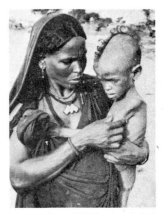

A starving child in the Sahel region of North Africa. (Courtesy Agency for International Development)

CONDITIONS BETWEEN TIME 1 AND TIME 2		BODY PROTEIN (N) POOL SIZE	
	NI = NO	Time 1	Time 2
Nitrogen equilibrium Body size and composition constant		☐	☐
	NI > NO		
Positive nitrogen balance Growth, tissue development		☐	▨ more N in pool
	NI < NO		
Negative nitrogen balance Loss of body tissue		☐	⬚ less N in pool

FIGURE 27-6   A negative nitrogen balance is a sign of malnutrition. When the amount of nitrogen taken in by the body (NI) is equal to the amount put out (NO), the nitrogen requirement of an adult is being met. The person is then neither gaining nor losing body protein. A growing child should have NI greater than NO, since body proteins are being built. If NO is greater than NI, the body is using proteins for energy and depleting the body tissues to do so.

TABLE 27–2 PERCENTAGE OF ESSENTIAL AMINO ACIDS IN FOOD
PROTEINS COMPARED WITH FAO/WHO REFERENCE PATTERNS

| Protein Food | The most common limiting amino acids | | | | Amino acids usually adequate in the diet | | | |
	Lysine	Methionine and Cysteine	Threo-nine	Trypto-phan	Iso-leucine	Leucine	Phenylalanine and Tyrosine	Valine
Reference pattern (in mg) amino acid per g of protein (=100%)	55	35	40	10	40	70	60	50
Percentage of reference pattern in 1 g of protein from:								
Eggs	127	166	128	150	155	126	165	136
Cow's milk	131	98	110	140	160	179	218	148
Beef	162	114	115	110	120	116	133	100
Soybeans	116	74	98	130	112	111	135	96
Peanuts (ground)	65	69	65	100	85	91	148	84
Cassava meal	74	77	65	110	70	56	68	66
Potatoes, white	87	54	95	160	95	86	112	94
Wheat, whole grain	53	114	72	110	82	96	125	88
Wheat, processed	38	114	68	110	90	100	120	82
Corn, whole grain	49	100	90	70	92	179	145	96
Rice, brown	69	97	98	120	95	117	143	110
Rice, polished white	65	106	82	130	105	117	133	116

Values adapted from Briggs, G.M., and Calloway, D.H., *Bogert's Nutrition and Physical Fitness,* 10th edition, Philadelphia, W.B. Saunders, 1979, Table 5-3.

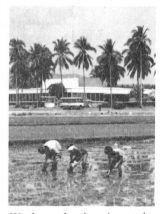

Workers planting rice at the International Rice Research Institute, Los Baños, Philippines. The search for high-yield, high-protein grains has produced several varieties of "miracle rice."

teins. The most deficient amino acid is usually lysine (wheat, corn, and rice in Table 27–2). Since these grains represent the principal food for most of the world's population, the world food problem is very largely a "lysine problem." Some cultures use potatoes, cassava, or beans as the diet staple. In such cases, a methionine or leucine deficiency may be the problem.

Rats fed a diet of incomplete protein suffer serious health problems (Figure 27–7). Fad diets are often constructed in such a way that protein malnutrition results. The worst such diet is the "Zen macrobiotic" diet (which should not be confused with Zen Buddhism), in which the "ideal" is to subsist on rice alone. Some people using such a diet have starved to death even though they were getting adequate energy calories; others have suffered permanent kidney damage.

Intensive studies are under way in various research institutes around the world to improve the yield and hardiness of cereal crops, as well as to increase the proportion of lysine in these grains. The "Green Revolution" holds great promise—if it works. Alternate sources of protein, such as fish meal, seaweed, bacteria colonies on oil, and "soyaburgers," are also being pursued.*

---

* Difficulties in solving the food problems of malnourished populations are not limited to producing enough protein. For example, in addition to finding high-yield, high-protein rice strains that can cope with plant disease, insects, and a variety of soil and weather conditions, the International Rice Research Institute must also take into account the cultural traditions of each country. Some countries are accustomed to short-grain rice, others to the long-grain variety. If the taste, texture, or smell of a new "miracle rice" variety is too different from the traditional type, people will be slow to accept the new product and malnutrition will persist. This type of problem is obviously much greater with novel foods, like fish meal, algae steaks, and seaweed.

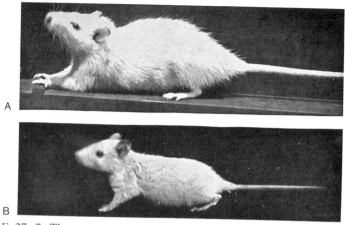

FIGURE 27-7 The top rat was grown on a complete protein (casein from milk), but the bottom rat received an incomplete protein (gliadin from wheat). Both quality *and* quantity of dietary protein are nutritionally important.

Even in the "rich" American diet, ways must be found to provide adequate nutrition for the entire population without depending solely on expensive cuts of meat. One way to do this is to *combine* two or more incomplete proteins so that the *total* of each essential amino acid is adequate for the body's needs. Some combinations that do an excellent job of providing amino acid balance are a peanut butter sandwich with milk, potato with egg, and a grilled cheese sandwich (wheat plus milk protein).

Another health factor is related to the *amount* of protein in a food; for example, rice contains only 7 to 8% protein, soybeans about 40%. In order to build up an adequate amino acid pool, you would have to eat more rice than soybeans and thus take in many more calories in the form of carbohydrates; this could lead to an obesity problem.

In terms of amino acid intake alone, animal protein is probably better than wheat, corn, or rice as the body's major source.*

Active and inactive body proteins

On p. 632, we discussed some enzymes that are synthesized by the cell in an inactive or precursor (*proenzyme*) form (a form that doesn't work as an enzyme). The same is true of other proteins, such as insulin. The synthesis of an inactive form serves as a way of storing a protein until it is needed in its **active protein** form.

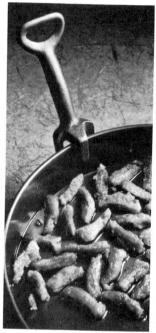

Soybean flour can be used to make a high-protein substitute for ground beef. (Courtesy Archer Daniels-Midland Co.)

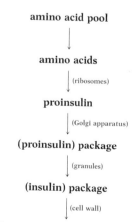

amino acid pool
↓
amino acids
↓ (ribosomes)
proinsulin
↓ (Golgi apparatus)
(proinsulin) package
↓ (granules)
(insulin) package
↓ (cell wall)
free insulin in blood stream

---

* Although meats in general provide the maximum amount of protein for a given mass of food, some meats (and eggs) contain very high levels of cholesterol and saturated fats, which may be related in some people to heart and circulatory disease. Taking this into account, the best sources of protein for adults might be fish (baked or poached rather than fried) and skim milk. An astounding 61% of the calories of fish is protein, and fish contains much less fat than beef or chicken.

As an example of a biologically inactive protein, we will consider *proinsulin*. The entire production process for insulin occurs in the islet cells of the pancreas, starting with the synthesis of proinsulin on the ribosomes (Section 20.5). The proinsulin molecules are then carried to the Golgi apparatus (Figure 20-5), where they are wrapped inside neat packages called *storage granules*. As these granules migrate through the cytoplasm, the proinsulin is converted to active insulin. When insulin is required by the body, these granules reach the cell membrane and secrete active insulin hormone into the blood.

Other cells in the body are responsible for the synthesis of proenzymes, other prohormones, and precursors of the essential blood plasma proteins.

SELF-CHECK

27.3) If corn meal were the only source of protein in a child's diet, would health problems result? Explain.

27.4) A child is brought into a hospital with negative nitrogen balance. What probably caused this state? How do we measure it? How can we cure it?

27.5) How would your metabolism be affected if, for some reason, your pancreas cells could not split away the inactive part of the proinsulin molecule to produce insulin?

27.3 CATABOLISM OF AMINO ACIDS

LEARNING GOAL 27F: Describe the process of transamination.
27G: Describe how oxidative deamination produces ammonia or ammonium ion.

The diets of most North Americans contain adequate amounts of carbohydrates, fats, and proteins. Generally, the body prefers glucose for brain and nervous system activity and for energy. Fat takes care of energy needs between meals or during fasting. When eaten by adults, protein yields amino acids that are no longer needed for growth and can be broken down to produce energy. This process is not so efficient as that for glucose and much less efficient than that for fats. If you can afford the cost, a high-protein, low-carbohydrate, low-fat diet is very effective for losing weight.

Transamination

The major process by which the body removes nitrogen from amino acids is by transferring the amino group to α-ketoglutaric acid, a compound that is made in ample amounts in the Krebs cycle. One example of this process is

$$
\underset{\substack{\text{aspartic} \\ \text{acid}}}{\underset{\displaystyle \text{COOH}}{\overset{\displaystyle \text{COOH}}{\overset{\displaystyle | }{\underset{|}{\overset{|}{\text{CH}_2}}}}}}
\;\; \overset{\displaystyle \text{HCNH}_2}{} \;\; + \;\;
\underset{\substack{\alpha\text{-ketoglutaric} \\ \text{acid}}}{}
$$

(Structures, left to right:)

aspartic acid: COOH — CH$_2$ — HCNH$_2$ — COOH

+ α-ketoglutaric acid: COOH — CH$_2$ — CH$_2$ — C=O — COOH

$\xrightarrow[\substack{\text{pyridoxal} \\ \text{phosphate}}]{\substack{\text{aspartate} \\ \text{transaminase}}}$

oxaloacetic acid: COOH — CH$_2$ — C=O — COOH

+ glutamic acid: COOH — CH$_2$ — CH$_2$ — HCNH$_2$ — COOH

The general name for this process is **transamination,** and it is common to most amino acids. There are **transaminase** enzymes for many amino acids. Two important ones useful in medical diagnosis are alanine and aspartate transaminases, shown in Table 23–1 and on the blood test form in Figure 24–1 (as "transferases"). Because of the breakdown of heart muscle, both of these enzymes are found at higher levels in cases of myocardial infarction (heart attack).

Oxidative deamination

The glutamic acid produced in transamination can give up its amino group, which is neutralized and excreted as NH_4^+ ion in the urine:

glutamic acid: COOH — CH$_2$ — CH$_2$ — H—C—NH$_2$ — COOH

$+ H_2O \; \underset{\substack{\text{NAD}^+ \quad \text{NADH}}}{\overset{\substack{\text{glutamate} \\ \text{dehydrogenase}}}{\rightleftharpoons}}$

α-ketoglutaric acid: COOH — CH$_2$ — CH$_2$ — C=O — COOH

$+ NH_4^+$

This process is the reverse of transamination and returns us to α-ketoglutaric acid, which can then accept new amino groups from other amino acids. This process is called **oxidative deamination.**

Acids other than glutamic acid can undergo the same process:

$$
\underset{\substack{\text{amino acid}}}{\text{R}-\underset{\underset{\text{NH}_2}{|}}{\text{CH}}-\text{COOH}} \;\; \xrightarrow[\substack{\text{FAD} \quad \text{FADH}_2}]{\substack{\text{amino acid} \\ \text{oxidase}}} \;\; \underset{\substack{\text{amino acid}}}{\text{R}-\underset{\underset{\text{NH}}{\|}}{\text{C}}-\text{COOH}} \;\; \xrightarrow[\text{H}_2\text{O}]{\text{hydrolysis}}
$$

$$
\underset{\substack{\text{keto acid}}}{\text{R}-\underset{\underset{\text{O}}{\|}}{\text{C}}-\text{COOH}} + NH_4^+
$$

The fate of the keto acid formed by transamination or oxidative deamination depends on the amino acid from which it came. The keto acids from over one half of the amino acids end up as acetyl CoA that feeds into the Krebs cycle for energy. The rest are converted to compounds such as oxaloacetate and α-ketoglutarate and similarly continue through the Krebs cycle. The specific reactions in the metabolism of each of the 20 amino acids are beyond the scope of this text.

We mentioned earlier that amino acids are not the best source of energy for the body. For example, if you eat hamburgers, steaks, and hot dogs to obtain a little over 100 grams of protein per day, the amino acids traveling through the reactions just described will provide only about 70 grams of glucose. A long period of starvation will deplete even the fat depots, forcing the body to use its protein as the main source of energy. At this point, a person would be in severe negative nitrogen balance, losing muscle tissue to stay alive.

SELF-CHECK

27.6) Why is α-ketoglutaric acid a key compound in amino acid catabolism?

27.7) What two enzymes are involved in the formation of NH_4^+ by oxidative deamination?

27.8) What coenzymes are used in the process of oxidative deamination?

27.4 FORMATION OF AMINO ACIDS

LEARNING GOAL 27H: Describe how amino acids are formed by reverse oxidative deamination and transamination.

We have already seen that the synthesis of tissue and organ proteins requires an adequate supply of essential amino acids, which must come from the diet. What about the nonessential amino acids, which are also required in protein synthesis? These can be formed by the reverse of the oxidative deamination and transamination process involving α-ketoglutaric and glutamic acids. In general, ammonia reacts with α-ketoglutaric acid to form glutamic acid, which then transfers its amino group by transamination to a keto acid to form a new amino acid:

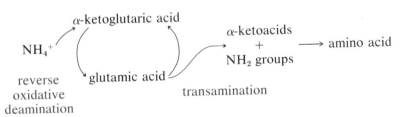

The Krebs cycle furnishes the α-ketoglutaric acid and the NH_4^+ comes from the deamination of excess amino acids. The glutamic acid that is formed then transfers amino groups to keto acids to synthesize needed nonessential amino acids.

For example, pyruvic acid forms alanine and oxalacetic acid forms aspartic acid by this process. The body thus has a mechanism for removing amino groups from an amino acid it has in excess and using them to synthesize another amino acid it needs for specific protein molecules.

It is reasonable to assume that not all of the nonessential amino acids are formed by the process just described. The simple amino acid serine is made from 3-PO_4- glyceric acid from the Embden-Meyerhof pathway. Serine is readily converted to glycine. As mentioned earlier, cysteine is formed from the essential amino acid methionine and tyrosine is made by adding a hydroxyl group to phenylalanine.

27.9) Describe the role of glutamic acid in the formation of nonessential amino acids.

SELF-CHECK

27.5 FORMATION OF UREA

LEARNING GOAL 27I: *Explain the importance of carbamyl phosphate to the urea cycle.*

27J: *Describe the functions of ornithine and arginine in the urea cycle.*

27K: *Describe how glutamine is formed in the liver and how it produces ammonia in the kidneys.*

As discussed in the last section, the amino groups from amino acids may be collected by α-ketoglutaric acid to form glutamic acid or they may be converted to NH_4^+ by oxidative deamination. It is not difficult for aspartic acid or alanine to form glutamic acid or for glutamic acid to transfer its amino group to form aspartic acid, alanine, or other amino acids. This process, however, does not use up very much of the daily load of amino acids. Remember that adults are normally in nitrogen balance. Each day, we excrete the same amount of nitrogen we take in. Most of the nitrogen is excreted as urea. Some of it is excreted as uric acid, which will be discussed in the next section, and a small amount leaves the body in the form of ammonia.

We have already seen that metabolism runs in cycles, so it should be no surprise that the body has a **urea cycle.** A molecule of carbon dioxide and two amino groups from the breakdown of amino acids enter this cycle by combining with *ornithine* to form *citrulline* and eventually the amino acid arginine. Arginase in the liver splits urea away from arginine to form the starting compound ornithine and the cycle continues (Figure 27–8). Both ornithine and citrulline are amino acids not found in proteins but present in the liver. Recall that the body often activates molecules before starting a synthesis, as in the activation of acetyl CoA for the Krebs cycle. In the urea cycle, the CO_2 from the Krebs cycle and the ammonia from the catabolism of amino acids are activated through the formation of *carbamyl phosphate.*

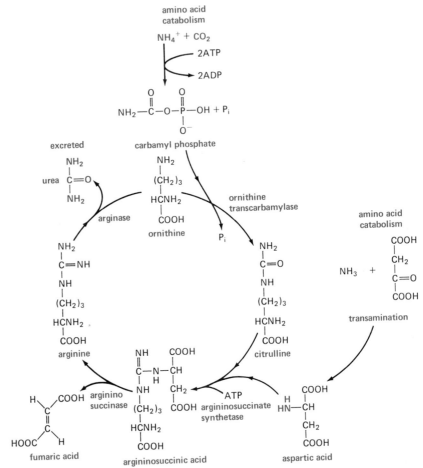

FIGURE 27–8 The urea cycle.

$$NH_2-\underset{\overset{\parallel}{O}}{C}-O-\underset{\overset{\parallel}{\underset{\underset{O^-}{|}}{}}}{\overset{\overset{O}{\parallel}}{P}}-OH$$

carbamyl phosphate

The activated CO_2 and ammonia are transferred to ornithine, which acts as a carrier on the way to arginine, in a manner similar to the way oxaloacetic acid carries acetyl groups in the Krebs cycle. (It is not necessary for you to learn all the details of this cycle.)

The product excreted from the body is urea.

$$NH_2$$
$$|$$
$$C=O$$
$$|$$
$$NH_2$$

urea

One amino group of urea comes from carbamyl phosphate, the other enters the cycle in aspartic acid formed in transamination. Urea is a neutral, water-soluble molecule that, after being formed by the liver, is carried in the blood to the kidneys and excreted in the urine. It is the main end product of amino acid catabolism and accounts for 80 to 90 per cent of the daily excretion of nitrogen in the urine. About 30 grams of urea are excreted each day.

Recall that one of the body's defenses against acidosis is the formation of ammonia by the kidney tubule cells (p. 669). This ammonia combines with ketone bodies to form ammonium salts for excretion and to recover sodium ion. Ammonia does not circulate in the blood except in very small amounts. If a large amount of ammonia were present in the blood, it would produce severe alkalosis. In aquatic animals that excrete ammonia instead of urea, and to a small extent in our bodies, ammonia formed in the liver by trans-amination can combine with glutamic acid to form *glutamine,* which can be carried to the kidneys by the blood without changing the pH. There it is converted to ammonia by the enzyme *glutaminase.* We use the ammonia to combat acidosis.

Aquatic animals such as tadpoles excrete their nitrogen as ammonia in the urine. After tadpoles become frogs, their livers form all the enzymes and other compounds necessary for the urea cycle. They then excrete urea instead of ammonia.

Note that both ammonia and ammonium ion are present in the kidneys and in urine, with proportions depending on the pH. Therefore, in describing many of the processes covered in this chapter, biochemists tend to use the two terms interchangeably.

SELF-CHECK

27.10)   How are the two amino groups of urea fed into the urea cycle?
27.11)   Does ornithine function in the urea cycle pretty much the way oxaloacetate functions in the Krebs cycle? Explain.
27.12)   How is glutamic acid in the liver related to ammonia production by the kidneys?

27.6 METABOLISM OF NUCLEOPROTEINS

LEARNING GOAL 27L: Describe what happens to the hydrolysis products of nucleoproteins after digestion.
        27M: Describe the steps leading to the formation of uric acid.

Nucleoproteins are essential constituents of the nucleus of all cells and are composed of a protein combined with a nucleic acid. The most important nucleic acids, DNA and RNA, are essential constituents of chromosomes and viruses and are involved in the synthesis of proteins. Nucleoproteins in the food we eat are first digested (hydrolyzed) to nucleic acids and proteins, and the proteins are then split into amino acids. Nucleic acids are broken down into their constituents by a series of digestive enzymes:

$$nucleoprotein \longrightarrow nucleic\ acid + protein$$
$$\downarrow$$
$$nucleotides$$
$$\downarrow$$
$$nucleosides + H_3PO_4$$
$$\downarrow$$
$$purines + pyrimidines + ribose$$

In metabolism, the amino acids and ribose follow the normal processes for proteins and carbohydrates. The phosphoric acid may be used to form other phosphate compounds (such as glucose-6-PO_4 or ATP), or it may be excreted in the urine as phosphates.

Purine metabolism

The body must have a way of synthesizing purines for the production of AMP, ATP, and nucleic acids. The synthesis is carried out by several complex reactions that are beyond the scope of this discussion. In brief, the process starts with ribose-5-PO_4, which first adds an amino group on carbon 1. This is followed by the addition of glycine and other nitrogen and carbon atoms and a closing of the rings to form inosinic acid, which can be readily converted to adenine or guanine (Figure 20–8).

The purines formed by the hydrolysis of nucleic acids either in digestion or in the tissues are not broken down to NH_3, CO_2, and H_2O as the amino acids are. Instead, they are progressively oxidized from adenine to hypoxanthine (6-oxypurine) and from guanine to xanthine (2,6-dioxypurine), with final oxidation to *uric acid* (2,6,8-trioxypurine). In most mammals (but not in humans and apes), the uric acid is converted to *allantoin,* a water-soluble compound:

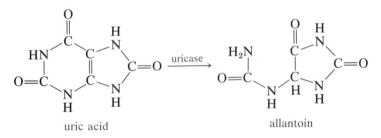

uric acid   allantoin

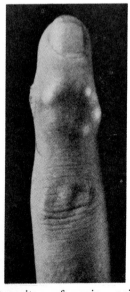

Deposits of uric acid crystals, shown in the joints of this finger, cause the painful condition known as "gout."

Uric acid is the end product of purine catabolism in humans and is excreted in the urine. In a way, it is unfortunate that humans have lost the enzyme uricase over the years because without it uric acid, a very insoluble compound, must be carried to the kidneys by the blood. If the concentration of uric acid in the blood rises much above 7 mg/dL (normal is 5 to 7 mg/dL), a saturation level is reached and uric acid crystals form in the tissues, especially in the joints of the fingers and the big toe. The pointed, needle-shaped crystals can cause considerable pain when the joints move.

This painful condition, called *gout,* has an interesting history. For many years, men with gout (it's most common in males) were associated with high intellect or a high station in life (for example, kings, princes, and college professors). Recent research on a group of young adult males strongly suggests that those with high levels of uric acid in their blood have greater drive and ambition than their friends with normal levels, but not necessarily a higher intellect.

Pyrimidine metabolism

The synthesis of pyrimidines in the body starts with carbamyl phosphate, which combines with the amino acid aspartic acid to form carbamyl aspartic acid. Ring closure then occurs, and orotic acid (6-carboxyluracil) is formed. Orotic acid combines with ribose and phosphoric acid to form a nucleotide that readily loses its carboxyl group, and the result is uridylic acid. Other pyrimidine nucleotides use uridylic acid as a starting compound for their synthesis.

Fortunately, the catabolism of pyrimidines does not follow the same path as that of purines. Cytosine loses ammonia to form uracil (p. 553), which is first reduced and then has its ring split open to form β-alanine, ammonia, and CO_2. These products are converted to urea for excretion in the urine. Since the product of the catabolism of pyrimidines is urea rather than uric acid, development of gout is not promoted.

Carbohydrate, lipid, and protein metabolism

Now that we have completed our discussion of the metabolism of the basic food nutrients, it may help to look at Figure 27–9, a chart relating the

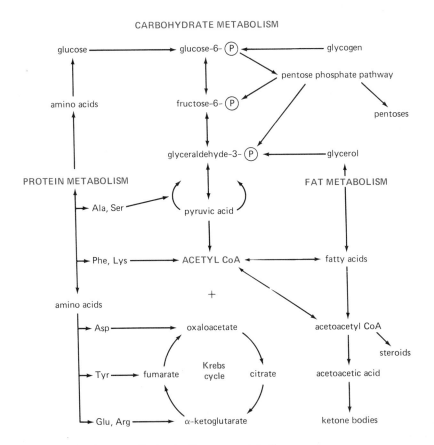

FIGURE 27–9 An overall chart of human metabolism.

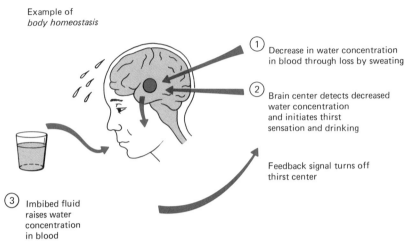

Example of
body homeostasis

1 Decrease in water concentration
in blood through loss by sweating

2 Brain center detects decreased
water concentration
and initiates thirst
sensation and drinking

Feedback signal turns off
thirst center

3 Imbibed fluid
raises water
concentration
in blood

FIGURE 27–10 An example of homeostasis, the tendency of an organism to keep all aspects of its internal environment constant by a system of regulation and control. ①In hot weather, the blood becomes more concentrated as a result of the loss of body fluids in sweat. This increases the oncotic pressure (Section 24.1). ② The brain senses the change in the body's internal system of checks and balances and sends a signal for a hormone that makes us thirsty and also causes the kidneys to excrete less water. ③ After we drink some water, the oncotic pressure goes down. The brain, sensing that "all has returned to normal," stops producing the hormone (in this case, vasopressin).

three pathways. As you now know, hormonal control and other "feedback" mechanisms provide a way for the body to regulate the amount of reactant that enters each path.

Homeostasis

The French physiologist Claude Bernard found that the blood sugar concentration and, in fact, all the levels listed in the blood and urine report forms of Chapter 24, are kept relatively constant in a normal body. The American physiologist Walter Cannon called this process **homeostasis,** the operation of body processes that are coordinated with each other to maintain constant levels of reactants and products. An example of homeostasis is provided in Figure 27–10. Human physiology and biochemistry are largely a science of finding out how the body maintains itself in this manner. You have seen many examples of homeostasis in these final three chapters on metabolism.

SELF-CHECK

27.13) Name the products of the complete hydrolysis of nucleoproteins.

27.14) What are the symptoms of gout? What is the cause? What is one possible "advantage" of having gout?

27.15*) Use Figure 25–6 (p. 686) to explain the concept of *homeostasis* in the human body.

CHAPTER TWENTY-SEVEN IN REVIEW ■ Protein Metabolism

GLOSSARY FOR CHAPTER TWENTY-SEVEN

active protein A protein molecule, such as an enzyme or hormone, that has been changed from an inactive precursor (proenzyme or prohormone). (p. 719)

amino acid pool The assortment of amino acid molecules in the blood plasma and cytoplasm available to the body for all phases of protein metabolism. (p. 712)

complete protein A food protein containing adequate amounts of all essential amino acids. (p. 717)

essential amino acid An amino acid that is essential for growth and cannot be synthesized from other materials in the body. (p. 715)

homeostasis The tendency of the body to keep constant all aspects of its internal environment (concentrations, osmotic pressures) through feedback and control mechanisms and especially through the hormonal regulation of metabolic processes. (p. 728)

nitrogen balance A comparison of the amount of nitrogen entering the body through food with the amount excreted; a growing child should have positive nitrogen balance; an adult should generally be in equilibrium; negative nitrogen balance is a sign of malnutrition. (p. 717)

oxidative deamination The removal of amino groups from amino acids. (p. 721)

transaminase An enzyme that catalyzes transamination. (p. 721)

transamination The conversion of keto acids to amino acids, effectively transferring the amino group from one molecule to another; often uses glutamic or aspartic acid as the source of the amino group. (p. 721)

urea cycle A series of reactions in the liver that use CO_2 and NH_3 from protein metabolism to produce urea for excretion. (p. 723)

QUESTIONS AND PROBLEMS FOR CHAPTER TWENTY-SEVEN ■

Protein Metabolism

SECTION 27.1 THE AMINO ACID POOL

27.16) What happens to the amino acids formed by the hydrolysis of proteins during digestion?

27.17*) Name three important enzymes used in protein digestion.

27.32) Some of the amino acids in blood are made into tissue proteins. How stable are tissue proteins once they are made?

27.33*) Where would you suppose the enzyme pepsin is synthesized? Why?

SECTION 27.2 FOOD AND PROTEIN SYNTHESIS

27.18) List the amino acids that are essential for growth in a human infant.

27.19) Very seldom are students in a negative nitrogen balance. Explain.

27.20) Insulin may be stored in the cell in an inactive form. Explain.

27.34) What would happen to cows fed a tryptophan-deficient diet from birth?

27.35) A child in a very poor family failed to grow at a normal rate. What would you suspect as the cause?

27.36) Why is insulin stored in an inactive form? When is it activated?

SECTION 27.3 CATABOLISM OF AMINO ACIDS

27.21) What keto acid is formed from alanine by transamination?

27.22) What reaction in catabolism is catalyzed by glutamate dehydrogenase?

27.23) How do most amino acids lose their amino groups during catabolism?

27.37) Why is glutamic acid often emphasized in the transamination process?

27.38) What is the advantage to the body of forming NH_3 from amino acids during catabolism?

27.39) What happens to the keto acids that result from amino acid catabolism?

SECTION 27.4 FORMATION OF AMINO ACIDS

27.24) What is meant by reverse oxidative deamination?

27.40) What amino acid is formed in the reverse transamination from pyruvic acid and glutamic acid?

SECTION 27.5 FORMATION OF UREA

27.25) Ammonia and CO_2 from the complete breakdown of amino acids are combined into what compound for entry into the urea cycle?

27.26) Why are ornithine and citrulline unusual amino acids?

27.27) The concentration of glutamine in the kidneys increases in a patient with diabetic acidosis. Explain.

27.41) Additional ammonia molecules are fed into the urea cycle in the form of an amino acid. Explain.

27.42) How is citrulline involved in the entrance of ammonia into the urea cycle?

27.43) Why is it safer to have glutamine rather than ammonia carried by the blood?

SECTION 27.6 METABOLISM OF NUCLEOPROTEINS

27.28) Name the digestive enzyme that splits a nucleotide into a nucleoside.

27.29) What would be a disadvantage of a high concentration of uric acid in the blood?

27.30*) Enzyme therapy is in the future. How might injections of uricase help a person with gout?

27.31) How is carbamyl phosphate involved in pyrimidine metabolism?

27.44) Of what importance to the body are nucleoproteins?

27.45) What would be an advantage to the body of the synthesis of allantoin instead of uric acid?

27.46) Describe the cause of gout.

27.47) Explain what happens to the end products of pyrimidine catabolism.

27.48*) How are the demands on the amino acid pool different in adults and in growing children?

27.49*) If a person ate nothing but proteins and sufficient vitamins for a month, from where would the energy for normal brain and heart function be obtained?

DNA and the Future

28

As you have progressed through this textbook, you have come closer and closer to the frontiers of research in molecular biology. Most of the general and organic chemistry you have studied has been known for many decades. However, our knowledge of *biochemistry* is quite recent and is still undergoing substantial change.

At the beginning of the 1980's, scientists and the general public alike were excited by the implications of the events recorded by such newspaper headlines as

Scientists clone mice in laboratory
Human growth hormone made by bacteria
Blood tests detect some forms of cancer

The subjects of genetic engineering, cancer, and viruses represent present-day fields of scientific research that are constantly changing and have immense importance to the future of humanity. Each month through the end of the twentieth century will doubtless bring stories of new developments.

This chapter will provide some background in these subjects so that you can begin to understand the importance of some of these events. For the most current information, you will have to consult magazines and scientific journals. We would particularly recommend that you make every effort to look regularly at the pages of *Scientific American*, as well as the publications of the American Association for the Advancement of Science.

One factor links many of the frontiers of biological research—the importance of DNA, the carrier of hereditary information. The central role of DNA will thus provide a constant theme for the various parts of this final chapter.

The AAAS publishes *Science*, a semitechnical journal, much of which you will be able to understand, as well as *Science 81* (. . . *82*, . . . *83*, etc.), an excellent survey for laypersons. Several British journals, such as *Nature* and *New Scientist*, are also very good. Some interesting and very well-illustrated articles with less technical content will be found in the more popularized science magazines, such as *Science Digest* and *Discovery*.

28.1 DNA REPLICATION AND GENES

LEARNING GOAL 28A: *Briefly describe the replication of DNA.*

The human body contains two different kinds of cells: *haploid* cells and *diploid* cells. The haploid cells are also called *germ cells*, because these are the cells, as ova (eggs) in women and sperm cells in men, that give rise to new human beings.

Haploid comes from the Greek word *haploos*, meaning "single or simple." A haploid cell, therefore, contains a single set of chromosomes. *Diploid*, meaning "twofold," describes a cell having *twice as many* chromosomes as a haploid cell. Just remember that the haploid cells are the ova and sperm cells, the "sex" cells, and the diploid cells are all other cells in the body.

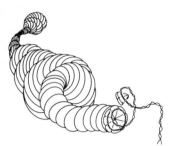

FIGURE 28–1 A chromosome consists of a single DNA double-helix molecule tightly packed with the aid of protein segments, such as histone. The chromosome strand itself is coiled to save space, so a tremendous amount of genetic information (in the form of base pairs) is stored in a minute volume in the nucleus of the cell. (After DuPraw, E. J., *DNA and Chromosomes,* New York, Holt, Rinehart & Winston, 1970)

The same genetic information is also, in some *cases, repeated in several genes. It has been reported that about 30% of human DNA consists of sequences that are repeated at least 20 times.*

Each human haploid (germ) cell contains, in its nucleus, 23 special DNA packages called chromosomes. As a sperm cell and an ovum combine at conception, the 23 chromosomes from the sperm cell and the 23 chromosomes from the ovum pair up to provide the 46 chromosomes found in every *diploid cell* of the body. The diploid cells include all body cells except the ova and sperm cells. (In this text, we will sometimes refer to diploid cells as "tissue cells," to remind you that these cells are what make up all the tissues, organs, and membranes of the body.) The nucleus of each cell of the body except the germ cells thus contains a full set of hereditary information. Each time a new cell is formed, the existing chromosomes must divide in such a way that this information is passed on in the process known as *DNA replication.*

The nature of a chromosome

Each **chromosome** contains a single, very long DNA molecule. This double-stranded chain is tightly coiled and held in place by protein, as shown in Figure 28–1. The diameter of a typical diploid cell is perhaps five to ten millionths of a meter, yet the DNA contained in the nucleus of that cell, if stretched out, might have a total length of two meters!

As you know from Section 20.3, the DNA structure involves a polynucleotide backbone to which are attached base pairs that involve adenine, guanine, cytosine, and thymine units. The DNA in the chromosomes of one cell may involve 5.5×10^9 base pairs. The order of the four bases in these chains provide *all* of the hereditary information passed on from parents to offspring.

The gene

A gene was first defined as a unit of inheritance, that is to say, something that controls the appearance of a specific trait, such as blue eyes, red hair, or musical ability. To a chemist, a **gene** is simply a region of chromosome DNA that provides, through transcription (Section 20.4) and translation (Section 20.5), the code for a particular protein molecule:

genetic information   transfer of hereditary
    (gene)   information

      DNA $\longrightarrow$ messenger RNA $\longrightarrow$ transfer RNA $\longrightarrow$ protein

in chromosomes of   in cytoplasm
  cell nucleus

The end product of this pattern is a specific protein molecule with a particular function to perform. We may see the result of this function in the form of hair or eye color, special abilities, or, in some cases, abnormalities called *hereditary diseases.*

We know from Chapter 20 that a sequence of three nucleotides in DNA provides the "message" that will result in a particular amino acid residue being inserted into the protein chain. The gene that codes for *proinsulin,* a molecule with 81 amino acid residues, would thus make up at least $3 \times 81 = 243$ nucleotide units on the DNA chain of a chromosome. Various polypeptide chains in the cells have from 100 to 2000 residues. Thus, a gene might have from 300 to 6000 nucleotide base pairs. Some proteins (hemoglobin, for example) involve more than one polypeptide chain, in which case several genes must work together to produce a functional molecule.

The exact location of a specific gene on a particular chromosome is often very difficult to establish, but biochemists have been successful in charting some of them. Fortunately, the genes that code for the individual enzymes of a pathway are often located next to each other on chromosomes and may be transcribed and translated as a group. Any attempt at surgical change of the genes inside a human embryo, one of the possible developments in the field of *genetic engineering,* must necessarily involve very detailed knowledge about the exact location of a gene along the 46 DNA coils of a cell nucleus.

Since all body cells other than germ cells contain the same 46 chromosomes and thus the same genes, all start with the same basic hereditary information. Specialization of these cells into skin, muscle, organs, and other types must result in most of the genes in the diploid cell becoming inactive and *not* producing proteins; otherwise, every cell would be filled by the same protein "mix." Only those genes needed for a particular cell are "activated." A relatively complex process provides the means by which a cell *induces* (turns on) or *represses* (turns off) the ability of a gene to make messenger RNA, and thus to manufacture proteins.

Replication of DNA

Each tissue cell of the human body normally contains *all* of the genetic material and information that was present in the fertilized ovum. The DNA in that original cell therefore had to be reproduced 75 trillion times (the number of cells in the body) in order to be found in each cell nucleus. The manner in which each DNA strand creates a duplicate of itself is called **replication.**

Watson and Crick, who developed the double-helix model for DNA (p. 556), also proposed a mechanism for the duplication of the DNA base pair sequence when a cell divides into two. The two interwoven strands of DNA are held together by hydrogen-bonding between *complementary* bases. The two strands thus contain complementary base-pair sequences. Duplication of DNA thus can occur through the separation of the two strands in such a way that each becomes a pattern on which a *replica* of the other strand can be built. Figure 28–2 shows how this process might occur. Just as transcription requires an "unraveling" enzyme, replication requires DNA polymerase to catalyze the process.

The result of replication is *two* DNA strands, each identical to the original.

Cloning

As already mentioned, each haploid (germ) cell in humans contains only 23 chromosomes. When a sperm and an ovum combine, the two nuclei merge to give a total of 46 chromosomes, so that *all* of the genetic information is available to produce the offspring. This information has come from *two* parents.

Cloning is the process in which a *diploid,* that is, a 46-chromosome cell, divides and produces a whole new organism. In higher animals, this simply

The road to successful cloning is very long and difficult. Not every body cell nucleus necessarily has the ability to produce an entirely new individual. In January 1981, the first scientific report appeared of successful cloning of mammals (mice). Earlier reports (and a book) claiming cloning of a male child have not yet been backed by any scientific evidence.

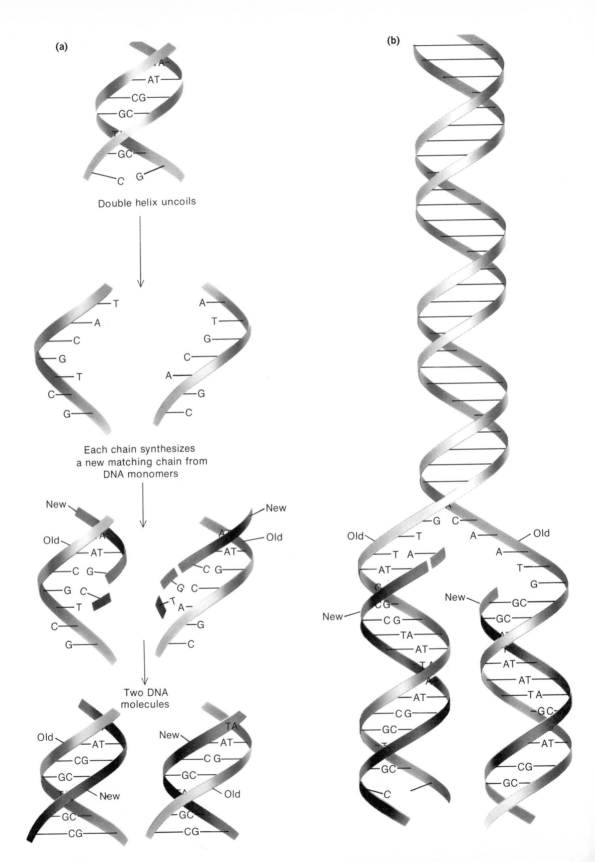

(a)

Double helix uncoils

Each chain synthesizes
a new matching chain from
DNA monomers

Two DNA
molecules

Old — New

Old — New

(b)

Old

New

Old

New

FIGURE 28-2   Replication of a DNA molecule: (a) As part of the DNA strand unwinds, RNA and enzymes are busy building new complementary DNA strands, using the originals as templates; the replicas are together identical to the original DNA double helix. (b) The process occurs gradually as part of the complex process of cell division. (After Watson, J., *Molecular Biology of the Gene*, 2nd edition, W. A. Benjamin, 1970, p. 267.)

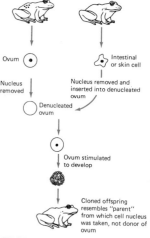

does not happen. The only cells that are "geared" to divide and form new organisms are the haploids, in the form of fertilized ova.

However, there is a way of cloning animals that works in some cases. The nucleus from an ovum (which contains the haploid number of chromosomes) is removed and replaced with a diploid nucleus (containing twice the haploid number of chromosomes) from a tissue cell. If the ovum is already fertilized, or if it can be stimulated to divide, then the resultant animal will have the characteristics of the *animal that provided the diploid nucleus*, not those of the donor of the ovum. The nucleus in the developing ovum determines the result, as shown in Figure 28-3. Of course, it is also necessary to have the cloned ovum develop to maturity.

Techniques for removing human ova and then reimplanting them in the uterus (so-called "test-tube babies") have been developed. Therefore, the potential exists for combining these two methods to produce a human clone. This idea has caught the public imagination. Visions of marching armies of identical, mindless semihumans have served fantasy buffs. Nothing could be further from the truth. Cloning raises serious ethical problems,* but a clone would be a normal and unique individual.

Have you ever known a set of identical twins? They are as alike as a clone would be to its parent, except that identical twins are the same age but a clone would necessarily be much younger than its parent. Identical twins are very much alike in *some* respects. However, they develop substantial personality differences, partly because of their upbringing and partly because the cell environment inside two developing embryos is never identical. Messenger RNA, in particular, has an important effect on development.

FIGURE 28-3   The technique of cloning. Long applied to frogs, this method has only recently and with great difficulty been applied to mammals. The offspring are genetically identical to the parent, although the effects of environment will produce a distinct individual.

SELF-CHECK

28.1)   Compare DNA *replication*, described in Figure 28-2, with the *transcription* of the genetic code to messenger RNA shown in Figure 20-15. How are these two processes alike? How do they differ?

28.2 INBORN ERRORS OF METABOLISM

*LEARNING GOAL 28B: Describe several possible causes of a gene defect.
28C: Describe a method by which a hereditary disease may be detected early in pregnancy.*

---

* Some scientists feel that research on cloning and on test-tube babies should proceed at full speed. Others are much more cautious about the implications of such research. One ethical problem is the possible use of surrogate (substitute) mothers as "wombs for hire" to carry a pregnancy to term. The effects of extensive cloning on marriage, family, and child-raising practices are also unknown. Many years ago, Aldous Huxley in *Brave New World* gave a futuristic scenario of a society in which children were conceived, developed, and raised by artificial means. If his predictions of the resulting emotionless, rigid, and dehumanized society were valid, perhaps we would be better off to abandon this field!

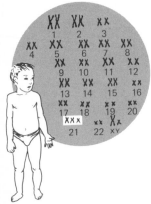

FIGURE 28–4 Detection of a disease caused by an incorrect number of chromosomes (Down's syndrome). The chromosomes in a cell ready to divide are stained and then photographed through a microscope. The photograph is then cut up and the chromosomes arranged in a known order, as shown. In this disease, which strikes one in every 700 U.S. births, an extra chromosome is found in the 21st pair.

In most instances, the rules of heredity give us strong hints as to whether children will have brown eyes or blue, dark skin or light, the stature of a basketball player or that of a jockey. Sometimes, however, problems arise when genes make a mistake. A child may inherit one or two defective genes that produce such hereditary diseases as diabetes mellitus, sickle cell anemia, and phenylketonuria.

If the parents are close blood relatives, there is an increased chance that a child might develop a disease that only occurs when *both* parents carry the defective gene. Other genetic diseases may result from the incorrect duplication of chromosomes, chance mutations, or the destruction of genes.

Chromosome errors

Some genetic diseases arise from errors in the number of chromosomes or errors in gene arrangement caused in the process of cell division. In some cases, such a biological error may be spotted by analysis of a karyotype, which is a map of the chromosomes of a body cell obtained by enlarging and cutting up a photograph of the chromosomes in a nucleus. Figure 28–4 shows such an analysis in a case of Down's syndrome, the production of a "mongoloid" child.

Mutation

A **mutation** is a change in the nucleotide sequence of a gene. Some mutations make a gene useless, possibly killing the organism; others have no obvious effect. If the gene is one that is duplicated many times in the chromosomes, its loss may not be very serious.

If a mutation occurs in a mature diploid cell, the change might be visible (Figure 28-5) but will not be passed along to the offspring. If it affects the germ cells, then the offspring may be seriously affected.

Chromosomes have always been subject to mutations, since the living organisms on earth are constantly bombarded by cosmic rays and other sources of radiation. Certain chemical agents (Table 28–1) and high temperatures may also cause mutations. The modern version of Darwin's theory of natural selection presumes that mutations caused by radiation are responsi-

TABLE 28–1 SOME KNOWN MUTAGENIC CHEMICALS

Aflatoxin (from mold)
Benzo(α)pyrene (cigarette smoke)
Caffeine (coffee, tea, cola)
Captan (a fungicide)
Dimethyl sulfate (industrial)
LSD (psychedelic drug)
Maleic hydrazide ("Slo-Gro" plant agent)
Mustard gas (chemical warfare)
Nitrous acid, HNO_2 (from nitrites)
Ozone, O_3 (in upper atmosphere)
Glue solvents ("glue sniffing")

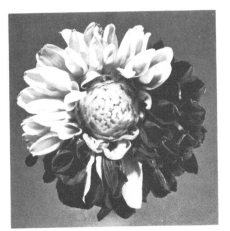

FIGURE 28–5 A mutation in a diploid cell affects living cells but not future generations. This dahlia bloom has been exposed to gamma radiation from a cobalt-60 source. Half the petals of the normally red flower are white. (Brookhaven National Laboratory)

ble for the bulk of the natural variations in primitive organisms. These variations, of course, were necessary for evolution.

If the chromosomes are subject to high levels of radiation, a larger number of mutations will result. The successful campaign for the abolition of atmospheric tests of nuclear weapons was based on the fact that such tests will produce many mutations and many cases of cancer.

Fortunately, individual cases of mutation-caused genetic disease are rather rare. For each million germ cells, perhaps 150 will have defects that appear immediately, and about 100 will contain *recessive* defects, which will appear only if two individuals with the same defect have children. Instances of recessive defects include roughly 30 cases each of albinism, total color blindness, and hemophilia per million germ cells. However, as the victims of these injurious, but not lethal, mutations have children, the defect is passed along.

Inborn errors of metabolism

In the preceding chapters, we saw numerous important metabolic processes that require enzymes and, in some cases, hormones. A gene defect can cause a metabolic problem by failing to provide necessary cell biochemicals. In 1906, Garrod, a British physician, described metabolic defects that he considered to be problems of heredity and named them "inborn errors of metabolism." Garrod knew of six such diseases, including albinism and alkaptonuria, but we now know of many more diseases of this type, some of which are extremely rare.

Table 28–2 lists some hereditary diseases and also indicates whether some of them may be detected early in pregnancy or only after birth. The most common technique for detecting birth defects and possible genetic disease is **amniocentesis,** the withdrawal of a small amount of fluid from the amniotic sac inside the uterus of a pregnant woman. The fetal cells floating in this fluid may be karyotyped (Figure 28–4) to check for chromosome defects. The fetal blood and urine may also be examined to detect defects. The diagnostic procedure of withdrawing amniotic fluid itself carries risk of damage to the fetus and of miscarriage. It is therefore not used on a wide scale since the potential benefits must outweigh the risks. Amniocentesis is

TABLE 28–2   SOME INBORN ERRORS OF METABOLISM

Disease	Missing protein	Physiological effect	Early detection
Albinism	Tyrosinase	No pigmentation	After birth
Alkaptonuria	Homogentisic acid oxidase	Faulty tyrosine metabolism	After birth
β-Thalassemia	Hemoglobin defect	Anemia	Fetal blood
Fabry's disease			
Gaucher's disease		Degeneration of nervous system	
Niemann-Pick disease	Lipid-hydrolyzing enzymes	through buildup of lipids	Amniocentesis
Tay-Sachs disease			
Galactosemia	Galactose-to-glucose enzyme	Cannot tolerate lactose	Amniocentesis
Hemophilia	Clotting factor	Poor blood clotting	Fetal blood
Phenylketonuria	Phenylalanine hydroxylase	Phenylalanine buildup	At birth
Sickle cell anemia	Hemoglobin defect	Deficient red blood cell O_2 capacity	Amniocentesis
Tyrosinemia	Hydroxyphenylpyruvate oxidase	Kidney and liver defects	After birth

useful only when it may provide specific information to help the prospective parents choose among possible courses of action.

Sickle Cell Anemia

On p. 661 we described the effect of having one incorrect base-pair in the gene that is coded to make one of the protein chains of the hemoglobin molecule. Perhaps one in every ten black Americans, along with many people from Mediterranean countries, is a "carrier" of a gene defect for sickle cell anemia. Such a person will be perfectly normal, except possibly during heavy exercise or at high altitudes. However, if a baby receives defective genes from both parents, the sickle cell anemia will appear, crippling and eventually killing the child. If oxygen is removed from a blood sample of a person with the defective gene, the red blood cells will sickle. This provides an easy test for carriers of the disease.

Tay-Sachs Disease

In a note on p. 520, we mentioned three genetic diseases caused by the absence of enzymes that hydrolyze specific lipid molecules. The Tay-Sachs defective gene, like that for sickle cell anemia, may be carried by persons who are unaware of that fact. Carriers are often persons of Eastern European Jewish descent, although the disease is found elsewhere, including the Lac St-Jean region of Quebec. Since carriers have only one-fourth the normal level of the deficient enzyme in their blood, there is, as for sickle cell anemia, a simple blood test for Tay-Sachs carriers.

Diabetes Mellitus

This disease, described in Section 25.2, is a result of an insulin deficiency. However, studies by J. Vallence-Owen have indicated that, in many cases, the actual formation of insulin and its concentration in the blood are normal. It seems that an abnormal blood protein, *synalbumin*, works against the action of insulin, thus creating a lack of hormone effect. Excessive synalbumin in the blood is inherited. This may explain how diabetes mellitus is passed on from one generation to another as an inborn error of metabolism.

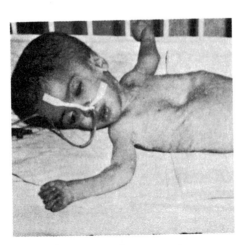

Tay-Sachs disease, one of the inborn errors of metabolism. This three-year-old child has the enlarged head and atrophied muscles characteristic of the disease. (From Volk, B. W., (ed.), *Tay-Sachs Disease*, New York, Grune & Stratton)

Hemophilia

On p. 650 we discussed the symptoms of hemophilia, a group of diseases that result in improper clotting of the blood. Although hemophiliacs are usually males, females can carry the disease. The most famous carrier was Queen Victoria, who passed the disease down to at least six of her great-grandsons.

Phenylketonuria

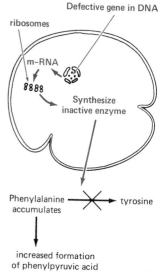

The major symptom of phenylketonuria, associated with mental retardation, is the excretion in the urine of large amounts of phenylpyruvic acid, up to as much as 2 grams each day. The gene that would normally code for the synthesis of the enzyme *phenylalanine hydroxylase,* which converts phenylalanine to tyrosine, is defective. The result is an accumulation of phenylalanine in the blood, spinal fluid, and urine (Figure 28–6).

Today, the practical problem in fighting PKU is to identify babies with the disease and to begin proper treatment immediately. The most foolproof method is to test for increased phenylalanine concentrations in a drop of blood from a newborn baby's heel. Several states require the screening of all babies immediately after birth by this technique because treatment must be started within a few days of birth to prevent mental retardation. In the United States, roughly 200 babies are born annually with this disease and must undergo a rigid dietary regime for several years to prevent brain damage. The treatment is simple, but very difficult to carry out: restrict the amount of phenylalanine in the diet.*

This single gene defect causes other problems. Women with PKU often give birth to deformed babies that do not survive, as do about 10 000 U.S. women who have higher-than-normal blood concentrations of phenylalanine but have not been diagnosed as having PKU. Consideration is now being given to screening expectant mothers for high levels of blood phenylalanine.

FIGURE 28–6 In phenylketonuria, the gene for the synthesis of the enzyme that converts phenylalanine to tyrosine is defective. Phenylalanine then accumulates in the body fluids and can lead to mental retardation.

Alkaptonuria

A rare gene defect causes lack of *homogentisic acid oxidase,* which plays a role in the metabolism of tyrosine. Instead of normal oxidation to fumaric acid and then to acetoacetic acid, the conversion to fumaric acid is blocked (Figure 28–7). This condition may be recognized in early infancy by diapers that are darkly stained with urine.

In adults, alkaptonuria may first be detected in a routine urinalysis, in which the urine shows stronger-than-usual reducing properties. As patients grow older, their ligaments and cartilage tend to become dark blue in color, and arthritis of the bones may develop. At present, there is no specific treatment for this rare condition.

---

* The diet for a PKU child has been called a "nutritionist's nightmare" because the child may eat no meat, fish, wheat, or dairy products. Only specified amounts of vegetables and fruits, such as rice cereal and applesauce, are allowed. A commercially available protein powder with low phenylalanine has been developed. With the proper diet, a child diagnosed as having PKU can develop normally.

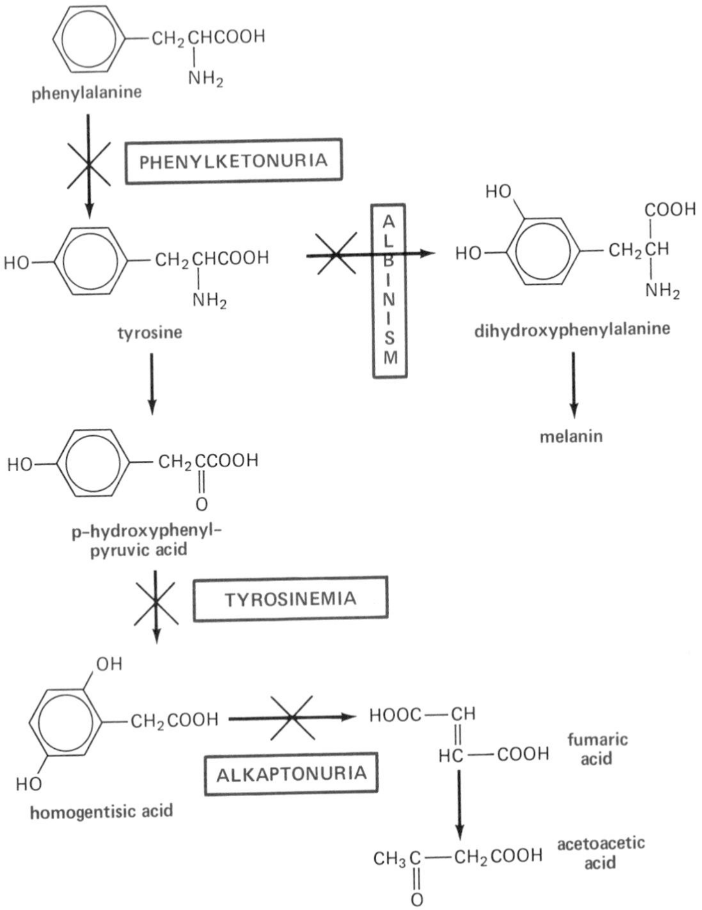

FIGURE 28–7 Four genetic diseases discussed in this chapter are caused by a lack of the enzymes needed for amino acid metabolism.

Tyrosinemia

This is another rare error of tyrosine metabolism, in which the enzyme necessary for the reaction that produces homogentisic acid is lacking. The symptoms are kidney defects and cirrhosis of the liver, found primarily in premature infants. The disease may be acute or chronic. The acute cases usually die of liver failure within seven months of birth.

Ascorbic acid (vitamin C) is the coenzyme of the enzyme missing in cases of tyrosinemia, and the symptoms may be reduced by taking large amounts of ascorbic acid. Long-term treatment for chronic cases consists of a diet low in tyrosine and phenylalanine. If the diet is started early enough, both kidney and liver damage may be avoided.

Albinism

Albinism is yet another rare error in tyrosine metabolism, in which the metabolic pathway to the production of the skin pigment *melanin* is blocked, as shown in Figure 28–7. A person with this genetic condition has very fair skin, white hair, and pink eyes that are quite sensitive to light. The great white whale of the novel *Moby Dick* was probably an albino.

At present, there is no treatment for albinism. However, it does not present nearly as great a threat to life and health as the other metabolic errors we have discussed.

Genetic counseling

Despite great advances in our understanding of the causes and possible treatments of many genetic diseases, it is very difficult to educate both doctors and the general public regarding the more than 1600 recognizable gene defects. Genetic counseling is available at some hospitals, particularly to people from high-risk groups or families.* A couple who have had one defective child are most likely to seek advice about the probability that a subsequent birth will be abnormal.

However, we each carry from six to eight lethal recessive genes, and by the process of random mutations or chromosome damage, we may contain germ cells that are defective. Genetic diseases may thus crop up in any family.

The job of counselors is to provide information regarding possible risk factors and to explain the nature of the disease that might result. The couple may also require assistance in setting out the possible options to obtain more information about the child (for example, whether or not to undergo amniocentesis, which may show a defect but which may also terminate a perfectly normal pregnancy) and about other choices, such as abortion or sterilization. It is the present opinion of most medical societies that diagnostic screening techniques should only be used hand-in-hand with full counseling, or we might create more human suffering than we alleviate.

28.2) List two ways in which a gene might be damaged and cause a genetic disease.

28.3) Under what conditions is it possible to detect the existence of a genetic defect in the fetus early in pregnancy?

28.4*) Which do you think would be likely to create a more serious problem, the substitution of one base for another on the DNA chain or the addition or subtraction of a base? (After you have thought about this question, see note on p. 559. You should also be aware that the body has a means of repairing damaged DNA strands, through the use of special enzymes, and thus the mutations that affect us represent only a tiny fraction of the number that actually occur. See Clark, M., *Contemporary Biology,* 2nd edition, Philadelphia, W.B. Saunders, 1979, Chapter 16a.)

SELF-CHECK

28.3 VIRUSES AND CANCER

LEARNING GOAL 28D: *Give a chemical description of a virus.*
28E: *Describe in general terms the different kinds of treatment that can stop the spread of cancer.*

---

* Three devastating diseases, cystic fibrosis, muscular dystrophy, and multiple sclerosis, all have some genetic component. Neural tube defects, which result in spina bifida (an open spinal column) or an abnormal brain, are also gene defects but cannot be predicted. Such defects can be detected by the presence of a special protein in the mother's blood. See the excellent articles in *Science 81,* Vol. 2 (Jan.–Feb. 1981), pp. 32–41.

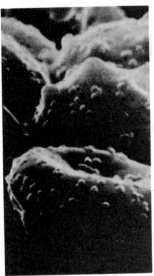

FIGURE 28–8 Human red blood cells infected with influenza virus particles (the small dotlike bumps on the blood cells). (Courtesy R. F. Baker, University of Southern California School of Medicine, Los Angeles)

We are all familiar with the effects of being infected by a virus. Such particles cause the common cold, influenza, measles, chickenpox, mumps, and perhaps multiple sclerosis. We might tend to classify viruses with bacteria as "germs" that cause human disease. However, this would be incorrect. A virus is not really a living organism. It cannot grow, divide, metabolize nutrients, or perform any other life function by itself. Only in a living cell can a virus become active and multiply.

The nature of a virus

A **virus** is basically a set of genes packaged inside a protein coat. Inside the coat, there is nothing but a single strand of DNA or RNA, coded to reproduce itself, to make more coat protein, and perhaps to make some enzymes. There are no ribosomes and no capability to make proteins. These must be *borrowed* from the host organism. Figure 28–8 shows influenza viruses on red blood cells. From this you can judge the relative sizes and shape of virus particles.

DNA viruses function by entering living cells and forming small circles of DNA. These DNA segments multiply many times. The viral DNA then borrows RNA polymerase, the enzyme for transcribing the DNA message onto messenger RNA, from the host cell and makes m-RNA coded to produce the virus coat proteins. Such molecules are dutifully synthesized by the host cell on its own ribosomes. These molecules then surround the newly formed viral DNA to make new virus particles.

Eventually the cell breaks and releases the viruses, which may then infect other cells. Infected cells are thus normally killed within a few hours or days of viral entry, depending on the rate of multiplication of the virus.

Several other kinds of virus particles, each with its own mechanism, are known. Each acts as a *parasite,* using the protein-building machinery of the host cell to build new virus particles.

Latent viruses

Sometimes a cell infected with a virus shows no sign of infection for a long time, and even continues to divide and produce daughter cells. Then, suddenly, the virus is triggered into activity (often by an agent such as x-rays, ultraviolet light, or a chemical such as those in Table 28–1), multiplying quickly in *every* daughter cell, breaking each open and invading the tissue.

One way this could occur is if the viral DNA were to merge with the chromosomal DNA of the host cell and replicate with it each time the cell divides. Both the fusion of latent virus DNA with host DNA and its release depend on special enzymes coded by viral genes.

The implications of this ability of a virus to merge with host genetic material are striking. Viruses could be used to bring desired genes into cells. Work of this type is indeed being carried out by researchers working in the field of gene splicing. Also, if the viral DNA carries genes that cause cancer, this might explain some of the mysteries surrounding the appearance of cancer in a previously normal cell.

Interferon

The human cell, as you might expect, is not defenseless against invasion by viruses. The body has an immune system that gradually "shakes off" a viral disease. This immune system is the basis for the very successful vaccines against smallpox and polio.

However, in addition to the specific antibodies (bodies that work *against* a virus) produced by the body, an infection by one virus in a tissue may produce a temporary immunity in *other* cells against infection, even by different, unrelated viruses. This effect is called the "interference phenomenon." In 1957, Alick Isaacs and Jean Lindenmann in London discovered that **interferon** was the protein responsible.

The role of interferon is shown in Figure 28–9. It seems to keep viral DNA from using the ribosomes of the host cell. It prevents translation of the viral genetic message while permitting the synthesis of host-cell proteins to proceed normally. This substance is released several *days* before the appearance in the body of large numbers of antibodies from the immune system.

Medical scientists hope to test interferon on a large scale as an antiviral and anticancer drug. However, interferon produced by one species will not work in another. Only human interferon will function in humans. A course of treatment (when interferon could be obtained) cost about $50 000 in 1981, and the greatest problem was preparing enough interferon for clinical trials. Several companies are therefore making substantial efforts to produce human interferon by recombinant DNA, opening up tremendous possibilities for medical treatment.*

The nature of cancer

Cancer is not simply one disease; it is really a hundred or more diseases with some factors in common. It may strike in virtually any tissue of the body, as shown in Figure 28–10. In nearly all cases, the cancerous cells

---

* A method for accomplishing this has been patented by Charles Weissmann of the University of Zurich. Unlike most previous scientific discoveries, recombinant DNA research is likely to make its pioneers wealthy. Many scientists working in this field have established corporations to license gene splicing methods (*Life,* May 1980, p. 57).

Another approach to using interferon is to somehow stimulate the body to produce more of the material. There are at least four different kinds of interferon, from different kinds of cells. The major type comes from white blood cells, but the most useful types may be those from the cells of the thymus gland. Various forms of double-stranded RNA have been tested as "pretend viruses" to try to stimulate interferon production. A third promising line of antivirus research is the synthesis of interferon-like compounds.

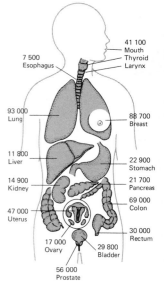

FIGURE 28–10 Estimated new U.S. cases of cancer in 1976, by site (American Cancer Society). Of an estimated 785 000 Americans who were diagnosed in 1980 as having cancer, only about one third will survive past 1985.

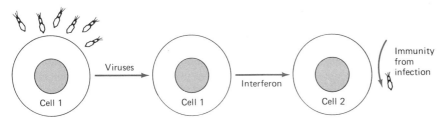

FIGURE 28–9 Interferon, a small polypeptide, prevents a virus from multiplying in both cell 1 and cell 2 by keeping the virus from using the cell's RNA.

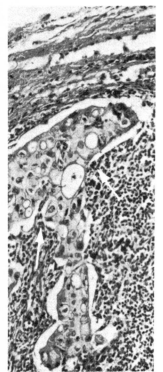

FIGURE 28–11   A human breast cancer that has metastasized to the brain of the patient. The larger brain cells are being pushed aside (arrows) by the rapid growth of the cancerous breast-type cells.

exhibit a wild, uncontrolled growth. While normal cells "recognize" their neighbors and stop growing when in contact with them, cancer cells show no such recognition. They grow and divide, piling over one another in a disorderly arrangement and pushing aside the normal cells of a tissue.

Another common factor in cancer—the one that makes it so deadly—is the ability of a cancer cell to metastasize, that is, to spread to other parts of the body. Cancer cells carried by the blood stream and lymph nodes to other parts of the body continue the growth patterns seen in the originally infected tissue! For example, breast cancer cells, if not completely eliminated by treatment and by filtering through lymph nodes, often form **metastasis** in the brain (Figure 28–11).

As shown in Figure 28–12, several factors seem to combine to create the conditions that produce cancer. Among them:

1) The genetic factor. The tendency to develop certain cancers can be inherited. For example, some women from families with a history of breast cancer are considered to have a greater chance of developing the same condition than the general female population.
2) A hormonal factor. The steroid sex hormones have been linked to the development of cancers in the reproductive systems of both men and women. Such hormones normally activate certain genes in the cells they stimulate. Excessive or abnormal activation of genes may thus lead to cancer in some cases.

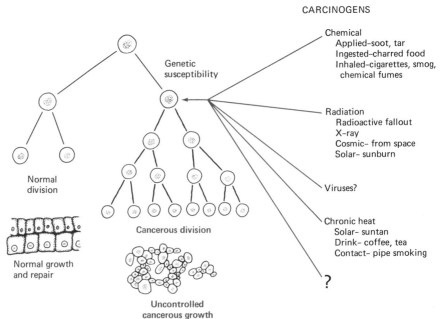

CARCINOGENS

Genetic susceptibility

Chemical
   Applied–soot, tar
   Ingested–charred food
   Inhaled–cigarettes, smog, chemical fumes

Radiation
   Radioactive fallout
   X–ray
   Cosmic– from space
   Solar– sunburn

Viruses?

Chronic heat
   Solar– suntan
   Drink– coffee, tea
   Contact– pipe smoking

?

Normal division

Cancerous division

Normal growth and repair

Uncontrolled cancerous growth

FIGURE 28–12   Some factors in cancer. The basic cause is a defective gene, caused by an inherited faulty chromosome or a mutation; this provides the susceptibility to cancer. The defective gene generally does not express itself unless *triggered* by an environmental factor, such as those listed to the right. Nonsusceptible cells may also become cancerous if subjected to enough carcinogenic "insult." Sunbathers are prone to develop skin cancer, habitual use of scalding drinks is linked to cancer of the esophagus, and the hot stem of a pipe can cause cancer of the lip.

3) An environmental factor. Cancers seem to be "triggered" by exposure to something in the environment that may damage genes. This triggering agent is called a **carcinogen** and is what is meant when scientists or officials refer to a chemical, food dye, cigarette smoke, asbestos fibers, or other substances as "capable of causing cancer." Most carcinogens are also mutagens.

Cancer is, above all, the result of altered or abnormal genes inside the cell. The exact role of the cell DNA in replacing the "normal" cell instructions with cancerous ones is not known. However, abnormal numbers of chromosomes are characteristic of cancer cells, and the appearance of the chromosomes often also changes.

Since cancer is caused by abnormal genes and since viruses bring abnormal genes into the cell, it is logical to look for some relationship between viruses and cancer. More than 70 years ago, Peyton Rous demonstrated that a chicken sarcoma, a cancer of muscles or connective tissues, could be caused by a virus containing a single strand of RNA. Since then, we have discovered many animal tumors that are caused by DNA and RNA viruses. The method by which a DNA virus might cause a cell to become cancerous, shown in Figure 28–13, is very similar to the situation we discussed with regard to *latent viruses.*

Viral DNA may remain latent in the host for months or even years before producing a tumor. In some cases, it may be transmitted as a "silent gene" through the ova or sperm of an infected host to the next generation. This could explain the genetic factor in cancer.

In spite of a tremendous suspicion on the part of scientists that there is a link between viruses and cancer, there is no solid evidence that any specific human cancer is caused by a virus. Almost all animal cancers (which are often virus-induced) are *sarcomas,* tumors of muscle or connective tissue, while most cancers in humans are *carcinomas,* tumors of the *epithelial* tissues that form the skin and the linings of the internal organs (digestive system, lung, endocrine glands, and, in fact, most of the locations shown in Figure 28–10). It is difficult to find evidence of viral involvement in cancer if the virus acts as shown in Figure 28–13, hiding its own identity in the chromosomes of the host.

The human cancer that has been most closely linked with viruses is Burkitt's lymphoma, a rare cancer of the lymph glands. A type of herpes DNA virus can be obtained from cancer cells of this type. However, this may be a meaningless coincidence, since this same virus commonly causes mononucleosis throughout the world but is linked with Burkitt's lymphoma only in Africa!

The task of establishing a link between a virus and a type of cancer is made even more difficult by the possibility of the genetic, hormonal, and environmental factors already discussed. The role of the aging process in cancer is also an unknown factor.

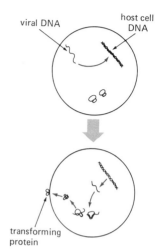

FIGURE 28–13 How a DNA virus might cause cancer. The viral DNA combines with that of the host cell and remains latent *except for* coding a small piece of m-RNA for "transforming protein." This protein then somehow converts the cell from normal to cancerous. It is shown here acting at the cell membrane, but it could be elsewhere, perhaps altering the regulation of the genes of the host cell.

Cancer and the immune system

According to one theory, just as cells and the body have (through interferon and antibodies) a defense against viruses, there is also a defense against cancer cells. In this theory, the cancer cells have abnormal proteins on their surfaces, and this condition makes the immune system of the body search them out and destroy them. In that case, only when the immune

Hormone regulation in the body is very complicated. Cortisone, which was once commonly prescribed for a large number of allergic and other symptoms, is now considered a rather dangerous drug because of its supression of the natural immune system. Lawrence Burton has found that lack of a particular protein in the serum of cancer patients may be related to a weakening of the immune system. Injections of the protein have benefitted some cancer patients.

system loses its capability to cope with the number of cancer cells produced do such cells escape destruction and begin to invade neighboring tissues.

This theory implies that people with inadequate immune systems should more easily develop cancer, and this is indeed the case. Likewise, prolonged stress in animals increases the number of tumors, presumably because the cortisone released by the stress supresses the immune system.

This might provide an explanation for two somewhat puzzling aspects of cancer, (a) the very long period that is often seen between exposure to a cancer-causing agent (such as asbestos fibers) and the appearance of the symptoms and (b) the fact that cancers occasionally regress spontaneously. The latter factor causes much confusion in the general public if the regression (temporary disappearance) occurs while some "miracle cure" is being tried.

The higher incidence of cancer in aged persons may be a result of the loss of immune ability.

One problem in designing cancer treatment is the fact that most types of treatment, including surgical removal of cancers and other types of therapy, *also* suppress the body's natural immune system that might itself be able to help. In addition, such suppression of the natural defenses of the body makes it easy prey for viral infections.

If it can be obtained in large enough quantities, the natural "defense" protein *interferon* (Figure 28–9) may serve two important roles in cancer therapy. First of all, it could help ward off viral diseases that the (suppressed) body immune system has not been able to defeat. Second, there is some clinical evidence that interferon may be effective in the treatment of some cancers.

Blood tests for cancer

Hundreds of research teams in all parts of the world are seeking to isolate proteins produced exclusively by cancer cells and not by normal cells. In some cases, such proteins have been found, and they may be used to test for the presence of a cancer in its very early, highly treatable stage. Once the symptoms of a cancer are so evident that a clear diagnosis is made through x-rays or biopsy, it may be too late to prevent its spread. Workers at McGill University have found a way to test for the presence of colon cancer cells; others have reported a way to detect lung cancer through simple tests. This is a research field that offers great promise for somewhat relieving the trauma that often accompanies the news that cancer has been detected.

Cancer treatment

The various forms of cancer cause about one of every six deaths each year in the Western countries, second only to heart disease. Most of the deaths are due to metastases, which are much harder to treat (since the cells may be anywhere in the body) than a cancer that is localized in one particular place.

See *Life*, November 1980, p. 112, for a well-illustrated account of some modern methods of diagnosis and treatment.

If the cancer is localized, the treatment is aimed at killing the cancer cells while leaving alive as many normal cells as possible. Surgical removal and irradiation using radioactive isotopes (Section 3.5 and Table 3–6) are the usual methods. In addition, even in tumors that are probably localized, chemotherapy is often started, just in case metastases exist.

If the cancer has spread, chemotherapy is always used. The biochemical treatment of cancer is based largely on the fact that cancer cells are constantly dividing, while normal cells divide only occasionally in most tissues. Any chemical agent that blocks cell division, such as *vinblastine,* a natural alkaloid from the periwinkle plant, will be useful. This particular chemical is effective in treatment of *choriocarcinoma,* a type of uterine tumor.

Nitrogen-containing compounds related to a World War I chemical warfare agent known as *mustard gas* (dichloroethyl sulfide) are alkylating agents. *Cyclophosphamide,* for example, removes purines (adenine and guanine) from DNA and causes cross-linking, which prevents DNA replication.

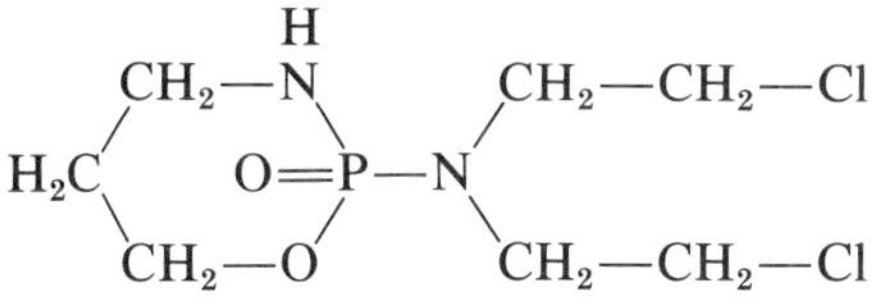

cyclophosphamide

Any compound that prevents replication will keep cancer cells from multiplying. Cyclophosphamide has been of use in treating leukemia, Hodgkins disease, and lymphosarcoma.

Several antibiotics, such as *adriamycin,* inhibit both replication and transcription and are thus useful in cancer therapy. A purine-like compound, *6-mercaptopurine,* is one of several drugs that masquerade as essential intermediates in the synthesis of purines and pyrimidines in the cell. It is very useful in the treatment of acute leukemia. *Fluorouracil,* a pyrimidine-like compound, serves a very similar role in the treatment of advanced carcinoma. These drugs act by blocking DNA and RNA synthesis at an early stage.

An *antibiotic* is a substance produced by one organism that blocks the metabolism of another organism. What works against bacteria can sometimes work against cancer cells. Such antibiotics can be rather toxic to humans but may be particularly valuable against tumors caused by RNA viruses.

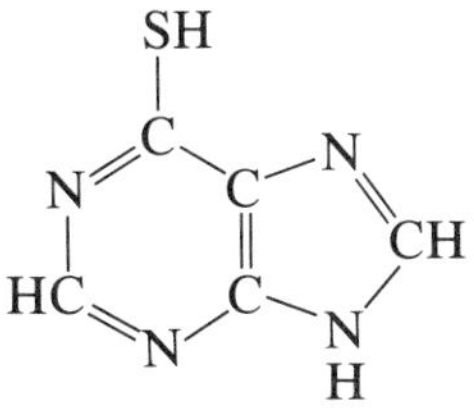

6-mercaptopurine 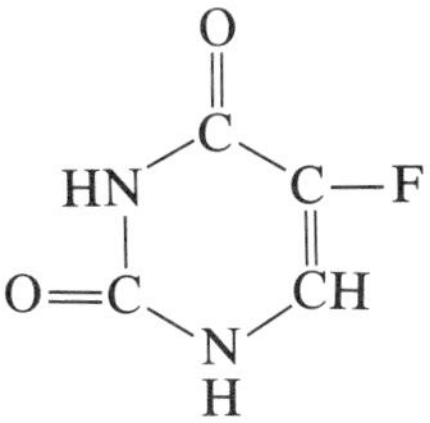   fluorouracil

Methotrexate is a drug that acts like folic acid (p. 636) and, like 6-mercaptopurine, blocks the synthesis of purine nucleotides. It can produce dramatic temporary remissions in leukemia, and long-lasting remissions in choriocarcinoma.

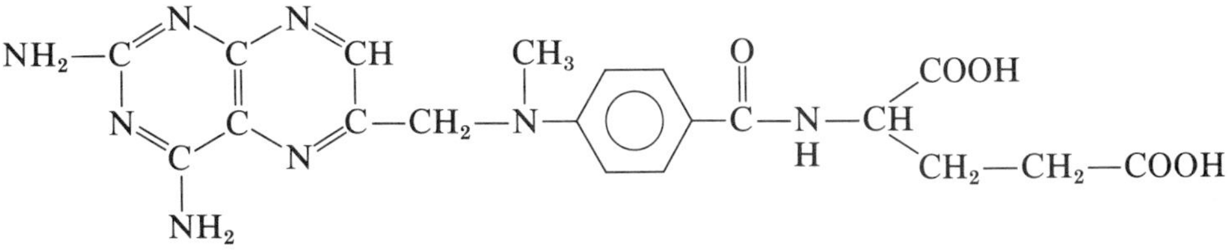

methotrexate

Some active ingredients in marijuana are very effective in reducing nausea and vomiting from cancer chemotherapy.

Some inorganic compounds are also effective in drug therapy against cancer (Figure 28–14).

Chemotherapeutic drugs being used today have two major disadvantages. First of all, at best, they are only able to control the spread of cancer and produce remission; they are usually unable to "cure." Second, the side effects of chemotherapy (and also radiotherapy) are extremely uncomfortable; some patients may sometimes feel that the treatment is almost worse than the disease.

Only recently have cancer researchers begun to draw together all of the evidence regarding viruses, interferon, the immune system, and the manner of cancer cell division. There is some hope that by combining all available information, medical scientists will be able to get the upper hand against this dread complex of diseases.

SELF-CHECK

28.5)   Chemically, what is present in a cell that is not present in a virus?

28.6)   In what manner is chemotherapy effective in treating various forms of cancer?

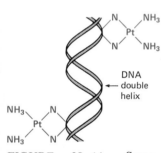

FIGURE 28–14 Some metal complexes (p. 657) have ligands (electron donor groups) that can be lost, allowing the metal to bond to nitrogens on DNA. This then causes the double helix to unwind. In the ligand shown here, the *cis* isomer is effective in cancer therapy, but the *trans* isomer is not. (See *Chemical and Engineering News,* Jan. 21, 1980, p. 35.)

28.4 GENETIC ENGINEERING

LEARNING GOAL 28F: List some of the possible benefits to humanity of recombinant DNA research. List one major hazard.

We have discussed several ways in which nature itself interferes with the normal process of DNA replication. This has inspired geneticists to wonder if there might be ways to manipulate the genetic material, for example, to fix a defective gene in a human ovum or to force bacteria to produce proteins that they would not normally synthesize.

While the correcting of errors in the genetic material of a human germ cell does not seem likely in the immediate future, *gene splicing,* forcing bacteria to function with foreign DNA strands, has moved in a few short years from vision to reality.

Recombinant DNA

Gene splicing or **recombinant DNA** work usually involves three properties of bacteria:

1) A special bacterial enzyme, called a *restriction enzyme,* is capable of cutting the DNA double helix, leaving the ends that are exposed "sticky" and capable of joining with other strands. Each particular restriction enzyme always breaks DNA at the same point in the base-pair sequence.
2) A second bacterial enzyme, called a *ligase,* is capable of joining up sticky ends, thus permitting a foreign DNA to join up with the natural DNA of the bacterium.
3) Bacteria contain tiny pieces of DNA in the form of rings, which are independent of the chromosomes and which can easily enter bacterial cells. These DNA segments, called *plasmids,* closely resemble certain types of viruses.

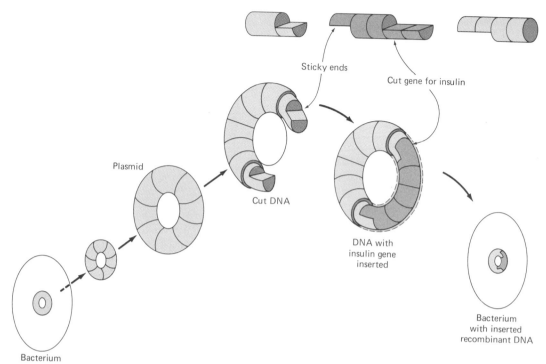

FIGURE 28–15 Gene splicing or recombinant DNA involves the insertion of a foreign gene (here, the DNA coded for production of insulin) into a bacterial plasmid. This method may eventually be used to set up bacterial "factories" that can produce any proteins of interest to us. Also see the illustrations in *Life*, May 1980, p. 48.

A particular kind of bacterium known as *Escherichia coli* (*E. coli* for short) has been the biggest contributor to our knowledge of genetics. Common in the intestines of humans and other higher animals, the genetic material of *E. coli* has served for thousands of highly significant experiments.

Figure 28–15 shows a typical gene splicing process. In this case, we wish to insert a gene from a rat pancreas cell that has the information to make a form of *insulin* hormone that can be used by human diabetics. A plasmid is isolated and opened up by the restriction enzyme. The DNA from the rat pancreas is broken by the same enzyme. This assures that the "sticky" ends of the two types of DNA will contain complementary base pair sequences and will join properly. The cut gene for insulin is then inserted into the opened plasmid, and ligase enzymes seal it in place. Since the DNA fragments have *recombined*, we now have a *recombinant DNA* plasmid. The plasmid is inserted back into a bacterium, which then multiplies normally, copying both its usual genes and the gene we inserted for insulin. As this bacterium cell divides and multiplies, so does the plasmid carrying the insulin gene. As a result, we have turned the one cell into a bacterial colony that cooperates with us in producing insulin.

See also *Scientific American*, Vol. 245, No. 3 (September 1981), a special issue on "Industrial Microbiology."

Proteins from bacterial factories

One researcher in the recombinant DNA field, David Baltimore of the Massachusetts Institute of Technology, has predicted that just about any protein molecule of medical interest can be manufactured in unlimited quantities within the next 15 years. One pharmaceutical company, Eli Lilly, is already producing insulin from bacteria for wide-scale testing. Once full production begins on a commercial scale, this source of human insulin should be a safe and relatively cheap alternative to the present method of isolating the hormone from animal pancreas glands.

In early 1981, testing on humans of bacterial-produced *growth hormone* was begun. Until then, because of its scarcity, this pituitary hormone had been limited to the treatment of children with severe growth problems. It used to take all of the hormone from 50 human pituitary glands to treat one child for a year. However, there are many other possible uses of this hormone, which seems to stimulate protein production and DNA and RNA synthesis. This hormone was first produced in 1979, and the short period between discovery and testing on humans demonstrates the fast-moving nature of recombinant DNA work.

In the research stage as of 1981 were attempts to produce vaccines for hepatitis and the common cold by gene splicing. A recombinant DNA that may correct sickle cell anemia is also the subject of active research.

Applications of such research are not limited to human proteins. Ralph Hardy, a plant biologist, is hoping to apply gene splicing techniques to plant breeding. The crossbreeding of plants to improve yields and resistance to insects and weather ordinarily takes many months. The process might be carried out more rapidly by splicing one plant's desirable genes into another species. There are also attempts being made to increase the yield of alcohol from corn and to produce antibiotic drugs through genetic research.

Human "designed genes"

As we mentioned earlier, it is one thing to make living protein factories out of bacteria colonies and quite something else to change the DNA makeup of a higher animal. However, research is continuing with the eventual goal of curing diseases such as diabetes, sickle cell anemia, hemophilia, and Tay-Sachs disease.

The first step has already been taken. A team of Yale University scientists injected viral genes into mouse fertilized ova, which were then transferred to the wombs of female mice. A few newborns were shown to have portions of the injected genes in their tissue cells. This experiment suggests that we may some day be able to change the genetic material in a human ovum, then reimplant it to develop to full term.*

---

* A research group at the University of California at Los Angeles has approached human gene splicing from a different angle. They isolated genes that help produce an enzyme resistant to methotrexate (Section 28.4), a cancer-fighting drug that, as a side effect, kills bone marrow cells. When a suspension of such genes was injected into mouse bone marrow, cells that carried the resistant gene developed. Methotrexate could then be given to combat cancer with less harmful side effects on red blood cell production in the bone marrow.

Since then, Martin Cline of the same group has treated two women whose bone marrow was not producing hemoglobin. The treatment consisted of mixing bone marrow cells with hemoglobin-producing genes and implanting the mixture in the patients. Cline has been very strongly criticized for prematurely beginning experiments on human patients. On the other hand, the human patients were sure to die if untreated. This case points out some of the ethical questions associated with medical research.

Possible dangers

This all sounds like a miraculous solution to many medical problems. Perhaps it is. Yet there are unknown dangers attached to such "tinkering" with nature's information system.

For example, the host bacterium *E. coli* coexists very nicely with us in our intestines. By tinkering with plasmids, it is possible that someone might unintentionally create a highly dangerous and infective mutation of *E. coli* that could cause serious disease among the general population. The debate over such possibilities, which has inspired some cities and towns to ban recombinant DNA research within their borders, has also led to the creation of very strict rules for conducting gene splicing research. Only specially weakened strains of *E. coli* that cannot survive outside the laboratory may be used. Also, the laboratories must be carefully designed to prevent any escape of bacteria.

Even with all these precautions, many geneticists are disturbed about the ethical implications of "designed genes." They are not sure that such interference with nature will necessarily be beneficial to the human race.

SELF-CHECK

28.7) Some proteins, such as vasopressin, a polypeptide hormone that regulates the thirst response, may have value in increasing our ability to think and remember. Suppose a drug company is considering producing such a protein through recombinant DNA research. List some advantages. Can you think of any possible disadvantages?

28.8) Why have some towns attempted to ban recombinant DNA research within their borders?

EPILOGUE

The material discussed in this chapter is full of promise and hope, with a good measure of caution. In a way, all of modern science is like that. Beneficial industrial processess are often accompanied by pollution problems that must be overcome. Raising the standard of living of people in some areas of the world has adversely affected the welfare of people in other areas. To be well fed, well housed, well heated, and well air conditioned means the eventual depletion of agricultural reserves, the world's lumber supply, and reserves of fossil fuels. The science of chemistry must increase its efforts to produce satisfactory substitutes for food and fossil fuels while world organizations strive to increase the welfare of all people.

Our knowledge of foods and nutrition has over the years resulted in taller, stronger, and healthier children. To preserve and protect food products for widespread distribution, many chemical compounds have been incorporated as "food additives." A few of these compounds have been found to cause cancer in rats when fed in large doses. This has resulted in extensive searches for, and the frantic reporting of, ingested substances that are carcinogenic. Further knowledge through chemistry may moderate our thinking and cause us to reexamine our current view of foods and nutrition.

The more we know about human genetics, viruses, and cancer, the more we are aware of what can go wrong with the body. As medical science increases our life span, and as its skills at diagnosing diseases increase, our knowledge of medical problems such as cancer improves. On the whole, our health is better and our food and environment are safer than in other eras, which had to contend with plagues, epidemics, and devastating natural disasters.

At one time people thought that science "has all the answers." As chemical and medical research produces better products and solutions to problems, it also raises new questions that must be answered by further research. Our technology is in a constant state of change, with a slow, continual improvement in our standard of living the result. Just as the body has a magnificent system of metabolic regulation and control equipped to fight infections, repair damaged genes, and destroy cancer cells up to the limit of its ability, so will our society, by becoming better informed and better equipped, be able to overcome the obstacles to a better life.

CHAPTER TWENTY-EIGHT IN REVIEW ■ DNA and the Future

GLOSSARY FOR CHAPTER TWENTY-EIGHT

amniocentesis Removal of a small sample of amniotic fluid through the mother's abdominal wall; usually used to detect genetic defects in the fetus. (p. 739)

cancer Abnormal growth of transformed body cells that invade and destroy normal tissues; may be caused by a combination of genetic factors and carcinogens. (p. 745)

carcinogen An agent that induces cancer in a normal cell; includes certain chemicals, radiations, and probably viruses. (p. 747)

chromosome Long structures in the nucleus, which contain DNA in a protein support; there are 46 in a human diploid cell and 23 in a human haploid cell carrying genetic information in the form of *genes*. (p. 734)

cloning The division of a diploid cell nucleus, a normal occurrence in some species but difficult to achieve in the higher animals. (p. 735)

gene A section of the DNA base-pair sequence in a chromosome that produces m-RNA coded for a specific protein; the "unit" of inheritance. (p. 734)

interferon A protein released in a

cell in response to viral infection; it can protect that cell and others from further infection by any viruses; a leading candidate for production through recombinant DNA work because of the extremely high cost of current production techniques. (p. 745)

metastasis A group of cancer cells that have broken away from the initial tumor and spread, through the blood stream, to a new site. (p. 746)

mutation A change in the base-pair sequence of a gene, which may be repaired by enzymes in the cell or may cause an error in metabolism; can be caused by a *mutagen*, such

as certain chemicals, viruses, and radiations. (p. 738)

recombinant DNA Gene splicing; a technique by which selected genes from one organism can be introduced into the DNA of another organism and be replicated with that of the host. (p. 750)

replication In cell division, the formation of two identical daughter double-helix strands of DNA from a single parent strand. (p. 735)

virus An infective agent composed of a nucleic acid strand and a protein coat; requires the machinery of a host cell in order to reproduce; may be involved in cancer. (p. 744)

QUESTIONS AND PROBLEMS FOR CHAPTER TWENTY-EIGHT ■
DNA and the Future

28.1 DNA REPLICATION AND GENES

28.9) When does replication occur in a cell?

28.10) What raw materials must be available in the cell nucleus, in addition to DNA and enzymes, in order for replication to occur?

28.11*) Can a haploid cell be cloned to create a new person? Explain.

28.12*) What unusual ethical problem arises if we try to clone a human being?

28.37) Describe the process of replication for one DNA strand.

28.38) What is the role of enzymes in replication?

28.39*) Certain cells in the body have become so specialized that some of their genes have become useless. Can such cells be used to clone a new person? Explain.

28.40*) One science fiction story concerns a group of women who reject all men and populate a planet. They will reproduce by cloning and therefore have no need of the male sex. Could this be *scientifically* possible? Explain.

28.2 INBORN ERRORS OF METABOLISM

28.13) Name two factors that could cause a genetic mutation.

28.14*) Sickle cell anemia or Tay-Sachs disease may show up in a child whose parents do not carry the gene for the disease. How?

28.41) Gamma radiation is often used to treat cancer (Section 3.5), yet there is some chance it may create new gene defects. Explain.

28.42*) Describe the value of screening parents who may be carriers of recessive genes that could cause metabolic defects.

28.15) How might a pregnant woman over 35 years of age find out if her child will have Down's syndrome?

28.16*) How may carriers of the sickle cell anemia trait be detected?

28.17*) Which is more likely to lead to a decision by parents to terminate pregnancy, the knowledge that the fetus has albinism or the knowledge that it has Tay-Sachs disease? Explain.

28.18*) What do diabetes mellitus and hemophilia have in common?

28.3 VIRUSES AND CANCER

28.19) Do viruses contain glucose? Explain. Are viruses "alive"?

28.20*) Describe the manner in which the body defends itself against a viral infection.

28.21*) How might a *latent* virus possibly cause cancer in a later generation?

28.22*) What kind of control that keeps a normal cell from dividing is not present in a cancer cell?

28.23*) Why is it very dangerous if any cancerous cells reach the blood stream?

28.24*) Why is it impossible to detect the presence of latent viruses in a cancer cell?

28.25*) Why might cortisone be an unwise treatment for a person with suspected cancer?

28.26*) Scientists consider it to be a fact that "cigarette smoking causes cancer." Why doesn't *every* smoker eventually develop lung cancer?

28.43*) Down's syndrome is not caused by a gene mutation, yet it is really a kind of "inborn error of metabolism." Explain.

28.44*) If two sickle cell anemia carriers have children, will *all* of the children have the disease?

28.45) How might a set of parents who know they both carry the gene for Tay-Sachs disease find out if the fetus has the disease?

28.46*) What do albinism and phenylketonuria have in common?

28.47) Do viruses contain fatty acids? Explain.

28.48*) Describe the manner in which a DNA virus infects a cell. What organelles of the host cell does the virus "borrow"?

28.49*) Describe the ways in which viral infection of a cell resembles recombinant DNA work.

28.50*) In what ways may a cluster of cancer cells be distinguished from normal cells?

28.51*) Cancer cells, in small amounts, may be caught and destroyed in the lymph nodes. Why are lymph nodes often removed along with the primary tumor in surgery?

28.52*) Explain why scientists are almost completely convinced that there is a link between viruses and human cancer.

28.53*) Why might a weakened immune system cause problems in a person who is working with radioactive materials?

28.54*) Australia has the highest proportion of people who tan themselves on beaches. It also has the highest rate of skin cancer in the world. Is there a relationship between these two facts?

28.27*) How *might* the presence of lung cancer be detected early enough to provide for a cure in the great majority of cases?

28.28) What is the role of gamma radiation (Section 3.5) in the treatment of cancer?

28.29) Why will a chemotherapy agent that blocks cell division be useful?

28.30) Why will a chemotherapy agent that "pretends" to be a purine be useful?

28.31*) Can cancer be *cured* by the agents currently available?

28.4 GENETIC ENGINEERING

28.32) Why will it be very important if gene splicing succeeds in producing low-cost insulin that is effective in humans?

28.33*) Can recombinant DNA be used to produce a vitamin?

28.34*) What is the role of a *restriction enzyme* in gene splicing? Do you suppose normal human cells contain such enzymes?

28.35) Why are only specially weakened strains of *E. coli* used in recombinant DNA experiments?

28.36*) How might gene splicing be used, eventually, to cure Tay-Sachs disease in an embryo?

28.55*) If an early screening test should become available for breast cancer, who do you think should be selected to undergo the test? What criteria should be used?

28.56) What is the reason for implanting a capsule of radioactive material inside a cancerous tumor?

28.57) Why will a chemotherapy agent that blocks DNA replication be useful?

28.58) Why will a chemotherapy agent that "pretends" to be a pyrimidine base be useful?

28.59*) Someday it will be announced that "all cancers can be cured." What kinds of discoveries might this involve?

28.60) Why will it be very important if gene splicing succeeds in producing low-cost human growth hormone?

28.61) Can recombinant DNA be used to produce a steroid hormone?

28.62*) What is the role of a *ligase* in gene splicing? Do you suppose normal human cells contain ligase?

28.63) Why have biologists reached international agreements to carry out gene splicing only under certain extremely well-controlled conditions?

28.64*) How might gene splicing eventually be used to cure sickle cell anemia in a one-year-old child?

Answers to Self-Checks, Questions, and Problems

This section of the text contains answers to the questions in the self-checks and in the left-hand column of questions and problems at the end of each chapter. All such questions have colored numbers, such as 11.17. The answers to questions in the right-hand column at the end of each chapter (black numbers) will be found in the *Instructor's Manual*.

In many cases, where the question asks for an explanation or example, the answer given here is a "suggested" response. Your own answer might differ from ours and still be correct. Check with your instructor if in doubt.

For number problems, a complete setup has been shown for at least the *first* problem of each type.

CHAPTER ONE SELF-CHECKS

1.1   sodium Na   calcium Ca   iron Fe   potassium K   phosphorus P chromium Cr

1.2   H hydrogen   F fluorine   Cu copper   Cl chlorine   Sn tin Mg magnesium   Si silicon   Co cobalt   I iodine   Zn zinc

1.3   **a** O_3: oxygen (3)   **b** $CaCO_3$: calcium (1), carbon (1), oxygen (3) **c** H_2O_2: hydrogen (2), oxygen (2)   **d** $C_{16}H_{32}O_2$: carbon (16), hydrogen (32), oxygen (2)   **e** $C_9H_{11}O_3N$: carbon (9), hydrogen (11), oxygen (3), nitrogen (1)   **f** NH_3: nitrogen (1), hydrogen (3)   **g** Fe_2O_3: iron (2), oxygen (3) **h** $C_{12}H_{22}O_{11}$: carbon (12), hydrogen (22), oxygen (11)   **i** NH_4NO_3: nitrogen (2), hydrogen (4), oxygen (3)   **j** $C_3H_5O_3(NO_2)_3$: carbon (3), hydrogen (5), nitrogen (3), oxygen (9)

1.4   **a** $C_5H_{10}O_5$ has no nitrogen, could be a carbohydrate   **b** $C_5H_{13}NO_2$ contains nitrogen, so could be a protein segment (amino acid)

1.5   All Calories, of any kind, count equally, so you might *gain* weight. Such an unbalanced diet can also be quite dangerous to health.

1.6   The primary role of proteins is to build new tissues.

CHAPTER ONE QUESTIONS AND PROBLEMS (Left-hand column)

1.7   oxygen O   zinc Zn   iron Fe   tin Sn   magnesium Mg

1.8   potassium K

1.9   Ni nickel   S sulfur   P phosphorus   Si silicon   Na sodium Cr chromium

1.10   Mn manganese   1.11   fluorine F

1.12   H hydrogen, C carbon, N nitrogen, and O oxygen

1.13   as water   1.14   iron Fe

1.15 N_2O: nitrogen (2), oxygen (1)

1.16 Na_3PO_4: sodium (3), phosphorus (1), oxygen (4)

1.17 $Ca(OH)_2$: calcium (1), oxygen (2), hydrogen (2)

1.18 CH_3OH: carbon (1), hydrogen (4), oxygen (1)

1.19 $(NH_2)_2CO$: nitrogen (2), hydrogen (4), carbon (1), oxygen (1)

1.20 $C_6H_{12}O_6$: carbon (6), hydrogen (12), oxygen (6)

1.21 $C_5H_{10}NO_2$: carbon (5), hydrogen (10), nitrogen (1), oxygen (2)

1.22 $C_{63}H_{88}CoN_{14}O_{14}P$: carbon (63), hydrogen (88), cobalt (1), nitrogen (14), oxygen (14), phosphorus (1)

1.23 $(C_{738}H_{1166}FeN_{203}O_{208}S_2)_4$: carbon (2952), hydrogen (4664), iron (4), nitrogen (812), oxygen (832), sulfur (8)

1.24 C carbon, H hydrogen, and O oxygen

1.25 hydrogen (H_2) and oxygen (O_2)   **1.26**   primarily for energy

1.27 to work with enzymes and otherwise make body reactions possible

1.28 Too much of any nutrient can be injurious to body functioning.

CHAPTER TWO SELF-CHECKS

2.1   **a** $173 \text{ cm} \times \dfrac{1 \text{ m}}{1 \text{ m}} = 173 \text{ cm} \times \dfrac{10^3 \text{ mm}}{10^2 \text{ cm}} = 1730 \text{ mm} = 1.73 \times 10^3 \text{ mm}$

   b 1.73 m   **c** 0.00173 km   **d** 68.1 in.

   e $173 \text{ cm} \times \dfrac{1 \text{ m}}{100 \text{ cm}} \times \dfrac{1 \text{ km}}{1000 \text{ m}} \times \dfrac{0.6214 \text{ mile}}{1 \text{ km}} = 0.00108 \text{ mile}$

2.2   **a** $3.4 \text{ mi} \times \dfrac{1.609 \text{ km}}{1 \text{ mi}} = 5.47 \text{ km} = 5.5 \text{ km}$ to proper significant digits

   b $1.5 \text{ mil} \times \dfrac{0.0254 \text{ mm}}{1 \text{ mil}} = 0.0381 \text{ mm} = 3.8 \times 10^{-2} \text{ mm}$

   c $50 \text{ yd} \times \dfrac{3 \text{ ft}}{1 \text{ yd}} \times \dfrac{1 \text{ m}}{3.281 \text{ ft}} = 45.7 \text{ m} = 46 \text{ m}$

2.3   **a** $5.81 \text{ L} \times \dfrac{1000 \text{ mL}}{1 \text{ L}} = 5810 \text{ mL} = 5.81 \times 10^3 \text{ mL}$

   b $45.6 \text{ cm}^3 \times \dfrac{1 \text{ mL}}{1 \text{ cm}^3} = 45.6 \text{ mL}$

   c $0.75 \text{ pint} \times \dfrac{0.4732 \text{ L}}{1 \text{ pint}} \times \dfrac{1000 \text{ mL}}{1 \text{ L}} = 354.9 \text{ mL} = 3.5 \times 10^2 \text{ mL}$

2.4   12 in. × 30 in. × 12 in. = 30.5 cm × 76.2 cm × 30.5 cm = $7.09 \times 10^4 \text{ cm}^3$

   $7.09 \times 10^4 \text{ cm}^3 = 7.09 \times 10^4 \text{ mL} = 7.09 \times 10^1 \text{ L} \times \dfrac{0.2642 \text{ gal}}{1 \text{ L}} = 19 \text{ gal}$

2.5   Brand A: $48 \text{ fl oz} \times \dfrac{29.57 \text{ mL}}{1 \text{ fl oz}} = 1419 \text{ mL}$; $\dfrac{93¢}{1419 \text{ mL}} = 0.0655¢/\text{mL}$

   Brand B: 1.50 L = 1500 mL; $\dfrac{100¢}{1500 \text{ mL}} = 0.0667¢/\text{mL}$

   Brand A is slightly more economical.

2.6 $0.77 \times 10^{-10} \text{ m} \times \dfrac{100 \text{ cm}}{1 \text{ m}} = 7.7 \times 10^{-9} \text{ cm} = 0.077 \text{ nm} = 0.77 \text{ Å}$

2.7 $1069 \text{ lb} \times \dfrac{1 \text{ kg}}{2.205 \text{ lb}} = 485 \text{ kg}$ $\left(or\ 1069 \text{ lb} \times \dfrac{0.454 \text{ kg}}{1 \text{ lb}} = 485 \text{ kg}\right)$

2.8   approximately 473 grams for the well-nourished animal, 233 grams for the other

2.9 $0.090 \text{ oz} \times \dfrac{28.3 \text{ g}}{1 \text{ oz}} = 2.5 \text{ grams}$ **2.10**   324 mg of ASA

2.11   six times as much; $6 \times 286 \text{ lb} = 1716 \text{ lb}$, or almost 1 ton; lower weight

2.12 $\text{density} = \dfrac{\text{mass}}{\text{volume}} = \dfrac{30.39 \text{ g}}{30.00 \text{ cm}^3} = 1.013 \text{ g/cm}^3$; specific gravity = 1.013

This is somewhat outside the normal range, and so other tests should be taken to check for possible kidney disease.

2.13 $1 \text{ qt milk} \times \dfrac{0.9463 \text{ L}}{1 \text{ qt}} \times \dfrac{1000 \text{ cm}^3}{1 \text{ L}} \times \dfrac{1.03 \text{ g milk}}{1 \text{ cm}^3} = 975 \text{ grams}$

2.14   Graphite and diamond both contain individual atoms of carbon, which are arranged in different fashions. All carbon atoms act identically when they combine with oxygen to form CO_2.

2.15   **a** neutron   **b** electron   **c** proton   **d** neutron, proton

2.16   **a** Ca^{2+}, K^+ **b** Cl^- **c** Ca^{2+}/Cl^-, K^+/Cl^- **d** Ca^{2+}/K^+

2.17   A law is a statement that something has always been observed to happen in the same way. If the experiments have been carried out properly, the law will not be "incorrect" but might have exceptions that have not yet been noticed.

2.18   A theory is an explanation of observed facts. Several theories can be developed to explain the same facts. Even accepted theories are often revised to better explain the observations. A theory *may* be incorrect.

2.19   **a** $^{26}_{11}\text{Na}$: 11 protons, 15 neutrons ($26 - 11 = 15$); sodium-26   **b** $^{28}_{15}\text{P}$: 15 protons, 13 neutrons; phosphorus-28   **c** $^{40}_{20}\text{Ca}$: 20 protons, 20 neutrons; calcium-40   **d** $^{58}_{26}\text{Fe}$: 26 protons, 32 neutrons; iron-58   **e** $^{79}_{35}\text{Br}$: 35 protons, 44 neutrons; bromine-79

2.20   **a** $^{16}_{8}\text{O}$ **b** $^{235}_{92}\text{U}$ **c** $^{30}_{13}\text{Al}$ **d** $^{197}_{79}\text{Au}$ (gold)

2.21   **a** $\dfrac{(50.54\% \times 79.0) + (49.46\% \times 81.0)}{100.00\%} = \dfrac{3993 + 4006}{100.00} = 80.0 \text{ amu}$

b 35.5 amu for Cl   **c** 31.0 amu for P   **d** 63.6 amu for Cu
e 52.06 amu = 52.1 amu for Cr

There are several alternative ways to proceed, including that of Example 2v; all give the same answers, which match the atomic weights within the precision given (three significant digits), which is ± 0.1 amu.

CHAPTER TWO QUESTIONS AND PROBLEMS
(Left-hand column)

2.22   **a** $100 \text{ mm} \times \dfrac{1 \text{ m}}{1 \text{ m}} = 100 \text{ mm} \times \dfrac{100 \text{ cm}}{1000 \text{ mm}} = 10.0 \text{ cm}$

b $10 \text{ km} = 1.0 \times 10^6 \text{ cm}$ **c** $2.0 \text{ m} = 2.0 \times 10^2 \text{ cm}$ **d** $145 \ \mu\text{m} = 1.45 \times 10^{-2} \text{ cm}$

2.23   **a** 172 cm   **b** $1.72 \times 10^{-3} \text{ km}$ **c** $1.72 \times 10^6 \ \mu\text{m}$ **d** $1.72 \times 10^{10} \text{ Å}$

2.24 $6500 \text{ Å} \times \dfrac{1 \times 10^{-10} \text{ m}}{1 \text{ Å}} = 6.5 \times 10^3 \times 10^{-10} = 6.5 \times 10^{-7} \text{ m}$

2.25 $1.0 \text{ nm} = 1.0 \times 10^{-9} \text{ m}$

2.26   **a** 15 000 volts   **b** 1 pfd = 10^{-12} farad   **c** 1 mA = 0.001 ampere

2.27   **a** 2.5 mL = 0.0025 L   **b** 2.5 cm³   **c** $2.5 \times 10^3 \ \mu\text{L}$

2.28 $100 \text{ yd} \times \dfrac{3 \text{ ft}}{1 \text{ yd}} \times \dfrac{0.305 \text{ m}}{1 \text{ ft}} = 91.5 \text{ m}$ $\left(or\ 300 \text{ ft} \times \dfrac{1 \text{ m}}{3.281 \text{ ft}} = 91.4 \text{ m} \right)$

2.29   29.9 in. = 75.9 cm   2.30   0.078 in. = 2.0 mm

2.31   **a** 8.0 fl oz = 0.25 qt   **b** 0.24 L   **c** 2.4×10^2 mL

2.32   Since liters are most easily related to cubic centimeters, change the measurements to cm: $(30.5 \text{ cm})^3 = 2.84 \times 10^4 \text{ cm}^3 = 2.84 \times 10^1 \text{ L} = 28.4 \text{ L}$.

2.33   33¢/750 mL = 0.044¢/mL; 41¢/946 mL = 0.043¢/mL; the quart bottle!

2.34   There is no change in mass, only in weight (which depends on gravity).

2.35   **a** $9.5 \text{ mg} \times \dfrac{0.001 \text{ g}}{1 \text{ mg}} = 9.5 \times 10^{-3}$ g

  b 9.5×10^{-5} g   **c** 6.5×10^{-8} g   **d** 0.355 g Cl^-

2.36   17.5 g = 0.0175 kg   2.37   80 mg = 0.080 g

2.38   13 lb 14 oz = $(13 \times 454) + (14 \times 28.3)$ = 5902 g + 396 g = 6298 g
  $= 6.30 + 10^3$ g

2.39 $150 \text{ lb body} \times \dfrac{0.454 \text{ kg body}}{1 \text{ lb body}} \times \dfrac{150 \text{ mg heroin}}{1 \text{ kg body}} \times \dfrac{0.001 \text{ g heroin}}{1 \text{ mg heroin}} = 10.2 \text{ g}$
  Remember to always include the *substance* in each conversion factor.

2.40 $1000 \text{ cm}^3 \text{ ice} \times \dfrac{0.92 \text{ g ice}}{1 \text{ cm}^3 \text{ ice}} = 920 \text{ g ice} = 9.2 \times 10^2 \text{ g ice}$

2.41 $31.1 \text{ g Au} \times \dfrac{1 \text{ cm}^3 \text{ Au}}{19.3 \text{ g Au}} = 1.61 \text{ cm}^3$ (not much, for a cost of many hundreds
  of dollars!)

2.42   No, only the metals with densities over 1.0 g/cm³ will sink. From Table 2-4, the metal potassium (density = 0.86 g/cm³) will float as it reacts with water.

2.43 $1 \text{ lb oil} \times \dfrac{454 \text{ g oil}}{1 \text{ lb oil}} \times \dfrac{1 \text{ cm}^3 \text{ oil}}{0.92 \text{ g oil}} \times \dfrac{1 \text{ mL}}{1 \text{ cm}^3} = 493 \text{ mL olive oil}$

2.44 $\dfrac{7.7 \text{ lb whiskey}}{1 \text{ gal whiskey}} \times \dfrac{454 \text{ g}}{1 \text{ lb}} \times \dfrac{0.2642 \text{ gal}}{1 \text{ L}} \times \dfrac{1 \text{ L}}{1000 \text{ cm}^3} = 0.92 \text{ g/cm}^3 \text{ whiskey}$; specific gravity = 0.92

2.45   When chemical reaction occurs, the atoms of carbon remain unchanged but only pass from one chemical form (alcohol) to another (CO_2). No carbon atoms may be lost or produced in the process.

2.46   neutron has *no* charge; mass = 1.0 amu; is in the nucleus

2.47   **a** cations Na^+, Fe^{3+} **b** anion OH^- **c** Na^+/OH^-, Fe^{3+}/OH^- attract

2.48   a statement about an experimental result that is always observed to occur; a law is confirmed by repeated experiments of the same type

2.49   masses of a Ca atom and a Ca^{2+} cation are essentially the same, averaging 40.1 amu; they differ by the mass of two electrons, or only 0.001 amu

2.50   Possible answers include water balance, nerve action, and movement across cell membranes.

2.51   No. We cannot describe an electron orbit because an electron does *not* simply travel around the nucleus as does a planet around the sun; see Figure 2-5.

2.52   **a** $^{112}_{50}$Sn: tin; atomic number 50; mass number 112; 50 protons; 62 neutrons
  b $^{20}_{11}$Na: sodium; $Z = 11$; $A = 20$; 11 protons; 9 neutrons
  c $^{52}_{26}$Fe: iron; $Z = 26$; $A = 52$; 26 protons; 26 neutrons

2.53 $^{60}_{27}$Co (cobalt-60)

2.54   no; yes, for example: $^{14}_{6}C$, $^{14}_{7}N$, $^{14}_{8}O$

2.55
$$\frac{(95.0\% \times 32.0 \text{ amu}) + (0.76\% \times 33.0) + (4.22\% \times 34.0) + (0.014\% \times 36.0)}{100.000\%}$$

$$= \frac{3040 + 25 + 143.5 + 0.5}{100} = 32.09 \text{ amu} = 32.1 \text{ amu for sulfur}$$

2.56   Since $1 \text{ Å} = 10^{-10} \text{ m} = 10^{-8} \text{ cm}$, $0.50 \text{ Å} = 5.0 \times 10^{-9} \text{ cm}$; then $(0.50 \text{ Å})^3 = (5.0 \times 10^{-9} \text{ cm})^3 = 1.25 \times 10^{-25} \text{ cm}^3$ for the volume; mass of one hydrogen atom (average) $= 1.008 \text{ amu} \times \dfrac{1.66 \times 10^{-24} \text{ g}}{1 \text{ amu}} = 1.67 \times 10^{-24} \text{ g}$; density $=$ mass/volume $= 13.4 \text{ g/cm}^3$

Hydrogen gas occupies much more space than this, so is much less dense.

CHAPTER THREE SELF-CHECKS

3.1   **a** $_6$C: $1s^2\ 2s^2\ 2p^2$ **b** $_{18}$Ar: $1s^2\ 2s^2\ 2p^6\ 3s^2\ 3p^6$ **c** $_{20}$Ca: $1s^2\ 2s^2\ 2p^6\ 3s^2\ 3p^6\ 4s^2$
  d $_{13}$Al: $1s^2\ 2s^2\ 2p^6\ 3s^2\ 3p^1$

3.2 $_{16}$S: $[_{10}\text{Ne}]\ 3s^2\ 3p^4$

3.3   configurations which involve completed s and p outer sublevels; $ns^2\ np^6$

3.4   An electron in the 1s sublevel has lower energy and is closer to the nucleus (on the average) than an electron in the 2s sublevel.

3.5   **a** halogen: $ns^2\ np^5$ **b** Group 2: ns^2 **c** noble gas: $ns^2\ np^6$

3.6   **a** K: alkali metals, Group 1   **b** Cl: halogens, Group 7   **c** Ar: noble gases, Group 8 (sometimes called Group 0)

3.7   **a** $\cdot\dot{C}\cdot$ **b** Mg   **c** $:\ddot{F}:$ **d** $\cdot$Ca$\cdot$

3.8   **a** 2+   **b** 1−   **c** 2−

3.9 Mg^{2+} is formed when Mg loses two electrons to arrive at the Ne configuration (10 electrons); I^- is formed when I gains one electron to attain the xenon stable configuration (54 electrons); S^{2-} results when the S atom gains two electrons to achieve the argon noble-gas configuration (18 electrons).

3.10   The ionization energy of a metal is *low,* since an electron is easily lost.

3.11   The oxidation states of metals are always *positive* (+) or zero.

3.12   **a** Pb is more metallic than Sb, being closer to the bottom left of the table.
  b S is more metallic than F (although both are classified as nonmetals).
  c Cs is more metallic than Ba (although both are metals).

3.13   **a** Mg: 0   **b** Ca^{2+}: +2   **c** H_2: 0   **d** Fe^{3+}: +3   **e** Cl^-: −1

3.14   The ionization energy of a nonmetal is relatively high.

3.15   Negative oxidation states (−1, −2, −3) are more typical of nonmetals, although most nonmetals can be found in positive oxidation states as well.

3.16   Fluorine, chlorine, and oxygen are the most ''nonmetallic''; another acceptable answer would be fluorine, chlorine, and bromine, all of which easily form 1− ions.

3.17   No to both questions; our thyroid gland requires iodine to make a necessary hormone; too much iodine is poisonous.

3.18   Group 1: alkali metals; Group 2: alkaline earth metals
  Group 7: halogens; Group 8: noble gases

3.19   If we let ''X'' stand for a nonmetal element symbol:

   a $ns^2\ np^3$ $:\dot{X}\cdot$ **b** $ns^2\ np^6$ $[:\ddot{X}:]^-$

3.20   **a** Gamma (γ) rays involve electromagnetic radiation, not particles with mass.   **b** Alpha (α) particles are nuclei of helium atoms.   **c** Gamma rays are very similar to x-rays.   **d** Beta (β) rays are electrons, just like those in a TV set.   **e** Gamma rays can pass through the body.

3.21   When a gamma ray strikes a chromosome in the nucleus of a cell, it can break bonds; this can cause changes in the hereditary information.

3.22   A scanner can be used to determine which part of the lungs is receiving air, and how quickly; it can easily detect lung blockage.

3.23   **a** Ionizing radiation can break bonds inside cells and in various ways cause the cells to die; this is true of both normal and cancerous cells.   **b** The gold might not be removed if its decay product is stable and not injurious; most of the radiation from the gold itself would be gone after a week.

3.24   Astatine (Z-85) is similar to iodine (Z-53) and will be absorbed into the thyroid gland, where it could damage cells.

3.25   The dosage is far too low to cause the symptoms. Hair loss is very common in men as they age ("pattern baldness").

3.26   **a** At exactly one half-life later, we would have half of the original amount left; 0.50 millicurie.   **b** At 64 hours after administration, five half-lives have passed. The amount left is $1/2 \times 1/2 \times 1/2 \times 1/2 \times 1/2 = 0.031$ of the original; thus: 0.031 millicurie.

3.27   Iodine is taken up from food into the thyroid gland. Radioactive iodine, chemically identical to ordinary iodine, will enter the gland in this manner and damage cells. If the body has already taken in considerable amounts of iodine, it is less likely to retain small amounts of additional iodine that comes from radioactive sources; the more iodine available to the body, the less chance that any particular I^- ion will find its way to the gland.

CHAPTER THREE QUESTIONS AND PROBLEMS

3.28   The electron does not follow a known path; it should be treated as a "cloud," as in Figures 2-5 and 3-1.

3.29   One; an orbital may contain zero, one, or two electrons at any one time.

3.30 $_{13}$Al: (↑↓)   (↑↓)   (↑↓)(↑↓)(↑↓)   (↑↓)   (↑)( )( )
             1s   2s   2p   3s   3p

3.31   **a** $_3$Li: $1s^2\ 2s^1$ **b** $_{14}$Si: $1s^2\ 2s^2\ 2p^6\ 3s^2\ 3p^2$ **c** $_9$F: $1s^2\ 2s^2\ 2p^5$

3.32   The argon core $[_{18}Ar]$ contains 18 electrons, arranged $1s^2\ 2s^2\ 2p^6\ 3s^2\ 3p^6$.
        a $_{19}$K: $[_{18}Ar]\ 4s^1$ **b** $_{20}$Ca: $[_{18}Ar]\ 4s^2$ **c** $_{33}$As: $[_{18}Ar]\ 4s^2\ 3d^{10}\ 4p^3$

3.33   **a** The helium atom contains only two electrons; the configuration shows three!   **b** A p sublevel can hold a maximum of *six* electrons, not seven as shown.   **c** The 2s sublevel is shown twice, but can only appear once.

3.34   **a** Group 3   **b** Group 2   **c** Group 7

3.35   In the periodic table of Figure 3–14, those elements which are   **a** halogens: Q, M   **b** alkali metals: D, E   **c** in Period 4: D, G, L, M   **d** *not* representative elements: J, L, W

3.36   **a** 2 + in Mg^{2+} **b** 2 − in S^{2-} **c** 1 − in I^-

3.37   **a** Na^+ sodium ion   **b** O^{2-} oxide ion   **c** Te^{2-} telluride ion

3.38   **a** ·C·   **b** K·   **c** :Br: **d** Ca

3.39   As each electron is removed, the remaining particle becomes more positively charged and attracts even more tightly the electrons that are left.

3.40 **a** positive (+) charges   **b** left half (or bottom right) of table   **c** low ionization energy   **d** positive (+) oxidation states

3.41 potassium K^+ 3.42 magnesium Mg^{2+}

3.43 cobalt Co   3.44 iron Fe (in the form of Fe^{2+} and Fe^{3+})

3.45 **a** +3   **b** 0   **c** −1   3.46 carbon C

3.47 No; nitrogen in its zero oxidation state (as N_2) cannot be used. The body uses nitrogen in its −3 oxidation state.

3.48 chlorine, needed as Cl^- ion, but poisonous as Cl_2 gas (oxygen can cause illness and death if breathed in high concentrations for an extended period)

3.49 to strengthen bones and teeth

3.50 **a** alpha particle mass is relatively high   **b** 2+ charge   **c** more dangerous inside body, since it has low penetrating power

3.51 by ionizing atoms and breaking bonds, especially in chromosomes (genes)

3.52 phosphorus-32 emits beta particles, which are electrons

3.53 Small amounts of radioiodine can be used to measure how quickly the gland absorbs iodine; large amounts will produce enough radiation to kill cells, especially those that are rapidly dividing (such as cancer cells).

3.54 Small amounts of injected radiosodium will be distributed throughout the blood stream and then taken up by the body in the same manner as normal Na^+.

3.55 The chromium-51 atoms will emit gamma rays from the sites where they are attached to red blood cells. By monitoring radiation from the various regions of the uterus, we can tell where the red blood cells (and therefore the placenta) are located.

3.56 Strontium-90 acts like Ca^{2+} (since both are in Group 2) and lodges in bones; it thus can cause bone cancer. Cesium-137 will end up in body fluids in the same manner as the other Group 1 ions, Na^+ and K^+. Iodine-131 will be taken up by the thyroid gland, like normal I^- ions.

3.57 According to Table 3–6, a dose of 22 rem would have no observable health effect. However, it would be unwise to repeat such a series of x-rays unless absolutely essential.

3.58 The half-life of cobalt-60 is 5.3 years. After that time, a 16.0-curie source would have 8.0 curies left. After 10.6 years, only 4.0 curies would remain.

3.59 *Curies*, which measure the number of emissions per second; *rem* tell you what effect those emissions will have on body tissues.

3.60 **a** alpha source—less penetrating power, since it is stopped by the outer layer of skin   **b** source blocked by layer of lead—the lead stops most of the radiation   **c** cobalt-60—since the half-life (5.3 years) is longer than that of cobalt-57 (0.75 year), in any given time period, fewer ^{60}Co atoms will disintegrate

CHAPTER FOUR SELF-CHECKS

4.1 Opposite charges attract each other.

4.2 **a** KI   **b** SnF_2 **c** $CaSO_4$ [*not* $Ca_2(SO_4)_2$ since we use the simpler ratios]   **d** $(NH_4)_2CO_3$ **e** $FePO_4$ **f** ZrO_2 **g** Zn_3P_2

4.3 **a** K^+ potassium ion   **d** CO_3^{2-} carbonate ion
b OH^- hydroxide ion   **e** Fe^{3+} iron(III) ion
c NH_4^+ ammonium ion   **f** $H_2PO_4^-$ dihydrogen phosphate ion

      g Zn^{2+} zinc ion   **i** Mn^{2+} manganese (II) ion
      h $C_2O_4^{2-}$ oxalate ion   **j** S^{2-} sulfide ion

4.4   **a** Ag^+ **b** Cu^{2+} **c** Br^- **d** PO_4^{3-} **e** Mn^{2+} **f** Mg^{2+}
      g Al^{3+} **h** CN^- **i** HSO_4^- **j** CH_3COO^- (or $C_2H_3O_2^-$)

4.5   **a** HCO_3^- hydrogen carbonate ion   **b** Fe^{3+} iron(III) ion   **c** Cu^+ copper(I) ion

4.6   **a** $FeSO_4$ **b** $Al(OH)_3$ **c** $K_2C_2O_4$ **d** $Mg(C_6H_5COO)_2$
      [or $(C_6H_5COO)_2Mg$]   **e** $ZnCl_2$ **f** $Zn_3(PO_4)_2$ **g** $HgCl_2$ **h** $NaHCO_3$
      i NH_4NO_3

4.7   Each iodine atom, with electron configuration $_{53}I$: $[_{36}Kr]5s^2\,4d^{10}\,5p^5$, seeks one
      electron to fill its valence-level octet. By sharing two electrons, each atom then
      has an octet and a more stable configuration.

4.8   **a** F_2 :F̈:F̈:   **e** NI_3 :Ï:N̈:Ï:
                                          :Ï:

                                                H
      b HBr H:B̈r: **f** CH_4 H:C:H
                                                H

                                            H H
      c H_2S H:S̈:H   **g** C_2H_6 H:C:C:H
                                              H H

                                            H
      d OCl_2 :C̈l:Ö:C̈l: **h** CH_3OH H:C:Ö:H
                                              H

                                                             H
                      (*also correct:* H_2CO H:C::Ö:)

4.9   **a** nitrogen dioxide   **d** iodine monochloride
      b diphosphorus pentasulfide   **e** diphosphorus trioxide
      c silicon tetrachloride   **f** iodine heptafluoride

4.10   **a** I_2O_5 **b** CS_2 **c** ClF_3 **d** SF_6 **e** Si_3N_4

4.11   **a** methane   **b** propane   **c** ethyl alcohol

4.12   **a** CH_3OH **b** C_4H_{10} **c** HCHO *or* H_2CO

4.13   **a** C_4H_{10}: (4) (12.0 amu) + (10) (1.0 amu) = 58.0 amu   **b** 58.5 amu
      c 46.0 amu   **d** $Fe_3(PO_4)_2$ 358 amu   **e** N_2O 44.0 amu

4.14   Those for butane, ethyl alcohol, and N_2O are molecular weights.

4.15   **a** C_2H_5OH total weight of one molecule: 46.0 amu

      carbon: $\dfrac{2 \times 12.0\ \text{amu}}{46.0\ \text{amu}} \times 100 = 52.2\%$ carbon

      hydrogen: $\dfrac{6 \times 1.0\ \text{amu}}{46.0\ \text{amu}} \times 100 = 13.0\%$ hydrogen

      oxygen: $\dfrac{1 \times 16.0\ \text{amu}}{46.0\ \text{amu}} \times 100 = 34.8\%$ oxygen

      (Check: 52.2% + 13.0% + 34.8% = 100.0%)
      b 46.8% iron, 17.3% phosphorus, 35.8% oxygen in $Fe_3(PO_4)_2$

4.16 $10.0 \text{ g } C_2H_5OH \times \dfrac{34.8\% \text{ oxygen}}{100.0\% \text{ total}} = 3.48 \text{ g oxygen}$

4.17 Formulas (b) and (f) are simplest formulas.   **a** $C_6H_{14} \rightarrow$ "C_3H_7"
c $C_2H_4O_2 \rightarrow$ "CH_2O"   **d** $N_2O_4 \rightarrow$ "NO_2"   **e** $C_{18}H_{22}O_2 \rightarrow$ "$C_9H_{11}O$"

4.18 **a** Assume we have 100.0 amu of compound. That gives us 23.8 amu carbon, 5.9 amu hydrogen, and 70.3 amu chlorine. How many atoms of each element?

$23.8 \text{ amu C} \times \dfrac{1 \text{ atom C}}{12.0 \text{ amu}} = 1.98 \text{ atoms C}$

$5.9 \text{ amu H} \times \dfrac{1 \text{ atom H}}{1.0 \text{ amu}} = 5.9 \text{ atoms H}$

$70.3 \text{ amu Cl} \times \dfrac{1 \text{ atom Cl}}{35.5 \text{ amu}} = 1.98 \text{ atoms Cl}$

Divide all three numbers of atoms by the lowest, here 1.98 atoms.

$\dfrac{1.98 \text{ atoms C}}{1.98} = 1 \text{ C}$ $\dfrac{5.9 \text{ atoms H}}{1.98} = 3 \text{ H}$ $\dfrac{1.98 \text{ atoms Cl}}{1.98} = 1 \text{ Cl}$

The simplest formula is "CH_3Cl."
b We start with 100.0 amu of compound, containing 93.7 amu of C and 6.3 amu of H. Dividing: 93.7 amu C/12.0 = 7.81 atoms C; 6.3 amu H/1.0 = 6.3 atoms H. Dividing again by 6.3, we obtain 1.24 carbons to 1.00 hydrogen. This cannot be the final ratio, since we must be working with whole atoms. There must then be five carbons to every four hydrogens, or "C_5H_4." The actual molecular formula of naphthalene is $C_{10}H_8$.   **c** Morphine is "$C_{17}H_{19}NO_3$."

4.19 Calculate first the percentage of carbon in aspirin, $C_9H_8O_4$. The molecular weight is 180 amu, of which $(9)(12.0) = 108$ amu is carbon. The carbon makes up $108/180 = 0.600 = 60.0\%$ of aspirin. Assume we have a tablet weighing 1.00 gram. Then 25.0% of 1.00 gram is 0.250 gram carbon. This same carbon comes entirely from aspirin. Then $0.250 \text{ g C} \times \dfrac{100.0\% \text{ aspirin}}{60.0\% \text{ C}} = 0.417 \text{ g as-}$ pirin, or 41.7% of the tablet.

CHAPTER FOUR QUESTIONS AND PROBLEMS

4.20 A cation (with a + charge) attracts an anion (with a − charge); NH_4CN

4.21 **a** NaC_6H_5COO *or* C_6H_5COONa **d** NH_4HSO_4 (do not combine the hydrogens)
b $MnSO_4$ **e** $K_2Cr_2O_7$
c $Ca(OH)_2$ **f** $Cu_3(PO_4)_2$

4.22 **a** copper(I) oxide   **b** sodium phosphate   **c** barium permanganate
d aluminum nitrate   **e** iron(III) hydroxide

4.23 **a** $AgBr$ **b** $MgHPO_4$ **c** $FeCO_3$ **d** ZnS **e** $NaC_{17}H_{35}COO$ *or*
$C_{17}H_{35}COONa$ **f** $NH_4C_2H_3O_2$ *or* CH_3COONH_4

4.24 Since oxygen (as oxide ion) carries a 2 − charge, and since there are two oxide ions, we must be working with a Ti^{4+} cation; titanium (IV) ion.

4.25 Since the potassium ion is K^+, cyanate must be NCO^-.

4.26 Each Ca^{2+} contributes 2 +, each PO_4^{3-} gives 3 −, and each OH^- gives 1 −; adding them, we obtain $(10)(2+) + (6)(3-) + (2)(1-) = 20+ 20- = 0$.

4.27 The ions are K^+, Ag^+, and two CN^- anions; potassium silver cyanide; no!

4.28 A covalent bond is created by electron sharing between neutral atoms; an ionic bond is formed by attraction between a cation and an anion.

4.29   Metals do not have covalence numbers, since they do not form covalent bonds.

4.30   **a** $:\ddot{Br}:\ddot{Br}:$ **b** $H:\ddot{I}:$ **c** $:\ddot{Cl}:\ddot{N}:\ddot{Cl}:$ **d** $:\ddot{F}:\ddot{C}:\ddot{F}:$
with $:\ddot{Cl}:$ below N, and $:\ddot{F}:$ above and $:\ddot{F}:$ below C

4.31   **a** $:\ddot{Br}:\ddot{P}:\ddot{Br}:$ with $:\ddot{Br}:$ below   **b** $H:\ddot{Si}:H$ with H above and H below   **c** $:\ddot{F}:\ddot{C}:\ddot{C}:\ddot{C}:\ddot{F}:$ with $:\ddot{F}:$ atoms above and below the carbons

4.32   **a** nitrogen monoxide (*or* mononitrogen monoxide)   **b** carbon tetra-fluoride   **c** chlorine dioxide   **d** chlorine trifluoride   **e** iodine penta-fluoride   **f** diarsenic pentoxide (the "a" in "pentaoxide" is dropped)

4.33   **a** SO_2 **b** Si_2Br_6 **c** Mn_3C **d** P_2I_4 **e** BrF **f** $MoCl_5$

4.34   The two compounds CH_4 and $C_{10}H_8$ contain both carbon and hydrogen, nothing else.

4.35   **a** ethane   **b** propane   **c** ammonia   **d** methyl alcohol

4.36   **a** C_2H_5OH **b** C_4H_{10} **c** $HCHO$ **d** CH_4

4.37   refrigerants (as in air conditioners) and propellants (spray cans)

4.38   **a** C_2H_6 30.0 amu   **b** $Al_2(CO_3)_2$ $2 \times 27.0 + 3 \times 60.0 = 234$ amu   **c** CH_3OH 32.0 amu   **d** NH_4NO_3 80.0 amu   **e** C_4H_9Cl 92.5 amu   **f** $C_{28}H_{44}O$ 396 amu   **g** $C_3H_7NO_2$ 89.0 amu

4.39   **a** The molecular weight of CH_3OH is 32.0 amu, of which 12.0 amu is carbon. Then $12.0/32.0 = 0.375 = 37.5\%$ carbon in methyl alcohol.   **b** 48.0/92.5 gives 51.9% C   **c** 336/396 gives 84.8% C in vitamin D   **d** 36.0/89.0 gives 40.4% C   **e** 36.0/234 gives 15.4% C in $Al_2(CO_3)_3$

4.40   Ethane, C_2H_6, has the simplest formula "CH_3"; the rest are already simplest.

4.41   10.0 g $Al_2(CO_3)_3$ contain $9 \times 16 = 144$ amu oxygen in one molecule, which has a molecular weight of 234 amu; percent $O = (144/234) \times 100 = 61.5\%$; then 61.5% of 10.0 g gives *6.15 grams* of oxygen in 10.0 g of aluminum carbonate.

4.42   In 100.0 amu of amphetamine sulfate we will have 46.3 amu C, 6.0 amu N, 6.5 amu H, 13.8 amu S, and 27.5 amu O. How many atoms of each?

$$\frac{46.3 \text{ amu C}}{12.0 \text{ amu/atom}} = 3.86 \text{ atoms C} \qquad \frac{6.0 \text{ amu N}}{14.0 \text{ amu/atom}} = 0.429 \text{ atom N}$$

$$\frac{6.5 \text{ amu H}}{1.0 \text{ amu/atom}} = 6.5 \text{ atoms H} \qquad \frac{13.8 \text{ amu S}}{32.1 \text{ amu/atom}} = 0.430 \text{ atom S}$$

$$\frac{27.5 \text{ amu O}}{16.0 \text{ amu/atom}} = 1.72 \text{ atoms O} \qquad \text{Divide all numbers by 0.43, the smallest!}$$

$$\frac{3.86 \text{ C}}{0.43} = 9 \text{ C} \quad \frac{6.5 \text{ H}}{0.43} = 15 \text{ H} \quad \frac{1.72 \text{ O}}{0.43} = 4 \text{ O} \quad \frac{0.43 \text{ N}}{0.43} = 1 \text{ N} \quad \frac{0.43 \text{ S}}{0.43} = 1 \text{ S}$$

simplest formula: "$C_9H_{15}NSO_4$" (note: the order of O, N, S is *not* important)

4.43   Using the same procedure as for Problem 4.42, we obtain $76.4/12.0 = 6.37$ atoms C, 9.2 atoms H, and 0.906 atom O; dividing by 0.906, we get 7 C, 10 H, 1 O; the simplest formula is "$C_7H_{10}O$."

4.44   The total weight of the simplest formula unit, "$C_7H_{10}O$," is 110 amu; this is one third of the real molecular weight; the molecule actually has the formula $C_{21}H_{30}O_3$.

CHAPTER FIVE SELF-CHECKS

5.1   **a** $2 K + F_2 \rightarrow 2 KF$ **b** $2 Ca + O_2 \rightarrow 2 CaO$ **c** $N_2 + 3 H_2 \rightarrow$ $2 NH_3$ **d** $C + 2 H_2 \rightarrow CH_4$ **e** $2 N_2 + 5 O_2 \rightarrow 2 N_2O_5$ **f** $4 Al + 3 O_2 \rightarrow 2 Al_2O_3$

5.2   **a** $3 C + 4 H_2 \rightarrow C_3H_8$ **b** $4 Na + O_2 \rightarrow 2 Na_2O$ **c** $2 Fe + 3 F_2 \rightarrow$ $2 FeF_3$ **d** $2 C + 2 H_2 + O_2 \rightarrow 2 HCHO$

5.3   **a** $KClO_4 \rightarrow KCl + 2 O_2$ **b** $H_2SO_4 \rightarrow H_2O + SO_3$ **c** $2 HgO \rightarrow 2 Hg + O_2$ **d** $NH_4NO_2 \rightarrow 2 H_2O + N_2$

5.4   **a** $Al_{(s)} + 3 Fe(NO_3)_{2(aq)} \rightarrow 2 Al(NO_3)_{3(aq)} + 3 Fe_{(s)}$ **b** $K_2O_{(s)} + H_2O_{(\ell)} \rightarrow$ $2 KOH_{(aq)}$ **c** $2 NaOH_{(aq)} + H_2C_2O_{4(s)} \rightarrow 2 H_2O_{(\ell)} + Na_2C_2O_{4(aq)}$ **d** $Ca(OH)_{2(aq)} + H_2SO_{4(aq)} \rightarrow 2 H_2O_{(\ell)} + CaSO_{4(aq)}$

5.5   The first equation contains only formula units of molecules and ionic salts; it shows what overall substances react, but is poor for indicating which particles really exist in solution. The second is an *ionic* equation, which shows which particles are really present for each substance.

5.6   In a chemical equilibrium, as many reactant molecules are becoming products in each second as product molecules are becoming reactants, and so there is no net change in the amount of any substance present. In the case shown, as many H_2CO_3 molecules dissociate each second as are formed by the reverse reaction.

5.7   **a** $C_2H_5OH + 3 O_2 \rightarrow 2 CO_2 + 3 H_2O$ **b** $C_3H_8 + 5 O_2 \rightarrow 3 CO_2 + 4 H_2O$ **c** $2 C_2H_2 + 5 O_2 \rightarrow 4 CO_2 + 2 H_2O$ **d** $C_6H_{12}O_6 + 6 O_2 \rightarrow 6 CO_2 + 6 H_2O$

5.8   The weight of one mole of fluorine atoms is 19.0 g, and one mole of F_2 molecules has a mass of $(2)(19.0) = 38.0$ grams. Then:

a $190 \text{ g F} \times \dfrac{1 \text{ mole F}}{19.0 \text{ g F}} = 10.0$ moles of F atoms

b $190 \text{ g } F_2 \times \dfrac{1 \text{ mole } F_2}{38.0 \text{ g } F_2} = 5.00$ moles of F_2 molecules

c Sodium fluoride has a weight of $(23.0 + 19.0) = 42.0$ grams per mole.

$190 \text{ g NaF} \times \dfrac{1 \text{ mole NaF}}{42.0 \text{ g NaF}} = 4.52$ moles of NaF formula units

d Fluoromethane has a weight of $(12.0 + 3.0 + 19.0) = 34.0$ grams per mole.

$190 \text{ g } CH_3F \times \dfrac{1 \text{ mole } CH_3F}{34.0 \text{ g } CH_3F} = 5.59$ moles of CH_3F molecules

5.9   **a** $17.5 \text{ moles } CH_3F \times \dfrac{34.0 \text{ g } CH_3F}{1 \text{ mole } CH_3F} = 595$ grams CH_3F

b $55.5 \text{ moles } H_2O \times \dfrac{18.0 \text{ g } H_2O}{1 \text{ mole } H_2O} = 999$ grams H_2O

Thus, one liter of water contains just about 55.5 moles of liquid H_2O.

c $0.0125 \text{ mole HCl} \times \dfrac{36.5 \text{ g HCl}}{1 \text{ mole HCl}} = 0.456$ grams HCl

d $1.27 \text{ moles I} \times \dfrac{126.9 \text{ g I}}{1 \text{ mole I}} = 161$ grams of iodine atoms

5.10   **a** $10 \text{ atoms C} \times \dfrac{1 \text{ mole C}}{6.02 \times 10^{23} \text{ atoms C}} = 1.66 \times 10^{-23}$ mole of carbon atoms

b 6.02×10^{24} molecules $H_2 \times \dfrac{1 \text{ mole } H_2}{6.02 \times 10^{23} \text{ molecules } H_2} = 10.0$ moles H_2

5.11 **a** 0.890 mole $O_2 \times \dfrac{6.02 \times 10^{23} \text{ molecules } O_2}{1 \text{ mole } O_2} = 5.36 \times 10^{23}$ molecules O_2

b 18.5 moles $Ag \times \dfrac{6.02 \times 10^{23} \text{ atoms } Ag}{1 \text{ mole } Ag} = 1.11 \times 10^{25}$ atoms Ag

c 24.0 g $C \times \dfrac{1 \text{ mole } C}{12.0 \text{ g } C} \times \dfrac{6.02 \times 10^{23} \text{ atoms } C}{1 \text{ mole } C} = 1.20 \times 10^{24}$ atoms C

d 3.50 g $CH_4 \times \dfrac{1 \text{ mole } CH_4}{16.0 \text{ g } CH_4} \times \dfrac{6.02 \times 10^{23} \text{ molecules } CH_4}{1 \text{ mole } CH_4} \times$

$\dfrac{1 \text{ atom } C}{1 \text{ molecule } CH_4} = 1.32 \times 10^{23}$ atoms C

5.12 **a** One formula unit of $CaCO_3$ solid reacts with two formula units of aqueous HCl to produce one molecule of CO_2 gas, one molecule of liquid H_2O, and one formula unit of aqueous $CaCl_2$.   **b** One mole of $CaCO_3$ solid reacts with two moles of aqueous HCl to produce one mole of CO_2 gas, one mole of liquid H_2O, and one mole of aqueous $CaCl_2$.

5.13 **a** 1.0 mole $HCl \times \dfrac{1 \text{ mole } CaCO_3}{2 \text{ moles } HCl} = 0.50$ mole $CaCO_3$

b 1.0 g $HCl \times \dfrac{1 \text{ mole } HCl}{36.5 \text{ g } HCl} \times \dfrac{1 \text{ mole } CaCO_3}{2 \text{ moles } HCl} \times \dfrac{100 \text{ g } CaCO_3}{1 \text{ mole } CaCO_3} =$
1.37 g $CaCO_3$

c 1.0 g $CaCO_3 \times \dfrac{1 \text{ mole } CaCO_3}{100 \text{ g } CaCO_3} \times \dfrac{1 \text{ mole } CO_2}{1 \text{ mole } CaCO_3} \times \dfrac{44.0 \text{ g } CO_2}{1 \text{ mole } CO_2} =$
0.440 g CO_2

d 1.5 L acid $\times \dfrac{0.010 \text{ mole } HCl}{1 \text{ liter acid}} \times \dfrac{1 \text{ mole } CaCO_3}{2 \text{ moles } HCl} \times \dfrac{100 \text{ g } CaCO_3}{1 \text{ mole } CaCO_3} =$
0.75 g $CaCO_3$

e This is a limiting-reagent problem; find how many moles of CO_2 would be produced by *complete* reaction of each reactant:

5.0 g $CaCO_3 \times \dfrac{1 \text{ mole } CaCO_3}{100 \text{ g } CaCO_3} \times \dfrac{1 \text{ mole } CO_2}{1 \text{ mole } CaCO_3} = 0.050$ mole CO_2 using up $CaCO_3$

0.080 mole $HCl \times \dfrac{1 \text{ mole } CO_2}{2 \text{ moles } HCl} = 0.040$ mole CO_2 if HCl is all used up

The maximum amount of CO_2 we can possibly get is 0.040 mole, which is the product if HCl is the limiting reagent; $CaCO_3$ is in excess.

CHAPTER FIVE QUESTIONS AND PROBLEMS

5.14 **a** Two formula units of $KClO_3$ decompose to give two formula units of KCl and three molecules of O_2 gas.   **b** Two molecules of CH_3OH react with three molecules of O_2 gas to give two molecules of CO_2 and four molecules of H_2O.

5.15 **a** $Ca + F_2 \rightarrow CaF_2$ **b** $2 C + O_2 \rightarrow 2 CO$ **c** $2 Na + I_2 \rightarrow 2 NaI$
d $3 C + 4 H_2 \rightarrow C_3H_8$

5.16 **a** $2 NaCl \rightarrow 2 Na + Cl_2$ **b** $H_2SO_3 \rightarrow H_2O + SO_2$

5.17 **a** $^{99}_{42}Mo \rightarrow ^{99}_{43}Tc + ^{0}_{-1}e$ **b** $^{3}_{1}H \rightarrow ^{3}_{2}He + ^{0}_{-1}e$ **c** $^{238}_{92}U \rightarrow ^{234}_{90}Th + ^{4}_{2}He^{2+}$

5.18 **a** $4 P + 3 O_2 \rightarrow 2 P_2O_3$ **b** $P_2O_3 + 3 H_2O \rightarrow 2 H_3PO_3$ **c** $2 Al + Fe_2O_3 \rightarrow 2 Fe + Al_2O_3$ **d** $2 NaBr + F_2 \rightarrow 2 NaF + Br_2$ **e** $2 H_2O_2 \rightarrow 2 H_2O + O_2$ **f** $MgCO_3 \rightarrow MgO + CO_2$ **g** $NH_4NO_2 \rightarrow N_2 + 2 H_2O$

5.19 **a** $2 Na_{(s)} + 2 H_2O_{(\ell)} \rightarrow H_{2(g)} + 2 NaOH_{(aq)}$ **b** $Al_2O_{3(s)} + 6 HCl_{(aq)} \rightarrow 2 AlCl_{3(aq)} + 3 H_2O_{(\ell)}$ **c** $H_{2(g)} + FeO_{(s)} \rightarrow H_2O_{(\ell)} + Fe_{(s)}$ **d** $Fe_2O_{3(s)} + 3 CO_{(g)} \rightarrow 2 Fe_{(s)} + 3 CO_{2(g)}$ **e** $ZnCO_{3(s)} + 2 HCl_{(aq)} \rightarrow ZnCl_{2(aq)} + CO_{2(g)} + H_2O_{(\ell)}$ **f** $FeS_{(s)} + 2 HBr_{(aq)} \rightarrow FeBr_{2(aq)} + H_2S_{(aq)}$ **g** $3 AgNO_{3(aq)} + AlCl_{3(aq)} \rightarrow 3 AgCl_{(s)} + Al(NO_3)_{3(aq)}$

5.20 **a** $NaOH_{(aq)} + HNO_{3(aq)} \rightarrow H_2O_{(\ell)} + NaNO_{3(aq)}$ **b** $Ca(OH)_{2(s)} + 2 HI_{(aq)} \rightarrow 2 H_2O_{(\ell)} + CaI_{2(aq)}$ **c** $Ba(OH)_{2(aq)} + H_2C_2O_{4(s)} \rightarrow 2 H_2O_{(\ell)} + BaC_2O_{4(aq)}$ **d** $Mg(OH)_{2(s)} + 2 HCl_{(aq)} \rightarrow 2 H_2O_{(\ell)} + MgCl_{2(aq)}$

5.21 The first is an ionic equation, which shows which particles are really present in solution for the reactants and the products. The second is a *net* ionic equation, which eliminates ions that are present on both sides (spectators) of the ionic equation and therefore do not participate in the chemical change. The clear advantage of the net ionic equation is that it shows us that the natures of the cation (Na^+) and anion (NO_3^-), in the base and acid that are combining here, are not important.

5.22 When calcium phosphate solid is in equilibrium with calcium ions and phosphate ions, the rate at which the solid calculus dissolves is equal to the rate at which solid is formed by precipitation.

5.23 **a** $2 Ag^+_{(aq)} + SO^{2-}_{4(aq)} \rightarrow Ag_2SO_{4(s)}$ **b** $Cu^{2+}_{(aq)} + 4 NH_{3(aq)} \rightarrow Cu(NH_3)^{2+}_{4(aq)}$

5.24 **a** $CaC_2 + 2 H_2O \rightarrow Ca(OH)_2 + C_2H_2$ **b** $CH_4 + Cl_2 \rightarrow CH_3Cl + HCl$

5.25 **a** $C_2H_4 + 3 O_2 \rightarrow 2 CO_2 + 2 H_2O$ **b** $2 C_6H_{14} + 19 O_2 \rightarrow 12 CO_2 + 14 H_2O$ **c** $C_4H_9OH + 6 O_2 \rightarrow 4 CO_2 + 5 H_2O$ **d** $CH_3COCH_3 + 4 O_2 \rightarrow 3 CO_2 + 3 H_2O$ **e** $C_{12}H_{22}O_{11} + 12 O_2 \rightarrow 12 CO_2 + 11 H_2O$

5.26 $0.25 \text{ mole Fe} \times \dfrac{55.8 \text{ g Fe}}{1 \text{ mole Fe}} = 14 \text{ g Fe}$

5.27 **a** $36.0 \text{ g C} \times \dfrac{1 \text{ mole C}}{12.0 \text{ g C}} = 3.00 \text{ moles C atoms}$

b $0.00471 \text{ g Mg} \times \dfrac{1 \text{ mole Mg}}{24.3 \text{ g Mg}} = 1.94 \times 10^{-4} \text{ mole Mg atoms}$

c $4.0 \text{ g H}_2 \times \dfrac{1 \text{ mole H}_2}{2.0 \text{ g H}_2} = 2.0 \text{ moles H}_2 \text{ molecules}$

d $3.69 \times 10^4 \text{ g N} \times \dfrac{1 \text{ mole N}}{14.0 \text{ g N}} = 2.64 \times 10^3 \text{ moles N atoms}$

e $5.00 \text{ g HF} \times \dfrac{1 \text{ mole HF}}{20.0 \text{ g HF}} = 0.250 \text{ mole HF molecules}$

f $0.0593 \text{ g NaCl} \times \dfrac{1 \text{ mole NaCl}}{58.5 \text{ g NaCl}} = 1.01 \times 10^{-3} \text{ mole NaCl formula units}$

g $17.6 \text{ g CHCl}_3 \times \dfrac{1 \text{ mole CHCl}_3}{119 \text{ g CHCl}_3} = 0.148 \text{ mole CHCl}_3 \text{ molecules}$

5.28 **a** $0.0875 \text{ mole K} \times \dfrac{39.1 \text{ g K}}{1 \text{ mole K}} = 3.42 \text{ g K}$

b $3.75 \text{ moles O}_2 \times \dfrac{32.0 \text{ g O}_2}{1 \text{ mole O}_2} = 120 \text{ g O}_2$

c $31.4 \text{ moles CaCl}_2 \times \dfrac{111 \text{ g CaCl}_2}{1 \text{ mole CaCl}_2} = 3.49 \times 10^3 \text{ g CaCl}_2$

d $1.74 \text{ moles C}_8H_{18} \times \dfrac{114 \text{ g C}_8H_{18}}{1 \text{ mole C}_8H_{18}} = 198 \text{ g C}_8H_{18}$

5.29   **a** 0.539 mole $CH_3OH \times \dfrac{32.0 \text{ g } CH_3OH}{1 \text{ mole } CH_3OH} = 17.2$ g CH_3OH

    b 0.539 mole $CH_3OH \times \dfrac{6.02 \times 10^{23} \text{ molecules}}{1 \text{ mole } CH_3OH} = 3.24 \times 10^{23}$ molecules

    c 3.24×10^{23} molecules $CH_3OH \times \dfrac{1 \text{ atom } O}{1 \text{ molecule } CH_3OH} = 3.24 \times$
10^{23} atoms O

    d 3.24×10^{23} molecules $CH_3OH \times \dfrac{4 \text{ atoms } H}{1 \text{ molecule } CH_3OH} = 1.30 \times$
10^{24} atoms H

5.30   **a** 392 molecules sucrose $\times \dfrac{22 \text{ atoms } H}{1 \text{ molecule sucrose}} = 8624$ atoms H

    b 392 molecules sucrose $\times \dfrac{1 \text{ mole sucrose}}{6.02 \times 10^{23} \text{ molecules}} = 6.51 \times 10^{-22}$ mole
sucrose

    c 6.51×10^{-22} mole sucrose $\times \dfrac{342 \text{ g sucrose}}{1 \text{ mole sucrose}} = 2.23 \times 10^{-19}$ g sucrose

    d 6.51×10^{-22} mole sucrose $\times \dfrac{11 \text{ moles } O}{1 \text{ mole sucrose}} = 7.16 \times 10^{-21}$ mole
O atoms

5.31   **a** One molecule of urea reacts with one molecule of water to give two molecules of ammonia and one molecule of carbon dioxide.   **b** One mole of
urea reacts with one mole of water to give two moles of ammonia and one
mole of carbon dioxide.

    c 3.00 moles urea $\times \dfrac{2 \text{ moles } NH_3}{1 \text{ mole urea}} = 6.00$ moles ammonia

    d 3.00 moles urea $\times \dfrac{1 \text{ mole } H_2O}{1 \text{ mole urea}} = 3.00$ moles water

    e 10.0 g urea $\times \dfrac{1 \text{ mole urea}}{60.0 \text{ g urea}} \times \dfrac{2 \text{ moles } NH_3}{1 \text{ mole urea}} \times \dfrac{17.0 \text{ g } NH_3}{1 \text{ mole } NH_3} = 5.67$ g NH_3

5.32   **a** 125 g $KO_2 \times \dfrac{1 \text{ mole } KO_2}{71.1 \text{ g } KO_2} \times \dfrac{3 \text{ moles } O_2}{4 \text{ moles } KO_2} \times \dfrac{32.0 \text{ g } O_2}{1 \text{ mole } O_2} = 42.2$ g O_2

    b 1.00 kg $CO_2 \times \dfrac{1000 \text{ g } CO_2}{1 \text{ kg } CO_2} \times \dfrac{1 \text{ mole } CO_2}{44.0 \text{ g } CO_2} \times \dfrac{4 \text{ mole } KO_2}{2 \text{ mole } CO_2} \times \dfrac{71.1 \text{ g } KO_2}{1 \text{ mole } KO_2} =$
3.23×10^3 g KO_2

    c 5.00 moles $O_2 \times \dfrac{4 \text{ moles } KO_2}{3 \text{ moles } O_2} \times \dfrac{71.1 \text{ g } KO_2}{1 \text{ mole } KO_2} = 474$ g KO_2

    d Find the number of grams each reactant could produce;

       150 g $KO_2 \times \dfrac{1 \text{ mole } KO_2}{71.1 \text{ g } KO_2} \times \dfrac{3 \text{ moles } O_2}{4 \text{ moles } KO_2} \times \dfrac{32.0 \text{ g } O_2}{1 \text{ mole } O_2} = 50.6$ g O_2

       60.0 g $CO_2 \times \dfrac{1 \text{ mole } CO_2}{44.0 \text{ g } CO_2} \times \dfrac{3 \text{ moles } O_2}{2 \text{ moles } CO_2} \times \dfrac{32.0 \text{ g } O_2}{1 \text{ mole } O_2} = 65.5$ g O_2

    The limiting reagent is KO_2, giving a yield of 50.6 g O_2; CO_2 is in excess.

5.33   **a** To simplify writing the compounds, let citric acid be "CA" and baking soda
"BK." How much CO_2 could each give, if used up completely?

    6.00 g CA $\times \dfrac{1 \text{ mole CA}}{192 \text{ g CA}} \times \dfrac{3 \text{ moles } CO_2}{1 \text{ mole CA}} \times \dfrac{44.0 \text{ g } CO_2}{1 \text{ mole } CO_2} = 4.13$ g CO_2

$$20.0 \text{ g BK} \times \frac{1 \text{ mole BK}}{84.0 \text{ g BK}} \times \frac{3 \text{ moles CO}_2}{3 \text{ moles BK}} \times \frac{44.0 \text{ g CO}_2}{1 \text{ mole CO}_2} = 10.5 \text{ g CO}_2$$

Then $NaHCO_3$ is in excess, and only 4.13 g of CO_2 can be formed.

b $6.00 \text{ g CA} \times \frac{1 \text{ mole CA}}{192 \text{ g CA}} \times \frac{3 \text{ moles CO}_2}{1 \text{ mole CA}} \times \frac{39.2 \text{ L CO}_2}{1 \text{ mole CO}_2} = 3.68 \text{ L CO}_2$

c Some of the released CO_2 gas may escape from the cake (as when a cake "falls"), and some may dissolve in the water present; the reaction also does not go to completion.

CHAPTER SIX SELF-CHECKS

6.1 The element closer to the upper right of the table will have the higher EN.
   a Cl   **b** Mg   **c** Br   **d** S

6.2 $^{\delta+}$H—O$^{\delta-}$, polar, $\Delta EN = 1.4$ 6.3 $K^+ Cl^-$, ionic, $\Delta EN = 2.2$

6.4 C—H, essentially nonpolar; $\Delta EN = 0.4$ 6.5 $^{\delta+}$S—O$^{\delta-}$, polar, $\Delta EN = 1.0$

6.6 Selenium (EN = 2.4) has a higher electronegativity than silicon (EN = 1.8); the Se—F bond should thus be stronger than the Si—F bond, based on the degree of polarity; similarly, the Si—F bond should be longer.

6.7 **a** C_2H_5OH; 20 valence e$^-$;

$$\begin{array}{cc} H & H \\ H:\overset{\cdot\cdot}{\underset{\cdot\cdot}{C}}:\overset{\cdot\cdot}{\underset{\cdot\cdot}{C}}:\overset{\cdot\cdot}{\underset{\cdot\cdot}{O}}:H \\ H & H \end{array}$$

b C_3H_8; 20 valence e$^-$;

$$\begin{array}{ccc} H & H & H \\ H:\overset{\cdot\cdot}{\underset{\cdot\cdot}{C}}:\overset{\cdot\cdot}{\underset{\cdot\cdot}{C}}:\overset{\cdot\cdot}{\underset{\cdot\cdot}{C}}:H \\ H & H & H \end{array}$$

c C_3H_4; 16 valence e$^-$;

$$\begin{array}{c} H \\ H:C:::C:\overset{\cdot\cdot}{\underset{\cdot\cdot}{C}}:H \\ H \end{array}$$

(the diagram $H:\overset{}{\underset{\overset{\cdot\cdot}{H}}{C}}::C::\overset{}{\underset{\overset{\cdot\cdot}{H}}{C}}:H$ is acceptable)

d CH_3CHO; 18 valence e$^-$;

$$\begin{array}{c} H \\ H:\overset{\cdot\cdot}{\underset{\cdot\cdot}{C}}:C::\overset{\cdot\cdot}{\underset{\cdot\cdot}{O}}: \\ H \quad H \end{array}$$

e PO_4^{3-}; 5 + 24 + 3 = 32 valence e$^-$;

$$\begin{array}{c} :\overset{\cdot\cdot}{\underset{\cdot\cdot}{O}}: \\ :\overset{\cdot\cdot}{O}:\overset{\cdot\cdot}{\underset{\cdot\cdot}{P}}:\overset{\cdot\cdot}{O}: \\ :\overset{\cdot\cdot}{\underset{\cdot\cdot}{O}}: \end{array}$$

(may also be seen with a double bond to one oxygen and 10 e$^-$ around P)

f NO_2^-; 18 valence e$^-$; $:\overset{\cdot\cdot}{O}::\overset{\cdot\cdot}{N}:\overset{\cdot\cdot}{\underset{\cdot\cdot}{O}}:$ *or* $:\overset{\cdot\cdot}{\underset{\cdot\cdot}{O}}:\overset{\cdot\cdot}{N}::\overset{\cdot\cdot}{O}:$

g CO; 10 valence e$^-$; $:C:::O:$

h C_8H_{12}; 44 valence e$^-$; many possible Lewis diagrams, each containing three double bonds *or* one triple bond and one double bond. Typical examples:

$$\begin{array}{c}\text{H}\quad\text{H}\quad\ \ \text{H}\ \ \text{H}\ \ \ \text{H}\ \text{H}\ \ \text{H}\ \text{H}\\ \text{H}:\overset{..}{\text{C}}:\text{C}::\text{C}:\text{C}::\text{C}:\text{C}::\text{C}:\overset{..}{\text{C}}:\text{H}\\ \text{H}\qquad\qquad\qquad\qquad\ \text{H}\end{array}$$

$$\begin{array}{c}\text{H}\qquad\qquad\quad\ \text{H}\ \text{H}\ \ \ \text{H}\ \text{H}\ \text{H}\\ \text{H}:\overset{..}{\text{C}}:\text{C}:::\text{C}:\text{C}:\text{C}::\text{C}:\text{C}:\overset{..}{\text{C}}:\text{H}\\ \text{H}\qquad\qquad\text{H}\qquad\qquad\text{H}\ \text{H}\end{array}$$

i SO_3; 24 valence e$^-$; $:\overset{..}{\underset{..}{\text{O}}}:\overset{..}{\underset{..}{\text{S}}}:\overset{..}{\underset{..}{\text{O}}}:$ *or* $:\overset{..}{\text{O}}::\overset{..}{\underset{..}{\text{S}}}:\overset{..}{\underset{..}{\text{O}}}:$ *or* $:\overset{..}{\underset{..}{\text{O}}}:\overset{..}{\underset{..}{\text{S}}}::\overset{..}{\text{O}}:$

$\qquad\qquad\qquad\qquad\quad:\overset{..}{\underset{..}{\text{O}}}:\qquad\qquad\quad:\overset{..}{\underset{..}{\text{O}}}:\qquad\qquad\quad:\overset{..}{\underset{..}{\text{O}}}:$

j HCN; 10 valence e$^-$; $\text{H}:\text{C}:::\overset{..}{\text{N}}:$

6.8   In the diagrams for NO_2^- and SO_3, we find that there is no one electron distribution that is clearly correct; we have in fact written several "resonance" forms. The actual electron distribution is somewhere between those shown and is delocalized for those two cases.

6.9   Compare the Lewis diagrams: $\text{H}:\text{C}:::\overset{..}{\text{N}}:$ and $\begin{array}{c}\text{H}\ \text{H}\\ \text{H}:\overset{..}{\text{C}}:\overset{..}{\text{N}}:\text{H}.\\ \text{H}\end{array}$

In HCN the carbon-nitrogen link is a triple bond. In CH_3NH_2 it is a single bond. The CN bond should be stronger in HCN; the two nuclei should be farther apart in CH_3NH_2.

6.10   *All* of the bonds in CH_3NH_2 (there are six bonds) are *sigma* bonds. Every single bond is a sigma bond. In HCN, the H—C and one C—N bond are *sigma* bonds; there are also two *pi* bonds between the C and the N, since a triple bond consists of one sigma and two pi bonds.

6.11   In a molecular orbital, the forces that create the orbital come from two or more atoms in a molecule; in an atomic orbital, we take into account only the forces in that single atom. In either case, the orbital is simply a possible "place" with a particular energy which can hold up to two electrons. If there are two electrons in a bonding molecular orbital, we have a covalent bond. If there are no electrons in the orbital, there is nothing holding the atoms together.

6.12   The following diagrams are typical for single-bonded Lewis pictures:

$\qquad\qquad\qquad\qquad\qquad\qquad\qquad\qquad\qquad:\overset{..}{\underset{..}{\text{X}}}:$

$:\overset{..}{\underset{..}{\text{X}}}:\overset{..}{\underset{..}{\text{X}}}:\qquad:\overset{..}{\underset{..}{\text{X}}}:\overset{..}{\underset{..}{\text{X}}}:\overset{..}{\underset{..}{\text{X}}}:\qquad:\overset{..}{\underset{..}{\text{X}}}:\overset{..}{\text{X}}:\overset{..}{\underset{..}{\text{X}}}:\qquad:\overset{..}{\underset{..}{\text{X}}}:\overset{}{\text{X}}:\overset{..}{\underset{..}{\text{X}}}:\qquad:\overset{..}{\underset{..}{\text{X}}}:\overset{..}{\underset{..}{\text{X}}}:\overset{..}{\underset{..}{\text{X}}}:\overset{..}{\underset{..}{\text{X}}}:\overset{..}{\underset{..}{\text{X}}}:$

$\qquad\qquad\qquad\qquad\qquad\qquad\qquad\quad:\overset{}{\underset{..}{\text{X}}}:\qquad\qquad\quad:\overset{}{\underset{..}{\text{X}}}:$

14 e$^-$ 20 e$^-$ 26 e$^-$ 32 e$^-$ 38 e$^-$

If the total of valence electrons reaches one of these numbers, there are no double or triple bonds.

6.13   [*See Figure 6–17 for various ways to draw a tetrahedron.*]

6.14   **a** ClCCH; 16 valence e$^-$; one triple bond; $:\overset{..}{\underset{..}{\text{Cl}}}:\text{C}:::\text{C}:\text{H}$; linear, 180°

b H_2S; 8 valence e$^-$; no multiple bonds; $\text{H}:\overset{..}{\underset{..}{\text{S}}}:\text{H}$; bent, 109°, like H_2O

c H_2CCH_2; 12 valence e$^-$; one double bond; $\begin{array}{c}\text{H}:\text{C}::\text{C}:\text{H}\\ \ \ \text{H}\quad\text{H}\end{array}$; planar triangular, 120°

d PH_3; 8 valence e$^-$; no multiple bond; $\begin{array}{c}\text{H}:\overset{..}{\text{P}}:\text{H}\\ \ \text{H}\end{array}$; pyramidal, 109°, like NH_3

e NO_3^-; 24 valence e^-; one double bond; $: \overset{..}{O} :: N : \overset{..}{O} :$;   planar triangular, 120°

$: \overset{..}{O} :$

(delocalized electrons are actually involved, but the final geometry is the same as that calculated using any of the three "resonance" forms)

6.15 Ethane, C_2H_6, is truly three-dimensional since the bonds around each of the two carbon atoms are directed to the corners of a tetrahedron; a planar molecule like $H_2C{=}O$ or a linear molecule like $HC{\equiv}CH$ has a shape that can accurately be shown in two dimensions.

6.16 **a** H_2CO is polar.   **b** C_4H_{10} is nonpolar.   **c** $HC{\equiv}CH$ is nonpolar. **d** H_2O is polar.   **e** $HC{\equiv}CF$ is polar.   **f** CF_4 is nonpolar, since its polar bonds cancel out.   **g** PH_3 is nonpolar, although shaped like NH_3, since $\Delta EN = 0$.   **h** $C_8H_{17}O$ is polar.   **i** CH_3I is polar.   **j** BeH_2 is nonpolar, since it is linear.

6.17 CH_2F_2 is polar. Use Figure 6-21, putting the two fluorines at the lower right and the two hydrogens at the top and left. The lower right is then δ^-, the upper left is clearly δ^+.

CHAPTER SIX QUESTIONS AND PROBLEMS

6.18 **a** N   **b** Na   **c** I

6.19 **a** $Na^+ F^-$ ionic   **b** $^{\delta+}C{-}F^{\delta-}$ polar covalent   **c** $H{-}S$ is essentially nonpolar by our cutoff point of $\Delta EN = 0.6$.

6.20 The $C{-}O$ bond is polar covalent and thus should be shorter than if that same bond were nonpolar. The length should be less than 1.225 Å.

6.21 The electronegativity of a metal must be quite low.

6.22 **a** A has a larger size.   **b** Z has the higher electronegativity.

6.23 in order of increasing size: Ca^{2+} Ca^+ Ca K

6.24 There is some charge separation; the electrons in the covalent bond are located closer to one atom than to the other, leaving one atom with slightly more negative charge around it than the other atom.

6.25 **a** ionic: Rb_2O, K_2S, CsF **b** all the rest

6.26 **a** NH_4^+ and NO_3^-; the $N{-}H$ bonds in NH_4^+ and the $N{-}O$ bonds in NO_3^- are covalent   **b** Cu^{2+} and HPO_4^{2-}; the $P{-}O$ and $O{-}H$ bonds in HPO_4^{2-} are covalent   **c** Al^{3+} and CH_3COO^-; the $C{-}H$ and $C{-}O$ bonds in acetate ion are covalent
The formulas of the three salts are NH_4NO_3, $CuHPO_4$, and $Al(CH_3COO)_3$.

6.27 **a** N_2; 10 valence e^-; $: N ::: N :$ (or $: N{\equiv}N :$ which is a structural formula of the type that may be used for any of these answers).

b ClO^-; 14 valence e^-; $: \overset{..}{\underset{..}{Cl}} : \overset{..}{\underset{..}{O}} :$

c $HOPO_3^{2-}$; 32 valence e^-; $H : \overset{..}{\underset{..}{O}} : \overset{\overset{\displaystyle : \overset{..}{O} :}{..}}{\underset{\underset{\displaystyle : \overset{..}{O} :}{..}}{P}} : \overset{..}{\underset{..}{O}} :$

d SiO_2; 16 valence e^-; $: \overset{..}{O} :: Si :: \overset{..}{O} :$

e ONONO; 28 valence e⁻; this is four short of the number (32) required to have only single bonds (see Self-Check 6.12), and so there are two double bonds (or one triple bond); *many* possible diagrams and resonance forms,

including $:\!\overset{..}{O}\!:\!\overset{..}{N}\!::\!\overset{..}{O}\!:\!\overset{..}{N}\!::\!\overset{..}{O}\!: \longleftrightarrow :\!\overset{..}{O}\!:\!\overset{..}{N}\!:\!\overset{..}{O}\!::\!\overset{..}{N}\!:\!\overset{..}{O}\!: \quad :\!\overset{..}{O}\!::\!\overset{..}{N}\!:\!\overset{..}{O}\!:\!\overset{..}{N}\!:\!\overset{..}{O}\!:$,

and so forth; a triple-bonded diagram may be correct, although unlikely to make a strong contribution to the actual electron distribution

f C_3H_8; 20 valence e⁻ (no multiple bonds);

$$
\begin{array}{ccc}
\text{H} & \text{H} & \text{H} \\
\text{H}:\text{C}:\text{C}:\text{C}:\text{H} & & \text{(propane)} \\
\text{H} & \text{H} & \text{H}
\end{array}
$$

g C_3H_4; 16 valence e⁻ (two double bonds or one triple bond);

$$
\begin{array}{cc}
\text{H} & \\
\text{H}:\text{C}:::\text{C}:\overset{..}{\text{C}}:\text{H} \quad \textit{or} \quad \text{H}:\text{C}::\text{C}::\text{C}:\text{H} \\
\text{H} & \text{H} \quad\quad \text{H}
\end{array}
$$

h $C_2H_5COCH_3$; 30 valence e⁻ (one double bond);

$$
\begin{array}{cccc}
\text{H} & \text{H} & & \text{H} \\
\text{H}:\text{C}:\text{C}:\text{C}:\text{C}:\text{H} \\
\text{H} & \text{H} & \overset{..}{\text{O}} & \text{H}
\end{array}
$$

6.28 Ethane, C_2H_6, has a longer C—C bond because it is a single bond; the bond between the carbons in ethene, C_2H_4, is a double bond.

6.29 There may be a single, double, or triple bond between two atoms; in each case, there is *one* sigma bond; zero, one, or two pi bonds may be formed.

6.30 In both the molecular orbital and atomic orbital descriptions of an electron, the electron probability "cloud" is located in space and associated with a particular energy level. Each can hold up to 2 electrons.

6.31 An atomic orbital description of an electron implies that the electron is attached to only *one* atom; delocalization means that the electron is associated with more than one atom.

6.32 A triple bond contains one sigma and two pi bonds.

6.33 SO_2; 18 valence e⁻ (one double bond); $:\!\overset{..}{O}\!::\!\overset{..}{S}\!:\!\overset{..}{O}\!: \longleftrightarrow :\!\overset{..}{O}\!:\!\overset{..}{S}\!::\!\overset{..}{O}\!:$ Each

S—O bond is between a single bond and a double bond and contains roughly three electrons; the pi-bonding electrons are delocalized.

6.34 We need an anion that contains three octets with only 18 valence electrons. One possibility is NO_2^- (nitrite anion). Others can perhaps be found.

$$
\left[:\!\overset{..}{O}\!::\!\overset{..}{N}\!:\!\overset{..}{O}\!:\right]^- \longleftrightarrow \left[:\!\overset{..}{O}\!:\!\overset{..}{N}\!::\!\overset{..}{O}\!:\right]^- \quad \text{(nitrite)}
$$

6.35 The environment of delocalized electrons around every metal nucleus is the same; if we deform (push) the metal atoms, we do not change the charges on the surroundings. An ion in an ionic solid is held in place by attractions from oppositely charged ions; if we push it too far, it starts to be repelled by ions with the same charge as its own; this shatters the crystal.

6.36 [*See Figure 6–17*]

6.37 **a** SF_2; 20 e⁻; $:\!\overset{..}{F}\!:\!\overset{..}{S}\!:\!\overset{..}{F}\!:$ bent, 109°, like H_2O

b $CHBr_3$; 26 e⁻;

$$
\begin{array}{c}
\text{H} \\
:\!\overset{..}{\text{Br}}\!:\text{C}:\!\overset{..}{\text{Br}}\!: \\
:\!\overset{..}{\text{Br}}\!:
\end{array}
$$
tetrahedral, 109°, like CH_4

c CaH_2; 4 e$^-$; H:Ca:H linear, 180°

d H_2CNH; 12 e$^-$; H:C::N̈:H triangular planar, 120°
 H

e $SO_4{}^{2-}$; 32 e$^-$; :Ö:
 :Ö:S:Ö: tetrahedral, 109°, like CH_4
 :Ö:

f F_2CO; 24 e$^-$ (one double bond); :F̈:
 :F̈:C::Ö: triangular planar, 120°

g BF_3; 24 e$^-$; :F̈:
 :F̈:B:F̈: triangular planar, 120°

h NSF; 18 e$^-$; :N̈::S:F̈: bent, 120°, like SO_2

6.38 Each of the molecules (CH_4, NH_3, H_2O) has a central atom surrounded by four electron pairs, which repel each other and get as far apart as possible. These electron pairs are then arranged tetrahedrally around each central atom. When any two electron pairs are involved in bonding, the bond angle is about 109°.

6.39 **a** ClO_2; 19 e$^-$, a bit short of an octet around the central atom. With seven electrons, the central atom will act much as though it had three pairs around it, thus the bond angles are close to 120°, although the extra electron repels all of the pairs and makes the angle slightly smaller. **b** FNNF; 24 e$^-$ (one double bond); :F̈:N̈::N̈:F̈: each nitrogen acts as though it had three electron pairs around it; thus triangular planar, 120° **c** CH_3Br; structure similar to that shown in Question 6.37b; tetrahedral, 109°

6.40 **a** SF_2 (bent) polar **b** $CHBr_3$ (tetrahedral) polar **c** CaH_2 (linear) non-polar **d** H_2CNH (triangular) polar **e** $SO_4{}^{2-}$ (tetrahedral) nonpolar (dipoles cancel) **f** F_2CO (triangular) polar **g** BF_3 (triangular) nonpolar **h** NSF (bent) polar

6.41 **a** NCO^-; 16 e$^-$; :N:::C:Ö: linear, 180°, polar

b HNNN; 16 e$^-$; H:N̈::N::N̈: linear, 180°, polar

c $(NC)_2CC(CN)_2$; 44 e$^-$; :N:::C:C::C:C:::N: N—C—C bond angles 180°
 C C
 ⋮⋮ ⋮⋮ C—C—C bond angles 120°
 N N

6.42 This corresponds to the situation in Question 6.39a. The $CH_3\cdot$ fragment should be triangular planar.

CHAPTER SEVEN SELF-CHECKS

7.1 **a** heptane, C_7H_{16};
 H H H H H H H
H—C—C—C—C—C—C—C—H
 H H H H H H H

b decane, $C_{10}H_{22}$;

$$H-\overset{\overset{\displaystyle H}{|}}{\underset{\underset{\displaystyle H}{|}}{C}}-\overset{\overset{\displaystyle H}{|}}{\underset{\underset{\displaystyle H}{|}}{C}}-\overset{\overset{\displaystyle H}{|}}{\underset{\underset{\displaystyle H}{|}}{C}}-\overset{\overset{\displaystyle H}{|}}{\underset{\underset{\displaystyle H}{|}}{C}}-\overset{\overset{\displaystyle H}{|}}{\underset{\underset{\displaystyle H}{|}}{C}}-\overset{\overset{\displaystyle H}{|}}{\underset{\underset{\displaystyle H}{|}}{C}}-\overset{\overset{\displaystyle H}{|}}{\underset{\underset{\displaystyle H}{|}}{C}}-\overset{\overset{\displaystyle H}{|}}{\underset{\underset{\displaystyle H}{|}}{C}}-\overset{\overset{\displaystyle H}{|}}{\underset{\underset{\displaystyle H}{|}}{C}}-\overset{\overset{\displaystyle H}{|}}{\underset{\underset{\displaystyle H}{|}}{C}}-H$$

c 3-ethyl-4,4-dimethyloctane, $C_{12}H_{26}$;

d 3-methylpentane
e 3-ethyl-2-methylpentane
f 4-ethyloctane

7.2 First name each compound, then decide which are identical.   **a** 3-methylhexane   **b** 3,3-dimethylpentane   **c** 2-methylhexane   **d** 2,2,3-trimethylbutane   None are identical, since no two have the same name. All are isomers with the molecular formula C_7H_{16}.

7.3   **a** 1-hexene   **b** 4-methyl-1-pentene   **c** 4-methyl-1-hexyne   **d** 4-nonyne

7.4   **a** Six different compounds with molecular formula C_5H_{10} and one double bond:

1-pentene $H_2C{=}CHCH_2CH_2CH_3$

trans-2-pentene

cis-2-pentene

3-methyl-1-butene $H_2C{=}CHCHCH_3$
$\quad\quad\quad\quad\quad\quad\quad\quad\quad\quad\quad\quad |$
$\quad\quad\quad\quad\quad\quad\quad\quad\quad\quad\quad CH_3$

2-methyl-1-butene $H_2C{=}CCH_2CH_3$
$\quad\quad\quad\quad\quad\quad\quad\quad\quad\quad\quad\quad |$
$\quad\quad\quad\quad\quad\quad\quad\quad\quad\quad CH_3$

2-methyl-2-butene $H_3CC{=}CHCH_3$
$\quad\quad\quad\quad\quad\quad\quad\quad\quad |$
$\quad\quad\quad\quad\quad\quad\quad\quad CH_3$

b *trans*-3-hexene

7.5 Only (b) would have *cis* and *trans* isomers; (a) has identical (methyl) groups on one of the two carbons of the double bond; (c) similarly has identical hydrogens on one of those carbons.

7.6 **a** $(CH_3)_2CHCH{-}CH_3$ **b** $(CH_3)_2C{-}CH_2CH_2CH_3$ **c** $H_3C{-}CHCl$
$\quad\quad\quad\quad\quad\quad\quad\quad |$ $\quad\quad\quad\quad\quad\quad\quad\quad\quad\quad\quad |$ $\quad\quad\quad\quad\quad\quad\quad |$
$\quad\quad\quad\quad\quad\quad\quad\quad F$ $\quad\quad\quad\quad\quad\quad\quad\quad\quad\quad Cl$ $\quad\quad\quad\quad\quad\quad Cl$

7.7   Only (b) would have geometrical isomers; for (a) and (c) two identical groups
are on carbon 1 of the ring.

CHAPTER SEVEN QUESTIONS AND PROBLEMS

7.8   **a** heptane   **b** ethyl   **c** 2-methylhexane   **d** 2,4-dimethylhexane
e 2,2-dimethylbutane   **f** 3-ethyl-pentane

7.9   **a**

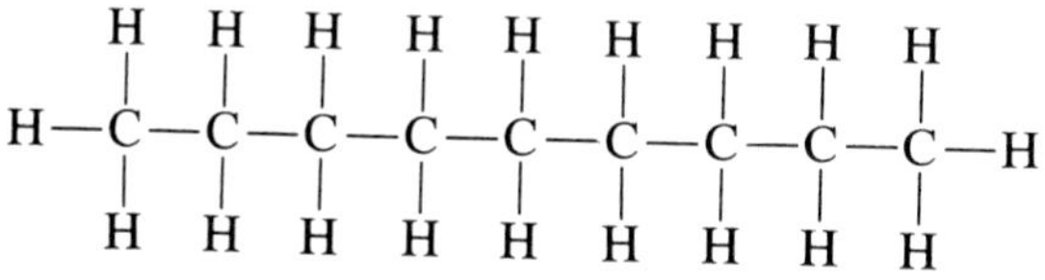

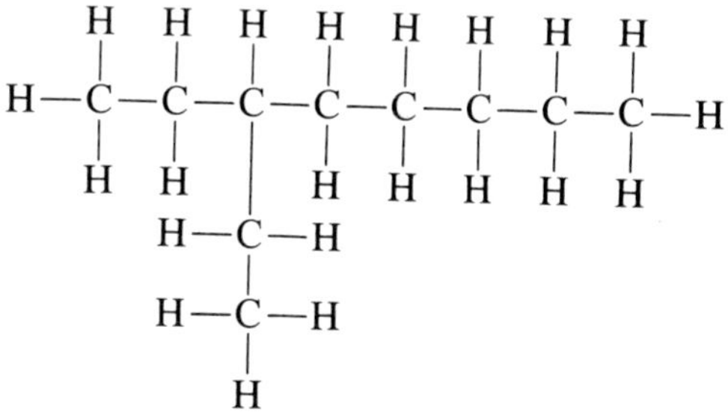

b $CH_3CH_2CH_2CH_2—$

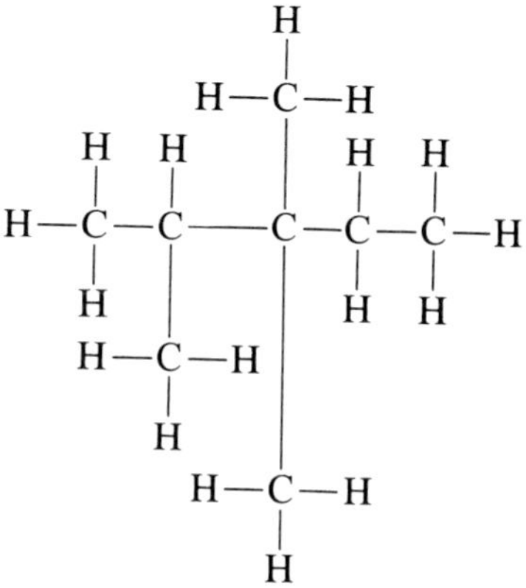

c

d

e

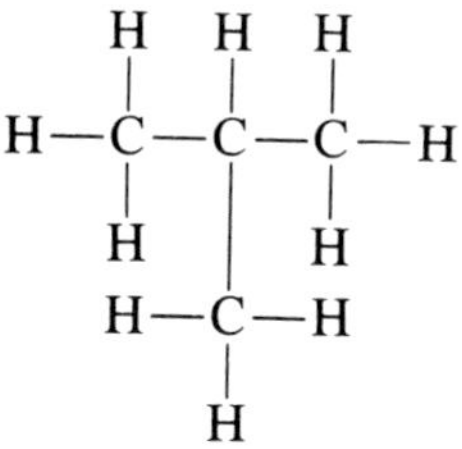

7.10   **a** identical compounds   **b** identical compounds

7.11

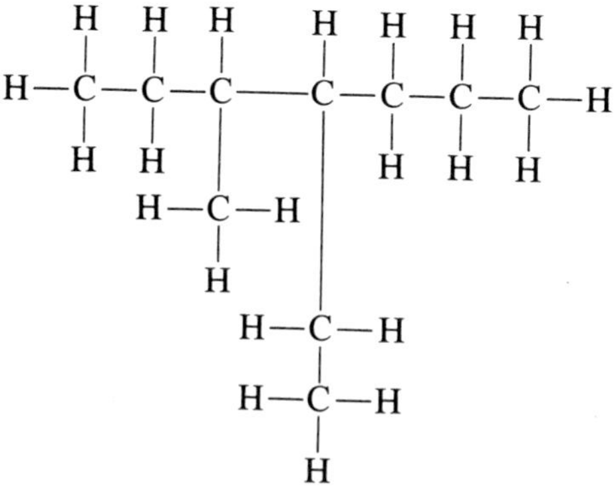

it obeys the octet rule; $C_{10}H_{22}$; 142 g/mole

7.12   a 1-hexene   **b** 3-ethyl-3-hexene   **c** 3-hexyne

7.13   a

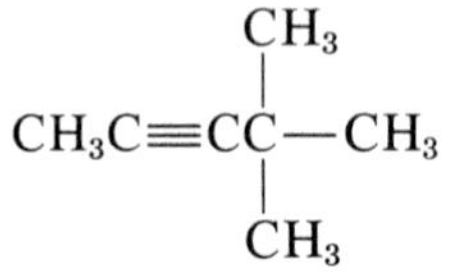

$$CH_3C{\equiv}CC{-}CH_3$$

with CH_3 above and CH_3 below the fourth carbon

b

CH_3 and H on left/top, $C{=}C$, H and CH_2CH_3 on bottom/right

7.14

$CH_3CH_2CH_2CH_2$ and H on top, $C{=}C$, H and CH_2CH_3 on bottom   *trans*-3-octene

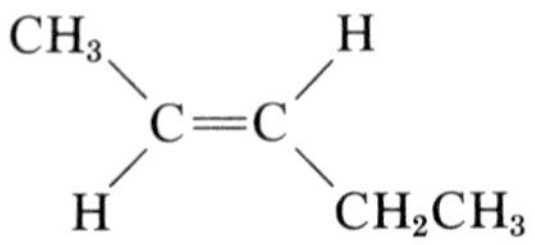

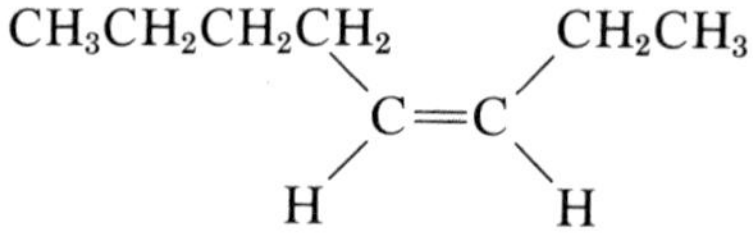

$CH_3CH_2CH_2CH_2$ and CH_2CH_3 on top, $C{=}C$, H and H on bottom   *cis*-3-octene

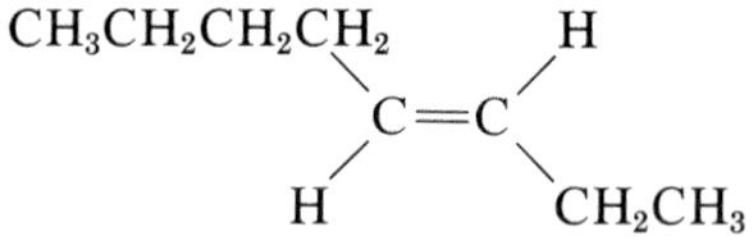

7.15

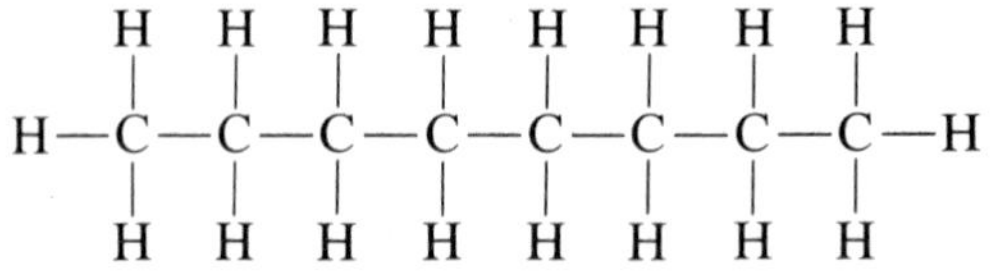

$$H{-}C{-}C{-}C{-}C{-}C{-}C{-}C{-}C{-}H$$

with H above and below each carbon (8 carbons)   octane

7.16   a

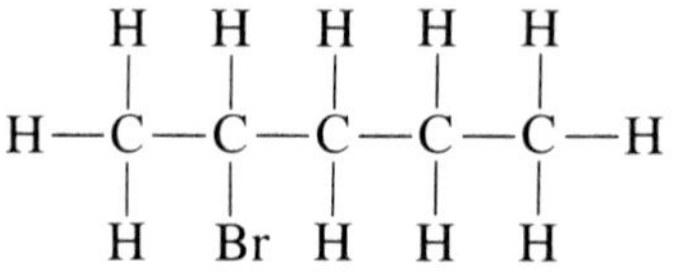

$$H{-}C{-}C{-}C{-}C{-}C{-}H$$

with H, H, H, H, H on top and H, Br, H, H, H on bottom

b

$$H{-}C{-}C{-}C{-}H$$

with H, F, H on top; H, H on bottom; and H$-$C$-$H below the middle carbon with H beneath

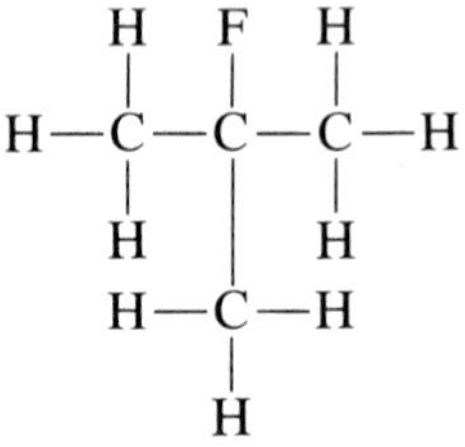

c

$$H{-}C{-}C{-}C{-}C{-}H$$

with H, H, Br, H on top; H, H, H on bottom; and H$-$C$-$H below the third carbon with H beneath

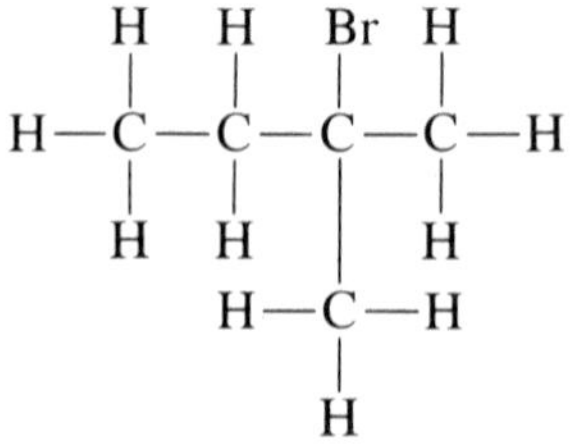

7.17   a

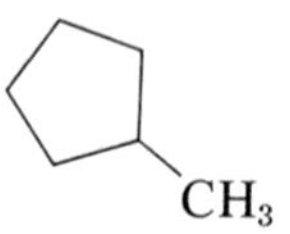

cyclopentane ring with CH_3

b

cyclopropane ring with CH_3 and CH_3

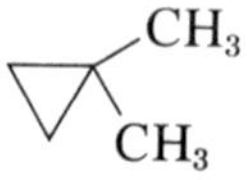

7.18   a ethylcyclopropane   **b** *cis*-1,2-dimethylcyclopentane

7.19

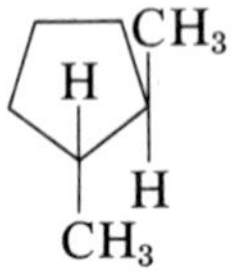

cyclopentane ring with CH_3, H, H, CH_3

7.20

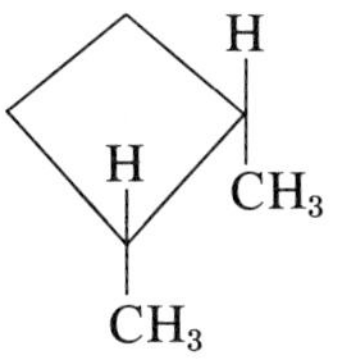

cis-1,2-dimethylcyclobutane

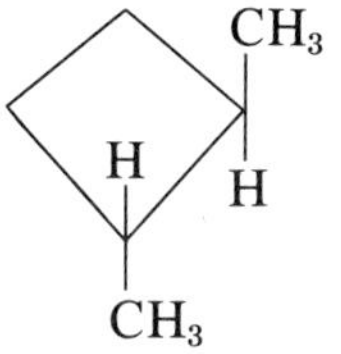

trans-1,2-dimethylcyclobutane

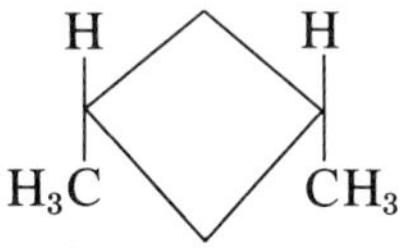

cis-1,3-dimethylcyclobutane

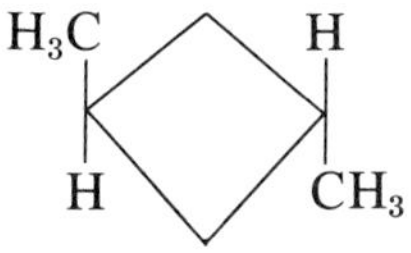

trans-1,3-dimethylcyclobutane

CHAPTER EIGHT SELF-CHECKS

8.1 Remember that the oxidation states must add up to the charge on the species.   **a** Mn: $+4$, O: -2 **b** Fe: $+3$, S: $+6$, O: -2 **c** Pb: $+4$, O: -2 **d** C: $+4$, O: -2 **e** Cl: $+1$, O: -2 **f** P: $+3$, O: -2 **g** S: $+4$, O: -2 **h** H: $+1$, P: $+5$, O: -2 **i** Cl: $+5$, O: -2 **j** Cl: $+7$, O: -2

8.2 $2\,Cl^- \rightarrow Cl_2$; oxidation states: -1 to 0; Cl is oxidized (loses electrons) $MnO_2 \rightarrow Mn^{2+}$; oxidation states $+4$ to $+2$ for Mn, which is reduced (gains electrons; Cl^- is the reducing agent, since it reduces MnO_2 to Mn^{2+}; MnO_2 is the oxidizing agent, since it oxidizes Cl^- to Cl_2

8.3 Yes, it is a redox reaction since two hydrogens are lost from 1-butanol (the reduced form) to yield $CH_3CH_2CH_2CHO$, 1-butanal (the oxidized form).

8.4 Yes, it is a redox reaction since CrO_3 (the oxidizer, or oxidizing agent) oxidizes menthol (the reduced form) to menthone (the oxidized form); the reducer, or reducing agent, is menthol; the oxidation level has been increased (more carbon-oxygen bonds).

8.5 Yes, it is a redox reaction, with 2-butanone as oxidizer and $NaBH_4$ as reducer; 2-butanone (oxidized form) has been reduced to 2-butanol; oxidation level has been decreased; hydrogens have been added; the number of carbon-oxygen bonds has gone down.

CHAPTER EIGHT QUESTIONS AND PROBLEMS

8.6 reduction (gain of electrons)   **8.8** reduction

8.7 reduction (gain of electrons)   **8.9** oxidation

8.10 Electrons are transferred from the atoms being oxidized to the atoms being reduced.

8.11   Reduction is the gain of electrons.

8.12   Oxidation; the number of carbon-oxygen bonds has increased.

8.13   **a** Cl: -1 in $AlCl_3$ **b** Cl: -1 in Cl^- **c** Cl: $+7$ in $HClO_4$

8.14   Yes, Cl goes from -1 in NaCl to $+3$ in $NaClO_2$ and is thus oxidized.

8.15   N: $+3$ **8.16**   Chlorine is oxidized, manganese is reduced.

8.17   Oxidation is an increase in oxidation state to a more positive number.

8.18   oxidation, two C—O bonds instead of one; fewer C—H bonds

8.19   reduction, one C—O bond instead of two; more C—H bonds

8.20   Oxidation occurs if the number of C—O bonds increases from reactants to products; reduction occurs if the number of C—O bonds decreases.

8.21   Reduction (fewer C—O bonds); 2-butanone (oxidized form) to 2-butanol (reduced form).

8.22   Suggested answers: **a** chromic oxide, chromium(VI) oxide, CrO_3
b potassium permanganate, MnO_4^-, $KMnO_4$ **c** potassium dichromate, $Cr_2O_7^{2-}$, $K_2Cr_2O_7$

8.23   An oxidizer (or oxidizing agent) *removes* electrons from another reactant.

8.24 CrO_3 is the oxidizer; CH_3CH_2CHO is the reducer.

8.25 $NaBH_4$ is the reducer.

8.26   In any air combustion (burning), O_2 gas is the oxidizer.

8.27   Hydrogen (H_2) gas is the reducer.

8.28   No; an alcohol, with one C—O bond, is already at a higher oxidation level than the alkane.

8.29   An aldehyde with *two* C—O bonds is oxidized to a carboxylic acid with *three* C—O bonds.

8.30   An alkane with *no* C—O bond is oxidized to an alcohol with *one* C—O bond.

8.31   yes; from one C—O bond to three C—O bonds; lower to higher oxidation level

8.32   Oxidation; oxidizer is $KMnO_4$; alcohol group has gone from one C—O bond to three (a change of two levels); aldehyde group has gone from two C—O bonds to three (a change of one level).

CHAPTER NINE SELF-CHECKS

9.1   **a** Choose one alcohol and one ether for $C_4H_{10}O$, which has no double bonds; alcohols:

ethers:

$$H-\underset{\underset{H}{|}}{\overset{\overset{H}{|}}{C}}-\underset{\underset{H}{|}}{\overset{\overset{H}{|}}{C}}-O-\underset{\underset{H}{|}}{\overset{\overset{H}{|}}{C}}-\underset{\underset{H}{|}}{\overset{\overset{H}{|}}{C}}-H \qquad H-\underset{\underset{H}{|}}{\overset{\overset{H}{|}}{C}}-\underset{\underset{H}{|}}{\overset{\overset{H}{|}}{C}}-\underset{\underset{H}{|}}{\overset{\overset{H}{|}}{C}}-O-\underset{\underset{H}{|}}{\overset{\overset{H}{|}}{C}}-H$$

$$H-\underset{\underset{H}{|}}{\overset{\overset{H}{|}}{C}}-\underset{\underset{\underset{H}{|}}{\overset{\overset{H}{|}}{C}}-\underset{H}{\overset{|}{H}}}{\overset{\overset{H}{|}}{C}}-O-\underset{\underset{H}{|}}{\overset{\overset{H}{|}}{C}}-H$$

b similarly for C_3H_8O, which has no double bonds; ether:

$$H-\underset{\underset{H}{|}}{\overset{\overset{H}{|}}{C}}-\underset{\underset{H}{|}}{\overset{\overset{H}{|}}{C}}-O-\underset{\underset{H}{|}}{\overset{\overset{H}{|}}{C}}-H$$

alcohols:

$$H-\underset{\underset{H}{|}}{\overset{\overset{H}{|}}{C}}-\underset{\underset{O-H}{|}}{\overset{\overset{H}{|}}{C}}-\underset{\underset{H}{|}}{\overset{\overset{H}{|}}{C}}-H \qquad or \qquad H-\underset{\underset{H}{|}}{\overset{\overset{H}{|}}{C}}-\underset{\underset{H}{|}}{\overset{\overset{H}{|}}{C}}-\underset{\underset{H}{|}}{\overset{\overset{H}{|}}{C}}-O-H$$

c $C_2H_4O_2$ has two oxygens, one double bond; various possibilities:

$$H-\underset{\underset{H}{|}\;\overset{}{O}}{\overset{\overset{H}{|}}{C}}-C-O-H \qquad H-C-O-\underset{\underset{H}{|}}{\overset{\overset{H}{|}}{C}}-H \qquad H-\underset{\underset{O}{\|}}{\overset{\overset{H}{|}}{C}}-\underset{\underset{H}{|}}{\overset{\overset{H}{|}}{C}}-O-H \qquad H-O-\underset{\underset{H}{|}}{\overset{\overset{H}{|}}{C}}=\underset{\underset{H}{|}}{\overset{\overset{H}{|}}{C}}-O-H$$

acetic acid   methyl formate   glycolaldehyde   (unstable—doesn't exist)

9.2   The isomer must have two double bonds (thus the same number of pi bonds):

$$H-\underset{H}{\overset{H}{C}}=\underset{H}{\overset{H}{C}}-\underset{H}{\overset{H}{C}}=\underset{H}{\overset{H}{C}}-H \qquad or \qquad H-\overset{H}{C}=C=\underset{H}{\overset{H}{C}}-\underset{\underset{H}{|}}{\overset{\overset{H}{|}}{C}}-H$$

9.3   **a** $-\overset{\overset{H}{|}}{C}=O$ aldehyde

b $-\overset{|}{\underset{|}{C}}-O-\overset{|}{\underset{|}{C}}-$ ether   and $-\overset{|}{\underset{|}{C}}-Br$ alkyl halide

c $-C\equiv C-$ alkyne   and $-\overset{|}{\underset{|}{C}}-O-H$ alcohol   and $-\overset{\overset{O}{\|}}{C}-O-H$ carboxylic acid

d $-\overset{|}{C}=\overset{|}{C}-$ alkene   and $-\overset{\overset{O}{\|}}{C}-O-H$ carboxylic acid

e $-\overset{|}{\underset{|}{C}}-\overset{|}{\underset{\|}{C}}-\overset{|}{\underset{|}{C}}-$ ketone and $-\overset{|}{\underset{|}{C}}-\overset{|}{\underset{\|}{C}}-H$ aldehyde

f $-\overset{|}{\underset{|}{C}}-O-H$ alcohol   and $-\overset{|}{\underset{|}{C}}-\overset{O}{\overset{\|}{C}}-H$ aldehyde

9.4   **a** 3-methyl-2-pentanol   **b** 3-methyl-1-pentanol   **c** 2-methyl-2-pentanol

9.5   **a** secondary (two other carbons bonded to the carbon that carries the hydroxyl group)   **b** primary   **c** tertiary

9.6   **a** $CH_3CH_2\overset{OH}{\overset{|}{CH}}CHCH_3$ + oxidizer $\longrightarrow$ $CH_3CH_2\overset{}{\underset{|}{CH}}-\overset{O}{\overset{\|}{C}}CH_3$ a ketone

with CH_3 below each.

b $CH_3CH_2\overset{}{\underset{|}{CH}}CH_2CH_2OH$ + oxidizer $\longrightarrow$

with CH_3 below.

$CH_3CH_2\overset{}{\underset{|}{CH}}CH_2\overset{}{\underset{|}{C}}{=}O$ an aldehyde

with CH_3 and H below.

c tertiary alcohol + oxidizer $\rightarrow$ no reaction

9.7   **a** $CH_3CH_2CH_2CH_2OH$ (alcohol)

b $(CH_3)_2\overset{}{\underset{|}{C}}CH_3$ (tertiary alcohol)

with OH below.

c $(CH_3)_3\overset{H}{\overset{|}{C}}C{=}O$ (aldehyde)

d $(CH_3CH_2)_2C{=}O$ (ketone)

9.8   **a** 3-ethyl-5-methylheptanal   **b** 2,7-dimethyl-4-octanone

9.9   **a** $(CH_3)_2CHCH_2\overset{O}{\overset{\|}{CH}}$ **b** $CH_3\overset{}{\underset{\|}{C}}CH_2C(CH_3)_3$ **c** $CH_3CHCH(CH_3)_2$

with O below b's carbonyl, and $\overset{CH}{\underset{O}{}}$ group with $CH{=}O$ at c.

9.10 CH_3CH_2OH

9.11   **a** 3-methylbutanoic acid   **b** 2-methylbutanoic acid
   c 4,4-dimethylpentanoic acid

9.12   **a** $H-\overset{O}{\overset{\|}{C}}-ONa$ **b** $CH_3CH_2\overset{O}{\overset{\|}{C}}-H$ **c** CH_3CH_2OH

9.13   **a** methylpropanoate   **b** ethylpropanoate

9.14   **a** CH_3COONa and CH_3CH_2OH **b** $HCOONa$ and CH_3OH

CHAPTER NINE QUESTIONS AND PROBLEMS

9.15 $CH_3CH_2CH_2OH$ and $CH_3CHOHCH_3$

9.16
$$H_2C—CH_2$$
$$|\quad\quad|$$
$$H_2C—CH_2$$

9.17 $HC\equiv CCH_2CH_3$ and $CH_3C\equiv CCH_3$ **9.18** alkene and aldehyde

9.19 isomers of $C_5H_{10}O$ (one double bond) many possibilities, such as:

$$CH_3CH_2CH_2CH_2\overset{\overset{\textstyle H}{|}}{C}=O \quad\text{(aldehyde)};\quad CH_3CH_2CH_2\overset{\overset{\textstyle O}{\|}}{C}CH_3 \quad\text{(ketone)};$$

$CH_3CH_2\overset{\overset{\textstyle O}{\|}}{C}CH_2CH_3$ (ketone); $CH_3CH=CHCH_2CH_2OH$ (alkene and alcohol);
$CH_3CH_2CH=CHCH_2OH$ (alkene and alcohol); $CH_2=CHCH_2CH_2CH_2OH$
(alkene and alcohol); $CH_3CH=CH—OCH_2CH_3$ (alkene and ether);
$CH_2=CHCH_2OCH_2CH_3$ (alkene and ether); $CH_3CH=CHCH_2OCH_3$ (alkene
and ether);

(aldehyde); $(CH_3)_2CH\overset{\overset{\textstyle O}{\|}}{C}CH_3$ (ketone); $H_2C=CCH_2CH_2OH$ (alkene and
$$\quad\quad\quad\quad\quad\quad\quad\quad\quad\quad\quad\quad\quad\quad\quad\quad\quad\quad\quad\quad | $$
$$\quad\quad\quad\quad\quad\quad\quad\quad\quad\quad\quad\quad\quad\quad\quad\quad\quad\quad\quad CH_3$$
alcohol); $(CH_3)_3CCHO$ (aldehyde); $CH_3CH_2CH(CH_3)CHO$ (aldehyde);
$H_2C=C(CH_3)OCH_2CH_3$ (alkene and ether)

9.20 5-methyl-2-hexanol

9.21 $CH_3CHCH_2CH_2CH_2CH_3$
$$\quad\quad\quad\quad | $$
$$\quad\quad\quad\quad OH$$

9.22 4-ethyl-3-hexanol

9.23 9.20: secondary
9.22: secondary

9.24 $CH_3CH_2CH_2OH$

9.25 $CH_3CH_2CHCH_2CH_3$
$$\quad\quad\quad\quad | $$
$$\quad\quad\quad\quad OH$$

9.26 $CH_3CH_2CH_2CH_2OH$ 1-butanol (primary)

$CH_3CH_2CHCH_3$ 2-butanol (secondary)
$$\quad\quad | $$
$$\quad\quad OH$$

$CH_3—CHCH_2OH$ 2-methyl-1-propanol (primary)
$$\quad\quad\quad\quad | $$
$$\quad\quad\quad\quad CH_3$$

$$\quad\quad\quad\quad CH_3$$
$$\quad\quad\quad\quad | $$
$CH_3—C—OH$ 2-methyl-2-propanol (tertiary)
$$\quad\quad\quad\quad | $$
$$\quad\quad\quad\quad CH_3$$

9.27 $CH_3CH_2\overset{\overset{\textstyle O}{\|}}{C}CH_3$

9.28 aldehyde

9.29 3-hexanone

9.30 2-methylpentanal

9.31 CH_3CHCH_2OH
$\ \ \ \ \underset{\displaystyle CH_3}{|}$

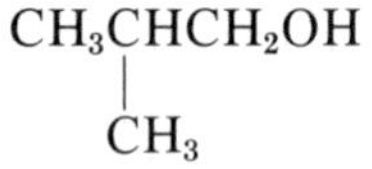

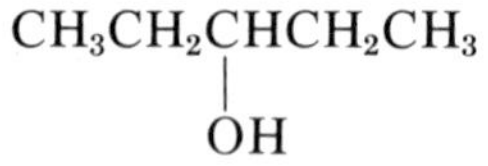

9.32 $CH_3CH_2CHCH_2CH_3$
$\ \ \ \ \ \ \ \ \ \ \underset{\displaystyle OH}{|}$

9.33 $CH_3CH{=}CHCH_3 + H_2O \xrightarrow{\ H^+\ } CH_3\underset{\displaystyle \underset{|}{H}}{\overset{\displaystyle \overset{|}{OH}}{C}}CH_2CH_3 \xrightarrow{\ CrO_3\ }$

$CH_3\overset{\displaystyle O}{\overset{\displaystyle \|}{C}}CH_2CH_3 \xrightarrow[\text{2) hydrolysis}]{\text{1) } CH_3MgI} CH_3{-}\underset{\displaystyle \underset{|}{CH_3}}{\overset{\displaystyle \overset{|}{OH}}{C}}CH_2CH_3$

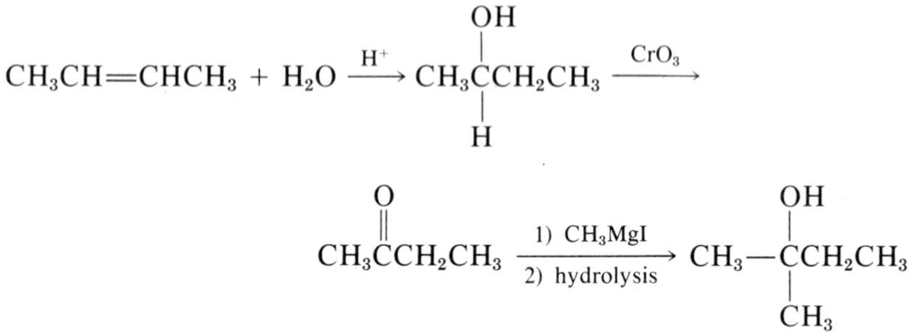

9.34 pentanoic acid

9.35 $CH_3CH_2OH, CH_3COOH, HCHO, CH_3\overset{\displaystyle O}{\overset{\displaystyle \|}{C}}CH_3$

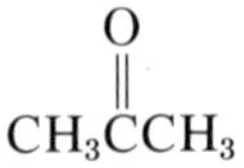

9.36 $H{-}\underset{\displaystyle \underset{|}{H}}{\overset{\displaystyle \overset{|}{H}}{C}}{-}\overset{\displaystyle O}{\overset{\displaystyle \|}{C}}{-}ONa$

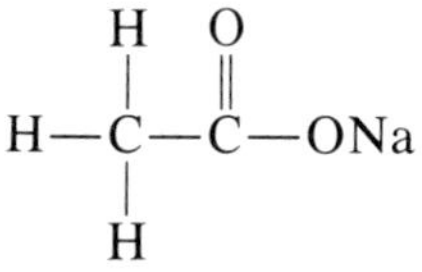

9.37 sodium ethanoate

9.38 methyl butanoate

9.39 $H{-}\overset{\displaystyle O}{\overset{\displaystyle \|}{C}}{-}O{-}CH_3$

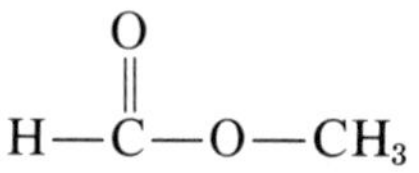

9.40 $CH_3CH_2CO_2Na$ and CH_3OH

9.41 some possibilities: CH_3CH_2OH (alcoholic beverages); $HOCH_2CH_2OH$ (anti-freeze); CH_3OH (commercial uses); $(CH_3)_2CHOH$ (rubbing alcohol); CH_2OH-$CHOHCH_2OH$ (glycerol)

CHAPTER TEN SELF-CHECKS

10.1 The four measurable properties are temperature, volume, amount, and pressure.

10.2 [See summary; compare with your answer.]

10.3 If a gas has a definite volume, it must be inside a container of some kind; the wall is the inner surface of that container that "holds in" the gas molecules.

10.4 Gas particles strike the wall and then bounce back; the force of these collisions provides the pressure.

10.5 No.

10.6 A gas is mostly empty space.

10.7 $105.0°F = 40.6°C$

10.8 $82°C = 180°F = 355$ K; no

10.9 293 K $= 20°C = 68°F$, much lower than normal body temperature of $37°C = 98.6°F$

10.10 Temperature is a measure of the average energy of motion; to measure a meaningful temperature, there must be enough molecules at equilibrium to maintain a fixed "average" energy of motion—this is not possible in space.

10.11 $2.00 \text{ L} \times 273 \text{ K}/293 \text{ K} = 1.86 \text{ L}$; as the temperature goes down, so does the volume

10.12 $2.00 \text{ torr} \times 1 \text{ atm}/760 \text{ torr} = 0.00263 \text{ atm}$

10.13 $736 \text{ mm Hg} = 736 \text{ torr} \times \dfrac{1 \text{ atm}}{760 \text{ torr}} = 0.968 \text{ atm}$

10.14 $0.151 \text{ atm} \times 760 \text{ mm Hg/atm} = 115 \text{ mm Hg}$

10.15 $P_2/P_1 = 25.0/16.0 = 1.56$; so $T_2/T_1 = 1.56 = T_2/293 \text{ K}$; $T_2 = 458 \text{ K} = 185°C$ or $457 \text{ K} = 184°C$

10.16 The total pressure must be just about atmospheric pressure (actually, slightly higher); approximately $760 = 115 \text{ torr} + P$, $P = $ about 645 torr

10.17 $P_2/P_1 = 1.00/5.00 = 0.200$; then $V_1/V_2 = 0.200 = 2.50 \text{ mL}/V_2$; $V_2 = 12.5 \text{ mL}$

10.18 $P = (1.00 \text{ atm}) (1000/3500) = 0.286 \text{ atm}$

10.19 $PV = nRT$, so $n = PV/RT = (749 \text{ torr}) (0.250 \text{ L})/(62.4) (398 \text{ K}) = 0.00754$ mole; $1.67 \text{ g}/0.00754 \text{ mole} = 221 \text{ g/mole}$

10.20 No, the liquid mercury would splatter out into the weightless environment of the cabin; a barometer will work only if the weight of mercury at sea level is being compared with the weight of an air column of the atmosphere.

10.21 No.

10.22 The air inside the tire exerts pressure on the walls as a result of collisions; we must do work to push more molecules into the tire so that there will be more collisions, thus more pressure.

10.23 When work is done, some of the energy lost is converted to heat.

10.24 **a** The same number, 3.1×10^{21} molecules of SO_2 or atoms of He   **b** 3.1×10^{21} molecules is 5.1×10^{-3} mole $= n$. $V = 0.100 \text{ L}$; $P = 1.00 \text{ atm}$; $R = 0.0821 \text{ L-atm/mole-K}$. $PV = nRT$; $T = PV/nR = 237 \text{ K} = -36°C$.

10.25 **a** $0.335 \text{ mole } Cl_2 \times 22.4 \text{ L ideal gas at STP/mole} = 7.50 \text{ liters } Cl_2$
b $100 \text{ g } CO_2 \times 1 \text{ mole}/44.0 \text{ g} \times 22.4 \text{ L/mole} = 50.9 \text{ liters } CO_2$ **c** $H_2O_{(\ell)}$ is *not* an ideal gas! The density of liquid water is very close to 1.00 g/mL, so 10.0 g liquid water occupy *10.0 mL* at 0°C.   **d** You need the balanced equation: $N_2 + 3 H_2 \rightarrow 2 NH_3$; 2.00 liters of H_2 will react with 0.67 liter of N_2 to give 1.33 liters of NH_3, with 3.33 liters of N_2 left over as excess reactant; the total volume would then be $3.33 \text{ L } N_2 + 1.33 \text{ L } NH_3 = 4.66$ liters of gas. Limiting-reagent problems are discussed in Section 5.4.

10.26 Oxygen represents 21% of air molecules, or roughly 0.21 atm.

10.27 nitrogen (N_2) and argon (Ar); *see Table 10-2;* no effect on the body

10.28 [*See text to check answers.*]

10.29 *Lead* particles interfere with hemoglobin production; *CO* reduces the efficiency of the hemoglobin in the blood stream; *oxides* of nitrogen and sulfur form strong acids when they dissolve in water and damage lung tissue; *ozone* also causes direct damage; *particles* clog the lungs and interfere with gas exchange; some *hydrocarbons* in smoke can cause lung cancer.

10.30 O_2 molecule breathed in, enters alveoli of lungs, passes into blood stream, adsorbed onto hemoglobin molecule of a red blood cell; no

10.31 Even after you breathe out, the lungs retain some air (residual volume, *see Figure 10-15*), which can be used to create extra pressure to force an object out of the throat.

CHAPTER TEN QUESTIONS AND PROBLEMS

10.32 **a** very small; negligible in comparison with the total volume   **b** Collisions are assumed to be *elastic*, with no energy lost as heat.   **c** Gases are mostly empty space.

10.33 volume and pressure

10.34 Gas molecules are in constant motion, colliding with each other and with the walls of the container; if solid particles are present in smoke, collisions with the gas molecules knock them in random directions.

10.35 **a** 115°F = 46.1°C   **b** 30°C = 86°F   **c** 311 K = 100°F

10.36 2.5 C deg × 9/5 = 4.5 F deg   (do *not* add 32F° to a temperature *difference!*)

10.37 0 K = −273°C = −459°F = 0°R, so 212°F = 671°R

10.38 15°C = 288 K; 30°C = 303 K; 4.00 × 303/288 = 4.21 liters

10.39 Density = mass/volume; the same mass occupies greater volume at higher temperature and thus has lower density (at constant pressure).

10.40 Helium molecules are smaller than air (N_2, O_2) molecules and move much faster; they escape more quickly from the small holes in the rubber balloon.

10.41 The air pressure (the weight of the atmosphere) is pressing down on the part of the board that is on the table, keeping it in place; unless the board is raised slowly (allowing air molecules time to get underneath), no such force pushes *up* on the board.

10.42 **a** 78.9 torr + 1 atm/760 torr = 0.104 atm   **b** 30 psi = 1551 torr   **c** 145 mm Hg = 19.3 kPa

10.43 Mercury freezes at −39°C (−38°F) and cannot be used at very cold temperatures in an instrument that involves reading the height of a column of liquid mercury.

10.44 Not necessarily, since the force would be pushing in a different direction.

10.45 43 psi × 248/273 = 39 psi (or a gauge pressure of 39 − 15 = 24 psi from 28)

10.46 For each three O_2 molecules that react, we obtain only two O_3 molecules to exert pressure on the walls of the flask; the result is lower total pressure.

10.47 As the temperature increases for an ideal gas at constant volume, the molecules hit the walls more often, and with greater speed; the result is greater force against the walls, and thus higher pressure.

10.48 1824 mm Hg of O_2 and 456 mm Hg of N_2O

10.49 **a** The pressure on the gas is suddenly lowered (to 1 atm), and so its volume increases quickly to that of the room; the force of the gas escaping from the container to fill the room results in the movement of the cylinder.
b Yawning puts slightly higher pressure on the gas inside the lungs; the lungs can respond to this by increasing the alveoli volume, thus relieving the extra pressure.   **c** By reducing the pressure on the air in the straw, we make the force pressing down on that air less than the force pressing up from the liquid; the air can return to an equilibrium of forces by occupying a smaller volume, thus allowing liquid to travel up the straw.

10.50 3.0 L × 1.0 atm/0.90 atm = 3.3 L

10.51 The butane gas (above the butane liquid) in the lighter is pressing out against the case, but that case has 1.0 atm pressure pressing it back at sea level; in a high-altitude airplane cabin, the air pressure is lower but the butane pressure is the same, and so the case might break.

10.52 $PV = nRT$, $n = PV/RT$ = 312 moles O_2; 312 moles × 32.0 g/mole = 9.98 × 10^3 g O_2

10.53 $(9.00/3.00) \times 7.4 \times 10^{22} = 2.2 \times 10^{23}$ helium atoms

10.54 3.7 L ethene $\times$ (3 L O_2)/(1 L ethene) = 11.1 liters O_2 needed

3.7 L ethene $\times$ (2 L CO_2)/(1 L ethene) = 7.4 liters CO_2 formed

10.55 8.00 g $NaHCO_3 \times \dfrac{1 \text{ mole } NaHCO_3}{84.0 \text{ g } NaHCO_3} \times \dfrac{1 \text{ mole } CO_2 \text{ formed}}{1 \text{ mole } NaHCO_3 \text{ used}} =$

0.0952 mole CO_2

$V = nRT/P = (0.0952)(0.0821)(310)/1.00 = 2.42$ liters of CO_2

10.56 10 g $C_3H_8 \times \dfrac{1 \text{ mole } C_3H_8}{44.0 \text{ g } C_3H_8} \times \dfrac{22.4 \text{ L ideal gas at STP}}{1 \text{ mole } C_3H_8} = 5.09$ liters C_3H_8

10.57 N_2 and O_2

10.58 **a** automobile-related smog   **b** industrial smokestacks   **c** smokestacks

10.59 SO_3 dissolves in the water of mucous membranes to give sulfuric acid.

10.60 to lead air into the alveoli and to carry CO_2 from the alveoli; constriction of the bronchioles leads to discomfort and possibly to inadequate gas exchange

10.61 a patient having difficulty breathing or a diver who has decompressed too quickly

10.62 900 g Hb $\times \dfrac{1 \text{ mole Hb}}{68\ 000 \text{ g Hb}} \times \dfrac{4 \text{ moles } O_2}{1 \text{ mole Hb}} \times \dfrac{22.4 \text{ L } O_2 \text{ at STP}}{1 \text{ mole } O_2} = 1.19$ L O_2

CHAPTER ELEVEN SELF-CHECKS

11.1 easily compresses; diffuses throughout volume available; obeys ideal laws; liquids do not share these properties because of intermolecular forces, high density

11.2 **a** *solid* shortening has greater forces than *liquid* oil   **b** *gelatin* dessert known to have higher viscosity than *water*   **c** *water* boils at higher temperature, less volatile than *alcohol*

11.3 **a** water at 10°C, molecules moving more slowly, more time for forces to act   **b** gelatin dessert—higher forces, greater viscosity, greater surface tension   **c** liquid soap, lower vapor pressure (you can't smell it as well), higher intermolecular forces so higher normal boiling point

11.4 the blood pressure resulting from a heart beat (as opposed to diastolic pressure, the lower pressure which is found between heart beats)

11.5 muscle action, coupled with a system of valves to prevent back flow

11.6 Blood pressure higher in arteries than in veins means that weak spots may bulge and break; higher artery pressure also results in greater loss of blood through any opening in a given time period; blood loss from veins is slower.

11.7 Extra blood pressure caused by force of gravity increases blood flow.

11.8 polar liquids; each molecule has a charge separation between δ^+ and δ^- ends

11.9 temporary shifts in electron clouds creating momentary dipoles

11.10 **a** CHF_3, since it is polar; dipoles in CF_4 cancel out and so CF_4 is nonpolar   **b** octane—greater dispersion forces owing to larger size, number of electrons   **c** perhaps butanal—dipole force due to oxygen being at one end of molecule   **d** NO—polar, whereas N_2 is nonpolar

11.11 hydrogen-bonding in a, b, d, e, and g; NOT in CH_3F or in *ionic* NH_4NO_3

11.12 glucose, because of more hydrogen-bonding

11.13 hydrogen-bonding between hydroxyl group and water molecules

11.14 **a** endothermic—requires heat to break liquid attractions

b exothermic—loses heat to surroundings to reach solid state
c exothermic—solid has less heat than original gas   **d** endothermic—
you are receiving heat from your surroundings

11.15   Liquid is present; the partial pressure of the gas is equal to the vapor pressure of the substance at that temperature, and no vapor is entering or leaving the system.

11.16   The lattice points in a molecular solid are occupied by molecules; in an ionic solid, alternate points hold cations and anions.

11.17   The intermolecular forces (dipole, dispersion) are generally much weaker than the ionic bonds holding an ionic crystal together.

11.18   **a** Salt (NaCl) is crystalline.   **b** Sugar (sucrose, $C_{12}H_{22}O_{11}$) is crystalline.   **c** Glass is amorphous.

11.19   In each crystal, lattice positions are occupied by Co^{2+} cations and Cl^- anions attracting each other by ionic bonds; water occupies some of the spaces between the ions, with more water in the red form than in the blue form; high humidity favors the red form.

11.20   It is easy for water to become trapped inside the lattice, since the crystal is forming in a water solution.

11.21   We may add solutions of the two soluble salts to each other, to get a precipitate: $AgNO_{3(aq)} + NaBr_{(aq)} \rightarrow AgBr_{(s)} + NaNO_{3(aq)}$

CHAPTER ELEVEN QUESTIONS AND PROBLEMS

11.22   Intermolecular forces are holding the liquid molecules together; most of the vapor is empty space.

11.23   The liquid molecules exert pressure because of their weight, not because of the speed with which they strike the walls.

11.24   Higher attractions result in greater forces holding the outer layer of molecules to the rest, thus greater surface tension.

11.25   Lower viscosity means that it passes *more* easily through a needle.

11.26   300 mm Hg = 0.395 atm

11.27   Clot in artery can cause bursting of artery as a result of high blood pressure, or can cut off supply of oxygenated blood to cells, causing cell death; vein is less likely to burst; if a vein is blocked, the returning blood can often use alternative veins.

11.28   Extra pressure due to heart pumping is not being measured.

11.29   The pressure becomes distributed through the water, and so the entire body is supported evenly, rather than at only a few points.

11.30   The fluid in the brain prevents the brain itself from moving to the same extent as does the bony skull; the result is first the movement of the skull followed later by the brain moving back; the impact of the brain against the *back* of the skull then causes injury.

11.31   temporary dipoles, caused by normal movement of electron clouds, causing and attracting other temporary dipoles

11.32   Dispersion forces are more important in molecules with large numbers of electrons and large sizes; this usually goes along with high molecular weight.

11.33   **a** heptane—larger, so greater dispersion forces   **b** H_2CCHF because of dipole forces, which are not present in H_2CCH_2 **c** BN because of dipole forces   **d** pentane, with greater overall size, since it is long whereas the other molecule (with identical molecular weight) is spherical

11.34 Kr because of larger size, more electrons

11.35 NH_3 gas, of course (*not* H_2 and N_2)

11.36 **a** yes; hydrogen-bonding between hydroxyl groups **b** no; no N, O, or F **c** no **d** yes; hydrogen-bonding between —NH groups

11.37 forces in H_2O much greater, due to small size of oxygen, creating hydrogen-bonding

11.38 The covalent N—H bond is much stronger than the hydrogen-bonding attraction.

11.39 Hydrogen-bonding between the —OH group of one molecule and the C=O group of the neighboring molecule creates two such attractions in the dimer.

11.40 only alcohols, since in ethers the hydrogens do *not* have δ^+ partial charges

11.41 five

11.42 Ice is less dense than water and occupies more volume for the same mass.

11.43 Melting ice requires heat to break attractions in the solid; at higher temperature, more ice will melt.

11.44 sublimation; endothermic

11.45 at a higher temperature; since the external pressure is over 1.00 atm, the vapor pressure must reach over 1.00 atm before boiling will start

11.46 The particles are fixed in position.

11.47 It is soft, black, powdery.

11.48 molecular, shown by the low melting point

11.49 **a** ionic (high MP, dissolves in water) **b** macromolecular (high MP, does not dissolve), but could be ionic

11.50 hardness, ability to withstand use in fluids without corrosion

11.51 $Na_2SO_4 \cdot 10\ H_2O$

11.52 iron(III) chloride hexahydrate; 270 amu

11.53 **a** $HCl_{(aq)} + AgNO_{3(aq)} \rightarrow AgCl_{(s)} + HNO_{3(aq)}$
 b $MgI_{2(aq)} + 2\ NaOH_{(aq)} \rightarrow Mg(OH)_{2(s)} + 2\ NaI_{(aq)}$

11.54 If only small amounts of F^- and Ca^{2+} ions are present in the final solution, the rate of dissolution of any crystal that forms is greater than the rate of crystal formation, and so no precipitate results.

CHAPTER TWELVE SELF-CHECKS

12.1 **a** solution **b** colloid **c** colloid **d** suspension

12.2 **a** foam **b** aerosol **c** emulsion

12.3 NaCl (solute); water (solvent)

12.4 **a** Add less than 24.6 grams of Na_2SiF_6 to one liter of boiling water or add less than 6.5 grams of Na_2SiF_6 to one liter of cold water. **b** Add 24.6 g Na_2SiF_6 to one L boiling water; add 6.5 g to one L cold water. **c** Add *more than* 6.5 g Na_2SiF_6 to one liter of boiling water, then cool slowly and carefully to 12°C.

12.5 **a** no **b** yes **c** yes

12.6 **a** higher in water (ionic salt) **b** higher in hexane (nonpolar hydrocarbon) **c** higher in water (hydrogen-bonds with water, polar) **d** higher in hexane (nonpolar) **e** higher in water (polar, hydrogen-bonds) **f** higher in hexane (nonpolar) **g** higher in hexane (hydrocarbon-like) **h** higher in water (polar, short carbon chain) **i** higher in hexane (nonpolar)

12.7   need apparatus like that shown in Figure 12–15; test to see if electric current is passed strongly, weakly, or not at all by noting the intensity of the light in the bulb

12.8   The tetraethyl lead additive in gasoline is part of the exhaust emission and dissolves in the water of lakes and rivers.

12.9   Aeration provides O_2 to aid the oxidation of the dissolved organic waste.

12.10   The ion-exchange resin in the water softener exchanges Ca^{2+} and Mg^{2+} ions for Na^+ ions, thus preventing precipitation of insoluble calcium and magnesium salts.

12.11   In a case where the osmotic pressure of body fluids is too high.

12.12   The salt concentration in the salt water is higher than in the fluid of the fish cells; the external solution is hypertonic—water will drain out of the fish cell, and the fish will become dehydrated.

12.13   No; it contains solute particles, which cause a freezing point depression.

12.14 $CaCl_2$; it gives a greater number of dissolved particles on ionization.

12.15   NaCl; it gives two moles of dissolved particles on ionization; glucose does not ionize and gives only one mole of particles.

CHAPTER TWELVE QUESTIONS AND PROBLEMS

12.16   roughly 10 Å to 1000 Å

12.17, 12.18   [*See text or check answer with instructor.*]

12.19   foam—small amount of gas dispersed in larger amounts of solid rock

12.20   acetic acid (solute); water (solvent)

12.21   oxygen

12.22   Add 128 grams of KI to 100 mL of water at 20°C.

12.23   Add an amount greater than 209 grams of CaI_2 to water at 100°C and slowly cool to 20°C.

12.24   raises the concentration of oxygen in the blood, since the solubility of O_2 in the blood increases as the partial pressure increases

12.25   a, formic acid, and c, hydrazine, will be more soluble in water since they can hydrogen-bond to water.

12.26   weak electrolyte; low degree of ionization at this concentration

12.27   Forces holding the ether molecules together and forces holding the water molecules together must be overcome; forces of attraction between the ether and water are created.

12.28   should be nonpolar and relatively insoluble in water

12.29   by a separatory funnel; the denser liquid will settle to the bottom of the funnel and can be removed; or, by skimming or decanting off the top layer

12.30   industrial waste from chemical industries   **12.31**   phosphates

12.32   from industrial wastes, especially electroplating

12.33   to allow suspended particles to settle out

12.34   exchanges Ca^{2+} for Na^+ ions   **12.35**   by evaporation; yes

12.36   could be designed so that less phosphate and nitrate are carried off into rivers and streams

12.37 $(CH_3)_2Hg$ or similar compounds

12.38   Small concentrations of fluoride ion in drinking water make children's teeth more resistant to decay.

12.39 Pure water would be hypotonic with the blood in the patient's vein and would cause extra water to enter red blood cells, which will burst.

12.40 It will shrink and shrivel up, losing water to the hypertonic sea.

12.41 lowers the freezing point   **12.42** higher temperature

12.43 They contain higher concentrations of solute in body fluids, and so the freezing point of the fluids is lowered.

CHAPTER THIRTEEN SELF-CHECKS

13.1 **a** $HNO_{3(aq)} \rightarrow H^+_{(aq)} + NO^-_{3(aq)}$ **b** $KOH_{(aq)} \rightarrow K^+_{(aq)} + OH^-_{(aq)}$

13.2 $Ca(OH)_{2(aq)} + 2\ HCl_{(aq)} \rightarrow CaCl_{2(aq)} + 2\ H_2O_{(\ell)}$

13.3 While these strong bases do dissociate almost 100% in water, the solids $Mg(OH)_2$ and $Ca(OH)_2$ are only slightly soluble, and not enough solid enters water solution to provide a dangerous concentration of OH^- ion.

13.4 It is insoluble in water.

13.5 $Zn_{(s)} + H_2SO_{4(aq)} \rightarrow H_{2(g)} + ZnSO_{4(aq)}$

13.6 A pH above 7.0 is basic.   **a** basic   **b** basic   **c** acidic   **d** neutral   **e** acidic   **f** acidic   **g** acidic

13.7 in order of *decreasing* pH: a, b, d, e, g, f, c

13.8 **a** $CH_3COOH_{(aq)} \rightleftharpoons H^+_{(aq)} + CH_3COO^-_{(aq)}$
b $HOOCCH_2CH_2COOH_{(aq)} \rightleftharpoons H^+_{(aq)} + HOOCCH_2CH_2COO^-_{(aq)}$
c $H_2SO_{3(aq)} \rightleftharpoons H^+_{(aq)} + HSO^-_{3(aq)}$
d $NH^+_{4(aq)} \rightleftharpoons H^+_{(aq)} + NH_{3(aq)}$
e $C_5NH_4COOH \rightleftharpoons H^+_{(aq)} + C_5NH_4COO^-_{(aq)}$

13.9 **a** The conjugate bases are CH_3COO^-, $HOOCCH_2CH_2COO^-$, HSO_3^-, NH_3, and $C_5NH_4COO^-$, as shown as products of the equations.   **b** acetate ion; hydrogen succinate ion; hydrogen sulfite ion; ammonia; nicotinate ion

13.10 The *lower* the pK_a, the more acidic will be a solution of given concentration: H_2SO_3 is most acidic, then succinic, then acetic; least acidic is ammonium ion.

13.11 **a** yes   **b** yes   **c** no (only one —COOH)   **d** no

13.12 The stronger acid and stronger base (anion) will react to produce the weaker acid and weaker base; since you know that the product will include the weaker acid, you need only compare the two acids: **a** ascorbic acid and NaF (ascorbic acid weaker than HF)   **b** phenol and potassium formate (phenol weaker than formic acid)   **c** sodium sulfate and CO_2 ($NaHSO_4$ and $NaHCO_3$ acceptable)

13.13 Water has a $pK_a = 14.0$ at 25°C, so look for any with $pK_a < 14.0$: a and c.

13.14 **a** 2-chloropropanoic acid (chlorine draws electron from hydrogen)
b chloroacetic acid (chlorine more electronegative than iodine)
c $HClO_4$ (oxygen is highly electronegative, has same effect as chlorine)

13.15 **a** $C_6H_5O^-_{(aq)} + H_2O_{(\ell)} \rightleftharpoons C_6H_5OH_{(aq)} + OH^-_{(aq)}$
b $CH_3COO^-_{(aq)} + H_2O_{(\ell)} \rightleftharpoons CH_3COOH_{(aq)} + OH^-_{(aq)}$
c $CH_3NH_{2(aq)} + H_2O_{(\ell)} \rightleftharpoons CH_3NH^+_{3(aq)} + OH^-_{(aq)}$
d $C_6H_5NH_{2(aq)} + H_2O_{(\ell)} \rightleftharpoons C_6H_5NH^+_{3(aq)} + OH^-_{(aq)}$

13.16 knowing that $pK_b = 14.00 - pK_a$ of the conjugate acid: **a** 11.0   **b** 13.90   **c** 6.5   **d** 12.1

13.17 **a** $H_3C_6H_5O_6 + CO_3^{2-} \rightarrow H_2C_6H_5O_6^- + HCO_3^-$
b $HNO_2 + CH_3NH_2 \rightarrow NO_2^- + CH_3NH_3^+$
c $HNO_3 + CH_3CHOHCOO^- \rightarrow NO_3^- + CH_3CHOHCOOH$

13.18   An agonized trip to the hospital! The CO_3^{2-} ion is a *much* stronger base than the bicarbonate HCO_3^- ion and gives a serious chemical burn to the esophagus, mouth, and stomach lining if the concentration is high enough.

13.19   **a** secondary amine (one —H on nitrogen)   **b** primary amine (—NH_2 group)   **c** two secondary amines (—NH— groups)   **d** primary amine (—NH_2 group)   **e** and **f**: none, only *amide* groups   **g** primary amine (—NH_2 group)   **h** one primary amine (—NH_2 group) and one quaternary ammonium salt situation

13.20 $CH_3CH_2COOH + H_2NCH_3 \longrightarrow CH_3CH_2{-}\underset{\underset{O}{\|}}{C}{-}\underset{\underset{H}{|}}{N}{-}CH_3 + H_2O$

13.21   The active portion of the antihistamine competes with histamine for the "receptor sites" that trigger allergic reaction symptoms.

13.22   From the acids in Table 13-4, those that are amphoteric are HSO_4^-, $H_2PO_4^-$, HCO_3^-, and HPO_4^{2-} ions; several of the conjugate bases, such as dihydrogen citrate and hydrogen oxalate, are also amphoteric.

13.23   **a** zwitterion form of threonine: $^+H_3N{-}\underset{\underset{COO^-}{|}}{\overset{\overset{CHOHCH_3}{|}}{CH}}$

   b $CH_3CHOHCH(COO^-)NH_3^+ + H^+ \rightarrow CH_3CHOHCH(COOH)NH_3^+$
   c $CH_3CHOHCH(COO^-)NH_3^+ + OH^- \rightarrow CH_3CHOHCH(COO^-)NH_2 + H_2O$

13.24   **a** $C_6H_7O_6^- + H^+ \rightarrow HC_6H_7O_6$ (ascorbic acid produced)
   b $HC_6H_7O_6 + OH^- \rightarrow C_6H_7O_6^- + H_2O$ (ascorbate ion produced)

13.25   You would seek to use equal concentrations of a weak acid and its conjugate base, such that the weak acid has $pK_a = 12.0$; an equal mixture of HPO_4^{2-} and PO_4^{3-} would do the job; these could come from solutions of Na_2HPO_4 and Na_3PO_4, respectively.

13.26   This statement is illustrated by the answer to Self-Check 13.24; in the case of blood plasma, HCO_3^- reacts with H^+ in aqueous solution to give the weak acid H_2CO_3.

13.27   As for the preceding question, we see that the number of moles of conjugate acid increases and the number of moles of conjugate base decreases as the buffer copes with added H^+; the pH depends on the acid-base ratio, which goes up; the pH then goes down, but not as much as it would if only H^+ and water were present.

13.28   on the basis of price, odor, or other qualities you like; not on the basis of pH since, after dilution with water, all will have essentially neutral pH and minimal effect on skin

13.29   No; a depilatory uses a relatively strong base (high pH) to break the ionic bonds (salt bridges) in hair and make it easily removed; it can also affect the outer layer of skin in the same manner.

13.30   **a** in blood: bicarbonate/CO_2 buffer and hemoglobin buffer
   b inside cells: phosphate ion buffer and protein buffers

CHAPTER THIRTEEN QUESTIONS AND PROBLEMS

13.31   typical equations:
   $KOH_{(aq)} \rightarrow K^+_{(aq)} + OH^-_{(aq)}$
   $Ca(OH)_{2(aq)} \rightarrow Ca^{2+}_{(aq)} + 2\ OH^-_{(aq)}$

13.32 strong acids: HNO_3 only

13.33 strong bases: $Ca(OH)_2$ and KOH

13.34 No; a very dilute solution of NaOH would be safer than concentrated $NH_{3(aq)}$.

13.35 $2\ HNO_{3(aq)} + Mg(OH)_{2(s)} \rightarrow Mg(NO_3)_{2(aq)} + 2\ H_2O_{(\ell)}$

13.36 A pH of 9.2 is basic (higher than pH 7.0).

13.37 Both are acidic; carrot juice is more acidic (lower pH).

13.38 Acids *react* with zinc, as shown in the answer to Self-Check 13.5.

13.39 The bottle of 16 M HNO_3 is ''concentrated'' nitric acid.

13.40 **a** pH = 3.0   **b** pH = 9.0

13.41 If the battery explodes, the splattered sulfuric acid (a strong acid in a relatively high concentration) can cause severe chemical burns.

13.42 the equation for use of *Tums:*
$CaCO_{3(s)} + 2\ HCl_{(aq)} \rightarrow CaCl_{2(aq)} + H_2O_{(\ell)} + CO_{2(g)}$
High blood calcium levels (which would be caused by the dissolved $CaCl_2$, a product of the neutralization) can damage kidneys.

13.43 $HF_{(aq)} \rightleftharpoons H^+_{(aq)} + F^-_{(aq)}$; $HNO_{2(aq)} \rightleftharpoons H^+_{(aq)} + NO^-_{2(aq)}$;
$CH_3COOH_{(aq)} \rightleftharpoons H^+_{(aq)} + CH_3COO^-_{(aq)}$; HCl is a strong acid.

13.44 that of bromoacetic acid, with a lower pK_a

13.45 **a** F^- **b** SO_4^{2-} **c** $C_6H_5COO^-$ **d** PO_4^{3-}

13.46 Only (b), adipic acid, is polyprotic.

13.47 **a** F^- and HCO_3^- **b** CH_3COOH and HSO_3^- as given

13.48 using the equation of Section 13.2: $pH \approx \frac{1}{2}pK_a - \frac{1}{2}\log_{10}[HA]$ **a** for $HCOOH$, $pK_a = 3.7$, so $\frac{1}{2}(3.7 + 1.0) = 2.35$ **b** for NH_4^+, $pK_a = 9.3$, so $\frac{1}{2}(9.3 + 2.0) = 5.65$

13.49 Lower pK_a means more acidic; tribromoacetic acid; the greater the number of highly electronegative atoms, the more electrons are drawn out of the acidic hydrogen, allowing it to be released as $H^+_{(aq)}$.

13.50 **a** $CH_3CH_2NH_{2(aq)} + H_2O_{(\ell)} \rightleftharpoons CH_3CH_2NH^+_{3(aq)} + OH^-_{(aq)}$
b $HCOONa_{(aq)} + H_2O_{(\ell)} \rightleftharpoons HCOOH_{(aq)} + NaOH_{(aq)}$
or $HCOO^-_{(aq)} + H_2O_{(\ell)} \rightleftharpoons HCOOH_{(aq)} + OH^-_{(aq)}$

13.51 **a** $2\ HC_6H_7O_{6(aq)} + Na_2CO_{3(aq)} \rightarrow 2\ NaC_6H_7O_{6(aq)} + CO_{2(g)} + H_2O_{(\ell)}$
Other equations are possible, with products HCO_3^- or H_2CO_3.
b $2\ HNO_{2(aq)} + Mg(OH)_{2(aq)} \rightarrow Mg(NO_2)_{2(aq)} + 2\ H_2O_{(\ell)}$

13.52 $pK_b = 14.00 - pK_a$ of conjugate acid; $14.00 - 8.26 = 5.74$; basic

13.53 $C_6H_5CH_2CH(CH_3)NH_2 + HC_6H_7O_6 \rightarrow C_6H_5CH_2CH(CH_3)NH_3^+ + C_6H_7O_6^-$

13.54 **a** $NaNO_3$ is neutral (no pK_a for strong acid, no pK_b for strong base).
b NH_4Cl is acidic.   **c** KF is basic.   **d** CH_3NH_3Br is acidic.
e $NaHCO_3$ is basic (although amphoteric, $pK_b < pK_a$).

13.55 any answer with —NH— such as $(CH_3)_2NH$

13.56

13.57 the products are the acid anion and the amine (two bases):

$$\overset{\displaystyle H}{\underset{\displaystyle |}{\overset{\displaystyle |}{-N:}}} + CH_3COO^-$$

13.58 Because of the carbon rings and chains, drugs containing amine groups are generally insoluble in water; they can be dissolved in the form of *ionic salts*, such as the chlorides or sulfates, and thus absorbed into the body through the digestive system and blood stream.

13.59 Aspirin reduces inflammation, acetaminophen does not.

13.60 Generally no; a combination of ingredients is really suitable only for a (relatively unusual) combination of symptoms that require those ingredients, such as a headache due to allergy; even so, caffeine and the antacid work against each other with regard to stomach acidity.

13.61 Antihistamines often cause drowsiness and other side effects; since the effects differ for different people, you should be very much aware of the exact side effects you encounter.

13.62 $H_2NC_6H_4COOH + H^+ \rightarrow {}^+H_3NC_6H_4COOH$ acting as a base
$H_2NC_6H_4COOH + OH^- \rightarrow H_2NC_6H_4COO^- + H_2O$ acting as an acid

13.63 Since there is a 20/1 ratio of base to acid in the buffer, more base is being removed; the body would suffer from too low a pH (acidosis).

13.64 $HCO_{3(aq)}^- + HC_4H_4O_{6(aq)} \rightarrow H_2O_{(\ell)} + CO_{2(g)} + C_4H_4O_{6(aq)}^-$

13.65 The HPO_4^{2-} ions can react with excess acid to form $H_2PO_4^-$; the $H_2PO_4^-$ ions can react with excess base to form water and HPO_4^{2-}; the ratio of the two remains relatively constant, so long as no large amounts of acid or of base must be neutralized.

13.66 Strong base converts $-NH_3^+$ to $-NH_2$ and thus breaks ionic bonds in proteins of hair.

13.67 $2\ HNO_{3(aq)} + CaCO_{3(s)} \rightarrow CO_{2(g)} + H_2O_{(\ell)} + Ca(NO_3)_{2(aq)}$; marble artwork dissolves.

CHAPTER FOURTEEN SELF-CHECKS

14.1 **a** $0.100\ L \times \dfrac{0.100\ \text{mole}\ KNO_3}{L} \times \dfrac{101\ g\ KNO_3}{\text{mole}\ KNO_3} = 1.01\ g\ KNO_3$

Take 1.01 g KNO_3, dissolve in water in a 100-mL volumetric flask, and fill to mark. **b** Dissolve 2.71 g $HgCl_2$ and use a 50-mL volumetric flask. **c** Dissolve 5.22 g lactic acid and use a 25-mL volumetric flask. **d** Dissolve 1.52 g $CaSO_4 \cdot {}^1\!/_2H_2O$ and use a 500-mL volumetric flask.

14.2 **a** 3% of 50.00 g is 1.5 g; take 1.5 g $NaNO_2$, use a 50-mL volumetric flask **b** 2.5 g of boric acid in a 250-mL flask **c** 0.40 g of tannic acid in a 10-mL flask **d** 0.0050 g of epinephrine in a 5-mL flask

14.3 **a** $1.5\ g\ NaNO_2 \times \dfrac{1\ \text{mole}\ NaNO_2}{69.0\ g\ NaNO_2} = 0.022\ \text{mole}\ NaNO_2$ in 0.0500 L = 0.44 *M*

b 0.040 mole boric acid in 0.250 L = 0.16 *M*
c 0.00024 mole tannic acid in 0.0100 L = 0.024 *M*
d 2.3×10^{-5} mole epinephrine in 0.0050 L = 0.0046 *M*

14.4 **a** 0.030% w/v KCl

b $0.083 \text{ g CaCl}_2 \times \dfrac{1 \text{ mole CaCl}_2}{111 \text{ g CaCl}_2} \times \dfrac{1 \text{ mole Ca}^{2+}}{1 \text{ mole CaCl}_2} \times \dfrac{1000 \text{ mL}}{250 \text{ mL}} = 0.0030 \ M$

c From CaCl_2, we obtain Cl^- concentration of $0.0060 \ M$ Cl^-.
From KCl, we get $0.075/74.6 \times 4 = 0.0040 \ M$ Cl^-.
From NaCl, we have $2.15/58.5 \times 4 = 0.147 \ M$ Cl^-; adding we get
$0.157 \ M$ Cl^-.

14.5 $1/2000 \times 5000$ g solution $= 2.50 \text{ g HgCl}_2$; $0.0018 \ M$

14.6 $1.00 \text{ g Mg} \times \dfrac{1 \text{ mole Mg}}{24.3 \text{ g Mg}} \times \dfrac{1 \text{ mole Mg}^{2+}}{1 \text{ mole Mg}} \times \dfrac{1 \text{ liter water}}{0.0520 \text{ mole Mg}^{2+}} = 0.791 \text{ L}$

14.7   **a** $1.1 \text{ mg/L} = 0.0011 \text{ g/L} = 0.00011 \text{ g/100 mL} = 0.00011\%$ ($1.1 \times 10^{-4}\%$)   **b** $2.0 \times 10^{-5} \ M$ **c** 3.3×10^{-3} g of Fe^{3+} in 3.0 L blood

14.8   **a** $454 \text{ g NaCl} \times \dfrac{0.100 \text{ L}}{0.9 \text{ g NaCl}} = 50$ liters of 0.9% w/v saline

b $454 \text{ g NaCl} \times \dfrac{1 \text{ mole NaCl}}{58.5 \text{ g NaCl}} \times \dfrac{1 \text{ L sea water}}{0.457 \text{ mole NaCl}} = 17.0$ liters of sea water

c 78 L of blood plasma   **d** 1.24 L of saturated brine

14.9   **a** need $0.0250 \text{ L} \times 1.50 \ M = 0.0375 \text{ mole H}_2\text{SO}_4 \times \dfrac{1000 \text{ mL conc.}}{18.0 \text{ mole}} =$
2.08 mL conc. *or* $25.0 \text{ mL} \times 1.50 \ M/18.0 \ M = 2.08$ mL concentrated solution in a 25-mL flask   **b** 5.74 mL of stock solution in a 500-mL flask to make 0.17 M NH_3 **c** 8.62 mL of HCl stock solution in a 100-mL flask
d 0.953 mL of HNO_3 stock solution in a 10-mL flask
e 8.62 mL of acetic acid stock solution in a 50-mL flask

14.10   From our answer to Self-Check 14.4c, we already know that the solution contains $0.157 \ M$ Cl^- and $0.0030 \ M$ Ca^{2+}; we can quickly calculate Na^+ at $0.147 \ M$ and K^+ at $0.0040 \ M$ from the same data; adding them all up we obtain 0.311 mole of particles per liter of solution = 311 mOs/L, roughly isotonic with blood plasma (average value 304 mOs/L).

14.11   The ionic concentrations add up to 1.09 moles of particles per liter of sea water, or 1090 mOs/L; higher than that of blood plasma (hypertonic); yes, water is lost from skin cells immersed in a hypertonic solution; when a shipwrecked sailor drinks sea water, more urine must be excreted to eliminate the excess salts than the amount of sea water consumed, so that the net effect is to *dehydrate* the body!

14.12   We want 300 mOs/L, or a total ionic concentration of $0.30 \ M$; if there are two ions, then each should be at about $0.15 \ M$, thus the molarity of each salt would be $0.15 \ M$.

14.13   **a** pH = 12.46   **b** pH = 3.13   **c** pH = 6.82   **d** pH = 10.62

14.14   **a** $[\text{H}^+] = 7.4 \times 10^{-4} \ M$ **b** $[\text{H}^+] = 2.4 \times 10^{-12} \ M$ **c** $[\text{H}^+] = 1.3 \times 10^{-3} \ M$ **d** $[\text{H}^+] = 3.1 \times 10^{-8} \ M$

14.15   **a** pK_a for H_2PO_4^- is 7.2; $pH = pK_a + \log \dfrac{\text{base}}{\text{acid}} = 7.2 + \log 4 = 7.8$

b $pH = 3.7 + \log 3 = 4.2$ **c** $pH = 10.2 + \log 2/3 = 10.0$
d $pH = 3.9 + \log 1/2 = 3.6$ **e** $pH = 6.4 + 1.30 = 7.7$

14.16   **a** $\text{H}^+_{(aq)} + \text{OH}^-_{(aq)} \rightarrow \text{H}_2\text{O}_{(\ell)}$ **b** same as for (a)
c $\text{H}^+_{(aq)} + \text{CH}_3\text{NH}_{2(aq)} \rightarrow \text{CH}_3\text{NH}^+_{3(aq)}$
d $\text{CH}_3\text{CHOHCOOH}_{(aq)} + \text{NH}_{3(aq)} \rightarrow \text{CH}_3\text{CHOHCOO}^-_{(aq)} + \text{NH}^+_{4(aq)}$

14.17   **a** The two substances we are mixing must be soluble, since they are already in solution; all sodium salts are soluble; check Fe(OH)_3—it is

insoluble; you know that an iron(III) hydroxide precipitate is formed:
$Fe^{3+}_{(aq)} + 3\ OH^-_{(aq)} \rightarrow Fe(OH)_{3(s)}$ **b** $Ag^+_{(aq)} + I^-_{(aq)} \rightarrow AgI_{(s)}$
c $Cu^{2+}_{(aq)} + S^{2-}_{(aq)} \rightarrow CuS_{(s)}$ **d** no reaction—all substances are soluble
e $Ba^{2+}_{(aq)} + SO^{2-}_{4(aq)} \rightarrow BaSO_{4(s)}$ *and* $2\ H^+_{(aq)} + S^{2-}_{(aq)} \rightarrow H_2S_{(aq)}$

14.18   **a** $37.51\ mL\ OH^- \times \dfrac{0.2079\ mole\ OH^-}{1000\ mL\ OH^-} \times \dfrac{1\ mole\ H^+}{1\ mole\ OH^-} = 7.798 \times 10^{-3}$ mole
H^+ dividing by $25.00\ mL = 0.02500\ L$ gives $[H^+] = 0.3119\ M$
b 1.228×10^{-3} mole lactic acid is 0.1105 g out of $5.00\ mL = 2.21\%$ w/v
c 5.97×10^{-6} mole $MnO_4^- \times 5/2 = 1.49 \times 10^{-5}$ mole oxalate in
$0.1000\ L$ or $1.49 \times 10^{-4}\ M$ oxalate in urine   **d** 0.004415 mole OH^- for
0.004415 mole H^+ for 0.002207 mole H_2SO_4 in 0.0100 liter, so $0.2207\ M$

14.19   **a** $34.03/17.85 \times 0.100\ N = 0.191\ N$ **b** $0.0897\ N$ **c** $0.439\ N$

14.20   **a** Zn loses *two* electrons when a reducing agent; $65.37/2 = 32.7$ g/eq Zn
b H_2NNH_2 has two basic sides; $32.0/2 = 16.0$ g/eq H_2NNH_2
c C_6H_5COOH has only one acidic hydrogen; $122/1 = 122$ g/eq
C_6H_5COOH **d** HPO_4^{2-} has a $2-$ charge as an electrolyte; $96/2 = 48$
g/eq HPO_4^{2-}

CHAPTER FOURTEEN QUESTIONS AND PROBLEMS

14.21   **a** $0.02500\ L \times \dfrac{0.100\ mole\ AgNO_3}{L} \times \dfrac{170\ g\ AgNO_3}{1\ mole} = 0.425$ g $AgNO_3$ into a
25-mL flask, then dissolve in water, then add water until mark on flask is
reached and mix   **b** 0.0050 g methyl orange in a 5-mL volumetric
flask   **c** 12.6 g $NaHCO_3$ (0.150 mole) in a 100-mL volumetric flask
d 12.5 g procaine (2.5×5 g) in a 250-mL volumetric flask

14.22 $(454/4000) \times 100 = 11.4\%$ w/v; 7.77 moles in $4.00\ L = 1.94\ M$

14.23 $(1/10^5) \times 100\ mL = 10^{-3}\ mL$ or $10^{-3}\%$ w/v $= 10^{-3}$ g in $100\ mL$
$(10^{-3}\ g/100\ mL) \times 1\ mole/183\ g = 5 \times 10^{-6}$ mole in $100\ mL = 5 \times 10^{-5}\ M$

14.24   **a** $3.0\ L \times 2.2 \times 10^{-5}$ mole $NH_3/L \times 17.0$ g $NH_3/mole = 1.1 \times 10^{-3}$ g (or
1.1 mg) NH_3 **b** $3.0\ L \times (0.0010\ g\ SO_4^{2-})/(0.100\ L) = 0.030$ g (or 30 mg)
SO_4^{2-} **c** 40 nanomoles/L $= 40 \times 10^{-9} g\ H^+/L \times 3.0\ L = 1.2 \times 10^{-7} g\ H^+$
d $3.0\ L$ is $30\ dL$, so 600 ng/dL $\times 30\ dL = 18\ 000$ ng $= 1.8 \times 10^{-5}$ g

14.25   **a** $(1.50/11.6) \times 50.00\ mL = 6.47\ mL$ stock HCl solution mixed in a 50-mL
volumetric flask with enough distilled water to reach the mark
b $15.8\ mL$ stock HCl in a 250-mL volumetric flask

14.26   a volumetric flask, filled with final solution up to its calibration mark

14.27   **a** NH_3 does not dissociate, and so we want $0.30\ M\ NH_3$; this requires a
total volume of $(6.00/0.30) \times 50\ mL = 1000\ mL$; we must then add 950
mL of water.   **b** $CaCl_2$ dissociates into $Ca^{2+} + 2\ Cl^-$, three ions in all;
we need $0.10\ M\ CaCl_2$; the 10.0% w/v solution has $(0.10)(5.00) = 0.50$ g $=$
0.0045 mole; total volume should be $0.0045/0.10 = 0.045\ L = 45\ mL$;
we must add 40 mL of water.

14.28   Acetic acid dissociates only slightly; for the purposes of this problem, let us assume no dissociation; then osmotic pressure in torr $= 19\ 300 \times$ molarity $=$
760 torr, so that molarity $= 760/19\ 300 = 0.0394\ M$; use any appropriate
method for preparing such a solution of CH_3COOH from a stock solution,
since acetic acid is not available in solid form.

14.29   **a** pH $= 2.40$ **b** pH $= 9.49$ **c** pH $= 4.41$ **d** pH $= 6.92$

14.30   **a** $[H^+] = 7.8 \times 10^{-6}\ M$ **b** $[H^+] = 3.0 \times 10^{-4}\ M$ **c** $[H^+] = 1.8 \times 10^{-10}\ M$ **d** $[H^+] = 3.2 \times 10^{-11}\ M$

14.31 using $pH = pK_a + \log$ base/acid: **a** $pH = pK_a = 4.1$ **b** $pH = 4.1 - 0.7 = 3.4$ **c** $pH = 4.1 + .48 = 4.6$

14.32 The solution initially contains 0.010 mole each of acid and base; we have added 0.0050 mole OH^-; this reacts with 0.0050 mole of acid to give 0.0050 mole of conjugate base, leaving 0.005 M acid, 0.015 M base; base/acid ratio is now 3/1, so that $pH = 4.6$ as in Question 14.31c; if only 0.0050 mole OH^- were present in 1 L of solution, $pH = 11.70$.

14.33 **a** $H^+_{(aq)} + OH^-_{(aq)} \rightarrow H_2O_{(\ell)}$ **b** $Fe^{3+}_{(aq)} + PO^{3-}_{4(aq)} \rightarrow FePO_{4(s)}$ **c** no reaction (two acids involved) **d** $HSO^-_{4(aq)} + OH^-_{(aq)} \rightarrow SO^{2-}_{4(aq)} + H_2O_{(\ell)}$ **e** $Ba^{2+}_{(aq)} + SO^{2-}_{4(aq)} \rightarrow BaSO_{4(s)}$ **f** $2\,OH^-_{(aq)} + Mg^{2+}_{(aq)} \rightarrow Mg(OH)_{2(s)}$ **g** no reaction (all substances soluble) **h** $HCO^-_{3(aq)} + H^+_{(aq)} \rightarrow H_2CO_3 \rightarrow H_2O_{(\ell)} + CO_{2(g)}$ **i** $H_2NCH_2COOH_{(aq)} + OH^-_{(aq)} \rightarrow H_2NCH_2COO^-_{(aq)} + H_2O_{(\ell)}$

14.34 **a** $(15.67/10.00) \times 0.100\ M = 0.157\ M$ HNO_3 **b** 2 moles KOH required for one mole H_2SO_4; 1.58 M KOH

14.35 Titration of a strong acid with weak base gives an end point on the acidic side; methyl orange or methyl red might be chosen.

14.36 **a** 0.10 N HCl **b** 0.0050 N NH_3 **c** H_3PO_4 has three acidic hydrogens; $1.50\ M \times 3 = 4.50\ N$ H_3PO_4

14.37 **a** $0.100\ N \times 37.69/15.78 = 0.239\ N$ acid **b** $0.0790\ N \times 17.79/10.00 = 0.140\ N$ reducing agent

14.38 **a** oxalic acid is diprotic; 90.0 g/mole $\div 2 = 45.0$ g/eq HOOCCOOH **b** Fe^{3+} carries a 3+ charge; 55.8 g/mole $\div 3 = 18.6$ g/eq Fe^{3+} **c** F_2 gains two electrons to become 2 F^-; 38.0 g/mole $\div 2 = 19.0$ g/eq F_2

14.39 **a** K^+: 4.2 meq/L = 0.0042 eq/L = 0.0042 M **b** $CH_3CHOHCOO^-$: 1.3 meq/L = 0.0013 eq/L = 0.0013 M **c** Mg^{2+}: 1.9 meq/L = 0.0019 eq/L $\times$ 1 mole/2 eq = 0.00095 M

CHAPTER FIFTEEN SELF-CHECKS

15.1 **a** fluorobenzene **b** p-dinitrobenzene **c** propylbenzene **d** o-chlorotoluene **e** m-bromonitrobenzene **f** m-xylene **g** p-chloroethylbenzene **h** 2-chloro-2-nitrotoluene

15.2

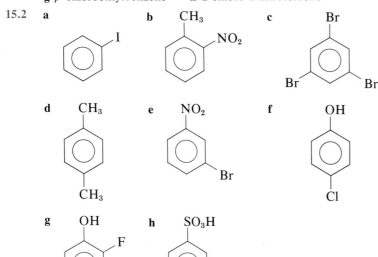

15.3   CH$_2$CH$_3$

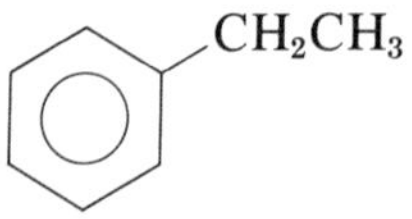

15.4   (a) and (b) are fused-ring hydrocarbons

15.5   3-methylfuran   15.6

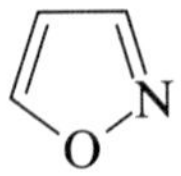

CHAPTER FIFTEEN QUESTIONS AND PROBLEMS

15.7   They undergo substitution reactions rather than addition reactions; the pi bonds are delocalized around a ring.

15.8   and   15.9

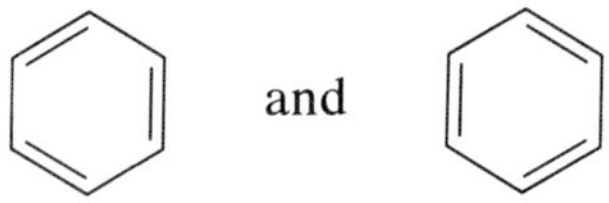

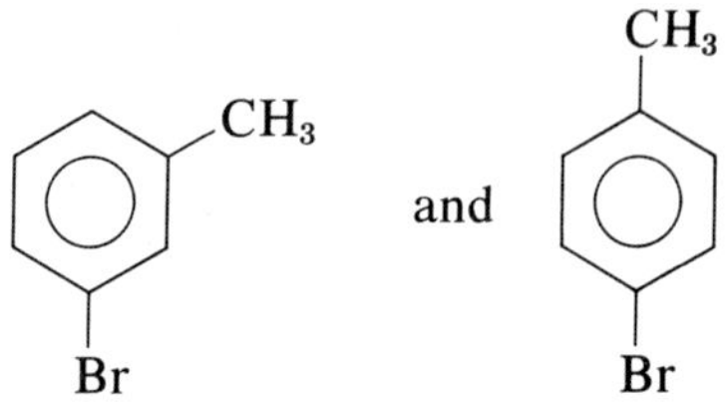

15.10   o-bromotoluene; m-bromotoluene; p-bromotoluene

15.11   o-dichlorobenzene; m-dichlorobenzene; p-dichlorobenzene

15.12 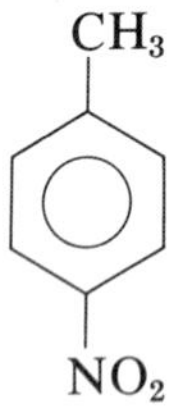   15.13   m-nitrobenzaldehyde

15.14 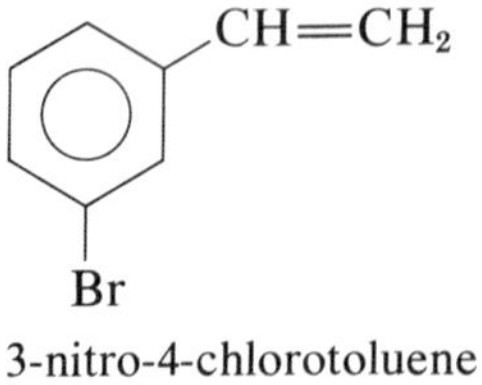   15.15   butylbenzene

15.16   3-nitro-4-chlorotoluene   15.17

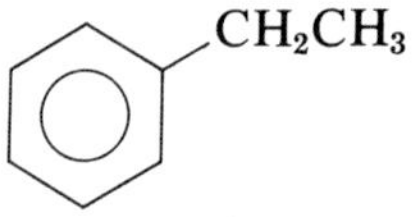

15.18 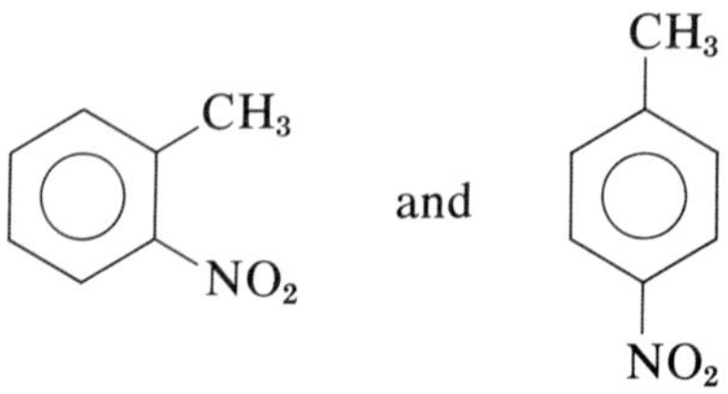   15.19

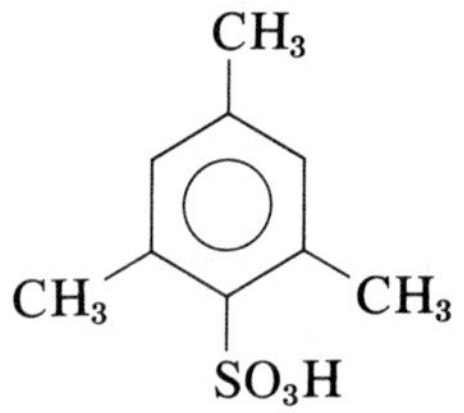

15.20

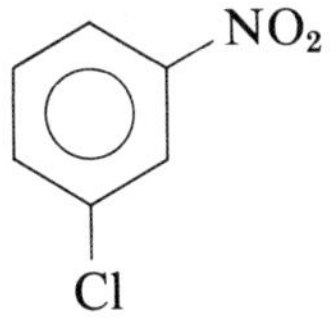

15.21

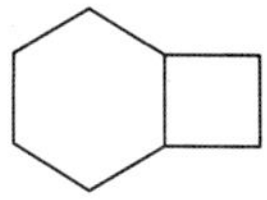

15.22

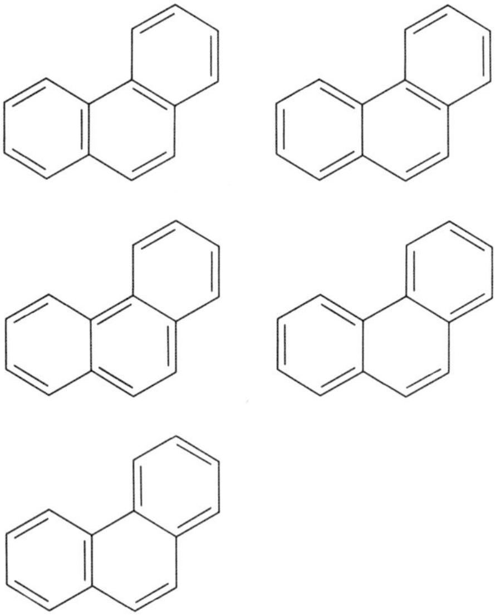

15.23

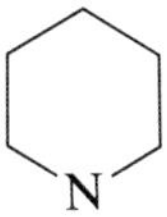

15.24

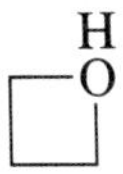

15.25 heterocyclic

15.26 carbocyclic

15.27

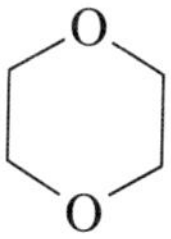

15.28

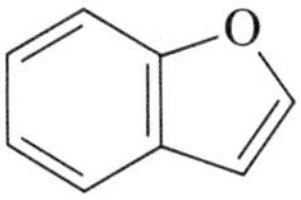

15.29

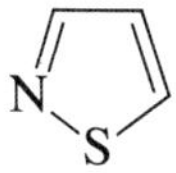

CHAPTER SIXTEEN SELF-CHECKS

one possibility:

16.1   **a** A—A—A—A—A—A—B—B—B—A—A—A—A—A—A—B—B—B
       b —A—B—A—A—B—A—B—B—B—A—
       c —A—A—A—A—A—A—A—A *or* —B—B—B—B—B—B—B

16.2   *initiation:*

$$R-\overset{\overset{\displaystyle O}{\|}}{C}-O-O-\overset{\overset{\displaystyle O}{\|}}{C}-R \xrightarrow{\text{heat}} 2\ CO_2 + 2R\cdot$$

propagation: $R\cdot + CH_2{=}CHCl \longrightarrow RCH_2\overset{\cdot}{C}HCl$

$RCH_2\overset{\cdot}{C}HCl + CH_2{=}CHCl \longrightarrow RCH_2CHClCH_2\overset{\cdot}{C}HCl$, etc.

termination: $2\ RCH_2\dot{C}HCl \longrightarrow RCH_2CHClCHClCH_2R$

or $R[CH_2CHCl]_{n+1}\ CH_2\dot{C}HCl + R\cdot \longrightarrow$

$R[CH_2CHCl]_{n+1}\ CH_2CHClR$

16.3 Too much initiator will supply too many R·radicals, which can cause premature termination by combining with the propagating radicals.

16.4 Ethene, propene, and tetrafluoroethene are some possibilities.

16.5 Each monomer must contain at least two functional groups capable of entering into the reaction that builds up the polymer chain.

16.6 $H_2N—\overset{\overset{\displaystyle O}{\|}}{C}—\overset{\displaystyle H}{N}—CH_2OH$

16.7

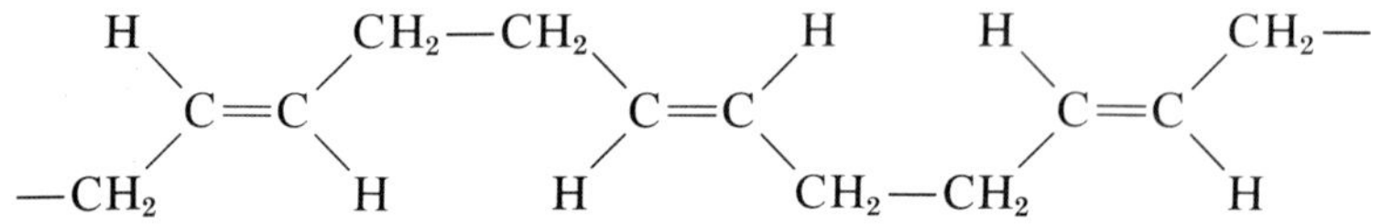

16.8 The plasticizers added to the polymer are lost by evaporation.

CHAPTER SIXTEEN QUESTIONS AND PROBLEMS

16.9 —A—A—A—B—B—A—A—A—B—B—A—A—A—B—B—

16.10 $—CH_2—CCl_2—CH_2—CCl_2—CH_2—CCl_2—$

16.11 $—CF_2—CFCl—CF_2—CFCl—CF_2—CFCl—$

16.12 $H_2C{=}CHCN$

16.13 $—CH_2—\underset{\underset{\displaystyle CO_2CH_3}{|}}{CH}—CH_2—\underset{\underset{\displaystyle CO_2CH_3}{|}}{CH}—CH_2—\underset{\underset{\displaystyle CO_2CH_3}{|}}{CH}—$

16.14 $R—\overset{\overset{\displaystyle O}{\|}}{C}—O—O—\overset{\overset{\displaystyle O}{\|}}{C}—R \xrightarrow{\text{heat}} 2R\cdot + 2\ CO_2$ (initiation)

$R\cdot + CH_2{=}CHCH_3 \longrightarrow RCH_2—\dot{C}HCH_3$

$RCH_2\dot{C}HCH_3 + H_2C{=}CHCH_3 \longrightarrow RCH_2\underset{\underset{\displaystyle CH_3}{|}}{C}HCH_2\underset{\underset{\displaystyle CH_3}{|}}{\dot{C}H}$ (propagation)

$R[CH_2\underset{\underset{\displaystyle CH_3}{|}}{C}H]_{n+1}\dot{C}HCH_3 + R\cdot \longrightarrow R[CH_2\underset{\underset{\displaystyle CH_3}{|}}{C}H]_{n+1}\overset{\overset{\displaystyle R}{|}}{C}HCH_3$ (termination)

16.15

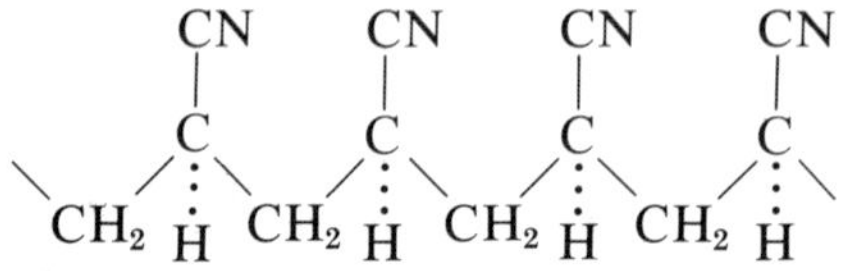

16.16 $HOOC(CH_2)_6COOH$ and $H_2N(CH_2)_6NH_2$

16.17 $HOOC(CH_2)_3COOH + H_2NCH_2CH_2NH_2 \longrightarrow$

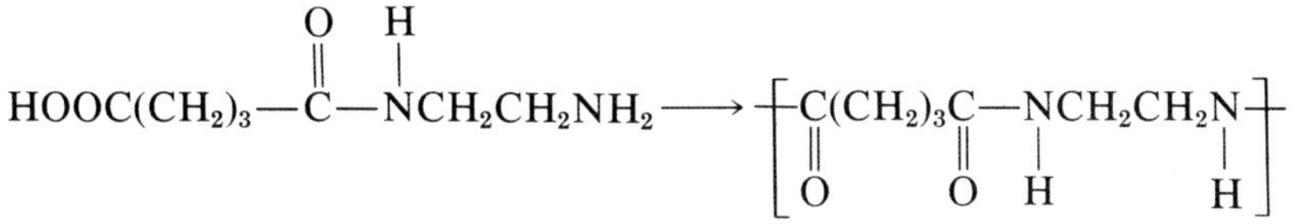

$$HOOC(CH_2)_3-\overset{\overset{\displaystyle O}{\|}}{C}-\overset{\overset{\displaystyle H}{|}}{N}CH_2CH_2NH_2 \longrightarrow \left[C(CH_2)_3\overset{\overset{\displaystyle O}{\|}}{C}-\overset{\overset{\displaystyle H}{|}}{N}CH_2CH_2\overset{\overset{\displaystyle H}{|}}{N} \right]$$

16.18 amide $\left(-\overset{\overset{\displaystyle O}{\|}}{C}-\overset{\overset{\displaystyle H}{|}}{N}- \right)$

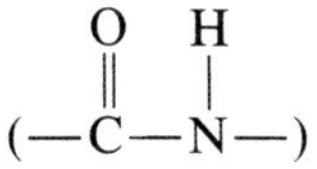

16.19 (b) and (c) contain difunctional monomers; in (a) the monomers can react to form an ester group, but the initial reaction cannot proceed any farther.

16.20

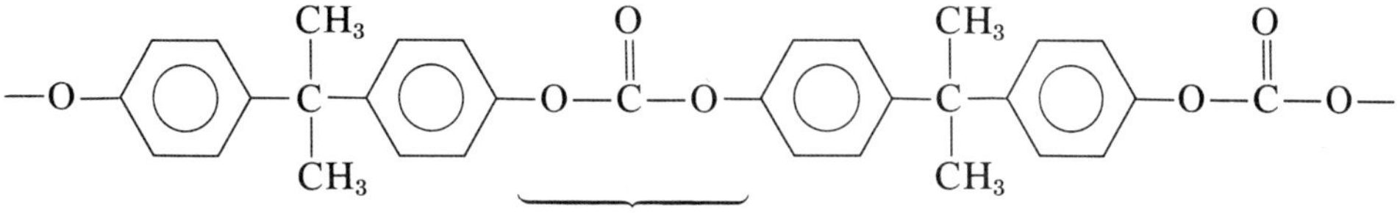

carbonate
group

16.21 $H_2N(CH_2)_3COOH$ or $O{=}C(CH_2)_3NH$

16.22 The acid and alcohol groups can form a polyester condensation polymer; the third acid group can serve as a cross-linking group between the polymer strands.

16.23 Thermosetting polymers undergo a permanent change when melted and cannot be remelted; thermoplastic polymers can be softened without any permanent change and can be remelted and reformed many times.

16.24

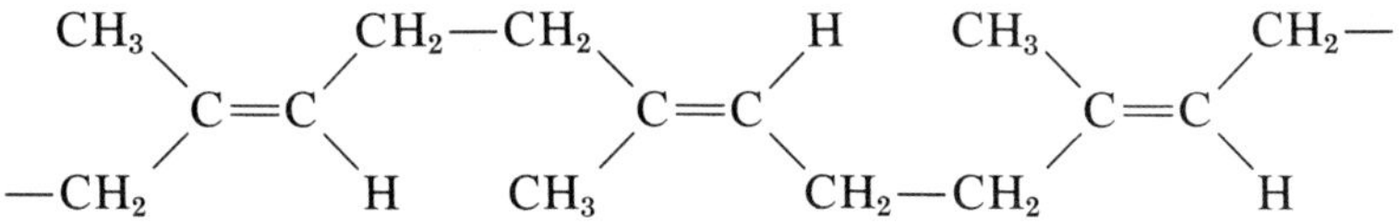

16.25 The plasticizer molecules fit into the spaces between the polymer strands and reduce the attractive forces between the strands, thus increasing the flexibility of the polymer.

CHAPTER SEVENTEEN SELF-CHECKS

17.1 Example:

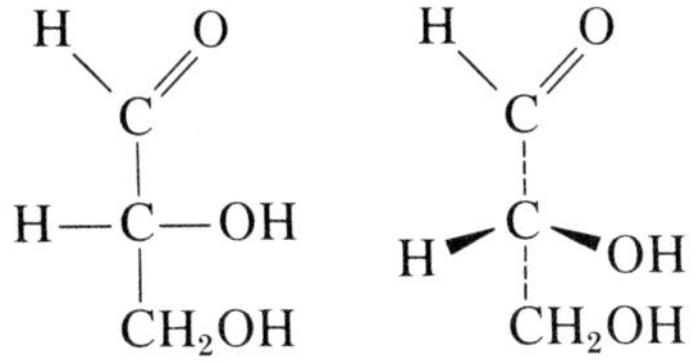

17.2

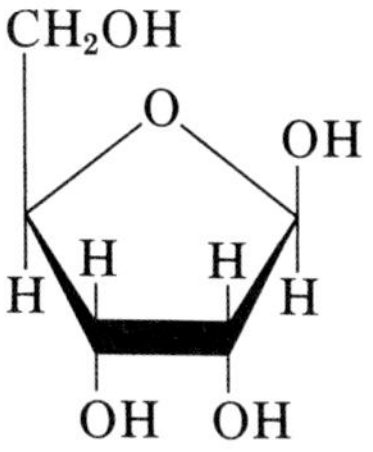

a   a pentose
b   beta
c   monosaccharide

d

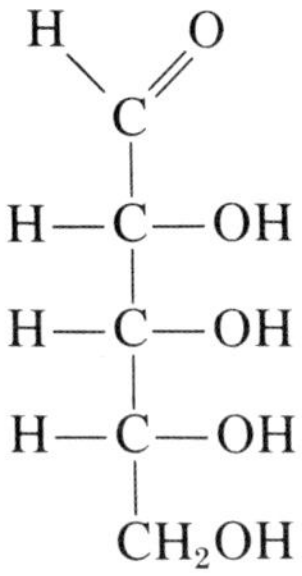

e   aldose

17.3

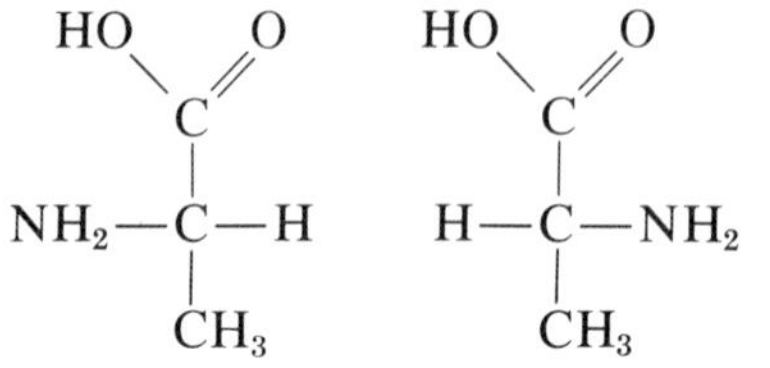

L form   D form

alanine

mirror images cannot be superimposed on each other; structural arrangement differs on the next-to-last carbon; the NH_2 group either on the left (L form) or right (D form); only the L form is used by the body to build proteins

17.4

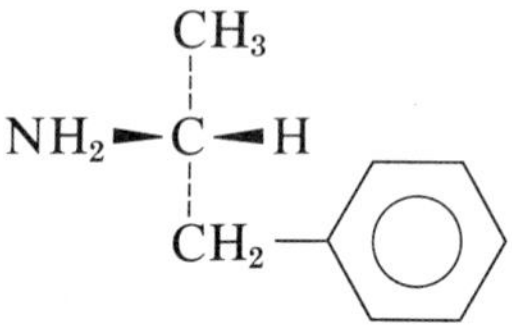

17.5   molecules (b) and (e)

17.6   The solution of L-mannose would rotate the plane of polarized light in a polarimeter; the racemic mixture would not.

17.7   The body can only use the D form of glucose; the student would not gain Calories or raw materials.

17.8   The carbonyl groups in the open-chain form are readily oxidized.

17.9   It forms hydrogen peroxide, which can be converted into a colored compound; the intensity of the color is proportional to the amount of glucose present.

17.10

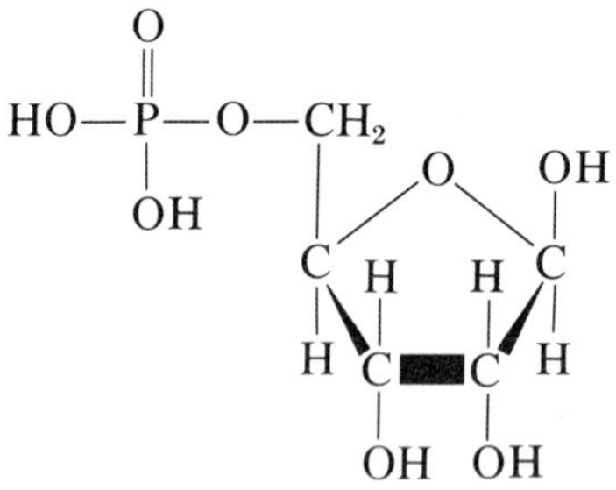

17.11

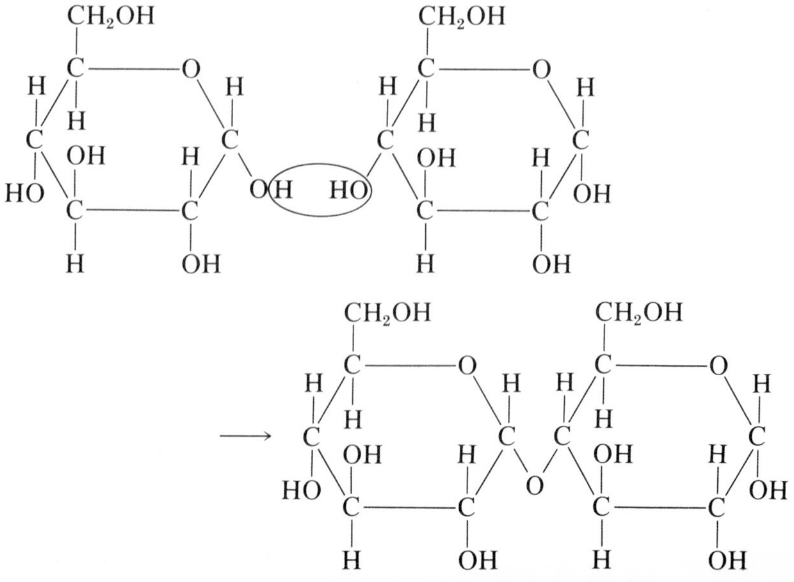

17.12 Each contains an aldehyde group that is not tied up in an acetal linkage.

17.13 starch and glycogen

17.14 **a** amylose   **b** cellulose

CHAPTER SEVENTEEN QUESTIONS AND PROBLEMS

17.15 Glyceraldehyde is an aldose and triose; dihydroxyacetone is a ketose and triose.

17.16

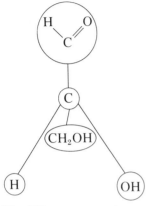

17.17 The OH group on carbon 1 in the Haworth structure (Figure 17–2) is below the ring.

17.18

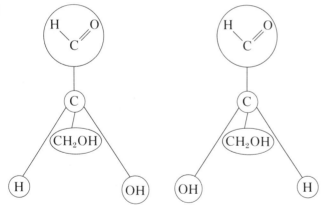

D-glyceraldehyde   L-glyceraldehyde

17.19 In a solution, each rotates the plane of polarized light either to the right or left.

17.20 It contains an equal mixture of D and L forms, and the L form tastes sweet to most people.

17.21 the open-chain isomer

17.22

17.23

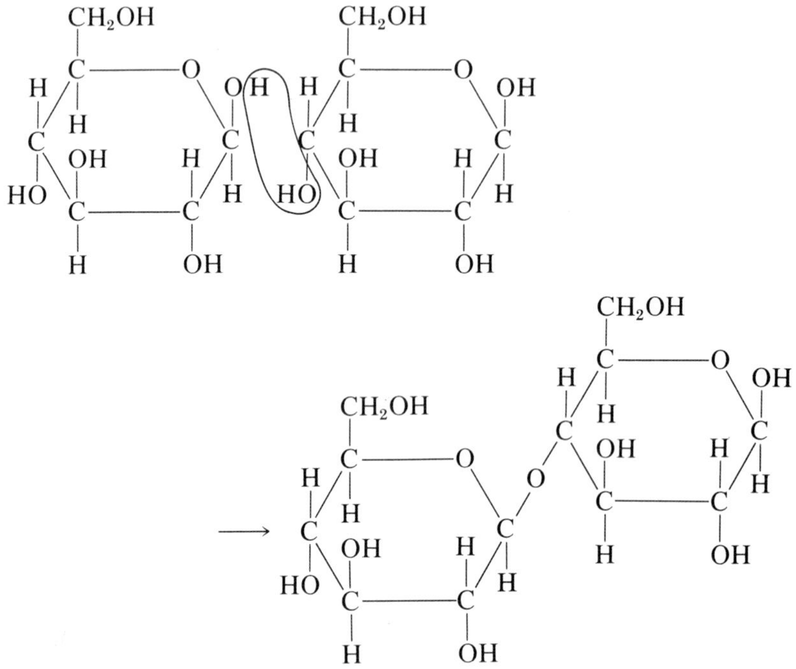

17.24

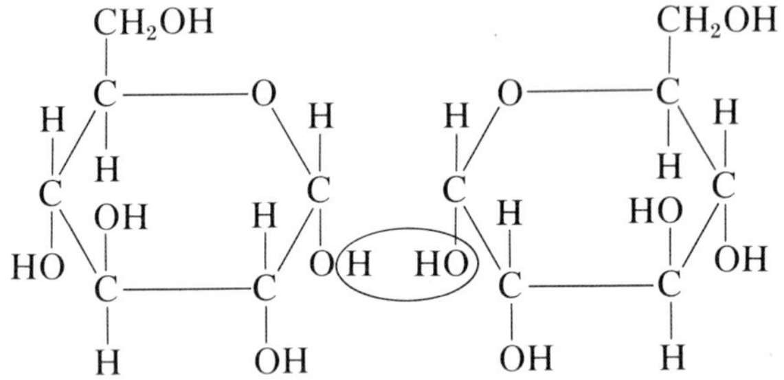

Join the α OH's on carbon 1 and split out a molecule of water; no aldehyde groups in the hemiacetal form remain to reduce Benedict's solution.

17.25 One is an amylose compound made up of a continuous chain of glucose monomers joined with C-1-alpha linkages; the other is amylopectin, a branched-chain polymer of glucose with both C-1-alpha and alpha-1,6 linkages.

17.26 They differ in the kind of linkage between glucose units: C-1-alpha in starch and C-1-beta in cellulose.

CHAPTER EIGHTEEN SELF-CHECKS

18.1 $CH_3(CH_2)_6CH{=}CH(CH_2)_6COOH$ is one possible answer.

18.2 A fat is an ester of fatty acids and glycerol; a wax is an ester of fatty acids and a high-molecular-weight monohydroxy alcohol.

18.3 Compared with solid fats, oils and margarine are high in unsaturated fatty acids.

18.4 Both types of hydrolysis produce glycerol; fatty acids result from acid hydrolysis; salts of fatty acids or soap are produced from base hydrolysis.

18.5 A cerebroside contains an amino alcohol and a carbohydrate not present in a fat.

18.6 A membrane involved in facilitated diffusion—for example, of glucose— would contain a greater proportion of protein.

18.7 It consists of a steroid ring system with an OH on carbon 3, unsaturation between carbons 5 and 6, methyl groups on carbons 18 and 19 and a hydrocarbon chain starting with carbon 20.

18.8 It has a similar ring system and a methyl group on carbon 19; it differs by having an alternate-double-bond ring, with an OH on carbon 3, no methyl group on carbon 18, and a carbonyl group (C=O) on carbon 20.

CHAPTER EIGHTEEN QUESTIONS AND PROBLEMS

18.9
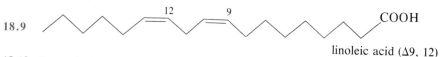
linoleic acid (Δ9, 12)

18.10 Instead of glycerol in a fat, a wax contains a 24 to 36 carbon atom monohydroxy alcohol.

18.11 cholesterol

18.12 to produce soap; the base used in saponification produces a salt of the fatty acid, such as sodium stearate.

18.13 A phospholipid is soluble in both lipid and water (head and tail portions).

18.14 They are involved in the diffusion of water-soluble molecules across the membrane and the facilitated diffusion of substances such as glucose into the cell.

18.15 Yes, it has the same ring system, plus side groups.

18.16 the OH on carbon 3, methyl groups on carbons 18 and 19, and a hydrocarbon chain on carbon 20

CHAPTER NINETEEN SELF-CHECKS

19.1 [See Table 19-1 to check your answers.]

19.2 CH_2—COO^- The zwitterion form is isoelectric since it has an equal number
  | of + and − charges; the pH at which only the zwitterion exists
  NH_3^+ is called the isoelectric point.

19.3 If a drop of solution of a mixture of amino acids is placed on a strip of filter paper and the paper is dipped into a mixture of solvents, the solvent moves upward, carrying the amino acids to different positions on the paper; by using a sample of known amino acids for comparison, each amino acid can be identified by its position.

19.4
$$CH_2-\overset{\overset{\textstyle O}{\|}}{C}-N-CH_2-\overset{\overset{\textstyle O}{\|}}{C}-N-CH-COOH$$
 | | | |
 NH_2 H   H CH_3

glycylglycylalanine

19.5

gives an example

19.6 Each molecule of an individual protein has the same amino acid sequence characteristic of that protein.

19.7 The two disulfide groups that connect the two polypeptide chains are essential for the biological action of insulin; the third affects the geometry of one chain.

19.8 long polypeptide chains of amino acids joined by peptide bonds

19.9 The α helix is a three-dimensional structure; the hydrogen-bonds are not all in the same plane as in the pleated sheet structure.

19.10 Salt linkages would be on the surface (they require extra charges found in acidic or basic amino acids); hydrophobic attractions occur in the interior; disulfide bonds could occur any place in the molecule where cysteine residues are on nearby polypeptide chains.

19.11 The acetic acid in vinegar is not dissociated enough to affect the protein; stock nitric acid denatures and precipitates skin proteins.

19.12 Have them swallow milk or an egg white solution to precipitate the mercury salt; then give an emetic to induce vomiting to remove the mercury from the body.

CHAPTER NINETEEN QUESTIONS AND PROBLEMS

19.13 amino acid molecules

19.14 The formula should be that of lysine, arginine, or histidine.

19.15 the pH at which the amino acid in solution has an equal number of + and − charges

19.16 Add a drop of known tyrosine solution to the paper and carry it through the exact procedure; the spots should move to the same position on the paper.

19.17 two peptide linkages

19.18 four alpha carbons, four carbonyl carbons, and four amino nitrogens

19.19 Yes; it would contain three peptide linkages; any number over two linkages will give a positive test.

19.20 cysteine

19.21

19.22 Polar amino acid residues are found mainly on the surface (where they interact with polar water molecules); nonpolar amino acid residues are mainly inside the globular structure.

19.23 Covalent bonds may be formed between two cysteine residues; salt linkages are formed between acidic and basic amino acid units.

19.24 A 70 per cent solution of alcohol kills any bacteria on the skin and prevents an infection.

19.25 A visible precipitate would be formed by the addition of mercury(II) chloride or of a solution of tungstic acid; or color tests may be used.

CHAPTER TWENTY SELF-CHECKS

20.1 Nucleus, mitochondria, Golgi apparatus, ribosome, lysosome, and endoplasmic reticulum; synthesis of such proteins occurs on the ribosomes of the rough endoplasmic reticulum.

20.2 They produce energy for the cell and the tissues.

20.3 Deoxyribose, phosphoric acid, adenine, guanine, cytosine, and thymine; RNA would yield ribose instead of deoxyribose and uracil instead of thymine.

20.4 esterification reactions using three molecules of phosphoric acid for each molecule of adenosine

20.5 The base pairs are adenine and thymine (A—T) and guanine and cytosine (G—C).

20.6 hydrogen-bonding between the base pairs A—T and G—C

20.7 DNA, nucleoside triphosphates, and the enzyme RNA polymerase

20.8 The m-RNA is a single long polynucleotide strand, whereas the t-RNA molecule is folded into a cloverleaf shape as a result of hydrogen-bonding; also, m-RNA is larger than t-RNA.

20.9 They are attached to a t-RNA that has a specific anticodon that combines with a codon on m-RNA to attach the amino acid in the proper sequence to a growing polypeptide chain on a ribosome.

20.10 Only random polypeptide chains would then be formed; t-RNA and m-RNA are required to form specific proteins with exact amino acid sequences.

20.11 The codons UUU and UUC on m-RNA would fit anticodons AAA and AAG on t-RNA to add phenylalanine to a growing peptide chain.

CHAPTER TWENTY QUESTIONS AND PROBLEMS

20.12 [See Figure 20–2.]

20.13 Mitochondria produce energy from glucose; ribosomes are involved in the synthesis of proteins.

20.14 The R in RNA stands for "ribo," as in ribose.

20.15 adenine and ribose

20.16 The five-carbon sugar is attached to the individual bases; the phosphoric acid joins the sugar molecules together to form the chain.

20.17 To make a complete double helix of DNA, equal numbers of hydrogen-bonded pairs of A—T and G—C are required.

20.18 m-RNA, r-RNA, and t-RNA molecules with many different sequences

20.19 t-RNA; carries individual amino acids onto the m-RNA

20.20 tryptophan; codon is UGG

20.21 It connects by pairing bases, anticodon sequence to codon sequence on m-RNA.

20.22 It codes for methionine and initiates (starts) the formation of the polypeptide chain.

CHAPTER TWENTY-ONE SELF-CHECKS

21.1 **a** 0.250 kg Al × +75 K × 0.21 kcal/kg-K = +3.9 kcal
b 0.0500 kg O_2 × −30 K × 0.219 kcal/kg-K = −0.329 kcal
c 0.454 kg NaCl × +124 kcal/kg = +56.3 kcal (fusion)
d 5.00 × 10^{-4} kg Hg × −71 kcal/kg = −0.0355 kcal (condensation)
e 1.00 g CH_4 × (1 mole/16.0 g) × −213 kcal/mole = −13.3 kcal (combustion)
f 30.0 g $C_{15}H_{31}COOH$ × (1 mole/256 g) × −2385 kcal/mole = −279 kcal

21.2 Turn around the equation for burning acetic acid and add it to the first:

$$C_2H_5OH_{(\ell)} + 3\ O_{2(g)} \longrightarrow 2\ CO_{2(g)} + 3\ H_2O_{(\ell)} \qquad \Delta H = -327\ \text{kcal}$$
$$\underline{2\ CO_{2(g)} + 2\ H_2O_{(\ell)} \longrightarrow CH_3COOH_{(\ell)} + 2\ O_{2(g)} \qquad \Delta H = +209\ \text{kcal}}$$
$$C_2H_5OH_{(\ell)} + O_{2(g)} \longrightarrow CH_3COOH_{(\ell)} + H_2O_{(\ell)} \qquad \Delta H = -118\ \text{kcal}$$

Since water, O_2, and CO_2 appear on both sides of the equation, eliminate extra molecules equally on both sides to reach the final form.

21.3   in hot coffee; a greater amount of heat is available to break up the crystals; heat is considered a reactant in this equation (Le Chatelier's Principle)

21.4   protein: 2.5 g × 4.0 kcal/g = 10 kcal; fat: 0.8 g × 9.0 kcal/g = 7.2 kcal; carbohydrate: 12 g × 4.0 kcal/g = 48 kcal; total: 65 kcal = 65 Calories

21.5   Exposed skin can more easily radiate heat, evaporate sweat, and allow air to carry away heat by convection, all of which help cool the body; ordinary exercise produces less heat than metabolic processes.

21.6   Process (b)—boiling—is endothermic but happens naturally at 100°C only because the gas molecules can diffuse to fill the volume available; the other two processes give off heat (exothermic).

21.7   The reaction converting graphite to diamonds is nonspontaneous in nature; if we wait long enough, the reverse reaction (diamond to graphite) will happen, since it is spontaneous (however, the time involved might be quite great, so we continue to wear and use diamonds).

21.8   The molecules may not have had the proper orientation in space (proper position to break bonds), and so only a "glancing" collision occurred.

21.9   Refer to Figure 21–9: going from C + D to A + B is an endothermic process since A + B have more energy; this process requires more activation energy to reach the top of the "hill" (needing E_a + P.E.) than does the reverse process starting with A + B, which needs only E_a.

21.10 Refer to Figure 21–10: at lower temperatures, fewer molecules have high enough collision energies to overcome E_a, so fewer collisions each second can result in formation of products.

21.11 Your graph should be the *reverse* of Figure 21–12; the catalyst lowers the activation energy in both directions.

21.12 Digestive enzymes are needed to make the rate of hydrolysis of food materials high enough to serve the nutritional needs of the body; in the absence of such enzymes, foods would decompose quite slowly.

CHAPTER TWENTY-ONE QUESTIONS AND PROBLEMS

21.13 0.255 kg acetone × +25 K × 0.51 kcal/kg-K = +3.25 kcal

21.14 0.500 kg iron × ΔT × 0.106 kcal/kg-K = +2.81 kcal, so $\Delta T = \dfrac{2.81}{0.053} =$ +53 K, then 23°C + 53 = 76°C

21.15 1000 kg × +49 kcal/kg = +4.9 × 10⁴ kcal (fusion of copper)

21.16 2.00 kg × −80 kcal/kg = −160 kcal for freezing of water

21.17 0.200 kg naphthalene × ΔH_{fus} = +7.20 kcal; $\Delta H_{fus} = \dfrac{7.20}{0.200}$ = +36 kcal/kg

21.18 As the liquid water freezes, it releases heat (the heat of fusion), which serves to keep the grape vines slightly warmer than if the water were not there.

21.19 Silver filling, with low specific heat, heats up much faster.

21.20 There are two processes to calculate:
cooling copper (ℓ and s) from 1550°C to 25°C; $\Delta T = -1525$ K
0.150 kg Cu $\times -1525$ K $\times$ 0.092 kcal/kg-K $= -21.0$ kcal
then freezing copper at 1083°C: 0.150 kg $\times -49$ kcal/kg $= -7.35$ kcal
adding together, $-21.0 - 7.35 = -28.4$ kcal in all for ΔH

21.21 $C_3H_{8(g)} + 5\ O_{2(g)} \rightarrow 3\ CO_{2(g)} + 4\ H_2O_{(\ell)} + $ heat

21.22 3.45 kg propane $\times \dfrac{1 \text{ mole}}{0.0440 \text{ kg}} \times \dfrac{-531 \text{ kcal}}{\text{mole}} = -4.16 \times 10^4$ kcal

21.23 8 hr $\times \dfrac{60 \text{ min}}{\text{hour}} \times 25.0 \text{ kg} \times \dfrac{5 \times 10^{-7} \text{ mole ATP}}{\text{kg muscle-minute}} \times \dfrac{-9.0 \text{ kcal}}{\text{mole ATP}} = -0.054$ kcal
(this is only the heat output for the ATP-to-ADP conversion, not the total heat produced by muscle action)

21.24 20 g carbohydrate $\times$ 4.0 kcal/g = 80 kcal; 0.3 g protein $\times$ 4.0 kcal/g = 1.2 kcal; 0.8 g fat $\times$ 9.0 kcal/g = 7.2 kcal; total = 88.4 kcal = 88 Calories

21.25 50 kcal $\times$ 1 g carbohydrate/4.0 kcal = 12.5 g carbohydrate

21.26 Some of the hydrogen is already combined with oxygen (in —OH groups) in the carbohydrate molecule, whereas in fats, more of the hydrogen is bonded to carbon and remains to be oxidized; carbohydrates also contain a higher percentage (by weight) of oxygen, which does not contribute to the heat output on combustion.

21.27 Evaporation of water from the skin requires heat energy, which comes from the skin surface and thus helps to cool the skin; sweating under conditions of 100% humidity is, in fact, not cooling at all!

21.28 The extra heat produced inside the body by exercise requires greater cooling, and so the body responds by providing sweat.

21.29 Exercise uses up some of the energy (Calories) available to the body for use or storage, and thus reduces the "unused" amount of energy that is kept in fat depots; however, limitations on food consumption have a more dramatic effect on body weight.

21.30 the amount of energy required to maintain life in a resting person

21.31 spontaneous above 77°C, nonspontaneous below 77°C, equilibrium at 77°C

21.32 **a** spontaneous   **b** nonspontaneous   **c** equilibrium

21.33 **a** minus   **b** plus   **c** zero

21.34 **a** negative   **b** positive   **c** positive

21.35 The overall process has a negative ΔG ($+61.6 - 74.18 = -12.6$), so would be spontaneous; that does *not* mean that the process would necessarily work efficiently or at a high enough rate to be useful.

21.36 wrong position of colliding atoms to form activated complex

21.37 [See Figure 21–8.]

21.38 more molecules have adequate energy to break bonds; see Figure 21–10

21.39 [See Figure 21–12.]

21.40 to speed up metabolic reactions

21.41 an enzyme that catalyzes the hydrolysis of a carbohydrate into simple sugars

CHAPTER TWENTY-TWO SELF-CHECKS

22.1 The cell cannot use heat as does an electrical power plant because the cell must operate at a constant temperature and pressure.

22.2 AMP + $H_2O \rightarrow$ adenosine + H_3PO_4, $\Delta G_h = -2.2$ kcal/mole; the energy stored in AMP is released on hydrolysis to adenosine and H_3PO_4.

22.3 The reaction will *not* occur spontaneously; the cell reaction could be written A + B $\rightarrow$ C, $\Delta G = +2.0$ kcal/mole; since ATP $\rightarrow$ ADP + H_3PO_4, $\Delta G_h = -7.3$ kcal/mole by coupling: ATP + A + B $\rightarrow$ ADP + C + H_3PO_4, $\Delta G = -5.3$ kcal/mole, which would make the cell reaction work.

22.4 no, because that would represent a reverse flow of phosphate group transfer *up* Table 22-1; it would also require the formation of a higher energy compound, creatine phosphate, from ADP

22.5 1,3-diphosphoglycerate; it would liberate less energy than ATP $(11.8 + 2.4 = 14.2$ kcal/mole)

22.6 Glucose is changed to fructose 1,6-diphosphate, which is split into two molecules of glyceraldehyde phosphate, each of which produces one pyruvate.

22.7 The molecular weight of glucose equals 180 amu, and so 1.00 gram equals $\frac{1}{180}$, or 0.00555, moles; produces $2 \times 0.00555 = 0.0111$ mole of ATP or $0.0111 \times 6.02 \times 10^{23}$ equals 6.69×10^{21} molecules of ATP; an equal number, 6.69×10^{21}, of energy carrier NADH molecules are produced.

22.8 The nicotinamide portion of the molecule is reduced with a shift of double bonds, hydrogenation of the top carbon in the ring, and the release of H^+.

22.9 a cofactor, usually an organic molecular group bound to the enzyme protein, that is essential to the activity of the enzyme

22.10 Glycolysis occurs in the cytoplasm; it is followed by the Krebs cycle in the mitochondria; energy carriers feed into the electron transport chain in the mitochondria.

22.11 The "priming" is a complex reaction in which the pyruvate from glycolysis reacts with coenzyme A and NAD^+ to form acetyl coenzyme A + NADH + CO_2.

22.12 In the Krebs cycle NAD^+ and FAD are converted into NADH and $FADH_2$ molecules, which feed into the electron transport chain where the ATP molecules are formed.

23.13 to provide an adequate supply of this essential nutrient or to prevent oxidation the six-carbon citrate eventually to four-carbon oxaloacetate so that it can recycle through the Krebs cycle.

22.14 It is a key compound because it originally reacts with acetyl coenzyme A (from pyruvate) to start the cycle and is then recycled.

22.15 In the electron transport chain NADH loses H atoms while being oxidized to NAD^+ by a flavoprotein.

22.16 Cytochrome c is a protein bound to heme, which contains a central iron atom; the iron atom is readily reduced from a $3+$ to a $2+$ form, a property important in the electron transport chain.

22.17 The reversible change from a $3+$ to $2+$ iron in the cytochrome molecules is essential for the normal action of electron transport.

22.18 Coenzyme Q is a special transfer molecule that carries electrons from flavoprotein to the first cytochrome in the electron transport chain.

22.19 $FADH_2$ enters the electron transport chain after the flavoprotein step, which has already produced a molecule of ATP from NADH.

22.20 Both processes take place in the mitochondria, which can thus process energy carriers much more efficiently than in the cytoplasm.

CHAPTER TWENTY-TWO QUESTIONS AND PROBLEMS

22.21

$$HO—\overset{\overset{O}{\|}}{\underset{\underset{OH}{|}}{P}}—O—\overset{\overset{O}{\|}}{\underset{\underset{OH}{|}}{P}}—OH$$

22.22 It stores more energy and releases more energy on hydrolysis than a low-energy compound, due to phosphorus-oxygen bonds.

22.23 Glucose + fructose to form sucrose will not occur spontaneously unless glucose is coupled with ATP → ADP to drive the reaction to completion.

22.24 no, because the ATP → ADP system provides only −7.3 kcal/mole, which would not overcome the +8.9 kcal/mole to make the reaction work

22.25 It serves as the middle agent, or "broker," in many cell reactions by coupling with energy-producing systems and systems that need energy to work in the cell.

22.26 conversion of glucose to glucose-6-PO_4 and conversion of glucose-6-PO_4 to fructose 1,6-di-PO_4; the two reactions require two ATP molecules

22.27 two molecules of ATP for each pyruvate formed in these steps

22.28 From Figure 22–4 it can be seen that ADP is the left-hand portion of the NAD^+ structure.

22.29 Our cells rely mostly on glucose as a source of energy, and the process of glycolysis converts glucose into pyruvate, which enters the energy-producing Krebs cycle.

22.30 An active acetyl group must be formed from pyruvate to combine with oxaloacetate and start the cycle.

22.31 in reaction 6 while α-keto glutarate is converted to succinate

22.32 the five-carbon compound α-ketoglutarate

22.33 the formation of acetyl coenzyme A from pyruvate

22.34 They feed into the electron transport system at either the flavoprotein or the coenzyme Q stage.

22.35 Two ATP molecules are formed.

22.36 A quinone structure is reduced to a hydroquinone structure in coenzyme Q, but iron 3+ is reduced to iron 2+ in cytochrome.

22.37 The NADH first reduces a flavoprotein molecule, with the production of one ATP molecule; the $FADH_2$ enters the system at the next step to reduce coenzyme Q; then they both send electrons through the cytochromes to produce two ATP molecules (NADH → 3ATP, $FADH_2$ → 2ATP).

CHAPTER TWENTY-THREE SELF-CHECKS

23.1 Inorganic catalysts do not increase reaction rate nearly as much as the enzymes, which are "tailored" to fit biological substrates.

23.2 The shape of an enzyme (at its active site) must exactly fit the three-dimensional geometric structure of a substrate before it can show enzymatic activity.

23.3 It would have a high value of K_m, indicating that the enzyme can gain and lose a substrate molecule very rapidly.

23.4 It works best in a basic medium; it would not work in the acid contents of the stomach but would in the small intestine (basic medium).

23.5   Like all chemical processes, body reactions speed up with an increase of temperature up to about 50°C; above 50°C the enzyme proteins will become denatured and cause a decrease in activity.

23.6   A competitive inhibitor competes with the substrate molecules in forming the enzyme-substrate complex, thereby decreasing the activity of the enzyme; a noncompetitive inhibitor combines with some group at the active site of an enzyme, destroying its activity permanently.

23.7   It reacts with the —SH groups of enzymes, destroying their activity.

23.8   It resembles p-aminobenzoic acid (Figure 23–10), which is essential to the life of bacteria; by replacing this acid on the active site of the bacterial enzyme it inhibits enzyme activity and destroys the bacterium.

23.9   A proenzyme is a protein molecule that can react to form an active enzyme; a coenzyme is an organic molecule that is necessary as part of the enzyme for catalysis to occur.

23.10   The enzymes in the cells and tissues all act in an aqueous solution.

23.11   Niacin is associated with NAD^+, riboflavin with FAD, and pantothenic acid with coenzyme A.

23.12   Folic acid and vitamin B_{12} are used to treat anemia.

23.13   to provide an adequate supply of this essential nutrient or to prevent oxidation of the food

23.14   Their molecules contain long carbon chains or steroid rings, which are fat-soluble but not water-soluble.

23.15   People who live on country farms absorb more sunshine daily than do people who live in urban ghettos, and this absorbed sunshine is used by the body in producing vitamin D.

23.16   a part of rhodopsin, the visual pigment of the eye; in the visual cycle, vitamin A is required to regenerate this pigment; the blood must have an adequate supply of this vitamin

23.17   There is no experimental evidence that taking vitamin E will increase sex drive.

CHAPTER TWENTY-THREE QUESTIONS AND PROBLEMS

23.18   Enzymes are protein molecules whose shapes are determined by the sequence of amino acids in the polypeptide chain; they have active sites in definite positions on the chain.

23.19   The protein structure of an enzyme may be folded in such a way that it exactly fits the geometric structure of only a single substrate.

23.20   The active site on an enzyme consists of amino acids in the proper position to fit the shape of the substrate and to combine with it to form an active intermediate complex.

23.21   It equals one half the concentration of substrate required to reach maximum activity in an enzyme reaction.

23.22   The pH of most cell contents ranges between 7.2 and 7.6.

23.23   a reduction in reaction rate

23.24   Cyanide rapidly reacts with the iron atom in cytochrome c and effectively shuts off the electron transport system of the cells and stops their respiration.

23.25   As one example: Sulfanilamide is a competitive inhibitor that competes with p-aminobenzoic acid for the active site of bacterial enzymes, thus decreasing the action of the enzymes; this can kill the bacteria; if large amounts of p-aminobenzoic acid are added to the system, it replaces sulfanilamide on the active site and the bacteria live.

23.26   Proenzymes are not active; if some active digestive enzymes were formed by a gland, they could digest the protein structure of the gland and destroy it.

23.27   One type is a metal cation, such as Zn^{2+}, which serves as an essential cofactor for the activity of the enzyme; a coenzyme is a small organic molecule like NAD^+ that is essential for the action of several enzymes.

23.28   It is an essential component of the structure of the coenzymes NAD^+ and $NADP^+$.

23.29   Pantothenic acid is part of coenzyme A (acetyl coenzyme A in the Krebs cycle).

23.30   It is an essential part of the visual cycle in the eye and also functions to maintain the health of mucous membranes in the ear, nose, throat, and sex glands.

23.31   Children develop rickets, which leads to poor bone and tooth formation.

23.32   It is needed for the proper clotting of blood because it is used in the synthesis of prothrombin.

CHAPTER TWENTY-FOUR SELF-CHECKS

24.1   **a** white blood cells   **b** red blood cells   **c** plasma proteins, especially albumin

24.2   They probably inject an anticoagulant into the cattle blood before feeding.

24.3   It decreases the oncotic pressure and the ability to pull water into the capillaries from the interstitial space; therefore more water would move into the interstitial spaces, causing edema.

24.4   A diabetic not being treated with insulin would develop acidosis; a major symptom would be hyperventilation to excrete the extra CO_2 that is formed.

24.5   Acidosis causes a decrease in the oxygen-carrying ability of hemoglobin (see Figure 24–10).

24.6   The O_2 is carried mainly as oxyhemoglobin in the red blood cells; the CO_2 is carried mainly as bicarbonate in the plasma and the red blood cells.

24.7   An enzyme, carbonic anhydrase, which converts CO_2 to bicarbonate, is located only in the red blood cells.

24.8   It carries oxygen to the tissues; the excess base combines with carbonic acid in the tissues to form bicarbonate to carry CO_2 back to the lungs with little change in pH (isohydric).

24.9   It stores oxygen in the muscles for use during muscular activity and carries oxygen inside cells to evenly distribute oxygen in all areas of the cell.

24.10   The Cl^- shifts to accommodate the movement of HCO_3^- both in the tissues and in the lungs to balance electrical charge.

24.11   The kidneys will respond by excreting the excess NaCl in the urine; they will also excrete an excess of water needed to dilute the salt and so the urine volume will increase (see also Self-Check 14.11).

24.12   This may result from a kidney disease called nephritis or in the later stages of problem pregnancies (toxemia of pregnancy).

24.13   by the process of urine acidification, exchanging Na^+ for H^+ across the tubule walls

24.14   The Group 1 cation is K^+, and the Group 2 cation is Mg^{2+}.

CHAPTER TWENTY-FOUR QUESTIONS AND PROBLEMS

24.15 erythrocytes (red blood cells) and leucocytes; erythrocytes carry oxygen and serve as blood buffers, and leucocytes (white blood cells) fight infection

24.16 a decrease in plasma protein concentration or an increase in blood pressure (which forces water out into the tissues)

24.17 Blood clotting efficiency would be decreased since Ca^{2+} ions are essential for clotting, so clotting time would increase.

24.18 the fluid or blood pressure exerted by the action of the heart

24.19 By losing gastric acid from the body, the child would develop a condition of alkalosis and the blood pH would rise above 7.4.

24.20 The P_{O_2} of the lungs results in the taking up of O_2 by hemoglobin, which carries the O_2 to the tissues in the form of basic oxyhemoglobin.

24.21 It decreases the ability of hemoglobin to carry oxygen and results in an increased release of oxygen to the body cells.

24.22 Both forms are essential for buffering action in the cells; basic oxyhemoglobin carries O_2 and base to the tissues, and acidic oxyhemoglobin neutralizes bicarbonate in the lungs to form CO_2 for excretion.

24.23 from the plasma into the cells to allow HCO_3^- to move into the plasma

24.24 to have an immediate supply in case of rapid muscle activity

24.25 Only about 1% of the O_2 and 8% of the CO_2 carried by the blood is dissolved in the plasma; without hemoglobin, O_2 and CO_2 transport would be greatly impaired.

24.26 The kidney will excrete a larger volume of urine and electrolytes will be lost from the plasma; also, temporary edema of the tissues will occur.

24.27 Continuous alcohol intake may have made the kidney cells more permeable to protein or produced a type of nephritis.

24.28 Paper test strips with bromphenol blue on their surface are used to test for protein.

24.29 They would excrete the excess base from the body as bicarbonate to adjust the pH of the plasma.

24.30 It will be abnormal, with accumulation of fluid in the blood and tissues and occurrence of edema.

24.31 The anions of the plasma are mainly Cl^- and HCO_3^-, versus HPO_4^{2-} and protein anions in the cytoplasm.

24.32 It is necessary for the movement of CO_2 from the tissues to the lungs for excretion and to maintain the proper pH.

24.33 We would have to drink an extra 8.2 liters of fluid each day (Table 24–7).

CHAPTER TWENTY-FIVE SELF-CHECKS

25.1 Anabolism is the process that synthesizes complex molecules from simple nutrients, whereas catabolism is a breaking-down process that converts large molecules to small molecules and energy.

25.2 It liquifies the food by mixing it with gastric juice and starts the digestion of proteins.

25.3 acetyl coenzyme A

25.4 Yes, there is a mild hyperglycemia after a meal containing carbohydrates; eating several candy bars will also produce hyperglycemia.

25.5 Excessive amounts of insulin remove glucose from the blood and produce the *condition* of hypoglycemia (not a disease).

25.6 insulin; there is no other hormone that can take its place

25.7 The liver contains an enzyme required to convert glycogen to glucose; this enzyme is not present in muscle tissue, and so muscle glycogen does not yield glucose.

25.8 Glycogenesis is the conversion of glucose to glycogen (blood sugar to liver glycogen); gluconeogenesis means "the formation of new glucose," which occurs in the liver and uses amino acids and glycerol as source.

25.9 Resting muscles can obtain most of their energy from the oxidation of fatty acids; actively working muscles also obtain energy from glucose.

25.10 The lactic acid returns to the liver, where it enters the Cori cycle, being changed into glucose by gluconeogenesis; this glucose can enter the blood and be used for energy by the muscle, or it can be converted into liver glycogen.

25.11 The metabolism of the brain requires glucose as its major fuel and therefore is dependent on a normal glucose level.

25.12 Photosynthesis forms glucose and O_2 from CO_2 and H_2O.

CHAPTER TWENTY-FIVE QUESTIONS AND PROBLEMS

25.13 The large complex food molecules must be broken down to smaller molecules that can be used by the body.

25.14 It produces pyruvate, which forms acetyl coenzyme A, a key compound in anabolism.

25.15 mostly storage of glucose as glycogen or fat and oxidation by the tissues to produce energy

25.16 The pancreas produces less insulin than is required for normal glycogen formation and oxidation of glucose by the tissues.

25.17 epinephrine secreted by the adrenal gland; in emotional situations extra epinephrine is secreted, causing breakdown of liver glycogen with the liberation of glucose that produces hyperglycemia

25.18 During periods of fasting the glycogen content decreases so that after breakfast more glycogen is formed, which decreases until lunch, when it builds up again and then drops until dinner, which usually stores the largest amount of liver glycogen; high-carbohydrate meals build up glycogen; long periods of fasting decrease the amount stored.

25.19 Glucose-6-PO_4 is formed from glucose to start the process of glycogenesis by being converted to glucose-1-PO_4.

25.20 production of lactic acid, which causes fatigue and an oxygen lack

25.21 glucose is required for brain metabolism and the formation of ATP

25.22 Although the alternate pathways do oxidize glucose, the main purpose is to form the coenzyme NADPH used in the metabolism of other foodstuffs, such as fatty acids.

25.23 No; our carbohydrate supply and that of animals whose meat we consume would disappear; without the O_2 added by plants to the air, respiration would stop.

CHAPTER TWENTY-SIX SELF-CHECKS

26.1 fats, phospholipids, and cholesterol

26.2 Lipase splits away the outer two fatty acids from a triglyceride, leaving a monoglyceride with the fatty acid on the central carbon atom of glycerol.

26.3   By being converted into lipoproteins, they can be transported in a more water-soluble form.

26.4   pyruvate and acetyl coenzyme A

26.5   Pyruvate formed in the cytoplasm by glycolysis moves into the mitochondria and forms acetyl coenzyme A; when not needed in the Krebs cycle the coenzyme migrates back into the cytoplasm to form fatty acids.

26.6   Yes; fat that yields the same energy as ATP is only one fifth the mass of a comparable glycogen storage unit.

26.7   may have inadequate cushioning around vital organs (to protect against a blow) and would be less able to stand prolonged periods without eating

26.8   The activated form of glycerol is glycerol-3-PO_4, a key compound in glycolysis.

26.9   essential constituents of cell membranes; form lipoproteins for lipid transport; essential components of the blood clotting mechanism

26.10   from three molecules of acetyl coenzyme A

26.11   You have a normal blood cholesterol level.

26.12   Change the diet by reducing the intake of fat and perhaps by substituting unsaturated fats for animal fats; if a smoker, cut down on cigarettes and drink lesser amounts of caffeine-containing beverages.

26.13   Instead of acetic acid, the key compound in the oxidation scheme is acetyl coenzyme A.

26.14   They feed into the Krebs cycle to produce energy in the form of ATP.

26.15   Yes; they are normally formed from acetoacetyl CoA, an intermediate in the beta-oxidation of fatty acids; acetoacetic acid formed in this reaction is converted to acetone or β-hydroxybutyric acid in the liver.

26.16   It can be formed from acetoacetyl CoA or from the condensation of two molecules of acetyl CoA, which is converted to acetoacetic acid by a liver enzyme.

26.17   They are neutralized by the bicarbonate buffer and may be excreted as carboxylate anions or as ammonium compounds formed by the kidney.

CHAPTER TWENTY-SIX QUESTIONS AND PROBLEMS

26.18   The fat molecules are converted into a water-based emulsion by the action of bile salts.

26.19   They can be acted on directly by lipase without the assistance of bile salts.

26.20   They increase in concentration and the level is then returned to normal by processes of storage, oxidation, and excretion.

26.21   Pyruvate formed in the cytoplasm can move into the mitochondria and be converted to acetyl coenzyme A, which then moves back into the cytoplasm for fatty acid synthesis.

26.22   acetoacetyl coenzyme A

26.23   It has more fat (90 per cent) and higher density than connective tissue but has a similar blood supply and network of nerves.

26.24   Hunger pangs would probably wake the animal long before its normal hibernation period was over.

26.25   It combines with two fatty acid coenzyme A derivatives to form a diglyceride phosphate as a step in the synthesis; it is formed from dihydroxyacetone-PO_4.

26.26   they share some common reactions; dihydroxyacetone-PO_4 forming glycerol-3-PO_4 and two fatty acid coenzyme A molecules plus glycerol-3-PO_4 forming diglyceride phosphate

26.27 It uses acetyl coenzyme A, with three molecules forming mevalonic acid.

26.28 Cholesterol plaques that become deposited in the arterial walls, especially in the aorta and arteries of the heart, may lead to arteriosclerosis (hardening of the arteries) and circulatory problems that end in coronary heart disease; a high intake of animal fats, excessive weight, smoking, and high caffeine intake may be among the factors in heart disease.

26.29 The glycerol forms glycerophosphate and dihydroxyacetone phosphate, two compounds that can proceed through the Embden-Meyerhof pathway of glycolysis.

26.30 β-oxidation means that the fatty acid molecules are oxidized on the beta carbon (second carbon from the carboxyl group) with the splitting off of two-carbon fragments.

26.31 coenzyme A, FAD, and NAD^+

26.32 It is a ketone rather than a keto acid.

26.33 It is involved in the synthesis of fatty acids on the way to the formation of butyryl coenzyme A; it is also formed in the complete oxidation of a fatty acid like palmitic as two-carbon fragments are split off on the way to form the last molecule of acetyl coenzyme A that feeds into the Krebs cycle.

26.34 by starvation the body would oxidize more fatty acids for energy, producing more acetoacetic acid; by feeding a diet high in fat and low in carbohydrates

CHAPTER TWENTY-SEVEN SELF-CHECKS

27.1 in the amino acid pool; from food protein (digestion and absorption) and tissue proteins (breakdown)

27.2 a gradual decrease in muscle protein that would be noticed after several months; without the amino acid pool, the muscle would not be able to regain all the lost protein

27.3 Yes; corn is an incomplete protein lacking the essential amino acid lysine; failure to develop and grow normally would result.

27.4 It was probably caused by a diet inadequate in complete proteins; by measuring food nitrogen intake (on the child's regular diet) and nitrogen output, a negative balance would be established; the cure would be feeding adequate amounts of good-quality proteins to support growth.

27.5 You would develop diabetes mellitus with hyperglycemia and glycosuria and require injections of insulin to regain normal metabolism.

27.6 It is involved in the two essential reactions of amino acid catabolism: transamination and oxidative deamination.

27.7 transaminase and glutamate dehydrogenase

27.8 NAD^+ and FAD

27.9 Glutamic acid is formed from ammonia and α-ketoglutaric acid and then transfers its amino group by transamination to a keto acid to form a new amino acid.

27.10 One enters the cycle in carbamyl phosphate; the other enters in the form of aspartic acid.

27.11 Yes, it starts the cycle by combining with carbamyl phosphate and formed again when urea is split off arginine to be recycled.

27.12 Ammonia formed in the liver combines with glutamic acid to form glutamine, which is carried to the kidneys and converted into ammonia by the enzyme glutaminase.

27.13 purines, pyrimidines, ribose, deoxyribose, phosphoric acid, and proteins

27.14 Painful conditions develop as a result of the deposit of uric acid crystals in the joints; the possible "advantage" is increased drive and ambition that accompany gout.

27.15 Homeostasis means that all essential constituents of the blood are maintained at a fairly constant normal concentration; from Figure 25–6 it is seen that organs such as the liver and kidney, the intestines, fat and muscle tissue, and many hormones act in concert to maintain blood glucose level.

CHAPTER TWENTY-SEVEN QUESTIONS AND PROBLEMS

27.16 They enter the temporary amino acid pool, where they can be used for synthesis of proteins or be broken down by catabolism to provide energy.

27.17 pepsin, trypsin, and polypeptidase (best answers)

27.18 arginine, methionine, histidine, phenylalanine, isoleucine, threonine, leucine, tryptophan, lysine, and valine

27.19 Students generally eat a diet fairly high in protein, which supplies an adequate amount of essential amino acids; they have also completed most of their growth.

27.20 Insulin is synthesized in the cell as proinsulin, an inactive form stored in granules; the insulin is not activated until the granules move to the cell membrane.

27.21 pyruvic acid

27.22 oxidative deamination; glutamic acid gives up its NH_2 group to form NH_4^+ and α-ketoglutaric acid

27.23 by transamination

27.24 taking the normal end product NH_4^+ and reacting it with α-ketoglutaric acid to form glutamic acid, which transfers its amino group by transamination to a keto acid to form a new amino acid

27.25 carbamyl phosphate

27.26 They are not found in food proteins but only in the liver, where they are used in the urea cycle.

27.27 Glutamine is used to form ammonia in the kidney; in diabetic acidosis more acidic molecules (ketone bodies) must be neutralized and excreted; ammonia is used to save Na^+ from the increased amount of acids, and therefore more glutamine is required to form the ammonia.

27.28 a nucleotidase

27.29 Insoluble crystals of uric acid may collect in the joints, causing the painful condition of gout.

27.30 Uricase could convert uric acid to allantoin, a more soluble compound that can be excreted in the urine.

27.31 The synthesis of pyrimidines in the body starts with the combining of carbamyl phosphate with aspartic acid.

CHAPTER TWENTY-EIGHT SELF-CHECKS

28.1 Both processes involve the unraveling of the DNA strands and the use of one strand as a template for joining together nucleic acid units in the proper sequence; after translation, the DNA recoils into its original form, but after replication the two original DNA strands have separated, each with a new complementary partner strand; different polymerase enzymes are needed and different products (m-RNA and daughter DNA) are made.

28.2   any two sources of ionizing radiation; or chemical damage from sources like ozone, benzo(a)pyrene, or LSD; or mechanical damage in cell division

28.3   If the fetal cells can be examined to find the defect, thorough chemical tests, chromosome observation, or other methods, then amniocentesis may lead to positive diagnosis of diseases such as Tay-Sachs and sickle cell anemia.

28.4   Addition or subtraction of a base, if inside a genetic code, will throw every codon off by one letter and generate a useless protein; if one base is simply substituted for another, it may have serious effects (as in some types of hemoglobin defects, such as sickle cell anemia) or may pass unnoticed, especially since there are several different codons that can result in the *same* amino acid residue.

28.5   A virus has no organelles (nucleus, ribosomes, mitochondria) and thus cannot carry out metabolic processes or synthesize proteins (or replicate) except through the use of cell machinery; there are many chemical substances that are only found in cells, not in viruses.

28.6   Cancer cells cause damage by dividing in a rapid and uncontrolled manner; a chemical that prevents or slows cell division may slow the cancer; a chemical that kills cells, but is more lethal to dividing cells than to normal cells, may also be effective.

28.7   A memory-increasing drug may have value in cases of amnesia, in helping psychotherapists discover hidden traumas that patients have forgotten, or perhaps in helping professionals and students remember what they want to remember; possible disadvantages are that such a drug might raise false expectations, flood the mind with details which are not useful and which interfere with the ''search'' for what we really want to remember or force us to recall events we might prefer to forget.

28.8   In spite of all precautions, a mutant form of *E. coli* bacteria might be released to cause an uncontrolled epidemic, especially since the normal *E. coli* is ''at home'' in the human gastrointestinal tract.

CHAPTER TWENTY-EIGHT QUESTIONS AND PROBLEMS

28.9   during cell division (mitosis)

28.10   deoxyribose, phosphoric acids, and the proper bases

28.11   not using presently understood methods; only a diploid (46-chromosome) cell contains all of the basic genetic information; a haploid cell contains only half of the information

28.12   The pregnancy would have to be carried to term by a substitute mother. (Test-tube babies do *not* mature in a test tube; they are only conceived there.)

28.13   ionizing radiation; chemical interference with replication (as from ozone)

28.14   The mutation may have *first* arisen in one of the two germ cells that produced the child.

28.15   Some amniotic fluid is withdrawn by amniocentesis, and fetal cell chromosomes are mapped and inspected to see if there is an extra chromosome.

28.16   A blood sample from the potential parent is deoxygenated; if some cells sickle, then the faulty gene is present.

28.17   A Tay-Sachs diagnosis is traumatic because the child is doomed to an early death; albinism is a relatively minor defect.

28.18   Both diseases are hereditary, and family histories have long been used to predict the chance of disease.

28.19   No; a virus is not a cell but simply nucleic acid with a protein coat; no.

28.20   Cells quickly produce interferon which blocks virus use of host cell ribosomes; antibodies enter bloodstream to fight viral attack.

28.21   The latent virus may incorporate its DNA into the genes of the host cell and viral DNA will then be replicated with that of the host. At some future time the viral DNA may be triggered into activity.

28.22   Proteins on surface of normal cells signal cell to stop dividing when in contact with other cells. Cancer cells keep dividing in an uncontrolled manner.

28.23   Cancerous cells may metastasize to other tissues and organs, spreading the cancer.

28.24   The viral DNA may be "hidden" within chromosomes of the host cell.

28.25   Cortisone suppresses the body's natural immune system which defends tissues against cancerous cells.

28.26   The genetic tendency to develop lung cancer is not equally present in every smoker; it takes a long period for cancer to develop, perhaps by weakening of the immune system, and the period may vary for different people.

28.27   by blood tests for proteins produced by cancer cells

28.28   Gamma rays are used to kill cancer cells, since they are most lethal to cells that are dividing rapidly.

28.29   Cancer cells divide frequently; the agent might be able to block the growth of a tumor, while having much less effect on normal tissues.

28.30   It will be incorporated into the DNA or RNA of rapidly-dividing cells, and will disrupt the genetic code, since it is chemically different from the "natural" base.

28.31   no, only held in remission in some cases

28.32   Many diabetics rely on daily, expensive, insulin injections; bacteria offer some promise of providing much cheaper insulin in a form closer to the natural human hormone.

28.33   No, since DNA produces proteins; vitamins are not proteins.

28.34   to break the DNA strand; yes, since repair of cell DNA occurs naturally

28.35   to reduce the possibility of an epidemic caused by release of a mutant strain of bacterium

28.36   A normal gene for the missing enzyme might be spliced into the DNA of fetal cells.

Working with Numbers— A Brief Review

As you have seen in most chapters of this text, much chemical work involves *measurement* of mass, volume, concentrations, pH, pressure, or temperature. Since the results of these measurements are numbers, we must often be able to do simple calculations with them. These computations rarely involve more than simple addition, subtraction, multiplication, or division.

The purpose of this appendix is to make sure you have the tools, both mental and physical, which *you* need to handle the numbers of chemistry.

We have divided these into six parts:

B.1.   The rules of arithmetic, including powers, roots, and logs
B.2.   Scientific notation, using powers of ten
B.3.   The electronic calculator, how to use one to advantage
B.4.   Significant digits and precision, how many digits to keep
B.5.   Percent and parts per million, how to calculate them
B.6.   Reading a graph, if you do not yet know how

None of these skills are difficult. All are needed, at some time or other, to understand scientific results. The ability to work with numbers should be combined with the techniques for setting up and solving the problems presented at various points in your course.

Before we go into the skills of arithmetic, one final word about "solving problems." The most important skill of all is the ability to use common sense. If someone told you that a newborn baby weighed 3.5 grams, you should be able to recognize this as nonsense. A baby is more likely to weigh 3.5 *kilo*grams! The ability to see that a given "measured result" is wrong but another "makes sense" comes from your own experience with the world around you, not from the numbers themselves.

If you encounter any difficulty in setting up and solving problems of any type, ask yourself the following questions:

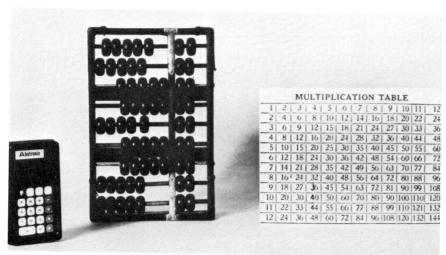

MULTIPLICATION TABLE											
1	2	3	4	5	6	7	8	9	10	11	12
2	4	6	8	10	12	14	16	18	20	22	24
3	6	9	12	15	18	21	24	27	30	33	36
4	8	12	16	20	24	28	32	36	40	44	48
5	10	15	20	25	30	35	40	45	50	55	60
6	12	18	24	30	36	42	48	54	60	66	72
7	14	21	28	35	42	49	56	63	70	77	84
8	16	24	32	40	48	56	64	72	80	88	96
9	18	27	36	45	54	63	72	81	90	99	108
10	20	30	40	50	60	70	80	90	100	110	120
11	22	33	44	55	66	77	88	99	110	121	132
12	24	36	48	60	72	84	96	108	120	132	144

What *information* is given in the problem?

What should be the *units* of the final answer?

From my knowledge of the world, what kind of number would be *reasonable* for the final answer?

Can I draw a *picture* of the problem situation and reach some conclusions?

You may find that one of these four questions provides a key that leads to the solution of the problem. Each numerical answer should also be *checked* to make sure it makes sense.

B.1. THE RULES OF ARITHMETIC

If you feel very comfortable with arithmetic, you probably do not need this review. However, and especially if English is a second language for you, it may be useful to review the words and symbols we use to show the operations of addition, subtraction, multiplication, division, grouping, raising to a power, taking a root, and, for some students, finding a common logarithm.

Addition   symbol: +

EXAMPLE: $1 + 6 = 7$ "One plus six equals seven."

EXAMPLE: $-13 + 9 = -4$ "Minus thirteen plus nine equals minus four."   or   "Negative thirteen plus positive nine equals negative four."

Subtraction   symbol: −

EXAMPLE: $5 - 2 = 3$ "Five minus two equals three."

EXAMPLE: $25 - 72 = -47$ "Twenty-five minus seventy-two equals negative forty-seven."

EXAMPLE: $-33 - 59 = -92$

EXAMPLE: $-27 - (-47) = -27 + 47 = +20$

When you *subtract* a *negative* number, the two minus signs cancel out and the effect is to add a positive number.

Multiplication   symbol: ×   or   ·   or   ( )( )

EXAMPLE: $5 \times 6 = 30$ "Five times six equals thirty."

EXAMPLE: $5 \times -6 = -30$

EXAMPLE: $-5 \times 6 = -30$

EXAMPLE: $-5 \times -6 = +30$

Each number that is being multiplied is called a *factor*. If there is one negative factor, the answer to the multiplication will be negative. If there are two negative factors, then their minus signs cancel out and the answer is positive, since $(-1) \times (-1) = +1$.

EXAMPLE: $33 \cdot -79 = -2607$

EXAMPLE: $-73.5 \times -22.7 = +1668.45$

EXAMPLE: $(0.079)(342) = 27.018$

Division symbol: a/b or $a \div b$ or $\dfrac{a}{b}$

EXAMPLE: $36/6 = 6$ "Thirty-six divided by six equals six."

EXAMPLE: $-36/6 = -6$

EXAMPLE: $(-36) \div (-6) = +6$

EXAMPLE: $144 \div -12 = -12$

EXAMPLE: $\dfrac{17 + 8}{-3 - 2} = \dfrac{+25}{-5} = -5$

The answer to a division problem with negative numbers will be negative or positive on exactly the same basis as described for multiplication.

EXAMPLE: $-9/4 = -2.25$

EXAMPLE: $23/11 = 2.090909 \ldots$

The answer to an addition problem is often called the *sum,* that for a multiplication is the *product,* and the result for a division is the *quotient.*

Unlike addition, subtraction, or multiplication, division may lead to a continuing decimal, rather than an exact answer.

Grouping symbol: parentheses ( )

We use parentheses either to clarify which number is meant or to group numbers which should be handled together.

EXAMPLE:
NOT $+6 - -7 + -5 = +8$ BUT $(+6) - (-7) + (-5) = +8$

EXAMPLE: $3 \times 4 + 6 = ?$ is ambiguous. It is unclear which operation comes first. You must write

$$(3 \times 4) + 6 = 12 + 6 = 18$$

or

$$3 \times (4 + 6) = 3 \times 10 = 30$$

The same principle applies to writing chemical formulas such as $Ca_3(PO_4)_2$, as described at the beginning of Chapter 5.

You should use parentheses whenever needed to clarify what you are doing.

Raising to a power symbol: small superscript, as "b" in a^b

EXAMPLE: $2^2 = 4$ "Two to the power two equals four."
$2^2 = 2 \times 2 = 4$ "Two to the second power equals four."
"Two squared equals four."

EXAMPLE: $7^3 = 7 \times 7 \times 7 = 343$ "Seven to the third power equals three hundred and forty-three."

Raising to the third power is also called "cubing." Four cubed is 64.

> EXAMPLE: $(0.5)^6 = (0.5)(0.5)(0.5)(0.5)(0.5)(0.5) = 0.015625$
> or $(1/2)^6 = 1/2 \cdot 1/2 \cdot 1/2 \cdot 1/2 \cdot 1/2 \cdot 1/2 = 1/64 = 0.015625$

In its simplest form, raising a number to a positive power means multiplying the number by itself, using the number of factors shown in the power. The most useful power, or *exponent*, in science is the power of ten.

> EXAMPLE: $10^0 = 1$ $10^1 = 10$ $10^2 = 100$ $10^3 = 1000$ $10^6 = 1\ 000\ 000$

The power (exponent) of ten gives the number of zeros after the 1 in the answer: $10^{23} = 100\ 000\ 000\ 000\ 000\ 000\ 000\ 000$.

Use of a *negative* power means taking the *reciprocal* of a number, thus dividing the number into one: $a^{-b} = 1/a^b$.

> EXAMPLE: $5^{-1} = 1/5 = 0.2$ $2^{-2} = 1/2^2 = 1/4 = 0.25$ $10^{-3} = 1/1000 = 0.001$

Ten to a negative power gives the number of places to move the decimal point *to the left* from the number 1.00000. . . .

Taking a root (fractional power)   symbol: $\sqrt{}$ or $\sqrt[3]{}$ or a^b where b is not a whole number

> EXAMPLE: $\sqrt{49} = 49^{1/2} = 49^{0.5} = 7$ "The square root of forty-nine is seven." "Forty-nine to the one-half power is seven."
>
> EXAMPLE: $\sqrt[3]{729} = 729^{1/3} = 729^{0.333} = 9$
> "The cube root of seven hundred and twenty-nine is nine."
> "Seven hundred and twenty-nine to the one-third power is nine."
> "Seven hundred and twenty-nine to the 0.33333 . . . power is nine."

Roots are the most difficult operation in arithmetic. Luckily, we do not use them in this textbook, and you will rarely need them in most fields of science.

Logarithms   symbol for common logarithm: log or $\log_{10}$

The logarithm most commonly used in chemistry is the "common," or base-ten, logarithm, $\log_{10}$. It has a very important application in Chapter 13 on acidity. The logarithm of a number is simply the power to which ten must be raised to equal that number.

> EXAMPLE: Since $10^2 = 100$, $\log_{10} 100 = 2$
> Since $10^6 = 1\ 000\ 000$, $\log_{10} 1\ 000\ 000 = 6$
> Since $10^{-2} = 0.01$, $\log_{10} 0.01 = -2$
> Since $10^0 = 1$, $\log_{10} 1 = 0$

If you are already given a power of ten, you simply use that power as the logarithm.

> EXAMPLE: $\log_{10} 10^{-23} = -23$

Since pH $= -\log_{10}$(concentration of H$^+$), the pH is simply the negative of the power of ten of the molarity of hydrated H$^+$ ions, as discussed in Section 13.1 and shown in Table 13.2. For the most general applications, the logarithm is as simple as the above example.

If you must calculate a pH with one or two decimal places, such as pH $= 7.42$, this skill is provided in Section 14.2, which teaches you to perform the calculation using either a calculator or a two-place logarithm table, provided as Table 14–1.

If you are given a logarithm, the number that has that logarithm is known as the *anti*logarithm. Logarithms can be very handy in doing multiplication and division and in taking powers and roots. The "old" engineer's slide rule is based on this fact. However, electronic calculators are even handier, as we will discuss in Section B.3.

SELF-CHECK
EXERCISE B–1

Perform each of the following calculations in your head, and write down the answers on a sheet of paper. Then check your answers against those written upside down at the bottom of this box.

a) $7 + 94 = ?$

b) $-13 + 49 = ?$

c) $-27 - 57 = ?$

d) $(-3) - (-2) = ?$

e) $7 \times 8 = ?$

f) $6 \times -7 = ?$

g) $(3 - 5)(3) = ?$

h) $36 \div 12 = ?$

i) $96 \div -16 = ?$

j) $-42 \div -6 = ?$

k) $\dfrac{(-5 + 19)}{(9 - 2)} = ?$

l) $^1/_3 = ?$ (in decimal form)

m) $\sqrt{81} = ?$

n) $16^{1/4} = ?$

o) $5^2 = ?$

p) $2^{-3} = ?$

ANSWERS B–1

a) $+101$ b) $+36$ c) -84 d) -1 e) $+56$ f) -42

g) -6 h) $+3$ i) -6 j) $+7$ k) $14/7 = +2$

l) $0.3333 \cdots$ m) $+9$ (or -9)   n) $+2$ (or -2)

o) $+25$ p) $+0.125$

A calculator with a *log* key can be used to find common logarithms, and if there is a "10^x" key, the antilogarithm can be found. Do *not* confuse "log" with "ln," which is a different kind of function called a "natural logarithm."

B.2 SCIENTIFIC NOTATION

Quite early in this text, you encounter Avogadro's number: 6.02×10^{23}. We write the number in this fashion to save space, since it would be extremely awkward to write 602 000 000 000 000 000 000 000 each time we wished to convert molecules to moles. It would also be misleading with regard to the precision with which this number is known (Section B.4) to write it with 24 digits.

Since Avogadro's number can be written $6.02 \times$ 100 000 000 000 000 000 000 000, we compress the "power of ten" part of the number and write it 10^{23}. This shortened form is called "scientific notation." If you count, you will find 23 zeros after the number 1, as discussed in the previous section. The same is done for any very large number.

EXAMPLES: The speed of light is 2.998×10^8 meters/second.
The volume of the earth is 1.083×10^{12} cubic kilometers.
The estimated geological age of the oldest rocks is 3.6×10^9 years.

It may help to remember that "one million" is 10^6 and "one U.S. billion" is 10^9.

Given a very small number, we similarly use scientific notation. The mass of a proton could, in Table 2–5, have been written

one proton = 0.000 000 000 000 000 000 000 001 673 grams

However, this can also be written

$$1.673 \times 0.000\ 000\ 000\ 000\ 000\ 000\ 000\ 001 \text{ grams}$$

or

$$1.673 \times 10^{-24} \text{ grams}$$

When numbers are written in standard scientific, or *exponential*, notation, there is always one digit (1 through 9) to the left of the decimal point, and then a power of ten.

EXAMPLES: The charge on an electron is 1.60×10^{-19} coulombs.
The mass of an electron is 9.107×10^{-31} kilograms.
In Figure 24–1, we find that the normal blood level of thyroxine (thyroid gland hormone) is about 8 μg/dL, or 8×10^{-6} grams in 100 mL. The metric prefixes (mega, kilo, deca, centi, milli, etc.) given in Table 2–1 are all based on this type of exponential (power of ten) notation. One *pico*second is defined as 10^{-12} second.

When given a large number in the "long" (written-out) form, you convert it to scientific notation by counting how many digits you must move the decimal point to the *left* to obtain a standard number.

EXAMPLE: There are normally about 5 000 000 000 white blood cells in a liter of blood. Convert this to scientific notation.

$$5\ 000\ 000\ 000 = 5. \times 1\ 000\ 000\ 000. = 5. \times 10^9$$

9 digits

When given a small number in the "long" form, you convert it to scientific notation by counting how many digits you must move the decimal point to the *right*.

EXAMPLE: A cell membrane (Section 18.3) is approximately 0.000 000 008 meters thick. Convert this to scientific notation.

$$0.000\ 000\ 008 \text{ m} = 8. \times 0.000\ 000\ 001 = 8. \times 10^{-9}$$

9 digits

On occasion, you may have to multiply or divide two numbers written in exponential form. You then follow these rules:

When multiplying two powers of ten, you *add* the exponents.

EXAMPLE: $10^5 + 10^9 = 10^{5+9} = 10^{14}$
$10^{13} + 10^{-3} = 10^{13-3} = 10^{10}$

When dividing one power of ten by another power of ten, the simplest way to avoid errors is to take the denominator (under the line) and turn it around by finding its reciprocal. The reciprocal of $10^n = 10^{-n}$ and vice versa.

EXAMPLE: $\dfrac{10^7}{10^{-4}} = 10^7 \times \dfrac{1}{10^{-4}} = 10^7 \times 10^{+4} = 10^{7+4} = 10^{11}$

You are much less likely to add or subtract scientific numbers than to multiply and divide them. In fact, the *conversion-factor method* for solving problems, presented in Section 2.1, works only for multiplication and division.

However, if you should indeed have to add or subtract exponential numbers, avoid one common pitfall! Make sure the powers of ten of the two numbers are the *same*, and then keep the same power of ten in the answer.

EXAMPLE: One cubic millimeter of blood normally contains 5000 white blood cells and 5×10^6 red blood cells. How many cells are present in all? The wrong way! 5×10^3 white + 5×10^6 red = 10×10^9 cells in all?

A *million* red blood cells, which outnumber the white blood cells, can not possibly give a *billion* cells in all! This student has multiplied the powers of ten, instead of adding the two numbers together.
The right way! $5 \times 10^3 + 5 \times 10^6 = 0.005 \times 10^6 + 5 \times 10^6 = 5.005 \times 10^6$
OR, equally correct: $5 \times 10^3 + 5 \times 10^6 = 5 \times 10^3 + 5000 \times 10^3 = 5005 \times 10^3$
In these two cases, we correctly come up with five million and five thousand cells. As you will see in Section B.4, and as common sense will tell you, the correct answer is 5×10^6, or five million total cells, to the precision with which cells are counted in the blood.

SELF-CHECK
EXERCISE B–2

Convert each of the following numbers to correct scientific notation.

a) 96 494   (coulombs in one mole of electrons)
b) 1 067 500   (osmotic pressure of water in the blood stream, in mm Hg)
c) 0.000 005   (meters, farthest distance from a typical cell to the nearest capillary)

Convert each of the following numbers from scientific to long form.

d) 7.5×10^{13} (approximate number of cells in the human body)
e) 1.0×10^{-7} (cm, diameter of a sucrose molecule)

ANSWERS B–2:
a) 9.6494×10^4 Keep all digits, please!
b) $1.067\ 500 \times 10^6$ mm Hg
c) 5×10^{-6} m
d) $75\ 000\ 000\ 000\ 000$ cells
e) $0.000\ 000\ 1$ cm

B.3 THE ELECTRONIC CALCULATOR

The arithmetic operations of Section B.1 can all be done most easily with a hand-held electronic calculator, although the easiest of these operations can be done in your head. These calculators dropped in price and rose in reliability during the 1970's, and so the models for the 1980's offer good value and excellent capabilities.

Type of calculator

You should estimate how much calculation will be required of you in this course, and also what will be expected in other courses. If your program does not involve much mathematics and physics, you will probably do best by purchasing a very simple calculator in the $10 to $20 range. Such a calculator should be able to add, subtract, multiply, and divide and should preferably have a memory. It will suffice for the kinds of calculations needed for this text, and any calculations involving multiplication and division of powers of ten may be done by the methods shown in Section B.2.

If you expect to do considerably more calculating, then you should consider a "scientific" calculator in the $20 to $35 range, which can work with numbers from 1×10^{-99} to $1 \times 10^{+99}$ (look for a button marked "EE" or "EXP") and can calculate logarithms directly (see if it has a button marked "LOG" and preferably one marked "10^x" for antilogs).

Even more powerful calculators, with several memories, statistical functions, and programming ability, are available. Although these are very useful for engineers, they are probably too complex and too expensive for your purposes, since you are unlikely to use more than a fraction of their capabilities. Always also consider the possibility of loss or theft, and what that would do to your budget planning.

For either the simple calculator or a scientific version, we would strongly recommend obtaining one with a liquid-crystal display (LCD) rather than one with a light-emitting diode (LED). The LCD uses small amounts of current to change the color of bits of material, so that the batteries last a long time. If you purchase an LED type, you are more likely to find yourself in a panic in the middle of an exam, exclaiming "My battery just ran out!"

It is wise for every *student who uses a calculator in a test to have a spare set of batteries* immediately *available!*

Checking the operation of the calculator

After you purchase your calculator, go through the instruction manual and be sure you understand how to use the basic keys. Remember to turn your calculator off each time after using it!

When a calculator is first turned on, an easy way to check that it is working properly is to press the following keys: $\boxed{1}\boxed{.}\boxed{1}\boxed{1}\boxed{1}\boxed{1}\boxed{1}\boxed{1}\boxed{1}$ so that this number (1.1111111) appears in the display. Then square it. Your calculator should read "1.23456789" or "1.2345679," depending on how many digits are shown in the display.

Simple operations

Your instruction manual will tell you how to add, subtract, multiply, and divide two numbers. Be sure you know how to do these things. You will use these operations 99% of the time you use your calculator. Then branch out into "chain" operations, where three or four numbers are involved.

Scientific notation on a calculator

Most calculators work in the manner described here. A few, especially those made by Hewlett-Packard, use a different kind of logic and require different (but just as efficient) procedures.

If you have a simple calculator, skip this paragraph. Given a number such as "6.02×10^{23}", you will simply punch the "6.02" into the calculator and separately, using pencil and paper, determine the power of ten of the answer.

If your calculator has scientific capabilities, it has a key marked "EE" or "EXP." You can then punch in Avogadro's number by pushing the following keys: $\boxed{6}\boxed{.}\boxed{0}\boxed{2}\boxed{EE}\boxed{2}\boxed{3}$

Remember that EE or EXP means "times ten to the power ____." Do *not* go the route of pressing $\boxed{6}\ \boxed{.}\ \boxed{0}\ \boxed{2}\ \boxed{\times}\ \boxed{1}\ \boxed{0}\ \boxed{\text{EE}}\ \boxed{2}\ \boxed{3}$, since that will give you a number ten times as high as you want.

Digits to keep

A calculator gives you a false sense of precision. By pressing only a few keys, you can obtain an answer with eight or nine digits! Pretty good? Not really. The answer is only as good as the data fed into the calculator. The other digits are meaningless, as we will discuss further in Section B.4. The computer experts have a saying for this: "Garbage in? Garbage out!"

SELF-CHECK
EXERCISE B–3

Perform the following arithmetic operations using the same methods *you plan to use throughout the school year in this course. If you are using a calculator, write down all of the digits you get at this stage. We will discuss how to round off results in the next section. Your answer should agree with those given upside down, at least up to the final one or two digits.*

a) $3.069 + 93.87 = ?$

b) $5.797 - 19.87 = ?$

c) $0.2304 \times 6.375 = ?$

d) $1.481 \div 4.397 = ?$

e) $11^3 = ?$

f) $\dfrac{(-3.124 - 9.985)}{(1.508)(410.83)} = ?$

g) $(3.769 \times 10^{-7})(6.02 \times 10^{23}) = ?$

h) $\dfrac{(7.854 \times 10^{-10})}{(9.22 \times 10^{-6})} = ?$

And now try this one, which cannot *be completed on your calculator.*

i) $\dfrac{(1.025 \times 10^{37})(4.433 \times 10^{29})}{(1.236 \times 10^{-36})}$

i) $3.676\ 233\ 8 \times 10^{-37+29+36} = 3.676\ 233\ 8 \times 10^{102}$
h) $8.518\ 438\ 2 \times 10^{-5}$ g) $2.268\ 938 \times 10^{17}$ f) $-2.115\ 953\ 3 \times 10^{-2}$
e) 1331 f) $-0.021\ 159\ 533$ or
a) 96.939 b) -14.073 c) 1.4688 d) $0.336\ 820\ 56$ or

ANSWERS B–3

> Some calculators have a way to set the number of digits in the displayed answer. **If yours does, set it to show the maximum number of digits.**

B.4 SIGNIFICANT DIGITS AND PRECISION

Scientists use two different kinds of numbers. An *exact* number is known to be "right on." There is no question about its value.

EXAMPLES: The following are *exact* numbers:
A normal person has *two* ears   (2.000 000 000 000 . . .)
A cube has *eight* corners   (8.000 000 000 000 . . .)
A kilometer contains *1000* meters (1000.000 000 000 . . .)
A cubic centimeter is *0.001* liter   (0.001 000 000 000 . . .)

The first two examples are exact because we are counting something that is *well* known. A count of the red blood cells in one cubic millimeter of your blood is *not* exact because it will vary from one sample to another, and from one time of day to another. A count of the number of floors in Chicago's Sears Tower (110 stories) is exact, although the height of that building (443 meters) is *not* exact.

The second two examples are exact because the measurements are *defined* relative to each other. In the same way, there are *exactly* 12 inches in one foot, *exactly* 5280 feet in one statute mile, and *exactly* $60 \times 60 \times 24 = 86\ 400$ seconds in one day.

You can perform any kinds of calculations on exact numbers, and obtain more exact numbers. There are *exactly* $12 \times 5280 = 63\ 360$ inches in one mile.

MEASURED NUMBERS

Any number value that must be obtained by measurement is, by its very nature, an inexact number. The time of a swimmer crossing the finish line, the weight of a person, the distance from the earth to the moon—these are all measured quantities with a measurement error that may be estimated.

Consider the iron rod being measured in Figure B–1. There is certainly "an exact length" of that iron rod, but no one will ever be in a position to tell us what it is. Instead, we must use some kind of ruler or measuring apparatus to estimate its length. Assuming the ruler is accurate, the iron rod could be estimated to be 2.53 units long.

Is that *exactly* 2.53 units? What do you estimate, as you look at Figure B–1? It might really be 2.52 units. We just cannot be sure whether that final digit is correct, or is perhaps one number off.

Now you can understand what scientists mean when they say, as on p. 24 of Section 2.1:

If the quantity has been measured, the last digit written down is considered to be uncertain.

Another way of saying the same thing is, "Human ability to measure the real world is limited; thus there is a limit to the number of meaningful digits we can use to express such a measurement." The height of the Sears Tower reported in an almanac is 443 meters. It is highly unlikely that we know the measurement much better than that. There would certainly be no point in using the number "443.000 000 meters" in a calculation.

SIGNIFICANT DIGITS IN CALCULATIONS

The *precision* of a measurement tells you two things. It gives you first some information about how carefully a measuring instrument is calibrated and how closely it can be read. In Figure B–1, as in all types of direct-reading instruments, you should be able to read to one tenth of one marked division. Since the ruler is marked at each 0.1 division, we should be able to estimate a length within 0.01 unit, which is one tenth of the distance between 2.5 and 2.6 units. A reading of 2.53 units expresses this, since the last digit (the 0.01-place digit) is uncertain.

Second, the precision of a measurement tells you how *repeatable* that value should be. If five different people look at Figure B–1, they should all agree that the length is between 2.5 and 2.6 units. There might be disagreement on the next digit, the uncertain digit.

Whenever we take any kind of measurement, there is error involved. You cannot look at a result and know what kind of error should be attached to it unless you are familiar with the measuring instrument: the ruler, balance, thermometer, or apparatus. We must count on the person who took the measurement to tell us what errors might be involved. We therefore report any measurement we take in such a

FIGURE B–1 Measurement of length. Estimate the length of the iron rod shown, using the units given on the ruler. You are expected to write down an answer which is precise to one tenth of one ruler division.

If you use data provided by measurements taken by another person, you are assuming that person to be honest and knowledgeable about the apparatus. A scientist takes great pains to build a reputation for carrying out experiments by the *scientific method*, so that other workers will trust his or her results.

way that the last digit is understood to be uncertain. The number of digits in a measured value, including this uncertain digit, tells you the number of *significant digits*.

Multiplication and division

The use of significant digits becomes important when we make calculations that use measured values. For example, suppose we have measured the length of the iron rod in Figure B–1 to be 2.53 centimeters. Suppose its diameter is measured to be 0.22 centimeters. We can look up the formula for the volume of a cylinder, $V = \pi d^2 h/4$. If we work this calculation on an electronic calculator, we obtain:

$$(3.141\ 592\ 7)(0.22)(0.22)(2.53)/4 = 0.096\ 173\ 576\ cm^3$$

By this point, you certainly realize that to keep so many figures in the answer would be absurd. How many significant digits have we written? Not ten. The two zeros in the answer serve only to tell us where to start writing numbers. They are *not* significant digits. We can see this if we write the above answer in scientific notation: $9.617\ 357\ 6 \times 10^{-2}$. Now it is clear that there are eight significant digits.

But should there be eight? No! If we look at the numbers in the problem, the *least precise* value is 0.22 cm, the diameter of the rod. That has *two* significant digits.

Remember the following rule:

In multiplication and division, an answer contains no more significant digits than the least number of significant digits used in the operation.

Our answer to this problem should thus have *two* digits, just as many as in our least precise measurement. We must round off 0.096 173 576 from eight digits to two digits. To do this, we follow the rule (on p. 25):

If the digits *after* the uncertain digit are . . . 499 999 . . . or less, drop them. If the digits *after* the uncertain digit are . . . 500 000 . . . or more, raise the uncertain digit by one, and drop the rest.

The result for the previous calculation would be an answer of 0.096 cm³.

EXAMPLE: Let us round the following measured numbers to *three* significant digits.
a) 973.89 **b)** 0.092 75 **c)** 43.009 **d)** 3.783 99 × 10⁵
ANSWERS: **a)** 974 **b)** 0.0928 **c)** 43.0 **d)** 3.78 × 10⁵

Check over these examples to be sure you understand the principles of rounding off to a specified number of significant digits.

Addition and subtraction

The rules for significant figures in addition and subtraction are different from those we have just used. A simple example will illustrate why.

EXAMPLE: From the iron rod, which is 2.53 units long (Figure B–1), we cut a piece that is 2.512 units long. How much will we have left? To how many digits should we express our answer?

ANSWER: On an electronic calculator: 2.53 − 2.512 = 0.018; even on the calculator, we have subtracted a number with four significant digits from a value with three significant digits and gotten an answer with only two digits. Even that is too precise, however. We should line up the two numbers:

Or, the extra zeros only serve to tell us where to place the decimal point. Although the *point* (a period, .) is commonly used in North America, much of the world uses a decimal *comma*. They would write not 2.53 cm, but 2,53 cm.

$$\begin{array}{r} 2.53 \\ -2.512 \\ \hline 0.018 = 0.02 \end{array}$$

The *column of uncertainty* is shown in color and is set by the least precise measurement, the value 2.53. The result is good only to *one* significant figure

In addition or subtraction, line up the numbers one above the other. Find the column with the first uncertain digit. That column also contains the uncertain digit in the answer.

If two numbers are written with powers of ten, they cannot be added or subtracted properly in a column unless the powers of ten are *the same*. This may require changing one or more numbers. For example, $3.0 \times 10^3 + 4.0 \times 10^2$ cannot be added directly. Rewrite the problem in the form $3.0 \times 10^3 + 0.40 \times 10^3 = 3.4 \times 10^3$.

EXAMPLE: Add the following column of measurements, and round off the answer to the proper number of significant digits.

$$\begin{array}{rl} 8.379 & \text{meters} \\ +\ 19.52 & \text{centimeters} \\ +\ 0.068\ 30 & \text{millimeters} \\ \hline = & ? \end{array}$$

Stop! We can't do this problem because the units are not the *same.* You can't add apples to oranges, or meters to millimeters, or (numbers $\times 10^2$) to (numbers $\times 10^{-2}$). To be added or subtracted in a column, values must have the same units. Rewrite the problem in centimeters: 8.379 meters = 837.9 cm and 0.068 30 mm = 0.006 830 cm. *Now* you can set up a column of figures.

$$\begin{array}{rl} 837.9 & \text{cm} \\ +\ 19.52 & \text{cm} \\ +\ 0.006\ 830 & \text{cm} \\ \hline 857.426\ 83 & \text{cm} = 857.4 \text{ cm} \end{array}$$

SELF-CHECK
EXERCISE B–4

Round each of the following values to two *significant digits:*

a) 1.4752 g **b)** 0.007 611 m **c)** 1.0198×10^{-7} sec
d) 0.0394 mg **e)** 4.55×10^4 cm **f)** 2.000×10^{-22} kg

Solve each of the following calculations, assuming that every number is a measured value. Express the answer to the proper significant digits.

g) $(56.98)(139) = ?$ **h)** $(4.826 \times 10^{-5})(0.000\ 74) = ?$

i) $\dfrac{(2.86 \times 10^4)(3.163 \times 10^{-2})}{1.8} = ?$ **j)** $\dfrac{(8.712 - 7.9)}{0.001\ 32} = ?$

ANSWERS B–4:
a) 1.5 g **b)** 0.0076 m **c)** 1.0×10^{-7} sec **d)** 0.039 mg
e) 4.6×10^4 cm **f)** 2.0×10^{-22} kg **g)** 7.92×10^3 (not 7920, which is ambiguous) **h)** 3.6×10^{-8} **i)** 5.0×10^2
j) 6×10^2 (only one significant digit after subtraction)

B.5. PER CENT AND PARTS PER MILLION

We use the term "per cent" frequently in our daily lives. A store has a sale at "20% off." Food prices have gone up 1.2% in a month. The failure rate in a course may be expressed as so many percent.

The word "per" is also used in English quite commonly. A speed limit may be 55 miles *per* hour. A baseball pitcher may strike out an average of eight batters *per* game.

"Per" actually means "divided by." The speed of a car is determined by dividing the number of miles traveled by the number of hours it took to cover the distance. If you drive 4 hours to go 200 miles, your average speed is (200 miles) ÷ (4 hours) = 50 miles *per* hour.

Per Cent

The term "per cent" means "divided by 100," since "centum" is Latin for "one hundred." It is used to indicate how many parts of something are present in a *total* of 100 parts. If you receive 20%, 20 per cent, of a pie, that means if the pie were divided into 100 equal pieces, you would receive 20 of them.

A fraction of a whole, such as 0.20 or $1/4$, is converted to a per cent value by multiplying by 100:

$$\frac{0.20 \text{ part}}{1 \text{ total}} \times 100\% = 20\% \text{ of the total}$$

$$\frac{1 \text{ part}}{4 \text{ total}} \times 100\% = 25\% \text{ of the total}$$

EXAMPLE: In a particular chemistry test, there were 32 students writing and 24 passed. What was the pass rate in per cent?

ANSWER: $\dfrac{24 \text{ students passed}}{32 \text{ students total}} \times 100\% = 75\%$ of the total passed

Using Per Cent

Per cent may be used as a conversion factor if you recognize that 100% is equivalent to a "whole" thing.

EXAMPLE: Oxygen makes up 21.0% of inhaled air molecules. A person inhales 2.00×10^{25} molecules. How many of them are oxygen?
ANSWER: Use the *conversion-factor method* of Section 2.1, p. 18. We have a total number of molecules. This must be equivalent to 100%.

$$2.00 \times 10^{25} \text{ molecules total} \times \frac{21.0\% \text{ oxygen}}{100\% \text{ total}} = 4.20 \times 10^{24} \text{ molecules } O_2$$

EXAMPLE: A closed jar contains $5.0 \times 10^{21} \, O_2$ molecules. Oxygen makes up 21.0% of the air molecules in the jar. How many total molecules of air are in the jar?
ANSWER: Again use the conversion-factor method, but be careful. We are given not the total but the part that is oxygen. We want the total!

$$5.0 \times 10^{21} \text{ molecules } O_2 \times \frac{100\% \text{ total}}{21.0\% \, O_2} = 2.4 \times 10^{22} \text{ total air molecules}$$

In this case, we had to turn the previous conversion factor upside down.

For each problem involving per cent, be sure you know whether it refers to per cent by *weight*, or per cent by *volume* of a gas (or by numbers of molecules). The same two possibilities exist for parts per million.

EXAMPLE: For an average man, fluids make up about 70% of his body weight (Chapter 24). If this man has a total body weight of 148 pounds, how many pounds of body fluids does he have?

ANSWER: $148 \text{ pounds total} \times \dfrac{70\% \text{ fluid}}{100\% \text{ total}} = 104 \text{ pounds}$

Since the 70% figure is a measured quantity (Appendix B.4) we should report the answer to only one or two significant figures, or perhaps 1.0×10^2 pounds.

Parts Per Million (ppm)

If you understand the use of "per" in per cent, you should be able to do calculations in parts per million in the same fashion. If an impurity is present in the amount of 2.5 ppm, there are two possible conversion factors:

$$\frac{2.5 \text{ parts impurity}}{1\ 000\ 000 \text{ parts total}} \quad \text{or} \quad \frac{1\ 000\ 000 \text{ parts total}}{2.5 \text{ parts impurity}}$$

EXAMPLE: The U.S. federal air quality standard for sulfur dioxide gas requires an average, over the whole year, of not more than 0.03 ppm SO_2. An SO_2 level of 5.0 ppm for 1 hour is enough to cause breathing difficulty. Pollution from smokestacks should thus be controlled as described in Section 10.5. An average adult takes in 1.3×10^{22} air molecules with each breath. If the air contains the dangerous level of 5.0 ppm SO_2, how many molecules of SO_2 are in each breath?

In this and the following examples, we will assume that the total *amount is the same as the amount of air or water present. This approximation is true for very small amounts of impurities.*

ANSWER: $1.3 \times 10^{22} \text{ total molecules} \times \dfrac{5.0\ SO_2 \text{ molecules}}{1\ 000\ 000 \text{ total molecules}}$

$= 6.5 \times 10^{16}\ SO_2 \text{ molecules}$

EXAMPLE: The maximum allowable level of mercury (Hg) in water supplies of the U.S. and Canada is 0.50 ppm by weight. If we have 0.200 gram of mercury (in a dangerous form, such as methyl mercury), with how much water should it be diluted to reach the allowable level?

ANSWER: $0.200 \text{ g Hg} \times \dfrac{1\ 000\ 000 \text{ parts total}}{0.50 \text{ part Hg}} = 400\ 000 \text{ g total}$

To reach a total weight of 400 000 grams, we must add 400 liters of water.

EXAMPLE: A dose of 50 micrograms (5.0×10^{-5} g) of LSD may take the user on a "trip" of more than 8 hours. If the LSD is placed in a glass containing 250 g of water, what is the LSD level in ppm by weight?

ANSWER: Start with a million parts by weight of water, thus 1.0×10^6 grams.

$1.0 \times 10^6 \text{ g total} \times \dfrac{5.0 \times 10^{-5} \text{ g LSD}}{250 \text{ g total}} = 0.20 \text{ g LSD in 1 million g total}$

The level is thus, using the definition of parts per million, 0.20 ppm LSD.

SELF-CHECK
EXERCISES B–5

a) A radiation dose of 500 rem (p. 80) will kill about 50% of exposed humans within 30 days, and is thus symbolized $LD_{50}/30 = 500$ rem. If 2500 people were each equally exposed to 500 rem on July 1, how many would we expect to be alive on July 31?

b) In Figure 1–1 on p. 2 we find that carbon makes up 0.27% of the mass of the universe. If we take a section of the universe that has a mass of 1.99×10^{33} grams (equal to the mass of the sun), on the average how many grams will be carbon? Be careful! The value 0.27% is not the same as the *fraction* 0.27.

c) An underwater diver breathes air that is at a total pressure of 3000 torr and is 21.0% oxygen. What is the oxygen partial pressure (p. 282) in this breathing mixture?

d) Ethyl alcohol at a blood level of 0.30% may cause death. If the blood volume is 5.0 liters, what volume of alcohol circulating through the system could cause death? How many liters of 100-proof vodka, which is 50% alcohol, would provide this amount? (See p. 419).

e) Approximately 5.0×10^9 grams of mercury are released each year into the environment from U.S. industrial use (p. 359). How much water should be used to disperse this poisonous material to a level of 0.50 ppm by weight?

ANSWERS B–5

a) about 1250   **b)** 5.3×10^{30} g C   **c)** 630 torr   **d)** 0.015 L; 0.030 L = 30 mL, or about 1 oz, if all absorbed at once   **e)** 1.0×10^{16} g H_2O, or about 2.5 trillion gallons, the size of one very large lake.

B.6 READING A GRAPH

In this text, we use several dozen graphs to transmit information. Other graphs are seen frequently in newspapers and magazines. The graph is a way of telling you facts so that you can see any *patterns,* or *trends,* that are present. These patterns then may be used to predict the results of experiments which have not yet been done, or data which have not yet been gathered.

Bar Graphs

The simplest type of graph is a bar graph, shown in Figure B–2. The vertical (up and down) axis, often called the "*y* axis," is a scale of values that shows something we wish to emphasize. On this particular graph, it gives the world population in various years, with the purpose of showing the tremendous growth of the human race in the years since 1850. We can gain information from such a graph simply by reading directly to the left from the top of a bar, in a manner similar to the way we measured the height of the steel bar in Figure B–1.

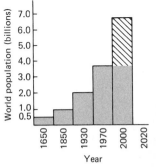

FIGURE B–2 A bar graph of total world population in various years.

EXAMPLE: The cross-hatched part of the bar for the year 2000 shows the predicted increase in world population between 1970 and 2000. How many people will be involved?

ANSWER: From the top of the 1970 bar, we can estimate the world population at that time to be about 3.8 billion. The top of the 2000 bar is at about 6.8 billion. The difference is $6.8 - 3.8 = 3.0$ billion.

This particular bar graph shows where zero population would fall, the lowest point on the vertical axis. Not every bar graph will necessarily have zero as a data point. For example, Figure 24–5 on p. 656 shows the effect of various body conditions on the blood stream pH. The vertical scale there ranges from pH = 7.0 to pH = 7.8. The scale is carefully chosen to be of maximum informational value.

The horizontal (bottom, left-to-right) axis on a bar graph may or may not have any significance at all. In Figure B–2, the points on this axis, often called the "x axis," are in order of increasing years, but are not otherwise related to each other. In Figure 24–5, there is *no* particular information transmitted by the distance of a bar along the horizontal axis.

Two-Dimensional Graphs

If the distance along the *x* axis (horizontal direction) is given a specific meaning, then we transmit information not by bars but by points, usually represented as dots along a smooth curve. Each point on the curve represents a set of *two* values, the distance along the vertical (*y*) axis, and the distance along the horizontal (*x*) axis.

In Figure B–3, the mass of a sample of magnesium (in grams) is plotted against the volume of the sample. Any particular point along the white line corresponds to some volume in cubic centimeters (*x*) and to the mass of that sample (*y*). By taking the mass and dividing it by the volume, we could obtain the density of magnesium, as discussed in Section 2.3. Since a sample of zero volume would have a mass of zero, the value "0" falls at one end of each scale. This point is called the "origin" of the graph.

In Figure B–4, we have a graph of temperature in Fahrenheit degrees (*y* axis) versus the same temperature in Celsius degrees (*x* axis). Point *a* shows that 0°C is the same temperature as 32°F. Point *b* shows the normal boiling point of water, 212°F and 100°C. The remainder of the curve could be used to convert a °F reading to °C and vice versa. For example, a fever temperature of 104°F corresponds to 40°C. The curve thus gives the same information as the formulas of Section 10.2.

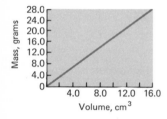

Mass of magnesium
vs volume of magnesium

FIGURE B–3   A graph of mass of a magnesium metal sample against volume in cubic centimeters. The slope of this curve gives the density.

In Figure B–3, the actual data points are not shown as dots and must be assumed to lie along the white line. In reports on experimental work, the data points are shown.

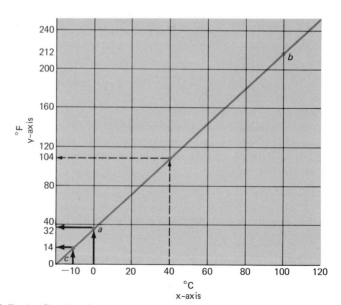

FIGURE B–4   Graph of temperature in °F against °C. The curve may be used to convert from one temperature scale to the other. However, it has its limitations. It does *not* tell you, as is true, that −40°F = −40°C.

A curve will not always give us all of the information we need. In some cases, we would have to extrapolate beyond the borders of the graph. In that situation, we would have to know if we were dealing with a linear, or straight-line, graph such as those in Figures B–3 and B–4, or with a more complicated curve, such as that in Figure 21–10 on p. 585.

When reading a graph, you are expected to use a ruler or straight-edge to find the y value and x value of any given point, and to be able to read the scale to within one tenth of one division, just as with Figure B–1. Be careful not to try to obtain more information from a graph than it can provide. Figure B–3, for example, has its y axis marked in divisions that have three significant digits, and yet you could not possibly read that scale to better than the nearest gram.

> EXAMPLE: What will be the mass of 8.0 cm³ of magnesium, using Figure B–3?
> ANSWER: Try it yourself with a ruler, then see how our answers compare.
>
> – .
>
> It seems to be about 13 grams. This would give a density of 13 g/8.0 cm³ = 1.6 g/cm³. The "handbook" value is 1.74 g/cm³. Clearly, this graph cannot be read to better than two significant digits.

Drawing Your Own Graphs

If in preparing a laboratory report or project you are expected to produce graphs, follow these six steps.

1) Choose the x and y axes carefully. The x axis should show the values you are controlling in your experiment; the y axis values should be out of your control (independent variable) and should be numbers you read from a measuring instrument.
2) Make a table of values for each variable.
3) Choose the scales on the x and y axes in such a way that your data points will cover most of the graph. The origin (value = 0) will *not* necessarily appear on a scale. Put these scales on graph paper.
4) Put a dot at each data point, and *circle* it.
5) When your data points are all graphed, see if any points should be rejected because of a very high probable error.
6) Excluding any rejected points, draw a smooth curve (with a ruler or a French curve) that best indicates the trend shown by your points.

The shape of the curve, in theory, will often be known in advance. You may thus be instructed to draw "the best straight line" that lies closest to the data points.

These instructions are necessarily very brief and limited. For a much more detailed discussion of graphing methods, see W. L. Masterton and E. J. Slowinski, *Elementary Mathematical Preparation for General Chemistry*, Philadelphia, W.B. Saunders, 1974, Chapter 10.

> SELF-CHECK
> EXERCISES B–6
>
> a)   In the bar graph of Figure 24–18 on p. 672, estimate the concentration in meq/liter of HCO_3^- ion in interstitial fluid.
> b)   In Figure 3–9 on p. 66, which is essentially a bar graph, which has a higher first ionization energy, N or Cl?
> c)   In Figure 6–9 on p. 159 what electronegativity difference corresponds to a bond with 50% ionic character?

d) In Figure 10–15 on p. 294, where the x axis corresponds to time, what normal lung volume in mL corresponds to the *vital capacity?*

e) In Figure 23–7 on p. 626, at what pH will trypsin have its maximum activity?

f) In Figure 24–10 on p. 660, at what oxygen tension in torr will hemoglobin be 90% saturated at a pH of 7.4?

ANSWERS B-6

a) 30 meq/L   **b)** nitrogen   **c)** about 1.8 = ΔBN
d) 4600 mL   (or better, 4.6×10^3 mL)   **e)** pH = 8.0
f) roughly 58 torr

Illustration Credits

The following list acknowledges sources not already credited in the illustration legends throughout the text.

PREFACE

Page vii Stamp photo by Peter P. Berlow.
Page ix From Toon, Ernest R., and George L. Ellis, *Foundations of Chemistry,* 2d ed., 1978, Holt, Rinehart & Winston of Canada, Ltd., Toronto.
Page x From Cohen, Robert S., *Physical Science,* 1976, Holt, Rinehart & Winston, New York. Engraving from The Bettmann Archive.

CHAPTER 1

Page 1 From Clark, Mary E., *Contemporary Biology,* 2d ed., 1979, Saunders College Publishing, Philadelphia.
Figure 1-1 After Jones, Mark, M., J. T. Netterville, D. O. Johnston, and J. L. Wood, *Chemistry, Man and Society,* 3d ed., 1980, Saunders College Publishing, Philadelphia.
Page 4 Upper photo from Masterton, William L., E. J. Slowinski, and E. T. Walford, *Chemistry,* 1980, Holt, Rinehart & Winston, New York.
Middle photo from Turk, Amos, J. Turk, J. T. Wittes, and R. E. Wittes, *Environmental Science,* 2d ed., 1978, Saunders College Publishing, Philadelphia.
Bottom photo from Masterton, Slowinski & Walford, *op. cit.,* 1980.
Page 5 Photo from Brescia, Frank, S. Mehlman, F. C. Pellegrini, and S. Stambler, *Chemistry, a Modern Introduction,* 2d ed., 1978, Saunders College Publishing, Philadelphia.
Page 6 Photo from Masterton, Slowinski & Walford, *op. cit.,* 1980.
Page 7 Upper left diagram after Harvard Project Physics (Holton, Rutherford and Watson, editors), *Project Physics Text,* 1975, Holt, Rinehart & Winston, New York.
Figure 1-5 After Briggs, George M., and D. H. Calloway, *Bogert's Nutrition and Physical Fitness,* 10th ed., 1979, Saunders College Publishing, Philadelphia.
Page 10 Photo from Briggs & Calloway, *op. cit.,* 1979.
Table 1-3 After Briggs & Calloway, *op. cit.,* 1979.

CHAPTER 2

Page 17 Stamp photo by Peter P. Berlow.
Middle photo from Highsmith, Phillip, *Physics, Energy and Our World,* 1975, Saunders College Publishing, Philadelphia.
Diagram after Cherim, Stanley M., and L. E. Kallan, *Chemistry, an Introduction,* 2d ed., 1980, Saunders College Publishing, Philadelphia.
Figure 2-1 After Cherim & Kallan, *op. cit.,* 1980.
Page 23 Stamp photo by Peter P. Berlow.
Page 24 After Masterton, Slowinski & Walford, *op. cit.,* 1980
Page 26 From Whitten, Kenneth W., and K. D. Gailey, *General Chemistry,* 1981, Saunders College Publishing, Philadelphia.
Page 27 From Peters, Edward I., *Introduction to Chemical Principles,* 2d ed., 1978, Saunders College Publishing, Philadelphia.
Figure 2-2 From Briggs & Calloway, *op. cit.,* 1979.
Page 29 Diagram after Toon & Ellis, *op. cit.,* 1978.

Page 31 Photo from Kuhn, Karl F., and J. S. Faughn, *Physics in Your World,* 2d ed., 1980, Saunders College Publishing, Philadelphia.
Page 33 Stamp photos by Peter P. Berlow.
Page 34 Lower diagrams after Jones et al., *op. cit.,* 1980.
Page 35 Upper photo from Lahaie, René, L. Papillon and P. Valiquette, *Elements of Experimental Chemistry,* 1978, Holt, Rinehart & Winston of Canada, Ltd., Toronto. Courtesy of the Radio Times Hulton Picture Library.
Bottom photo from Cohen, *op. cit.,* 1976. Courtesy of the American Institute of Physics, Niels Bohr Library.
Page 36 Stamp photo by Peter P. Berlow.
Figure 2-3 After Peters, *op. cit.,* 1978.
Figure 2-4 After Cherim & Kallan, *op. cit.,* 1980.
Page 38 From Highsmith, *op. cit.,* 1975.
Page 39 After Cherim & Kallan, *op. cit.,* 1980.
Page 41 Stamp photo by Peter P. Berlow.
Page 43 From Highsmith, *op. cit.,* 1975.

CHAPTER 3

Page 52 Stamp photo by Peter P. Berlow.
Figure 3-5 After Peters, *op. cit.,* 1978.
Figure 3-6 From Peters, *op. cit.,* 1978.
Page 61 Stamp photo by Peter P. Berlow.
Figure 3-8 From Peters, *op. cit.,* 1978.
Figure 3-9 After Peters, *op. cit.,* 1978.
Figure 3-10 After Peters, *op. cit.,* 1978.
Page 68 Stamp photo by Peter P. Berlow.
Page 69 From Briggs & Calloway, *op. cit.,* 1979.
Page 70 From Turk, Jonathan, *Introduction to Environmental Studies,* 1980, by Saunders College Publishing, Philadelphia.
Figure 3-11 From Masterton, Slowinski & Walford, *op. cit.,* 1980.
Page 73 From Briggs & Calloway, *op. cit.,* 1979.
Page 75 From Lahaie et al, *op. cit.,* 1978. Courtesy Neon Products Ltd.
Figure 3-12 After Peters, *op. cit.,* 1978.
Page 79 From Lahaie et al., *op. cit.,* 1978. Courtesy Brookhaven National Laboratory.
Page 80 After Turk et al., *op. cit.,* 1978.
Table 3-6 From Masterton, William L., E. J. Slowinski, and C. L. Stanitski, *Chemical Principles,* 5th ed., 1981, Saunders College Publishing, Philadelphia.
Figure 3-13 After Brescia et al., *op. cit.,* 1978.
Page 83 From Highsmith, *op. cit.,* 1975.
Page 84 Diagram from J. Turk, *op. cit.,* 1980. Photo from Jones et al., *op. cit.,* 1980.
Figure 3-14 From Peters, *op. cit.,* 1978.
Page 93 From Highsmith, *op. cit.,* 1975.

CHAPTER 4

Figure 4-2 From Masterton, Slowinski & Stanitski, *op. cit.,* 1981.
Figure 4-3 From Masterton, Slowinski & Stanitski, *op. cit.,* 1981.
Figure 4-5 From Peters, *op. cit.,* 1978.

CHAPTER 5

Figure 5-1	From Lahaie et al, *op. cit.,* 1978. Photo by T. P. Schmitter.
Figure 5-2	After Masterton, Slowinski & Walford, *op. cit.,* 1980.
Figure 5-3	After Peters, *op. cit.,* 1978.
Figure 5-4	After Cherim & Kallan, *op. cit.,* 1980.
Figure 5-5	After Toon & Ellis, *op. cit.,* 1978.

CHAPTER 6

Figure 6-1	After Masterton, Slowinski & Stanitski, *op. cit.,* 1981.
Figure 6-2	After Masterton, Slowinski & Stanitski, *op. cit.,* 1981.
Figure 6-3	After Jones et al., *op. cit.,* 1980.
Figure 6-4	After Cherim & Kallan, *op. cit.,* 1980.
Figure 6-5	After Peters, *op. cit.,* 1978.
Figure 6-6	After Peters, *op. cit.,* 1978.
Figure 6-7	After Newell, Sydney B., *Chemistry, an Introduction,* 2d ed., 1980, Little, Brown and Company, Boston.
Figure 6-8	After Brescia et al., *op. cit.,* 1978.
Figure 6-9	After Peters, *op. cit.,* 1978.
Figure 6-10	After Toon & Ellis, *op. cit.,* 1978.
Figure 6-12	After Brescia et al., *op. cit.,* 1978.
Figure 6-13	After Routh, Joseph I., D. P. Eyman, and D. J. Burton, *Essentials of General, Organic and Biochemistry,* 3d ed., 1977, Saunders College Publishing, Philadelphia.
Figure 6-14	After Brescia et al., *op. cit.,* 1978.
Figure 6-15	After Jones et al., *op. cit.,* 1980.
Figure 6-16	After Brescia et al., *op. cit.,* 1978.
Page 172	Upper diagram after Toon & Ellis, *op. cit.,* 1978. Lower diagram after Routh, Eyman & Burton, *op. cit.,* 1977.
Figure 6-18	After Toon & Ellis, *op. cit.,* 1978.
Figure 6-19	After Jones et al., *op. cit.,* 1980.
Figure 6-20	After Peters, *op. cit.,* 1978.
Figure 6-21	After Masterton, Slowinski & Stanitski, *op. cit.,* 1981.
Page 183	From Brescia et al., *op. cit.,* 1978.

CHAPTER 7

Figure 7-1	From Cherim & Kallan, *op. cit.,* 1980.
Figure 7-2	From Peters, *op. cit.,* 1978.
Page 198	After Routh, Eyman & Burton, *op. cit.,* 1977.
Page 202	After Toon & Ellis, *op. cit.,* 1978.
Page 204	Upper diagram after Brescia et al., *op. cit.,* 1978.
Page 205	Photo from Toon & Ellis, *op. cit.,* 1978. Diagram after Routh, Eyman & Burton, *op. cit.,* 1977.
Page 208	After Routh, Eyman & Burton, *op. cit.,* 1977.
Figure 7-3	After Routh, Eyman & Burton, *op. cit.,* 1977.

CHAPTER 8

Figure 8-1	After Toon & Ellis, *op. cit.,* 1978.
Figure 8-2	From Brescia et al., *op. cit.,* 1978.
Figure 8-3	From Masterton, Slowinski & Walford, *op. cit.,* 1980.
Figure 8-4	After Toon & Ellis, *op. cit.,* 1978.

CHAPTER 9

Figure 9-1	After Lee, Garth L., H. O. Van Order, and R. O. Ragsdale, *General and Organic Chemistry,* 1971, W. B. Saunders Company, Philadelphia.
Page 252	Stamp photo by Peter P. Berlow.
Figure 9-2	From Whitten & Gailey, *op. cit.,* 1981.
Figure 9-3	From Masterton, Slowinski & Walford, *op. cit.,* 1980.

CHAPTER 10

Page 266	From Masterton, Slowinski & Walford, *op. cit.,* 1980.
Page 267	From Harvard Project Physics, *op. cit.,* 1975.

Figure 10-1	After Toon & Ellis, *op. cit.,* 1978.
Page 269	After Toon & Ellis, *op. cit.,* 1978.
Page 271	Photo from Harvard Project Physics, *op. cit.,* 1975. Courtesy of Macmillan and Company, London.
Figure 10-2	After Routh, Eyman & Burton, *op. cit.,* 1977.
Page 273	From Cohen, *op. cit.,* 1976. Courtesy of Westinghouse, Inc.
Figure 10-3	After Peters, *op. cit.,* 1978.
Figure 10-4	From Masterton, Slowinski & Walford, *op. cit.,* 1980.
Page 277	From Highsmith, *op. cit.,* 1975.
Page 278	From Masterton, Slowinski & Walford, *op. cit.,* 1980.
Figure 10-5	From Masterton, Slowinski & Walford, *op. cit.,* 1980.
Page 279	Stamp photo by Peter P. Berlow. Lower photo from Highsmith, *op. cit.,* 1975.
Figure 10-6	After Peters, *op. cit.,* 1978.
Page 280	Photo from Harvard Project Physics, *op. cit.,* 1975.
Page 281	Stamp photo by Peter P. Berlow.
Figure 10-7	After Peters, *op. cit.,* 1978.
Figure 10-8	After Peters, *op. cit.,* 1978.
Figure 10-9	After Masterton, Slowinski & Walford, *op. cit.,* 1980.
Figure 10-10	After Guyton, Arthur C., *Physiology of the Human Body,* 5th ed., 1979, Saunders College Publishing, Philadelphia.
Figure 10-11	Copyright by The Montreal Gazette. Used by permission.
Page 288	From Highsmith, *op. cit.,* 1975.
Figure 10-12	After Toon & Ellis, *op. cit.,* 1978.
Figure 10-13	After Peters, *op. cit.,* 1978.
Page 290	Stamp photo by Peter P. Berlow.
Figure 10-14	From Brescia et al., *op. cit.,* 1978.
Figure 10-15	After Clark, *op. cit.,* 1979.
Figure 10-16	From Clark, *op. cit.,* 1979.
Page 294	Lung diagrams after Clark, *ibid.*
Figure 10-17	From J. Turk, *op. cit.,* 1980.
Figure 10-18	From Jones et al., *op. cit.,* 1980.
Figure 10-19	From J. Turk, *op. cit.,* 1980.
Table 10-3	From Jones et al., *op. cit.,* 1980.
Page 297	Upper photo from Highsmith, *op. cit.,* 1975. Lower photo from J. Turk, *op. cit.,* 1980.
Page 298	From Routh, Joseph I., *20th Century Chemistry,* 3d ed., 1963, W. B. Saunders Company, Philadelphia.
Page 299	Upper photo from J. Routh, *op. cit.,* 1963. Lower photo from Harvard Project Physics, *op. cit.,* 1975. Courtesy of NASA.
Figure 10-20	After Cherim & Kallan, *op. cit.,* 1980.

CHAPTER 11

Figure 11-1	After Peters, *op. cit.,* 1978.
Page 309	Bottom diagram, after Highsmith, *op. cit.,* 1975.
Figure 11-2	After Brescia et al., *op. cit.,* 1978.
Page 310	Photo from Highsmith, *op. cit.,* 1975.
Figure 11-3	From Brescia et al., *op. cit.,* 1978.
Figure 11-4	From Brescia et al., *op. cit.,* 1978.
Figure 11-5	After Peters, Edward I., *Problem Solving for Chemistry,* 2d ed., 1976, Saunders College Publishing, Philadelphia.
Page 313	After Cohen *op. cit.,* 1976.
Figure 11-6	After Highsmith, *op. cit.,* 1975.
Page 314	After Rushmer, R. F., *Cardiovascular Dynamics,* 1976, W. B. Saunders Company, Philadelphia.
Page 315	Left diagrams after Sackheim, George I., *Practical Physics for Nurses,* 1962, W. B. Saunders Company, Philadelphia. Right diagrams after Fitch, Kenneth L., and P. G. Johnson, *Human Life Science,* 1977, Holt, Rinehart & Winston, New York.
Page 316	From Fitch & Johnson, *op. cit.,* 1977.
Figure 11-7	After Masterton, Slowinski & Walford, *op. cit.,* 1980.
Figure 11-8	From Brescia et al., *op. cit.,* 1978.
Figure 11-9	After Toon & Ellis, *op. cit.,* 1978.
Figure 11-10	After Routh, Eyman & Burton, *op. cit.,* 1977.
Page 322	After Brescia et al., *op. cit.,* 1978.
Figure 11-12	From Jones et al., *op. cit.,* 1980.
Figure 11-13	After Cherim & Kallan, *op. cit.,* 1980.
Figure 11-14	From Peters, *op. cit.,* 1978.

Page 327	From Masterton, Slowinski & Walford, *op. cit.*, 1980.
Page 329	Upper photo from Jones et al., *op. cit.*, 1980. Lower photo from Peters, *op. cit.*, 1978.
Figure 11-15	From Peters, *op. cit.*, 1978.
Figure 11-16	After Toon & Ellis, *op. cit.*, 1978.
Page 330	Central diagram from Brescia et al., *op. cit.*, 1978.
Table 11-9	From Masterton, Slowinski & Walford, *op. cit.*, 1980.
Figure 11-17	After Toon & Ellis, *op. cit.*, 1978.
Page 332	Upper photo from Brescia et al., *op. cit.*, 1978. Lower photo from J. Routh, *op. cit.*, 1963.
Page 333	After Toon & Ellis, *op. cit.*, 1978.

CHAPTER 12

Figure 12-1	After Masterton, Slowinski & Walford, *op. cit.*, 1980.
Figure 12-2	From Peters, *op. cit.*, 1978.
Figure 12-3	After Toon & Ellis, *op. cit.*, 1978.
Figure 12-4	From Brescia et al., *op. cit.*, 1978.
Figure 12-5	After Lee, Van Order & Ragsdale, *op. cit.*, 1971.
Figure 12-6	After Brescia et al., *op. cit.*, 1978.
Figure 12-7	After Peters, *op. cit.*, 1978.
Figure 12-8	After Masterton, Slowinski & Walford, *op. cit.*, 1980.
Figure 12-9	From Peters, *op. cit.*, 1978.
Page 348	Left diagrams after Masterton, Slowinski & Walford, *op. cit.*, 1980.
Page 349	From Masterton, Slowinski & Walford, *op. cit.*, 1980.
Figure 12-10	After Routh, Eyman & Burton, *op. cit.*, 1977.
Page 352	After Clark, *op. cit.*, 1979.
Figure 12-12	From Peters, *op. cit.*, 1978.
Figure 12-13	After Masterton, Slowinski & Stanitski, *op. cit.*, 1981.
Figure 12-14	From Peters, *op. cit.*, 1978.
Figure 12-15	From Peters, *op. cit.*, 1978.
Figure 12-16	After Jones et al., *op. cit.*, 1980.
Page 357	From Jones et al., *op. cit.*, 1980.
Figure 12-17	After Jones et al., *op. cit.*, 1980.
Figure 12-18	After Eastman, Richard H., *General Chemistry: Experiment and Theory,* 1970, Holt, Rinehart & Winston, New York.
Page 361	After Jones et al., *op. cit.*, 1980.
Figure 12-19	From Jones et al., *op. cit.*, 1980.
Figure 12-20	After Lee, Van Order & Ragsdale, *op. cit.*, 1971.
Figure 12-21	After Routh, Eyman & Burton, *op. cit.*, 1977.
Figure 12-22	After Clark, *op. cit.*, 1979.
Figure 12-23	After Clark, *op. cit.*, 1979, from Friedman, E. A., *Strategy in Renal Failure,* 1978, John Wiley & Sons, New York.
Figure 12-24	After Brescia et al., *op. cit.*, 1978.

CHAPTER 13

Page 373	From Brescia et al., *op. cit.*, 1978.
Figure 13-1	From Cherim & Kallan, *op. cit.*, 1980.
Page 379	After Toon & Ellis, *op. cit.*, 1978.
Figure 13-2	From Jones et al., *op. cit.*, 1980.
Page 381	From Peters, *op. cit.*, 1978.
Page 397	From J. Routh, *op. cit.*, 1963.
Page 401	From Jones et al., *op. cit.*, 1980.

CHAPTER 14

Figure 14-1	From Peters, *op. cit.*, 1978.
Figure 14-3	After Fitch & Johnson, *op. cit.*, 1977.
Figure 14-4	From Cherim & Kallan, *op. cit.*, 1980.
Page 420	Photo from J. Routh, *op. cit.*, 1963.
Page 421	After Toon & Ellis, *op. cit.*, 1978.
Page 423	From Peters, *op. cit.*, 1978.
Figure 14-5	From Toon & Ellis, *op. cit.*, 1978.
Figure 14-6	After Routh, Eyman & Burton, *op. cit.*, 1977.
Table 14-3	After Brescia et al., *op. cit.*, 1978.
Page 432	From Lahaie et al., *op. cit.*, 1978. Photo by Clara Aich and George Senty.
Page 434	From Fitch & Johnson, *op. cit.*, 1977.

CHAPTER 15

Page 443	Stamp photo by Peter P. Berlow.
Figure 15-1	After Ternay, Andrew L. Jr., *Contemporary Organic Chemistry,* 2d ed., 1979, Saunders College Publishing, Philadelphia.
Figure 15-2	After Routh, Eyman & Burton, *op. cit.*, 1977.
Page 450	Stamp photo by Peter P. Berlow.

CHAPTER 16

Figure 16-1	After Masterton, Slowinski & Walford, *op. cit.*, 1980.
Figure 16-2	After Masterton, Slowinski & Stanitski, *op. cit.*, 1981.
Figure 16-3	After Routh, Eyman & Burton, *op. cit.*, 1977.
Page 475	From Masterton, Slowinski & Walford, *op. cit.*, 1980.
Figure 16-4	After Jones et al., *op. cit.*, 1980.
Figure 16-5	After Routh, Eyman & Burton, *op. cit.*, 1977.
Figure 16-6	After Toon & Ellis, *op. cit.*, 1978.
Figure 16-7	After Jones et al., *op. cit.*, 1980.
Figure 16-8	After Jones et al., *op. cit.*, 1980.

CHAPTER 17

Page 488	From J. Routh, *op. cit.*, 1963.
Page 489	From J. Routh, *op. cit.*, 1963.
Page 490	From Clark, *op. cit.*, 1979. Courtesy of Grant Heilman, Lititz, Pa.
Page 494	Stamp photo by Peter P. Berlow.
Figure 17-3	After Merken, Melvin, *Physical Science with Modern Applications,* 2d ed., 1980, Saunders College Publishing, Philadelphia.
Figure 17-5	After Harvard Project Physics, *op. cit.*, 1975.
Figure 17-6	From Masterton, Slowinski & Stanitski, *op. cit.*, 1981.
Page 499	From J. Routh, *op. cit.*, 1963.
Figure 17-10	After Jones et al., *op. cit.*, 1980.
Page 506	From J. Routh, *op. cit.*, 1963.

CHAPTER 18

Page 510	From Briggs & Calloway, *op. cit.*, 1979.
Table 18-2	From Jones et al., *op. cit.*, 1980.
Page 515	From Whitten & Gailey, *op. cit.*, 1981.
Page 516	From Toon & Ellis, *op. cit.*, 1978.
Figure 18-1	Tracing supplied by Joseph I. Routh.
Figure 18-2	After McGilvery, Robert W., *Biochemical Concepts,* 1975, Saunders College Publishing, Philadelphia.
Figure 18-3	From Villee, C. A., and V. G. Dethier, *Biological Principles and Processes,* 2d ed., 1976, Saunders College Publishing, Philadelphia.
Figure 18-4	After Clark, *op. cit.*, 1979.
Figure 18-5	From DeWitt, William, *Biology of the Cell: An Evolutionary Approach,* 1977, Saunders College Publishing, Philadelphia.
Figure 18-6	After Villee & Dethier, *op. cit.*, 1976.
Figure 18-7	After Villee & Dethier, *op. cit.*, 1976.
Figure 18-8	After Clark, *op. cit.*, 1979.
Figure 18-10	After Clark, *op. cit.*, 1979.
Figure 18-11	After Villee & Dethier, *op. cit.*, 1976.
Figure 18-12	After Routh, Eyman & Burton, *op. cit.*, 1977.
Page 528	Photo from Fitch & Johnson, *op. cit.*, 1977.

CHAPTER 19

Figure 19-1	From Routh, Eyman & Burton, *op. cit.*, 1977.
Figure 19-2	From Routh, Eyman & Burton, *op. cit.*, 1977.
Figure 19-3	From Routh, Eyman & Burton, *op. cit.*, 1977.
Figure 19-4	After Brescia et al., *op. cit.*, 1978.
Figure 19-6	After Jones et al., *op. cit.*, 1980.

Figure 19-7	Top: after Routh, Eyman & Burton, *op. cit.,* 1977. Bottom: after Toon & Ellis, *op. cit.,* 1978.
Figure 19-8	From Jones et al., *op. cit.,* 1980.
Figure 19-9	After Routh, Eyman & Burton, *op. cit.,* 1977.
Figure 19-11	From Routh, Eyman & Burton, *op. cit.,* 1977.
Page 543	Diagram after Toon & Ellis, *op. cit.,* 1978. Photo from J. Routh, *op. cit.,* 1963.

CHAPTER 20

Figure 20-1	From Guyton, *op. cit.,* 1979.
Figure 20-2	From Jones et al., *op. cit.,* 1980.
Figure 20-3	From Guyton, *op. cit.,* 1979.
Figure 20-4	From Guyton, *op. cit.,* 1979.
Figure 20-5	From Clark, *op. cit.,* 1979.
Figure 20-6	From Clark, *op. cit.,* 1979.
Page 552	From Clark, *op. cit.,* 1979. Courtesy of Dr. E. T. Weier.
Figure 20-9	After Brescia et al., *op. cit.,* 1978.
Figure 20-11	From Clark, *op. cit.,* 1979.
Figure 20-12	After Jones et al., *op. cit.,* 1980.
Figure 20-13	After Jones et al., *op. cit.,* 1980.
Page 556	From Jones et al., *op. cit.,* 1980.
Figure 20-14	After W. DeWitt, *op. cit.,* 1977.
Figure 20-15	From Clark, *op. cit.,* 1979.
Figure 20-16	From Jones et al., *op. cit.,* 1980.
Figure 20-18	After Jones et al., *op. cit.,* 1980.
Figure 20-19	After Jones et al., *op. cit.,* 1980.
Figure 20-20	After Shepro, D., F. Belamarich, and C. Levy, *Human Anatomy and Physiology, a Cellular Approach,* 1974, Holt, Rinehart & Winston, New York.

CHAPTER 21

Figure 21-3	From Briggs & Calloway, *op. cit.,* 1979.
Figure 21-4	From Gerking, Shelby D., *Biological Systems,* 2d ed., 1974, Saunders College Publishing, Philadelphia.
Figure 21-5	From Guyton, *op. cit.,* 1979.
Figure 21-6	After Briggs & Calloway, *op. cit.,* 1979.
Page 581	From Toon & Ellis, *op. cit.,* 1978.
Page 582	From Toon & Ellis, *op. cit.,* 1978.
Figure 21-7	From Brescia et al., *op. cit.,* 1978.
Figure 21-8	After Peters, *op. cit.,* 1978.
Figure 21-9	After Cohen, *op. cit.,* 1976.
Figure 21-10	After M. Merken, *op. cit.,* 1980.
Figure 21-11	After Villee & Dethier, *op. cit.,* 1976.
Figure 21-12	After Peters, *op. cit.,* 1978.
Figure 21-13	After Masterton, Slowinski & Stanitski, *op. cit.,* 1981.

CHAPTER 22

Figure 22-1	After Clark, *op. cit.,* 1979.
Figure 22-2	After Clark, *op. cit.,* 1979.
Figure 22-3	After Gerking, *op. cit.,* 1974.
Table 22-2	From Clark, *op. cit.,* 1979.
Table 22-3	From DeRobertis, E.D.P., and E.M.F. DeRobertis, *Cell and Molecular Biology,* 7th ed., 1980, Saunders College Publishing, Philadelphia.
Figure 22-7	Adapted from Dickerson, Richard E., and I. Geis, *Chemistry, Matter and the Universe,* 1976, W. A. Benjamin, Inc., Menlo Park.
Figure 22-8	From DeRobertis, *op. cit.,* 1980.

CHAPTER 23

Page 620	After DeRobertis, *op. cit.,* 1980.
Figure 23-1	After Routh, Eyman & Burton, *op. cit.,* 1977.
Figure 23-2	After Clark, *op. cit.,* 1979.
Figure 23-3	After DeRobertis, *op. cit.,* 1980.
Figure 23-7	After Gerking, *op. cit.,* 1974.

Figure 23-8	After Gerking, *op. cit.,* 1974.
Page 628	After Jones et al., *op. cit.,* 1980.
Figure 23-9	After Jones et al., *op. cit.,* 1980.
Figure 23-10	After Clark, *op. cit.,* 1979.
Page 633	Photo from Briggs & Calloway, *op. cit.,* 1979.
Page 634	Photo from J. Routh, *op. cit.,* 1963.
Page 635	Photo from Briggs & Calloway, *op. cit.,* 1979.
Figure 23-11	After Brescia et al., *op. cit.,* 1978.
Page 638	From Briggs & Calloway, *op. cit.,* 1979.
Page 639	Photo from J. Routh, *op. cit.,* 1963.
Figure 23-13	After Briggs & Calloway, *op. cit.,* 1979.
Figure 23-14	After Briggs & Calloway, *op. cit.,* 1970.

CHAPTER 24

Figure 24-2	After Shepro et al., *op. cit.,* 1974.
Figure 24-3	Diagram from Routh, Eyman & Burton, *op. cit.,* 1977. Photo from Silverstein, Alvin, *The Biological Sciences,* 1974, the Rinehart Press/Holt, Rinehart & Winston, San Francisco. Courtesy of Abbott Laboratories.
Page 651	Upper photo from J. Routh, *op. cit.,* 1963.
Figure 24-4	After Guyton, *op. cit.,* 1979.
Figure 24-5	After Guyton, *op. cit.,* 1979.
Figure 24-7	From Whitten & Gailey, *op. cit.,* 1981.
Page 657	Upper drawings after Clark, *op. cit.,* 1979.
Figure 24-8	From Jones et al., *op. cit.,* 1980.
Figure 24-9	After Jones et al., *op. cit.,* 1980.
Figure 24-12	From Brescia et al., *op. cit.,* 1978.
Table 24-4	From Jones et al., *op. cit.,* 1980.
Figure 24-15	After Clark, *op. cit.,* 1979.
Figure 24-18	After Routh, Eyman & Burton, *op. cit.,* 1977.

CHAPTER 25

Figure 25-1	After Clark, *op. cit.,* 1979.
Figure 25-2	After Briggs & Calloway, *op. cit.,* 1979.
Figure 25-4	From Briggs & Calloway, *op. cit.,* 1979.
Figure 25-5	After Fitch & Johnson, *op. cit.,* 1977.
Page 684	From Fitch, Kenneth L., H. C. Elliott and P. B. Johnson, *Life Science and Man,* 1973, Holt, Rinehart & Winston, New York.
Figure 25-6	After Clark, *op. cit.,* 1979.
Page 691	Photo from J. Routh, *op. cit.,* 1963.
Page 692	Photo from J. Routh, *op. cit.,* 1963.

CHAPTER 26

Page 697	Photo from J. Routh, *op. cit.,* 1963.
Page 700	Photo from Briggs & Calloway, *op. cit.,* 1979.
Page 702	Photo from Fitch & Johnson, *op. cit.,* 1977.

CHAPTER 27

Figure 27-1	After Routh, Eyman & Burton, *op. cit.,* 1977.
Figure 27-2	After Briggs & Calloway, *op. cit.,* 1979.
Page 712	Photo from J. Routh, *op. cit.,* 1963.
Page 714	From Briggs & Calloway, *op. cit.,* 1979.
Figure 27-4	After Clark, *op. cit.,* 1979.
Figure 27-5	From Briggs & Calloway, *op. cit.,* 1979.
Figure 27-6	From Briggs & Calloway, *op. cit.,* 1979.
Page 717	Photo from J. Turk, *op. cit.,* 1980.
Page 718	Photo from J. Turk, *op. cit.,* 1980.
Figure 27-7	From Briggs & Calloway, *op. cit.,* 1979. Courtesy of Yale University Press.
Page 719	Right photo from Turk et al., *op. cit.,* 1978.
Page 726	Photo from J. Routh, *op. cit.,* 1963.
Figure 27-10	After Shepro et al., *op. cit.,* 1974.

CHAPTER 28

Figure 28-1	After Fitch & Johnson, *op. cit.,* 1977.
Figure 28-2	From Brescia et al., *op. cit.,* 1978.
Figure 28-3	After Silverstein, *op. cit.,* 1974.
Figure 28-4	After Shepro et al., *op. cit.,* 1974.
Figure 28-5	From Toon & Ellis, *op. cit.,* 1978
Page 740	From Clark, *op. cit.,* 1979.
Figure 28-8	From Fitch & Johnson, *op. cit.,* 1977.
Figure 28-9	After Shepro et al., *op. cit.,* 1974.
Figure 28-10	After Fitch & Johnson, *op. cit.,* 1977.
Figure 28-11	From Clark, *op. cit.,* 1979, from Willis, R. A., *The Spread of Tumours in the Body,* 3d ed., 1973, Butterworths, London.

Figure 28-12	After Fitch & Johnson, *op. cit.,* 1977.
Figure 28-13	After Clark, *op. cit.,* 1979.
Figure 28-14	After Masterton, Slowinski & Stanitski, *op. cit.,* 1981.

APPENDIX B

Figure B-0	From Brescia et al., *op. cit.,* 1978.
Figure B-1	After Toon & Ellis, *op. cit.,* 1978.
Figure B-2	After Toon & Ellis, *op. cit.,* 1978.
Figure B-3	After Toon & Ellis, *op. cit.,* 1978.
Figure B-4	After Brescia et al., *op. cit.,* 1978.

INDEX

Entries in italics indicate illustrations; page numbers followed by t indicate tables; those in boldface number are in chapter glossaries.

INTERNATIONAL TABLE OF ATOMIC WEIGHTS (1973)

Based on relative atomic mass of $^{12}C = 12$. Includes 1975 corrected values.

The following values apply to elements as they exist in materials of terrestrial origin and to certain artificial elements. When used with the due regard to footnotes, they are reliable to ±1 in the last digit, or ±3 when followed by an asterisk (*). Value in parentheses is the mass number of the isotope of longest half-life.

	Symbol	Atomic number	Atomic weight		Symbol	Atomic number	Atomic weight
Actinium	Ac	89	(227)	Mercury	Hg	80	200.59*
Aluminum	Al	13	26.98154*	Molybdenum	Mo	42	95.94
Americium	Am	95	(243)	Neodymium	Nd	60	144.24*
Antimony	Sb	51	121.75*	Neon	Ne	10	20.179*,c,*
Argon	Ar	18	39.948b,c,d,g	Neptunium	Np	93	237.0482f
Arsenic	As	33	74.9216*	Nickel	Ni	28	58.70
Astatine	At	85	(210)	Niobium	Nb	41	92.9064*
Barium	Ba	56	137.33	Nitrogen	N	7	14.0067b,c
Berkelium	Bk	97	(247)	Nobelium	No	102	(255)
Beryllium	Be	4	9.01218*	Osmium	Os	76	190.2g
Bismuth	Bi	83	208.9804*	Oxygen	O	8	15.9994b,c,d
Boron	B	5	10.81c,d,*	Palladium	Pd	46	106.4
Bromine	Br	35	79.904c	Phosphorus	P	15	30.97376*
Cadmium	Cd	48	112.41	Platinum	Pt	78	195.09*
Calcium	Ca	20	40.08g	Plutonium	Pu	94	(244)
Californium	Cf	98	(251)	Polonium	Po	84	(209)
Carbon	C	6	12.011b,d	Potassium	K	19	39.0983*
Cerium	Ce	58	140.12	Praseodymium	Pr	59	140.9077*
Cesium	Cs	55	132.9054*	Promethium	Pm	61	(145)
Chlorine	Cl	17	35.453c	Protactinium	Pa	91	231.0359*,f
Chromium	Cr	24	51.996c	Radium	Ra	88	226.0254f,g
Cobalt	Co	27	58.9332*	Radon	Rn	86	(222)
Copper	Cu	29	63.546*,c,d	Rhenium	Re	75	186.207c
Curium	Cm	96	(247)	Rhodium	Rh	45	102.9055*
Dysprosium	Dy	66	162.50*	Rubidium	Rb	37	85.4678*,c
Einsteinium	Es	99	(254)	Ruthenium	Ru	44	101.07*
Erbium	Er	68	167.26*	Samarium	Sm	62	150.4
Europium	Eu	63	151.96	Scandium	Sc	21	44.9559*
Fermium	Fm	100	(257)	Selenium	Se	34	78.96*
Fluorine	F	9	18.998403*	Silicon	Si	14	28.0855*,d
Francium	Fr	87	(223)	Silver	Ag	47	107.868*
Gadolinium	Gd	64	157.25*	Sodium	Na	11	22.9877*
Gallium	Ga	31	69.72	Strontium	Sr	38	87.62g
Germanium	Ge	32	72.58*	Sulfur	S	16	32.06d
Gold	Au	79	196.9665*	Tantalum	Ta	73	180.9479*,b
Hafnium	Hf	72	178.49*	Technetium	Tc	43	(97)
Helium	He	2	4.00260b,c	Tellurium	Te	52	127.60*
Holmium	Ho	67	164.9304*	Terbium	Tb	65	158.9254*
Hydrogen	H	1	1.0079b,d	Thallium	Tl	81	204.37*
Indium	In	49	114.82	Thorium	Th	90	232.0381f,g
Iodine	I	53	126.9045*	Thulium	Tm	69	168.9342*
Iridium	Ir	77	192.22*	Tin	Sn	50	118.69*
Iron	Fe	26	55.847*	Titanium	Ti	22	47.90*
Krypton	Kr	36	83.80*	Tungsten	W	74	183.85*
Lanthanum	La	57	138.9055*,b	Uranium	U	92	238.029b,c,e,g
Lawrencium	Lr	103	(260)	Vanadium	V	23	50.9415 b,c
Lead	Pb	82	207.2d,g	Wolfram	W	74	183.85*
Lithium	Li	3	6.941*,c,d,e,g	Xenon	Xe	54	131.30*
Lutetium	Lu	71	174.967 *	Ytterbium	Yb	70	173.04*
Magnesium	Mg	12	24.305c,g	Yttrium	Y	39	88.9059*
Manganese	Mn	25	54.9380*	Zinc	Zn	30	65.38
Mendelevium	Md	101	(258)	Zirconium	Zr	40	91.22

a Elements with only one stable nuclide.

b Element with one predominant isotope (about 99 to 100% abundance).

c Element for which the atomic weight is based on calibrated measurements.

d Element for which known variation in isotopic abundance in terrestrial samples limits the precision of the atomic weight given.

e Element for which users are cautioned against the possibility of large variations in atomic weight due to inadvertent or undisclosed artificial isotopic separation in commercially available materials.

f Most commonly available long-lived isotope.

g In some geological specimens this element has a highly anomalous isotopic composition, corresponding to an atomic weight significantly different from that given.

Whitten & Gailey, General Chemistry, 1981